FOUNDATIONS OF

Maternal-Newborn
AND Women's Health
Nursing

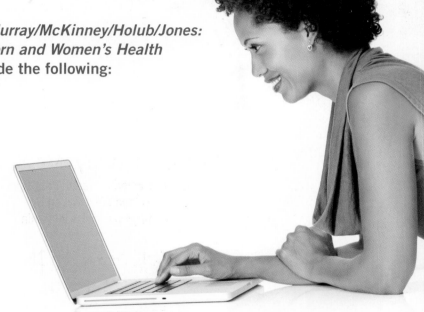

7th EDITION

FOUNDATIONS OF
Maternal-Newborn
AND Women's Health
Nursing

Sharon Murray, MSN, RN
Professor Emerita, Health Professions
Golden West College
Huntington Beach, California

Emily McKinney, MSN, RN, C
(deceased)
Nurse Educator and Consultant
Dallas, Texas

Karen Shaw Holub, MS, RNC-OB
Assistant Clinical Professor
Baylor University
Louise Herrington School of Nursing
Dallas, Texas

Renee Jones, DNP, RNC-OB, WHNP-BC
Assistant Clinical Professor
Baylor University
Louise Herrington School of Nursing
Dallas, Texas

ELSEVIER

ELSEVIER

3251 Riverport Lane
St. Louis, Missouri 63043

FOUNDATIONS OF MATERNAL-NEWBORN AND WOMEN'S
HEALTH NURSING, SEVENTH EDITION

ISBN: 978-0-323-39894-7

Notices

Library of Congress Cataloging-in-Publication Data
Names: Murray, Sharon Smith, author. | McKinney, Emily Slone, author. |
   Holub, Karen, author. | Jones, Renee, author.
Title: Foundations of maternal-newborn and women's health nursing / Sharon Smith Murray, Emily Slone
   McKinney, Karen Holub, Renee Jones.
Description: 7th edition. | St. Louis, Missouri : Elsevier, [2019] | Includes bibliographical references and index.
Identifiers: LCCN 2017050406 | ISBN 9780323398947 (pbk. : alk. paper)
Subjects: | MESH: Maternal-Child Nursing | Family Health | Women's Health
Classification: LCC RG951 | NLM WY 157.3 | DDC 618.2/0231--dc23 LC record available at
https://lccn.loc.gov/2017050406

Senior Content Strategist: Sandra Clark
Director, Content Development: Laurie Gower
Content Development Specialist: Betsy McCormac
Publishing Services Manager: Jeff Patterson
Senior Project Manager: Tracey Schriefer
Design Direction: Amy Buxton

Printed in China

Last digit is the print number: 9   8   7   6   5   4   3   2

CONTRIBUTORS AND REVIEWERS

CONTRIBUTORS

Lynn Callister, RN, PhD, FAAN
Professor Emeritus - College of Nursing
Brigham Young University
Provo, Utah

Kathryn Corso, MSN, RNC-OB, C-EFM
Supervisor - Labor and Delivery
Baylor University Medical Center
Dallas, Texas

Becky Cypher, MSN, PNNP
Chief Nursing Officer
PeriGen
Princeton, New Jersey

Kristine DeButy, BSN, RNC-OB
Nurse Manager II - Labor & Delivery
Baylor University Medical Center
Dallas, Texas

Stephanie Fassett, MSN, RNC-OB
Nurse Educator - Medical City Plano
Plano, Texas;
Adjunct Faculty
Baylor University
Louise Herrington School of Nursing
Dallas, Texas

Vanessa Flannery, BSN, MSN
Associate Professor - Nursing
Morehead State University
Morehead, Kentucky

Tania Lopez, MS, CNM
Adjunct Faculty
Baylor University
Louise Herrington School of Nursing
Dallas, Texas;
Adjunct Faculty - School of Public Health
University of North Texas Health Science Center
Advanced Practice Nurse - Perinatal Services
John Peter Smith Hospital
Fort Worth, Texas

Kari Mau, DNP, APRN-BC, RNFA, C-EFM
Instructor - College of Nursing
Medical University of South Carolina
Charleston, South Carolina;
Nurse Practitioner - The Breast Health Center
Bluffton, South Carolina

Jessica McNeil, MSN, RNC-OB, C-EFM
Nurse Manager - Labor & Delivery & Mother/Baby Units
Texas Health Presbyterian Hospital Flowermound
Flowermound, Texas;
Clinical Educator - Clinical Education & Professional Practice
UT Southwestern Medical Center
Adjunct Faculty
Baylor University
Louise Herrington School of Nursing
Dallas, Texas

Cathy Miller, RN, PhD
Associate Professor
College of Nursing and Health Sciences
Texas A&M University Corpus Christi
Corpus Christi, Texas

Grace Moodt, DNP, MSN
Associate Professor/Interim Director
School of Nursing
Austin Peay State University
Clarksville, Tennessee

Sandra Nasr, MS, RNC-OB
Adjunct Faculty
Texas Woman's University
School of Nursing
Dallas, Texas
Adjunct Faculty
Baylor University
Louise Herrington School of Nursing
Dallas, Texas

Susan Peck, MSN, APN, WHNP
Cedar Knolls, New Jersey

Dawn Piacenza, MSN
Clinical Nurse Specialist
Wesley Medical Center
Wichita, Kansas

Catherine Paige Pollard, BSN, RN
Adjunct Faculty
Baylor University
Louise Herrington School of Nursing
Dallas, Texas

Jennifer Rodriguez, RN, MSN
Faculty OB/PEDS
Kellogg Community College
Battle Creek, Michigan

Cheryl Roth, PhD, WHNP-BC, RNC-OB, RNFA
Nurse Practitioner - Labor & Delivery/Couplet
Honor Health Scottsdale Shea & Osborn
Scottsdale, Arizona

Kristin Scheffer, BSN, RNC-OB, C-EFM
Labor & Delivery/Antepartum
Professional Development Educator
Baylor University Medical Center
Dallas, Texas

Karen Stanzo, MSN, RN, IBCLC
Supervisor - Lactation and Family Services
Baylor Scott and White Medical Center at McKinney
McKinney, Texas

Mary Suzanne White, MSN, RN, PHCNS-BC
Associate Professor - Nursing
Morehead State University
Morehead, Kentucky

Della Wrightson, BS, MSN, RNC-NIC
Neonatal Clinical Nurse Specialist
Levine Children's Hospital
Charlotte, North Carolina

INSTRUCTOR AND STUDENT ANCILLARIES

Jennifer T. Alderman, MSN, RNC-OB, CNL
Assistant Professor, School of Nursing
University of North Carolina at Chapel Hill
Chapel Hill, North Carolina
PowerPoint Slides

Barbara Pascoe, RN, BA, MA
Director - Maternity, Gynecology, and Pediatrics
Concord Hospital
Concord, New Hampshire
Test Bank

Shannon E. Perry, RN, PhD, FAAN
Professor Emerita, School of Nursing
San Francisco State University
San Francisco, California
Review Questions

REVIEWERS

Marcia A. Clevesy, MSN, NCC, RNC, APRN
Instructor - School of Nursing
University of Nevada - Las Vegas
Las Vegas, Nevada

Kari Mau, DNP, APRN-BC, RNFA, C-EFM
Instructor - College of Nursing
Medical University of South Carolina
Charleston, South Carolina;
Nurse Practitioner - The Breast Health Center
Bluffton, South Carolina

Grace Moodt, DNP, MSN
Associate Professor/Interim Director
School of Nursing
Austin Peay State University
Clarksville, Tennessee

Aimee Ortiz, DHSc, MSN, RN
Assistant Professor
Rio Hondo College
Whittier, California

Rebecca Padgett, MSN, RN
Nursing Faculty
Jefferson Davis Community College
Brewton, Alabama

Christina M. Rutledge, RN, MN, CNE
Module Leader - Practical Nurse Course
Amedd Center and School, Madigan Army Medical Center
Tacoma, Washington

To our families: Jamie, Hannah, and Cole Jones; Bill, Amanda, and
Jill Holub for the sacrifices you made for this book and
for your love and support every day.

PREFACE

Our challenge as educators and providers of nursing care in many settings is to keep up with the rapid changes in health care while preparing students to stay focused on the *care* of nursing. Nursing faculty teach the student ways to use the nursing process, drugs, and technology that are beneficial while imparting the values of patient-centered care. Our text tries to help the student learn to balance "high-touch" care with "high-tech," often lifesaving, care in different settings.

Although health care delivery has changed dramatically, with greater emphasis on outcome management, the family's need for education and support does not lessen. Nurses have responded to families' needs by developing alternative means of education that use every possible moment before admission and during their stay in the health care facility. Women's health care extends over many more years than just the childbearing years, often from adolescence to old age. The women's health nurse may need to understand how to best teach the 15-year-old girl and the 80-year-old woman on the same day. Women's health content is covered in Chapter 27. Family planning (Chapter 25) and infertility (Chapter 26) are also part of women's health care in our book.

An effective textbook must present comprehensive content that can be read with ease because nursing students differ in learning abilities, experience, and primary language. Documentation of care in the office, clinic, or acute care setting is primarily in the electronic medical record. Many of our learners have grown up using computers and may be less familiar with their patients who do not have the same computer literacy. Our objective for the seventh edition of *Foundations of Maternal-Newborn and Women's Health Nursing* continues to be presenting complex material as simply and clearly as possible. We again provide step-by-step instruction in assessments and interventions so that students can function quickly in the clinical area at a beginning level. To this end, proven learning aids, such as summaries, illustrations, and tables, are used generously throughout the book.

CONTENT

Nurses should be flexible to accommodate women and their families from different cultures and who communicate in different languages and hold different health beliefs. Nurses use critical thinking skills to devise culture-specific care that includes providing necessary education and support. The six elements we consider most important are a scientific base of information, nursing process, communication, client teaching, critical thinking, and cultural diversity.

Scientific Base

Effective nursing care depends on having a sound understanding of the basis for medical treatments and nursing actions. Although anatomy and physiology courses are part of every curriculum, students often need a review, particularly of the specific content related to childbearing. Because of this, we have incorporated principles of physiology and pathophysiology throughout the book. We have presented these scientific concepts in a clear and understandable manner so that the reader can comprehend the forces underlying both health and dysfunction.

We have included research evidence that supports specific nursing care methods when available. In several chapters is a short summary of a published research article. At the end of the research summary we ask a mix of questions to challenge readers' thought processes. We want readers to think about how they might apply the article's information now, identify what else we need to know about the topic, or think of how the information might apply outside the maternal-newborn and women's health specialties.

Chapters 3, 4, and 5 provide general information about reproductive physiology, genetics, and the process of conception and fetal development. Chapters 6, 12, 17, and 19 explain physiologic adaptations during pregnancy, birth, and the postpartum period and in the newborn. Chapters 10, 11, 16, 23, and 24 describe the pathophysiologic, psychological, and social bases of complications in the mother and in the newborn. Women's health includes many of the cascade of problems that result from obesity, now a problem of epidemic proportions in the United States. Other chapters in the book include the impact of obesity when it is applicable.

The Nursing Process

The nursing process is the accepted framework for assessment and analysis of the patient's needs. It is used to plan and provide nursing care and evaluate the person's response to care. A person's needs often are a mixture of those for which nurses have the primary accountability and those for which another discipline provides definitive therapy yet for which nurses have some responsibility. Therefore for analyzing patient needs, we have chosen either a *patient problem* or a *collaborative problem,* depending on whether nurses are primarily responsible for helping the person meet those needs.

The reader is led through the five steps of the nursing process. Basic information about the condition is presented, and general nursing care follows, organized by the steps of the nursing process. Interventions are general rather than patient specific and are explained by rationales. Case studies with patient-specific nursing care plans are available in the online resources.

Communication

Although they seldom are included as core content in maternal-newborn nursing texts, communication skills are essential to providing adequate care for a childbearing family. We reinforce the student's previous learning and give practical examples of ways in which communication skills can be used in the maternity, newborn, and women's health settings.

Guidelines and examples of effective communication and potential blocks are reviewed in Chapter 1. In addition, dialogues throughout the text present realistic possible nurse–client interactions. As the interaction develops, we identify communication techniques and explain their rationales. Because no one is perfect, we occasionally insert communication blocks, identify them, and suggest alternative responses.

Teaching

Childbearing families are entitled to comprehensive information about how to achieve the best pregnancy outcome and how to best care for the mother and her baby after birth. Women of all ages need current information about maintaining their health. Nurses may be their primary instructors in many areas of maternal-newborn and women's health nursing, and they should be well prepared and well organized to be effective. We present patient teaching in three ways:

- Teaching-learning principles are discussed in Chapter 1.
- Chapters are organized to highlight key content so that the student can gather information and translate it into teaching that is individualized for the person or group of people. For example, Chapter 22, Infant Feeding, lays a foundation of basic information, discusses some common problems, identifies relevant assessments, and presents nursing interventions devoted to teaching parents ways to feed their infant successfully.
- Teaching guidelines are highlighted in *Patient Teaching* features, which give ideas on ways to answer the most common questions on a topic. These features are constructed to show students ways to present information in everyday language rather than in professional language so that the family will better understand the teaching. For instance, the feature "When to Go to the Hospital or Birth Center" (Chapter 15) addresses the concern of many expectant parents that they will not recognize the onset of labor.

Critical Thinking

Nurses must learn critical thinking skills to overcome habits or impulses that can lead to poor clinical decisions. Chapter 1 discusses steps in critical thinking and describes how critical thinking is used in each step of the nursing process. In addition, critical thinking exercises are presented in two ways. First, exercises based on clinical scenarios of common situations with questions to stimulate critical thinking are placed throughout the text. Answers to the questions are found in Appendix B and provide reinforcement for learning. Second, patient-specific nursing care plans (available online) contain critical thinking exercises that require participation by the learner. This makes the care plans interactive and reinforces the concept of critical thinking in clinical practice.

Cultural Diversity

Cultural values are among the most significant factors that influence a woman's perception of childbirth, and effective nursing care must be culture specific. This requires nurses to consider their own cultural values and examine how these values may create conflict with those whose values are different.

Chapter 2 offers an overview of Western cultural values and identifies some areas such as communication and health beliefs that may be sources of conflict. Because many different cultural groups exist in the United States and Canada, emphasis is placed on ways to do a cultural assessment. Plans for care then can show how understanding a family's culture helps nurses provide care that shows respect for cultural differences and traditional healing practices.

New information is integrated throughout the book in all areas, such as the antepartum period, nutrition, birth, the postpartum period, care of the newborn, and women's health.

The Internet is often used by lay people and professionals alike as a source of health information. We provide the addresses for many websites throughout our text that contain reliable, current information relevant to maternal, newborn, and women's health nursing. Examples of these sites are the March of Dimes, Centers for Disease Control and Prevention, National Institutes of Health, and American Cancer Society. Websites for professional associations and other reliable sources are included when appropriate.

ORGANIZATION

The seventh edition of *Foundations of Maternal-Newborn and Women's Health Nursing* is divided into five parts. Part I, Foundations for Nursing Care of Childbearing Families, presents an overview of contemporary nursing care of the family, including ethical, social, and legal aspects. A review of reproductive anatomy and physiology and the hereditary and environmental factors that affect care are also presented.

Part II, The Family Before Birth, begins with conception and prenatal development. These chapters also cover the physiologic and psychosocial adaptations to pregnancy and include a thorough explanation of recommended nutrition during pregnancy and after childbirth. A chapter that includes antepartum fetal assessments and their purpose and two chapters covering families with special needs and antepartum complications are included in Part II.

Part III, The Family During Birth, addresses the physiologic processes of birth, nursing care during labor, and birth and intrapartum complications. These chapters include intrapartum fetal monitoring, pain management, and obstetric procedures such as cesarean birth.

Part IV, The Family Following Birth, describes care of the normal new mother and infant, as well as infant feeding and postpartum and neonatal complications.

Part V, Women's Health Care, focuses on family planning, care of the infertile couple, and women's health care.

FEATURES

- *Visual Appeal.* The book is visually appealing, with numerous up-to-date, full-color illustrations and photographs that clarify concepts and reinforce learning.
- *Objectives.* Each chapter begins with a list of objectives that spell out the purposes of the chapter.
- *Glossary.* A glossary at the back of the book contains key terms and their definitions from all chapters and other terms related to this course.
- *Knowledge Check.* Questions to help students monitor their understanding of the material presented are placed at intervals throughout each chapter. Answers to questions are placed in Appendix A so that students can have immediate feedback.
- *Critical Thinking Exercises.* Clinical situations are boxed and set apart to stimulate critical thinking. We believe strongly that immediate feedback is a powerful learning tool, so answers to critical thinking exercises in the text appear in Appendix B.
- *Evidence-Based Practice:* These research reviews include the latest evidence-based guidelines for various topics and reinforce the importance of integrating research-based guidelines into nursing practice.
- *Critical to Remember* and *Safety Checks.* Condensed summaries of the essential facts to remember are boxed and set apart to reinforce critical information.
- *Patient Teaching.* This feature can be used by students who must begin patient teaching very early in their clinical rotations. These include answers to the most common questions asked by women and parents, often phrased in lay terms or as the nurse would actually answer a patient.
- *Procedures.* Illustrated procedures that are specific to maternity, newborn, and women's health nursing, such as assessment of the uterine fundus, are presented in a step-by-step format with rationales for each step.
- *Drug Guides.* Guides for medications often administered in maternal-newborn and women's health care are available in appropriate chapters.
- *Complementary and Alternative Therapies.* We have included content about these therapies when appropriate throughout the text.
- *Summary Concepts.* A concise review of content is provided at the end of each chapter. In addition, tables and flow charts are frequently used to summarize complex material.

ANCILLARIES

Materials that complement *Foundations of Maternal-Newborn and Women's Health Nursing* include:

For Students

- *Evolve:* Evolve is an innovative website that provides a wealth of content, resources, and state-of-the-art information on maternity nursing. Learning resources for students include Case Studies, Content Updates, Audio Glossary, Printable Key Points, and NCLEX-Style Review Questions.
- *Simulation Learning System (SLS):* The SLS is an online tool kit that helps instructors and facilitators effectively incorporate medium- to high-fidelity simulation into their nursing curriculum. Detailed patient scenarios promote and enhance the clinical decision-making skills of students at all levels. The SLS provides detailed instructions for preparation and implementation of the simulation experience, debriefing questions that encourage critical thinking, and learning resources to reinforce student comprehension. Each scenario in the SLS complements the textbook content and helps bridge the gap between lecture and clinical. The SLS provides the perfect environment for students to practice what they are learning in the text for a true-to-life, hands-on learning experience.
- *Study Guide:* This manual presents a variety of additional activities designed to help students master content and become more proficient in the clinical area. Review questions at various levels of difficulty are included.
- *Virtual Clinical Excursions: Virtual Hospital and Workbook Companion:* A Virtual Hospital and Workbook package has been developed as a virtual clinical experience to expand student opportunities for critical thinking. This package guides the student through a virtual clinical environment and helps the user apply textbook content to virtual patients in that environment. Case studies are presented that allow students to use this textbook as a reference to assess, diagnose, plan, implement, and evaluate "real" patients using clinical scenarios. The state-of-the-art technologies reflected in this virtual hospital demonstrate cutting-edge learning opportunities for students and facilitate knowledge retention of the information found in the textbook. The clinical simulations and workbook represent the next generation of research-based learning tools that promote critical thinking and meaningful learning.

For Instructors

Evolve includes these teaching resources for instructors:

- *Electronic Test Bank in ExamView format* contains more than 900 NCLEX-style test items, including alternative-format questions. An answer key with page references to the text, rationales, and NCLEX-style coding is included.

- **TEACH** *for Nurses* includes teaching strategies; in-class case studies; and links to animations, nursing skills, and nursing curriculum standards such as QSEN, concepts, and BSN Essentials.
- *Electronic Image Collection,* containing more than 350 full-color illustrations and photographs from the text, helps instructors develop presentations and explain key concepts.

- *PowerPoint Slides,* with lecture notes for each chapter of the text, assist in presenting materials in the classroom. *Case Studies* and *Audience Response Questions* for i-clicker are included.
- A *Curriculum Guide* that includes a proposed class schedule and reading assignments for courses of varying lengths is provided. This gives educators suggestions for using the text in the most essential manner or in a more comprehensive way.

ACKNOWLEDGMENTS

Many people made the seventh edition of *Foundations of Maternal-Newborn and Women's Health Nursing* a reality. Thank you to the Elsevier team who brought us together and kept us focused and assisted throughout the publication process: Laurie Gower, Director; Betsy McCormac, Content Development Specialist; Tracey Schriefer, Project Manager; and Amy Buxton, Designer.

Thank you to the chapter contributors who shared their passion. Their clinical expertise and commitment to the future of nursing are deeply appreciated.

We will be forever grateful to Sharon Murray and Emily McKinney, whose vision and endless work brought us the previous editions of this book and whose love for nursing and nursing students will live on in future editions.

Karen Holub and Renee Jones

IN MEMORY OF EMILY McKINNEY

Emily McKinney passed away in December 2013. It was my privilege to coauthor six editions of *Foundations of Maternal-Newborn and Women's Health Nursing* and four editions of *Maternal-Child Nursing* with Emily. She also coauthored study guides for several other obstetric nursing textbooks. In 1999, she was awarded the honor of being included in the Dallas Fort Worth's Great 100 Nurses list. She was on the editorial staff of *JOGNN* (*Journal of Obstetric, Gynecologic, and Neonatal Nursing*) and was named Reviewer of the Year in 2006.

Emily was an excellent obstetric nurse and a talented nursing educator in the hospital as well as the classroom setting. She had an impressive knowledge of the science and the art of maternal-newborn nursing and was able to pass that knowledge on to her students in an easily digestible fashion.

It was Emily's idea to write a textbook that would be comprehensive yet easy to read. She realized that students often juggle several roles other than just being students. They are often parents and hold jobs to pay for their education and support their families. Emily used to say that simple words and short sentences could be just as effective as long, complicated words and sentences and much more easily absorbed by busy learners. When Trula Gorrie and I first met her in 1990, we knew that we shared Emily's vision, and a wonderful partnership was formed.

Emily loved learning. She particularly looked forward to the yearly AWHONN (Association of Women's Health, Obstetric, and Neonatal Nursing) conventions. We met there each year and enjoyed hearing about the latest techniques and discoveries to advance obstetric nursing that were discussed. She was eager to find ways to apply new information to her clinical practice and teaching.

Throughout the years she was working on textbooks, Emily faced some difficult health problems. Yet she persevered in writing her chapters. She produced an amazing amount of quality work in short periods in spite of feeling ill. She was determined to do this as a way to advance nursing and nursing education.

Emily was also dedicated to her family. Her many interests included making clothes for her husband and two daughters, as well as knitting hats for premature infants. Her daughters are following in her footsteps and are planning to go into nursing.

As an inspired nurse, Emily offered encouragement and practical help to her students and patients each day. Her passion for nursing was obvious to all. Emily is missed by everyone who knew her.

Sharon Murray

CONTENTS

1

Maternity and Women's Health Care Today

Kari Mau

OBJECTIVES

After studying this chapter, you should be able to:

1. Describe changes in maternity care, from home birth with lay midwives to the emergence of medical management.
2. Identify trends that led to the development of family-centered care.
3. Explain choices in childbearing.
4. Describe current trends that affect perinatal nursing and women's health nursing, such as Healthy People 2020, focus on safety and quality, cost containment, community-based care, advances in technology, and increased use of complementary and alternative medicine.
5. Discuss the trends in infant and maternal mortality rates and compare current infant mortality rates among specific racial groups and nations.
6. Explain the roles of nurses with advanced preparation in maternal-newborn or women's health nursing, including the roles of nurse-midwives, nurse practitioners, and clinical nurse specialists.
7. Discuss the roles for nurses in maternity care and women's health care.
8. Discuss the importance of nursing research in clinical practice.
9. Explain the importance of critical thinking in nursing practice and describe how it may be refined.
10. Relate the five steps of the nursing process to maternal-newborn and women's health nursing.
11. Explain how the nursing process relates to critical thinking.

Major changes in maternity care occurred in the first half of the twentieth century as childbirth moved from the home to a hospital setting. Change continues and confusion abounds as health care providers and payers attempt to control the increasing cost of care and rapid growth of expensive technology. Despite these challenges, health care professionals are focused on patient safety and quality of care. Health problems such as obesity, diabetes, and hypertension may have health consequences not only during childbearing years but also throughout middle age and beyond.

Although improvements in health care have resulted in a significant decline in maternal and infant mortality rates in the United States, statistics show a wide disparity between outcomes among races.

HISTORICAL PERSPECTIVES ON CHILDBEARING

Granny Midwives

Before the twentieth century, childbirth occurred most often in the home with the assistance of a "granny" midwife whose training was obtained through an apprenticeship with a more experienced granny or lay midwife. Many women and infants fared well when a midwife assisted with birth in the home, but maternal and infant death rates from childbearing were high for both hospital and home births.

Emergence of Medical Management

In the late nineteenth century, developments that were available to physicians but not always to midwives led to a decline in home births and an increase in physician-assisted hospital births. By 1960, 90% of all births in the United States occurred in hospitals.

Maternity care became highly regimented for most women. Physicians managed all **antepartum** (before onset of labor), **intrapartum** (time of labor and birth), and **postpartum** (first 6 weeks after childbirth) care. Lay midwifery became illegal in many areas, and nurse-midwifery was not well established. The woman's role in childbirth was passive: the physician "delivered" her infant. The primary functions of nurses were to assist the physician and follow prescribed medical orders after childbirth. Despite technologic advances

TABLE 1.1	Federal Projects for Maternal Child Care
Program	**Purpose**
Title V of Social Security Act www.ssa.gov/OP_Home/ssact/title05/0500.htm	Provides funds for maternal and child health programs
National Institute of Child Health and Human Development www.nichd.nih.gov	Supports research and education of personnel needed for maternal and child health programs
Medicaid www.medicaid.gov	Provides funds to facilitate health care access by low income pregnant women and young children
Head Start www.acf.hhs.gov	Provides educational opportunities for low-income children of preschool age
Women, Infants, and Children (WIC) Program www.fns.usda.gov/wic/women-infants-and-children-wic	Provides supplemental food and nutrition information
Temporary Assistance to Needy Families (TANF) www.benefits.gov	Provides temporary money for basic living costs of poor children and their families, with eligibility requirements and time limits varying among states; tribal programs available for Native Americans; replaced the Aid to Families with Dependent Children (AFDC) program
National Center for Family Planning www.nationalfamilyplanning.org	A clearinghouse for information on contraception
Healthy Start www.nationalhealthystart.org	Enhances community development of culturally appropriate strategies designed to decrease infant mortality and causes of low birth weight

and the move from home to hospital, maternal and infant mortality rates declined slowly. Affluent families could afford comprehensive medical care early in the pregnancy, but poor families had very limited access to prenatal care or information about childbearing. Two concurrent trends, federal government involvement and consumer demands, led to additional changes in maternity care.

Government Involvement in Maternal-Infant Care

High rates of maternal and infant mortality among poor women provided the impetus for federal involvement in maternity care. The Sheppard-Towner Act of 1921, the first federally sponsored program, provided funds for state-managed programs for mothers and children. Although the Sheppard-Towner Act was later repealed, it set the stage for future allocation of federal funds. Today, the federal government supports several programs to improve the health of mothers, infants, and young children (Table 1.1). Although government funds partially solved the problem of maternal and infant mortality, the distribution of health care remains inequitable.

Effects of Consumer Demands on Health Care

In the early 1950s, consumers began to insist on their right to be involved in their own health care. Pregnant women were no longer willing to accept only what was offered. They wanted information about planning and spacing their children, and they wanted to know what to expect during pregnancy. Fathers, siblings, and grandparents wanted to be part of the extraordinary time of pregnancy and childbirth. Parents wanted more "say" in the way their child was born.

Early in the 1950s, Dr. Grantly Dick-Read proposed a method of childbirth that allowed the mother to control her fear and thus control her pain during labor, allowing for birth without pharmacologic intervention. Methods such as Lamaze and Bradley also gained favor. A growing consensus among child psychologists and nurse researchers affirmed that early parent-newborn

contact outweighed the risks for infection in most situations. Knowledgeable parents insisted that their infants remain with them. The practice of separating the infant from the family was abandoned when infections did not increase in nurseries, and family-centered maternity care became the standard.

Development of Family-Centered Care

Family-centered care describes safe, high-quality care that recognizes and adapts to both the physical and psychosocial needs of the family, including the newborn. The goal is to foster family unity while maintaining physical safety. Family-centered care greatly increased the responsibilities of nurses. Nurses now assume a major role in teaching, counseling, and supporting families in their decisions about childbirth.

The basic principles of family-centered care are as follows:
- Childbirth is usually a normal, healthy event in the life of a family.
- Childbirth affects the entire family, and family relationships will need to be restructured.
- Families can make decisions about care if they are given adequate information and professional support.
- Maintaining a focus on family or other support can benefit a woman as she seeks to maintain health.

CHOICES IN CHILDBIRTH

Most families now recognize that they have choices in the childbirth experience. These choices include the type of provider, birth setting, and support persons for labor and birth. Some insurance providers may limit the choices available to the woman and her family. The woman should be encouraged to verify insurance coverage of provider and birth setting.

Health Care Provider

Women contemplating pregnancy and birth may choose a certified nurse midwife (CNM), nurse practitioner (NP), or

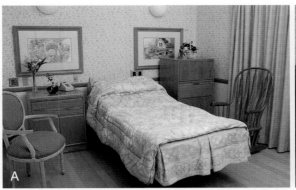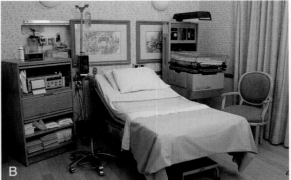

FIG. 1.1 Typical Labor, Delivery, and Recovery Room. Homelike furnishings **(A)** can be adapted quickly to expose the necessary technical equipment **(B)**.

physician to be their health care provider. They need to know what to expect from each of these practitioners.

A CNM cares for women at low risk for complications and refers them to a back-up physician if problems develop. A CNM provides well-woman as well as obstetric care. CNMs, NPs, and physicians treat women during pregnancy and the postpartum period, but NPs do not perform deliveries. NPs usually work in a physician's office and see women for routine prenatal care, but the delivery is performed by the physician. A CNM, NP, or family practice physician also may care for the newborn.

Some couples visit several different care providers before choosing the one they think is best for them. They may ask about the provider's usual practices and the provider's beliefs about areas that are important to them, such as medication, episiotomies, or aspects of infant care.

Birth Setting
Labor, Delivery, and Recovery Rooms
Today, the most common location for vaginal birth in a hospital is the labor, delivery, and recovery (LDR) room. In an LDR room, normal labor, birth, and recovery from birth take place in one setting (Fig. 1.1).

During labor, the woman's significant others can remain with her. These people may include relatives, friends, and her other children, depending on the policies of the agency and the mother's desires. After she has given birth, the mother typically remains in the LDR room for 1 to 2 hours, after which she is transferred to her postpartum room for the remainder of her hospital stay. The healthy infant may remain with the mother throughout her stay in the LDR room, receiving continuing evaluation for adaptation to neonatal life. When the mother is transferred to her postpartum room, the infant may be transferred to the nursery for more extensive assessment or may remain with the mother in a mother-baby postpartum room while being assessed.

Labor, Delivery, Recovery, and Postpartum Rooms
Some hospitals offer rooms like LDR rooms in layout and function, with the exception that the mother is not transferred to a postpartum unit after recovery. She and the infant remain in the labor, delivery, recovery, and postpartum (LDRP) room until discharge. The father or the woman's primary support person is encouraged to stay with the mother and the infant, and sleeping facilities for that person may be provided.

Birth Centers
Freestanding birth centers are designed to provide maternity care to low-risk women outside a hospital setting. Many centers also provide gynecologic services such as annual well-woman examination (WWE) and contraceptive counseling. The mother usually attends classes at the birth center or elsewhere to prepare for childbirth, breastfeeding, and infant care. Both the mother and the infant continue to receive follow-up care during the first 6 weeks after birth. This may include help for breastfeeding problems, a postpartum examination at 4 to 6 weeks, family planning information, and examination of the newborn. Birth is often assisted by the CNM who has provided care for the woman throughout her pregnancy and will continue to provide primary care for the mother and the infant.

Birth centers are less expensive compared with traditional hospitals, which provide advanced technology that may be unnecessary for low-risk women. Moreover, women who want a safe birth in a familiar, homelike setting with personnel they have known throughout their pregnancies often express satisfaction with birth centers.

The main disadvantage is that most independent birth centers are not equipped for major obstetric emergencies. If unforeseen difficulties develop during labor, the woman should be transferred by ambulance to a nearby hospital to the care of a back-up physician who has agreed to perform this duty. Although procedures have been designed for these situations, a sudden transfer is frightening for the family.

Home Births
In the United States only a small number of women give birth at home. Many CNMs have moved their practices to hospitals or birth centers and may be in practice with physicians. Mothers who once sought home births have found they can have many of the advantages of family-centered care in the safe environment of a hospital or birth center and yet retain the nurse-midwife's care and low-intervention approach they prefer.

Home birth provides the advantage of keeping the family together in its own familiar environment throughout the childbirth experience. When all goes well, birth at home can be a growth-enhancing experience for every family member. Bonding with the infant is unimpeded by hospital routines, and breastfeeding is highly encouraged and supported. Women who have their babies at home maintain a feeling of control because they actively plan and prepare for each detail of the birth.

Giving birth at home also has disadvantages. Women who plan a home birth should be screened carefully to make sure they have a very low risk for complications. If transfer to a nearby hospital becomes necessary, the time required may be an issue. Other problems associated with home birth include the need for the parents to provide a setting and adequate supplies for the birth. Moreover, the mother must take care of herself and the infant without the immediate help she would have in a hospital or birth center setting.

Support Person

During labor, the woman needs someone with her to help her through the experience. The support person is most often the father of her baby, but a relative or friend also may take this role. Some women wish to share the birth experience with several relatives and close friends. If the birth setting is traditional, only one or two people may be permitted to be present. In less traditional settings, more support people are usually allowed.

Some women hire a **doula** to provide support during labor. A doula is a trained labor support person who provides physical and emotional support throughout labor and sometimes during the postpartum period. Many doulas meet with the family before birth and offer pregnancy, childbirth, and parenting classes.

Siblings

The presence of children at birth is controversial. Some think children become closer to their new siblings when they are present at birth. Others think the sights of the birth process, blood, and their mothers in pain may be too frightening for children. Some debate focuses on the age of the child attending the birth.

Children who participate in the birth of a sibling may attend all or part of the labor and birth or may join the parents just after the birth to participate in the immediate celebration. An adult support person is necessary to stay with the child throughout the experience. The support person should have no role other than attending to the child. This role includes gauging the child's response, providing explanations and reassurance, and taking the child out of the room as needed.

Education

Perinatal education is important to help couples learn about pregnancy, birth, and parenting. Many classes not only focus on preparation for childbirth but also include information formerly received during the birth facility stay. There are options for perinatal education. New families make their choices based on the classes available in the area, costs, and types of information they need. Small classes of a few women and their partners are ideal but may be too expensive or unavailable (see Chapter 7).

? KNOWLEDGE CHECK

1. What led to federal government involvement in the health care of women and infants? Is today's health care equal among poor and more affluent women?
2. How does family-centered maternity care differ from maternity care during the first half of the nineteenth century?
3. How do labor, delivery, and recovery (LDR) rooms and labor, delivery, recovery, and postpartum (LDRP) rooms differ from birth centers and homes in their advantages and disadvantages?

CURRENT TRENDS IN PERINATAL AND WOMEN'S HEALTH CARE

Healthy People 2020

Healthy People 2020 (U.S. Department of Health and Human Services, 2010) is a set of 10-year objectives for improving the health of the people of the United States. It has four overarching goals, as follows:

- Attain high-quality, longer lives free of preventable disease, disability, injury, and premature death
- Achieve health equity, eliminate disparities, and improve the health of all groups
- Create social and physical environments that promote good health for all
- Promote quality of life, healthy development, and healthy behaviors across all life stages

Many of the specific objectives directly or indirectly pertain to maternity and women's health.

Safety and Quality
The Joint Commission

The Joint Commission (TJC) is an independent organization that accredits health care organizations. They defined a set of Perinatal Core Measures for best practice in perinatal care. Accredited organizations report their compliance with these measures each year. The five core measures for perinatal care are decrease the rate of elective deliveries, decrease the rate of cesarean births, increase the rate of antenatal administration of steroids in preterm labor, decrease the rate of newborns with septicemia or bacteremia, and increase the rate of exclusive breastfeeding (TJC, 2017).

Interprofessional Collaboration and Education

Interprofessional collaborative practice has been identified as a key to safe, high-quality, accessible, patient-centered care (Interprofessional Education Collaborative, 2016). To promote interprofessional team-based patient care and improve patient outcomes, the Interprofessional Education Collaborative (IPEC) has encouraged health professional schools to incorporate interprofessional learning experiences into their curricula and defined core competencies for inter-professional collaborative practice. In one study of prelicensure health profession students in a high-fidelity simulation, Rossler and Kimble (2016) found that interprofessional interactions during the simulation enhanced interprofessional communication, increased their appreciation for other disciplines, and delineated their discipline's contribution to the whole when providing care in practice.

Alliance for Innovation on Maternal Health

The Alliance for Innovation on Maternal Health (AIM) is a quality improvement alliance of professional organizations, patient representatives, and a health industry informational forum (Council on Patient Safety in Women's Health Care, 2017). AIM has developed patient safety bundles for maternal care that represent best practice and are supported by multidisciplinary professional organizations (American College of Obstetricians and Gynecologists, 2017).

Patient Safety Bundles. A bundle is a set of evidence-based practices performed together to improve patient outcomes. (Institute for Healthcare Improvement, 2017). Maternal safety bundles have been developed for maternal mental health: depression and anxiety, obstetric hemorrhage, severe hypertension in pregnancy, venous thromboembolism, safe reduction of primary cesarean birth, reduction of peripartum racial/ethnic disparities, and support after a severe maternal event (Council on Patient Safety in Women's Health Care, 2017). (See www.safehealthcareforeverywoman.org.)

Women's Health and Perinatal Nursing Care Quality Measures

Because the actions of nurses have a significant impact on patient outcomes, the Association of Women's Health, Obstetric and Neonatal Nurses (AWHONN) is in the process of developing nursing care quality measures to guide efforts to measure the quality of nursing care. These measures are currently being tested for feasibility, validity, and reliability, but currently include triage of a pregnant woman and her fetus(es); second stage of labor: mother-initiated, spontaneous pushing; skin-to-skin initiated immediately after birth; duration of uninterrupted skin-to-skin contact; eliminating supplementation of breast–fed healthy, term newborns; protection of maternal milk volume for premature infants admitted to the neonatal intensive care unit (NICU); initial contact with mothers after a neonatal transport; perinatal grief support; women's health and wellness coordination throughout the life span; labor support/partial labor support; and freedom of movement during labor (AWHONN, 2014).

Cost Containment

Government, insurance companies, health care facilities, and health care providers have made a concerted effort to control the increasing cost of health care in the United States.

The Patient Protection and Affordable Care Act was passed in 2010 with the intent to expand access to health insurance, increase consumer protections, emphasize prevention and wellness, improve quality and system performance, expand the health workforce, and curb rising health care costs (National Conference of State Legislatures, 2011) Updates can be found at www.HealthCare.gov.

Effects of Cost Containment on Maternity Care

Cost containment efforts have had major effects on maternity care, primarily regarding length of stay (LOS). Mothers who have a normal vaginal birth are typically discharged with their newborns from the hospital at 48 hours, and mothers who give birth by cesarean section leave at 96 hours. This is a short time to accomplish the teaching needed before discharge, particularly when the new mother is tired and uncomfortable from the birth. She may or may not have had prenatal classes to prepare her for the care she and her infant will need, and she may not have had prenatal care at all. Support of family or friends after discharge may not exist for all new mothers.

Reduced LOS has also affected caregivers, particularly nurses. Nurses are concerned about meeting the needs of families who leave the hospital a short time after the birth of an infant. It is especially difficult to provide adequate information about self-care and infant care when the mother is still recovering from childbirth.

Community-Based Perinatal and Women's Health Nursing

Community-based care has increased in perinatal and women's health nursing because an acute care setting is the most expensive for delivery of health care services. Advances in portable technology and wireless transmission allow nurses in many practice areas to perform procedures in the home that were once limited to the hospital. Documentation and data retrieval are available by secure wireless Internet connections. Additionally, women and their families are taught to manage less severe problems at home under the supervision of a nurse, entering the hospital only for possible worsening of the problem. Consumers often prefer home care because of decreased stress on the family when a woman or newborn does not need to be separated from the family support system for hospitalization.

The health care system of the future will likely be community oriented and involve care for greater numbers of patients in the home and through community agencies. Public health agencies have existed for many years, and many women obtain all antepartum, postpartum, and neonatal care in these clinics. Other community facilities such as neighborhood health centers, shelters for women and children, school-age mothers' programs, and nurse-managed postpartum centers also provide care to a variety of patients.

Nurses need a broad array of skills to function effectively in community-based care, whether that care takes place in individuals' homes or in large clinics. They should understand the communities in which they practice and the diversity within those communities. Nurses need skills to work with a multidisciplinary team. They are often responsible for assisting patients through high-technology choices and therefore need to be proficient in communication and teaching skills.

Perinatal nursing services delivered in a community setting encompass antepartum, postpartum, and neonatal care. Because care may be given in an environment physically separate from acute care settings, nurses should be able to function independently and have superior clinical and critical thinking skills. They should be proficient in interviewing, counseling, and teaching. They assume a leadership role in the coordination of the services a family may require in a complex case, and they frequently supervise the work of other care providers.

Common Types of Perinatal Home Care

Antepartum Home Care. Most preconceptional and low-risk antepartum care takes place in private offices or public clinics. High-risk conditions that may be seen in the home by a nurse include preterm labor, hyperemesis gravidarum (intractable vomiting during pregnancy), bleeding problems, preterm premature rupture of membranes, hypertension, and diabetes during pregnancy. Severity of these problems and gestational age affect how each will be managed.

Postpartum and Neonatal Home Care. Providing the necessary education to new mothers about their self-care, basic care of their infants, and signs of problems they should report after discharge is a challenge for health care professionals. Before the woman is discharged, hospitals may offer classes, closed-circuit television programs, written materials (often in multiple languages), individual teaching and demonstration, and videos with many relevant topics that a family can take home for later reference.

After the woman is discharged, various services may be offered for home care. These services may include telephone calls, home visits, information lines, and **lactation** consultations (breastfeeding assistance). In addition, nurse-managed outpatient clinics provide care for mothers and infants in some areas.

Home Care for High-Risk Neonates. Neonatal home care nurses may provide care to infants who are discharged from the acute care facility with serious medical conditions. Parents of preterm or low-birth-weight infants require a great deal of information and support. Infants with congenital anomalies such as cleft palate may require care adapted to their conditions. Increasing numbers of technology-dependent infants, such as those who require ventilator assistance, total parenteral nutrition, intravenous medications, and apnea monitoring, are now cared for at home.

The coordination of care for the high-risk newborn is a major challenge for home care nurses. Involvement of multiple specialty providers such as physicians, nurses, respiratory therapists, and equipment vendors may result in duplication or fragmentation of services. Duplication of services results in unnecessary costs, and fragmentation of services can result in dangerous gaps in care.

Advances in Technology

As with other areas of health care, perinatal care should keep pace with technologic advances. Health care professionals and patients have online access to information from a variety of databases that are often updated, and many of these include data used in this text. Verification of the source of information and appropriate interpretation of that information is essential. Telemedicine is used for consultation between professionals and may provide access to care for people in underserved areas. It is anticipated that the use of telemedicine will continue to evolve. Fetal monitoring data may be stored on electronic media rather than on paper. Video and digital imaging methods are used to preserve and recall crisp images and allow image overlay and computerized comparison, often at distant locations. Personal computer systems are linked to share information about staffing, scheduling, communication, and employee benefits. Electronic medical records are standard in most health care facilities. Electronic notebooks can be used to support nurses with drug information, send and receive wireless e-mail, maintain contacts, and download journal articles from publications such as the *Journal of Obstetric, Gynecologic, and Neonatal Nursing* and *Nursing for Women's Health.* Maintaining security is essential to ensure appropriate privacy for personal and professional information.

Complementary and Alternative Medicine

Complementary and alternative medicine (CAM) is common. CAM refers to health care approaches that differ from conventional "Western" medicine. When these practices are integrated with conventional treatments, they are complementary; when used in place of the mainstream practices, they are "alternative." Integrative medicine refers to the coordinated use of conventional and complementary approaches to health care (National Center for Complementary and Alternative Medicine, 2016) Table 1.2 gives examples of therapies for complementary or alternative care.

A press release from NCCAM (2011) described a survey conducted with the American Association of Retired Persons (AARP) and two-thirds of the people older than 50 years use some form of CAM but fewer than one-third have ever discussed it with their health care provider. The following are the most common reasons stated by those surveyed:

- The physician never asked.
- They did not know they should discuss CAM.
- There was not enough time during an office visit.

Safety is a major concern with the use of CAM. Many people who use these techniques or substances are self-referred. They may delay necessary care from a conventional physician or nurse-midwife, or the woman may ingest herbal remedies or other substances that are harmful during pregnancy or lactation. Some CAM therapies are harmful if combined with conventional medications or when taken in excess. Because herbs and vitamins are classified as foods rather than medications, they are not strictly regulated. Therefore people may consume variable amounts of active ingredients from these substances. Herbal therapies may be used for infertility, premenstrual syndrome, dysmenorrhea, menopausal symptoms, pregnancy and perineal discomforts, and lactation discomforts. Also, many people may not consider some therapies as "alternative" because they are considered mainstream in their

TABLE 1.2   Complementary and Alternative Medicine Categories

Category	Examples
Mind–body interventions: Behavioral, psychological, social, and spiritual approaches to health	Yoga, relaxation response techniques, meditation, tai chi, hypnotherapy, music therapy, spirituality, and biofeedback; some such as support groups and cognitive-behavioral therapy are now mainstream
Manipulative and body-based methods: Based on manipulation or movement of one or more parts of the body	Chiropractic or osteopathic manipulation; massage
Alternative medical systems: Systems developed outside the Western biomedical approach or that evolved apart from the early conventional medical approach in the United States	Examples of systems developed within Western cultures include homeopathy, naturopathic, and chiropractic medicine; non-Western approaches include traditional Chinese medicine, ayurveda, Native American medicine, and acupuncture
Biologically based therapies: Use of substances found in nature such as herbs, foods, and vitamins	Dietary supplements, herbal products, or medicinal plants such as ginkgo biloba, ginseng, echinacea, saw palmetto, witch hazel, bilberry, aloe vera, feverfew, and green tea; aromatherapy
Energy therapies: Two types involve the energy fields Biofield therapies: Presumed to affect energy fields that surround the body	Biofield therapies have not been scientifically proved; examples include qi gong, reiki, and therapeutic touch
Bioelectromagnetic-based therapies: Unconventional use of electromagnetic fields	Examples of bioelectromagnetic-based therapies include pulsed fields, magnetic fields, and alternating-current or direct-current fields

cultures, in which Western medicine is considered "alternative." Assessment for the use of CAM therapies is becoming more common for many patient assessment tools in medicine, nursing, pharmacy, and other health care specialties.

Nurses may find that their professional values do not conflict with many of the CAM therapies. As a profession, nursing supports a self-care and preventive approach to health care, in which individuals bear much of the responsibility for their health. Nursing practice has traditionally emphasized a holistic, or body–mind–spirit, model of health that fits with CAM. Nurses already may widely practice some CAM therapies such as therapeutic touch. The rising interest in CAM provides opportunities for nurses to participate in research related to the legitimacy of these treatment modalities.

Shortage of Nurses

Many current nurses are baby boomers (those born in the years 1946 to 1964), and they are nearing retirement age or have already retired. Baby boomers are a large population group, and their need for health care is expected to increase as they age.

Many nursing schools increased enrollment with the realization more registered nurses (RNs) will be needed for care of baby boomers in the future and large numbers of their faculty will likely retire soon. Studies have shown higher RN-to-patient ratios have reduced hospital mortality, reinforcing the need for an increase in their numbers as boomers retire. In the landmark report "*The Future of Nursing: Leading Change, Advancing Health*," the Institute of Medicine (IOM, 2011) identified the need for 80% of new RNs to be prepared at the baccalaureate or higher level by 2020. Despite this need, nursing schools are turning away qualified applicants to baccalaureate and graduate degree programs because of an insufficient number of faculty, clinical sites, classroom space, clinical preceptors, and budget constraints (American Association of Colleges of Nursing, 2016).

With inadequate nurse staffing and increasing patient loads as the population ages, nurses face greater work stress and fatigue, leading some to leave acute care or leave the profession. Lengthy shifts of 12 hours in most acute care facilities may be too much for the aging nurse, but these shifts also may be too demanding for the nurse who is a new parent, caregiver for an older adult, or trying to earn a higher degree while working. Fatigue of long work hours can affect both the nurse's health and the patient's safety. Many health care facilities continue not only to support education of new nurses but also to retain older nurses. Nursing scholarships from a facility may be available to their non-RN employees, usually after completion of the prerequisite courses. Joint appointment of RNs promotes sharing of the nurse's skills and knowledge between a school and a clinical facility. However, the school and clinical facility should clearly limit RN time demands for each facility. Hospitals earning "Magnet status" recognition from American Nurses Credentialing Center are often more attractive at acquiring and retaining nurses. Measures to maintain safety for both patients and working staff reduce the risks for injury and lost productivity. Greater flexibility in scheduling may be a way for acute care facilities to retain both younger and older nurses.

KNOWLEDGE CHECK

4. How can interprofessional education improve patient safety and quality of care?
5. What is a patient safety bundle?
6. What are AWHONN's Nursing Care Quality Measures?
7. What are possible dangers in the use of complementary and alternative medicine?

STATISTICS ON MATERNAL, INFANT, AND WOMEN'S HEALTH

Statistics is the science of collecting and interpreting numerical data. In the health and medical sciences, data often focus on mortality rates within a given population. **Mortality rates** indicate the number of deaths that occur each year by different categories. They are important sources of information about the health of groups of people within a country. They also may be an indication of the value a society places on health care and the kind of health care available to the people.

Maternal and Infant Mortality

Throughout history, mortality rates among women and infants have been high, especially in relation to childbirth. Infant and maternal mortality rates began to fall with the improved health of the general population, application of basic principles of sanitation, and increase in medical knowledge. Improvements in health care, including widely available antibiotics, public health facilities, and increased prenatal care, further reduced infant mortality.

Pregnancy-Related Maternal Mortality

In 2013, the **pregnancy-related mortality rate** was 17.3 per 100,000 live births among all women in the United States. This rate has steadily increased, and the reasons for this rise in pregnancy-related deaths is unclear. More pregnant women have chronic health conditions such as hypertension, diabetes, and chronic heart disease. These conditions place women at increased risk for pregnancy-related complications. Causes of pregnancy-related death include infection or sepsis, hemorrhage, and cardiovascular disease (CVD), including cardiomyopathy (Centers for Disease Control and Prevention [CDC], 2016). In addition, racial disparities exist. The pregnancy-related mortality for Black women is 41.1 deaths per 100,000, compared with White women, who experience 11.8 deaths per 100,000 (CDC, 2016).

Infant Mortality

The **infant mortality rate** (death before the age of 1 year) has decreased to 5.96 per 1000 in 2013. The **neonatal mortality rate** (death before 28 days of life) is 4.04 deaths per 1000 live births in 2013. The leading causes of infant mortality are congenital malformations, premature birth, and maternal complications of pregnancy (Mathews, MacDorman, & Thoma, 2015).

As in pregnancy-related mortality, racial disparities exist. Non-Hispanic black infants have the highest mortality rate, at 11.11 per 100,000 live births. Rates are also higher for American Indian or Alaska Native infants and infants of Puerto Rican descent (Mathews et al., 2015).

The following *Healthy People 2020* objectives relate to perinatal through infant mortality in the United States (U.S. Department of Health and Human Services, 2010):

- Reduce perinatal mortality (28 weeks to 7 days after birth) to 5.9 per 1000 live births and fetal deaths
- Reduce infant mortality from the 1998 rate of 7.2 per 1000 live births to 4.5 per 1000 live births
- Reduce neonatal mortality from the 1998 rate of 4.8 per 1000 live births to 2.9 per 1000 live births
- Reduce the percentage of low-birth-weight infants from 7.6 to 5
- Reduce the percentage of very-low-birth-weight infants from 1.4 to 0.9.

Infant Mortality across Nations

The United States has one of the highest gross national products in the world, and is expected to have one of the lowest infant mortality rates. Yet, the infant mortality rate in the United States ranked twenty-sixth among developed nations (MacDorman, Mathews, Moshangoo, & Zeitlin, 2014)

Preterm births in the United States increased for the first time in 8 years. In 2015, the preterm birth rate was 9.6% (March of Dimes, 2015). Late preterm births (34 to 36 completed weeks of gestation), that is, babies born 1 to 3 weeks short of term, have increased in recent years. Preterm birth is the greatest contributor to infant death (CDC, 2015).

Adolescent Pregnancy

Teen birth rates have decreased in the United States, and the 2014 teen birth rate fell to 24.2 per 1000 women in this age group. This may be attributed to use of birth control rather than reduction in sexually activity. The teen pregnancy rate in the United States is substantially higher than in other industrialized countries (CDC, 2014).

Women's Health

CVD is the leading cause of death in the United States, and 51% of the deaths occur in women. The epidemic of obesity contributes to the growing problems of hypertension, high blood cholesterol, and diabetes mellitus.

KNOWLEDGE CHECK

8. Why is the infant mortality rate so much lower today than at the beginning of the twentieth century?
9. How does the infant mortality rate in the United States compare with the rates in other countries?

STANDARDS OF PRACTICE FOR PERINATAL AND WOMEN'S HEALTH NURSING

Both community-based and acute care services should meet guidelines for practice established by the agency itself, appropriate specialty practice organizations, and accrediting agencies.

Agency Standards

Health care agencies are required to have policies, procedures, and protocols to define and guide all elements of care. These standards, which should comply with established national standards, should be kept current and accessible to the nursing personnel. Manuals for these agency standards are often available online within the agency for easier access. Updates and periodic reviews are required to maintain validity of care guidelines.

Organizational Standards

Organizational standards provide broader guidelines that are nationally recognized. AWHONN is recognized as the national professional organization for perinatal and women's health nursing services, publishing standards, education guides, monographs, professional issues, and nursing practice guidelines. Standards set by other professional organizations, such as the American Congress of Obstetricians and Gynecologists (ACOG), the American Academy of Pediatrics (AAP), and the National Association of Home Care and Hospice, may influence standards for perinatal and women's health nurses.

Legal Standards

Nurses who practice in any health care delivery system should understand the definition of nursing practice and the rules and regulations that govern its practice in their work settings. Nurses also should be aware of their scope of practice in varying locations as defined by state nurse practice acts.

Other regulatory bodies, such as the Occupational Safety and Health Administration (OSHA), the U.S. Food and Drug Administration (FDA), and the Centers for Disease Control and Prevention (CDC), also provide guidelines for practice in those areas. Accrediting agencies such as The Joint Commission (TJC) and the Community Health Accreditation Program (CHAP) give their approval after visiting facilities and observing whether standards are being met in practice. Approval from these accrediting agencies affects reimbursement and funding decisions as well.

THE NURSE'S ROLE

Nurses work in a variety of highly specialized areas; fetal diagnostic centers, infertility clinics, genetic counseling centers, and in acute care settings. Home-based care is an option for some perinatal conditions. Nurses have the primary responsibility to teach, counsel, and intervene for a wide variety of problems affecting the childbearing family.

Nurses should develop interpersonal skills to communicate, teach, and collaborate with patients, family, and other members of the health care team. Nurses are expected to base their practice on valid and current research and use critical thinking and the nursing process to identify and intervene for a variety of problems. The roles of the nurse include communicator, teacher, advocate, collaborator, researcher, and manager. Moreover, many nurses complete advanced programs of education and obtain licensure as an advanced practice nurse, allowing them to provide primary care to girls and women before, during, and after their childbearing years.

Communicator

Nurses use therapeutic communication. Unlike social communication, therapeutic communication is purposeful, goal directed, and focused. Although it may seem simple, therapeutic communication requires conscious effort and considerable practice.

Therapeutic Communication Techniques

Therapeutic communication involves responding and listening, and nurses should learn to use responses that facilitate rather than block communication. These facilitative responses, often called *communication techniques,* focus on both the content of the message and the feeling accompanying the message. Communication techniques include clarifying, **reflecting** (meditating or attentive consideration), maintaining silence, questioning, and directing. In addition, nurses should be aware of blocks to communication.

Teacher

Wellness and health improvement opportunities are common in maternity care, and thus teaching represents a major responsibility for nurses who work in these areas. Nurses teach in several settings, including one-on-one interactions, formal classes, and group discussions. To teach effectively, nurses should be familiar with the basic principles of teaching and learning, which include: (1) readiness of the learner affects the ability to learn, (2) active participation increases learning, (3) repetition of a skill increases retention and feelings of competence, (4) praise and positive feedback are powerful motivators, (5) role modeling is an effective methodology, (6) conflicts and frustration impede learning, (7) learning is enhanced when teaching is structured to present simple tasks before more complex material, (8) variety of teaching methods may maintain interest and illustrate concepts, and (9) retention is greater when material is presented in small segments over time. Many factors, including the family's developmental level, primary language, cultural orientation, and previous experiences, influence learning. In addition, the nurse should be aware that the physical environment and the organization and skill of the instructor will also effect learning.

Collaborator

Nurses collaborate with other members of the health care team, often coordinating and managing a woman's or infant's care. Care is improved by an interdisciplinary approach as nurses work together with dietitians, social workers, physicians, and others.

Managing the transition from an acute care setting to the home involves discharge planning and collaboration with other health care professionals. The nurse should be knowledgeable about community and financial resources to promote a smooth transition. Cooperation and communication are essential to best encourage women to participate in their care and meet the needs of newborns.

Researcher

Nurses use research when they follow clinical practice guidelines and professional standards. They participate in research when they are involved in structured quality improvement initiatives and when they search for a solution for a unique patient problem. Nursing care should be based on valid research findings rather than tradition. Evidence-based practice is expected.

Advocate

An advocate speaks on behalf of another person. As the health care environment becomes increasingly complex, care may become impersonal. The nurse is in an ideal position to humanize care and intercede on behalf of the patient and family. The nurse provides information to women and their families to ensure they are involved in decisions and activities related to their care. The nurse then incorporates those decisions into the planning and implementation of care. This may include communicating the family's decisions to other members of the health care team. On a community level, nurses should be advocates for health promotion of vulnerable groups such as victims of domestic violence or women unable to pay for low-cost preventive care such as yearly well woman exams.

Manager

The role of nurses includes that of manager. Nurses may delegate tasks such as ambulation or taking vital signs to unlicensed personnel. Thus nurses spend more time teaching women and families and supervising unlicensed personnel. Nursing case managers often provide coordination of care for many patients. Nurses are expected to understand the financial aspects of patient care. At the same time, they should continue to act as patient advocates and maintain standards of care.

> **KNOWLEDGE CHECK**
> 10. What are the roles of the nurse?
> 11. How does therapeutic communication differ from social communication?
> 12. What factors affect learning?

Advanced Preparation for Maternal-Newborn and Women's Health Nurses

Greater complexity of care and the need to contain costs have increased the need for nurses with various types of advanced preparation. Advanced practice nurses may practice as CNMs, nurse practitioners, clinical nurse specialists, nurse educators, and nurse researchers. Preparation for advanced practice involves obtaining a master's or doctoral degree. Prescriptive authority is often part of the advanced practice certification, but its extent may vary in different states. Nurses working in midlevel or higher management are often required to have an advanced degree in health care administration or the specialty that they lead.

Certified Nurse-Midwives

CNMs are RNs who have completed an extensive program of study and clinical experience. They have completed a graduate level (Master of Science [MS] or Doctor of Nursing Practice [DNP]) program and have passed a certification test

administered by the American College of Nurse-Midwives. CNMs are qualified to take complete health histories and perform physical examinations. They can provide complete care during pregnancy, childbirth, and the postpartum period. CNMs are committed to providing information to prevent problems during pregnancy and facilitate normal pregnancy and childbirth. The CNM provides annual well woman exams, gynecology services, family-planning information, and counseling. The practice approach of the CNM to childbirth is noninterventionist and supportive to low-risk patients. Pregnancy and birth are regarded as normal processes.

Nurse Practitioners

Nurse practitioners are RNs with advanced preparation at the master or doctoral level and certification who provide primary care for specific groups of patients. They obtain a complete health history, perform physical examinations, order and interpret laboratory and other diagnostic studies, and provide primary care for health maintenance and health promotion. Nurse practitioners may collaborate with physicians regarding administering treatments and medications, but depending on their scope of practice and the board of nursing mandates for practice in their state, they may work independently and prescribe medications.

The women's health nurse practitioner (WHNP) provides wellness-focused, primary, reproductive, and gynecologic care over a woman's life span, beginning from adolescence. Family nurse practitioners (FNPs) are prepared to provide preventive, holistic care for young as well as older family members. They may care for women during uncomplicated pregnancies and provide follow-up care to mothers and infants after childbirth. Unlike CNMs, nurse practitioners do not perform deliveries for the woman during childbirth.

Neonatal nurse practitioners (NNPs) assist in the care of high-risk newborns in the immediate post-birth care or in a NICU. Pediatric nurse practitioners (PNPs) provide health maintenance care to infants and children who do not require the services of physicians. They may see infants at well-baby visits and to provide treatment for common illnesses.

Clinical Nurse Specialists

Perinatal clinical specialists are RNs who, through study and supervised practice at the graduate level (master's or doctorate), have acquired expertise in the care of childbearing women with complex problems. Core competencies for the clinical nurse specialist (CNS) include direct care, consultation, systems leadership, collaboration, coaching, research, and ethical decision making (National Association of Clinical Nurse Specialists [NACNS], 2012). Unlike nurse practitioners and midwives, CNSs do not provide primary care.

NURSING RESEARCH

As maternal-newborn nursing and the health care system change, nurses are challenged to demonstrate that their work improves patient outcomes and is cost effective. To meet this challenge, nurses should generate, participate in, and use research. With the establishment of the National Institute of Nursing Research (NINR) in the National Institutes of Health (NIH) (www.ninr.nih.gov), nurses now have an infrastructure to ensure the support of nursing research and the education of well-prepared nurse researchers. The NINR seeks to establish a scientific basis for nursing care of patients throughout life. The translation of scientific advances into cost-effective, quality care is inherent to the mission of the NINR.

Evidence-Based Practice

Clinically based nursing research is increasing rapidly as nurse researchers strive to develop an independent body of knowledge that demonstrates the value of nursing interventions. This is achieved through evidence-based practice. Evidence-based practice is "a problem-solving approach to the delivery of health care that integrates the best evidence from studies and patient care data with clinician expertise and patient preferences and values." This approach promotes high-quality care and best patient outcomes (Melnyk, Fineout-Overholt, Stillwell, & Williamson, 2010).

AWHONN has an ongoing commitment to develop and disseminate evidence-based practice guidelines through the association's Research-Based Practice Program. Implementation of evidence-based guidelines promotes application of the best available scientific evidence for nursing care rather than care based on tradition alone.

Nurses contribute to their profession's knowledge base by systematically investigating theoretic or practice-related issues in nursing. Nursing generates and answers its own questions based on research of its unique subject matter. The responsibility for research within nursing is not limited to nurses with graduate degrees. It is important that all nurses apply valid research findings to their practices. Evidence-based practice is not just an ideal but also is an expectation of nursing practice. Nurses can contribute to the body of professional knowledge by demonstrating an awareness of the value of nursing research and assisting in problem identification and data collection to identify best practices. Nurses should keep their knowledge current by networking and sharing research findings at conferences, by publishing, and by reading research in professional journals. A minimal number of continuing education (CE) hours is needed for license renewal in each U.S. state and territory.

Students and inexperienced nurses may participate in nursing research planned by experts and use updated knowledge from research as they enter nursing practice. Refereed professional nursing journals such as *Journal of Obstetric, Gynecologic, and Neonatal Nursing; Nursing for Women's Health; Nursing Research; The Journal of Perinatal and Neonatal Nursing;* and *The Journal of Neonatal Nursing* are sources of verified information about maternal, newborn, and women's health nursing that help validate nursing actions and remove measures that have not proved valid.

The Agency for Healthcare Research and Quality (AHRQ), a branch of the U.S. Public Health Service, actively sponsors research in health issues facing mothers and children. From research generated through this agency, as well as others,

high-quality evidence can be accumulated to guide the best and lowest-cost clinical practices. Clinical practice guidelines are an important tool in developing parameters for safe, effective, and evidence-based care to mothers, infants, children, and families. The AHRQ has developed several guidelines related to adult and child care, as have other organizations and professional groups concerned with health care. Quality and safety improvements, enhanced primary care, access to high-quality care, and specific illnesses are addressed in available practice guidelines. Guidelines are available at www.guidelines.gov.

The Institute of Medicine (IOM) has published standards for developing practice guidelines to maximize the consistency within and among guidelines, regardless of guideline developers. The IOM recommends inclusion of information and process steps in every guideline. This includes ensuring diversity of members of a clinical guideline group; full disclosure of conflict of interest; in-depth systematic reviews to inform recommendations; provision of a rationale, quality of evidence, and strength of recommendation for each recommendation made by the guideline committee; and external review of recommendations for validity (IOM, 2011). Standardization of clinical practice guidelines will strengthen evidence-based care, especially for guidelines developed by nurses or professional nursing organizations.

Another resource for evidence-based practice in perinatal nursing is the Cochrane Collaboration (www.cochrane.org), which provides coordination of research results by an international network of individuals and institutions. The results in the Cochrane database do not prescribe policies, procedures, or protocols that a facility should follow. However, the evaluations of research identify and distill results from available research so best practices may be incorporated into facility practices.

CRITICAL THINKING

In recent years, critical thinking has received widespread attention in nursing. Clearly, nurses should be concerned with developing critical thinking skills, needed not only to pass the National Council Licensure Examination (NCLEX®) but also to function clinically. Nurses should be concerned with learning and refining the critical thinking skills needed to function in the rapidly changing clinical arena. Critical thinking is controlled and purposeful rather than undirected. It is outcome-focused toward finding solutions to problems.

For effective critical thinking, nurses should gain insight into their own thought processes and analyze their own thinking by taking it apart for examination and criticism. Critical thinking includes recognizing and acknowledging specific habits and responses that may interfere with productive thinking.

Critical thinking is based on reason rather than preference or prejudice. It also seeks to examine feelings to understand how emotions affect thinking. Finally, critical thinking requires the suspension of **judgment** (opinion) until evidence is adequate to support **inferences** or for drawing conclusions.

Purpose

The purpose of critical thinking is to help nurses make the best clinical judgments. The process begins when nurses realize that accumulating knowledge from texts and lectures is not enough. They also should be able to apply this knowledge to specific clinical situations and thus reach conclusions that provide the most effective care in each situation.

In addition, nurses should honestly examine their own thought processes for flaws that could lead to inaccurate conclusions or poor judgments. Although this examination requires self-analysis, a series of steps makes the process easier. Critical thinking exercises are presented throughout the book to help students develop skills in critical thinking and application of knowledge in possible real-life situations.

Steps

A series of steps may help clarify the way critical thinking is learned. These steps may be called the *ABCDEs of critical thinking.* They include recognition of *assumptions,* examination of personal *biases,* analysis of the amount of pressure for *closure,* examination of how *data* are collected and analyzed, and evaluation of how *emotions* may interfere with critical thinking.

Recognizing Assumptions

Assumptions are ideas, beliefs, or values that are taken for granted without basis in fact or reason. Such assumptions may lead to unexamined thoughts or unsound actions. For instance, the following assumptions may have negative consequences: "Anyone who wants a job can get one"; "Teenagers don't listen"; "Every woman wants a baby."

A list of everything known about a specific situation may help in the identification of assumptions. Each item on the list should be analyzed to determine whether it is true, whether it could be true, and whether it is untrue or evidence is insufficient to determine its truth.

Examining Biases

Biases are prejudices that sway the mind toward a particular conclusion or course of action on the basis of personal theories or stereotypes. Biases are based on unexamined beliefs, and many are widespread—for instance, "Fat people are lazy"; "Women are bad drivers"; "Men are insensitive."

People may be biased against those of different races, religions, or lifestyles. When faced with a predisposition to judge a person or a group of persons, it may be wise to ask oneself or a coworker a series of questions:
- "Why do you think that?"
- "What if this was a different person?"
- "What if there were different circumstances?"
- "What might someone who disagrees say?"
- "What is influencing my thinking?"

Determining the Need for Closure

Many people look for immediate answers and experience a great deal of anxiety until a solution is found for any problem. In other words, they have little tolerance for doubt or uncertainty, which is sometimes called **ambiguity**. As a result, they feel pressure to come to a decision or reach **closure** as early as possible. This is one of the most important aspects of critical thinking because those who feel pressure to reach an early decision or find a quick solution often do so with insufficient data.

To overcome pressure to reach an early conclusion, a conscious effort should be made to **suspend** (delay or bring to a stop) judgment. This is sometimes called *reflective* **skepticism**, or doubt in the absence of conclusive evidence. The first step is to acknowledge the anxiety created by postponed decisions. The next step involves deliberately waiting to make a decision. The "time-out" before a surgical procedure is an example of deliberately waiting; all staff members verify patient name, procedure, operative site, and implants, if applicable.

Some people who jump to conclusions often stop with one answer. To overcome this tendency, they should always look for a second "right" answer. They could also imagine the problem from the perspective of someone else. They might ask a series of questions:
- "What alternatives do we have?"
- "What else might work?"
- "What information supports this?"
- "What effect would that have?"
- "Is there good evidence to support that decision?"
- "Is there reason to doubt that evidence?"

On the other hand, some people can tolerate a great deal of doubt and uncertainty. They are comfortable with data collection and analysis but feel uncomfortable making decisions. They may procrastinate or postpone the decision for as long as possible.

Failure to make a decision in the clinical area may have serious consequences for patients and their families. Several questions may help overcome the tendency to postpone reaching a decision:
- "What signs indicate something is wrong?"
- "Do I need to do something about it?"
- "How much time do I have?"
- "What happens if I don't do something about this?"
- "What should I do first?"
- "What resources can help me?"

This step also might be called *priority setting,* and it is one of the most important aspects of critical thinking in nursing.

Becoming Skillful in Data Management

Expertise in collecting, organizing, and analyzing data involves developing an attitude of inquiry and learning to live with questions such as: "Why?" "What if?" "What else?" "Is this relevant?" "How does it relate to that?" "How can I organize the data?" "Do the data form patterns?" and "What can I infer from those patterns?"

Collecting Data. To obtain complete data, nurses should develop skill in verbal communication. Open-ended questions elicit more information than questions that require only a one-word answer. Follow-up questions often are needed to clarify information or pursue a particular thought.

Validating Data. Nurses should **validate** unclear or incomplete information to make certain that the information collected is accurate. This process may involve rechecking physical signs, collecting additional information, or determining whether a perception is accurate.

Organizing and Analyzing Data. Data are more useful when organized into patterns or clusters. The first step is to separate relevant data from data that may be interesting but are unrelated to the current situation.

The next step is to compare data with expected norms to determine what is within the expected range (normal) and what is not (abnormal). Abnormal results provide cues that can be grouped or clustered so that conclusions can be made. For example, all data that may indicate excessive bleeding, such as pulse rate, blood pressure, amount of vaginal bleeding, and skin color, may seem more meaningful when grouped. Organizing data into clusters often reveals that additional data are needed before a decision can be reached.

Acknowledging Emotions and Environmental Factors

Several emotions and environmental factors may influence critical thinking. For instance, the clinical area is often a noisy, fast-paced, and hectic environment with time limitations and distractions that make calm reflection and reasoning difficult. Fatigue also reduces the ability to concentrate during a 12-hour shift. Inexperienced nurses and students may lack confidence in their knowledge and often feel anxious, which may reduce the ability to think critically. Fatigue in older, experienced nurses reduces their ability to mentor new graduates or nurses with less experience in the specialty.

Many nurses, both experienced and inexperienced, have a strong need to protect their self-image. As a result, they may be unwilling to seek assistance and fail to communicate (Benner, Malloch & Sheets, 2010). Some nurses may become defensive when they have said or done something wrong. This response is a serious barrier to critical thinking, which requires that all health care professionals learn to acknowledge mistakes and become comfortable with constructive criticism.

Extreme emotions such as anger and frustration impede critical thinking by narrowing the focus to only data that support the intense feeling. For example, persons who are extremely frustrated often may repeat the perceived cause of their frustration and may be unable to move on to other information to address the problem.

The first step is to recognize and acknowledge factors or emotions that impede thinking. For example, nurses may find it necessary to say, "I feel flustered by all the activity and need to find a quiet spot for a few minutes of concentration." To develop critical thinking skills, the nurse should learn to admit mistakes and become comfortable saying, "I was wrong." Asking for assistance, verification, or validation is wise when fatigue is a problem or when lack of confidence creates anxiety.

The person who experiences intense frustration or anger should recognize these emotions and their influence on rational thought. A trusted colleague may be asked to point out signs of these emotions such as repetitive vehement comments. Some people use other methods of control such as visualizations, breathing exercises, and brief, self-imposed "time-outs" from the precipitating situation, if possible.

> ### ❓ KNOWLEDGE CHECK
> 13. What is the purpose of critical thinking?
> 14. What steps may be helpful in refining critical thinking?
> 15. What is meant by reflective skepticism?

◆ APPLICATION OF THE NURSING PROCESS

The nursing process forms the basis for maternal-newborn and women's health nursing, as for all nursing. The nursing process consists of five distinct steps: (1) assessment, (2) identification of patient problems or nursing diagnosis, (3) planning, (4) implementation, and (5) evaluation. In maternal-newborn and women's health nursing, the nursing process applies to a population that is often healthy and experiencing a life event that holds the potential for both growth and problems. Nursing activity in these settings is often devoted to the assessment and diagnosis of patient strengths and healthy functioning to achieve a higher or more satisfying level of wellness. This focus often differs from that of providing care for adults or children who are usually ill when the nurse encounters them.

The nursing process is written in the text as a linear, step-by-step process. However, with knowledge and experience, the nurse applies the nursing process in the clinical setting dynamically. For example, the nurse may discover that the woman has a full bladder early in a postpartum assessment. The nurse skips to an intervention and helps the woman to the restroom to urinate before completing the assessment. This action is taken by the nurse to prevent patient discomfort and possible excessive bleeding caused by a full bladder. In another example, the nurse goes to the woman's room to give her an injection of RhoGAM and discovers the woman nursing her baby, who is eagerly suckling for the first time in several hours. Based on critical thinking, the nurse delays the injection (an intervention), which would require the woman to change her position. The nurse realizes that the few minutes required for the infant to complete the feeding are more important than the short delay in giving the injection.

◆ Assessment

Nursing assessment should be accomplished systematically and deliberately and include objective and subjective data related to physiologic, psychologic, social, and cultural status of the patient. Although the woman or infant may be the primary patient, nurses should assess the belief systems, available support, perceptions, and plans of other family members to provide the best nursing care. Two levels of nursing

TABLE 1.3 **Examples of Actual and Increased Risk for Patient Problems and Wellness Opportunities**

ACTUAL PATIENT PROBLEMS		
Problem	Etiology	Signs and Symptoms
Inadequate nutrition	Lack of knowledge about nutritional needs during lactation	Weight loss of 5 kg and daily caloric intake <1500 calories
Inadequate breastfeeding	Nipple trauma	Cracked nipples and reports of discomfort during nursing
INCREASED RISK FOR A PATIENT PROBLEM		
Problem	Risk Factors	
Risk for inadequate nutrition	Lack of knowledge of nutritional needs during lactation issue	
Risk for inadequate breastfeeding	Lack of knowledge of correct positioning of infant and appropriate breast care	
WELLNESS OPPORTUNITIES		
Topic	Selected Defining Characteristics	
Opportunity for improved self-care	Expressed or observed desire to seek information for health promotion	
Opportunity for improved nutrition	Follows an appropriate standard for food intake such as MyPlate or American Diabetic Association guidelines	

assessment are used to collect comprehensive data: screening assessments and focus assessments.

Screening Assessment

The screening, or database, assessment is usually performed at the first contact with the person. Its purpose is to gather information about all aspects of the person's health. This information, called **baseline data**, describes their health status before interventions begin. It forms the basis for the identification of both strengths and problems.

A variety of methods are used to organize the assessment. For example, information may be grouped according to body systems or organized around nursing theory models such as Roy's adaptation to stress theory, Gordon's functional health patterns, the human response patterns of the North American Nursing Diagnosis Association International (NANDA-I), or Orem's self-care deficit theory.

Focused Assessment

A focused assessment is used to gather information specifically related to an actual health problem or a problem that the woman or family is at risk for acquiring. A focused assessment is often performed at the beginning of a shift and centers on areas relevant to childbearing, newborn, or women's health nursing. For instance, in care of the mother and infant after birth the nurse should assess the breasts and nipples because the mother is at risk for problems if she does not have adequate information about breastfeeding or care of the nipples. A focused assessment also may reveal strengths that nursing care will enhance.

◆ Identification of Patient Problems

The data gathered during assessment should be analyzed to identify existing or potential strengths or problems and their causes. Data are validated and grouped in a process of critical thinking to determine cues and inferences. The problems identified may be actual, or an increased risk for a problem or the nurse may identify wellness opportunities (Table 1.3).

Health needs for which nurses can provide **independent nursing interventions** and for which they are legally accountable are termed *nursing diagnoses.* At present, more than 200 nursing diagnoses have been identified by NANDA-I (www.nanda.org).

◆ Planning

The third step in the nursing process involves planning care for the problems identified. During this step, nurses set priorities, develop goals or outcomes, and plan interventions to accomplish these goals.

Setting Priorities

Setting priorities includes (1) determining which problems need immediate attention (life-threatening problems) and taking action; (2) determining whether potential problems call for a physician's order for diagnosis, monitoring, or treatment; and (3) discriminating actual problems that take precedence over an increased risk.

Establishing Goals and Expected Outcomes

Although the terms *goals* and *expected outcomes* are sometimes used interchangeably, they are different. Broad goals should be linked with specific and measurable outcome criteria. For example, if the goal is for the parents to demonstrate effective parenting by discharge, then the expected outcomes that serve as evidence might include prompt, consistent responses to infant signals and competence in bathing, feeding, and comforting the infant.

The following rules apply to written expected outcomes:

- Outcomes should be stated in patient-oriented terms, identifying who is expected to achieve the goal. This is usually the woman, the infant, or the family.
- Measurable verbs should be used. For example, *identify, demonstrate, express, walk, relate,* and *list* are observable and measurable verbs. Examples of verbs that are difficult to measure are *understand, appreciate, feel, accept, know,* and *experience.* For instance, "Ms. Brown will experience less anxiety about assuming care of her infant" poses a problem because determining whether she experiences less anxiety is difficult. This outcome can be reworded as "Ms. Brown will state that she feels less anxious about assuming care of her infant and will participate in infant care (umbilical cord, circumcision, bathing) before discharge."
- A time frame is necessary. When is the person expected to perform the action? By the first postpartum day? After teaching? By discharge? Within the second trimester?
- Goals and expected outcomes should be realistic and attainable. For instance, if the patient has pain as a result of a lack of knowledge about pain control, a realistic expected outcome might be "Sandra will state that her pain during labor is manageable using techniques taught by, her nurse." A goal such as "will remain free of pain throughout labor" is not attainable by nursing interventions only and is not realistic.
- Goals and expected outcomes are collaborated with the patient and family to ensure their participation in the plan of care.

Developing Nursing Interventions

After the goals and expected outcomes are developed, nurses write nursing interventions that will help the patient meet the established outcomes.

Interventions for Actual Patient Problems. Nursing interventions for actual patient problems are aimed at reducing or eliminating the causes or related factors. For instance, if the problem is ineffective attachment between the parents and the newborn resulting from separation from the infant because of illness, the desired outcome might be the parents will demonstrate progressive attachment behaviors such as touching, palming, eye contact, and participation in infant care within 1 week. Nursing interventions focus on role modeling attachment behaviors and increasing contact between parents and their baby.

Interventions for Risk for Patient Problems. Interventions are aimed at (1) monitoring for onset of the problem, (2) minimizing risk factors, and (3) preventing the problem. For example, if Baby Sam is at an increased risk for skin breakdown because of frequent, loose stools, the planned outcome is the skin remains intact. Nursing interventions include monitoring the condition of the skin at prescribed intervals for signs of skin impairment and initiating measures to keep the skin clean and dry to reduce the risk for skin impairment.

Wellness Interventions. Interventions also focus on opportunities for health enhancement. Nursing care seeks to promote patient success through the teaching of self-care measures. Examples of wellness interventions include teaching related to weight reduction, exercise to lower chronic hypertension, or reconditioning the body after birth.

◆ Implementing Interventions

Implementing nursing interventions may be a problem if written interventions are not specific. Nursing interventions should be as specific as physician's orders and may be formulated with computerized care plans. If a physician orders "hydrocodone with acetaminophen, 5 mg/500 mg, 1 tablet PO (orally) every 6 hours as needed for pain," the order specifies the combination drug to be given, the dose to be given, the route of administration, the time, and the reason. A well-written nursing intervention is equally specific: "Teach woman not to break, chew, or crush the drug tablet."

Conversely, poorly written interventions such as "Assist with breastfeeding" provide generalizations rather than specific interventions. Specific methods the nurse should use to assist breastfeeding are more effective. For example, "Demonstrate correct positioning in cradle and football hold at first attempt to breastfeed. Teach mother to elicit rooting reflex by stroking infant's lips with nipple. Demonstrate how to latch infant to nipple, and request a return demonstration before mother and baby are discharged."

◆ Evaluation

The evaluation determines the effectiveness of the plan and its goals or expected outcomes. The nurse should assess the status of the patient and compare the current status with the goals or outcome criteria developed during the planning step. The nurse then judges the person's progression toward goal achievement and makes a decision: Should the plan be continued? Modified? Abandoned? Are the problems resolved or the causes diminished? Is a different patient problem more relevant?

The nursing process is dynamic, and evaluation frequently results in expanded assessment and additional or modified patient problems and interventions. Nurses are cautioned not to view lack of goal achievement as a failure but as a signal to reassess and begin the process anew.

Individualized Nursing Care Plans

Nurses are responsible for documenting the patient problem or nursing diagnosis, expected outcomes, and interventions for each problem. This information is often communicated to colleagues through a written plan of care. Many institutions have standards of care for groups of patients such as those who have had normal spontaneous vaginal births. However, individual nursing care plans may be necessary based on needs or problems identified during the assessment step of the nursing process. When nurses write individualized plans of care, they implement the plans through interventions that direct the care (Box 1.1). Some patient situations end with a single office visit, whereas others progress over time such as normal or complicated birth. Specific planned nursing care may be documented by office, clinic, or hospital computer systems, and the systems may be linked to improve continuity.

The Nursing Process Related to Critical Thinking

Although the nursing process and critical thinking are similar and overlap in many respects, major differences exist. The

BOX 1.1   Developing Individualized Nursing Care through the Nursing Process

Although the nursing process is the foundation for nursing, initially it is a challenging process to apply in the clinical area. It requires proficiency in focused assessments of the new mother and infant and the ability to analyze data and plan nursing care for individual patients and families. Asking questions at each step of the nursing process may be helpful.

Assessment

1. Did some data not fit within normal limits or expected parameters? For example, the woman states that she feels "dizzy" when she tries to ambulate, or the postmenopausal woman describes vaginal bleeding at her annual well-woman examination.
2. If so, what else should be assessed? (What else should I evaluate? What might be related to this symptom? How do my assessments compare with previous assessments?) For example, what are the blood pressure, pulse rate, skin color, temperature, and amount of lochia if the woman feels dizzy? Is my assessment similar to earlier ones, or has there been a change?
3. Did the assessment identify the cause of the abnormal data? What are the laboratory values for her hemoglobin and hematocrit? What was her estimated blood loss at childbirth? Did she lose excessive blood during the hours and days after birth?
4. Are other factors present? Did she receive medication during labor? What kind of medication? Did she receive an anesthetic for labor pain? When? What medication is the woman now taking? How long has it been since she has eaten? Is the environment a related factor (crowded, warm, unfamiliar)? Is she reluctant to ask for assistance?

Identification of Patient Problems

1. Are adequate data available to reach a conclusion? What else is needed? (What do you wish you had assessed? What would you look for next time?)
2. What is the major concern? (On the basis of the data, what are your concerns?) The woman who is dizzy may fall as she ambulates to the bathroom, particularly if she does not ask for help. The woman with postmenopausal vaginal bleeding will need evaluation by a physician or nurse practitioner for possible cancer.
3. What might happen if no action is taken? (What might happen to the person if you do nothing?) She may suffer an injury or a complication.
4. Is there a NANDA-I–approved diagnostic category that reflects your major concern? How is it defined? Suppose

that during analysis you decide the major concern is that the patient will faint and suffer an injury. What diagnostic category most closely reflects this concern?
5. Does this diagnostic category "fit" this woman? Is she at greater risk for a problem than others in a similar situation? Why? What are the additional risk factors?
6. Is this a problem that nurses can manage independently? Are medical interventions also necessary?
7. If the problem can be managed by nurses, is it an actual problem (defining characteristics present) or a risk problem (risk factors present)?

Planning

1. What expected outcomes are desired? That the woman will remain free of injury during the hospital stay? That she will demonstrate position changes that reduce the episodes of vertigo?
2. Would the outcomes be clear, specific, and measurable to anyone reading them?
3. What nursing interventions should be initiated and carried out to accomplish these goals or outcomes?
4. Are your written interventions specific and clear? Are action verbs used (*assess, teach, assist*)? After you have written the interventions, examine them. Do they define exactly what is to be done (when, what, how far, how often)? Will they prevent the woman from suffering an injury?
5. Are the interventions based on sound rationale? For instance, dehydration possible during labor causes weakness that may result in falls; loss of blood during delivery often exceeds 500 mL, which results in hypotension that is aggravated when the woman stands suddenly. A woman who has recently delivered after receiving an epidural block may have lingering effects from this form of labor pain relief.

Implementing Nursing Interventions

1. What are the expected effects of the prescribed intervention? Are adverse effects possible? What are they?
2. Are the interventions acceptable to the woman and family?
3. Are the interventions clearly written so that they can be carefully followed?

Evaluation

1. What is the status of the woman at this time?
2. What were the goals and outcomes? Were they specific and measurable or should they be clarified?
3. Compare the current status of the woman with the stated goals and outcomes.
4. What should be done now?

NANDA-I, North American Nursing Diagnosis Association International.

KNOWLEDGE CHECK

16. How does screening assessment differ from focused assessment?
17. How do actual patient problems differ from risk patient problems?
18. How should goals and expected outcome criteria be stated?
19. Why are interventions sometimes difficult to implement? How can this difficulty be overcome?

five steps of the nursing process provide a logical method for problem solving. Problem solving begins with a specific problem and ends with a solution. Conversely, critical thinking is open ended; it goes before and beyond problem solving. Critical thinking may be triggered by a problem, a positive event, or an opportunity to improve. It focuses on appraisal of the way the individual thinks, and it emphasizes reflective skepticism. Critical thinking is used throughout each step of the nursing process (Table 1.4).

TABLE 1.4   Use of Critical Thinking in the Nursing Process

Nursing Process	Critical Thinking Skills
Assessment	Collecting complete data, validating data
	Clustering data (normal versus abnormal, important versus unimportant, relevant versus irrelevant)
	Identifying emotions
Analysis	Identifying cues and making inferences
	Reflecting and suspending judgment
	Examining thought processes for biases and assumptions
	Identifying alternatives
	Determining priorities
Planning	Examining need for closure
	Searching for alternative solutions
	Validating plan with patient or coworker
	Communicating plan
	Acknowledging defensive behavior
Implementation	Applying knowledge
	Testing plan
	Carrying out plan
Evaluation	Examining insights gained
	Recognizing new ways of thinking or acting
	Examining options and criteria for action
	Appraising self and others in the situation

SUMMARY CONCEPTS

- Technologic advances, increasing knowledge, government involvement, and consumer demands have changed maternity care in the United States.
- Family-centered maternity care, which is based on the principle that families can make decisions about health care if they have adequate information, has greatly enhanced the role of nurses.
- Women must make many decisions about childbirth, including choosing a birth attendant, a birth setting, a support person for labor, and the type of educational classes to attend.
- An emphasis on patient safety, quality of care, patient safety bundles, and Women's Health and Perinatal Nursing Care Quality measures, has balanced efforts for cost containment in the modern health care system.
- Reduced lengths of stay make it more difficult for the nurse to provide information regarding self-care and infant care to the woman who is recovering from the fatigue and discomfort of birth.
- Infant mortality rates have declined dramatically in the last 50 years. However, the United States continues to have a higher infant and maternal mortality rate than many other developed nations, and disparity of mortality rates across ethnic groups is still wide.
- The professional nurse should function as a communicator, patient and family educator, collaborator, patient advocate, researcher, and manager.
- Registered nurses with advanced education and licensure are prepared to provide primary care for women and children as certified nurse-midwives and nurse practitioners.
- Perinatal clinical nurse specialist roles include expert direct care, consultation, systems leadership, collaboration, coaching, research, and ethical decision making.
- Nurses should base their practices on the evidence generated by research. Professional journals are the best sources for the latest research.
- Nurses should refine their critical thinking abilities by examining their own thought processes for flaws that could lead to inaccurate conclusions or poor clinical judgments.
- The nursing process begins with assessment and includes analysis of data that may result in the identification of patient problems. Nurses are legally accountable for identifying and managing these problems.

REFERENCES & READINGS

American Association of Colleges of Nursing (AACN). (2016). *2015–2016 Enrollment and Graduations in Baccalaureate and Graduate Programs in Nursing.* Washington, DC: Author.

American College of Obstetricians and Gynecologists (ACOG). (2017). *Alliance for innovation on maternal health: AIM.* Retrieved from www.acog.org.

Association of Women's Health, Obstetric and Neonatal Nurses (AWHONN). (2014). *Women's Health and Perinatal Nursing Care Quality Refined Draft Measures Specification.* Washington, DC: Author. Retrieved from www.awhonn.org.

Benner, P., Malloch, K., & Sheets (2010). *V. Nursing pathways for patient safety.* St Louis, MO: Elsevier.

Centers for Disease Control and Prevention (CDC). (2014). *Teen pregnancy in the United States*. Retrieved from www.cdc.ogov/teenpregnancy.

Centers for Disease Control and Prevention (CDC). (2015). *Preterm birth*. Retrieved from www.cdc.gov/reproductivehealth/maternalinfanthealth/pretermbirth.htm.

Centers for Disease Control and Prevention (CDC). (2016). *Trends in pregnancy-related deaths*. Retrieved from www.cdc.gov/reproductivehealth/maternalinfanthealth/pmss.html.

Council on Patient Safety in Women's Health Care. (2017). *A Primer: Council on Patient Safety in Women's Health Care*. Washington, DC: Author. Retrieved from www.safehealthcareforeverywoman.org.

Institute for Healthcare Improvement. (2017). *Improvement stories: What is a bundle?* Retrieved from www.ihi.org/resources/Pages/ImprovementStories/WhatIsaBundle.aspx.

Institute of Medicine (IOM). (2011). *The future of nursing: Leading change, advancing health*. Washington, DC: National Academies Press.

Institute of Medicine (IOM). (2011). *Clinical practice guidelines we can trust*. Retrieved from www.nationalacademies.org/hmd/reports/2011/clinical-practice-guidelines-we-can-trust.

Interprofessional Education Collaborative. (2016). *Core competencies for interprofessional collaborative practice: 2016 update*. Washington, DC: Author.

MacDorman, M. F., Mathews, T. J., Mohangoo, A. D., & Zeitlin, J. (2014). *International comparisons of infant mortality and related factors: United States and Europe, 2010. National vital statistics reports; vol 63 no 5*. Hyattsville, MD: National Center for Health Statistics.

March of Dimes. (2015). *2015 prematurity birth report card*. Retrieved from www.marchofdimes.org.

Mathews, T. J., MacDorman, M. L., & Thomas, M. E. (2015). Infant mortality statistics from the 2013 period: Linked birth/infant death data set. *National Vital Statistics Reports, 64*(9).

Melnyk, B. M., Fineout-Overholt, E., Stillwell, S., & Williamson, K. M. (2010). Evidence-based practice: Step by step: The seven steps of evidence-based practice. *American Journal of Nursing, 110*(1), 51–53.

National Association of Clinical Nurse Specialists (NACNS). (2012). *Organizing framework and CNS core competencies*. Retrieved from www.nacns.org.

National Center for Complementary and Alternative Medicine (NCCAM). (2011). *CAM basics: What is CAM? Publication number D347*. Bethesda, MD: National Institutes of Health. Retrieved from www.nccam.nih.gov.

National Center for Complementary and Alternative Medicine (NCCAM). (2016). *Complementary, alternative or integrated health: What's in a name?* Retrieved from http://nccam.nih.gov.

National Conference of State Legislatures. (2011). *The affordable care act: A brief summary*. Retrieved from www.ncsl.org/portals/1/documents/health/hraca.pdf.

Rossler, K. L., & Kimble, L. P. (2016). Capturing readiness to learn and collaboration as explored with an interprofessional simulation scenario: A mixed-methods research study. *Nurse Education Today, 36*, 348–353.

The Joint Commission. (2017). *Specification Manual for Joint Commission National Quality Measures (v2017A)*. Retrieved from https://manual.jointcommission.org/releases/TJC2017A/PerinatalCare.html.

U.S. Department of Health and Human Services. (2010). *Healthy People 2020*. Retrieved from www.healthypeople.gov.

Social, Ethical, and Legal Issues

Lynn Clark Callister, Cathy L. Miller, Karen S. Holub

OBJECTIVES

After studying this chapter, you should be able to:

1. Explain family structure.
2. Describe characteristics of functional families and factors that interfere with family functioning.
3. Give examples of high-risk families.
4. Compare Western cultural values with those of differing cultural groups.
5. Explain cultural negotiation.
6. Relate how major social issues such as socioeconomic status, poverty, homelessness, and disparity in health care affect maternal-newborn and women's health nursing.
7. Describe the role of the nurse in assessment, prevention, and intervention of intimate partner violence.
8. Define human trafficking, also known as trafficking in persons.
9. Identify possible indicators ("red flags") of human trafficking.
10. Apply theories and principles of ethics to ethical dilemmas.
11. Describe how the steps of the nursing process can be applied to ethical decision making.
12. Discuss ethical conflicts related to reproductive issues such as elective pregnancy termination, forced contraception, and infertility therapy.
13. Discuss the maintenance of patient, institutional, and colleague confidentiality when using electronic communication.
14. Describe the legal basis for nursing practice.
15. Identify measures to prevent or defend malpractice claims.

The family forms the foundation of society. It is the first social institution a person knows in which one learns values, norms, and expected behaviors. The family exists within a culture. The culture affects the values, beliefs, and traditions of the family. The individual and family are part of a society. The American society is faced with social and ethical dilemmas that affect individuals and families for whom nurses provide care. Some ethical and social issues result in the passage of laws that regulate reproductive practice. The nurse should understand the legal basis for his or her scope of practice.

THE FAMILY

Family Structures

There are multiple family structures, including the most common nuclear or conjugal family with a husband, wife, and children. Extended family includes the nuclear family with grandparents, aunts, uncles, or cousins living together. One adult who is divorced, separated, or widowed living with a child or children is a single-parent family. Adolescent mothers constitute a type of family formation whether the mother is single or coupled, what her developmental age is, and whether she is living with her parents or living alone. These

mothers may have difficulty constructing their maternal identity (Macintosh & Callister, 2015). A blended or reconstituted family is one in which one or more parents bring into the union children from a previous relationship. Couples living without the legal bonds of marriage with or without children are in a cohabitative relationship. A communal family is a group of unrelated people who choose to live together, with the children the responsibility of the group. Foster or adoptive families are those who take responsibility for children who were not born to them. This may include foster or adoptive children from another country or of another cultural, ethnic, or racial group. Same gender families include two adults of the same sex living together, some with children (Polan & Taylor, 2015).

Differing family patterns of functioning are defined by how members of the family relate to each other. These include authoritarian or autocratic, authoritative or democratic, permissive or laissez-faire, or uninvolved. In an authoritarian family, the parents make the decisions and enforce rules. In democratic families, choices and responsibility are balanced in an atmosphere of respect for all family members. In the permissive family there is freedom with little accountability. Families are also either functional (healthy) or nonfunctional (unhealthy). Functional families exhibit characteristics which are helpful for a nurse to use to assess the way a specific family is functioning, including:

- Open communication, with family members expressing their needs and concerns
- Flexibility in role assignments, with family members working together to assist and support each other
- Agreement of adults on the basic principles of parenting with minimal discord
- Resiliency and adaptability

Factors interfering with healthy family functioning include lack of financial resources, absence of adequate family support, birth of an infant who requires specialized care, presence of unhealthy habits such as substance abuse or lack of anger management, and the inability to make mature decisions necessary to provide care to an infant.

High-risk families include those who live below the poverty level, those who live with chronic food insecurity, those headed by a single adolescent parent, and those with unanticipated stressors such as a preterm, ill, or disabled newborn. Families with lifestyle problems such as alcoholism, substance abuse, and family violence are considered at high risk for problems in providing adequate care for the infant. It is the responsibility of nurses to refer these families to social services agencies for financial assistance, crisis intervention, home visits, substance abuse rehabilitation, and anger management programs.

There are stages of families across the life span, from the beginning couple stage through the childbearing stage, the grown-child stage, and the older family stage. The childbearing phase creates some of the most powerful changes in a family as the relationship between the adults changes to include the care of a helpless infant. Family dynamics change when children must learn to share their parents' attention with a new sibling.

Cultural beliefs and practices influence what is considered normal or abnormal in family structure and relationships. Culture determines "learned patterns of behavior passed down through the generations" (Polan & Taylor, 2015, p. 18).

> ### ❓ KNOWLEDGE CHECK
> 1. What are characteristics of a functional family?
> 2. What factors may interfere with family functioning?

Family Demographics in the United States

In 2015, white non-Hispanics constituted 77.1% of the population, Hispanics/Latinos 17.6%, African-American/Black non-Hispanics 13.3%, Asian 5.6%. Those reporting having two or more races are 2.6%, American Indian/Alaska natives 1.2%, and Pacific Islanders 0.2%. In 2014 those who are foreign born constituted 13.1% of the population, with 14.8% of people living in poverty (U.S. Census Bureau, 2016a).

The number of children ages 0 to 17 in the United States in 2015 was 73.6 million, with children constituting 22.9% of the population. Children ages 0 to 17 years living with two married parents in 2015 was 65% (2015). Births to unmarried women ages 15 to 44 in 2014 was 43.9 per 1000 (2014), with 40.2% of births being to unmarried women. Adolescent (ages 15 to 17) births constitute 11 per 1000 births (2014). Of high

school students in 2013, 47% reported they had experienced sexual intercourse (Forum on Child and Family Statistics, 2016). African-American and Hispanic women are less likely to use a highly or moderately effective method of contraception (Dehlendorf et al., 2014).

In 2014 there were 3,988,076 live births in the United States, constituting a birthrate of 12.5 per 1000 population. The mean age at first birth is 26.3 years. The fertility rate per 1000 women ages 15 to 44 years of age was 62.9 births (Center for Disease Control, 2016a). The racial/ethnic fertility rates per 1000 women ages 15 to 44 is White, non-Hispanic: 60, African American/Black non-Hispanic: 65, Hispanic/Latino: 72, Asian 61, and American Indian/Alaska Native 45 (Child Trends, 2016). The 2013 birthrates by racial/ethnic groups of childbearing women were White, non-Hispanic 54.1%, Hispanic/Latino 22.9%, African American/Black non-Hispanic 19.8%, Asian/Pacific Islander 6.4%, and American Indian/Alaska Native 1.0% (Kids Count, 2016).

The cesarean birth rate for 2014 was 32.3%. Of live births, 8% were low-birth-weight (LBW) infants, with 9.6% being preterm (less than 37 weeks of gestation), with 6% of infants dying before their first birthday (Forum on Child and Family Statistics, 2016). There are racial and ethnic disparities in preterm birth, as noted by higher rates found in American Indian/Alaska Native women (Raglan, Lannon, Jones, & Schulkin, 2016). In 2014, 98.5% of births were in hospitals, with 84.8% of those births attended by physicians and 8.6% attended by certified nurse midwives (National Center for Health Statistics, 2016a).

CULTURE AND CHILDBEARING FAMILIES

Culture is the sum of beliefs and values that are learned, shared, and transmitted from generation to generation in a specific group of people. **Cultural values** guide the thinking, decisions, and actions of a group, particularly during pivotal life events such as childbirth and childrearing. **Ethnic** pertains to religious, racial, national, or cultural group characteristics such as speech patterns, social customs, and physical characteristics. **Ethnicity** is the condition of a group of people who share race, specific languages and dialects, religious faiths, traditions, values, and symbols. **Ethnocentrism** is when persons think their cultural beliefs and practices are superior to those of others and forms the basis for interpersonal conflicts. **Transcultural nursing** is concerned with the provision of nursing care with sensitivity for and respect of the needs of individuals, families, and groups of people.

Cultural Considerations
Cultural Values

Leininger (1978) identified dominant Western cultural values that may influence the thinking and action of nurses in the United States but may not be shared by culturally diverse childbearing women and their families, including the following:

- Democracy is a cultural value that may not be shared by families who think decisions should be made by the family, religious figures, or higher authorities in their cultural group. Fatalism, or the belief that events and results are predestined, also may affect health care decisions.

- Individualism conflicts with the values of many cultural groups.
- Cleanliness is considered by some groups to be an American "obsession."
- Preoccupation with time is a major source of conflict with those who mark time by different standards.
- Reliance on technology may be intimidating.
- The belief that optimal health is a right is in direct conflict with beliefs in many cultures in which health care is not a major expected right.
- Admiration for self-sufficiency and financial success may conflict with beliefs of other societies that place less value on wealth and more value on less tangible factors such as spirituality.

Differing cultures and lack of understanding of cultures (between the nurse and the childbearing family) may create communication difficulties related to communication style, decision making, touch, spirituality and religiosity, and time orientation.

Communication Style

Styles in communication differ among cultures. For example, among Asians, nodding and smiling may mean, "Yes, I hear you" but may not indicate agreement or even understanding. When presenting information, the nurse should validate understanding by asking the woman to repeat the information, saying: "Tell me what you understood" or "Show me what you learned."

Knowing communication principles helps nurses avoid making errors in communication. For example, Hispanics are traditionally diplomatic and tactful. They frequently engage in "small talk" before introducing questions about their care. Nurses should remember that small talk is a valuable use of time. It establishes rapport and helps accomplish the goals of care. It helps create an atmosphere of trust (confianza) in the relationship and helps the woman feel comfortable (Jones, 2014). Another example is American Indians/Alaska Natives often converse in a low tone that may be difficult to hear. They may consider note-taking taboo and expect the caregiver to remember what was said (Spector, 2017).

Decision Making

It is important to determine who makes decisions for the family. Is it the individual woman, the husband, other family members, or traditional authority figures? If decisions are collectively made or are beyond a woman's control, such as whether prenatal care is accessed and at what time during the pregnancy, the decision makers should be included in the conversation (Callister, 2014).

Eye Contact

Many Whites and African-Americans consider eye contact important to communication. Eye-contact avoidance sometimes frustrates health care personnel, who believe eye contact denotes honesty. In some cultures, such as American Indian/Alaska Natives cultures, avoiding eye contact is a sign of respect (Dillard & Olrun-Volkheimer, 2014). Eye-contact behavior is also an important consideration when nurses deal with Latino infants and children. *Mal ojo* (evil eye) is a sudden unexplained illness when an individual with special powers admires a child too openly. Eye contact between a woman and man may be considered seductive by those from Middle Eastern cultures.

Touch

Touch is also an important component of communication. In some cultures, such as those espousing Hinduism or the Islamic faith, touch by a woman other than the wife is offensive to men. Hispanics are more likely to appreciate touch, which is viewed as a sign of sincerity. Nurses should remain sensitive to the response of the person being touched and should refrain from touching if the person indicates it is not welcomed.

Spirituality and Religiosity

Many culturally diverse women may espouse deeply held religious and spiritual practices and beliefs and be reluctant to share these with their nurses. For example, Thai women described the adherence to practices and rituals associated with their beliefs about three essences: the body, mind-heart, and energy (Elter, Kennedy, Chesia, & Yimyam, 2016).

Time Orientation

Time orientation can create conflict between health care professionals and culturally diverse childbearing women. Native Americans, Middle Easterners, and Hispanics tend to emphasize the present moment rather than the future. If a woman does not place the same importance on keeping appointments, she may encounter anger and frustration in the health care setting that leaves her bewildered, ashamed, and unlikely to return for care. See Nursing Care Plan: Language Barrier during Pregnancy for an example of the issue of communication difficulties.

◎ NURSING CARE PLAN

Language Barrier during Pregnancy

Assessment

Diep T., a young Vietnamese primigravida at 16 weeks of gestation, speaks very little English. She listens quietly to the nurse's health care instructions, and although she appears confused, she asked no questions. Her husband, Bao N., nods and smiles frequently and speaks more English than his wife but has difficulty responding to questions about his wife's health.

Critical Thinking

Why should additional assessments be made before patient problems can be formulated? **Answer:** Nodding and smiling do not always mean that persons from another culture understand health teaching. Instead, such actions simply may indicate the information has been heard, or perhaps Mr. N. is being polite and does not want the nurse to feel inadequate. Before

Continued

◎ NURSING CARE PLAN—cont'd

Language Barrier during Pregnancy

assuming Mr. N. can translate health care teaching for his wife, the nurse should validate his learning by asking Mr. N. to explain what he has learned.

Patient Problem

Ineffective communication resulting from language barriers.

Planning: Expected Outcomes

Throughout the pregnancy the family will demonstrate adequate understanding of instructions by (1) keeping scheduled appointments, (2) following health care instructions, and (3) verbalizing basic needs and concerns at each prenatal visit

Interventions and Rationales

- Assess the couple's ability to speak, read, and write in English and determine whether they are fluent in other languages. *People who are not fluent in speaking a language may be more adept at reading it.*
- Obtain the assistance of a fluent interpreter, preferably a woman.
- Establish a list of bilingual staff members who are willing to interpret and understand the importance of confidentiality and exactness. Ensure staff members are knowledgeable about the phone interpreter services used by the clinical agency. Use a translator to develop written material in languages most commonly encountered in the facility. Develop communication aids about common teaching topics in various languages. Use communication cards with questions and answers printed in Vietnamese with Diep and her husband
- Use posters, pictures, and models to demonstrate anatomy, birth, or other concepts clearly.
- *A fluent interpreter is essential because Asians do not always reveal they do not understand instructions. This hinders follow-up questions. Printed materials help elicit basic information, reinforce information given verbally, and may answer unasked questions. Written materials and communication*

cards in the patient's language convey interest in communicating and provide a means of eliciting basic information. Pictures or models make information more understandable (Callister, 2016a).

- Face Diep and her husband rather than the interpreter when talking. Use quiet tones. Use the same interpreter whenever possible. Watch facial expressions for a clue to patients' understanding. *Talking directly to the patient while facing her shows respect and concern. Soft speech protects the patient's privacy and modesty. A natural response when people do not understand is to raise the voice. This may convey impatience or anger. A consistent interpreter enhances communication. Facial expressions may show confusion if the patient does not understand.*
- Ask the interpreter to explain exactly what the nurse says as much as possible instead of paraphrasing. *If the interpreter paraphrases the nurse's words, important information may be lost.*
- Consider nonverbal factors when communicating. Speak slowly and smile when appropriate. Keep an open posture. Do not cross the arms over the chest or turn away from the family. Listen carefully to what the family says. Nod, lean forward, or encourage continued talk with frequent "uh-huhs." Avoid fidgeting or watching a clock.
- Determine Diep's response to a light touch on the arm, and use or avoid touch depending on her response.
- Do not expect prolonged eye contact.
- *Even subtle body language can indicate interest and empathy or impatience, annoyance, or hurry. Touch and eye contact are sensitive cultural variables, and nurses should be aware they are not always welcomed.*
- Use phone interpreter services, which are provided in some clinical agencies, ensuring both the nurse and the woman receive accurate information.

Evaluation

Diep keeps each prenatal appointment. She follows all recommendations and gradually asks appropriate questions more often at each visit.

Culture and Health Beliefs in Childbearing

Childbirth is viewed by women as a meaningful life changing event, which is both "pivotal and paradoxical" (Prinds, Hvidtjørn, Mogensen, Skytthe, & Hvidt, 2014, p. 40). It is important to note that "childbirth is a time of transition and social celebration in all cultures . . . . Giving birth has the potential to be a rich and cultural spiritual experience facilitated by a [culturally competent] nurse" (Callister, 2014, pp. 41, 64).

There are more than 100 ethnocultural groups in the United States with traditional health beliefs (Callister, 2016a). But it is important to recognize that "culture" defined broadly means more than ethnocultural characteristics. "Culture" may include childbearing women who have been sexually abused as children, or others who have definite ideas about not using birth technologies but prefer traditional means of managing labor and birth that may even

include having a home birth. "Culture" may include poverty, low health literacy, having had female genital cutting, being disabled, or surrogate mothers. There are many cultures. Please note the following: "You may not know exactly what to expect when you walk into a woman's room in the clinic or the birthing unit, but being creative, flexible, and resilient in your approach to caring will bring many satisfying cultural experiences" (Callister, 2016a, p. 11).

Take the opportunity to learn about the uniqueness of each woman you care for and about her cultural beliefs and practices surrounding childbirth. For example, Asian women may believe health is the balance between "yin" and "yang." Those of African or Haitian origin may define health as "harmony with nature." Hispanics often consider health as a balance between "hot" and "cold."

Traditional methods to prevent illness are related to cultural beliefs such as the "evil eye" which causes injury, illness, or misfortune. Others are phenomena such as soul loss because of jealousy, environmental factors such as bad air, and natural events such as solar eclipses. Practices to prevent illness developed from beliefs regarding the cause of illness. This includes protective or religious objects such as amulets with magic powers or consecrated religious objects (such as talismans) frequently worn or carried to prevent illness.

Health Maintenance

The predominant culture in the United States may treat pregnancy as high risk, with frequent prenatal visits and multiple tests, hospitalization for giving birth, and significant use of technology, including epidural analgesia/anesthesia and induced labor. On the other hand, many cultures view pregnancy as a normal physiologic condition with little or no need for health care because the woman is not "sick."

Traditional practices may be used to maintain health during pregnancy and birth. For example, Mexican women may keep active to ensure a small newborn and easy birth and may continue sexual intercourse to lubricate the birth canal. East Indian women maintain a balance between "hot" (eggs, nuts, chili, garlic, mango, ginger) and "cold" foods (fresh fruit, yogurt, buttermilk) (Goyal, 2016). Prenatal care may not begin for Indonesian women until the second trimester, when the soul is believed to enter the unborn child. Korean women may practice Qi during pregnancy, which consists of physical postures, breathing techniques, and meditation. Native American women may not tie knots or make braids during pregnancy to prevent complications involving the umbilical cord. Some groups believe unclean things and strong emotions such as anger cause harm to the fetus or precipitate a difficult childbirth.

Immigrant and refugee childbearing women may have particular challenges, including vulnerability to being marginalized, low socioeconomic status, and lack of access to social resources, including prenatal care. Strategies have been suggested that may be helpful for nurses dealing with refugee women (Callister, 2016b). Somali immigrant mothers described the limitations of support they experienced because of separation from their families, which only highlighted for them the importance of cultural and religious beliefs and practices (Missal, Clark, & Kovaleva, 2016). In a research report focusing on Korean immigrant women's experiences giving birth in the United States, Seo, Kim, and Dickerson (2014) noted that the women developed distinct birth cultural practices that combined their Korean traditional beliefs and Western childbirth practices to promote positive outcomes. In a study of Hispanic childbearing women, they yearned (ef anhelo) to learn and understand more, but without sacrificing their ethnic and cultural identity (la identidad) (Fitzgerald, Cronin, & Boccella, 2015).

Belief in Fate

Some cultures believe in fate determining outcomes. This includes adverse events over which they have no personal control. This may mean in some instances they do not take personal responsibility for what happens when they bear a child.

Preventing Illness

Women may think they can ensure positive outcomes by observing cultural taboos. Advance preparation for the newborn is also avoided in some cultures. Arabic Muslim women believe preparing for the baby defies the will of Allah. Navajo families do not choose a name for the baby until after birth because they fear it will harm the infant if identified earlier. Russian women may not buy clothes or baby equipment until the fetus is born healthy. Women in many cultures eat raw garlic or onion or adhere to food taboos and prescribed combinations of foods.

Strict adherence to religious codes and moral conduct is also believed to prevent illness. The nurse should ask, "What do pregnant women take to protect themselves and the baby?" "What special foods and drinks are important?"

Use of Complementary and Other Therapies

Natural substances such as herbs and plants may be used to promote wellness and treat illness (National Center for Complementary and Alternative Medicine, n.d.). For example, Tongan mothers use *vaikita* made from orange peels and mango leaves to prevent postpartum illness *(kita)* (Reed, Callister, & Corbett, 2017). Dermabrasion, which is the rubbing or irritation of the skin to relieve discomfort, is a common health practice in Southeast Asia. This includes coining, in which an area is covered with an ointment and the edge of a coin rubbed over the area. These methods leave marks resembling bruises or burns on the skin, often mistaken for signs of physical abuse.

Women may use religious charms, holy words, prescribed acts, and traditional healers before seeking other health advice. Hispanics may consult *curanderas* for illness or a *partera* for care during pregnancy. Some Africans and Haitians may rely on folk medicine, including witchcraft, voodoo, or magic (Spector, 2017).

Modesty

Fear, modesty, and a desire to avoid examination by men may keep some women from seeking health care during pregnancy. In many cultures (such as Muslim, Hindu, Hispanic), exposure of the genitals to men is considered demeaning. In these cultures, the reputations of women depend on their demonstrated modesty. If possible, female health care providers should perform examinations. If this is not possible, the woman should be carefully draped with all areas of the body covered except those that must be exposed for examination. A female nurse should remain with these women at all times. Obtaining permission from the husband may be necessary before any examination or treatment can be performed. In addition, the woman's husband, a female friend, or a male relative should be allowed to be present during examinations.

Women who have experienced female genital cutting may be fearful and anxious about modesty issues, and nurses should be respectful and nonjudgmental (Little, 2015).

Culturally Competent Care

Nursing standards emphasize the importance of providing culturally competent care. The American Nurses Association (ANA) standards for professional nurses include the statement that registered nurses "demonstrate respect, equity, and empathy in actions and interactions with culturally diverse and vulnerable healthcare consumers" (ANA, 2015b) supported by guidelines for culturally competent care (Douglas et al., 2014). The U.S. Department of Health and Human Services (DHHS) released the enhanced National Standards for Culturally and Linguistically Appropriate Services (CLAS) in Health and Health Care (Koh, Gracia, & Alvarez, 2014). Standards of the Association of Women's Health, Obstetric, and Neonatal Nurses (AWHONN, 2009) also emphasizes the importance of culturally competent care.

In a study of pregnant Black women, childbearing experiences were enriched through quality interactions with their health care providers (Dahlem, Villarruel, & Ronis, 2014). Outcomes of culturally competent care include enhanced relationships between women and their providers, reduced complications, adherence to health care provider recommendations, improved quality of life, increased trust, and an appreciation of cultural diversity by providers (Lor, Crooks, & Tluczek, 2016). Assessing, developing, and using culturally appropriate health education for childbearing women is essential for the culturally competent nurse to improve patient outcomes (Callister, 2016a).

Culturally competent nursing care requires an awareness of, sensitivity to, and respect for the diversity of the women served. It involves assessment of the family's culture and cultural negotiation when necessary. Barriers to health care may include linguistic and sociocultural differences, socioeconomic barriers including lack of health insurance, a lack of health knowledge, a reluctance to question a health care provider, and the biomedical health care environment (Callister, 2014). For example, in a study of delayed health care seeking, American Muslim women with higher levels of modesty and religiosity were more likely to delay seeking prenatal care (Shahawy, Deshpande, & Nour, 2015; Vu, Milkie, Tala, & Aasim, 2016).

Cultural Assessment

The following questions might be considered when performing a cultural assessment, which should be used to develop plans for care that respect cultural differences and traditional health practices (Callister, 1995; Mattson, 2015).

- What is the family's ethnic affiliation?
- Is childbearing viewed as a normal physiologic process, a time of vulnerability and risk, or a state of illness?
- What are the prescribed practices, customs, and rituals related to diet, activity, and behavior during pregnancy and childbirth?
- How is childbirth pain managed, and what maternal and paternal behaviors are appropriate?
- What maternal restrictions or precautions are considered necessary during childbearing? Are any religious expectations required to be met after birth?
- Who provides support during pregnancy, childbirth, and beyond?
- What are the prescribed practices and restriction related to care of the newborn?
- Who in the family hierarchy makes health care decisions?
- What are the views of life and death, including predestination and fatalism?
- Do you need help understanding health care information?
- How can health care professionals be most helpful?

Cultural Negotiation

Cultural negotiation involves providing information while acknowledging the woman may hold views different from those of the nurse. A woman may not follow health care advice because of cultural beliefs. If the woman or her family indicates information is not helpful or is harmful in their opinion, the conflict should be acknowledged openly and clarified. "I sense that you are unsure about this. Tell me your concerns." After allowing the woman and her family to express their beliefs, the nurse explains why the recommendation was made and works with the family to find a compromise satisfactory to all.

Cultural negotiation also involves sensitivity to specific concerns. For example, nurses should be aware of Islamic laws governing modesty when caring for Muslim women. Some Muslim women must cover their hair, body, arms to the wrist, and legs to the ankles at all times when in the presence of men. A Muslim woman may be prohibited from being alone in the presence of a man other than her husband or a male relative.

"Perinatal nurses should seek to create a healthcare encounter with childbearing women that respects the sociocultural and spiritual context of life and moves beyond the superficial to understand the deeper meaning of childbearing. Perinatal nurses should never lose sight of the fact that a woman's childbirth experience is not only about making a baby but also about creating a mother—a mother who is strong and competent and who trusts her own capacities because she has been cared for by a culturally competent nurse" (Callister, 2014, p. 64).

TABLE 2.1	Impact of Socioeconomic Factors on the Family's Response to Pregnancy		
Affluent	**Middle Class**	**Working Poor and Unemployed**	**New Poor**
Resources			
Is confident of ability; has financial reserves to protect from economic fluctuations; owns or rents home in a safe neighborhood; has health insurance or can pay for health care; is able to provide enriched environment	Has relative security but fewer reserves and more debt; owns or rents home in relatively safe neighborhood; depends on employment for health insurance	Lacks skills and bargaining power; is most vulnerable to economic fluctuations; struggles to meet basic needs	Was previously self-sufficient but has lost prior resources; may have recently lost job and insurance; unused to public assistance
Value Placed on Health Care			
Values preventive care	Values health care but must rely on health insurance related to employment	May value health care but often does not see a way to improve situation	Values health care but may no longer have finances to access it
Time Orientation			
Is future oriented and seeks prenatal care early; expects best possible care and education for children	Is future oriented and seeks early prenatal care; makes plans to provide best possible care and education for children	Priority is to meet needs of present; often seeks prenatal care late; has an uncertain future	Has middle-class time orientation but must meet present needs; may begin prenatal care late

SOCIAL ISSUES

Nurses caring for patients and families must overcome social issues that influence health care. Some issues affecting maternity care include socioeconomic status, including poverty and homelessness; disparity in health care, allocation of health care resources, and care versus cure; and intimate partner violence and human trafficking.

Socioeconomic Status

The socioeconomic status of the family has significant influence on childbearing practices. The term *socioeconomic status* refers to the resources available for the family to meet the needs for food, shelter, and health care. Socioeconomic status can be divided into the affluent, the middle class, the working poor, and the new poor (Table 2.1).

The Affluent

Affluent families have resources to provide for their needs and purchase health care. They have a good income, secure shelter in a safe neighborhood, and the education and reserves to protect themselves from economic fluctuations. They can pay for health care through either private means or insurance.

Affluent families think they deserve the best in health care and respect from health care providers. They are future oriented and therefore value preventive care. In general, they seek early, regular antepartum care and comply with recommendations of the health care providers.

The Middle Class

The middle class constitutes the largest group of families in the United States. They usually are able to rent or own homes in relatively safe neighborhoods. They have adequate food and either education or skills that assist them to obtain and keep jobs for long periods.

Middle-class families rely on group insurance, obtained as a benefit of employment, to shield themselves from exorbitant health care costs. A major concern is loss of a job that results in loss of health insurance. They are future oriented and seek health care early in pregnancy.

The Working Poor and Unemployed

The working poor and unemployed include unskilled or unemployed workers. They work for low wages and are often the last hired and the first fired. They may live below the poverty level and have barely enough to survive. Some have difficulty meeting their basic needs for food and shelter, and some become homeless.

Because of economic uncertainty, these families place more emphasis on meeting present needs and less value on preventive (future-oriented) care. This often causes them to postpone prenatal care until the second or even the third trimester (see Nursing Care Plan: Socioeconomic Problems during Pregnancy).

◎ NURSING CARE PLAN

Socioeconomic Problems during Pregnancy

Assessment

Theresa, a 19-year-old primigravida, is seen for initial prenatal care at 24 weeks of gestation. She took the day off from work without pay in a factory and rode the bus to the clinic. She is currently living with her sister and brother-in-law, who receive Temporary Assistance for Needy Families. During the interview, Theresa states she will not be able to keep clinic appointments because she cannot afford to take more time off until the baby comes. She is unmarried and says the father of the baby is "gone." Physical assessment shows Theresa and her fetus are

Continued

◎ NURSING CARE PLAN—cont'd

Socioeconomic Problems during Pregnancy

healthy. She declares she does not need further prenatal care and only needs to find someone to deliver the baby.

Identification of Patient Problems

Potential for inadequate prenatal care because of lack of knowledge of the importance of prenatal care and lack of resources.

Planning: Expected Outcomes

During the first prenatal visit, Theresa will do the following:
1. Describe the benefits of prenatal care.
2. Verbalize a plan for obtaining regular prenatal care.

Interventions and Rationales

1. Use active listening to show concern and empathy with Theresa's difficulties in obtaining prenatal care. *Expressing interest in Theresa's situation may make her more likely to listen to health teaching.*
2. Emphasize why regular prenatal care is essential.
   a. To monitor the growth and development of the baby.
   b. To evaluate Theresa's health, which directly affects the health of the fetus.
   c. To detect problems and intervene before they become severe.
   Preventive care often is not a priority when the woman has conflicting needs for food and shelter. Many women are

unaware that complications such as preeclampsia or gestational diabetes, which may be identified and treated with routine care, are serious hazards if they remain undetected.
3. Assist Theresa in devising a plan to obtain regular prenatal care.
   a. Provide her with a list of prenatal clinics near her home or place of work and the hours they are open.
   b. Discuss transportation services and determine whether family or friends can help her keep prenatal appointments.
   c. Explore dates, times, and alternatives until she finds a schedule that works for her.
   d. Obtain a list of phone numbers (e.g., friends, family, employer) at which she can be reached for follow-up.
   Some clinics are open on weekends and evenings to accommodate working women. Unreliable transportation is a major reason for failure to keep scheduled appointments, and clinic schedules that allow some flexibility are helpful. Interest in a patient's individual situation is highly motivating for her to find a way to continue prenatal care.

Evaluation

Theresa is attentive as the nurse talks about the importance of health care. She shows interest in finding a way to have regular prenatal care and makes an appointment for the next visit. If she misses scheduled appointments, follow-up phone calls to arrange alternative appointments may be necessary.

The New Poor

The new poor constitute a group of individuals and families who were previously self-sufficient but are now without resources because of circumstances such as loss of a job or health care insurance. They must find their way in an unfamiliar and frightening health care system.

The values of the new poor are those of the middle class: self-sufficiency, hard work, and pride in the ability to succeed. Seeking public assistance is very difficult for this group. These families are devastated when they encounter the lack of respect that may occur when some health care workers interact with families unable to pay for health care.

Poverty

Poverty remains an underlying factor in problems such as homelessness and inadequate access to health care. Although poverty in the United States decreased from 2014 to 2015, it was still 13.5%, which means there were 43.1 million people living in poverty (U.S. Census Bureau, 2016b). Because of adverse living conditions, poor health care, and poor nutrition, infants born to women in low-income groups are more likely to begin life with problems such as low birth weight.

Poverty often breeds poverty. In poor families, children may leave the educational system early, making them less likely to learn skills necessary to obtain good jobs. Childbearing at an early age is common and further interferes with education and the ability to work. The cycle of poverty may continue from one generation to the next as a result of hopelessness and apathy (Fig. 2.1).

As health care costs have risen, the ability to pay for employer-sponsored health insurance has become more difficult for

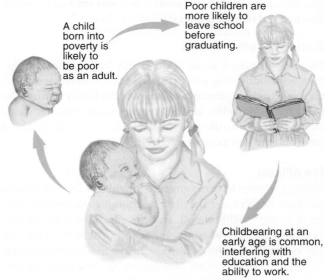

A child born into poverty is likely to be poor as an adult.

Poor children are more likely to leave school before graduating.

Childbearing at an early age is common, interfering with education and the ability to work.

FIG. 2.1 The cycle of poverty.

low- and middle-income workers. The working poor have jobs but receive wages barely adequate to meet their day-to-day needs or may work just under the full-time hours required to qualify them for employer insurance and other benefits. These jobs may not offer health insurance at all, or high premiums may be the only option. The working poor have little opportunity to save for emergencies such as serious illness.

Preliminary data for 2016 indicates 8.8% (28.2 million) of Americans do not have health insurance (National

Center for Health Statistics, 2017). Millions of other people have limited insurance and would not be able to survive financially in the event of serious illness. People without insurance seek care only when absolutely necessary. Health maintenance and illness prevention may seem costly and unnecessary to them. Some women receive no health care during pregnancy until they arrive at the hospital for birth.

Homelessness

A snapshot view from the National Alliance to End Homelessness (2017) reports 564,708 people were homeless on a given night in January 2015. Families make up 206,286 (36.5%) of this number, and individuals make up another 358,422 (64.4%). Homeless families are often composed of single women and their children, and domestic violence is often part of their history as they attempt to escape the violence. Homeless people may wait until health problems are severe because of shame at becoming homeless and inability to pay for the care needed. Care is delayed until the homeless person enters the emergency room, and the needed care is far more costly than the preventive care the homeless person could not afford.

The pregnant homeless woman is less likely to seek prenatal care that might identify complications such as maternal hypertension, diabetes, substance abuse, or inadequate maternal weight gain, which adds to the risk for prematurity and low birth weight (March of Dimes, 2014). Pregnancy interferes with one's ability to work and may reduce income to the point that housing is unattainable.

Disparity in Health Care

Health disparities exist in a population when different groups of people have "differences in health outcomes and their causes" (CDC, 2016b, p. 1). Circumstances such as education, income, and employment status; transportation; housing; public safety; available social support; access to and use of health care and preventive services; and behavioral risk factors affect health outcomes. Disparities exist across multiple lines, including racial, ethnic, age, gender, socioeconomic status, and geographic (rural, inner city, urban/suburban, as well as between states).

Between 1990 and 2013, maternal mortality rates significantly decreased in most countries; however, in the United States, they more than doubled (Center for Reproductive Rights, 2014). Racial variation is significant. From 2011 to 2013, the rate of maternal deaths among Black women was more than three times greater than among White women and more than double all other races (CDC, 2017a). The infant mortality rate gap between black and white more than doubled from 2005 to 2013 (Mathews, MacDorman, & Thoma, 2015). Variation in the rates of sexually transmitted diseases (STDs) across race and ethnic groups may be influenced by issues such as access to sexual health services and the ability to pay for them (CDC, 2017b). Black women are more likely to die of cancer than White women, even though they have a lower incidence (American Cancer Society, 2013).

BOX 2.1 Factors Related to Poor Access to Health Care

Poverty
Unemployment
Lack of medical insurance
Adolescence
Minority group
Inner city residence
Rural residence
Unmarried mother status
Less than high school education
Inability to speak English

Prenatal care is widely accepted as an important element in a good pregnancy outcome. Late or no prenatal care is associated with increased risks for maternal and infant morbidity and mortality. Utilization of prenatal care varies by race and age. In 2014, late or no prenatal care was most common among American Indian and Alaska Native women (11% of births). Black (10%) and Hispanic women (8%) were also more likely to receive late or no prenatal care compared with Asian or Pacific Islander women (6%) and White women (4%). Teenage women are the most likely to receive late or no prenatal care. The younger the mother, the less likely the mother will receive prenatal care: 25% under age 15 and 10% ages 15 to 19. This is in stark contrast to pregnant women in their 30s who received late or no prenatal care in 4.5% of births (Child Trends DataBank, 2015).

Factors limiting access to care should be addressed to increase the use of preconception and prenatal care. Box 2.1 summarizes some of the factors interfering with access to care. Many factors overlap.

Barriers to Prenatal Care

Women's access to prenatal care is limited by financial, systemic, and attitudinal barriers. Financial barriers are among the most important factors limiting prenatal care. Many women have no insurance or insufficient insurance to cover maternity care. Although Medicaid finances prenatal care for indigent women, the enrollment process is burdensome and lengthy. Some women do not know how to access this resource or do not qualify.

Systemic barriers include institutional practices that interfere with consistent care. For example, women must often wait weeks for their first visit.

Prenatal visits are usually scheduled during daytime hours that conflict with working women's schedules. Taking time off from work often means loss of wages and may put the woman's job in jeopardy. In addition, child care is rarely available at sites of care, and some women are unable to find affordable care. Lack of transportation may keep women from getting prenatal care. In addition, interpreters may not be available for women who do not speak English well.

An important barrier to health care results from the unsympathetic attitude of some health care workers toward those who are unable to pay for prenatal care. Poor families may experience long delays, hurried examinations, rudeness, and arrogance from some members of the health care team. Staff may be overworked and frustrated with the workloads they carry. Women may wait hours for an examination that lasts only a few minutes. Many never see the same health care provider more than once. These women may not keep clinic appointments because they do not see the importance of the hurried examinations.

Nurses should treat each family with respect and consideration. Nurses can work to determine which barriers apply to the patients with whom they work and find ways to meet the needs of the specific population being served. Scheduling prenatal visits in the evening or on weekends, setting aside times for walk-in prenatal visits, and offering other services such as applications for Medicaid and Women, Infants, and Children (WIC) programs may increase use of prenatal services. Decreasing waiting time before appointments as much as possible is important. Cultural sensitivity is important for all caregivers.

Some women do not obtain early prenatal care because they do not realize they are pregnant, do not want the pregnancy confirmed, do not want anyone to know about the pregnancy, or are considering an abortion. A woman with an unintended pregnancy may be too depressed to begin prenatal care early. Many women rely on advice from family and friends during pregnancy, and some believe prenatal care is unimportant, especially when they are healthy and have no obvious problems with the pregnancy.

Allocation of Health Care Resources

In addition to the social factors involved in health disparities, how the available health care money is spent is an issue to be addressed. In 2014 the United States spent $3 trillion on health care, an average of $9523 per person annually (National Center for Health Statistics, 2016b). Expenditures for health care continue to rise. Areas to be addressed include ways to provide care for indigent persons, the uninsured or underinsured, and those with long-term care needs. Distribution of the limited funds available for health care among all these areas is a major concern.

Care versus Cure

Another issue is whether the focus of health care should be on preventive and caring measures or cures for diseases. In the past, medicine has centered more on treatment and cure rather than on prevention and care. Yet prevention avoids suffering and is less expensive than treating diseases after diagnosis.

The focus on cure has resulted in technologic advances enabling some people to live longer, healthier lives. However, the costs of technology should be balanced against the benefits obtained and by the number of people who benefit.

Although LBW infants constitute a small percentage of all newborns, they require a large percentage of total hospital expenditures. The expenses of one preterm infant for a single day in an intensive care nursery are more than enough to pay for care of the mother throughout her pregnancy and birth.

Yet if the mother had received prenatal care early and regularly, the infant might have avoided intensive care.

Quality-of-life issues are important with regard to technology. Neonatal nurseries are able to keep very-low-birth-weight (VLBW) babies alive because of advances in high technology for this group. Some of these infants go on to lead normal or near-normal lives. Others gain time but not quality of life. Families and health care professionals face difficult decisions about when to treat, when to end treatment, and how to recognize when the suffering outweighs the benefits.

Solutions

An expert committee of the National Academies of Sciences, Engineering, and Medicine (2017) reported on measures to address the inequities. Their report, "Communities in Action: Pathways to Health Equity," stressed the importance of community solutions to address local issues influencing health. Their recommendations include the need for government agencies that make decisions regarding factors affecting the health of high-risk populations (land use, housing, transportation, etc.) consider intended and unintended effects of all policies. They stressed that partnerships among residents, businesses, and policy makers are required to address this issue.

Government Programs for Health Care. Government programs for health care are intended as a safety net for vulnerable populations such as women and children with low socioeconomic status.

Medicare, Medicaid, and Children's Health Insurance Program. Medicare provides health insurance for people over 65 years of age, with disabilities, or with end-stage renal disease. Medicare is federally funded and administered by the Centers for Medicare and Medicaid Services (CMS), a division of the DHHS. Medicaid provides health care for indigent persons, older adults, and persons with disabilities. Pregnant women and young children are especially targeted. Medicaid is funded by both the federal and individual state governments. The states administer the program and determine which services are offered. Although the qualifying level of poverty varies across states, all women with an income less than 133% of the current federal poverty level are eligible for perinatal care. The Children's Health Insurance Program provides health care for children up to age 19 years through Medicaid and other programs. Like Medicaid, it is funded by both the federal and state governments and administered by the state.

Public Clinics. Women who do not have private insurance or Medicaid may receive prenatal care at public clinics, which typically base their fees on the family's income. However, barriers to care such as limited staff, hours of operation, lack of transportation, and lack of childcare for other children may affect the feasibility of such care.

Temporary Assistance to Needy Families. Temporary Assistance to Needy Families (TANF) provides financial assistance for basic living costs for pregnant women and families with one or more dependent children. Eligibility requirements, income limits, allowances for homelessness, and time limitations vary across states.

Shelters and Health Care for the Homeless. Federal funding has assisted homeless people with shelter and health care. However, the homeless have additional difficulties in obtaining health care because of lack of transportation, inconvenient hours, and poor continuity of care.

Quality and quantity of care in clinics may be poor because of inadequate funding. Nurses have been instrumental in opening shelters, clinics, and outreach services for the homeless, with nurse practitioners often playing a major role. Clinics headed by nurse practitioners are often opened in underserved rural and inner city areas. Nurses also help inform the public and legislatures about the needs of the homeless and others with few health care options

Innovative Programs. Innovative programs to ensure all women receive good prenatal care are necessary to improve pregnancy outcomes. Some outreach programs are designed to improve health in women who traditionally do not seek prenatal care. Bilingual health care workers and bilingual educational classes are part of some programs. Programs may be located in schools, shopping centers, churches, workplaces, and neighborhoods that are easily accessible to people. Mobile vans outfitted with basic equipment bring prenatal care to women who are unable or unwilling to attend care at fixed locations or in more distant neighborhoods. The number of such neighborhood programs is insufficient to make adequate health care for women and children a reality.

KNOWLEDGE CHECK

9. How do poverty and inadequate prenatal care affect infant mortality and morbidity?
10. What is the effect of health care disparities in the United States?

Intimate Partner Violence

Intimate partner violence (IPV) is defined as abuse by a current or former partner or spouse. It includes physical, sexual, and emotional abuse (e.g., threatening a partner's loved ones or possessions or harming a partner's self-worth). Approximately 31.5% of women in the United States have experienced physical violence by an intimate partner; 8.8% have been raped by their partner, and 15.8% have experienced other forms of sexual violence from their partner (Breiding et al., 2014). Adolescents as well as older women are victims of IPV. Although some studies show an increased incidence in economically disadvantaged groups, IPV is seen at all socioeconomic levels.

Physical abuse may involve threats, slapping, and pushing. It may escalate to punching, kicking, and beating resulting in internal injury, wounds from weapons, or death. Sexual abuse, including rape, often is part of physical abuse, with many abused women reporting being forced into sex by their male partner.

Physical violence occurs within the context of continuous mental abuse, threats, and coercion, and the abuser blames the victim for causing the abuse. As a result, victims feel shame, loss of self-respect, and powerlessness. They are often isolated from friends and family. Abused women often report reproductive coercion, attempts by the abuser to interfere with contraception use and pregnancy (American College of Obstetricians and Gynecologists [ACOG], 2013).

Although IPV spans all demographic categories, some factors associated with an increased risk include low self-esteem, low income, heavy alcohol and drug use, depression, and history of abuse (CDC, 2016c).

Effects of Intimate Partner Violence during Pregnancy

Violence may start or escalate in frequency and severity during pregnancy and the postpartum period. Pregnancy adds more stress to the relationship. The partner may feel trapped in the relationship and under increased pressure to provide emotional and financial support for the woman and the infant. Up to 20% of women may be physically abused during pregnancy (American Academy of Pediatrics [AAP] & ACOG, 2012). Abuse occurs more often during pregnancy than any other commonly screened medical complication, with the possible exception of preeclampsia (AAP& ACOG, 2012). The risk for abuse continues into the postpartum period.

Abuse during pregnancy is correlated with health problems for the mother and the infant. Abused women are more likely than nonabused women to start prenatal care late. They have an increased risk for uterine rupture, placental abruption, preterm birth, LBW infants, and maternal and fetal death (Cunningham et al., 2014). They may have increased risk for STDs (Spiwak, Afifi, Halli, Garcia-Moreno, & Sareen, 2013) and peripartum depression (de Oliveira-Fonseca-Machado, Aives, Scotini Freitas, dos Santos Monteiro, & Gomes-Sponholz, 2014).

Physical abuse of the mother may be an indication of what life holds for the unborn child. Some men who batter women also batter children, and some women who are victims of violence abuse their children. Approximately 27% of abused women abuse their children. Child abuse occurs in 33% to 77% of homes where there is IPV (AAP & ACOG, 2012). Children who witness violence in the home may have psychological, social, emotional, and behavioral problems (Wathen & MacMillan, 2013). Adults who abuse others often were abused as children.

Factors That Promote Violence

Family violence occurs in families in which roles are gender based and little value is placed on the woman's role. Men hold the power, and women are viewed as less worthy of respect than are men. Women usually earn less than men do in the job market, and they are often victimized by marriage. They may remain in unhealthy relationships because they are financially dependent on their partners. If they divorce, women often become single parents with a standard of living lower than that of their former husbands.

The woman's role in her own culture is important. For example, in many cultures, women think they should be submissive to men and sacrifice for their families because it is their duty to keep the family together. They may not have the education to be able to access help or obtain a job to provide a means of support if they should leave their partners. If the woman is an illegal immigrant, she is less likely to seek help from authorities for fear of being deported.

Stereotyping males as powerful and females as weak and without value has a profound effect on the self-esteem of women. Many women internalize these messages and come to believe they are less worthy than their partners and they are the cause of their own punishment.

The woman may come to accept her partner's statements indicating she is the cause of the violence. She may minimize the abuse or indicate to others that it is unusual. Women often feel a need to help the abuser and hope the partner will change and the abuse will end. As the relationship becomes increasingly abusive, the woman may begin to look for help.

Although alcohol is often stated as a cause of violence against women, chemical dependence and IPV are two separate problems. Chemical dependence is a disease of addiction, but abuse is a learned behavior and can be unlearned. However, violence may become more severe or bizarre when alcohol or drugs are involved. See Table 2.2 for a summary of the myths and realities of violence against women.

Characteristics of the Abuser

Physical abuse is about power, and it is only one of many tactics abusive men use to control their partners. Other tactics include isolation, intimidation, and threats. Extreme jealousy and possessiveness are typical of the abuser. An abusive man often attempts to control every aspect of the woman's life, such as where she goes, to whom she speaks, and what she wears. He controls access to money and transportation and may force the woman to account for every moment spent away from him.

The abusive man often has a low tolerance for frustration and poor impulse control. He does not perceive his violent behavior as a problem and often denies responsibility for the violence by blaming the woman. Most abusive men come from homes in which they witnessed the abuse of their mothers or were themselves abused as children.

Cycle of Violence

Although IPV may be random, there is often a pattern. The violence occurs in a cycle consisting of three phases: (1) a tension-building phase, (2) a battering incident, and (3) a "honeymoon" or "calm phase." Being aware of the behaviors associated with each phase will enable the nurse to counsel the woman (Fig. 2.2).

Nurse's Role in Prevention of Abuse

Nurses can do a great deal to prevent physical abuse of women. First, they should examine their own beliefs to determine whether they accept the attitude that blames the victim: "Why was she wearing that?" "She shouldn't have flirted with someone else." "Why does she stay with him?" Second, nurses can consciously practice empowerment of women. They should make it clear that the woman owns her body and has the right to decide how it should be treated. Nurses should use language indicating the woman is an active partner in her care: "You understand your body; what do you think?"

During examinations, nurses can introduce aspects of care to increase the woman's control over the situation. For example, make sure when the woman first meets the physician or nurse practitioner who is to examine her, she is seated and clothed instead of being unclothed and in a lithotomy position.

TABLE 2.2 Myths and Realities of Violence against Women

Myths	Realities
The battered woman syndrome affects only a small percentage of the population.	Battering is a major cause of injury to women. Approximately 24.3% of women have experienced severe violence from IPV.
Violence against women occurs only in lower socioeconomic classes and minority groups.	Violence occurs in families from all social, economic, educational, racial, and religious backgrounds.
The problem is really "partner abuse," couples who assault each other.	Women experience IPV more often than men. Violence against women is about control and power.
Alcohol and drugs cause abusive behavior.	Substance abuse and violence against women are two separate problems. Substance abuse is a disease, but violence is a learned behavior and can be unlearned.
The abuser is "out of control."	He is not out of control. Instead, he is making a decision because he chooses who, when, and where he abuses.
The woman "got what she deserved."	No one deserves to be beaten. No one has the right to beat another person. Violent behavior is the responsibility of the violent person.
Women "like it," or they would leave.	Women are threatened with severe punishment or death if they attempt to leave. Many have no resources and are isolated, and they and their children are dependent on the abuser.
Couples' counseling is a good recommendation for abusive relationships.	Couples' counseling not only is ineffective for the couple but also can be dangerous for the abused woman.

IPV, Intimate partner violence.

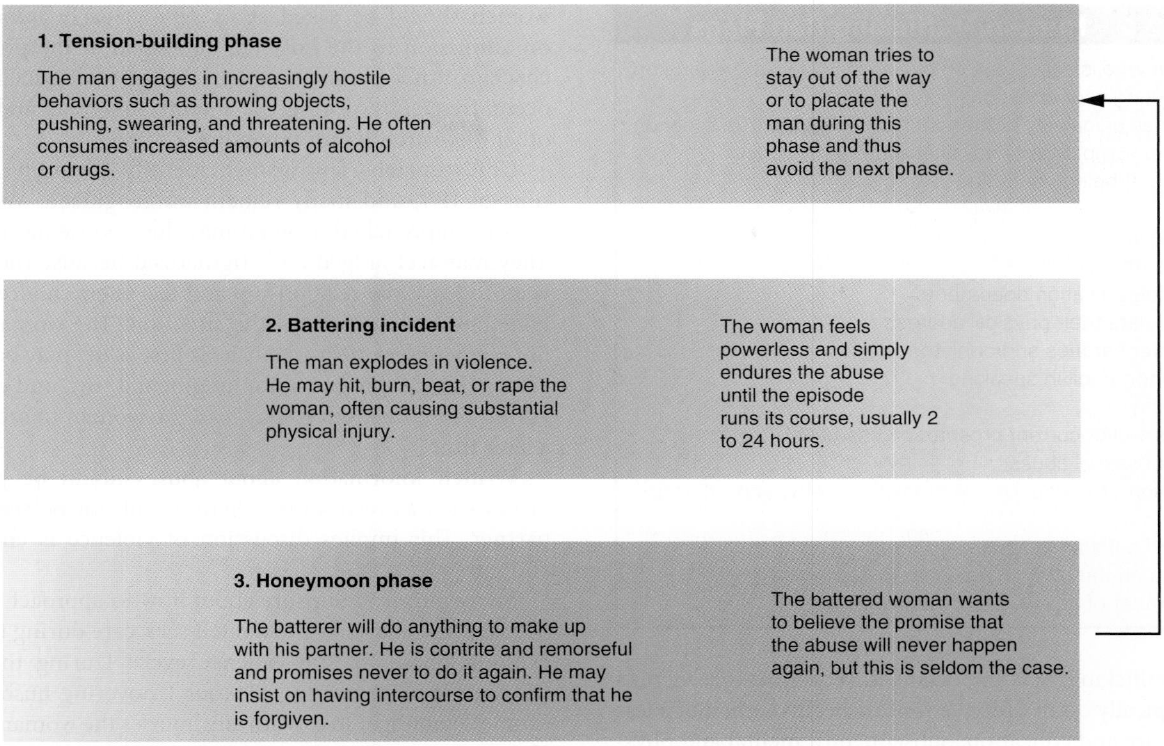

1. Tension-building phase

The man engages in increasingly hostile behaviors such as throwing objects, pushing, swearing, and threatening. He often consumes increased amounts of alcohol or drugs.

The woman tries to stay out of the way or to placate the man during this phase and thus avoid the next phase.

2. Battering incident

The man explodes in violence. He may hit, burn, beat, or rape the woman, often causing substantial physical injury.

The woman feels powerless and simply endures the abuse until the episode runs its course, usually 2 to 24 hours.

3. Honeymoon phase

The batterer will do anything to make up with his partner. He is contrite and remorseful and promises never to do it again. He may insist on having intercourse to confirm that he is forgiven.

The battered woman wants to believe the promise that the abuse will never happen again, but this is seldom the case.

FIG. 2.2 Types of behaviors that are evident in each step of the cycle of violence.

School nurses are in an excellent position to influence how teenagers define gender roles: "Real men don't beat up women." "Girls don't have to put up with verbal or physical abuse from anyone." "Use a condom; it's not cool to give STDs or an unwanted pregnancy to someone you care about."

Nurses should be familiar with national resources designed to provide health care workers with technical assistance, training materials, posters, bibliographies, and relevant articles. The National Domestic Violence Hotline offers information on crisis assistance throughout the United States. They have interpreters for 170 different languages and are available 24 hours a day. The other sources listed here provide information but are not crisis lines.

- National Domestic Violence Hotline: 800-799-SAFE, www.ndvh.org
- National Coalition against Domestic Violence: 303-839-1852, www.ncadv.org
- National Resource Center on Domestic Violence: www.nrcdv.org

Women who are being abused should be warned not to use their home computers to access the Internet for sources of information about abuse because their partners may be able to find out about recently used Internet sites.

KNOWLEDGE CHECK

11. What is the effect of pregnancy on battering behavior?
12. How can nurses alter their practice to help prevent violence against women?

Human Trafficking

Human trafficking is the recruitment and movement of individuals domestically and/or internationally for the purpose of exploitation. Trafficking in persons (TIP) takes many forms; however, the most common is sexual exploitation in sex trafficking and labor trafficking, which traffickers accomplish by means of force, coercion, and/or deception (United Nations, 2000). Although it is commonly recognized that there is no sound methodology for accurately generating the U.S. and global incidence of TIP, the International Labor Organization (ILO) estimates approximately 2.5 million persons are trafficked annually (ILO, 2005). This number is staggering considering estimates of only 1 in 100 victimizations are actually reported. The lack of scholarly evidence, accurate estimations of victimization, and best practices is commonly attributed in part to a lack of identification and reporting by health care providers (Miller, Duke, & Northam, 2016). De Chesnay (2013) recognized sex trafficking as a global pandemic.

Women and children of childbearing age make up the majority of reported TIP cases, with the average age of entry into sex trafficking reported to be between 12 to 14 years of age. Victims of TIP are subjected to an extensive myriad of abuses, including but not limited to sexual abuse, physical abuse, torture, psychological abuse, and the denial of basic human needs such as food and shelter (Miller et al., 2016). Further complicating the provision of care to this population is the isolation from support networks such as friends, family, and spiritual services.

Considering the abuses sustained by victims while under control of the trafficker and the inherently shadow nature of

BOX 2.2 Human Trafficking Red Flags

A person who is accompanied by an individual who insists on answering your questions

Reluctance or inability of the victim to reveal the true situation

Signs and symptoms of physical and mental abuse

Evidence of being controlled

Fearful

Submissive

Fear of authority figures

Lack of identification documents

Cannot relate their physical address

Inconsistent stories and/or histories

Foreign/non-English speaking

Homeless

Previous and/or current prostitution charges

History of sexual abuse

Possession of expensive electronics, jewelry, and other luxury items

History of substance abuse

Markings on the body that appear to be branding

High number of sex partners relative to age

human trafficking, it is important to recognize that victims of TIP typically do not receive routine health care, much less prenatal care and education. Subsequently, mental and physical health outcomes seen in this population include but are not limited to increased incidence of human immunodeficiency virus (HIV) infection, pelvic inflammatory disease, botched home abortions, retained products of conception, damage to reproductive organs, precipitous deliveries, anxiety, depression, suicidal ideation, and self-harm attempts.

Although the scope and magnitude of providing informed care to this population is beyond the scope of this chapter, it is important for nurses caring for women of child-bearing age to be aware and assess their patients for the red flags of TIP exploitation, recognizing victims of TIP rarely self-identify (Miller et al., 2016). A list of possible red flags found in victims of human trafficking is provided in Box 2.2. Although one red flag may not be indicative of the patient being a victim of TIP, the nurse should be assessing for patterns of red flags. For instance, a patient who is not English speaking would not necessarily raise suspicion, but a non–English speaking minor patient who does not know his or her address, and is accompanied by an older person who will not let the patient speak, may raise the nurse's index of suspicion. Maternal-newborn nurses are in a unique position to recognize victimized patients and begin the critical chain of recognition and intervention for this most vulnerable population (Miller, 2013).

◆ APPLICATION OF THE NURSING PROCESS: THE BATTERED WOMAN

◆ Assessment

During pregnancy, a woman is likely to have more frequent contact with health care providers than at any other time in her life. Because of the prevalence of IPV during pregnancy,

women should be asked about IPV at each prenatal visit, on admission to the hospital, and again at the postpartum checkup. After pregnancy, visits to the pediatrician usually occur frequently during the infant's first year and provide other opportunities for screening.

Unfortunately, few women identify themselves as victims of IPV, and many remain unrecognized. When they are first approached, women may deny abuse has occurred. They may feel judged and stigmatized because they do not want to leave the relationship and fear their children will be taken away if they reveal the situation. The woman who is not ready to seek help when she is first asked may be ready at a later time. Asking in a nonjudgmental way, and especially asking more than once, may lead the woman to seek help at a later time.

Written information about abuse should be placed in places such as restrooms, where it will not be seen by the partner. This implies discussion of violence is encouraged and safe.

Many nurses are unsure about how to approach the issue of suspected abuse. Women often seek care during the "honeymoon phase" of the violence cycle. During this phase, the man is often overly solicitous ("hovering husband syndrome") and eager to explain any injuries the woman exhibits. He often answers questions directed at the woman.

❓ CRITICAL THINKING EXERCISE 2.1

Mandy, a 28-year-old primigravida, is admitted to the labor, delivery, and recovery unit with contractions at 34 weeks of gestation. The right side of her face is swollen, old bruises shaped like fingerprints are present on her upper arms, and a large bruised area is apparent on her abdomen. She is accompanied by her husband, who is very solicitous. He verbalizes concern about her labor status and remains close beside her at all times. Mandy appears lethargic and avoids eye contact with the nurse who is admitting her. She states that she fainted at home and hurt herself when she fell against the bathtub. The nurse accepts the explanation and asks no further questions.

Questions

1. What assumptions has the nurse made?
2. What should make the nurse question whether the injuries resulted from falling?

At the change of shifts, Mandy is assigned to another nurse. The nurse waits for a time when Mandy's husband is out of the room and she can be alone with Mandy. The nurse asks, "Did you get these injuries from being hit?" Mandy appears extremely anxious and says, "Don't say anything to him! He got so mad when I was late getting home from shopping. It was my fault."

Questions

3. Why did the nurse wait for time alone with Mandy before asking questions?
4. How should the nurse respond? What bias should the nurse resist?
5. How can Mandy be protected?

Introducing the subject of violence in the presence of the man who may be responsible for it places the woman in danger. It is absolutely essential to separate the woman from the man for the discussion of violence. No other family members should be present during the interview. Even children may reveal the discussion of abuse to the partner or family members.

A common concern about discussing IPV is having time with the woman without her partner. Sometimes the partner can be sent to another area to give insurance information. Telling the partner that the nurse plans to discuss "feminine hygiene" and needs privacy also may be a way to have time alone with the woman.

Other reasons nurses cite for not discussing IPV include lack of time, not knowing what to do if IPV is discovered, and language barriers. If language barriers are present, a professional interpreter should be used to translate and never a family member or friend.

When a private, secure place has been found, explain that many women experience abuse. For example, "Because abuse is very common and can affect the woman's health, it is the policy at this hospital to ask every woman about abuse situations." This lets the woman know she is not being singled out for questioning. Reassure her privacy will be protected and confidentiality will be maintained.

Common screening questions include the following:
- Have you been threatened, hit, slapped, kicked, choked, or otherwise physically hurt by anyone within the last year?
- Has this happened since you have been pregnant?
- Has anyone forced you to have sexual activities?
- Are you ever afraid of anyone?

A "yes" answer should prompt questions about who hurt the woman and the frequency and kinds of abuse. If a woman has old or new signs of possible abuse, ask questions such as "Did someone hurt you?" and "Did you receive these injuries from being hit?"

The abused woman often appears hesitant, embarrassed, or evasive. She may speak in a low tone of voice, be unable to look the nurse in the eye, and appear guilty, ashamed, jumpy, or frightened. She may have a flat affect (absence of facial response) or one inappropriate for the situation.

CRITICAL TO REMEMBER

Cues Indicating Violence against Women

Nonverbal—Facial grimacing, slow and unsteady gait, vomiting, abdominal tenderness, absence of facial response

Injuries—Welts, swelling, burns, vaginal or rectal bleeding; bruises or lacerations in various stages of healing; evidence of old or new fractures of the nose, face, ribs, or arms; injuries to the face, breasts, abdomen, or genitals

Vague somatic complaints—Anxiety, depression, panic attacks, sleeplessness, anorexia

Discrepancy between history and type of injuries—Wounds that do not match the woman's story; multiple bruises in various stages of healing; bruising on the arms (which she may have raised while trying to protect herself); old, untreated wounds

---

Evaluate and document all signs of injury, both past and present. This includes areas of welts, bruising, swelling, lacerations, burns, and scars. Injuries are most commonly noted on the face, breasts, abdomen, and genitalia. Many women have new or old fractures of the face, nose, ribs, or arms. A photograph or a drawing may be used to record areas of injury. These may be important for future legal action.

If sexual abuse has occurred, a gynecologic examination is necessary because trauma to the labia, vagina, cervix, or anus often is present. Types of forced sex may include vaginal intercourse, anal intercourse, and insertion of objects into the vagina and anus.

Be particularly alert for nonverbal cues indicating abuse has occurred. Facial grimacing or a slow, unsteady gait may indicate pain. Vomiting or abdominal tenderness may indicate internal injury. A flat affect is indicative of women who mentally withdraw from the situation to protect themselves from the horror and humiliation they experience. Keep in mind the woman may fear for her life because abusive episodes tend to escalate. Open-ended questions help prompt full disclosure and the expression of feelings. Record direct quotes of what the woman says about her experience.

◆ Identification of Patient Problems

A variety of patient problems may be applicable, depending on assessment data. The most meaningful may be fearfulness secondary to the potential for injury to self or children.

◆ Planning: Expected Outcomes

The abused woman may have difficulty developing a long-term plan of care without a great deal of specialized assistance. She often is unwilling to leave the abusive situation, and nurses should focus on working with the woman to make short-term plans to protect her from future injury. The expected outcomes are that the woman will:
1. Acknowledge the physical assaults.
2. Develop a specific plan of action for when the abusive cycle begins.
3. Identify community resources that can provide protection for her and her children.

◆ Interventions

Listening. Use therapeutic communication techniques to listen and encourage the woman to share her feelings. Assure her you understand her situation is a difficult one and she has been surviving as well as she can. Praise even small positive steps she has taken to ensure safety for herself and her children. The woman should make her own decisions about whether to continue the relationship and should not feel coerced to end it.

Developing a Personal Safety Plan. Ask the woman what she does to decrease or avoid violence from her partner. Help her make concrete plans to protect her safety and that of her children. For example, if the woman insists on returning to the shared home, describe the cycle of behavior that culminates in physical abuse and factors such as drug or alcohol use that precipitate a violent episode. Discuss behaviors indicating the level of frustration and anger is increasing to the point at which the danger is escalating.

Assist her to do the following:

- Locate the nearest shelter, safe house, or another safe place and make specific plans to go there once the cycle of violence begins.
- Identify the safest, quickest routes out of the home.
- Hide extra keys to the car and house, money, personal information (social security numbers, birth certificates, insurance policy information, driver's license, bank account numbers, passport), medications, some clothes for herself and her children, and personal necessities. She should not hide them in the house but find another place such as the house of a friend or relative.
- Devise a code word and prearrange with someone to call the police when the word is used.
- Memorize the telephone number of the shelter or hotline because time is often a crucial element in the decision to leave. An easy number to remember is the one for the National Domestic Violence Hotline (1-800-799-SAFE), which provides immediate crisis assistance in the caller's community.
- Review the safety plan frequently because leaving the partner is one of the most dangerous times. Women are more likely to be injured or killed when they are leaving than at any other time.

Affirming She Is Not to Blame. The abused woman often believes she is responsible for the abuse. Let her know no one deserves to be hurt for any reason. The one who hurt her is the person responsible. She did not provoke it or cause it and could not have prevented it. Nurses are often responsible for teaching basic family processes such as the following:

- Violence is not normal.
- Violence usually is repeated and escalates.
- Battering is against the law.
- Abused women have alternatives.

She also needs nonjudgmental acceptance and recognition of the difficulties involved in making changes in her situation. Praise her for any actions she takes, even if they are only minor steps toward making her life safer. Reassure her that she is doing the right thing for herself and her children when she seeks help and makes plans for escape.

Providing Education. The pregnant woman is likely to worry about the effect of abuse on her pregnancy. Discuss the increased incidence of preterm labor with her and explain the signs. If she is using substances, explain the effects of smoking and of the use of alcohol and drugs and help her make plans to decrease or stop her use. Help her identify stressors and explore ways to reduce them wherever possible.

Providing Referrals. When contact with the battered woman is a short-term one, many interventions are outside the scope of nursing practice. Refer the family to community agencies such as the police department, legal services, community shelters, counseling services, and social service agencies, as needed. Include mental health referrals, if necessary, for treatment of depression or for counseling. Document referrals were made and whether the woman accepted them.

It is essential to accept the decisions of the battered woman and acknowledge she is on her own timetable. She may not take any actions at the time they are recommended. Therefore listening to her, believing her, and providing information about resources may be the only help the nurse can provide until the woman is ready to do more.

Do not become negative or pass judgment on the partner of an abused woman. She is often tied to the man by both economic and emotional bonds and may become defensive if her partner is criticized. Tell her resources are available for her partner, but he must first admit abuse and seek assistance before help can be offered. *Initiating referrals for the partner before he asks for help will increase the danger to the woman if he thinks he has been betrayed.*

◆ Evaluation

The plan of care can be deemed successful if the woman acknowledges the violent episodes in the home, makes concrete plans to protect herself and her children from future injury, and makes plans to use the community resources available to her.

? KNOWLEDGE CHECK

13. What major cues indicate a woman has been physically abused?
14. How can nurses intervene to help women protect their safety if they choose to remain in a home situation with a partner who physically abuses them?
15. What are possible indicators that a woman is a victim of human trafficking?

ETHICS AND BIOETHICS

Ethics involves determining the best course of action in a certain situation. Ethical reasoning is the analysis of what is morally right and reasonable. **Bioethics** is the application of ethics to health care. Ethical behavior for nurses is discussed in codes such as the ANA *Code of Ethics for Nurses with Interpretive Statements* (ANA, 2015a). Ethical issues have become more complex as technology has created more options in health care. These issues are controversial because agreement over what is right or best does not exist and because moral support is possible for more than one course of action.

Ethical Dilemmas

An **ethical dilemma** is a situation in which no solution is completely satisfactory. Opposing courses of action may seem equally desirable, or all possible solutions may seem undesirable. Ethical dilemmas are among the most difficult situations in nursing practice. To find solutions, nurses and other health care personnel should apply ethical theories and principles and determine the burdens and benefits of any course of action (Boggs, 2016).

Ethical Theories

Three models guide ethical decision making: deontologic, utilitarian, and human rights (Boggs, 2016). Few people use one decision-making model exclusively. Instead, they make decisions by examining models and determining which is most appropriate for the circumstances.

Deontologic Model. The **deontologic model** determines what is right by applying ethical principles and moral rules. It does not vary the solution according to individual situations. One example is the rule, "Life must be maintained at all costs and in all circumstances." Strictly used, the deontologic model would not consider the quality of life or weigh the use of scarce resources against the likelihood that the life maintained would be near-normal.

Utilitarian Model. The **utilitarian model** approaches ethical dilemmas by analyzing the benefits and burdens of any course of action to find one that will result in the greatest amount of good. Appropriate actions may vary with the situation when using the utilitarian model. The utilitarian approach is concerned more with the consequences of actions than the actions themselves. In its simplest form, the utilitarian approach is "The end justifies the means." If the outcome is positive, the method of arriving at that outcome is less important.

Human Rights Model. The belief that each person has human rights is the basis for the **human rights model** to making ethical decisions. The nurse may find personal difficulty in the right of a person to refuse care that the nurse and possibly other care providers believe is best. A nurse's goal is usually to save lives, but what if the person's life is intolerable or care is refused?

Ethical Principles

Ethical principles or rules are also important for solving ethical dilemmas. Four of the most important principles are beneficence, nonmaleficence, respect for autonomy, and justice. Other important ethical principles such as accountability, confidentiality, truth, and keeping promises are derived from these four basic principles (Box 2.3).

BOX 2.3   Ethical Principles in Health Care

Autonomy—People have the right to self-determination. This includes the right to respect, privacy, and information necessary to make decisions based on their personal values and beliefs.

Beneficence—Make a decision that produces greatest good or the least harm.

Nonmaleficence—Avoid risking or causing harm to others.

Justice—All people should be treated equally and fairly regardless of disease or social or economic status.

Fidelity—Keep promises, and do not make promises that cannot be kept.

Truth (veracity)—Tell the truth.

Confidentiality—Keep information private.

Accountability—Accept responsibility for actions as a health care professional.

From Alfaro-LeFevre, R. (2017). *Critical thinking, clinical reasoning and clinical judgment: A practical approach* (6th ed.). Philadelphia, PA: Elsevier; and Boggs, K. U. (2016). Clinical judgment and ethical decision making. In E. C. Arnold & K. U. Boggs (eds.), *Interpersonal relationships: Professional communication skills for nurses* (7th ed., pp. 40–56). Philadelphia, PA: Elsevier.

These principles guide decision making, but in some situations, the application of one principle conflicts with another. In such cases, one principle may outweigh another in importance.

Treatments designed to do good also may cause harm. For example, a cesarean birth may prevent permanent harm to a fetus in jeopardy. However, the surgery that saves the fetus also harms the mother, causing pain, temporary disability, and possible financial hardship. Also, certain basic surgical risks to the mother do exist. Both the mother and the health care providers may decide the principle of beneficence outweighs the principle of nonmaleficence. If the mother does not want surgery, the principles of autonomy and justice also should be considered. Is the mother's right to determine what happens to her body more or less important than the right of the fetus to fair and equal treatment?

Solving Dilemmas in Daily Practice

Nurses are often involved in supporting parents when tragedy strikes during a birth. They should be knowledgeable regarding the disease process and the appropriate nursing care in these situations and also be able to support family's needs when ethical dilemmas arise. However, ethical challenges often arise during day-to-day professional practice. Nurses and other professionals should learn to analyze and resolve these dilemmas. Personal values and cultural and language differences are some of the issues that often have an impact on the solving of ethical dilemmas.

Ethical dilemmas, a situation in which no solution seems completely satisfactory, also may have legal ramifications. For example, although the American Medical Association has stated anencephalic organ donation is ethically permissible, it may be illegal. In many states, the legal criteria for death include cardiopulmonary as well as brain death. Therefore donor organs from the baby with anencephaly are likely unusable for transplantation because of lengthy anoxia.

❓ CRITICAL THINKING EXERCISE 2.2

The parents of an infant with anencephaly state that they would like to donate the organs from their dying infant to another infant who might live as a result. They think in this way their own infant will live on as a part of another baby. Currently, opportunities for such transplantations are limited.

Questions
1. What is the deontologic view of this decision?
2. How would the utilitarian view differ?
3. Does the human rights model fit in this situation?
4. What ethical principles are involved? If such transplantations become routine, what problems might arise?

Greater understanding about conflicts and misunderstandings that may arise from the differences among people helps nurses find better solutions to ethical dilemmas and other problems common to daily life. Many approaches can be used to solve ethical dilemmas in nursing practice. No single approach guarantees a right decision, but it provides a logical, systematic method for decision making. Because the nursing process is also a method of problem solving, nurses can use a similar approach when faced with ethical dilemmas (Box 2.4).

Decision making in ethical dilemmas may seem straightforward, but it rarely results in answers acceptable to everyone. Health care agencies often have bioethics committees to formulate policies for ethical situations, provide education, and help make decisions in specific cases. The committees include a variety of professionals such as nurses, physicians, social workers, ethicists, and clergy members. The family members most closely affected by the decision also participate, if possible. A satisfactory solution to ethical dilemmas is more likely to occur when people work together.

? KNOWLEDGE CHECK

16. What is the difference between ethics and bioethics?
17. How do the deontologic, utilitarian, and human rights models differ within ethical theories?
18. When might two ethical principles conflict?
19. How do the steps of the nursing process relate to ethical decision making?

Ethical Issues in Reproduction

Many issues cross the boundary between ethics and legality and apply to all caregivers. These issues apply to many fields of care, including reproduction and women's health.

Reproduction issues often involve conflicts in which a woman's behaviors may cause harm to her fetus or be disliked by some or most members of society. Conflicts between a mother and fetus occur when the mother's needs, behavior, or wishes may injure the fetus. The most obvious instances involve abortion, substance abuse, and a mother's refusal to follow the advice of caregivers. Health care workers and society may respond to such a woman with anger rather than support. However, the rights of both mother and fetus should be examined.

BOX 2.4 Applying the Nursing Process to Solve Ethical Dilemmas

Assessment—Gather data to clearly identify the problem and the decisions necessary. Obtain viewpoints from all who will be affected by the decision and applicable legal, agency policy, and common practice standards.

Analysis—Decide whether an ethical dilemma exists. Analyze the situation using ethical theories and principles. Determine whether and how these conflict.

Planning—Identify as many options as possible, determine their advantages and disadvantages, and conclude which options are most realistic. Predict what is likely to happen if each option is followed. Include the option of doing nothing. Choose the solution.

Implementation—Carry out the solution. Determine who will implement the solution and how. Identify all interventions necessary and what support is needed.

Evaluation—Analyze the results. Determine whether further interventions are necessary.

Elective Pregnancy Termination

Abortion, or elective termination of pregnancy, was a volatile legal, social, and political issue even before the *Roe v. Wade* decision by the U.S. Supreme Court in 1973. Before then states could outlaw abortion within their boundaries. In *Roe v. Wade,* the Supreme Court stated abortion was legal in the United States and existing state laws prohibiting abortion were unconstitutional because they interfered with the mother's constitutional right to privacy. This decision stipulated (1) a woman could obtain an abortion at any time during the first trimester, (2) the state could regulate abortions during the second trimester only to protect the woman's health, and (3) the state could regulate or prohibit abortion during the third trimester, except when the mother's life might be jeopardized by continuing the pregnancy. Since 1973, many state laws have been upheld or rejected by Supreme Court decisions.

Some people believe abortion should be illegal at any time because it deprives the fetus of life. In contrast, others believe women have the right to control their reproductive functions and political discussion of reproductive rights is an invasion of a woman's most private decisions.

For many people the woman's constitutional right to privacy conflicts with the right to life of the fetus. However, the Supreme Court did not rule on when life begins. This omission provokes debate between those who think life begins at conception and those who think life begins when the fetus is viable, or capable of living outside the uterus. Those who think life begins at conception may be opposed to abortion at any time during pregnancy. Those who think life begins when the fetus is viable (20 to 24 weeks of gestation) may oppose abortion after that time. Nurses need to understand abortion laws and the conflicting beliefs that divide society on this issue.

Implications for Nurses. Nurses' responsibilities in the conflict about abortion cannot be ignored. First, they should be informed about the complexity of the abortion issue from legal and ethical standpoints and know the regulations and laws in their state. Second, they should realize that for many people, abortion is an ethical dilemma resulting in confusion, ambivalence, and personal distress. Next, they should also recognize that for many others, the issue is not a dilemma, but a fundamental violation of the personal or religious views that give meaning to their lives. Finally, nurses should acknowledge the sincere convictions and strong emotions of those on all sides of the issue, including themselves.

Professional Obligations. Nurses have no obligation to support a position with which they disagree. The nursing practice acts of many states allow nurses to refuse to assist with the procedure if it violates their ethical, moral, or religious beliefs. However, nurses are obligated to disclose this information before they are employed in an institution where abortions are performed. It is unethical for a nurse to withhold this information until assigned to care for a woman having an abortion and then refuse to provide care. As always, nurses should respect the decisions of women who look to nurses for care. If nurses think they are not able to provide compassionate care because of personal convictions, they should inform a supervisor so appropriate care can be arranged.

Mandated Contraception

The availability of contraception that does not require taking a regular oral dose, such as using a hormone-releasing patch or having hormone injections or an intrauterine device (IUD), has led to speculation about whether certain women should be forced to use this method of birth control. Requiring contraception has been used as a condition of probation, allowing women accused of child abuse to avoid jail terms.

Some people think mandated contraception is a reasonable way to prevent additional births in the case of women who are considered unsuitable parents and to reduce government expenses for dependent children. A punitive approach to social problems does not provide long-term solutions. Requiring poor women to use contraception to limit the money spent on supporting them is legally and ethically questionable and does not address the obligations of the children's father. Such a practice interferes with a woman's constitutional rights to privacy, reproduction, refusal of medical treatment, and freedom from cruel and unusual punishment. In addition, medication may pose health risks to the woman. Surgical sterilization (tubal ligation) also carries risks and should be considered permanent. Access to free or low-cost information on family planning would be more appropriate and ethical.

Fetal Injury

If a mother's actions cause injury to her fetus, the question of whether she should be restrained or prosecuted has legal and ethical implications. In some instances, courts have issued jail sentences to women who have caused or who may cause injury to the fetus. This response punishes the woman and places her in a situation in which she cannot further harm the fetus. In other cases, women have been forced to undergo cesarean births against their will when physicians have testified such a procedure was necessary to prevent injury to the fetus.

The state has an interest in protecting children, and the U.S. Supreme Court has ruled a child has the right to begin life with a sound mind and body. Many state laws require evidence of prenatal drug exposure be reported. Women have been charged with negligence, involuntary manslaughter, delivery of drugs to a minor, and child endangerment.

However, forcing a woman to behave in a certain way because she is pregnant violates the principles of autonomy, self-determination of competent adults, bodily integrity, and personal freedom. Because of fear of prosecution, this practice could impede, not advance, health care during pregnancy.

The punitive approach to fetal injury also raises the question of how much control the government should have over a pregnant woman. Laws could be passed to mandate maternal HIV testing with no right to refuse, fetal testing, intrauterine surgery, or even the foods the woman eats during pregnancy. The decision with regard to just how much control should be allowed in the interests of fetal safety is difficult.

Fetal Therapy

Fetal therapy is becoming more common as techniques improve and knowledge grows. Although intrauterine blood transfusions are relatively standard practice in some areas, fetal surgery is still relatively uncommon.

The risks and benefits of surgery for major fetal anomalies should be considered in every case. Even when surgery is successful, the fetus may not survive, may have other serious problems, or may be born severely preterm. The mother may require weeks of bed rest and a cesarean birth. Yet despite the risks, successful fetal surgery may result in birth of an infant who could not otherwise have survived.

Parents need help to balance the potential risks to the mother and the best interests of the fetus. They might feel pressured to have surgery or other fetal treatment they do not understand. As with any situation involving informed consent, women need adequate information before making a decision. They should understand if procedures are still experimental, the known chances of a procedure's success, and if any alternative treatments are available and their chances of success.

Issues in Infertility

Infertility Treatment. Perinatal technology has found ways for some previously infertile couples to bear children (see Chapter 26). Many techniques are more successful, but ethical concerns include the high cost and overall low success of some infertility treatments. Because many of these costs are not insured, their use is limited to the affluent. Techniques may benefit only a small percentage of infertile couples. Despite treatment, many couples never give birth, regardless of the costs or invasiveness of therapy. Successful treatment may lead to multiple gestations and complications related to maternal age.

Other ethical concerns focus on the fate of unused embryos. Should they be frozen for later use by the woman or someone else or used in genetic research? What if the parents divorce or die? Who should make these decisions? In multiple pregnancies with more fetuses than can be expected to survive intact, reduction surgery may be used to destroy one or more fetuses for the benefit of those remaining. The ethical and long-term psychological implications of this procedure are also controversial.

Assisted reproductive techniques now allow postmenopausal women to become pregnant. What are the ethical implications of conceiving and giving birth to children whose mother is several decades older than their friends' mothers and is more likely to die when the children are relatively young? Should the age and health of the parents be a factor in determining whether this treatment is offered? Should a consideration be the risk these women face for complications that might result in unhealthy infants? Should average life expectancy enter the decision?

Surrogate Parenting. In surrogate parenting, a woman agrees to bear an infant for another woman. Conception may take place outside the body using ova and sperm from the couple who wish to become parents. These embryos are then implanted into the surrogate mother, or the surrogate mother may be inseminated artificially with sperm from the intended father. Donated embryos also may be implanted into a surrogate mother.

Cases in which the surrogate mother has wanted to keep the child have created controversy. No standard regulations govern these cases, which are decided individually. Ethical concerns involve who should be a surrogate mother, what her role should be after birth, and who should make these decisions. Screening of parents and surrogates is necessary to determine whether they are suited for their roles. Who should perform the screening? Should it be left to the private interests of those involved, or should government become involved?

An issue closely related to surrogate parenting is the use of donor gametes or unused embryos from another infertile couple. Will the use of donor gametes or embryos violate religious or moral beliefs of the parents? Does the child thus conceived have a right to know the identity of the biologic parents? What are the rights of the biologic parents?

Privacy Issues

Many people are concerned about the possible misuse of their health information. They may fear that health information in the wrong hands, whether that information is accurate or not, may cost them a job, promotion, loan, or something equally valuable. Privacy concerns and fear of health care or other insurance loss may cause a person to withhold genetic or other medical history information from a provider. Quality of genetic counseling may be impaired if family members refuse to release their medical records.

Government Regulations

The Health Insurance Portability and Accountability Act (HIPAA) of 1996 was designed to reduce fraud in the insurance industry and make it easier for people to remain insured if they move from one job to another. Within HIPAA's provisions was the mandate for Congress to pass a law to protect the privacy of personal medical information by August 1999. Congress failed to do so, and the Secretary of the DHHS proposed interim regulations in October 1999 to protect personal medical privacy as required by HIPAA. The DHHS regulations provide consumers with significant new power over their records, including the right to see and correct their records, the application of civil and criminal penalties for violations of privacy standards, and protection against deliberate or inadvertent misuse or disclosure. See www.hhs.gov for additional information.

Electronic Communications. A person's health data are generally maintained in various computerized formats. Although this allows nearly instantaneous exchange of data among providers, it also may carry the potential for greater violation of privacy than data maintained on paper. Terminals may be placed in hallways or patient rooms to facilitate quick entry and retrieval of information for staff. The nurse should remember this information also may be easily accessed by a computer-savvy person despite the use of passcodes and other security measures. Nurses should take care to avoid violating patient confidentiality by promptly logging off terminals when finished and following facility protocols for protection of security pass codes.

Social media sites allow nurses to exchange information and nursing care tips that can improve practice. These forums also have the potential to allow lapses of patient or institutional confidentiality because their communications cannot be considered private. When participating in discussion lists or using e-mail, nurses should respect the confidentiality of patients, colleagues, and institutions. Institutional documents such as chart forms, policies, and procedures should not be shared without the facility's approval. A personal message should not be forwarded without the original sender's permission. The ANA and National Council for State Boards of Nursing provide resources for nursing regarding appropriate use of social media (www.nursingworld.org and www.ncsbn.org).

> ### ❓ KNOWLEDGE CHECK
>
> 22. What dangers are involved in punitive approaches to ethical and social problems?
> 23. What problems are involved in the use of advanced reproductive techniques?
> 24. Describe precautions the nurse should take to ensure the privacy of a person's medical records.

LEGAL ISSUES

The legal foundation for the practice of nursing provides safeguards for patients and sets standards by which nurses can be evaluated. Nurses need to understand how the law applies specifically to them. When nurses do not meet the standards expected, they may be held legally accountable.

Safeguards for Health Care

Three categories of safeguards determine the law's view of nursing practice: (1) nurse practice acts, (2) standards of care set by professional organizations, and (3) rules and policies set by the institution employing the nurse.

Nurse Practice Acts

The **nurse practice act** of each state determines the scope of practice of registered nurses in that state (ANA, 2015b). Nurse practice acts define what the nurse is allowed to do when caring for patients. The acts also specify what the nurse is expected to do when providing care. Some parts of the law may be very specific. Others are stated broadly to allow flexible interpretation of the role of nurses. Nurse practice acts vary across states, and nurses should understand these laws wherever they practice. Nurses should have a copy of the nurse practice act for their state and refer to it for questions about their scope of practice. Most state nurse practice acts are available on the Internet. The website of the National Council of State Boards of Nursing (NCSBN) (www.ncsbn.org) has information on nurse practice acts for all states, all territories, and the District of Columbia, as well as other information related to licensing and practice.

Laws relating to nursing practice also delineate methods, called **standard procedures** or *protocols*, by which nurses may assume certain duties commonly considered part of medical practice. The procedures are written by committees of nurses, physicians, and administrators. They specify the nursing qualifications required for practicing the procedures, define the appropriate situations, and state the education required. Standard procedures allow the role of the nurse to change to meet the needs of the community and expanding knowledge.

Standards of Care

Court decisions have generally held that nurses should practice according to established standards and health agency policies in addition to nurse practice acts. Standards of care are set by professional associations and describe the level of care that can be expected from practitioners. For example, perinatal nurses are held to the national standards published by AWHONN, which are based on research and the agreement of experts. AWHONN also publishes practice resources, position statements, and other guidelines for nurses. Nurses should be familiar with the latest standards of care that cover their own practices.

Agency Policies

Each health care agency sets specific policies, procedures, and protocols governing nursing care. Nurses are frequently involved in writing and revising nursing policies and procedures. Policies and procedures increase staff adherence to professional, legal, and regulatory standards, statutes, and accreditation requirements, decrease variation in practice, and provide a reference for staff, decreasing dependence on memory, which can be a major source of human errors or oversights (Irving, 2014). In the event of a malpractice claim, the applicable policy, procedure, or protocol is likely to be used as evidence. The case of the professionals is strengthened if all agency policies are followed properly. These policies should be revised and updated regularly.

Malpractice: Limiting Loss

Negligence is the failure to perform as a reasonable, prudent person of similar background would act in a similar situation. Negligence may consist of doing something that should not be done or failing to do something that should be done.

Malpractice is negligence by professionals such as nurses and physicians in the performance of their duties. Nurses may be accused of malpractice if they do not perform according to established standards of care and in the manner of a reasonable, prudent nurse with similar education and experience in a similar situation. Four elements must be present to prove negligence: duty, breach of duty, damage, and proximate cause.

CRITICAL TO REMEMBER
Elements of Negligence

Duty—The nurse must have a duty to act or give care to the patient. It must be part of the nurse's responsibility.
Breach of duty—A violation of that duty must occur. The nurse fails to conform to established standards in performing that duty.
Damage—An actual injury or harm to the patient as a result of the nurse's breach of duty must occur.
Proximate cause—The nurse's breach of duty must be proved to be the cause of harm to the patient.

Malpractice claims continue to be a major cost in health care. As a result of awards from such claims, the cost of malpractice insurance has risen for all health care workers. More health care workers practice defensively and accumulate evidence that their actions are in the patient's best interests.

Many reasons exist for perinatal malpractice claims. Complications are usually unexpected because parents view pregnancy and birth as normal. The birth of a child with a problem is a tragic shock, and parents may look for someone to blame. Although very small preterm infants may survive, some have long-term disabilities and require expensive care. Statutes of limitations vary across states, but plaintiffs often have more than 20 years to file lawsuits involving a newborn. Therefore the period during which a malpractice suit may be filed is longer.

Health care agencies and individual nurses should work together to prevent malpractice claims. Nurses are responsible and accountable for their own actions. Therefore they should be aware of the limits of their knowledge and scope of practice, and they should practice within those limits.

Prevention of claims is sometimes referred to as *risk management* or *quality assurance*. Although prevention of all malpractice claims is impossible, nurses can prevent malpractice judgments against themselves by following guidelines for informed consent, refusal of care, and documentation; acting as a patient advocate; and maintaining their levels of expertise.

Informed Consent

When patients receive adequate information, they are less likely to file malpractice suits. Informed consent is an ethical concept that has been enacted into law. Patients have the right to decide whether to accept or reject treatment options as part of their right to function autonomously. To make wise decisions, they need full information about treatments offered.

CRITICAL TO REMEMBER
Requirements of Informed Consent

Patient's competence to consent
Full disclosure of information needed
Patient's understanding of information
Patient's voluntary consent

Competence. Certain requirements should be met before consent is considered informed. First, the patient should be competent, or able to think through a situation and make rational decisions. Infants, children, and patients who are comatose or severely cognitively impaired are incapable of making such decisions. A patient who has received drugs that impair the ability to think is temporarily incompetent. In these cases, another person is appointed to make decisions for the patient.

In most states, the age of majority (the age at which a person can give consent to medical treatment) is 18 years. However, in some states, younger adolescents can consent independently to some treatments, such as those for mental illness, abortions, contraceptives, drug abuse, and STDs. An **emancipated minor** is younger than the age of majority, usually 18 years, and considered medically competent to make some medical decisions independent of a parent or guardian. Pregnant adolescents may be considered emancipated minors in some states. Nurses should be familiar with laws governing age of consent in their practice area.

Another exception to the usual requirement of informed consent is in emergency circumstances; in such situations, consent is considered implied. Treatment may proceed if there is no evidence the patient does not want the treatment. *Emergency* may be specifically defined by state law and is usually restricted to unforeseen conditions that, if uncorrected, would result in severe disability or death. Emergency consent applies only for the emergency condition and does not extend to any other nonemergency problem that coexists with the emergency condition.

Patient information about advance directives such as a living will, durable power of attorney for health care, and an alternative decision maker for the patient should be assessed on admission to the health care facility. Often, hospitals are required to inform patients about advance directives during the nursing admission assessment. The person who has not made advance directives should be offered the opportunity to make these choices.

Full Disclosure. The second requirement is full disclosure of information, including details of what the treatment entails, the expected results, and the meaning of those results. The risks, side effects, benefits, and other treatment options should be explained to patients. The person also should be informed about the consequences if no treatment is chosen.

Understanding of Information. The third requirement is that the person should comprehend information about proposed treatment. Health care professionals should explain the facts in terms the person can understand. If a patient does not speak English, an interpreter is required. A patient with hearing impairment should have a sign-language interpreter of the appropriate level to sign all explanations before consent is given. Interpreters should not be family or friends because these people may interpret selectively rather than objectively. Additionally, patient confidentiality is compromised when nonprofessional interpreters are used for sensitive information. Nurses should be advocates for the patient when they find the patient does not fully understand or has questions about a treatment. If it is a minor point, the

nurse may be able to explain it. Otherwise, the nurse should inform the physician of the need for clarification.

Voluntary Consent. The fourth requirement is that patients should be allowed to make choices voluntarily without undue influence or coercion from others. Although others may give information, the patient alone makes the decision. Patients should not feel pressured to choose in a certain way, and they should not think their future care depends on their decision.

Refusal of Care. Occasionally, some persons decline treatment offered by health care workers. Patients refuse treatment when they think the benefits of treatment are insufficient to balance the burdens of the treatment or their quality of life after treatment. Patients have the right to refuse care, and they can withdraw agreement to treatment at any time. When a person makes this decision, a number of steps should be taken (AAP & ACOG, 2012).

If the provider is unaware of the patient's decision, the nurse should notify that provider and document the notification accordingly. There should be verification that the patient understands the treatment and consequences of refusal. Opinions by other providers may be offered to the patient. A description of the treatment refused should be documented in the patient's chart, as well as the explanations given to the patient and her refusal.

Every effort should be made to obtain a written refusal from the patient indicating she has been informed of the risks and benefits of the treatment and the refusal of the treatment. The nurse should refer to the facility's procedure for patient refusal of treatment for other requirements. If no ethical dilemma exists, the patient's decision stands.

In cases of an ethical dilemma, a referral may be made to the hospital ethics committee. In rare situations, the physician may seek a court ruling to force treatment. For example, when a woman refuses a cesarean birth, her decision may gravely harm the fetus. This situation is the only legal instance in which a person is forced to undergo surgery for the health of another. However, court action is avoided, if possible, because it places the woman and her caregiver in adversarial positions. In addition, it invades the woman's privacy and interferes with her autonomy and right to informed consent. If legally mandated surgery were to become widespread and cause women to avoid health care during pregnancy, the resulting harm would affect more women and infants than those who would be protected by the surgery.

Coercion is illegal and unethical in obtaining consent. Even though the nurse may strongly think a woman should receive the treatment, she should not feel forced to submit to unwanted procedures. Nurses should not allow personal feelings to to adversely affect the quality of their care. People have the right to good nursing care, regardless of their decisions to accept or reject treatment.

Documentation

Nurses are expected to meet the **standard of care**, or the level of care expected of a professional as determined by laws, professional organizations, and health care agencies. Documentation is essential for collaborative patient care and is also the best evidence that a standard of care has been maintained. It includes nurses' notes, fetal monitoring strips, electronic data, flow sheets, care paths, consent forms, and any other data recorded on paper, recorded electronically, or both. In many instances, notations in hospital records are the only proof care has been given. When documentation is not present, juries may assume that care was not given.

Documentation should demonstrate thorough initial and ongoing assessments, identification of problems, interventions used, and evaluation of their effectiveness, as well as information reported to other members of the health care team.

Documenting Discharge Teaching. Discharge teaching is important to ensure patients know how to take care of themselves and their infants after they leave the facility. To prevent or defend against lawsuits, nurses should document the teaching they perform and the patient's understanding of that teaching. Various documentation forms verify teaching and the degree of understanding about important topics. The nurse also should note the need for reinforcement and the method of providing reinforcement.

Documenting Incidents. Another form of documentation used in risk management is the incident report, sometimes called a *quality assurance report* or *variance report*. The nurse completes a report when something occurs that might result in legal action—for example, injury to a patient, visitor, or staff member. The report alerts the agency's legal department that a problem may exist. It also identifies situations that might endanger patients in the future. Incident reports are not a part of the patient's chart and should not be referred to on the chart. When an incident occurs, documentation on the chart should include the same type of factual information about the patient's condition that would be recorded in any other situation.

Late entries in documentation may be necessary after an emergency in which the nurse should provide patient care quickly. Late entries should be accurate and objective rather than defensive, especially if the outcome was negative in the entry (Simpson, 2014).

The Nurse as Patient Advocate

Nurses are ethically and legally bound to act as the patient's advocate. When nurses think the patient's best interests are not being served, they are obligated to seek help from appropriate sources. This usually involves relaying the problem through the facility's chain of command. The nurse consults a supervisor and the patient's physician. If the results are not satisfactory, the nurse continues through administrative channels to the director of nurses, hospital administrator, and chief of the medical staff, if necessary. All nurses should know the chain-of-command process for their workplaces.

Nurses should document their efforts to seek help for patients. For example, when postpartum patients are experiencing excessive bleeding, nurses document the methods used to control the bleeding. They also document each time they call the physician, the information given to the physician, and the response received. When nurses cannot contact the physician or do not receive adequate instructions, they should document their efforts to seek instruction from others such as the supervisor. Nurses should continue their efforts until the patient receives the care needed.

Maintaining Expertise

The nurse also can reduce malpractice liability by maintaining expertise. To ensure nurses maintain their expertise in provision of safe care, states require proof of continuing education for renewal of nursing licenses. Nursing knowledge grows and changes rapidly, and all nurses should keep current. New information from classes, conferences, and professional publications can help nurses perform as would a reasonably prudent peer. Nurses should analyze research articles to determine whether changes in patient care are indicated by the research evidence.

Employers often provide continuing education classes for their nurses through conferences, satellite television systems, computer networks, and other means. Membership in professional organizations such as state branches of the ANA or in specialty organizations such as AWHONN gives nurses access to new information through publications, nursing conferences, and other educational offerings. Continuing nursing education is also widely available on the Internet.

Expertise is a concern when nurses are "floated," or required to work with patients whose needs differ from those of the nurses' usual patients. A nurse may be floated from one maternal-newborn setting to another or to a nonmaternity setting. In these situations, nurses need cross-training, which includes orientation and education to perform care safely in new areas. The employer should provide appropriate cross-training for nurses who float. Nurses who work outside their usual area of expertise should assess their own skills and avoid performing tasks or taking responsibilities in areas until they have been educated to be competent in those areas.

> ### ❓ KNOWLEDGE CHECK
>
> 25. How do state boards of nursing safeguard patients?
> 26. How do standards of care and agency policies influence judgments about malpractice?
> 27. How can standards of care be used to help defend malpractice claims against nurses?

COST CONTAINMENT AND DOWNSIZING

Measures to lower health care costs continue to directly and indirectly affect nurses' work. Two measures of special concern are the use of unlicensed assistive personnel and brief length of stay (LOS) for patients.

Delegation to Unlicensed Assistive Personnel

Delegation of care to an unlicensed person may allow the nurse to focus on greater needs within their group of patients. Orientation and education of unlicensed assistive personnel (UAP) should be completed and is competency based in both initial training and ongoing evaluations. UAP should be identified to the patient as a nonlicensed person.

Nurses should be aware that they remain legally responsible for patient assessments and make the critical judgments necessary to ensure patient safety when delegating tasks to UAP. Nurses should know the capabilities of each unlicensed person who is caring for patients and supervise them sufficiently to ensure competence. The ANA's *Principles for Delegation by Registered Nurses to Unlicensed Assistive Personnel (UAP), (ANA, 2012)* and AWHONN'S *The Role of Unlicensed Assistive Personnel (Nursing Assistive Personnel) in the Care of* Women and Newborns (2016) help nurses understand their roles in working with UAP.

Early Discharge

Regardless of the patient's diagnosis, the time from admission to discharge is as short as possible to keep costs in check and to reduce chances for a hospital-acquired infection. Because birth is considered a normal event that does not require a long LOS, care of new mothers and infants requires teaching from the earliest encounters. In 1996, federal legislation was passed to require insurance companies allow the option of a 48-hour hospital LOS after vaginal birth and a 4-day LOS after cesarean birth. Discharge may be earlier, if deemed appropriate, after discussion between the physician or midwife and the patient. Although it is not required by federal law, many states mandate prompt follow-up for early discharge in the patient's home, an office, or a clinic. Some third-party payers voluntarily cover home visits for mothers who opt for earlier discharge because of the lower total cost for the home visit plus a short hospital LOS.

Concerns about Early Discharge

Although advantages of early discharge include prompt ambulation and reduced risk for hospital-acquired infection, concerns exist for new mothers and their families. Women may be exhausted from a long labor or complicated birth and unable to absorb all the information nurses attempt to teach before discharge. Once home, many new mothers also must care for other children. Nurses may detect early signs of maternal or infant complications that may not be evident to parents while in the health care facility. Parents at home may not recognize the development of a serious maternal or neonatal infection or jaundice, and care may be delayed until the illness has become severe. The ethical and legal implications of sending a mother home before she is ready to adequately care for herself and her newborn are very real concerns for nurses who should balance cost constraints with patient needs.

Similar problems may occur in the older woman who must care for herself after an inpatient or outpatient procedure.

Sedating drugs given for a procedure may have prolonged effects, especially on older adults. Although the older woman may appear to understand all instructions and sign papers indicating her understanding, she may not remember what was taught after returning home. It is ideal for a trusted friend or family member to be taught with the patient and for printed or online instructions in simple language to be provided. Follow-up phone calls or visits are often scheduled to reevaluate the healing process after a procedure.

Methods to Deal with Short Lengths of Stay

Teaching begins at admission. Self-care during pregnancy or in women's health begins at first encounter. More teaching should occur during pregnancy when the mother's physical needs do not interfere with her ability to comprehend the new knowledge. In the facility, careful documentation and notification of the primary care provider are essential so patients are not discharged inappropriately if abnormal findings develop. Self-care and infant-care discharge instructions should be explained to the woman and her support person. A printed form, signed by both the patient and the nurse, is placed in the chart, with a copy given to the woman for later reference in self-care and care of the baby. Other methods for follow-up such as home visits, phone calls, and return visits to the birth facility for nursing assessments after discharge may identify complications early, when they can be addressed most effectively.

Nursing follow-up by phone calls is the least expensive of postdischarge methods. However, the nurse does not see or physically examine the patient or her infant, and specific protocols and procedures should be in place for nursing actions that should be taken if a potential problem is identified during the call. Documentation should be kept for follow-up phone calls. Any instructions given to the patient (recommended actions if problems arise, if a minor problem does not improve, or if a problem worsens) during the phone call should be documented.

? KNOWLEDGE CHECK

28. What concerns do nurses have about unlicensed assistive personnel?
29. Why is early discharge a concern for nurses?
30. What are the important points in follow-up phone call?

▍ SUMMARY CONCEPTS

- Families vary in their structures and patterns of functioning.
- Functional families are characterized by open communication, flexibility in role assignments, and adult agreement on basic principles of parenting, resiliency, and adaptability.
- Culture is the sum of beliefs and values that are learned, shared, and transmitted from generation to generation in a specific group of people.
- Dominant Western cultural values may influence the thinking and action of nurses in the United States but may not be shared by culturally diverse childbearing women and their families.

- Professional nurses are expected to provide culturally competent care, which requires an awareness of, sensitivity to, and respect for the diversity of patients served.
- Health care disparity is a major social issue that underlies adequacy of health care resources, access to prenatal care, government programs to increase health care to indigent women and children, and health care rationing.
- Multiple factors are associated with intimate partner violence, which is deliberate, severe, and generally repeated in a predictable cycle that often causes severe physical harm (or death) to the woman.
- Perinatal nurses should screen for intimate partner violence and provide appropriate education and resources.

- Human trafficking, also called trafficking of persons, is the recruitment and movement of individuals for the purpose of exploitation. Sex and labor trafficking are the most common forms.
- Women and children of childbearing age make up the majority of reported cases of human trafficking, with the average age of entry into sex trafficking reported to be between 12 to 14 years of age.
- Ethical dilemmas are a difficult area of practice and are best solved by applying common ethical methods and principles and the steps of the nursing process.
- When ethical principles of beneficence, nonmaleficence, autonomy, and justice result in ethical dilemmas, the nursing process may be used to guide ethical decision making.
- Punitive approaches to ethical and social problems may prevent women from seeking adequate prenatal care.
- Nurses are expected to perform in accordance with nurse practice acts, standards of care, and agency policies.
- Nurses can help defend malpractice claims by following guidelines for informed consent, refusal of care, and documentation and by maintaining their levels of expertise.
- Complete and timely documentation is the best evidence that the standard of care received by a patient was met.
- Continuing pressures on optimal nursing practice include use of unlicensed assistive personnel and short lengths of stay.

REFERENCES & READINGS

Alfaro-LeFevre, R. (2017). *Critical thinking, clinical reasoning and clinical judgment: A practical approach* (6th ed.) (pp. 121–142). Philadelphia, PA: Elsevier.

American Academy of Pediatrics (AAP) & American College of Obstetricians and Gynecologists (ACOG). (2012). *Guidelines for perinatal care* (7th ed.). Elk Grove Village, IL: Author.

American Cancer Society. (2013). *Cancer facts & figures for African Americans 2013-2014.* Atlanta, GA: Author. Retrieved from https://old.cancer.org/acs/groups/content/@epidemiologysurveilance/documents/document/acspc-036921.pdf.

American College of Obstetricians and Gynecologists (ACOG). (2013). *Reproductive and sexual coercion* (ACOG Committee Opinion Number 554). Washington, DC: Author.

American Nurses Association. (2012). *Principles for delegation by registered nurses to unlicensed assistive personnel* (UAP). Silver Spring, MD: Author.

American Nurses Association. (2015a). *Code of ethics for nurses with interpretive statements.* Silver Spring, MD: Author.

American Nurses Association. (2015b). *Nursing scope and standards of practice* (3rd ed.). Silver Spring, MD: Author.

Association of Women's Health, Obstetric & Neonatal Nurses (AWHONN). (2009). *Standards for professional nursing practice in the care of women and newborns* (7th ed.). Washington, DC: Author.

Association of Women's Health, Obstetric and Neonatal Nurses (AWHONN). (2016). Position statement: The role of unlicensed assistive personnel (nursing assistive personnel) in the care of women and newborns. *Journal of Obstetric and Gynecologic & Neonatal Nursing, 45*(1), 137–139.

Breiding, M. J., Smith, S. G., Basile, K. C., Walters, M. L., Chen, J., & Merrick, M. T. (2014). Prevalence and characteristics of sexual violence, stalking, and intimate partner violence victimization: National intimate partner and sexual violence survey, United States, 2011. *Morbidity and Mortality Weekly Report (MMWR) Surveillance Summaries, 63*(SS08), 1–18. Retrieved from www.cdc.gov/mmwr/preview/mmwrhtml/ss6308a1.htm?s_cid=ss6308a1_e.

Boggs, K. U. (2016). Clinical judgment and ethical decision making. In E. C. Arnold, & K. U. Boggs (Eds.), *Interpersonal relationships: Professional communication skills for nurses* (7th ed.) (pp. 40–56). Philadelphia, PA: Saunders.

Callister, L. C. (1995). Cultural meanings of childbirth. *Journal of Obstetric, Gynecologic, & Neonatal Nursing, 24*(4), 327–334.

Callister, L. C. (2014). Integrating cultural beliefs and practices when caring for childbearing women and families. In K. R. Simpson & P. A. Creehan (Eds.), *AWHONN perinatal nursing* (4th ed.) (pp. 41–64). Philadelphia, PA: Lippincott Williams & Wilkins.

Callister, L. C. (2016a). *Developing and assessing culturally appropriate health education for childbearing women.* White Plains, NY: March of Dimes Foundation.

Callister, L. C. (2016b). What do the childbearing women in your clinical practice look like? *Nursing and Women's Health, 20*(1), 9–11.

Centers for Disease Control and Prevention (CDC). (2016a). *National Center for Health Statistics: Births and Natality.* Retrieved from www.cdc.gov.

Center for Disease Control and Prevention (CDC). (2016b). *Strategies for reducing health disparities.* Retrieved from www.cdc.gov/minorityhealth/strategies2016/index.html.

Centers for Disease Control (CDC). (2016c). *Intimate partner violence: Risk and protective factors.* Retrieved from www.cdc.gov/violenceprevention/intimatepartnerviolence/riskprotectivefactors.html.

Center for Disease Control and Prevention (CDC). (2017a). *Pregnancy mortality surveillance system.* Retrieved from www.cdc.gov/reproductivehealth/maternalinfanthealth/pmss.html.

Centers for Disease Control and Prevention (CDC). (2017b). *2015 Sexually Transmitted Disease Surveillance: STDs in racial and ethnic minorities.* Retrieved from www.cdc.gov/std/stats15/minorities.htm.

Center for Reproductive Rights. (2014). *Reproductive injustice: Racial and gender discrimination in U.S. health care.* Retrieved from www.reproductiverights.org.

Child Trends DataBank. (2015). *Late or no prenatal care.* Retrieved from www.childtrends.org/?late-or-no-prenatal-care.

Child Trends DataBank. (2016). *Fertility and birth rates.* Retrieved from www.childtrends.org/?indicators=fertility-and-birth-rates.

Cunningham, F. G., Leveno, K. J., Bloom, S. L., Spong, C. Y., Dashe, J. S., Hoffman, B. L., . . . Sheffield, J. S. (2014). *Williams obstetrics* (24th ed.) (pp. 940–960). New York: McGraw-Hill.

Dahlem, C. H. Y., Villarruel, A. M., & Ronis, D. L. (2014). African American women and prenatal care: Perceptions of patient-provider interaction. *Western Journal of Nursing Research, 37*(2), 217–235.

Dehlendorf, C., Park, S. Y., Emeremni, C. A., Comer, D., Vincett, K., & Borrero, S. (2014). Racial/ethnic disparities in contraceptive use. *American Journal of Obstetrics and Gynecology, 10*(6), e1–e9.

de Chesnay, M. (2013). *Sex trafficking: A clinical guide for nurses.* New York: Springer.

de Oliveira Fonseca-Machado, M., Aives, L. C., Scotini Freitas, P., dos Santos Monteiro, J. C., & Gomes-Sponholz, F. (2014). Mental health of women who suffer intimate partner violence during pregnancy. *Investigacion & Educacion En Enfermeria, 32*(2), 291–305.

Dillard, D. M., & Olrun-Volkheimer, J. (2014). Providing culturally sensitive care for pregnant Alaska Native women and families. *International Journal of Childbirth Education, 29*(1), 62–66.

Douglas, M. K., Rosenkoetter, M., Pacquiao, D., Callister, L. C., Hattar-Pollara, M., Lauderdale, J., . . . Purnell, L. (2014). Guidelines for implementing culturally competent care. *Journal of Transcultural Nursing, 25*(2), 109–121.

Elter, P. T., Kennedy, H. P., Chesia, C. A., & Yimyam, S. (2016). Spiritual healing practices among rural postpartum Thai women. *Journal of Transcultural Nursing, 27*(3), 249–255, 2015.

Fitzgerald, E. M., Cronin, S. N., & Boccella, S. H. (2015). Anguish, yearning and identity: Toward a better understanding of the pregnant Hispanic woman's prenatal care experience. *Journal of Transcultural Nursing, 27*(5), 464–470.

Forum on Child and Family Statistics. (2016). *America's children: Key national indicators of well being 2016.* Retrieved from www.childstats.gov.

Goyal, D. (2016). Perinatal practices and traditions among Asian Indian women. *American Journal of Maternal/Child Nursing, 41*(2), 90–96.

International Labor Organization (ILO). (2005). *A global alliance against forced labour.* Geneva: Author.

Irving, A. V. (2014). *Policies and procedures for healthcare organizations: A risk management perspective. Patient Safety & Quality Healthcare.* Retrieved from www.psqh.com/analysis/policies-and-procedures-for-healthcare-organizations-a-risk-management-perspective/#sthash.OC3UaYpv.dpuf.

Jones, S. M. (2014). Making me feel comfortable: Developing trust in the nurse for Mexican Americans. *Western Journal of Nursing Research, 37*(11), 1423–1440.

Kids Count. (2016). *Total births by race.* Retrieved from www.datacenter.kidscount.org.

Koh, H. K., Gracia, J. N., & Alvarez, M. E. (2014). Culturally and linguistically appropriate service: Advancing with class. *New England Journal of Medicine, 371*(3), 198–201.

Leininger, M. (1978). *Transcultural nursing: Concepts, theories, practice.* New York: Wiley.

Little, C. M. (2015). Caring for women who have experienced female genital cutting. *American Journal of Maternal/Child Nursing, 40*(5), 291–297.

Lor, M., Crooks, N., & Tluczek, A. (2016). A proposed model of person-, family-, and culture-centered nursing care. *Nursing Outlook, 64*(4), 352–366.

Macintosh, J., & Callister, L. C. (2015). Discovering self: Childbearing adolescents' maternal identity. *American Journal of Maternal/Child Nursing, 40*(5), 245–248.

March of Dimes Birth Defects Foundation. (2014). *Low birthweight.* Retrieved from www.marchofdimes.com.

Mathews, T. J., MacDorman, M. F., & Thoma, M. E. (2015). Infant mortality statistics from the 2013 period linked birth/infant death data set. *National Vital Statistics Reports, 64*(9), 5.

Mattson, S. (2015). Ethnocultural considerations in the childbearing period. In S. Mattson, & J. E. Smith (Eds.), *AWHONN core curriculum for maternal-newborn nurses* (5th ed.). St. Louis, MO: Saunders.

Miller, C. L. (2013). Child sex trafficking in the emergency department: Opportunities and challenges. *Journal of Emergency Nursing, 39*(5), 477–478.

Miller, C. L., Duke, G., & Northam, S. (2016). Child sex trafficking recognition, intervention and referral: An educational framework for the development of health care provider education programs. *Journal of Human Trafficking.* http://dx.doi.org/10.1080/223322705.2015.1133990.

Missal, B., Clark, C., & Kovaleva, M. (2016). Somali immigrant new mothers' childbirth experiences in Minnesota. *Journal of Transcultural Nursing, 27*(4), 359–367.

National Academies of Science, Engineering and Medicine. (2017). *Communities in action: Pathways to health equity.* Washington, DC: Author.

National Alliance to End Homelessness. (2017). *Snapshot of homelessness.* Washington, DC: Author. Retrieved from www.endhomelessness.org/pages/snapshot_of_homelessness.

National Center for Complementary and Alternative Medicine (NCCAM). (n.d.). *The use of complementary and alternative medicine in the United States.* Retrieved from http://nccam.nih.gov.

National Center for Health Statistics. (2016a). *Births: Final data for 2014.* Retrieved from www.cdc.gov.nchs.

National Center for Health Statistics. (2016b). *Health expenditures.* Retrieved from www.cdc.gov/nchs/fastats/health-expenditures.htm.

National Center for Health Statistics. (2017). *Health insurance coverage: Early release of estimates from the National Health Interview Survey, January–September 2016.* Retrieved from www.cdc.gov/nchs/data/nhis/earlyrelease/insur201702.pdf.

Polan, E. U., & Taylor, D. R. (2015). *Journey across the lifespan: Human development and health promotion* (5th ed.). Philadelphia: 2015, F.A. Davis.

Prinds, C., Hvidtjørn, N. C., Mogensen, D., Skytthe, A., & Hvidt, N. C. (2014). Making existential meaning in the transition to motherhood. *Midwifery, 30*(6), 733–741.

Raglan, G. B., Lannon, S. M., Jones, K. M., & Schulkin. (2016). Racial and ethnic disparities in preterm birth among American Indian and Alaska Native women. *Maternal and Child Health Journal, 20*(1), 16–24.

Reed, S., Callister, L. C., & Corbett, C. (2017, in press). Honoring motherhood: The meaning of childbirth to Tongan women. *American Journal of Maternal/Child Nursing.*

Seo, J. Y., Kim, W., & Dickerson, S. S. M. (2014). Korean immigrant women's lived experience of childbirth in the United States. *Journal of Obstetric, Gynecologic, & Neonatal Nursing, 43,* 305–317.

Shahawy, S., Deshpande, N. A., & Nour, N. (2015). Cross-cultural obstetric and gynecologic care of Muslim patients. *Obstetrics and Gynecology, 126*(5), 969–973.

Simpson, K. R. (2014). Perinatal patient safety and professional liability issues. In K. R. Simpson, & P. A. Creehan (Eds.), *AWHONN perinatal nursing* (3rd ed.) (pp. 1–28). Philadelphia: Lippincott.

Spector, R. E. (2017). *Cultural diversity in health and illness* (9th ed.). Upper Saddle River, NJ: Pearson Prentice Hall.

Spiwak, R., Afifi, T. O., Halli, S., Garcia-Moreno, C., & Sareen, J. (2013). The relationship between physical intimate partner violence and sexually transmitted infection among women in India and the United States. *Journal of Interpersonal Violence, 28*(13), 2770–2791.

United Nations. (2000). *Optional protocol to prevent, suppress and punish trafficking in persons, especially women and children, supplementing the United Nations Convention Against Transnational Organized Crime, G.A. Res. 55/25 (2000).* Geneva: United Nations.

United States Census Bureau. (2016a). *Quick facts (United States) 2016.* Retrieved from www.census.gov/quickfacts/table/PST045215/00.

United States Census Bureau. (2016b). Income, poverty and health insurance coverage in the United States: 2015. Release Number: CB16–158. Retrieved from www.census.gov.

Vu, H., Milkie, A. A., Tala, R., & Aasim, I. (2016). Predictors of delayed healthcare seeking among American Muslim women. *Journal of Women's Health, 25*(6), 586–593.

Wathen, C. N., & MacMillan, H. L. (2013). Children's exposure to intimate partner violence: Impacts and interventions. *Paediatrics and Child Health, 18*(8), 419–422.

Reproductive Anatomy and Physiology

Jennifer H. Rodriguez

An understanding of the structure and function of the reproductive organs is necessary for the effective nursing care of women during and after their reproductive years and for couples who require family planning or infertility care. This chapter reviews basic prenatal development, sexual maturation, and the structure and function of the female and male reproductive systems. Because of its emphasis in this book, the female reproductive system is discussed most extensively.

SEXUAL DEVELOPMENT

Sexual development begins at conception when the **genetic sex** is determined by the union of an ovum and a sperm. During childhood, the sex organs are inactive and then become active during puberty.

Prenatal Development

The mother's ovum carries a single X chromosome. Each of the father's spermatozoa carries either an X chromosome or a Y chromosome. If an X-bearing spermatozoon fertilizes the ovum, the offspring's genetic sex is female. If a Y-bearing spermatozoon fertilizes the ovum, a genetic male offspring results.

Although genetic sex is determined at conception, the reproductive systems of males and females are similar, or sexually undifferentiated, for the first 6 weeks of prenatal life. During the seventh week, differences between males and females appear in the internal structures. The external genitalia continue to look similar until the ninth week, when these outer structures begin to change. Differentiation of the external sexual organs is complete at approximately 12 weeks of gestational age.

During fetal life, both ovaries and testes secrete their primary hormones, which are estrogen and testosterone, respectively. Testosterone causes development of male sex organs and external genitalia, and its absence results in development of female sex characteristics. Although estrogen is secreted by the fetal ovary, the hormone is not required to initiate development of female sex structures.

Childhood

The sex glands of girls and boys are inactive during infancy and childhood. At sexual maturity the hypothalamus stimulates the anterior pituitary gland to produce hormones that in turn stimulate sex hormone production by the **gonads**, the reproductive (sex) glands.

Sexual Maturation

Puberty refers to the time during which the reproductive organs become fully functional. It is not a single event but a series of changes occurring over several years during late childhood and early adolescence. Primary sex characteristics relate to the maturation of the organs directly responsible for reproduction. Examples of primary sex characteristics are maturation of ova in the ovaries and production of sperm in the testes. **Secondary sex characteristics** are changes in other systems that differentiate females and males but do not directly relate to reproduction. Examples of secondary sex characteristics in the female include breast development; selective distribution of fat in breasts, buttocks, and thighs; pubic and axillary hair; and higher pitched voice. Secondary sex characteristics in the male include increased muscle mass, growth of hair on the face and body as well as pubic and axillary hair, and development of a deeper voice.

Initiation of Sexual Maturation

Changes of puberty occur in an orderly sequence in the **somatic cells** (body cells other than the gametes) of both genders. Not all factors involved in the initiation of sexual maturation are known. Secretions of the hypothalamus, anterior pituitary, and gonads all play a role. The hypothalamus can secrete gonadotropin-releasing hormone (GnRH) to initiate puberty during infancy and early childhood, but it does not do so in significant amounts until late childhood. Production of even tiny quantities of sex hormones by the young child's ovaries or testes inhibits secretions of the hypothalamus, preventing premature onset of puberty. Maturation of another brain area, as yet unknown, probably triggers the hypothalamus to initiate puberty (Hall, 2016).

The maturing child's hypothalamus gradually increases production of GnRH beginning at age 9 to 12 years (Blackburn, 2013; Hall, 2016). The level of GnRH increases slowly until it reaches a level adequate to stimulate the anterior pituitary to increase its production of follicle-stimulating hormone (FSH) and luteinizing hormone (LH). The ovaries and testes increase production of sex hormones and begin maturing **gametes** (reproductive cells, an ovum in females and a sperm in males) in response to higher levels of FSH and LH. Sex hormones also induce development of secondary sex characteristics. Table 3.1 lists the major hormones that play a role in reproduction.

Puberty varies among individuals; these variances include the age puberty begins and the time required to complete these changes. Hormonal changes of puberty begin approximately 6 months to 1 year earlier in girls than in boys. The growth spurt associated with puberty also begins earlier for girls than for boys. The obvious changes of puberty in girls, such as breast development and height increase, begin an average of 2 years before changes in boys. Changes of puberty occur in an orderly sequence in both genders. Increases in height and weight are dramatic during puberty but slow after puberty until mature heights and weights are attained. Research has identified a link between early onset of puberty and obesity in girls, as well as a delay in puberty for those with less body fat (Maron, 2015).

Female Puberty Changes

As girls mature, the anterior pituitary gland secretes increasing amounts of FSH and LH in response to the hypothalamic secretion of GnRH. These two pituitary secretions stimulate secretion of estrogens and progesterone by the ovary, resulting in maturation of the reproductive organs and breasts and development of secondary sex characteristics. The first noticeable change of puberty in girls, development of the breasts, begins at approximately 8 to 13 years of age. Menstruation occurs about 2 to 2.5 years after breast development, with an average age range of 9 to 16 years.

Breast Changes. Initially, the nipple enlarges and protrudes. The areola surrounding the nipple also enlarges and becomes somewhat protuberant. These changes are followed by growth of the glandular and ductal tissue. Fat is deposited in the breasts to give them the characteristic rounded female appearance. During puberty, a girl's breasts often develop at different rates, resulting in a lopsided appearance until one breast catches up with the other.

Body Contours. The pelvis widens and assumes a rounded, basin-like shape that favors passage of the fetus during childbirth.

Fat is deposited selectively in the hips, giving them a rounder appearance than those of the male.

Body Hair. Pubic hair first appears downy and becomes thicker as puberty progresses. Axillary hair appears near the time of menarche. The texture and quantity of pubic and axillary hair vary among women and ethnic groups. Women of African descent usually have body hair that is coarser and curlier than that of White women. Asian women often have sparser body hair compared with women of other racial groups.

Skeletal Growth. Girls grow taller for several years during early puberty in response to estrogen stimulation. The growth spurt begins approximately 1 year after breast development begins. Estrogen also causes the epiphyses (growth areas of the bone) to unite with the shafts of the bones, which eventually stops growth in height.

Reproductive Organs. The girl's external genitalia enlarge as fat is deposited in the mons pubis, labia majora, and labia minora. The vagina, uterus, fallopian tubes, and ovaries grow larger. In addition, the vaginal mucosa changes, becoming more resistant to trauma and infection in preparation for sexual activity. Cyclic changes in the reproductive organs occur during each female reproductive cycle.

Menarche. Approximately 2 to 2.5 years after the beginning of breast development, girls experience their **menarche**, or first menstrual period. Early menstrual periods are often irregular and scant. These early menstrual cycles are not usually fertile because ovulation occurs inconsistently. Fertile reproductive cycles require preparation of the uterine lining precisely timed with ovulation. However, ovulation may occur during any female reproductive cycle, including the first. The sexually active girl can conceive even before her first menstrual period.

Delayed onset of menstruation is called *primary* **amenorrhea** if the girl's periods have not begun within 2 years after the onset of breast development or by 16 years of age or if the girl is more than 1 year older than her mother or sisters were when their menarche occurred. *Secondary amenorrhea* describes absence of menstruation for at least three cycles after regular cycles have been established or for 6 months. Both primary and secondary amenorrhea are more common in females who are thin. Women who are competitive athletes or dancers or who suffer from eating disorders (e.g., anorexia nervosa or bulimia) may have too little fat to produce enough sex hormones to stimulate ovulation and menstruation. Pregnancy is also a common cause of secondary amenorrhea. Both primary and secondary amenorrhea may result from inadequate pituitary stimulation of the ovary or failure of the ovary to respond to pituitary stimulation. Amenorrhea also may be caused by excessive androgenic hormones from the adrenal glands, which have a masculinizing effect.

Male Puberty Changes

Secretion of GnRH by the hypothalamus stimulates secretion of LH and FSH from the anterior pituitary. LH and FSH then stimulate secretion of testosterone and eventually cause

TABLE 3.1   Major Hormones in Reproduction

Produced By	Target Organs	Action in Female	Action in Male
Gonadotropin-Releasing Hormone			
Hypothalamus	Anterior pituitary	Stimulates release of FSH and LH, initiating puberty and sustaining female reproductive cycles; release is pulsatile.	Stimulates release of FSH and LH, initiating puberty; release is pulsatile.
Follicle-Stimulating Hormone			
Anterior pituitary	Ovaries (female) Testes (male)	Stimulates final maturation of follicle. Stimulates growth and maturation of graafian follicles before ovulation.	Stimulates Leydig cells of testes to secrete testosterone.
Luteinizing Hormone			
Anterior pituitary	Ovaries (female) Testes (male)	Stimulates final maturation of follicle. Surge of LH approximately 14 days before next menstrual period causes ovulation. Stimulates transformation of graafian follicle into corpus luteum, which continues secretion of estrogens and progesterone for about 12 days if ovum is not fertilized. If fertilization occurs, placenta gradually assumes this function.	Stimulates Leydig cells of testes to secrete testosterone.
Estrogens			
Ovaries and corpus luteum (female) Placenta (pregnancy) Formed in small quantities from testosterone in Sertoli cells of testes (male); other tissues, especially liver, produce estrogen in male	Internal and external reproductive organs Breasts (female) Testes (male)	Reproductive organs: a. Maturation at puberty b. Stimulation of endometrium before ovulation Breasts: Induce growth of glandular and ductal tissue; initiate deposition of fat at puberty. Stimulate growth of long bones but cause closure of epiphyses, limiting mature height. Pregnancy: Stimulate growth of uterus, breast tissue; inhibit active milk production; relax pelvic ligaments.	Necessary for normal sperm formation.
Progesterone			
Ovary, corpus luteum, placenta	Uterus, female breasts	Stimulates secretion of endometrial glands; causes endometrial vessels to become dilated and tortuous in preparation for possible embryo implantation. Pregnancy: Induces growth of cells of fallopian tubes and uterine lining to nourish embryo; decreases contractions of uterus; prepares breasts for lactation but inhibits prolactin secretion.	Not applicable.
Prolactin			
Anterior pituitary	Female breasts	Stimulates secretion of milk (lactogenesis); estrogen and progesterone from placenta have an inhibiting effect on milk production until after placenta is expelled at birth; suckling of newborn stimulates prolactin secretion to maintain milk production.	Not applicable.
Oxytocin			
Posterior pituitary	Uterus, female breasts	Uterus: Stimulates contractions during birth and stimulates postpartum contractions to compress uterine vessels and control bleeding. Stimulates let-down, or milk-ejection reflex, during breastfeeding.	Not applicable.
Testosterone			
Leydig cells of the testes (male) Adrenal glands (female) Ovaries (female)	Sexual organs (male) Male body conformation after puberty	Small quantities of androgenic (masculinizing) hormones from adrenal glands cause growth of pubic and axillary hair at puberty; most androgens, such as testosterone, are converted to estrogen.	Induces development of male sex organs in fetus. Induces growth and division of cells that mature sperm. Induces development of male secondary sex characteristics.

FSH, Follicle-stimulating hormone; *GnRH,* gonadotropin-releasing hormone; *LH,* luteinizing hormone.

spermatogenesis, or formation of male gametes, or sperm, in the maturing adolescent. Testosterone stimulates development of a boy's reproductive organs and secondary sex characteristics. The first outward sign of male puberty is growth of the testes, which may begin as early as 9.5 years of age. Penile growth begins approximately 1 year later as the circumference and length of the penis increase. The skin of the scrotum thins and darkens as the sexual organs mature. Final male sexual maturation is complete at approximately 17 years of age (Blackburn, 2013).

Nocturnal Emissions. Often called *wet dreams,* nocturnal emissions commonly occur during the teenage years. The boy experiences a spontaneous ejaculation of seminal fluid during sleep, often accompanied by dreams with sexual content. Boys should be prepared for this normal occurrence so they do not feel abnormal or ashamed or fear they have an infection or other problem.

Body Hair. Pubic hair growth begins at the base of the penis. Gradually, the hair coarsens and grows upward and in the midline of the abdomen. Approximately 2 years later, axillary hair appears. Facial hair begins as a fine, downy mustache and progresses to the characteristic beard of the adult male. In most boys, chest hair develops, and some boys have hair on their upper backs. The amount and character of body hair vary among men of different racial groups, with Asian and Native American men often having less than white or African men. The quantity and character of body hair among men of the same racial group also vary.

Body Composition. Because of the influence of testosterone, men develop a greater average muscle mass than women. At maturity a man's muscle mass exceeds the woman's by an average of 50% (Hall, 2016), explaining the biologic advantage of men in tasks requiring muscle strength.

Skeletal Growth. Testosterone causes boys to undergo a rapid growth spurt, especially in height. A boy's linear growth begins approximately 1 year later than a girl's and may continue into his twenties. Testosterone eventually causes union of the epiphysis with the shaft of long bones, as estrogen does in girls. The height-limiting effect of testosterone is not as strong as that of estrogen in females, with the result that boys grow in stature for several years longer than girls. The male's greater average height at maturity is the combined result of beginning the growth spurt at a slightly later age and continuing it for a longer time.

A boy's shoulders broaden as his height increases. His pelvis assumes a more upright shape, with narrower diameters and heavier composition than the female pelvis. A man's pelvis is structurally suited for tasks requiring load bearing.

Voice Changes. Hypertrophy of the laryngeal mucosa and enlargement of the larynx cause the male's voice to deepen. Before reaching their lower tones at maturity, many boys experience embarrassing "cracking" or "squeaking" of their voices when they speak.

Decline in Fertility

The **climacteric** is a transitional period that starts as female fertility declines and extends through menopause and the postmenopausal period. In most women, the climacteric occurs between ages 40 and 50 years. Maturation of ova and production of ovarian hormones gradually decline. The external and internal reproductive organs atrophy somewhat as well. **Menopause** is the term used to describe the final menstrual period. However, *menopause* (permanent cessation of menstruation) and *climacteric* are often used interchangeably to describe the entire gradual process of change. Perimenopause is the time from the onset of changes associated with the climacteric, continuing for approximately 2 to 5 years after the last menstrual period (Blackburn, 2013). (See Chapter 27 for more information about the woman's needs during this phase of her life.)

Men do not experience a distinct marker event like menopause. Production of testosterone and sperm gradually declines, and sexual function decreases in the late forties and fifties.

❓ KNOWLEDGE CHECK

1. What are the first noticeable changes of puberty in girls and boys?
2. What are basic differences between the mature male and female pelvis?
3. Why do males generally attain greater mature height than females?
4. What are common male and female secondary sex characteristics?

FEMALE REPRODUCTIVE ANATOMY

The nurse needs a basic knowledge of the structure and function of the external and internal reproductive organs to understand their roles in pregnancy and childbirth (Table 3.2).

TABLE 3.2   Functions of Female Reproductive and Accessory Organs

Organ	Function
Vagina	1. Passageway for menstrual flow
	2. Female organ for coitus; receives male penis during coitus
	3. Passageway for fetus during birth
Uterus	1. Houses and nourishes fetus to sufficient maturity to function outside mother's body; propels fetus to outside
Fallopian tube	1. Passageway for ovum as it travels from ovary to uterus
	2. Site of fertilization
Ovaries	1. Secrete estrogens and progesterone
	2. Contain ova within follicles for maturation during woman's reproductive life
Breasts	
Alveoli	1. Secrete milk after childbirth (acinar cells within alveoli)
Lactiferous ducts	2. Collect milk from alveoli and conduct it to outside

External Female Reproductive Organs

Collectively, the external female reproductive organs are called the *vulva*. These structures include the mons pubis, labia majora and minora, clitoris, structures of the vestibule, and perineum (Fig. 3.1).

Mons Pubis

The mons pubis is the rounded, fleshy prominence over the symphysis pubis that forms the anterior border of the external reproductive organs. It is covered with varying amounts of pubic hair.

Labia Majora and Minora

The labia majora are two rounded, fleshy folds of tissue that extend from the mons pubis to the perineum. They have a slightly deeper pigmentation than surrounding skin and are covered with pubic hair. The labia majora protect the more fragile tissues of the external genitalia.

The labia minora run parallel to and within the labia majora. The labia minora extend from the clitoris anteriorly and merge posteriorly to form the fourchette, which is the posterior rim of the vaginal introitus, or vaginal opening. The labia minora do not have pubic hair. They are highly vascular and respond to stimulation by becoming engorged with blood.

Clitoris

The clitoris is a small projection at the anterior junction of the two labia minora. This structure is composed of highly sensitive erectile tissue similar to that of the penis. The labia majora merge to form a prepuce over the clitoris.

Vestibule

The *vestibule* refers to structures enclosed by the labia minora. The urinary meatus, vaginal introitus, and ducts of Skene and

Bartholin glands lie within the vestibule. Skene, or periurethral, glands provide lubrication for the urethra. Bartholin glands provide lubrication for the vaginal introitus, particularly during sexual arousal.

The vaginal introitus is surrounded by erectile tissue. During sexual stimulation, blood flows into the erectile tissue, allowing the introitus to tighten around the penis. This adds a massaging feeling that heightens the male's sexual sensations and encourages ejaculation.

The hymen is a thin fold of mucosa partially separating the vagina and the vestibule. The intactness, or lack thereof, of the hymen is not a criterion of virginity. The hymen may be broken by injury, tampon use, intercourse, or childbirth.

Perineum

The perineum is the most posterior part of the external female reproductive organs. The perineum extends from the fourchette anteriorly to the anus posteriorly. It is composed of fibrous and muscular tissues that provide support for pelvic structures.

Internal Female Reproductive Organs

The internal reproductive structures are the vagina, uterus, fallopian tubes, and ovaries (Figs. 3.2 and 3.3). These organs are supported and contained within the bony pelvis.

Vagina

The vagina is a tube of muscular and membranous tissue approximately 8 to 10 cm long between the bladder anteriorly and the rectum posteriorly. The vagina connects the uterus above with the vestibule below. The vaginal lining has multiple folds, or **rugae**, and a muscular layer capable of marked distention during childbirth. The vagina is lubricated by secretions of the cervix (the lowermost part of the uterus) and Bartholin glands.

The vagina does not end abruptly at the uterine opening, but arches to form a pouch-like structure called the *vaginal fornix*. Each fornix is described by its location: anterior, posterior, and lateral.

The vagina has three major functions: (1) it allows discharge of the menstrual flow; (2) it is the female organ of **coitus** (male–female sexual union); and (3) it allows passage of the fetus from the uterus to outside the mother's body during childbirth.

Uterus

The uterus is a hollow, thick-walled, muscular organ shaped like a flat, upside-down pear. The uterus houses and nourishes the fetus until birth and then contracts rhythmically during labor to expel the fetus. Each month the uterus is prepared for a pregnancy, regardless of whether conception occurs.

The uterus measures approximately 7.5 × 5 × 2.5 cm and is larger in women who have borne children. It is suspended above the bladder and is anterior to the rectum. Its normal position is anteverted (rotated forward over the bladder) and slightly anteflexed (flexed forward).

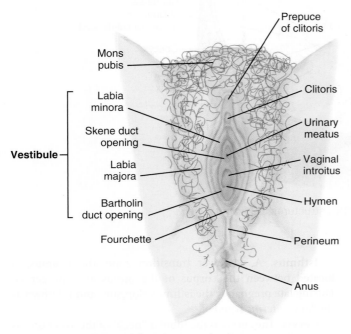

FIG. 3.1 External female reproductive structures.

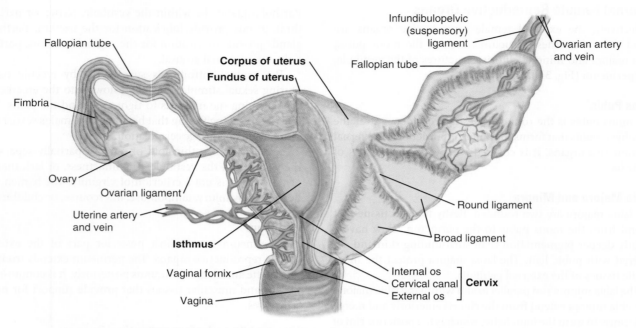

FIG. 3.2 Internal female reproductive structures, anterior view.

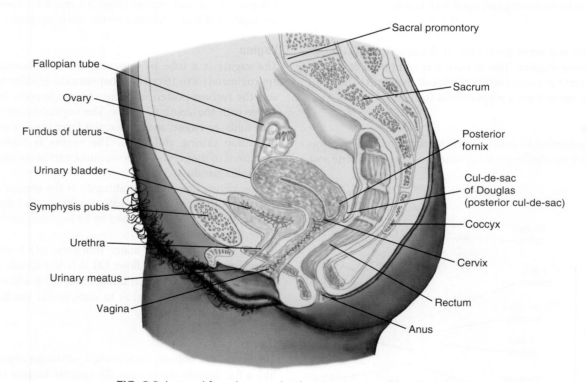

FIG. 3.3 Internal female reproductive structures, midsagittal view.

Divisions of the Uterus. The uterus has three divisions: the corpus, the isthmus, and the cervix.

Corpus. The corpus, or body, is the upper division of the uterus. The uppermost part of the uterine corpus, above the area where the fallopian tubes enter the uterus, is the fundus of the uterus.

Isthmus. A narrower transition zone, the isthmus, is located between the corpus of the uterus and the cervix. During late pregnancy the isthmus elongates and is known as the *lower uterine segment*.

Cervix. The cervix is the tubular "neck" of the lower uterus and is approximately 2 to 3 cm in length. During labor, the

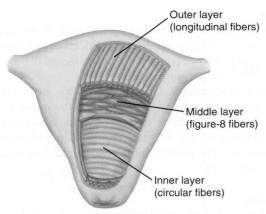

FIG. 3.4 Layers of the myometrium showing the three types of smooth muscle fiber.

Outer layer (longitudinal fibers)

Middle layer (figure-8 fibers)

Inner layer (circular fibers)

cervix effaces (thins) and dilates (opens) to allow passage of the fetus. The os is the opening in the cervix between the uterus and vagina. The upper cervix and lower cervix are marked by the internal os and external os, respectively. The external os of a childless woman is round and smooth. After vaginal birth the external os has an irregular, slit-like shape and may have tags of scar tissue.

Layers of the Uterus. The uterus has three layers: the perimetrium, the myometrium, and the endometrium.

Perimetrium. The perimetrium is the outer peritoneal layer of serous membrane that covers most of the uterus. Laterally the perimetrium is continuous with the broad ligaments on both sides of the uterus.

Myometrium. The myometrium is the middle layer of thick muscle. Most muscle fibers are concentrated in the upper uterus, and their number diminishes progressively toward the cervix. The myometrium contains three types of smooth muscle fiber, each suited to specific functions in childbearing (Fig. 3.4):

1. Longitudinal fibers are found mostly in the fundus and are designed to expel the fetus efficiently toward the pelvic outlet during birth.
2. Interlacing figure-8 fibers constitute the middle layer. These fibers contract after birth to compress blood vessels that pass between them to limit blood loss.
3. Circular fibers form constrictions where the fallopian tubes enter the uterus and surround the internal cervical os. Circular fibers prevent reflux of menstrual blood and tissue into the fallopian tubes, promote normal implantation of the fertilized ovum by controlling its entry into the uterus, and retain the fetus until the appropriate time of birth.

Endometrium. The endometrium is the inner layer of the uterus. It responds to the cyclic variations of estrogen and progesterone during the female reproductive cycle (see Fig. 3.7) The endometrium has two layers:

1. The basal layer is the area nearest the myometrium that regenerates the functional layer of the endometrium after each menstrual period and after childbirth.
2. The functional layer lies above the basal layer. Endometrial arteries, veins, and glands extend into the functional

layer and are shed during each menstrual period and after childbirth in the lochia, the vaginal drainage after childbirth.

Fallopian Tubes

The fallopian tubes, also called *oviducts,* are 8 to 14 cm long and quite narrow (2 to 3 mm at their narrowest and 5 to 8 mm at their widest). They form a pathway for the ovum between the ovary and uterus. Fertilization occurs in the fallopian tubes. Each fallopian tube enters the upper uterus at the cornu, or horn, of the uterus.

The fallopian tubes are lined with folded epithelium containing hairlike processes called **cilia** that beat rhythmically toward the uterine cavity to propel the ovum through the tube. The rough, folded surface of its lining and small diameter make the fallopian tube vulnerable to blockage from infection or scar tissue. Tubal blockage may result in sterility or a tubal (ectopic) pregnancy because the fertilized ovum cannot enter the uterus for proper implantation.

The fallopian tubes have four divisions:

1. The interstitial portion runs into the uterine cavity and lies within the uterine wall.
2. The isthmus is the narrow part adjacent to the uterus.
3. The ampulla is the wider area of the tube lateral to the isthmus, where fertilization occurs.
4. The infundibulum is the wide, funnel-shaped terminal end of the tube. Fimbriae are finger-like processes that surround the infundibulum.

The fallopian tubes are not directly connected to the ovary. The ovum is expelled into the abdominal cavity near the fimbriae at ovulation. Wavelike motions of the fimbriae draw the ovum into the tube. However, the tubal isthmus remains contracted until 3 days after conception to allow the fertilized ovum to develop within the tube. Initial growth of the fertilized ovum within the fallopian tube promotes its normal implantation in the upper uterus.

Ovaries

The ovaries are the female gonads, or sex glands. There are two functions of the ovary: (1) sex hormone production and (2) maturation of an ovum during each reproductive cycle.

The ovaries secrete estrogen and progesterone in varying amounts during a woman's reproductive cycle to prepare the uterine lining for pregnancy. Ovarian hormone secretion gradually declines to very low levels during the climacteric.

At birth, the ovary contains all the ova it will ever have. Approximately two million immature ova are present at birth. Many of these degenerate during childhood, and at puberty approximately 200,000 to 400,000 viable ova remain. Many ova begin the maturation process during each reproductive cycle, but most never reach maturity. During a woman's reproductive life, only about 400 of the ova ever mature enough to be released and fertilized. By the time a woman reaches the climacteric, almost all her ova have been released during ovulation or have regressed. The few remaining ova are unresponsive to stimulating hormones and do not mature (Blackburn, 2013; Moore & Persaud, 2013).

5. What is the vulva? Describe the location of each of these external female organs: labia majora and minora, clitoris, urinary meatus, vaginal introitus, hymen, and perineum.
6. What are the three divisions of the uterus? Where is the fundus located?
7. Describe the three myometrial layers of the uterus. What is the function of each layer?
8. How do the fallopian tubes propel the ovum from the ovary to the uterus? Why does the fertilized ovum first grow within the fallopian tube?
9. What are the two functions of the ovaries?

Support Structures

The bony pelvis supports and protects the lower abdominal and internal reproductive organs. Muscles and ligaments provide added support for the internal organs of the pelvis against the downward force of gravity and increases in intraabdominal pressure.

Pelvis

The bony pelvis is a basin-shaped structure at the lower end of the spine (Fig. 3.5). Its posterior wall is formed by the sacrum. The side and anterior pelvic walls are composed of three fused bones: the ilium, ischium, and pubis.

The linea terminalis, also called the *pelvic brim* or *ileopectineal line,* is an imaginary line dividing the upper, or false, pelvis from the lower, or true, pelvis. The false pelvis provides support for the internal organs and the upper part of the body. The true pelvis is most important during childbirth (see Chapter 12).

Muscles

Paired muscles enclose the lower pelvis and provide support for internal reproductive, urinary, and bowel structures (Fig. 3.6). In addition, a fibromuscular sheet, the pelvic fascia, provides support for the pelvic organs. Vaginal and urethral openings are located in the pelvic fascia.

The levator ani is a collection of three pairs of muscles: the pubococcygeus, which is also called the *pubovaginal muscle*

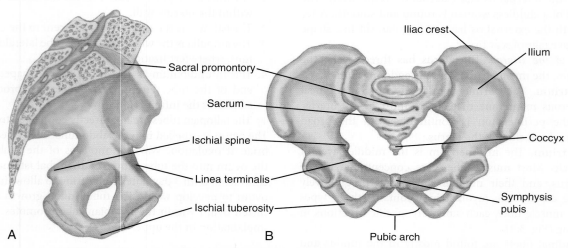

FIG. 3.5 Structures of the bony pelvis, shown in lateral (A) and anterior (B) views.

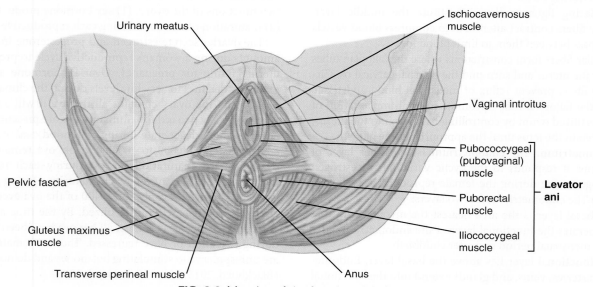

FIG. 3.6 Muscles of the female pelvic floor.

in the female; the puborectal; and the iliococcygeus. These muscles support internal pelvic structures and resist increases in the intraabdominal pressure.

The ischiocavernosus muscle extends from the clitoris to the ischial tuberosities on each side of the lower bony pelvis. The two transverse perineal muscles extend from fibrous tissue of the perineum to the two ischial tuberosities, stabilizing the center of the perineum.

Ligaments

Seven pairs of ligaments maintain the internal reproductive organs and their nerve and blood supplies in their proper positions within the pelvis (see Fig. 3.2).

Lateral Support. Paired ligaments stabilize the uterus and ovaries laterally and keep them in the midline of the pelvis. The broad ligament is a sheet of tissue extending from each side of the uterus to the lateral pelvic wall. The round ligament and fallopian tube mark the upper border of the broad ligament, and the lower edge is bounded by the uterine blood vessels. Within the two broad ligaments are the ovarian ligaments, blood vessels, and lymphatics.

The right and left cardinal ligaments provide support to the lower uterus and vagina. They extend from the lateral walls of the cervix and vagina to the side walls of the pelvis.

The two ovarian ligaments connect the ovaries to the lateral uterine walls. The infundibulopelvic (suspensory) ligaments connect the lateral ovary and distal fallopian tubes to the pelvic side walls. The infundibulopelvic ligament also carries the blood vessel and nerve supply for the ovary.

Anterior Support. Two pairs of ligaments provide anterior support for the internal reproductive organs. The round ligaments connect the upper uterus to the connective tissue of the labia majora. These ligaments maintain the uterus in its normal anteflexed position and help direct the fetal presenting part against the cervix during labor.

The pubocervical ligaments support the cervix anteriorly. They connect the cervix and interior surface of the symphysis pubis.

Posterior Support. The uterosacral ligaments provide posterior support, extending from the lower posterior uterus to the sacrum. These ligaments also contain the sympathetic and parasympathetic nerves of the autonomic nervous system.

Blood Supply

The uterine blood supply is carried by the uterine arteries, which are branches of the internal iliac artery. These vessels enter the uterus at the lower border of the broad ligament near the isthmus of the uterus. The vessels branch downward to supply the cervix and vagina and upward to supply the uterus. The upper branch also supplies the ovaries and fallopian tubes. The vessels are coiled to allow for elongation as the uterus enlarges and rises from the pelvis during pregnancy. Blood drains into the uterine veins and from there into the internal iliac veins.

Additional ovarian and tubal blood supply is carried by the ovarian artery, which arises from the abdominal aorta.

The ovarian blood supply drains into the two ovarian veins. The left ovarian vein drains into the left renal vein, and the right ovarian vein drains directly into the inferior vena cava.

Nerve Supply

Most functions of the reproductive system are under involuntary, or unconscious, control. Nerves of the autonomic nervous system from the uterovaginal plexus and inferior hypogastric plexus control automatic functions of the reproductive system.

Sensory and motor nerves that innervate the reproductive organs enter the spinal cord at the T12 through L2 levels. These nerves are important for pain management during childbearing (see Chapter 13).

> **❓ KNOWLEDGE CHECK**
>
> 10. Where is the true pelvis located?
> 11. What are the purposes of the muscles of the pelvis? What are the purposes of the ligaments?

FEMALE REPRODUCTIVE CYCLE

The term *female reproductive cycle* refers to the regular and recurrent changes in the anterior pituitary secretions, ovaries, and uterine endometrium designed to prepare the body for pregnancy (Fig. 3.7). Associated changes in the cervical mucus promote fertilization during each cycle. The female reproductive cycle is often called the *menstrual cycle* because menstruation provides a marker for each cycle's beginning and end if pregnancy does not occur.

The female reproductive cycle is driven by a feedback loop between the anterior pituitary and ovaries. A feedback loop is a change in the level of one secretion in response to a change in the level of another secretion. The feedback loop may be positive, in which rising levels of one secretion cause another to rise, or negative, in which rising levels of one secretion cause another to fall.

The duration of the cycle is approximately 28 days, although it may range from 20 to 45 days (Hall, 2016). Significant deviations from the 28-day cycle are associated with reduced fertility. The first day of the menstrual period is counted as day 1 of the woman's cycle. The female reproductive cycle is further divided into two cycles reflecting changes in the ovaries and uterine endometrium.

Ovarian Cycle

In response to GnRH from the woman's hypothalamus, the anterior pituitary secretes FSH and LH. These secretions stimulate the ovaries to mature and release an ovum and secrete additional hormones to prepare the endometrium for implantation of a fertilized ovum. The ovarian cycle consists of three phases: follicular, ovulatory, and luteal.

Follicular Phase

The follicular phase is the period during which an ovum matures. It begins with the first day of menstruation and ends

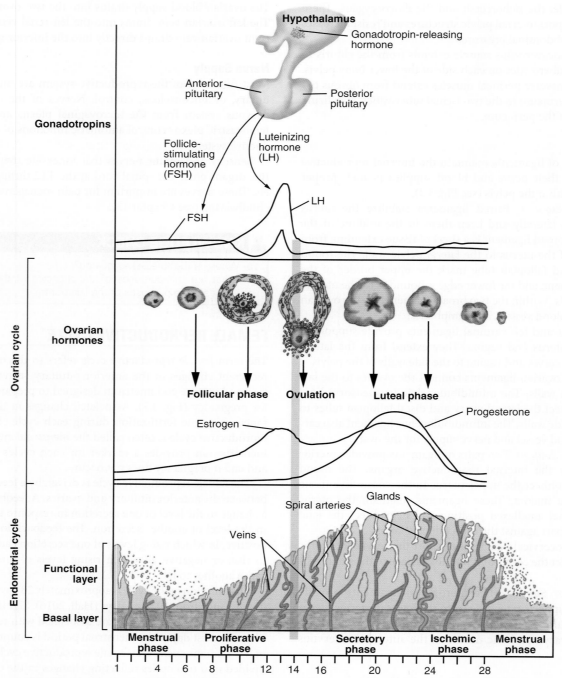

FIG. 3.7 The Female Reproductive Cycle. This figure illustrates the changes in hormone secretion from the anterior pituitary and interrelated changes in the ovary and uterine endometrium.

approximately 14 days later in a 28-day cycle. The length of this phase varies more among different women than do the lengths of the other two phases. The fall in estrogen and progesterone secretion by the ovary just before menstruation stimulates secretion of FSH and LH by the anterior pituitary. As the FSH and LH levels rise slightly, 6 to 12 **graafian follicles** (sacs within the ovary), each containing an immature ovum, begin to grow. Each follicle secretes fluid containing high levels of estrogen, which accelerates maturation by making

the follicle more sensitive to the effects of FSH. Eventually, one follicle outgrows the others to reach maturity. The mature follicle secretes large amounts of estrogen, which depresses FSH secretion. The dip in FSH secretion just before ovulation blocks further maturation of the less-developed follicles. Occasionally, more than one follicle matures and releases its ovum, which can lead to a multifetal pregnancy. Women who take fertility drugs may release multiple mature ova that are used for assisted reproductive techniques (Chapter 26).

Ovulatory Phase

Near the middle of a 28-day reproductive cycle and about 2 days before ovulation, LH secretion rises markedly. Secretion of FSH also rises but to a lesser extent than that of LH. These surges in LH and FSH levels cause a slight fall in follicular estrogen production and a rise in progesterone secretion, which stimulates final maturation of a single follicle and release of its ovum. Ovulation marks the beginning of the luteal phase of the female reproductive cycle and occurs 14 days before the next menstrual period.

The mature follicle is a mass of cells with a fluid-filled chamber. A smaller mass of cells houses the ovum within this chamber. At ovulation a blister-like projection called a *stigma* forms on the wall of the follicle, the follicle ruptures, and the ovum with its surrounding cells is released from the surface of the ovary, where it is picked up by the fimbriated end of the fallopian tube for transport to the uterus.

Luteal Phase

After ovulation and under the influence of LH, the remaining cells of the old follicle persist for approximately 12 days as a corpus luteum. The corpus luteum secretes estrogen and large amounts of progesterone to prepare the endometrium for a fertilized ovum. During this phase, levels of FSH and LH decrease in response to higher levels of estrogen and progesterone. If the ovum is fertilized, it secretes a hormone (chorionic gonadotropin) that causes persistence of the corpus luteum to maintain an early pregnancy. If the ovum is not fertilized, FSH and LH fall to low levels, and the corpus luteum regresses. Decline of estrogen and progesterone levels along with corpus luteum regression results in menstruation as the uterine lining breaks down.

The loss of estrogen and progesterone from the corpus luteum at the end of one cycle stimulates the anterior pituitary to again secrete more FSH and LH, initiating a new female reproductive cycle. The old corpus luteum is replaced by fibrous tissue called the *corpus albicans*.

Endometrial Cycle

The uterine endometrium responds to ovarian hormone stimulation with cyclic changes. Four phases mark the changes in the endometrium: proliferative, secretory, ischemic, and menstrual.

Proliferative Phase

The proliferative phase occurs as the ovum matures and is released during the first half of the ovarian cycle. After completion of a menstrual period, the endometrium is very thin. The basal layer of endometrial cells remains after menstruation. These cells multiply to form new endometrial epithelium and endometrial glands under the stimulation of estrogen secreted by the maturing ovarian follicles. Endometrial spiral arteries and endometrial veins elongate to accompany thickening of the functional endometrial layer and nourish the proliferating cells. As ovulation approaches, the endometrial glands secrete thin, stringy mucus that aids entry of sperm into the uterus.

Secretory Phase

The secretory phase occurs during the last half of the ovarian cycle as the uterus is prepared to receive a fertilized ovum. The endometrium continues to thicken under the influence of estrogen and progesterone from the corpus luteum, reaching its maximum thickness of 5 to 6 mm. The blood vessels and endometrial glands become twisted and dilated.

Progesterone from the corpus luteum causes the thick endometrium to secrete substances to nourish a fertilized ovum. Large quantities of glycogen, proteins, lipids, and minerals are stored within the endometrium, awaiting arrival of the ovum.

Ischemic and Menstrual Phases

If fertilization does not occur, the corpus luteum regresses, and its production of estrogen and progesterone falls. About 2 days before the onset of menstruation, vasospasm of the endometrial blood vessels causes the endometrium to become ischemic and necrotic. The necrotic areas of endometrium separate from the basal layers, resulting in the menstrual flow. The durations of the menstrual phase, from the first day of flow to the last is approximately 5 days.

During a menstrual period, women lose approximately 40 mL of blood. Because of the recurrent loss of blood, many women are mildly anemic during their reproductive years, especially if their diets are low in iron.

Changes in Cervical Mucus

During most of the female reproductive cycle, the mucus of the cervix is scant, thick, and sticky. Just before ovulation, cervical mucus becomes thin, clear, and elastic to promote passage of sperm into the uterus and fallopian tube, where they can fertilize the ovum. **Spinnbarkeit** refers to the elasticity of cervical mucus. A woman may assess the elasticity of her cervical mucus to either avoid or promote conception (Chapter 25).

? KNOWLEDGE CHECK

12. Which ovarian structures secrete estrogen and progesterone during the female reproductive cycle?
13. What three ovarian phases occur during each female reproductive cycle?
14. How does the uterine endometrium change during a woman's reproductive cycle?
15. Why does the cervical mucus become thin, clear, and elastic around the time of ovulation?

THE FEMALE BREAST

Structure

The breasts, or mammary glands, are not directly functional in reproduction, but they secrete milk after childbirth to nourish the infant. The small, raised nipple is located at the center of each breast (Fig. 3.8). The nipple is composed of sensitive erectile tissue and may respond to sexual stimulation. A larger circular areola surrounds the nipple. Both the nipple and areola are darker than surrounding skin.

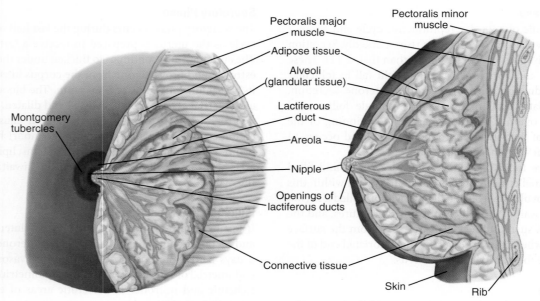

FIG. 3.8 Structures of the female breast.

Montgomery's tubercles are sebaceous glands in the areola. They are inactive and not obvious except during pregnancy and lactation, when they enlarge and secrete a substance that keeps the nipple soft.

Within each breast lobes of glandular tissue secrete milk. These lobes are arranged in a pattern similar to spokes of a wheel around the hub. Between 15 and 20 of these lobes are arranged around and behind the nipple and areola. Fibrous tissue and fat in the breast support the glandular tissue, blood vessels, lymphatics, and nerves.

Alveoli are small sacs containing acinar cells to secrete milk. The acinar cells extract the necessary substances from the mammary blood supply to manufacture milk when the breasts are properly stimulated by the anterior pituitary gland. Myoepithelial cells surround the alveoli to contract and eject the milk into the ductal system when signaled by secretion of the hormone oxytocin from the posterior pituitary gland. The alveoli drain into lactiferous ducts, which connect at the nipple to drain milk from all areas of the breast.

Function

The breasts are inactive until puberty, when rising estrogen levels stimulate growth of the glandular tissue. In addition, fat is deposited in the breasts, resulting in the mature female contour. The amount of fat is the major determinant of breast size; the amount of glandular tissue is similar for all mature women. Therefore breast size is unrelated to the amount of milk a woman can produce during lactation.

During pregnancy, high levels of estrogen and progesterone produced by the placenta stimulate growth of the alveoli and ductal system to prepare them for lactation. Prolactin secretion by the anterior pituitary gland stimulates milk production during pregnancy, but this effect is inhibited by estrogen and progesterone produced by the placenta. Inhibiting effects of estrogen and progesterone stop when the placenta

is expelled after birth, and active milk production occurs in response to the infant's suckling while breastfeeding.

KNOWLEDGE CHECK

16. What is the function of Montgomery's tubercles?
17. How is a woman's breast size related to the amount of milk she can produce?
18. Why is milk not actively secreted during pregnancy?

MALE REPRODUCTIVE ANATOMY AND PHYSIOLOGY

External Male Reproductive Organs

The male has two external organs of reproduction: the penis and scrotum (Fig. 3.9).

Penis

The penis has two functions. As part of the urinary tract, it carries urine from the bladder to the exterior during urination. As a reproductive organ, the penis deposits semen into the female vagina during coitus.

The penis is composed mostly of erectile tissue, which is spongy tissue with many small spaces inside. The three areas of erectile tissue are the corpus spongiosum, which surrounds the urethra, and two columns of the corpus cavernosum on each side of the penis.

The penis is flaccid most of the time because the small spaces within the erectile tissue are collapsed. During sexual stimulation, arteries within the penis dilate and veins are partly occluded, trapping blood in the spongy tissue. Entrapment of blood within the penis causes erection and enables penetration of the vagina during sexual intercourse.

The glans is the distal end of the penis. The urinary meatus is centered in the end of the glans. The loose skin

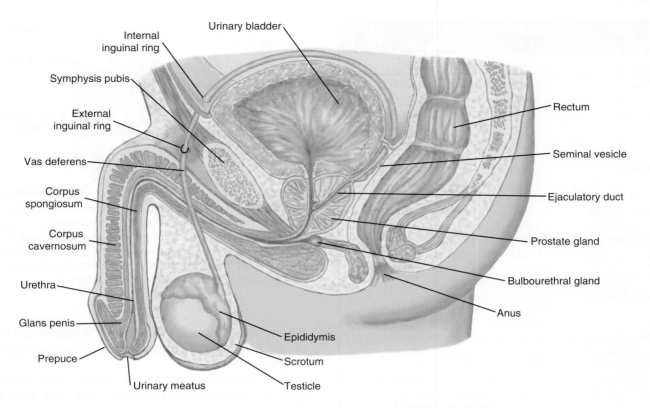

FIG. 3.9 Structures of the male reproductive system, midsagittal view.

of the prepuce, or foreskin, covers the glans. The prepuce may be removed during circumcision, a surgical procedure usually performed during the newborn period, although it may be performed later. The glans is very sensitive to tactile stimulation, which adds to the male's sensation during coitus.

Scrotum
The scrotum is a pouch of thin skin and muscle suspended behind the penis. The skin of the scrotum is somewhat darker than the surrounding skin and is covered with small ridges called *rugae.* The scrotum is divided internally by a septum. One of the male gonads (testicle) is contained within each pocket of the scrotum.

The scrotum's main purpose is to keep the testes cooler than the core body temperature. Formation of normal male sperm requires that the testes not be too warm. A cremaster muscle is attached to each testicle. Contraction of the cremaster muscles draws the testicles closer to the body for warming, and relaxation of these muscles allows the testicles to move away from the body for cooling.

Internal Male Reproductive Organs
The functions of the male external and internal reproductive organs are summarized in Table 3.3.

Testes
The male gonads, or testes, have two functions: they serve as endocrine glands, and they produce male gametes, or sperm,

also called *spermatozoa.* Androgens (male sex hormones) are the primary endocrine secretions of the testes. Androgens are produced by Leydig cells of the testes. The primary androgen produced by the testes is testosterone.

Unlike females, who experience a cyclic pattern of hormone secretion, males secrete testosterone in a relatively even pattern. A feedback loop with the hypothalamus and anterior pituitary stabilizes testosterone levels. A small amount of testosterone is converted to estrogen in males and is necessary for sperm formation.

Spermatogenesis occurs within tiny coiled tubes, the seminiferous tubules of the testes (Fig. 3.10). Leydig cells are interstitial cells supporting the seminiferous tubules and secrete testosterone, which is necessary to form new cells that will mature into sperm. Sertoli cells within the seminiferous tubules respond to FSH secretion by nourishing and supporting sperm as they mature. Unlike females, who have a lifetime supply of ova in their gonads at birth, males do not begin producing sperm until puberty. Normal males produce new sperm throughout life, although production declines with age.

At ejaculation, approximately 35 to 200 million sperm are deposited in the vagina (Blackburn, 2013; Hall, 2016). This large number is needed for normal fertility, although a single sperm fertilizes the ovum. Only a few sperm ever reach the fallopian tube, where an ovum may be available for fertilization. When the first sperm penetrates the ovum, changes within the ovum prevent other sperm from also fertilizing it (Chapter 5).

TABLE 3.3 Functions of Male Reproductive and Accessory Organs

Organ	Function
Penis	1. Conduit for urine from bladder 2. Male organ of sexual intercourse
Scrotum	1. Housing of testes and maintenance of their temperature at a level cooler than trunk of the body, thus promoting normal sperm formation
Testes	1. Endocrine glands that secrete primary male hormone (testosterone) 2. Sperm formation
Seminiferous tubules	1. Location of spermatogenesis within testes
Epididymis	1. Storage of some sperm 2. Final sperm maturation 3. Location where sperm develop ability to be motile
Vas deferens	1. Storage of sperm 2. Conduction of sperm from epididymis to urethra
Seminal vesicles, prostate, and bulbourethral glands	1. Secretion of seminal fluids that carry sperm and provide the following: • Nourishment of sperm • Protection of sperm from hostile acidic environment of vagina • Enhancement of motility of sperm • Washing of all sperm from urethra

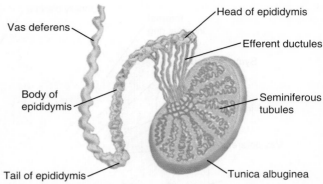

FIG. 3.10 Internal Structures of the Testis. Initial production of sperm begins within the tiny, coiled seminiferous tubules. Immature sperm pass from the seminiferous tubules to the epididymis and then to the vas deferens. During their passage through these structures, sperm mature and acquire the ability to propel themselves after ejaculation.

Accessory Ducts and Glands

From the seminiferous tubules, sperm pass into the epididymis within the scrotum for storage and final maturation. In the epididymis, sperm develop the ability to be motile, although secretions within the epididymis inhibit actual motility until ejaculation occurs.

The epididymis empties into the vas deferens, where larger numbers of sperm are stored. The vas deferens leads upward into the pelvis and then downward toward the penis through the internal and external inguinal rings. Within the pelvis the vas deferens joins the ejaculatory duct before connecting to the urethra.

Three glands—the seminal vesicles, the prostate, and the bulbourethral gland—secrete seminal fluids that carry sperm into the vagina during intercourse. The seminal fluid has four functions: (1) nourishing the sperm, (2) protecting the sperm from the hostile pH (acidic) environment of the vagina, (3) enhancing the motility of the sperm, and (4) washing the sperm from the urethra to maximize the number deposited in the vagina.

KNOWLEDGE CHECK

19. What are the two functions of the penis?
20. What two types of erectile tissue are in the penis? What is their function?
21. Why is it important for the testes to be contained within the scrotum?
22. What are the two functions of the testes?

SUMMARY CONCEPTS

- Initial prenatal development of the reproductive organs is similar for both males and females. If a critical part of the Y chromosome is not present at conception, female reproductive structures will develop.
- During puberty the reproductive organs become fully functional, and secondary sex characteristics develop.
- Puberty begins approximately 6 months to 1 year earlier in girls than in boys, although the early growth spurt in girls makes it seem they begin puberty much earlier compared with boys.
- Females are generally shorter than males at the completion of puberty because they begin their growth spurt at an earlier age and complete it more quickly than boys.

- Girls often do not ovulate in early menstrual cycles, although they can ovulate even before the first cycle. Therefore a girl can become pregnant before her first menstrual period if she is sexually active.
- The onset of puberty is more subtle in boys than in girls, beginning with growth of the testes and penis.
- Boys may have nocturnal emissions of seminal fluid, which may be distressing if the boy has not been educated that these events are normal and expected.
- At birth, a girl has all the ova she will ever have. New ova are not formed after birth; most are depleted when the woman reaches the climacteric.

- The female reproductive cycle is often called the *menstrual cycle*. It includes changes in the anterior pituitary gland, ovaries, and uterine endometrium to prepare for a fertilized ovum. The character of cervical mucus also changes during the cycle to encourage fertilization.
- Breast size is unrelated to glandular tissue or the quantity or quality of milk a woman can produce for her infant after birth. Breast size is primarily related to the amount of fat present.

- For normal sperm formation, a man's testes must be cooler than his core body temperature.
- Seminal fluids secreted by the seminal vesicles, the prostate, and the bulbourethral glands nourish and protect the sperm, enhance their motility, and ensure most sperm are deposited in the vagina during sexual intercourse.

REFERENCES & READINGS

Blackburn, S. T. (2013). *Maternal, fetal, and neonatal physiology: A clinical perspective* (4th ed.). St. Louis, MO: Saunders.

Hall, J. C. (2016). *Guyton and Hall textbook of medical physiology* (13th ed.). Philadelphia, PA: Saunders.

Maron, D. F. (2015). Why girls are starting puberty earlier. *Scientific America, 312*(5), 28–30.

Moore, K. L., Persaud, T. V. N., & Torchia, M. G. (2013). *Before we are born: Essentials of embryology and birth defects* (8th ed.). Philadelphia, PA: Saunders.

Hereditary and Environmental Influences on Childbearing

Tania Lopez

After studying this chapter, you should be able to:

1. Describe the structure and function of normal human genes and chromosomes.
2. Give examples of ways to study genes and chromosomes.
3. Explain benefits and ethical implications of the Human Genome Project.
4. Describe the characteristics of single gene traits and their transmission from parent to child.
5. Relate chromosomal abnormalities to spontaneous abortion and birth defects in the infant.
6. Explain characteristics of multifactorial birth defects.
7. Identify environmental factors that can interfere with prenatal development and ways to prevent or reduce their negative effects.
8. Describe genetic counseling.
9. Explain the role of the nurse in caring for individuals or families with concerns about birth defects.

Hereditary and environmental forces shape a person's development from before conception until death. As people learn more about genes and their influences on the body's function, they are discovering genes have more influence on health, disease, and medication effectiveness than was previously thought. The nurse needs a basic knowledge of these forces to better understand disorders evident at birth *(congenital)* and those that develop later in life. This chapter reviews the basics of hereditary influences on development and the impact of environmental factors in causing *birth defects*. The nursing role in relation to genetic knowledge is also discussed.

HEREDITARY INFLUENCES

Hereditary, or **genetic**, influences pertain to development results that direct cellular functions provided by genes that constitute the 46 chromosomes in every somatic cell. Disorders can result if too much or too little genetic material is present in the cells and if one or more genes are abnormal and provide incorrect directions.

Structure of Genes and Chromosomes

A review of the structure of genes and chromosomes aids in understanding the reasons for the occurrence of disorders. Chromosomes are composed of genes that in turn are composed of deoxyribonucleic acid (DNA) (Fig. 4.1).

Deoxyribonucleic Acid

DNA is the building block of genes and chromosomes. Its three units are (1) a sugar (deoxyribose), (2) a phosphate group, and (3) one of four nitrogen bases (adenine, thymine, guanine, and cytosine).

DNA resembles a spiral ladder, with a sugar and a phosphate group forming each side of the ladder and a pair of nitrogen bases forming each rung of the ladder. The four bases of the DNA molecule pair in a fixed way, allowing the DNA to be accurately duplicated during each cell division.

- Adenine pairs with thymine.
- Guanine pairs with cytosine.

The DNA also directs the manufacture of proteins needed for cell function. The sequence of bases within the DNA determines which amino acids will be assembled to form a protein and the order in which they will be assembled for cell processes. Some proteins form the structure of body cells, whereas others are enzymes that control metabolic processes within the cell. If the sequence of nitrogen bases in the DNA is incorrect or some bases are missing or added in critical places, a defect in body structure or function may result.

Bases are arranged in groups of three called *codons* for translation into a specific amino acid in the cell. For example, a triplet base codon may consist of the bases GCC (guanine, cytosine, cytosine), which tells the cell to produce the amino acid alanine. Other codons, known as *stop codons,* signal the end of a gene sequence.

Genes

A **gene** is a segment of DNA that directs the production of a specific product needed for body structure or function. Humans have 23,000 genes arranged on their chromosomes. Only a portion of the long strand of DNA that forms a chromosome makes a single gene. Some genes are active only during prenatal life, and others become functional at various times after birth. Gene regulation is the process of turning genes on

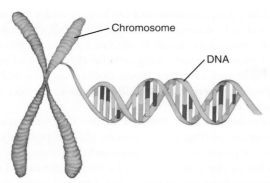

FIG. 4.1 The DNA helix is the building block of genes and chromosomes.

and off. During early development, cells begin to take on specific functions. Gene regulation ensures the appropriate genes are expressed at the proper times. Gene regulation also helps an organism respond to its environment. Gene regulation is accomplished by a variety of mechanisms, including chemical modification of genes and the use of regulatory proteins to turn genes on or off (Hall, 2016; Jorde, Carey, & Bamshad, 2016; National Human Genome Research Institute [NHGRI], 2016a).

Genes that code for the same trait often have two or more alternative forms, or **alleles**. Familiar examples of alleles are the ABO blood types. Normal alleles provide genetic variation and sometimes a biologic advantage. If an allele occurs at least 1% of the time in the population, it is called a **polymorphism**.

Some changed gene forms, or **mutations**, may be harmless, but many are harmful, such as those that cause the production of abnormal hemoglobin in sickle cell disease. Mutations may cause harm by the following actions:
- Substituting incorrect bases for the normal bases
- Interrupting the normal gene sequence or stopping it prematurely
- Duplicating some bases or entire gene sequences
- Adding or subtracting some bases within those making up a gene's sequence of bases, which will alter the amino acids it causes to be assembled

A mutation may occur in **gametes** (reproductive or germ cells) or **somatic cells** (other body cells). If the mutation occurs in a gamete, the mutation can be transmitted from one generation to the next. Mutations occurring in somatic cells are often associated with malignant change, but they are not transmitted from generation to generation.

Genes are too small to be seen under a microscope, but they can be studied in the following ways:
- By measuring the products they direct cells to produce, such as an enzyme or other substance
- By directly studying the gene's DNA
- By analyzing the gene's close association (linkage) with another gene that can be studied in one of the previous two ways

The tissue used for study of a gene depends on where the gene product is present in the body and the available technology. These tissues may include blood, skin cells, hair follicles, and fetal cells from the amniotic fluid or chorionic villi.

Genes that can be identified by direct analysis of DNA can be studied in any cells containing a nucleus, even if the gene product is not present in that tissue. Although not always used, DNA analysis of the blastomere (eight-cell stage of prenatal development) can be used to select embryos to be implanted in the uterus after in-vitro fertilization. This prevents implantation of embryos with a specific gene defect or common chromosome defects.

The National Human Genome Research Institute is part of the National Institutes of Health. The Human Genome Project is an international effort started in 1990 to identify all genes contained in the human body. Benefits of greater knowledge about specific human genes include the following:
- Performing genetic testing to determine the risk for a disorder or the actual or probable presence of the disorder
- Basing reproductive decisions on more accurate and specific information than has previously been available
- Identifying genetic susceptibility to a disorder so interventions to reduce risk can be instituted
- Using gene therapy to modify a defective gene
- Modifying therapy such as medication based on an individual's genetic code or the genetic makeup of tumor cells
- Individualizing treatment or medications for a specific person

The explosion of knowledge about the genetic basis for many diseases raises many legal and ethical issues for which we do not yet have answers (Box 4.1). As our knowledge base grows, new issues are likely to emerge:
- Genetic information has implications for others in the person's family, raising privacy issues.
- Knowledge about a genetic disorder often precedes knowledge about treatment of the disorder.
- Identification of genetic problems could lead to poor self-esteem, guilt, and excessive caution, or, conversely, a reckless lifestyle.
- Presymptomatic identification of genetically influenced illness would be a source of long-term anxiety.
- Genetic knowledge could affect one's choice of a partner.

Concern about employment or insurance coverage related to genetic tests was addressed in the United States in 2008 with the enactment of the Genetic Information Nondiscrimination Act (GINA). Insurance companies and employers are prohibited from discriminating on the basis of information from genetic tests. Insurance companies are prohibited from discriminating in ways such as canceling, denying, refusing to renew, or changing the terms or premiums based solely on a genetic predisposition toward a specific disease. Employers are prohibited from using genetic information when making employment decisions. A genetic test cannot be demanded by an employer or insurance company. The GINA document further clarified genetic information as part of an individual's health information, and this rule was implemented in 2013 (NHGRI, 2016b; White House Press Release, 2008).

Chromosomes

Genes are organized in 46 paired **chromosomes** in the nucleus of somatic cells. A gene can be likened to a single bead; a

BOX 4.1 Ethical Issues Created by Greater Genetic Knowledge

- Should testing be offered for a genetic disease for which no treatment is available? What if the disease is fatal? Should testing be required if a person may carry a diagnosable disorder that might be passed on to his or her children, even if the person does not want the test?
- Huntington's disease is an example of a genetic disease that can be diagnosed. It has serious effects, with a fatal outcome during midlife. Should testing be offered? Should it be required before the person is allowed to reproduce?
- Who should own and control genetic information? Does an insurer have the right to a person's genetic information to assess risk and therefore set more accurate rates? Or is this information private? Should this information be disregarded for everyone when insurance rates are set? Geneticists may have the ability to identify conditions that a person will develop in the future even if the problem is not present. Examples include hypertension, diabetes, and heart disease. If an insurance company knows the person will develop this disorder, rates would be higher or coverage would be denied. If an employer has this information, the person might not be hired, to avoid raising insurance costs for the company. Yet the reverse could be true. Genetic testing might prove a person *would not* develop a disorder, thereby gaining them lower rates. If genetic testing before being insured is not permitted, is it right that all persons insured by a company subsidize those who develop disorders that could have been determined before being insured by paying higher rates?
- How should issues of racial or ethnic identification be handled? What if a person's parentage is not what he or she has always believed? Discoveries in the process of genetic analysis may determine that a person is not of the racial identity previously thought, or a person might discover a parent is not the biologic parent. What should be done if information of this nature is uncovered? What are possible implications for self-image and identity? How might other members of the family be involved in the unexpected discovery?

chromosome is like a string of beads. Each chromosome is composed of varying numbers of genes. A total of 22 chromosome pairs are **autosomes** (non-sex chromosomes), and the twenty-third pair is composed of the **sex chromosomes**, XX (female) or XY (male). Added, missing, and structurally abnormal chromosomes are usually harmful. **Homologous** chromosomes carry matching genetic information; that is, they have the same genes in the same sequence.

Mature gametes have half the chromosomes (23) of other body cells. One chromosome from each pair is distributed randomly in the gametes, allowing variation of genetic traits among people. When the ovum and sperm unite at conception, the total is restored to 46 paired chromosomes.

Cells for full chromosome analysis must have a nucleus and be living. Chromosomes can be studied by using any of several types of cells: white blood cells, skin fibroblasts, bone marrow cells, and fetal cells from the chorionic villi of the placenta or suspended in amniotic fluid.

Unlike genes, chromosomes can be seen under the microscope but only during cell division for a full chromosome analysis. Specimens should be obtained and preserved carefully to provide enough living cells for chromosomal analysis. Temperature extremes, blood clotting, and the addition of improper preservatives can kill the cells and render them useless for analysis.

Chromosomes look jumbled before they are arranged into a karyotype (Fig. 4.2). Systematic study is possible using imaging of prepared chromosomes and then arranging them into a **karyotype** (Fig. 4.3). In a karyotype, autosomal pairs are arranged from largest to smallest. Letters describe groups of similar size and appearance. Sex chromosomes may be arranged in a separate group.

A person's karyotype is abbreviated by a combination of numbers and letters. The number describes the total number of chromosomes, followed by either an XX to indicate the sex chromosomes are female or an XY to indicate they are male. Therefore the chromosome complement is abbreviated as 46,XX for a normal female and as 46,XY for a normal male. If the chromosome number or structure is abnormal, as in Down's syndrome (trisomy 21), which has an extra 21 chromosome, an added abbreviation indicates the abnormality: 47 (total number of chromosomes), XY (male), + 21 (the number of the extra chromosome). Other abbreviations describe karyotypes with missing or structurally altered chromosomes.

Finer chromosome analysis uses fluorescent-labeled DNA probes that attach to specific chromosomes. This technique is called fluorescence in-situ hybridization (FISH) and permits testing for added, missing, or rearranged chromosome material that otherwise may not be visible microscopically. FISH analysis can be done rapidly because stimulation of cells to divide is not required as in other types of chromosome analysis. Another more specific chromosome analysis is the comparative genomic hybridization used to identify losses or duplications of specific chromosome regions, which often occur in tumor cells.

? KNOWLEDGE CHECK

1. What is the relationship among DNA, genes, and chromosomes?
2. Can genes be studied by examining them under a microscope? Why or why not? What methods are used to study them?
3. Why do cell specimens for chromosomal analysis have to be alive, regardless of the tissue used?
4. What do each of these abbreviations mean: 46XY and 46XX? How are chromosome abnormalities described?

Transmission of Traits by Single Genes

Inherited characteristics are passed from parent to child by the genes in each chromosome. These traits are classified according to whether they are **dominant** (strong) or **recessive** (weak) and whether the gene is located on one of the autosome pairs or on the sex chromosomes. Both normal and

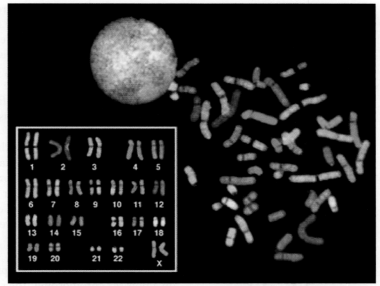

FIG. 4.2 Before arrangement in a karyotype, chromosomes appear jumbled. This photo is a spectral karyotype from a normal female. (From National Human Genome Research Institute. [2011]. Retrieved from www.genome.gov/).

abnormal hereditary characteristics are transmitted by these mechanisms.

Because humans have pairs of matched chromosomes, except for the sex chromosomes in the male, they have one allele for a gene at the same location on each member of the chromosome pair. The paired alleles may be identical (**homozygous**) or different (**heterozygous**).

Some genes, both normal and abnormal, occur more frequently in certain groups than in the population as a whole. For example, the gene that causes Tay-Sachs disease on chromosome 15 is carried by approximately 1 of every 30 U.S. Jews. This rate is also similar in persons of French-Canadian ancestry and members of the Cajun population in Louisiana and is approximately 100 times its occurrence in the general population (Jorde, et al., 2016; National Tay-Sachs and Allied Diseases Association [NTSAD], 2016). Because the abnormal gene occurs more frequently in these groups, their incidence of Tay-Sachs disease is also higher. Other disorders that are more common in certain ethnic groups are cystic fibrosis, which occurs primarily in whites of northern European descent, and sickle cell disease, which occurs more frequently in people of African descent.

Dominance

Dominance describes the way a person's **genotype** (genetic composition) is translated into the **phenotype**, or observable characteristics. In the case of a dominant gene, one copy is enough to cause the trait to be expressed. For example, in the ABO blood system, genes for types A and B are dominant. Therefore a single copy of either of these genes is enough for it to be expressed in the person's blood type.

Two identical copies of a recessive gene are required for the trait to be expressed. The gene for blood type O is recessive.

Laboratory testing identifies a person's blood type as O only if that person receives a gene for blood type O from both parents. If the person receives a gene for type O from one parent and type A from the other parent, blood type A is expressed in laboratory blood typing.

On the basis of dominant and recessive forms of a gene, a person with type A blood can have one of the following two possible combinations of gene alleles:

- Two type A alleles
- One type A allele and one type O allele

Other alleles are equally dominant. The person who receives a gene for blood type A from one parent and type B from the other will have type AB blood because both alleles are equally dominant and expressed in blood typing.

Dominance and recessiveness are relative qualities for many genes. Some people with a single copy of an abnormal recessive gene (carriers) may have a lower than normal level of the gene product (e.g., an enzyme) that can be detected by biochemical methods. These people often do not have overt disease because the normal copy of the gene produces enough of the required product to allow normal or near-normal function.

Chromosome Location

Genes located on autosomes are either autosomal dominant or autosomal recessive, depending on the number of identical copies of the gene needed to produce the trait. However, genes located on the X chromosome are paired only in females because males have one X chromosome and one Y chromosome.

A female with an abnormal recessive gene on one of her X chromosomes usually has a normal gene on the other X chromosome that compensates and maintains relatively normal

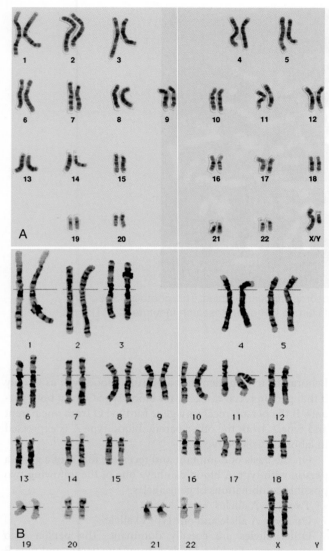

FIG. 4.3 Karyotypes of chromosomes that were stained, creating bands to distinguish each chromosome and identify missing or duplicated chromosome material. **A,** Normal male karyotype: 46,XY. **B,** Normal female karyotype: 46,XX. (**A,** from National Human Genome Research Institute. [2016]. *Digital media database: Karyotype.* Retrieved from www.genome. gov; **B,** from Jorde, L. B., Carey, J. C., & Bamshad, M. J. [2010]. *Medical genetics* [4th ed.]. Philadelphia, PA: Mosby.)

function. However, the male is at a disadvantage if his lone X chromosome has an abnormal gene. The male has no compensating normal gene because his other sex chromosome is a Y. The abnormal gene is expressed in the male because it is unopposed by a normal gene.

Patterns of Single Gene Inheritance

Three major patterns of single gene inheritance are autosomal dominant, autosomal recessive, and X-linked (Box 4.2). Few genes are found on the Y chromosome, primarily the one that causes the embryo to differentiate into a male (Jorde et al., 2016; Nussbaum, McInnes, & Willard, 2016). Because few Y-linked traits have been identified, these will not be discussed.

Although the word **pedigree** is widely used among genetic professionals, the nurse may need to interpret it for the patient. Be cautious when referring to the illustration of a family's genetic history as a *pedigree* because some associate the word only with animals. For example, when taking a genetic family history, the nurse might say, "I'm going to use several symbols to depict your family tree and its members' health histories. This diagram is called a *genogram*, but it's also often called a *pedigree*."

Single gene traits have mathematically predictable and fixed rates of occurrence. For example, if a couple has a child with an autosomal recessive disorder, the risk that future children will have the same disorder is 1 in 4 (25%) at every conception. The risk is the same at every conception, regardless of how many of a couple's children have been affected.

Autosomal Dominant Traits

An autosomal dominant trait is produced by a dominant gene on a non-sex chromosome. The expression of abnormal autosomal dominant genes may result in multiple and seemingly unrelated effects in the person. The gene's effects also may vary substantially in severity, leading a family to believe incorrectly that a trait skips a generation. A careful physical examination may reveal subtle evidence of the trait in each generation. In other cases, some people may carry the dominant gene but have no apparent expression of it in their physical makeup.

In some autosomal dominant disorders, such as Huntington's disease, those with the gene will always have the disease if they live to the age at which the disorder becomes apparent. In other disorders, only a portion of those carrying the gene ever exhibit the disease.

New mutations account for the introduction of abnormal autosomal dominant traits into a family with no history of the disorder. In this case, parents of the child are not affected because their body cells do not have the altered gene (Jorde et al., 2016; Nussbaum et al., 2016).

The person who is affected by an autosomal dominant disorder is usually heterozygous for the gene; that is, the person has a normal gene on one chromosome and an abnormal gene on the other chromosome of the pair. Occasionally, a person receives two copies of the same abnormal autosomal dominant gene. Such an individual is usually much more severely affected than someone with only one copy.

Autosomal Recessive Traits

An autosomal recessive trait occurs if a person receives two copies of a recessive gene carried on an autosome. Everyone is estimated to carry abnormal autosomal recessive genes without manifesting the disorder because everyone has a compensating normal gene. Because of the low probability of two unrelated people sharing even one of the same abnormal genes, the incidence of autosomal recessive diseases is relatively low in the general population.

Situations that increase the likelihood that two parents share the same abnormal autosomal recessive gene are as follows:
- Consanguinity (blood relationship of the parents): Blood relatives have more genes in common, including abnormal ones.

BOX 4.2 **Single Gene Traits**

Genogram (Pedigree) Symbols

A genogram symbolically represents a family's medical history and the relationships of its members to one another. It helps identify patterns of inheritance that may help distinguish one type of disorder from another.

☐ Male

◯ Female

◇ Sex not specified
(number indicates the number of persons represented by the symbol)

■ ● Affected

◧ ◐ Carriers (heterozygous) for an autosomal recessive trait

⊙ Female carrier of an X-linked recessive trait

⊘ Deceased

☐—◯ Mating/marriage

☐═◯ Consanguineous mating/marriage

I Roman numerals indicate generations

Autosomal Recessive
Characteristics

Two autosomal recessive genes are required to produce the trait.

Males and females are equally likely to have the trait.

There is often no prior family history of the disorder before the first affected child.

If more than one family member is affected, they are usually full siblings.

Consanguinity (close blood relationship) of the parents increases the risk for the disorder.

Disorders are more likely to occur in groups isolated by geography, culture, religion, or other factors.

Some autosomal recessive disorders are more common in specific ethnic groups.

Transmission of Trait from Parent to Child

Unaffected parents are carriers of the abnormal autosomal recessive trait.

Children of carriers have a 25% (1 in 4) chance for receiving both copies of the defective gene and thus having the disorder.

Children of carriers have a 50% (1 in 2) chance of receiving one copy of the gene and being carriers like the parents.

Children of carriers have a 25% (1 in 4) chance of receiving both copies of the normal gene. They are neither carriers nor affected.

Examples

Normal traits: Blood group O, Rh-negative blood factor.

Abnormal traits: Tay-Sachs disease, sickle cell disease, cystic fibrosis.

Genogram

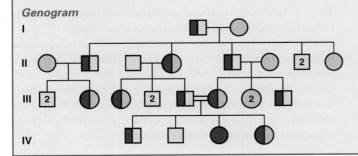

Autosomal Dominant
Characteristics

A single copy of the gene is enough to produce the trait.

Males and females are equally likely to have the trait.

Often appears in every generation of a family, although family members having the trait may have widely varying manifestations of it.

May have multiple and seemingly unrelated effects on body structure and function.

Transmission of Trait from Parent to Child

A parent with the trait has a 50% (1 in 2) chance of passing the trait to the child.

The trait may arise as a new mutation from an unaffected parent. The child who receives the mutated gene can then transmit it to future generations.

Examples

Normal traits: Blood groups A and B, Rh-positive blood factor.

Abnormal traits: Huntington's disease, neurofibromatosis.

Genogram

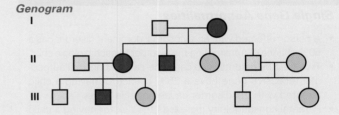

X-Linked Recessive
Characteristics

Although recessive, only one copy of the gene is needed to cause the disorder in males, who do not have a compensating X without the trait.

Males are affected, with rare exceptions.

Females are carriers of the trait but not usually adversely affected.

Affected males are related to one another through carrier females.

Affected males do not transmit the trait to their sons.

Transmission of Trait from Parent to Child

Males who have the disorder transmit the gene to 100% of their daughters and none of their sons.

Sons of carrier females have a 50% (1 in 2) chance of being affected. They also have a 50% chance of being unaffected.

Daughters of carrier females have a 50% (1 in 2) chance of being carriers like their mothers. They also have a 50% chance of being neither affected nor carriers.

A new X-linked recessive gene also may arise by mutation.

Examples

Colorblindness, Duchenne's muscular dystrophy, hemophilia A.

Genogram

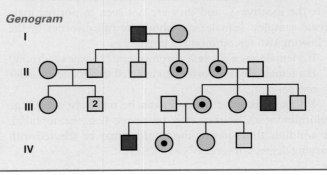

- Groups isolated by culture, geography, religion, or other factors: The isolation allows abnormal genes to become concentrated over the years and occur at a greater frequency than in more diverse groups.

Many autosomal recessive disorders are severe, and affected persons may not live long enough to reproduce. Two notable exceptions are phenylketonuria (PKU) and cystic fibrosis. Improved care of people with these disorders has allowed them to live into their reproductive years. If one member of the couple has the autosomal recessive disorder, all their children will be carriers. Their child's risk for having similarly affected children is also higher, depending on the prevalence of the abnormal gene in the general population and the likelihood that their mate is a carrier (American College of Obstetricians and Gynecologists [ACOG], 2015)

CRITICAL TO REMEMBER

Single Gene Abnormalities

- A person affected with an autosomal dominant disorder has a 50% chance of transmitting the disorder to each biologic child.
- Two healthy parents who carry the same abnormal autosomal recessive gene have a 25% chance of having a child affected with the disorder caused by this gene.
- Parental consanguinity increases the risk for having a child with an autosomal recessive disorder.
- One copy of an abnormal X-linked recessive gene is enough to produce the disorder in a male.
- Abnormal genes can arise as new mutations. If these mutations are in the gametes, they are transmitted to future generations.

X-Linked Traits

X-linked recessive traits are more common than X-linked dominant traits and are the only X-linked pattern discussed in this chapter. Gender differences in the occurrence of X-linked recessive traits and the relationship of affected males to one another are important factors distinguishing these disorders from autosomal dominant and recessive disorders. In general, males are the only ones to show full effects of an X-linked recessive disorder because their only X chromosome has the abnormal gene on it. One of the two X chromosomes is inactivated randomly in a normal female embryo. The active X chromosome in cells usually provides adequate cell function, although one of the two X chromosomes is inactivated. Barr bodies seen in female cells indicate the inactive X, and they are not seen in normal male tissue samples. Females can show the full disorder in the following two uncommon circumstances:

- If a female has a single X chromosome (Turner syndrome)
- If a female child is born to an affected father and a carrier mother

X-linked recessive disorders can be relatively mild (e.g., colorblindness), or they may be severe (e.g., hemophilia). In addition, those having the disorder may be affected with varying degrees of severity.

KNOWLEDGE CHECK

5. If a parent has an autosomal dominant disorder, what are the chances the child will have the same disorder?
6. Why would parents who are first cousins be more likely to have a child with an autosomal recessive disorder?
7. If each member of a couple carries the gene for an autosomal recessive disorder, what are the chances the children will have the disorder? What are the chances the children will be carriers? What are the chances the children will not receive the abnormal gene from either parent?
8. Why are males more often affected by X-linked recessive disorders? If a female carries an X-linked recessive disorder such as hemophilia, what are the chances her sons will have the disorder? What are the chances her daughters will be carriers?

Chromosomal Abnormalities

Chromosomal abnormalities can be numerical or structural. They are quite common (≥50%) in the embryo or fetus spontaneously aborted (miscarried). Chromosomal abnormalities often cause major defects because they involve deletion or duplication of many genes. The normal number of chromosomes in body cells other than reproductive cells is 46, referred to as **diploid**.

Numerical Abnormalities

Numerical chromosomal abnormalities involve added or missing single chromosomes or multiple sets of chromosomes. **Trisomy** and **monosomy** are numerical abnormalities of single chromosomes. The term **polyploidy** refers to abnormalities involving full sets of chromosomes.

Trisomy. A trisomy exists when each body cell contains an extra copy of one chromosome, bringing the total number to 47 (Fig. 4.4). Each chromosome is normal, but too many are present in each somatic cell. The most common trisomy is Down's syndrome, or trisomy 21, in which three copies of chromosome 21 are in each somatic cell. Trisomies of chromosomes 13 and 18 are less common and have more severe effects. The incidence of bearing children with trisomies increases with maternal age, so most women who are 35 years or older and become pregnant are offered prenatal diagnostic screening to determine whether the fetus has Down's syndrome or another trisomy.

Infants with Down's syndrome have characteristic features usually noticed at birth (Fig. 4.5). Chromosomal analysis is performed during the neonatal period to confirm the diagnosis and determine whether Down's syndrome is caused by trisomy 21 or a rarer chromosomal anomaly involving a structural rather than a numerical abnormality of chromosome 21.

Children with Down's syndrome reach developmental milestones more slowly than unaffected children. Their intellectual development is delayed, although the severity varies, just as intelligence varies in the general population. Early intervention programs and regular medical care help these children reach their full ability and manage the physical problems associated with Down's syndrome.

Klinefelter syndrome is a trisomy of the sex chromosomes. Males with Klinefelter syndrome (47,XXY) are taller than average, may have a lower intelligence and gynecomastia (larger breasts), and are usually sterile. Testosterone therapy and mastectomy for enlarged breasts may be done. Other sex chromosome trisomies possibly encountered include 47,XXX or 47,XYY (Jorde et al., 2016).

Monosomy. A monosomy exists when each body cell has a missing chromosome, with a total number of 45. The only monosomy compatible with postnatal life is Turner syndrome, or monosomy X (Fig. 4.6). Over 99% of conceptions with the 45,XO karyotype are lost in spontaneous abortion (Carlson, 2014; Jorde et al., 2016; Moore, Persaud, & Torcheria, 2016a).

The person with Turner syndrome has a single X chromosome and is always female.

Large cystic masses on either side of the neck (cystic hygromas) may be found on routine ultrasonography and lead to the diagnosis. Liveborn infants have excess skin around the neck left from the hygromas and edema most noticeable in the hands and feet during infancy. If Turner syndrome is not identified and treated during infancy or childhood, an affected girl will remain very short and will not have menstrual periods or develop secondary sex characteristics. Children with Turner syndrome usually have normal intelligence, although they may have difficulty with spatial relationships or with solving visual problems such as reading a map. The girl may have a broad, shieldlike chest with widely spaced nipples. Her kidneys may be joined at their upper poles (horseshoe kidney), and coarctation of the aorta may require corrective surgery. Treatment with estrogen at the age of puberty promotes development of secondary sexual characteristics. Continuing estrogen throughout life reduces development of osteoporosis (Jorde et al., 2016).

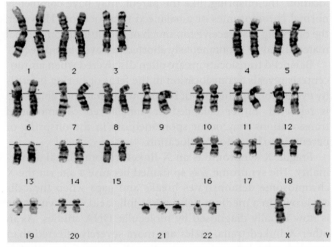

FIG. 4.4 Karyotype of a male with trisomy 21 (Down's syndrome: 47,XY,+ 21). (From Jorde, L. B., Carey, J. C., & Bamshad, M. J. [2016]. *Medical genetics* [4th ed., p. 107]. Philadelphia, PA: Elsevier.)

CRITICAL TO REMEMBER
Chromosome Abnormalities

Chromosome abnormalities are either numerical or structural.

Numerical	Structural
Entire single chromosome added (trisomy)	Part of a chromosome missing or added
Entire single chromosome missing (monosomy)	Rearrangements of material within chromosome(s)
One or more added sets of chromosomes, resulting in cells containing 69 (triploidy) or 92 (tetraploidy) chromosomes	Two chromosomes that adhere to each other
	Fragility of a specific site, such as on the X chromosome ("fragile X syndrome")

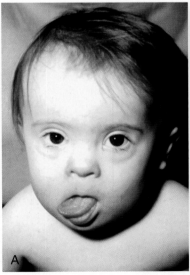
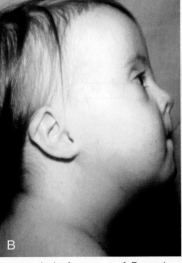
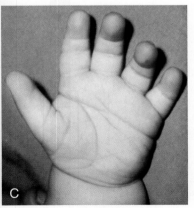

FIG. 4.5 Infant with several characteristic features of Down's syndrome, or trisomy 21. Note the infant has a flat face and occiput, low-set ears, and a protruding tongue. Also note the single transverse palm crease and a single crease on her fifth finger. (From Jones, K. L. [2013]. *Smith's recognizable patterns of human malformation* [7th ed.]. Philadelphia, PA: Saunders.)

Polyploidy. Polyploidy may occur when gametes do not halve their chromosome number during meiosis and retain both members of each pair or when two sperm fertilize an ovum simultaneously. The result is an embryo with one or more extra sets of chromosomes. The total number of chromosomes is a multiple of the **haploid** number of 23 (69 or 92 total chromosomes). Polyploidy usually results in an early spontaneous abortion but may occasionally be seen in a liveborn infant. This abnormality may be found in chorionic villus sampling (see Chapter 9) and may reflect an abnormality of the chorionic villi rather than of the fetus.

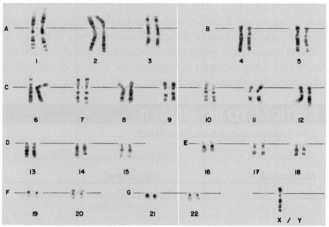

FIG. 4.6 Karyotype of a female with monosomy X (Turner syndrome: 45,X). (Courtesy Dr. Mary Jo Harrod, University of Texas Southwestern Medical Center, Dallas, TX.)

Structural Abnormalities

Chromosomal abnormalities may involve the structure of one or more chromosomes. Part of a chromosome may be missing or added, or DNA within the chromosome may be rearranged. Some of these rearrangements are common harmless variations. Others are harmful because important genetic material is lost or duplicated in the structural abnormality or the position of the genes in relation to other genes is altered so that their normal function is not possible.

Another structural abnormality occurs when all or part of a chromosome is attached to another (**translocation**) (Fig. 4.7). Many people with a translocation chromosomal abnormality are clinically normal because the total of their genetic material is normal or balanced. If a parent has a balanced translocation, the offspring, like the parent, may have completely normal chromosomes or a balanced translocation. However, the offspring may receive too much or too little chromosomal material and be spontaneously aborted or have birth defects.

Balanced translocations are often discovered when amniocentesis reveals a translocation in the fetus or during infertility evaluations if a history of recurrent spontaneous abortions is reported. Either balanced or unbalanced chromosomal translocations may occur spontaneously in the offspring of parents who have no translocation.

Fragile X syndrome is an X-linked chromosomal abnormality. The syndrome was so named because a site on the X chromosome demonstrates breaks and gaps when the cells are grown in a medium deficient in folic acid. The syndrome is now usually diagnosed by molecular DNA studies. As in other X-linked traits, males are more severely affected than females, who have a compensating X chromosome that is

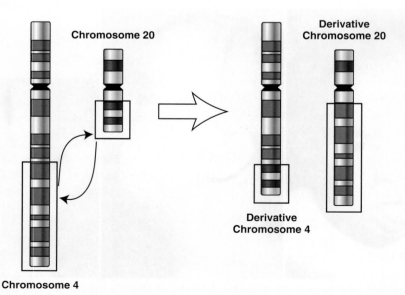

BEFORE TRANSLOCATION   **AFTER TRANSLOCATION**

Chromosome 20

Derivative Chromosome 20

Derivative Chromosome 4

Chromosome 4

FIG. 4.7 Illustration of a translocation of chromosome material between chromosomes 4 and 20. (National Institutes of Health, National Human Genome Research Institute. [2017], *Talking glossary of genetic terms.* Retrieved from www.genome.gov/).

usually normal. Fragile X syndrome is the most common inherited form of male intellectual disability (Jorde et al., 2016; Moore et al., 2016a).

KNOWLEDGE CHECK

9. What is a chromosomal trisomy? Describe a common trisomy.
10. What is a chromosomal monosomy? Which monosomy is compatible with life?
11. Why are structural chromosomal abnormalities often harmful?
12. What are the possible outcomes of the offspring of a parent who has a balanced chromosomal translocation?

MULTIFACTORIAL DISORDERS

Multifactorial disorders result from an interaction of genetic and environmental factors. The genetic tendency toward the disorder is modified by the environment. These interactions may either positively or negatively influence prenatal and postnatal development. For example, two embryos may have an equal genetic susceptibility for the development of a disorder such as spina bifida (open spine). However, the disorder will not occur unless an environment that favors its development, for example, deficient maternal intake of folic acid, also exists.

Characteristics

Multifactorial birth defects are typically present and detectable at birth and isolated defects rather than defects that occur with unrelated abnormalities. However, a multifactorial defect may cause a secondary defect. For example, infants with spina bifida often have hydrocephalus (abnormal collection of spinal fluid within the brain) as well. The hydrocephalus is not a separate defect but one that occurs because the primary defect—abnormal development of the spine and spinal cord—disrupts spinal fluid circulation, allowing the fluid to accumulate within the brain's ventricular system.

However, the infant who has defects other than those known to be associated with spina bifida probably does not have a multifactorial disorder. In this case the spina bifida is more likely to be part of a syndrome such as a chromosome defect, which may pose a different risk for recurrence in a future child.

Multifactorial disorders are some of the most common birth defects encountered. Examples include the following (Driscoll, Simpson, Holzgreve, & Otaño, 2017):

- Heart defects
- Neural tube defects such as anencephaly (absence of most of the brain and skull), spina bifida, and encephalocele
- Cleft lip and cleft palate
- Pyloric stenosis

Risk for Occurrence

Unlike single gene traits, multifactorial disorders are not associated with a fixed risk for occurrence or recurrence in a family. Presence of a trait in a family (**familial**) means risks are an average rather than a constant percentage. Factors affecting the risk are as follows:

1. Number of affected close relatives—Risk increases as the number of affected close relatives (parent, full sibling, or child) increases.
2. Severity of the disorder in affected family members—For example, bilateral cleft lip is associated with a higher risk for recurrence in a close relative than is a unilateral cleft lip on one side of the upper lip.
3. Gender of the affected person(s)—For example, pyloric stenosis occurs five times as often in males as in females. The couple who has a daughter with pyloric stenosis faces a higher risk for recurrence with future children because the genetic influence for development of the defect is greater if a female develops it.
4. Geographic location—The risk for some disorders, such as neural tube defects, is more prevalent in one population than another. Because a group at greater risk often lives near others with the same risk, occurrence of the disorder may be more frequent in that area (Driscoll et al., 2017; Jorde et al., 2016).

CRITICAL TO REMEMBER
Multifactorial Birth Defects

- Multifactorial defects are some of the most common birth defects encountered in maternity and pediatric nursing practice.
- They are a result of interaction between a person's genetic susceptibility and environmental factors during prenatal development.
- These are usually single, isolated defects, although the primary defect may cause secondary defects.
- Some occur more often in certain geographic areas and among more closely related population groups.
- A greater risk for occurrence exists with the following:
  - Several close relatives have the defect, whether mild or severe.
  - One close relative has a severe form of the defect.
  - The defect occurs in a child of the less frequently affected gender.
- Infants who have several major or minor defects that are not directly related probably do not have a multifactorial defect but have another syndrome such as a chromosomal abnormality.

If multifactorial disorders had no environmental component, the risk for occurrence and recurrence would be a precise percentage rather than a range. However, if no genetic component exists (if the disorder were totally related to environment), the ability to predict the risk for occurrence or recurrence would be minimal.

ENVIRONMENTAL INFLUENCES

Environment, for example, good nutrition that supplies all necessary raw materials for fetal growth and adequate folic acid intake before conception, may positively influence prenatal development. However, some environmental influences such as *teratogens* (environmental agents) or mechanical forces that can cause defects as the baby develops are harmful.

Environmental influences on childbearing are those not known to have a genetic component. At one time, the placenta was thought to be a shield against harmful agents within a pregnant woman's body. Now it is recognized that most agents can cross the placenta and affect the developing fetus.

Teratogens

Teratogens are agents in the fetal environment that either cause or increase the likelihood that a birth defect will occur. Some drugs have been definitely established as safe or harmful. With most agents, however, their potential for harming the fetus is not clear. Several factors make it difficult to establish the teratogenic potential of an agent:

1. Retrospective study—Investigators must rely on the mother's memory about substances she ingested or was exposed to during pregnancy. The conclusion that a specific agent is harmful and the ways in which it harms the fetus is possible only when many cases are collected in which the exposure history is similar and the birth defects are also similar.
2. Timing of exposure—Agents may be harmful at one stage of prenatal development but not at another. Exposure may be harmful but may vary with the prenatal development stage.
3. Different susceptibility of organ systems—Some agents affect only one fetal organ system, or they affect one system at one stage of development and another at a different stage of development.
4. Uncontrolled fetal exposure—Exposures cannot be controlled to eliminate extraneous agents or ensure a consistent dose. Interactions with other agents may reduce or compound the fetal effects. An agent toxic at one dose may have no apparent effect at another.
5. Placental transfer—Agents vary in their ability to cross the placenta.
6. Individual variations—Fetuses show varying susceptibility to harmful agents.
7. Nontransferability of animal studies—Results of animal studies cannot always be applied to humans. Agents that do not harm animal fetuses may damage the human embryo or fetus.
8. Risk for damage from an uncontrolled maternal disorder—Some maternal disorders, such as epilepsy or hypertension, may cause fetal damage if not controlled. A poorly controlled maternal disorder raises a question of whether the disorder itself or the medication used to control the disorder harms the fetus.

Teratogens typically cause more than one defect, which distinguishes teratogenic defects from multifactorial disorders. However, children affected by single gene and chromosome defects are also likely to have multiple defects. Therefore

clinicians consider single gene disorders, chromosomal abnormalities, and effects of teratogenic agents when trying to diagnose an infant born with multiple anomalies.

Hundreds of individual agents are either known or suspected teratogens (Box 4.3). Types of teratogens include the following:

- Maternal infectious agents (e.g., viruses, bacteria) that cross the placenta
- Drugs and other substances used by the woman (e.g., therapeutic agents, illicit drugs, tobacco, alcohol)
- Pollutants, chemicals, and other substances to which the mother is exposed in her daily life
- Ionizing radiation
- Maternal hyperthermia
- Effects of maternal disorders such as diabetes mellitus and PKU

Theoretically, all or some of the risk to the developing fetus can be eliminated by avoiding exposure to the agent or changing the fetal environment in some way (Chambers & Scialli, 2014).

Preventing Fetal Exposure

Ideally, prevention of exposure to harmful influences begins before conception because all major organ systems develop early in pregnancy, often before a woman realizes she is

---

BOX 4.3 Selected Environmental Substances Known or Thought to Harm the Fetus

- Alcohol
- Aminoglycosides
- Anticonvulsant agents
- Antihyperlipidemic agents (statins)
- Antineoplastic agents
- Antithyroid drugs
- Cocaine
- Diethylstilbestrol (DES)
- Folic acid antagonists
- Infections
  - Cytomegalovirus
  - Herpes simplex virus
  - Human immunodeficiency virus
  - Parvo
  - Rubella
  - Syphilis
  - Toxoplasmosis
  - Varicella
  - Zika
- Lithium
- Mercury
- Retinoic acid
- Tetracycline
- Tobacco
- Warfarin

The nurse should adhere to new information about adverse fetal effects from these or other drugs given during pregnancy.

pregnant. To avoid some agents such as alcohol and illicit drugs, some pregnant women must be committed to making substantial lifestyle changes. The Office of Teratology Information Specialists is a source of information about drug use (includes therapeutic, illicit, and herbal), infections and vaccines, and maternal medical conditions, as well as exposure to common things such as caffeine, suntan beds, or fish (www.mothertobaby.org). This website also has fact sheets nurses can provide to expectant mothers regarding various substance exposures that may be cause for concern.

Infections. Rubella immunization 28 days (1 month) before conception virtually eliminates the risk that the mother will contract this infection, which may damage the fetus severely. If a woman becomes pregnant within 28 days after immunization, fetal risk is considered unlikely (American Academy of Pediatrics [AAP] & American College of Obstetricians and Gynecologists [ACOG], 2012; March of Dimes Birth Defect Foundation, 2012). For infections that cannot be prevented by immunization, the nurse may counsel the woman to avoid situations in which acquiring the disease is more likely.

Drugs and Other Substances. The U.S. Food and Drug Administration (FDA) established pregnancy categories for therapeutic drugs based on their potential to harm the fetus. The categories ranged from A through D and X. Class A drugs have no demonstrated fetal risk in well-controlled studies. At the opposite end, pregnancy category X drugs are well established as being harmful. Using this system, the provider should balance the woman's need for the drug's therapeutic effects against the fetal need to avoid exposure to it. In December, 2014, the FDA published the Pregnancy and Lactation Labeling Rule, which changed the content and format of labeling information for prescription drugs and biologic products. The new rule requires removal of the pregnancy categories A, B, C, D, and X from drug labels and replace it with information to assist the health care provider evaluate benefit and risk of the drug and counsel pregnant women and nursing mothers and assist them to make informed and educated decisions regarding the drug. The rule went into effect on June 30, 2015 and is to be phased in (FDA, 2016). A woman's use of botanical preparations should be considered because some are harmful during pregnancy.

Establishing whether an illicit drug can cause prenatal damage is difficult because women who use these substances often have other problems that complicate analysis of fetal effects. For example, these women may use multiple drugs and may have poor nutritional status, untreated sexually transmitted diseases (STDs), inadequate prenatal care, and stressful lives. In addition, illicit drugs are unlikely to be pure, and substances used to dilute them may themselves be harmful. Legal drugs may be combined with illegal drugs, and users may abuse legal drugs.

Drugs are often metabolized and excreted in urine, including drugs in the fetal system. Fetal blood levels of drug often remain high because the fetus swallows amniotic fluid containing excreted drug products, even after the drug has been eliminated by the mother's body.

The best action is for the woman to eliminate use of non-therapeutic drugs and substances such as alcohol. If she requires certain therapeutic drugs, the physician may be able to prescribe an alternative drug with a lower risk to the fetus or may eliminate nonessential therapeutic drugs such as acne medications.

Ionizing Radiation. Nonurgent radiologic procedures may be done during the first 2 weeks after the menstrual period begins, before ovulation occurs. For urgent procedures during pregnancy, the lower abdomen should be shielded with a lead apron, if possible. The radiation dose is kept as low as possible to reduce fetal exposure. Ultrasonography and magnetic resonance imaging are the imaging techniques of choice for pregnant women (ACOG, 2016).

Maternal Hyperthermia. An important teratogen is maternal hyperthermia. The mother's temperature may rise unavoidably during illness. Nurses should caution pregnant women to avoid deliberate exposure to heat sources such as saunas and hot tubs. Temperatures vary widely among public hot tubs, and a specific guideline for duration of exposure is difficult. The important factor is how high the woman's body temperature rises and for how long, not just the sauna or hot tub temperature. She should remain in a sauna or hot tub no more than 10 minutes and should keep her head and chest out of the water. Exposure to temperatures of 37.8°C (100°F) or higher is not advised (AAP & ACOG, 2012; Cunningham et al., 2014).

Manipulating the Fetal Environment

Appropriate medical therapy can help a woman prevent fetal damage that could result from her illness. For example, a woman who has diabetes should try to keep her blood glucose levels normal and stable before and during pregnancy for the best possible fetal outcomes. A woman with PKU should return to her special phenylalanine-free diet before conception to prevent high levels of phenylalanine in her body that will damage the fetus.

Consuming folic acid before and during pregnancy can decrease the risk of neural tube defects in the fetus (CDC, 2017). Neural tube defects occur early in gestation, before many women realize they are pregnant. Because nearly half of the pregnancies in the United States are unplanned, all women of childbearing age should consume at least 0.4 mg (400 mcg) of folic acid daily. Women who have had a child with a neural tube defect may need a higher amount of folic acid, 4 mg (4000 mcg), after consulting with their health care providers (CDC, 2017). The Centers for Disease Control and Prevention (CDC), March of Dimes Birth Defects Foundation, and National Council on Folic Acid have initiated a national campaign to educate women about the importance of consuming adequate folic acid every day (CDC, 2017). The neural tube closes during the fourth week after conception, often before the woman knows she is pregnant. Nurses can help make women aware of their need for a supplement of folic acid before conception to help reduce this serious birth defect.

Mechanical Disruptions to Fetal Development

Mechanical forces that interfere with normal prenatal development include oligohydramnios and fibrous amniotic bands.

Oligohydramnios, an abnormally small volume of amniotic fluid, reduces the cushion surrounding the fetus and may result in deformations such as clubfoot. Prolonged oligohydramnios can interfere with fetal lung development by interfering with normal branching and development of the alveoli. Oligohydramnios may not be the primary fetal problem but related to other fetal anomalies. Oligohydramnios also may be a sign of reduced placental blood flow that may occur in certain complications of pregnancy.

Fibrous amniotic bands may result from tears in the inner sac (amnion) of the fetal membranes and can result in fetal deformations or intrauterine limb amputation. Fibrous bands are usually sporadic and unlikely to recur. Because these bands can cause multiple defects, they may be confused with birth defects from other causes such as chromosome and single gene abnormalities (Carlson, 2014).

❓ KNOWLEDGE CHECK

13. What are the usual characteristics of multifactorial disorders?
14. What factors can vary the likelihood that a multifactorial disorder will occur or recur?
15. How can a woman avoid exposing her fetus to teratogens?
16. Why should a woman with phenylketonuria adhere to a low-phenylalanine diet before and during pregnancy?
17. Why is adequate folic acid intake before conception important?

GENETIC COUNSELING

Genetic counseling provides information and support to help people understand the genetic disorder they are concerned about and the risk for its occurrence in their family, and make informed decisions about testing and treatment.

Availability

Genetic counseling is often available through facilities that provide maternal-fetal medicine services. State departments of mental health, intellectual disability, and rehabilitation services also may provide counseling services. Local chapters of the March of Dimes are an important source of information about birth defects and counseling services. Fact sheets and other information about birth defects and their prevention are available at the March of Dimes website www.marchofdimes.com. Organizations that focus on specific birth defects provide valuable support and assistance in obtaining needed services for individuals and families affected by the disorder.

Focus on the Family

Genetic counseling focuses on the family, not merely on the affected individual. One family member may have a birth defect, but study of the entire family is often needed for accurate counseling. This may involve obtaining medical records and performing physical examinations and laboratory studies on numerous family members. Counseling is impaired if family members are unwilling to provide medical records and will not agree to examinations and laboratory studies. In addition, those who seek counseling may be unwilling to request cooperation from other family members or share newly acquired genetic information.

Process of Genetic Counseling

Genetic counseling may be a slow process and is not always straightforward. Several visits spread over months may be needed. Multiple family members may be part of the process. Tests for rare disorders may be performed at only one or a few laboratories in the world, and several weeks may be needed to complete them. Despite a comprehensive evaluation, a diagnosis may never be established. An accurate diagnosis is crucial to provide families with the best information about the risks for a specific birth defect, prognosis for the person affected, and options available to prevent or manage the disorder (Box 4.4). Even if the counseling does not provide clear

---

BOX 4-4   Diagnostic Methods That May be Used in Genetic Counseling

Preconception Screening
Family history to identify hereditary patterns of disease or birth defects
Examination of family photographs
Physical examination for obvious or subtle signs of birth defects
Carrier testing
Persons from ethnic groups with a higher incidence of some disorders
Persons with a family history suggesting they may carry a gene for a specific disorder
Chromosomal analysis
DNA analysis

Prenatal Diagnosis for Fetal Abnormalities
Maternal serum tests to screen for abnormalities
  Maternal serum analytes (i.e., alpha-fetoprotein)
Noninvasive Prenatal Screening (NIPS or NIPT)
  Analysis of cell-free fetal DNA
Chorionic villus sampling
Amniocentesis
Ultrasonography
Percutaneous umbilical blood sampling

Postnatal Diagnosis for an Infant with a Birth Defect
Physical examination and measurements
Imaging procedures (e.g., ultrasonography, radiography, echocardiography)
Chromosome analysis
DNA analysis
Tests for metabolic disorders (phenylketonuria, cystic fibrosis)
Hemoglobin analysis for disorders such as sickle cell disease
Immunologic testing for infections
Autopsy

information, expanding knowledge may allow a definitive diagnosis later and families are encouraged to contact the center for updates.

Individuals or families may request genetic counseling before or during pregnancy or after a child has been born with a defect. A genetic evaluation may include many factors, such as:

- A complete medical history of the affected person, including prenatal and perinatal history
- The medical history of other family members
- Laboratory, imaging, and other studies
- Physical assessment of a child with the birth defect and other family members, as needed
- Examination of photographs, particularly for family members who are deceased or unavailable
- Construction of a genogram, or pedigree, to identify relationships among family members and their relevant medical history

If a diagnosis is established, genetic counseling educates the family about the following:
- What is known about the cause of the disorder
- The natural course of the disorder
- The likelihood the disorder will occur or recur in other family members
- Current availability of prenatal diagnosis for the disorder
- The ways a couple may be able to avoid having an affected child
- Availability of treatment and services for the person with the disorder

Genetic counseling is nondirective. The counselor does not tell the individual or parents what decision to make but educates them about options for dealing with the disorder. However, families often subjectively interpret the counseling. Some parents may regard a 50% risk for occurrence or recurrence as low, whereas others may think a 1% risk is unacceptably high. In addition, the family's values and beliefs influence whether they seek counseling and what they do with the information provided (Jorde et al., 2016; Lee, 2016).

When risks and probabilities are discussed, these numbers should be stated in terms the individual or parents can understand, and their understanding should be verified. A 1-in-100 risk may sound higher to many people than a 1-in-5 risk. However, when the same numbers are framed in terms of percentages, the 1% risk is obviously much lower than the 20% risk.

Supplemental Services

Comprehensive genetic counseling includes services of professionals from many disciplines, such as biology, medicine, nursing, social work, and education. These professionals provide family support and referrals to parent support groups, grief counseling personnel, and intervention for problems that accompany the birth of a child with a birth defect, for example, socioeconomic and family dysfunction.

PATIENT TEACHING

Birth Defects

1. *How can this birth defect be genetic? No one else in our family has ever had anything like it.*
   Autosomal recessive disorders are carried by parents who themselves are unaffected. The abnormal gene may have been passed down through many generations, but the risk for an affected child is nonexistent until two carrier parents mate.

2. *Isn't the chance this birth defect will happen to another of our children only one in a million?*
   Autosomal recessive disorders have a 25% (1 in 4) chance for recurring in children of the same parents. Autosomal dominant disorders may pose a 50% risk for recurrence unless they resulted from a new mutation in the parental germ cells.

3. *Isn't this birth defect very likely to recur? We'd better not have any more children.*
   Some birth defects are associated with a relatively high risk for recurrence; others have a low risk. Prenatal diagnosis may offer parents a way to avoid having an affected child, or some disorders may be treated before birth. New genetic knowledge may provide therapies not available just a short time ago. Parents' values and perceptions of risks for recurrence affect the final decision.

4. *Because we've already had a child with this birth defect (an autosomal recessive defect), will the next three be normal?*
   If both parents are carriers for an autosomal recessive disorder, a 25% (1 in 4) risk exists for their child to be affected that is constant with each conception. The chance their child will neither be affected nor be a carrier is constant with each conception. Each child has a 25% (1 in 4) chance for receiving both copies of the normal gene (unaffected and not a carrier) and a 50% (2 in 4) chance of receiving a single abnormal gene from one parent (a carrier but not affected with the disorder).

5. *If I undergo amniocentesis or another prenatal diagnostic test, can the test detect all birth defects?*
   Although many disorders can be prenatally diagnosed, not all can be diagnosed in the same fetus. Testing is offered for one or more specific disorders after a careful family history is taken to determine appropriate tests.

6. *If the prenatal test results are normal, will my baby be normal?*
   Normal results from prenatal testing exclude those specifically tested disorders. Every healthy couple has approximately a 5% risk of having a child with a birth defect, some of which are not obvious at birth. This baseline risk remains, even if all prenatal test results are normal.

7. *Will I have to have an abortion if my prenatal tests show my baby is abnormal?*
   Abortion may be an option for parents whose fetus is affected with a birth defect, but most parents are reassured by normal test results. If results are abnormal, some parents appreciate the time to prepare for a child with special needs. Better medical management can be planned for a newborn who is expected to have problems. Prenatal diagnosis gives many parents the confidence to have children despite their increased risk for having a child with a birth defect.

Nursing Care of Families Concerned about Birth Defects

Nurses have an important role in helping families concerned about birth defects. Some nurses work directly with family members who are undergoing genetic counseling. Many more nurses are generalists who bring their knowledge about birth defects and their prevention to those they encounter in everyday practice.

Nurses as Part of a Genetic Counseling Team

Many genetic counseling teams include nurses. Genetic nursing may include the following:

- Providing counseling after additional education in this area
- Guiding a woman or couple through prenatal diagnosis
- Supporting parents as they make decisions after receiving abnormal prenatal diagnostic results
- Helping the family deal with the emotional impact of a birth defect
- Assisting parents who have had a child with a birth defect to locate needed services and support
- Coordinating services of other professionals such as social workers, physical and occupational therapists, psychologists, and dietitians
- Helping families find appropriate support groups to help them cope with the daily stresses associated with a child who has a birth defect

Nurses in General Practice

Nurses who work in women's health care and those who work in antepartum, intrapartum, newborn, or pediatric settings often encounter families who are concerned about birth defects. These families may include a member with a birth defect. Other families may think they have an increased risk for having a child with a birth defect. Generalist nurses provide care and support that complements that given by nurses who work on a genetic counseling team.

Women's Health Nurses

The nurse who provides care in women's health may encounter families who should be referred for genetic counseling. The ideal time to provide counseling is before conception so the childbearing couple has more options if risks are identified. Personal and family histories are taken and updated during primary care visits, and the nurse may identify factors that could affect a future child before conception. For example, the nurse may identify a woman who belongs to a group in which the sickle cell gene is more frequent and subsequently arrange for testing to determine her carrier status. If testing reveals she is a carrier for the gene, the woman can be advised that she could conceive a child with sickle cell disease if her partner is also a carrier. If her partner has not been tested, the nurse can arrange for his testing. The carrier may want to advise blood relatives of the need for testing.

Antepartum Nurses

Antepartum nurses often identify those who may benefit from genetic counseling. The antepartum nurse also may assist families with decision making, teaching about tests, management of abnormal results, and needed emotional support.

THERAPEUTIC COMMUNICATIONS

Assisting a Woman Who May Benefit from Genetic Counseling

Paula is a 41-year-old White woman who is 8 weeks pregnant with her first child after more than 10 years of infertility. Barbara is a nurse who works with Paula's obstetrician.

Paula: I know all about the risks at my age. I'm not so much worried about my own health as the baby's.

Barbara: You seem to be concerned that the baby might not be all right. *(Clarifying)*

Paula: Sure, what woman wouldn't be? I know I'm more likely to have a baby with Down's syndrome at my age.

Barbara: Yes, the risks for having an infant with a chromosomal abnormality increase after the mother is 35 years old. Do you plan to have prenatal diagnosis to see if the fetus has this kind of problem? *(Paraphrasing and giving information. Barbara also uses a closed-ended question that tends to block communication because it is usually answered with a simple "yes" or "no.")*

Paula: Oh, yes. I know what's available from surfing the Internet, and my doctor has asked me if I want that blood test. When we waited so long to have children, I just assumed I'd have whatever tests were recommended. Now I just don't know.

Barbara: You're reconsidering prenatal testing now? *(Reflecting)*

Paula: Well, not exactly reconsidering. It's just that I've waited so long for a baby, and this may be our only one.

Barbara: [Waiting quietly but attentively because Paula seems to be thinking.] *(Using silence)*

Paula: I'm just worried about testing. I know blood tests aren't risky. I also know most prenatal tests have a low risk, but what if I lose a normal baby? It took me so long to finally get pregnant, and I'm running out of time. I might not get another chance.

Barbara: It must be a very difficult decision. *(Reflecting)*

Paula: It is. Even if I have testing and the baby has Down's syndrome, I'm not so sure I'd have an abortion. The outlook for people with Down's syndrome is much better than it used to be. Why have testing if I wouldn't do anything about an abnormal baby?

Barbara: You certainly have some valid concerns. How does your husband feel about testing? *(Questioning using an open-ended question)*

Paula: Oh, Bill is all for it. He keeps reminding me the baby is probably normal and I probably won't have a miscarriage if I have testing. His cousin had a child with Down's syndrome, and Bill doesn't think we should knowingly bring a child with a serious birth defect into the world. What would you do if you were in my place?

THERAPEUTIC COMMUNICATIONS—cont'd

Assisting a Woman Who May Benefit from Genetic Counseling

Barbara: I can't answer that question because I'm not in your place. Let's review some of the issues so you can make the best decision for yourself and your family. First, you know you have an increased risk for having a baby with a chromosomal defect such as Down's syndrome because of your age. Second, the odds the baby will be normal are higher than the risk the baby will be abnormal. Third, amniocentesis poses a small but real risk for causing a miscarriage. Fourth, you are undecided about whether you would end a pregnancy if the fetus were abnormal. Other issues to consider are time limitations and the option of screening with a sample of your blood. The blood test the doctor told you about is done on your blood 8 to 10 weeks from now. The results of that test may reassure you but they may result in the need to make decisions about more complex testing such as amniocentesis. *(Summarizing)*

Paula: I know. I'm running out of time in more ways than one.

Barbara: If you like, I can set up an appointment with a genetic counselor. The counselor can provide you with the most accurate assessment of your risk for having a child with a birth defect and also the risks of any indicated prenatal diagnosis procedure. Then you can decide whether to have testing.

Paula: I think I'd like that, as long as I don't have to be committed to a particular decision before I go.

BOX 4.5 Indications for Genetic Counseling Referral

Maternal age 35 years of age or older when the infant is born

Paternal age 40 years or older

Members of a group with an increased incidence of a specific disorder

Carriers of autosomal recessive disorders

Women who are carriers of X-linked disorders

Couples related by blood (consanguineous relationship)

Family history of birth defect or intellectual disability

Family history of unexplained stillbirth

Women who experience multiple spontaneous abortions

Pregnant women exposed to known or suspected teratogens or other harmful agents either before or during pregnancy

Pregnant women with abnormal prenatal screening results such as multiple-marker screen or suspicious ultrasound findings

---

BOX 4.6 Examples of Problems in Genetic Counseling and Prenatal Diagnosis

Inadequate medical records

Uncertain gestational age or inadequate prenatal care

Family members' refusal to share information

Records that are incomplete, vague, or uninformative

Inconclusive testing

Too few family members available when family studies are needed

Inadequate number of live fetal cells obtained during amniocentesis

Failure of fetal cells to grow in culture if other testing techniques are not useful

Ambiguous prenatal test results that are neither clearly normal nor clearly abnormal

Unexpected results from prenatal diagnosis

Finding an abnormality other than the one for which the person was tested

Nonpaternity revealed with testing

Inability to determine the severity of a prenatally diagnosed disorder

Inability to rule out all birth defects

Patient misunderstanding of the mathematical risk as it is presented

---

Identifying Families for Referral. Nurses in antepartum settings often identify a woman or family for whom referral for genetic counseling is appropriate at the first prenatal visit (Box 4.5). The personal and family history of the woman and her partner may disclose factors that increase their risks for having a child with a birth defect. In addition to the usual medical history about disorders such as hypertension and diabetes, the woman should be questioned about a family history of birth defects, diseases that seem to "run in the family," intellectual disability, and developmental delay.

Some people are reluctant to disclose that they have a family member with intellectual disability or a birth defect. The nurse can gently probe for sensitive information by asking questions about whether any family members have learning problems or are "slow." The use of words that are lay oriented and caring often elicits more information than clinical terms that may seem harsh, for example, "low IQ."

Helping the Family Decide about Genetic Counseling. If genetic counseling is appropriate, the physician or nurse-midwife discusses it with the woman and refers the family to an appropriate center. However, the final decision rests with the person affected. The nurse can help the woman and her family weigh issues that are important to them as they decide.

Genetic counseling can raise uncomfortable issues such as whether to undergo prenatal diagnosis, what to do if a condition cannot be prenatally diagnosed, and what options are acceptable if prenatal diagnosis shows abnormal results. Counseling may open family conflicts if information from other family members is needed or if family values differ on issues such as abortion of an abnormal fetus. In addition, the tests can show unexpected results (Box 4.6).

Teaching about Lifestyle. Nurses can teach a pregnant woman about harmful factors in her lifestyle that can be modified to reduce the risk for defects to offspring. The nurse can support the woman in making difficult lifestyle changes such as stopping alcohol consumption, reducing or eliminating smoking, and improving the diet. Use of liberal praise can motivate a woman to continue her efforts to promote an optimal outcome. However, a negative attitude from nurses or other professionals may make the woman feel like a failure, and she may abandon her efforts to create a healthier lifestyle.

Providing Emotional Support. Until they know prenatal test results are normal, possibly a period spanning several days or weeks, many women delay telling friends or family about their pregnancy or investing in it emotionally. When results are abnormal, women face more difficult decisions about whether to terminate or continue the pregnancy.

Helping the Family Deal with Abnormal Results. Because prenatal diagnostic tests are performed to detect disorders involving serious physical and often mental defects, the woman whose test results are abnormal must confront painful decisions. For many of these disorders, no effective prenatal or postnatal treatment exists. Only two choices may be available: continuing or terminating the pregnancy. In addition, the decision to terminate a pregnancy must be made in a short time. Making no decision is effectively a decision to continue the pregnancy. Although the physician or genetic counselor discusses abnormal results and available options, the nurse reinforces the information given to these anxious families and supports them.

When test results are abnormal, nurses should expect the couple to grieve. Even if a pregnancy was unplanned, the woman who undergoes prenatal diagnosis has already made the initial decision to continue the pregnancy. If results are abnormal, she must decide again if she will continue or end the pregnancy. Both parents will experience similar feelings of grief and loss when an abnormal diagnosis is detected prenatally (Fonseca, Nazaré, & Canavarro, 2013).

Intrapartum and Neonatal Nurses

Nurses working in intrapartum and neonatal settings encounter families who have given birth to an infant with a birth defect that may have been unexpected. Stillborn infants sometimes have birth defects that contributed to their intrauterine death. In addition to the loss of their baby, these parents face pain because of the associated abnormality. An autopsy may be performed to document all anomalies and establish the most accurate diagnosis of the birth defect for future counseling. Nursing care for families who experience a perinatal loss, whether a result of the infant's death or the loss of the expected normal infant, is addressed in Chapter 11.

Nurses who care for these families in the intrapartum and neonatal settings will find the parents anxious, depressed, and sometimes hostile because of the unexpected event. The

family's usual coping mechanisms may be inadequate for the situation, or new coping mechanisms may not have been developed. Diagnostic studies are often recommended soon after the birth of an infant with an abnormality to establish a diagnosis and give parents accurate information about the abnormality and the options available to them. However, a high anxiety level reduces their ability to understand the often massive amount of information received. The nurse is in a position to evaluate the family's perception of the problem, help them understand the diagnostic tests, reinforce correct information, and correct misunderstandings. In addition, the nurse is often most therapeutic by simply being an available, active listener, helping ease the family's pain over the event.

Nurses should encourage families to contact lay support groups, which are significant sources of support because members fully understand the daily problems encountered in the care of a child with a birth defect. Such groups can help the parents manage the stress and chronic grief associated with prolonged care of these children. Support groups also can help the parents see the positive aspects and victories when caring for their child with special needs. Internet sites regarding specific birth defects are often available to offer parent education and support.

Pediatric Nurses

Children with birth defects typically have numerous recurrent medical problems. They usually are hospitalized more often and for longer periods than children without birth defects. Travel to specialized hospitals may be needed for their care, adding to the family's stress. These families often incur substantial expenses for medical care and equipment not covered by insurance or public assistance programs. Transportation costs to reach distant health care facilities may be difficult to pay. Household income may be lost because one parent stops working to care for the child.

Family dysfunction is common, and the strain of caring for a child with a serious birth defect may lead to divorce. Siblings often feel left out of their parents' attention because the needs of this child demand so much of their parents' time.

The nurse case manager can reduce the family's stress by helping them locate appropriate support services. The nurse can contact social services departments to help the family find financial and other resources needed to care for the child. If parents have not connected with a lay support group, a nurse can encourage them to do so.

▌ SUMMARY CONCEPTS

- The 46 human chromosomes are long strands of DNA, each containing up to several thousand individual genes.
- With the exception of those genes located on the X and Y chromosomes in males, genes are inherited in pairs that may be identical or different. Some genes are dominant and some are recessive.
- Many genes can be analyzed by the products they produce, their DNA, or their close association with another gene that is more easily analyzed.

- Cells for chromosome analysis must be living cells. Specimens should be handled carefully to preserve viability if analysis of dividing cells in the metaphase of cell division is necessary. Other techniques, such as FISH, permit study of cells without requiring active cell division, allowing rapid test results.
- Chromosome abnormalities are either numerical, with the addition or deletion of an entire chromosome or chromosomes, or structural, with deletion, addition, rearrangement, or fragility of the chromosome material.

- Single gene disorders are associated with a fixed risk for occurrence or recurrence. The type of single gene abnormality (autosomal dominant, autosomal recessive, or X-linked) determines the risk.
- Multifactorial disorders occur because of a genetic predisposition combined with environmental factors.
- The risk for occurrence or recurrence of multifactorial disorders is not fixed, but varies according to the number of close relatives affected, severity of the defect in affected persons, gender of the affected person, and geographic location.
- Relatively few agents that can enter the fetal environment are known to be definitely teratogenic or definitely safe.

- The risk for fetal damage from environmental agents can be decreased by reducing exposure to the agent or manipulating the fetal environment.
- The purpose of genetic counseling is to educate individuals or families with accurate information so they can make informed decisions about reproduction and appropriate care for affected members.
- The nurse cares for people with concerns about birth defects by identifying those needing referral, teaching, coordinating services, and offering emotional support.

REFERENCES & READINGS

American Academy of Pediatrics (AAP) & American College of Obstetricians and Gynecologists (ACOG). (2012). *Guidelines for perinatal care* (7th ed.). Washington, DC: Author.

American College of Obstetricians and Gynecologists (ACOG). (2015). *Management of women with phenylketonuria. (ACOG Committee Opinion No. 636)*. Washington, DC: Author.

American College of Obstetricians and Gynecologists (ACOG). (2016). *Guidelines for diagnostic imaging during pregnancy and lactation. (ACOG Committee Opinion No. 656)*. Washington, DC: Author.

Carlson, B. M. (2014). *Human embryology and developmental biology* (5th ed.). Philadelphia, PA: Saunders.

Centers for Disease Control and Prevention (CDC). (2017). Folic acid. Retrieved from www.cdc.gov.

Chambers, C., & Scialli, A. R. (2014). Teratogenesis and environmental exposure. In R. K. Creasy, R. Resnik, M. F. Greene, J. D. Iams, C. J. Lockwood, & T. R. Moore (Eds.), *Creasy & Resnik's maternal fetal medicine: Principles and practice* (7th ed.) (pp. 465–472). Philadelphia, PA: Saunders.

Cunningham, F. G., Leveno, K. J., Bloom, S. L., et al. (2014). *Williams obstetrics* (24th ed.). New York: McGraw-Hill.

Driscoll, D. A., Simpson, J. L., Holzgreve, W., & Otaño, L. (2017). Genetic screening and prenatal genetic diagnosis. In S. G. Gabbe, J. R. Niebyl, J. L. Simpson, M. B. Landon, H. L. Galan, E. R. M. Jauniaux, D. A. Driscoll, V. Berghella, & W. A. Grobman (Eds.), *Obstetrics: Normal and problem pregnancies* (7th ed.) (pp. 193–218). Philadelphia, PA: Elsevier.

Fonseca, A., Nazaré, B., & Canavarro, M.C. (2013) Clinical determinants in parents' emotional reactions to the disclosure of a diagnosis of congenital anomaly. *Journal of Obstetric, Gynecologic, & Neonatal Nursing, 42*(2), 178–190.

Hall, J. E. (2016). *Textbook of medical physiology* (13th ed.). Philadelphia, PA: Elsevier.

Jones, K. L. (2013). *Smith's recognizable patterns of human malformation* (7th ed.). Philadelphia, PA: Saunders.

Jorde, L. B., Carey, J. C., & Bamshad, M. J. (2016). *Medical genetics* (5th ed.). Philadelphia, PA: Elsevier.

Lee, B. (2016). Genetic counseling. In R. M. Kliegman, B. F. Stanton, J. W. St. Geme, III, & N. F. Schor (Eds.), *Nelson textbook of pediatrics* (20th ed.) (pp. 580–584). Philadelphia, PA: Elsevier.

March of Dimes Birth Defects Foundation. (2012). Rubella and pregnancy. Retrieved from www.marchofdimes.com.

Moore, K. L., Persaud, T. V. N., & Torchia, M. G. (2016a). *Before we are born: Essentials of embryology and birth defects* (9th ed.). Philadelphia, PA: Elsevier.

National Human Genome Research Institute (NHGRI). (2016a). Educational resources: Chromosomal Abnormalities. Retrieved from www.genome.gov.

National Human Genome Research Institute (NHGRI). (2016b). Genetic Information Nondiscrimination Act of 2008. Retrieved from www.genome.gov/10002077/genetic-discrimination/genetic-discrimination/.

National Tay-Sachs and Allied Diseases Association (NTSAD). (2016). Tay-Sachs Disease. Retrieved from www.ntsad.org.

Nussbaum, R. L., McInnes, R. R., & Willard, H. F. (2016). *Thompson & Thompson genetics in medicine* (8th ed.). Philadelphia, PA: Elsevier.

Organization of Teratology Information Specialists. (2016). Retrieved online at www.mothertobaby.org.

U.S Food and Drug Administration. (2016). Pregnancy and Lactation Labeling (Drugs) Final Rule. Retrieved from www.fda.gov/Drugs/DevelopmentApprovalProcess/DevelopmentResources/Labeling/ucm093307.htm.

White House Press Release. (2008). *Genetic Information Nondiscrimination Act*. Washington: DC. Retrieved from www.whitehouse.gov.

5

Conception and Prenatal Development

Jennifer H. Rodriguez

OBJECTIVES

After studying this chapter, you should be able to:

1. Describe formation of the female and male gametes.
2. Explain the process of human conception.
3. Explain implantation and nourishment of the embryo before development of the placenta.
4. Describe normal prenatal development from conception through birth.
5. Explain structure and function of the placenta, the umbilical cord, and fetal membranes with amniotic fluid.
6. Describe prenatal circulation and the circulatory changes after birth.
7. Explain the mechanisms and trends in multifetal pregnancies.

THE FAMILY BEFORE BIRTH

A basic understanding of conception and prenatal development helps the nurse provide care to parents during normal childbearing and better understand problems such as infertility and birth defects. This chapter addresses formation of the gametes and the process of conception, prenatal development, and important auxiliary structures that support normal prenatal development. The reason for the occurrence of multifetal pregnancy (e.g., twinning) is also discussed.

GAMETOGENESIS

Gametogenesis is the development of ova in the woman and sperm in the man (Table 5.1). Production of **gametes** (reproductive or germ cells) requires a process different from formation of **somatic cells** or other body cells. Somatic cells reproduce by a process called *mitosis*. Each somatic cell has 46 paired chromosomes: 22 pairs of **autosomes** (non-sex chromosomes) and 1 pair of **sex chromosomes** (X or Y chromosomes). During mitosis, the cell divides into two new cells, each having 46 chromosomes like the parent cell.

Gametogenesis requires a special reduction division called *meiosis*. Unlike **mitosis**, in which the **diploid** number (46) of chromosomes is retained in the new cells, **meiosis** halves the number of chromosomes to arrive at the **haploid** number of 23. Only 1 of each chromosome pair (22 autosomes and 1

sex chromosome) is directed to the gamete. In addition, with the exception of the X and Y chromosomes in males, each chromosome exchanges some material with its mate so the new chromosome in the gamete contains some material from the mother and some from the father. This process, which is called *crossing over*, allows variation in genetic material while keeping constant the total amount of chromosome material from generation to generation. When the sperm and ovum unite at conception, the "halves" form a new cell and restore the chromosome number to 46.

Oogenesis

Oogenesis is the formation of female gametes (Fig. 5.1, *A*) within the ovary. Oogenesis begins during prenatal life when primitive ova (oogonia) multiply by mitosis. Each oogonium contains 46 chromosomes. Before birth, these oogonia enlarge to form primary oocytes, each surrounded by a layer of follicular cells. These are called *primary follicles.* The primary oogonium begins its first meiotic division during fetal life but does not complete the process until puberty. The primary follicle and its oogonium, which still contains 46 chromosomes, remain dormant throughout childhood.

By the 30th week of gestation, the female fetus has all the ova she will ever have. Many of these ova regress during childhood. When a girl's reproductive cycles begin at puberty, some of the primary follicles present at birth begin maturing. The process

TABLE 5.1 Comparison of Female and Male Gametogenesis

	Oogenesis	Spermatogenesis
Time during which primary germ cells are produced	Fetal life; no others develop after ~ 30 wk of gestation	Continuously after puberty
Hormones that control process	GnRH FSH LH Estrogen	GnRH FSH LH Testosterone Estrogen (small amounts converted from testosterone) Growth hormone
Number of mature germ cells that develop from each primary cell	One	Four
Quantity	One during each reproductive cycle of about 28 days	~35-200 million released with each ejaculation
Size	Large; visible to naked eye; abundant cytoplasm to nourish embryo until implantation	Tiny compared with ovum; little cytoplasm; head is almost all nuclear material (chromosomes)
Motility	Relatively nonmotile; transported by action of cilia and currents within fallopian tubes	Independently motile by means of whiplike tail; mitochondria in middle piece provide energy for motility
Chromosome complement	23 total: 22 autosomes plus 1 X sex chromosome	23 total: 22 autosomes, plus either an X or a Y sex chromosome

FSH, Follicle-stimulating hormone; *GnRH,* gonadotropin-releasing hormone; *LH,* luteinizing hormone.

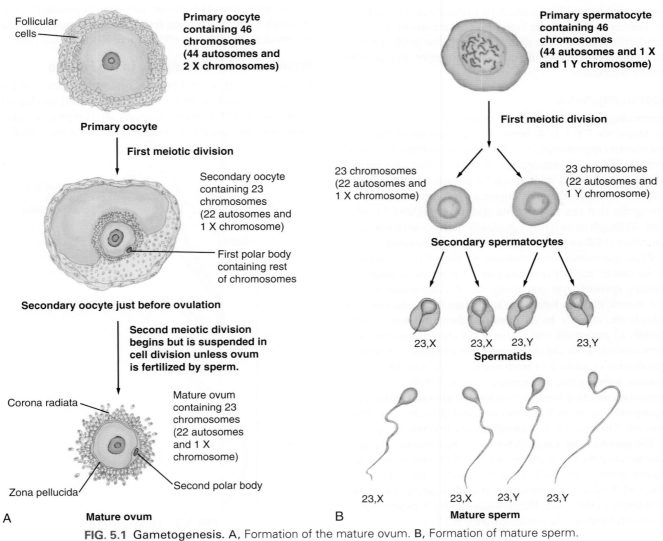

FIG. 5.1 Gametogenesis. A, Formation of the mature ovum. B, Formation of mature sperm.

of gamete maturation continues throughout her reproductive years until the climacteric. When the oocyte matures, two meiotic divisions reduce the chromosome number from 46 paired chromosomes to 23 unpaired chromosomes: 22 autosomes and 1 X chromosome. Shortly before **ovulation**, or release of the mature ovum from the ovary, the primary oocyte completes its first meiotic division, which began during fetal life. The result is a secondary oocyte containing 23 chromosomes. The primary cell's cytoplasm is divided unequally with this division, and most of it is retained by the secondary oocyte. The remainder of cytoplasm plus the other half of the chromosomes go into a tiny, nonfunctional polar body that soon degenerates.

At ovulation, the secondary oocyte begins to form a mature ovum (second meiotic division). Each of the 23 chromosomes divides without replication of the deoxyribonucleic acid (DNA). The second meiotic division is prolonged, and the mature ovum remains suspended in metaphase, the middle part of cell division. If fertilization occurs, the second meiotic division is completed, resulting in a mature ovum with 23 chromosomes and a second tiny polar body containing the 23 discarded chromosomes that degenerate. If the ovum is not fertilized, it does not complete the second meiotic division and degenerates. In oogenesis, one primary oocyte results in a single mature ovum.

When the mature ovum is released from the ovary, it is surrounded by two layers: the zona pellucida and the cells of the corona radiata. These layers protect the ovum and prevent fertilization by more than one sperm. For fertilization to occur, the sperm must penetrate these two layers to reach the ovum's cell nucleus.

Spermatogenesis

Spermatogenesis (formation of sperm, or male gametes, in the testes, see Fig. 5.1, *B*) begins during puberty in the male and requires approximately 70 days to be completed. Primitive sperm cells, or spermatogonia, develop during the prenatal period and begin multiplying by mitosis during puberty. Unlike the female, the male continues to produce new spermatogonia that can mature into sperm throughout his lifetime. Although male fertility gradually declines with age, men can father children in their fifties, sixties, and beyond.

Each spermatogonium contains 46 paired chromosomes. In the mature male, a spermatogonium enlarges to become a primary spermatocyte containing all 46 chromosomes. The first meiotic division forms two secondary spermatocytes and reduces the number to 23 unpaired chromosomes in each gamete: 22 autosomes and 1 X or Y sex chromosome in each spermatocyte. Each chromosome of the secondary spermatocyte divides to retain 23 chromosomes in the second meiotic division, forming two spermatids. Therefore 50% of the four spermatids resulting from the two meiotic divisions of the spermatogonium carry an X chromosome and 50% carry a Y chromosome. The spermatids gradually evolve into mature sperm.

The gamete from a male determines the gender of the new baby because the ovum carries only an X chromosome. Each mature sperm contains 23 chromosomes: 22 autosomes and either an X or a Y chromosome. If an X-bearing spermatozoon fertilizes the ovum, the baby is a girl. If a Y-bearing spermatozoon fertilizes the ovum, the baby is a boy.

The mature sperm has three major sections: a head, middle portion, and tail (Fig. 5.2). The head is almost entirely a cell nucleus and contains the male chromosomes that join the chromosomes of the ovum. The middle portion supplies energy for the tail's whiplike action. The movement of the tail propels the sperm toward the ovum.

> ## ? KNOWLEDGE CHECK
>
> 1. What is the purpose of meiosis in the gametes?
> 2. How many mature ova can be produced by each oogonium? When does meiosis occur in the female?
> 3. How many mature spermatozoa can be produced by each spermatogonium? When does meiosis occur in the male?

CONCEPTION

Natural conception is the interaction of many factors, including correct timing between release of a mature ovum at ovulation and **ejaculation** (semen expulsion) of enough healthy, mature, motile sperm into the vagina. Although exact viability is unknown, the ovum may survive no longer than 24 hours after its release at ovulation. Most sperm survive no more than 24 hours in the female reproductive tract, although a few may remain fertile in the woman's reproductive tract up to 80 hours (Blackburn, 2013; Hall, 2015).

Preparation for Conception in the Female

Before ovulation, several oocytes begin to mature under the influence of follicle-stimulating hormone (FSH) and luteinizing hormone (LH) from the woman's anterior pituitary gland. Each maturing oocyte is contained within a sac called the

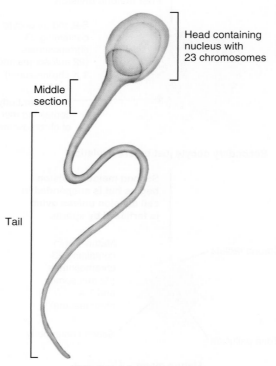

Head containing nucleus with 23 chromosomes

Middle section

Tail

FIG. 5.2 Mature sperm.

graafian follicle, which produces estrogen and progesterone to prepare the **endometrium** (uterine lining) for a possible pregnancy. Eventually, one follicle outgrows the others. The less mature oocytes permanently regress.

Release of the Ovum

Ovulation occurs approximately 14 days before a woman's next menstrual period would begin. The follicle develops a weak spot on the surface of the ovary and ruptures, releasing the mature ovum with its surrounding cells onto the surface of the ovary. The collapsed follicle is transformed into the **corpus luteum**, which maintains high estrogen and progesterone secretion necessary to make final preparation of the uterine lining for a fertilized ovum.

Ovum Transport

The mature ovum is released on the surface of the ovary, where it is picked up by the fimbriated (fringed) ends of the fallopian tube. The ovum is transported through the tube by the muscular action of the tube and movement of cilia within the tube. Fertilization normally occurs in the distal third of the fallopian tube (ampulla) near the ovary. The ovum, fertilized or not, enters the uterus approximately 4 days after its release from the ovary.

Preparation for Conception in the Male

The male preparation for fertilizing the ovum consists of ejaculation, movement of the sperm in the female reproductive tract, and preparation of the sperm for actual fertilization.

Ejaculation

When a male ejaculates during sexual intercourse, 35 to 200 million sperm are deposited in the upper vagina and over the cervix (Blackburn, 2013; Hall, 2015). The sperm are suspended in 2 to 5 milliliters (mL) of seminal fluid, which nourishes and protects the sperm from the acidic environment of the vagina (Blackburn, 2013; Hall, 2015). Many sperm are lost as the ejaculate drips from the vaginal introitus. Other sperm are inactivated by acidic vaginal secretions or digested by vaginal enzymes and phagocytes. The seminal fluid coagulates slightly after ejaculation to hold the semen deeply in the vagina. Many sperm are relatively immobile for approximately 15 to 30 minutes until other seminal enzymes dissolve the coagulated fluid and allow the sperm to begin moving upward through the cervix.

Transport of Sperm in the Female Reproductive Tract

The whiplike movement of the tails of spermatozoa propels them through the cervix, uterus, and fallopian tubes. Uterine contractions induced by prostaglandins in the seminal fluid enhance movement of the sperm toward the ovum. Only sperm cells enter the cervix. The seminal fluid remains in the vagina.

Many sperm are lost along the way. Some are digested by enzymes and phagocytes in the female reproductive tract, whereas others simply lose their direction, moving into the wrong tube or past the ovum and out into the peritoneal cavity.

Preparation of Sperm for Fertilization

Sperm are not immediately ready to fertilize the ovum when they are ejaculated. During the trip to the ovum, the sperm undergo changes enabling one of them to penetrate the protective layers surrounding the ovum, a process called *capacitation*. During capacitation, a glycoprotein coat and seminal proteins are removed from the acrosome, which is the tip of the sperm head. After capacitation, the sperm look the same but are more active and can better penetrate the corona radiata and zona pellucida surrounding the ovum.

Sperm must also undergo an acrosome reaction to further prepare them to fertilize the ovum. The sperm that reach the ovum release hyaluronidase and acrosin to digest a pathway through the corona radiata and zona pellucida. Their tails beat harder to propel them toward the center of the ovum. Eventually, one spermatozoon penetrates the ovum.

Fertilization

Fertilization occurs when one spermatozoon enters the ovum and the two nuclei containing the parents' chromosomes merge (Fig. 5.3).

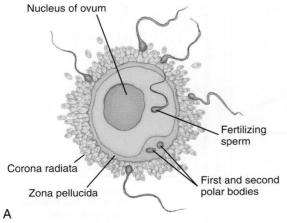
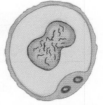
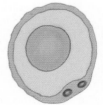

Nucleus of ovum

Fertilizing sperm

Corona radiata

Zona pellucida

First and second polar bodies

A

Mixing of cell nuclei and chromosomes of ovum and sperm

B

Fertilization complete

C

FIG. 5.3 **Process of Fertilization. A,** A sperm enters the ovum. **B,** The 23 chromosomes from the sperm mingle with the 23 chromosomes from the ovum, restoring the diploid number to 46. **C,** The fertilized ovum is now called a *zygote* and is ready for the first mitotic cell division.

Entry of One Spermatozoon into the Ovum

Entry of a spermatozoon into the ovum has three results. First is the zona reaction, in which changes in the zona pellucida surrounding the ovum prevent other sperm from entering. Second, the cell membranes of the ovum and sperm fuse and break down, allowing the contents of the sperm head to enter the cytoplasm of the ovum. Third, the ovum, which has been suspended in the middle of its second meiotic division since just before ovulation, completes meiosis. This results in a nucleus with 23 chromosomes and the expulsion of a second nonfunctional polar body. The mature ovum now contains 23 unpaired chromosomes (22 autosomes and 1 X chromosome) in its nucleus.

Fusion of the Nuclei of Sperm and Ovum

Once a spermatozoon has penetrated the ovum, fusion of their nuclei begins. The sperm head enlarges, and the tail degenerates. The nuclei of the gametes move toward the center of the ovum, where the membranes surrounding their nuclei touch and dissolve. The 23 chromosomes from the sperm mingle with the 23 from the ovum, restoring the diploid number to 46. Fertilization is complete, and cell division can begin when the nuclei of the sperm and ovum unite.

❓ KNOWLEDGE CHECK

4. Where does fertilization usually occur?
5. What are the functions of the seminal fluid?
6. What occurs when a spermatozoon penetrates the ovum?
7. When is fertilization complete and a new human conceived?

PREEMBRYONIC PERIOD

The preembryonic period is the first 2 weeks after conception (Fig. 5.4). Around the fourth day after conception, the fertilized ovum, now called a **zygote**, enters the uterus.

Initiation of Cell Division

The zygote divides into 2, then 4, then 8 cells, and so on until the 16-cell stage. The cells become tightly compacted with each division, so they occupy about the same amount of space as the original zygote. When the **conceptus** (cells and membranes resulting from fertilization of the ovum) is a solid ball of 16 cells, it is called a **morula** because it resembles a mulberry.

The outer cells of the morula secrete fluid, forming a *blastocyst,* a sac of cells with an inner cell mass placed off center within the sac. The inner cell mass develops into the **fetus**. Part of the outer layer of cells develops the fetal membranes and the **placenta**, or the fetal structure that provides nourishment, removes wastes, and secretes necessary hormones for continuation of the pregnancy.

Entry of the Zygote into the Uterus

When the blastocyst contains approximately 100 cells, it enters the uterus. It lingers in the uterus another 2 to 4 days before beginning implantation. The endometrium, now called the *decidua,* is in the secretory phase of the reproductive cycle, 1½ weeks before the woman would otherwise begin her menstrual period. The endometrial glands are secreting at their maximum, providing rich fluids to nourish the conceptus before placental circulation is established. The endometrial spiral arteries are well developed in the secretory phase, providing easy access for the development of the placental blood supply.

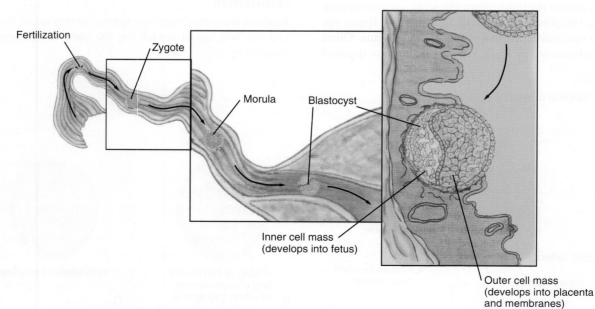

FIG. 5.4 Prenatal Development from Fertilization through Implantation of the Blastocyst. Implantation gradually occurs from day 6 through day 10. Implantation is complete on day 10.

Fertilization

Zygote

Morula

Blastocyst

Inner cell mass
(develops into fetus)

Outer cell mass
(develops into placenta
and membranes)

Implantation in the Decidua

The conceptus carries a small supply of nutrients for early cell division. However, implantation at the proper time and location in the uterus is critical for continued development. Implantation, or **nidation**, is a gradual process that occurs between days 6 and 10 after conception. During the relatively long process of implantation, embryonic structures continue to develop.

Maintaining the Decidua

Implantation and survival of the conceptus require a continuing supply of estrogen and progesterone to maintain the decidua in the secretory phase. The zygote secretes human chorionic gonadotropin (hCG) to signal the woman's body that a pregnancy has begun. Production of hCG by the conceptus causes the corpus luteum to persist and continue secretion of estrogen and progesterone until the placenta takes over this function.

Location of Implantation

The conceptus must be in the right place at the right time for normal implantation to occur. The site of implantation is important because it is where the placenta develops. Normal implantation occurs in the upper uterus, slightly more often on the posterior wall than the anterior wall (Moore, Persaud, & Torchia, 2013). The upper uterus is the best area for implantation and placental development for three reasons:

1. The upper uterus is richly supplied with blood for optimal fetal gas exchange, nutrition, and waste elimination.
2. The uterine lining is thick in the upper uterus, preventing the placenta from attaching too deeply into the uterine muscle and facilitating easy expulsion of the placenta after full-term birth.
3. Implantation in the upper uterus limits blood loss after birth because strong interlacing muscle fibers in this area compress open endometrial vessels after the placenta detaches.

Mechanism of Implantation

Enzymes produced by the conceptus erode the decidua, tapping maternal sources of nutrition. Primary chorionic villi are tiny projections on the surface of the conceptus extending into the endometrium, now called the *decidua basalis,* which lies between the conceptus and the wall of the uterus. The chorionic villi eventually form the fetal side of the placenta. The decidua basalis forms the maternal side of the placenta (see Fig. 5.7, *A*).

At this early stage, nutritive fluid passes to the embryo by *diffusion* (the passive movement across a cell membrane from an area of higher concentration to one of lower concentration) because the circulatory system is not yet established. The conceptus is fully embedded within the mother's uterine decidua by 10 days, and the site of implantation is almost invisible.

As the conceptus implants, usually near the time of the next expected menstrual period, a small amount of bleeding ("spotting") may occur at the site. Implantation bleeding may be confused with a normal menstrual period, particularly if the woman's menstrual periods are usually light.

KNOWLEDGE CHECK

8. When does implantation occur?
9. What are the advantages of implantation in the upper uterus?
10. How is the embryo nourished before the placenta develops?

EMBRYONIC PERIOD

The embryonic period of development extends from the beginning of the third week through the eighth week after conception (Fig. 5.5). Basic structures of all major body organs are completed during the embryonic period (Table 5.2).

Differentiation of Cells

The **embryo** (developing baby from the beginning of the third week through the eighth week after conception) progresses from undifferentiated cells with essentially identical functions to differentiated, or specialized, body cells. By the end of the eighth week, all major organ systems are in place, and many are functioning, although in a simple way.

Development of the specialized structures is controlled by three factors: (1) genetic information in the chromosomes received from the parents, (2) interaction between adjacent tissues, and (3) timing. Although basic instructions are carried within the chromosomes, one tissue may induce change toward greater specialization in another, but only if a signal between the two tissues occurs at a specific time during development. In this way, structures develop with appropriate sizes and relationships to each other.

During the embryonic period, structures are vulnerable to damage from **teratogens** because these structures are developing rapidly. Normal development of one structure often requires normal and properly timed development of another structure. Unfortunately, a woman may not realize she is pregnant during this sensitive time. For this reason, the possibility of pregnancy should be explored with her before the prescription of drugs or administration of diagnostic procedures such as radiography. Some agents may be damaging at one time during pregnancy but not at another. Others may be damaging at any time during pregnancy.

Weekly Developments

Development occurs simultaneously in all embryonic organ systems. Prenatal development proceeds in patterns that continue after birth:

- Cephalocaudal (head to toe)
- Central-to-peripheral direction (from center outward)
- Simple to complex (early cells may become any cell of the body before they become specialized into specific structures with specific functions)
- General to specific (upper extremities begin as limb buds before detailed development of bones, joints, muscles, ligaments, and fingers)

Full term ranges from 36 to 40 weeks of **fertilization age** calculated from date of conception or 38 to 42 weeks of **gestational**

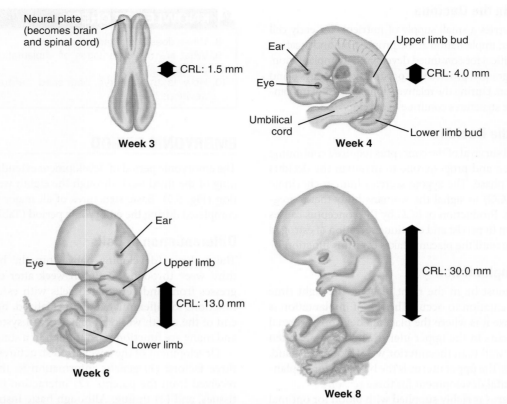

FIG. 5.5 Embryonic Development from Week 3 through Week 8 after fertilization. A, Week 3. B, Week 4. C, Week 6. D, Week 8. *CRL,* Crown–rump length.

age (after last menstrual period). Because conception occurs approximately 2 weeks after the first day of the last menstrual period in most women who have 4-week cycles, the fertilization age used in this chapter is approximately 2 weeks shorter than the gestational age. However, gestational age is most commonly used in practice because the last menstrual period provides a known marker, whereas most women do not know exactly when they conceived. Ultrasonography provides added information to identify the most accurate fetal age (see Chapter 9).

Week 2

Implantation is complete by the end of the second week after fertilization. The most growth occurs in the outer cells, or trophoblast, which eventually becomes the fetal part of the placenta. The inner cell mass becomes flattened into the embryonic disc and will later develop into the baby. Cells that eventually form part of the fetal membranes develop.

Week 3

Many women miss their first menstrual period during the third week after conception. The embryonic disc develops three layers, called *germ layers,* which, in turn, give rise to major organ systems of the body (Table 5.3). The three germ layers are the ectoderm, the mesoderm, and the endoderm.

The central nervous system (CNS) begins developing during the third week. A thickened, flat neural plate appears, extending toward the cephalic end of the embryonic disc. The neural plate develops a longitudinal groove that folds to form

the neural tube. At the end of the third week, the neural tube is fused in the middle but still open at each end.

Early heart development consists of a pair of parallel heart tubes that fuse longitudinally. The primitive, or tubular, heart begins beating at 22 to 23 days, resulting in a wavelike flow of blood. By the end of the fourth week, coordinated contractions result in the unidirectional flow of blood characteristic of the mature heart. Vessels developing in the chorionic villi and membranes join the heart tube. Primitive blood cells arise from the endoderm lining the distal blood vessels.

Week 4

The shape of the embryo changes during the fourth week after conception. It folds at the head and tail end and laterally, resembling a C-shaped cylinder. A "tail" is apparent during the embryonic period because the brain and spinal cord develop more rapidly than other systems. The tail disappears as the rest of the body catches up with growth of the CNS. The neural tube closes during the fourth week. If the neural tube does not close, defects such as anencephaly and spina bifida result.

Formation of the face and upper respiratory tract begins. Beginnings of the internal ear and the eye are apparent. The upper extremities appear as buds on the lateral body walls. Because the embryo is sharply flexed anteriorly, the heart is near the embryo's mouth. Partitioning of the heart into four chambers begins during the fourth week and is completed by the end of the sixth week.

TABLE 5.2	Timetable of Prenatal Development Based on Fertilization Age*				
Nervous/ Sensory System	Cardiorespiratory System	Digestive System	Genitourinary System	Musculoskeletal System	Integumentary System
3 Weeks: 1.5-mm CRL†					
Flat neural plate begins closing to form neural tube. Neural tube still open at each end.	Heart consists of two parallel tubes that fuse into a single tube. Contractions of heart tube begin. Chorionic villi of early placenta connect with heart.	Endoderm (inner germ layer) will become digestive tract.		Paired, cube-shaped swellings (somites) appear and will form most of head and trunk skeleton. Muscle, bone, and cartilage develop from mesoderm.	Epidermis (outer skin layer) will develop from ectoderm (outer germ layer). Dermis (deep skin layer) and connective tissue will develop from mesoderm (middle germ layer).
4 Weeks: 4-mm CRL					
Neural tube closed at each end. Cranial end of neural tube will form brain; caudal end will form spinal cord. Eye development begins as an outgrowth of forebrain. Nose development begins as two pits. Inner ear begins developing from hindbrain.	Heart begins partitioning into four chambers and begins beating. Blood circulating through embryonic vessels and chorionic villi. Tracheal development begins as a bud on upper gut and branches into two bronchial buds.	Development of primitive gut as embryo folds laterally. Stomach begins as a widening of tube-shaped primitive gut. Liver, gallbladder, and biliary ducts begin as a bud from primitive gut.	Primordial germ (reproductive) cells are present on embryonic yolk sac.	Upper limb buds are present and look like flippers. Lower limb buds appear.	Mammary ridges that will develop into mammary glands appear.
6 Weeks: 13-mm CRL					
Development of pituitary gland and cranial nerves. Head sharply flexed because of rapid brain growth. Eyelid development beginning. External ear development begins in neck region as six swellings.	Blood formation primarily in liver. Three right and two left lung lobes develop as outgrowths of right and left bronchi. Partitioning of heart into four chambers completed.	Most intestines are contained within umbilical cord because liver and kidneys occupy most of abdominal cavity. Stomach nearing final form. Development of upper and lower jaws.	Kidneys are near bladder in pelvis. Kidneys occupy much of abdominal cavity. Primordial germ cells incorporated into developing gonads. Male and female gonads are identical in appearance.	Arms are paddle shaped, and fingers webbed. Feet and toes develop similarly, but a few days later than arms and hands. Bones cartilaginous, but ossification of skull begins.	Mammary glands begin development. Tooth buds for primary (deciduous) teeth begin developing.
8 Weeks: 30-mm CRL					
Spinal cord stops at end of vertebral column. Taste buds begin developing. Eyelids fuse. Ears have final form but are low-set.	Heart partitioned into four chambers. Heartbeat detectable with ultrasound. Additional branching of bronchi.	Stomach has reached final form. Lips are fused. Intestines remain in umbilical cord.	Testes begin developing under influence of Y chromosome. Ovaries will develop if a Y chromosome is not present. External genitalia begin to differentiate but still appear quite similar.	Fingers and toes still webbed, but distinct by end of week 8. Bones begin to ossify. Joints resemble those of adults.	Auricles of ear low-set but beginning to assume final shape.

Continued

TABLE 5.2   **Timetable of Prenatal Development Based on Fertilization Age*—cont'd**

Nervous/ Sensory System	Cardiorespiratory System	Digestive System	Genitourinary System	Musculoskeletal System	Integumentary System
10 Weeks: 61-mm CRL; weight, 14 g†					
Head flexion still present, but straighter. Eyelids closed and fused. Top of external ear slightly below eye level.	May be possible to detect heartbeat with Doppler transducer. Blood produced in spleen and lymphatic tissue.	Intestines contained within abdominal cavity as growth of this cavity catches up with digestive system development. Digestive tract patent from mouth to anus.	Kidneys in their adult position. Male and female external genitalia have different appearance but are still easily confused.	Toes distinct; soles face each other.	Fingernails begin developing. Tooth buds for permanent teeth begin developing below those for primary teeth.
12 Weeks: 87-mm CRL; weight, 45 g					
Surface of brain is smooth, without sulci (grooves) or gyri (convolutions). Nasal septum and palate complete development.	Heartbeat should be detected with Doppler transducer.	Sucking reflex present. Bile formed by liver.	Kidneys begin producing urine. Male and female external genitalia can be distinguished by appearance.	Limbs are long and thin. Involuntary muscles of viscera develop.	Downy lanugo begins developing at end of this week.
16 Weeks: 140-mm CRL; weight, 200 g					
Face is human-looking because eyes face forward rather than to side.	Pulmonary vascular system developing rapidly.	Fetus swallows amniotic fluid and produces meconium (bowel contents).	Urine excreted into amniotic fluid.	Lower limbs reach final relative length, longer than upper limbs. A woman who has been pregnant before may begin to feel fetal movements.	External ears have enough cartilage to stand away from head somewhat Blood vessels easily visible through delicate skin. Fingerprints developing.
20 Weeks: 160-mm CRL; weight, 460 g					
Myelination of nerves begins and continues through first year of postnatal life.	Heartbeat should be detectable with regular fetoscope.	Peristalsis well developed.	More than 40% of nephrons are mature and functioning. Testes contained in abdomen but begin descent toward scrotum. Primordial follicles of ovary reach peak of 5-7 million and then gradually decline.	Fetal movements felt by mother and may be palpable by an experienced examiner.	Skin is thin and covered with vernix caseosa. Brown fat production complete. Nipples begin development.

TABLE 5.2   Timetable of Prenatal Development Based on Fertilization Age*—cont'd

Nervous/ Sensory System	Cardiorespiratory System	Digestive System	Genitourinary System	Musculoskeletal System	Integumentary System
24 Weeks: 230-mm CRL; weight, 820 g					
Spinal cord ends at level of first sacral vertebra because of more rapid growth of vertebral canal.	Primitive thin-walled alveoli (air sacs) have developed and are surrounded by capillary network. Surfactant production begins in lungs. Respiration possible, but many fetuses die or have disabilities if born at this time.		Testes descending toward inguinal rings.	Fetus is active. Fetal movements become progressively more noticeable to both mother and examiner.	Body appearance lean. Skin wrinkled and red. Fingerprints and footprints developed. Fingernails present. Eyebrows and lashes present.
28 Weeks: 270-mm CRL; weight, 1300 g					
Major sulci and gyri are present. Eyelids no longer fused after 26 weeks. Responds to bitter substances on tongue.	Erythrocyte formation completely in bone marrow. Sufficient alveoli, surfactant, and capillary network to allow respiratory function, although respiratory distress syndrome is common. Many infants born at this time survive with intensive care.		Testes descended through inguinal canal into scrotum by end of week 26.		Skin slightly wrinkled but smoothing out as subcutaneous fat is deposited under it.
32 Weeks: 300-mm CRL; weight, 2100 g					
Maturation of parasympathetic nears that of sympathetic nervous system, resulting in fetal heart rate variability on electronic fetal monitor tracing.	Surfactant production nears mature levels. Respiratory distress still possible if born at 32 weeks. Fetal heart rate variability gradually increases toward full term.				Skin smooth and pigmented. Large vessels visible beneath skin. Fingernails reach fingertips. Lanugo disappearing.
38 Weeks: 360-mm CRL, weight, 3400 g					
Sulci and gyri developed. Visual acuity ~20/600 at birth.	Newborn infant has ~1/8 to 1/6 number of alveoli of an adult. Well-developed ability to exchange gas.		Both testes usually palpable in scrotum at birth. The newborn girl's ovaries contain ~1 million follicles. No new ones are formed after birth; their numbers continue to decline after birth.		Fetus plump, and skin smooth. Vernix caseosa present in major body creases. Lanugo present on shoulders and upper back only. Fingernails extend beyond fingertips. Ear cartilage firm.

*Fertilization age is about 2 wk less than gestational age.
†*CRL*, Crown-rump length; *g*, gram(s).

TABLE 5.3 Derivatives of the Three Germ Layers		
Ectoderm	**Mesoderm**	**Endoderm**
Brain and spinal cord	Cartilage	Lining of gastrointestinal and respiratory tracts
Peripheral nervous system	Bone	
	Connective tissue	
Pituitary gland	Muscle tissue	Tonsils
Sensory epithelium of eye, ear, and nose	Heart	Thyroid
	Blood vessels	Parathyroid
	Blood cells	Thymus
Epidermis	Lymphatic system	Liver
Hair	Spleen	Pancreas
Nails	Kidneys	Lining of urinary bladder and urethra
Subcutaneous glands	Adrenal cortex	
	Ovaries	
	Testes	
Mammary glands	Reproductive system	Lining of ear canal
Tooth enamel	Lining membranes (pericardial, pleural, and peritoneal)	

The lower respiratory tract begins growth as a branch of the upper digestive tract, which is a simple tube at this time. Gradually, the esophagus and trachea complete separation. The trachea branches to form the right and left bronchi. These bronchi, in turn, branch to form the three lobes of the right lung and two lobes of the left lung. Continued branching of the bronchi eventually forms the terminal air sacs, or alveoli. The alveoli proliferate and become surrounded by a rich capillary network enabling oxygen and carbon dioxide exchange at birth.

Week 5

The head is very large because the brain grows rapidly during the fifth week after fertilization. The heart is beating and developing four chambers. Upper limb buds are paddle shaped with obvious notches between the fingers. Lower limbs form slightly later than upper limbs. Lower limbs are also paddle shaped, but the area between the toes is not as well defined as is the division between the fingers.

Week 6

The rapidly developing head is bent over the chest. The heart reaches its final four-chambered form. Upper and lower extremities continue to become more defined.

The eyes continue to develop, and the beginnings of the external ears appear as six small bumps on each side of the neck. Facial development begins with eyes, ears, and nasal pits widely separated and aligned with the body walls. Gradually the embryo grows such that the face comes together in the midline and the external ears assume their proper position on the sides of the head.

Week 7

General growth and refinement of all systems occur 7 weeks after conception. The face becomes more human looking. The eyelids begin to grow, and the extremities become longer and better defined. The trunk elongates and straightens, although a C-shaped spinal curve remains in the newborn at birth.

The intestines have been growing faster than the abdominal cavity during the embryonic period. The relatively large liver and kidneys also occupy much of the abdominal cavity. Therefore most of the intestines are contained within the umbilical cord while the abdominal cavity grows to accommodate them. The abdomen is large enough to contain all its normal contents by 10 weeks.

Week 8

The embryo has a definite human form, and refinements to all systems continue. The ears are low-set but approaching their final location. The eyes are pigmented but not yet fully covered by eyelids. Fingers and toes are stubby but well-defined. The external genitalia begin to differentiate, but male and female characteristics are not distinct until 10 weeks after conception, or 12 weeks after the woman's last menstrual period.

❓ KNOWLEDGE CHECK

11. Why is the embryo particularly susceptible to damage from teratogens?
12. How does the lower respiratory tract develop?
13. Why are the intestines mostly contained within the umbilical cord until the 10th week?

FETAL PERIOD

The fetal period is the longest part of prenatal development. It begins 9 weeks after conception and ends with birth. All major systems are present in their basic form. Dramatic growth and refinement in the structure and function of all organ systems occur during the fetal period (Fig. 5.6). Teratogens may damage already formed structures but are less likely to cause major structural alterations. The CNS is vulnerable to damaging agents through the entire pregnancy.

Weeks 9 through 12

The head is approximately half the total length of the fetus at the beginning of this period. The body begins growing faster than the head, changing the proportions. The extremities approach their final relative lengths, although the legs remain proportionately shorter than the arms. The first fetal movements begin but are too slight for the mother to detect.

The face is broad with a wide nose and widely spaced eyes. The eyes close at 9 weeks and reopen at 26 weeks after conception. The ears appear low-set because the mandible is still small.

The intestinal contents partly contained within the umbilical cord enter the abdomen by 11 weeks as the capacity of the abdominal cavity catches up with them in size. Blood formation occurs primarily in the liver during week 9 but shifts to the spleen by the end of week 12. The fetus begins producing urine during this period and excretes it into the amniotic fluid.

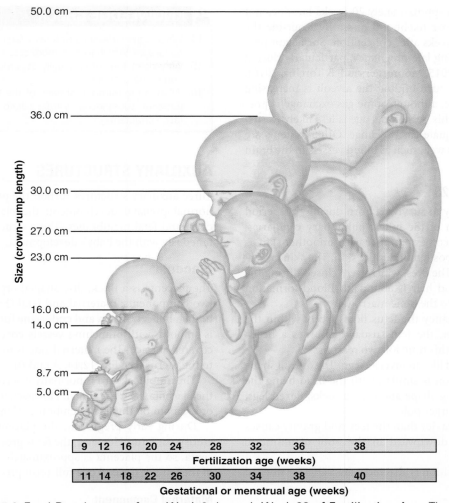

FIG. 5.6 Fetal Development from Week 9 through Week 38 of Fertilization Age. The gestational age, measured from the first day of the last menstrual period, is approximately 2 weeks longer than the fertilization age.

Internal differences in males and females begin to be apparent in the seventh week. External genitalia look similar until the end of the 9th week. By the end of week 12, the fetal gender can be determined by the appearance of the external genitalia.

Weeks 13 through 16

The fetus grows rapidly in length, so the head becomes smaller in proportion to the total length. Movements strengthen, and some women, particularly those who have been pregnant before, are able to detect them. This phenomenon is referred to as *quickening*. The face looks human because the eyes face fully forward. The ears approach their final position at the sides of the head and in line with the eyes.

Weeks 17 through 20

Fetal movements feel like fluttering or "butterflies." Some women may not recognize these subtle sensations. The fetus is unlikely to survive outside of the uterus at the age of 20 weeks.

Changes in the skin and hair are evident. *Vernix caseosa*, a fatty, cheeselike secretion of the fetal sebaceous glands, covers the skin to protect it from constant exposure to amniotic fluid. *Lanugo* is fine, downy hair covering the fetal body and helps the vernix adhere to the skin. Both vernix and lanugo diminish as the fetus reaches term. Eyebrows and head hair appear.

Brown fat is a special heat-producing fat deposited during this period. It is located on the back of the neck, behind the sternum, and around the kidneys (Chapter 19, Fig. 19.4).

Weeks 21 through 24

While continuing to grow and gain weight, the fetus still appears thin because of minimal subcutaneous fat. The skin is translucent and red because the capillaries are close to its fragile surface.

The lungs begin to produce surfactant, a surface-active lipid that makes it easier for the baby to breathe after birth. Surfactant reduces surface tension in the lung alveoli and prevents them from collapsing with each breath. Production of surfactant begins at approximately 20 weeks but does not reach levels that increase likelihood of survival outside the uterus until 26 to 28 weeks after conception. Surfactant production increases during late pregnancy, particularly during the last 2 weeks (Hall, 2015; Moore, Persaud, & Torchia, 2016). The capillary network surrounding the alveoli is increasing but still very immature, although some gas exchange is possible. A fetus born at this gestational age is less likely to survive because of inadequate gas exchange. Other systems are extremely immature as well, such as blood vessels in the brain that may bleed.

Weeks 25 through 28

The fetus is more likely to survive if born during this period because of maturation of the lungs, pulmonary capillaries, and CNS. The fetus becomes plumper with smoother skin as subcutaneous fat is deposited under the skin. The skin gradually becomes less red. The eyes, which were closed during the 9th week, reopen. Head hair is abundant. Blood formation shifts from the spleen to the bone marrow.

During early pregnancy the fetus floats freely within the amniotic sac. However, the fetus usually assumes a head-down position during this time for two reasons:

1. The uterus is shaped like an inverted egg. The overall shape of the fetus in flexion is similar, with the head being the small pole of the egg shape and the buttocks, flexed legs, and feet being the larger pole.
2. The fetal head is heavier than the feet, and gravity causes the head to drift downward in the pool of amniotic fluid.

The head-down position is also most favorable for normal birth.

Weeks 29 through 32

The skin is pigmented according to race and is smooth. Larger vessels are visible over the abdomen, but small capillaries cannot be seen. Toenails are present, and fingernails extend to the fingertips. The fetus has more subcutaneous fat, which rounds the body contours. If the fetus is born during this period, chances of survival are good with specialized neonatal care.

Weeks 33 through 38

Growth of all body systems continues until birth, but the rate of growth slows as full term approaches. The fetus is mainly gaining weight. The pulmonary system matures to enable efficient and unlabored breathing after birth.

The well-nourished term fetus at 38 or more weeks is rotund with abundant subcutaneous fat. At birth, boys are slightly heavier than girls. The skin is pink to brownish pink, depending on race. Lanugo may be present over the forehead, upper back, and upper arms. Vernix often remains in major creases such as the groin and axillae.

The testes are in the scrotum. Breasts of both male and female infants are enlarged, and breast tissue is palpable beneath the areola and nipple because of maternal hormone effects.

AUXILIARY STRUCTURES

Three auxiliary structures sustain the pregnancy and permit normal prenatal development: the placenta, the umbilical cord, and fetal membranes. These structures develop simultaneously with the baby's development.

Placenta

The placenta is a thick, disc-shaped organ. The placenta has two components: maternal and fetal (Fig. 5.7). It is involved in metabolic, transfer, and endocrine functions. The fetal side is smooth, with branching vessels covering the membrane-covered surface. The maternal side is rough where it attaches to the uterus (see Fig. 12.14, *A* and *B*).

The umbilical cord is normally inserted on the fetal side of the placenta, near the center. However, it may insert off center or even out on the fetal membranes (Fig. 5.8).

During early pregnancy, the placenta is larger than the embryo or fetus. However, the fetus grows faster than the placenta, so the placenta is approximately one-sixth the weight of the fetus at the end of a full-term pregnancy.

Maternal Component

Development. When conception occurs, cells of the endometrium undergo changes to promote early nutrition of the embryo and enable most of the uterine lining to be shed after birth. These changes convert endometrial cells into the decidua. In addition to providing nourishment for the embryo, the decidua may protect the mother from uncontrolled invasion of fetal placental tissue into the uterine wall.

The three decidual layers are (1) the decidua basalis, which underlies the developing embryo and forms the maternal side of the placenta; (2) the decidua capsularis, which overlies the embryo and bulges into the uterine cavity as the embryo and fetus grow; and (3) the decidua parietalis, which lines the rest of the uterine cavity. By approximately 22 weeks of gestation, the decidua capsularis fuses with the decidua parietalis, filling the uterine cavity.

Circulation on the Maternal Side. Maternal and fetal blood normally do not mix in the placenta, although they flow very close to each other. Exchange of substances between mother and fetus occurs within the intervillous spaces of the placenta. While in the intervillous space, the mother's blood is briefly outside her circulatory system. Approximately 150 mL of maternal blood is contained within the intervillous space. Blood in the intervillous space is changed approximately three to four times per minute, requiring circulation of 450 to 750 mL per minute for placental perfusion.

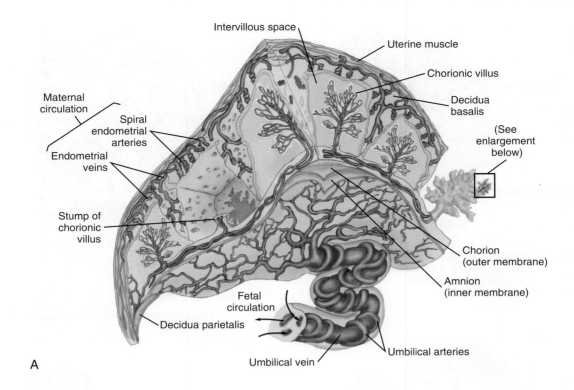

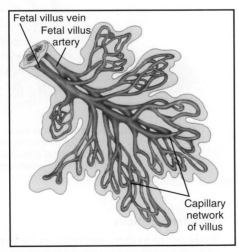

FIG. 5.7 **A,** Placental structure showing relationship of placenta. *Arrows* indicate the direction of blood flow between the fetus and placenta through the umbilical arteries and vein. Blood from the mother bathes the fetal chorionic villi within the intervillous spaces to allow exchange of oxygen, nutrients, and waste products without gross mixing of maternal and fetal blood. **B,** Structure of a chorionic villus; its fetal capillary network is illustrated.

Maternal blood spurts into the intervillous spaces through 80 to 100 spiral arteries in the decidua. After the oxygenated and nutrient-bearing maternal blood washes over the chorionic villi containing the fetal vessels, it returns to the maternal circulation through the endometrial veins for elimination of fetal waste products.

Fetal Component

Development. The fetal side of the placenta develops from the outer cell layer (trophoblast) of the blastocyst at the same time the inner cell mass develops into the embryo and fetus. The primary chorionic villi are the initial structures that eventually form the fetal side of the placenta.

Circulation on the Fetal Side. The umbilical cord contains the umbilical arteries and vein to transport blood between the fetus and placenta. Chorionic villi are bathed by oxygen- and nutrient-rich maternal blood in the maternal intervillous spaces. Each chorionic villus is supplied by a tiny fetal artery carrying deoxygenated blood and waste products from the fetus. The vein of the chorionic villus

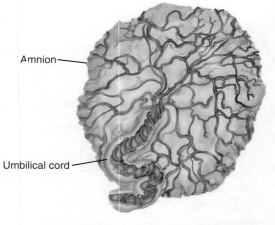

Amnion

Umbilical cord

Normal placenta with insertion of umbilical
cord near center and branching of fetal umbilical
vessels over the surface

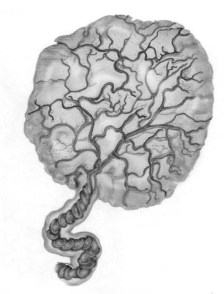

Placenta with cord inserted near margin
of placenta

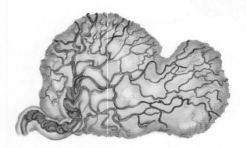

Placenta with a small accessory lobe

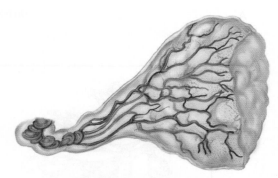

Velamentous insertion of umbilical cord.
Cord vessels branch far out on membranes.
When membranes rupture, fetal umbilical vessels
may be torn and the fetus can hemorrhage.

FIG. 5.8 Placental variations.

returns oxygenated blood and nutrients to the embryo and fetus.

Capillaries in the chorionic villi are separated from actual contact with the mother's blood by the membranes of each villus. This arrangement allows contact close enough for exchange and prevents mixing of maternal and fetal blood. The closed fetal circulation is important because the blood types of mother and fetus may not be compatible.

The placental arteries and veins converge in the blood vessels of the umbilical cord. Two umbilical arteries and one umbilical vein transport blood between the fetus and the fetal side of the placenta. Blood is circulated to and from the fetal side of the placenta by the fetal heart.

Metabolic Functions

The placenta produces some nutrients needed by the embryo and for placental functions. Substances synthesized include glycogen, cholesterol, and fatty acids (Moore et al., 2016).

Transfer Functions

Exchange of oxygen, nutrients, and waste products across the chorionic villi occurs through several methods (Table 5.4). Placental transfer of harmful substances also may occur. Most substances that enter the mother's bloodstream can enter the fetal circulation, and many agents enter it almost immediately.

Gas Exchange. Respiration is a key function of the placenta. Oxygen and carbon dioxide pass through the placental membrane by simple diffusion. The average oxygen partial pressure (Po_2) of maternal blood in the intervillous space is 50 mm Hg. The average blood Po_2 in the umbilical vein (after oxygenation) is approximately 30 mm Hg (Hall, 2015).

The following three reasons explain how the fetus can thrive in this low-oxygen environment:

1. Fetal hemoglobin can carry 20% to 50% more oxygen than adult hemoglobin.

TABLE 5.4	**Mechanisms of Placental Transfer**	
Mechanism	**Description**	**Examples of Substances Transferred**
Simple diffusion	Passive movement of substances across a cell membrane from an area of higher concentration to one of lower concentration	Oxygen and carbon dioxide Carbon monoxide Water Urea and uric acid Most drugs and their metabolites
Facilitated diffusion	Passage of substances across a cell membrane by binding with carrier proteins that assist transfer	Glucose
Active transport	Transfer of substances across a cell membrane against a pressure or electrical gradient or from an area of lower concentration to one of higher concentration	Amino acids Water-soluble vitamins Minerals: calcium, iron, iodine
Pinocytosis	Movement of large molecules by ingestion within cells	Maternal IgG class antibodies Some passage of maternal IgA antibodies

IgA, Immunoglobulin A; *IgG,* immunoglobulin G.

2. The fetus has a higher oxygen-carrying capacity because of a higher average hemoglobin level (14.5 to 22.5 g/dL) and hematocrit value (approximately 48% to 69%).

3. Hemoglobin can carry more oxygen at low carbon dioxide partial pressure (P_{CO_2}) levels than it can at high levels (Bohr effect). Blood entering the placenta from the fetus has a high P_{CO_2}, but carbon dioxide diffuses quickly to the mother's blood, where the P_{CO_2} is lower, reversing the levels of carbon dioxide in the maternal and the fetal blood. Therefore the fetal blood becomes more alkaline, and the maternal blood becomes more acidic. This allows the mother's blood to release oxygen and the fetal blood to combine with oxygen readily.

The fetal P_{CO_2} is only approximately 2 to 3 mm Hg higher than the P_{CO_2} of maternal blood. However, carbon dioxide is very soluble, allowing it to pass across the placental membrane into maternal blood at this low-pressure gradient.

Nutrient Transfer. The growing fetus requires a constant supply of nutrients from the pregnant woman. Glucose, fatty acids, vitamins, and electrolytes pass readily across the placenta. Glucose is the major energy source for fetal growth and metabolic activities.

Waste Removal. In addition to carbon dioxide, urea, uric acid, and bilirubin are readily transferred from fetus to mother for disposal. Because the normal placenta removes wastes for the fetus, metabolic defects such as phenylketonuria (PKU) are usually not evident until after birth.

Antibody Transfer. Many of the immunoglobulin G (IgG) class of antibodies are passed from mother to fetus through the placenta. This confers passive (temporary) immunity to the fetus against diseases to which the mother is immune, for example, measles. Passage of antibodies against disease is beneficial because the newborn does not produce antibodies for several months after birth. The preterm or small-for-gestational age infant has little protection from maternal antibodies because they are transferred during late pregnancy and are poorly transferred if placental function is inadequate.

Passage of antibodies from mother to fetus is not always beneficial. If maternal and fetal blood types are not compatible, the mother may already have or may produce antibodies against fetal erythrocytes. The mother's antibodies may then destroy the fetal erythrocytes, causing fetal anemia or even death. This situation may occur if the mother is Rh-negative and the fetus is Rh-positive.

Transfer of Maternal Hormones. Most maternal protein hormones do not reach the fetus in significant amounts. The female fetus exposed to androgenic hormones may have masculinization of her genitalia, and her true gender may be difficult to visually determine at birth.

Endocrine Functions. The placenta produces several hormones necessary for normal pregnancy. hCG causes the corpus luteum to persist for the first 6 to 8 weeks of pregnancy and secrete estrogens and progesterone. As the placenta develops further, it takes over estrogen and progesterone production, and the corpus luteum regresses. When a Y chromosome is present in the male fetus, hCG also causes the fetal testes to secrete testosterone, necessary for normal development of male reproductive structures.

Human placental lactogen, also called *human chorionic somatomammotropin,* promotes normal nutrition and growth of the fetus as well as maternal breast development for lactation. This placental hormone decreases maternal insulin sensitivity and glucose use, making more glucose available for fetal nutrition.

Steroid hormones secreted by the placenta include estrogens and progesterone. Estrogens cause enlargement of the woman's uterus, enlargement of the breasts, growth of the ductal system of the breasts, and enlargement of the external genitalia. Progesterone is essential for normal continuation of the pregnancy. It modifies and maintains the endometrium to receive and nourish the conceptus and forms the decidua. Progesterone also reduces muscle contractions of the uterus to prevent spontaneous abortions. (See Chapter 6 for a more detailed list of the functions of estrogen and progesterone during pregnancy). Other hormones produced by the placenta include human chorionic thyrotropin and human chorionic adrenocorticotropin.

Fetal Membranes and Amniotic Fluid

The two fetal membranes are the *amnion* (inner membrane) and the *chorion* (outer membrane). The two membranes are so close they seem to be one membrane (the "bag of waters"), but they can be separated. If the membranes rupture in labor, amnion and chorion usually rupture together, releasing the amniotic fluid within the sac.

The amnion is continuous with the surface of the umbilical cord, joining the epithelium of the abdominal skin of the fetus. Chorionic villi proliferate over the entire surface of the gestational sac for the first 8 weeks after conception. A conceptus observed at this time looks like a shaggy sphere with the embryo suspended inside. As the embryo grows, it bulges into the uterine cavity. The villi on the outer surface gradually atrophy and form the smooth-surfaced chorion. The remaining villi continue to branch and enlarge to form the fetal side of the placenta.

Amniotic fluid protects the growing fetus and promotes normal prenatal development. Amniotic fluid protects the fetus by the following actions:

- Cushioning against impacts to the maternal abdomen
- Maintaining a stable temperature
- Promoting normal prenatal development by the following actions:
  - Allowing symmetric development as the major body surfaces fold toward the midline
  - Preventing the membranes from adhering to developing fetal parts
  - Allowing room and buoyancy for fetal movement

Amniotic fluid is derived from fetal urine and fluid transported from the maternal blood across the amnion. Cast-off fetal epithelial cells and vernix are suspended in the amniotic fluid. The water of the amniotic fluid changes by absorption across the amnion, returning to the mother. The fetus also swallows amniotic fluid and absorbs it in the digestive tract. Waste products are returned to the placenta through the umbilical arteries.

The volume of amniotic fluid increases during pregnancy and is approximately 700 to 800 mL at term. An abnormally small quantity of fluid (less than 50% of the amount expected for gestation or under 400 mL at term) is called *oligohydramnios* and may be associated with the following (Blackburn, 2013; Carlson, 2014; Hall, 2015):

- Poor placental blood flow
- Preterm rupture of the membranes

- Failure of fetal kidney development
- Blocked urinary excretion
- Poor fetal lung development (pulmonary hypoplasia)
- Malformations such as skeletal abnormalities from compression of fetal parts

Hydramnios (also called *polyhydramnios*) is the opposite situation, in which the quantity may exceed 2000 mL. Hydramnios may be associated with the following (Blackburn, 2013):

- Imbalanced water exchange among mother, fetus, and amniotic fluid that has no known cause
- Poorly controlled maternal diabetes mellitus resulting in large quantities of fetal urine excretion having an elevated glucose level
- Malformations of the CNS, cardiovascular system, or gastrointestinal tract that interfere with normal fluid ingestion, metabolism, and excretion
- Chromosomal abnormalities
- Multifetal gestation

FETAL CIRCULATION

The course of fetal blood circulation is from the fetal heart to the placenta for exchange of oxygen, nutrients, and waste products and back to the fetus for delivery to fetal tissues (Fig. 5.9, *A*).

Umbilical Cord

The fetal umbilical cord is the lifeline between the fetus and placenta. It has two arteries carrying deoxygenated blood and waste products away from the fetus to the placenta, where these substances are transferred to the mother's circulation. The umbilical vein carries freshly oxygenated and nutrient-laden blood from the placenta back to the fetus. The umbilical arteries and vein are coiled within the cord to allow them to stretch and prevent obstruction of blood flow through them. The entire cord is cushioned by a soft substance called *Wharton's jelly* to prevent obstruction resulting from pressure.

Fetal Circulatory Circuit

Because the fetus does not breathe air, several alterations of the postnatal circulatory route are needed (see Fig. 5.9, *A*). Also, the fetal liver does not have the metabolic functions it will have after birth because the mother's body performs these functions. Three shunts in the fetal circulatory system allow blood with the highest oxygen content to be sent to the fetal heart and brain: the ductus venosus, foramen ovale, and ductus arteriosus.

Ductus Venosus

Oxygenated blood from the placenta enters the fetal circulation through the umbilical vein. About one-third of the blood is directed away from the liver into the ductus venosus, which connects to the inferior vena cava. The rest of the umbilical vein flow goes through the liver before entering the inferior vena cava. Near the end of pregnancy the liver needs more perfusion, and 70% to 80% of the oxygenated blood goes to the liver first and then to the ductus venosus (Blackburn, 2013).

Blood from the ductus venosus or the portal system of the liver enters the inferior vena cava and joins blood from the lower part of the body. Little mixing of blood from the ductus venosus and the lower body occurs because it travels to the heart in separate streams within the inferior vena cava. As blood flows into the right atrium, a flap of tissue directs the blood from the more highly oxygenated stream across the atrium to the foramen ovale.

Foramen Ovale

The foramen ovale is a flap valve in the septum between the right and left atria of the fetal heart. As blood flows into the right atrium, 50% to 60% crosses the foramen ovale to the left atrium (Blackburn, 2013). In the left atrium it mixes with the small amount of blood entering from the pulmonary veins, flows to the left ventricle, and leaves through the aorta. The majority of the blood in the ascending aorta flows to the coronary, left carotid, and subclavian arteries. Therefore most of the better-oxygenated blood bypasses the nonfunctioning lungs before birth and travels to the heart, brain, head, and upper body.

Blood that does not cross the foramen ovale moves to the right ventricle, but flow to the lungs is restricted by the narrow pulmonary artery and pulmonary blood vessels, causing a high pressure in the right side of the heart. Pressure is low on the left side of the heart because little resistance occurs as blood leaves the left ventricle to travel to the rest of the body and into the widely dilated placental vessels. This difference in pressures between the right and left atria allows blood to flow through the foramen ovale.

Pulmonary Blood Vessels

Blood from the superior vena cava and the less oxygenated blood from the inferior vena cava flow into the right atrium, to the right ventricle, and into the pulmonary artery. Most of the blood passes through the ductus arteriosus to the descending aorta, and 10% to 12% of the blood goes to the lungs. After 30 weeks of gestation, the amount of blood to the lungs increases (Blackburn, 2013). Blood flow to the lungs is limited because the pulmonary artery and other blood vessels are constricted, causing high pulmonary vascular resistance. Blood perfusing the lungs returns to the left atrium by the pulmonary veins.

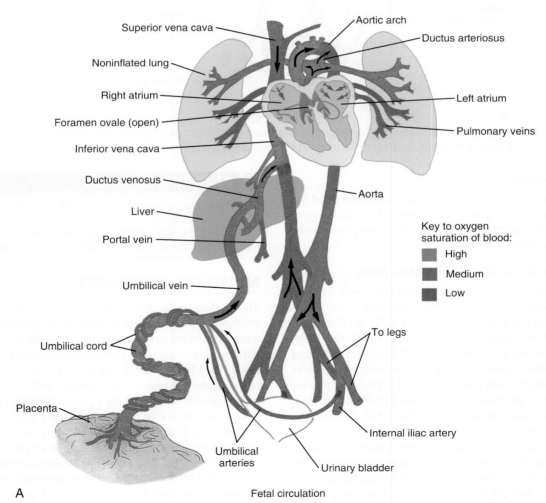

FIG. 5.9 A, Fetal circulation. Three shunts allow most blood from the placenta to bypass the fetal lungs and liver; they are the ductus venosus, ductus arteriosus, and foramen ovale.

Continued

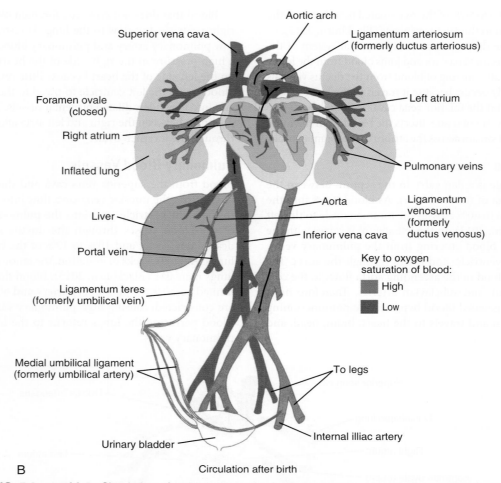

FIG. 5.9, cont'd B, Circulation after birth. Note the fetal shunts have closed. The umbilical vessels, ductus venosus, and ductus arteriosus will be converted to ligaments.

Ductus Arteriosus

The ductus arteriosus connects the pulmonary artery and the descending aorta during fetal life. Dilation of the ductus arteriosus is maintained by prostaglandins from the placenta and low oxygen content of the blood.

Changes in Blood Circulation after Birth

Fetal circulatory shunts are not needed after birth because the infant oxygenates blood in the lungs and is not circulating blood to the placenta (see Fig. 5.9, *B*). As the infant breathes and the lungs expand, blood flow to the lungs increases, pressure in the right side of the heart falls, and the foramen ovale closes. The ductus arteriosus constricts as the arterial oxygen level rises. Persistent hypoxia may cause the ductus arteriosus to remain open for a prolonged period. The ductus venosus constricts when flow of blood from the umbilical cord stops.

Transition to the postnatal circulatory pattern is gradual. Functional closure begins when the infant breathes and the cord is cut, removing the placenta from the circulation. The foramen ovale and ductus venosus are permanently closed as tissue proliferates in these structures. The ductus venosus becomes a ligament, as do the umbilical vein and arteries.

> **❓ KNOWLEDGE CHECK**
>
> 22. What are the purposes of the fetal membranes and amniotic fluid?
> 23. Trace the path of fetal circulation from the placenta through the fetal body and back to the placenta.

MULTIFETAL PREGNANCY

The incidence of multifetal pregnancy (multiple gestation) has increased in the United States. Much of the increase is a result of a rise in maternal age, when women naturally are more likely to have twins, and infertility treatments that induce multiple ovulation. Twin births in 2013 rose to 337 per 1000 live births. The rate of triplet and higher-order multiple births has fluctuated in the recent past. After reaching a peak in 1998, the rate declined to 119.5 per 100,000 births in 2013 (Martin et al., 2015).

Twinning is the most common form of multifetal pregnancy. The same processes that occur in twin pregnancies also may occur in higher-order multiple gestations. Twins are often called *identical* or *fraternal* by lay people but are more accurately described by their zygosity, or the number of ova and sperm involved. The two types of twins are *monozygotic* and *dizygotic* (Fig. 5.10).

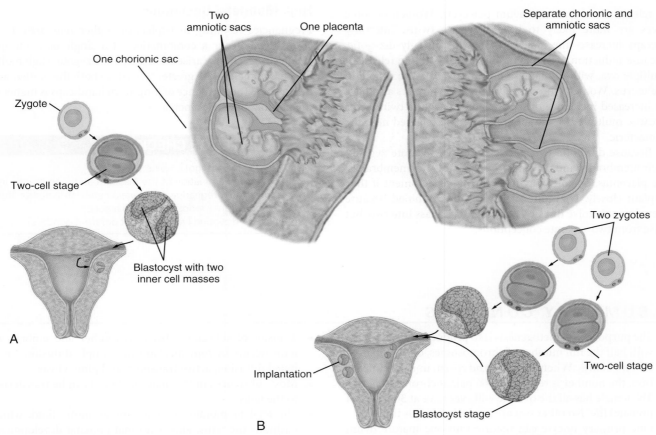

FIG 5.10 **A,** Monozygotic twinning. The single inner cell mass divides into two inner cell masses during the blastocyst stage. These twins have a single placenta and chorion, but each twin develops in its own amnion. **B,** Dizygotic twinning. Two ova are released during ovulation, and each is fertilized by a separate spermatozoon. The ova may implant near each other in the uterus, or they may be far apart.

Monozygotic Twinning

Monozygotic twins are conceived by the union of a single ovum and spermatozoon, with later division of the conceptus into two. Monozygotic twins have identical genetic complements and are the same gender. However, they may not always look identical at birth because one twin may have grown much larger than the other or one may have a birth defect such as a cleft lip. Monozygotic twins have a higher rate of birth defects, preterm births, and low birth weight. Monozygotic twinning occurs essentially at random (about 1 in 250 natural [nonassisted] pregnancies), and a hereditary or racial component is not well established (Newman & Unal, 2017).

Monozygotic twinning occurs when a single conceptus divides early in gestation. The blastocyst in most monozygotic twins is formed with two inner cell masses instead of one. If this occurs, the fetuses usually have two amnions (inner membranes) but a single chorion (outer membrane) (Blackburn, 2013; Cunningham et al., 2014; Newman & Unal, 2017).

If the conceptus divides earlier, two separate but identical morulas (and then blastocysts) develop and implant separately. These monozygotic twins have two amnions and two chorions. Although the placentas develop separately, they may fuse and appear as one at birth. The chorions also may fuse during prenatal development. Examination of the placenta and membranes after birth may not identify whether twins are monozygotic or dizygotic. Tests such as DNA analysis or detailed blood typing may be needed to determine whether twins are monozygotic or dizygotic.

Late separation of the inner cell mass may result in twins having a single amnion and a single chorion. These twins are more likely to die because their umbilical cords become entangled during pregnancy. Incomplete separation of the inner cell mass may result in conjoined twins.

Dizygotic Twinning

Dizygotic twins arise from two ova fertilized by different sperm. Dizygotic twins may be the same or different gender, and they may not have similar physical traits.

Dizygotic twinning may be hereditary in some families, presumably because of an inherited tendency of the females to release more than one ovum per cycle. Women of some races are more likely to have dizygotic twins. Infertility therapy increases the incidence of twins, usually dizygotic, because induction of ovulation often results in the release of multiple ova, with implantation of more than one zygote in the uterus. Women who conceive after age 40 years also have an increased incidence of spontaneous dizygotic twin births because multiple ova are more likely to be released near the climacteric.

Because dizygotic twins arise from two separate zygotes, their membranes and placentas are separate. The membranes, the placentas, or both may fuse during development if they implant closely. Dizygotic twins are not conjoined because they do not involve division of a single cell mass into two, but arise from two separate conceptions.

High Multifetal Gestations

Pregnancies resulting in triplets or higher may arise from a single zygote or a combination of a single and multiple zygotes, or each may arise from a separate zygote. High multifetal pregnancies pose greater hazards to both the mother and her fetuses. The incidence of long-term handicaps is higher as the number of fetuses increases.

❓ KNOWLEDGE CHECK

24. How do monozygotic twins occur?
25. Why can examination of the placenta and membranes in a multifetal pregnancy not always establish whether the newborns are monozygotic or dizygotic?
26. Why are dizygotic twins often of different genders?

SUMMARY CONCEPTS

- The purpose of gametogenesis is to produce ova and sperm with half the full number of chromosomes, or 23 unpaired chromosomes. When an ovum and sperm unite at conception, the number is restored to 46 paired chromosomes.
- The female has all the ova she will ever have at 30 weeks of prenatal life. No other ova are formed after this time.
- One primary oocyte can mature into one mature ovum with 23 unpaired chromosomes (22 autosomes and 1 X chromosome).
- Males can continuously produce new sperm from puberty through the rest of their life, although fertility gradually declines after age 40 years.
- One primary spermatocyte can result in production of four mature sperm. Two of the mature sperm have 22 autosomes and 1 X sex chromosome. Two have 22 autosomes and 1 Y sex chromosome.
- The male determines the baby's gender because sperm carry either an X or a Y sex chromosome. The female contributes only an X chromosome to the baby.
- The basic structures of all organ systems are established during the first 8 weeks of pregnancy. During this period, teratogens may cause major structural and functional damage to the developing organs.
- The fetal period is one of growth and refinement of already established organ systems. Teratogens are less likely to cause major structural damage to the fetus but may cause major functional damage.
- The placenta is an embryonic or a fetal organ with metabolic, respiratory, and endocrine functions.

- Transfer of substances between mother and embryo or fetus occurs by four mechanisms: simple diffusion, facilitated diffusion, active transport, and pinocytosis.
- Most substances in the maternal blood can be transferred to the fetus.
- The fetal membranes contain the amniotic fluid, which cushions the fetus, allows normal prenatal development, and maintains a stable temperature.
- The umbilical cord is the lifeline between the fetus and the placenta. Two umbilical arteries carry deoxygenated blood and waste products to the placenta for transfer to the mother's blood. One umbilical vein carries oxygenated and nutrient-rich blood to the fetus. Coiling of the vessels and enclosure in Wharton's jelly reduce the risk for obstruction of the umbilical vessels.
- Three fetal circulatory shunts are needed to partially bypass the fetal liver and lungs: the ductus venosus, foramen ovale, and ductus arteriosus. These structures close functionally after birth but are not closed permanently until several weeks or months later.
- Multifetal pregnancy may be monozygotic or dizygotic. Twins are the most common form of multifetal pregnancy.
- Examination of the placenta and membranes alone cannot conclusively establish whether multiple fetuses are monozygotic or dizygotic.
- Dizygotic twins are more likely to occur in certain families and racial groups and especially in mothers older than 40 years and women who take fertility treatments to induce ovulation.

REFERENCES & READINGS

Blackburn, S. T. (2013). *Maternal, fetal, & neonatal physiology: A clinical perspective* (4th ed.). Philadelphia, PA: Saunders.

Carlson, B. M. (2014). *Human embryology and developmental biology* (5th ed.). Philadelphia, PA: Mosby.

Cunningham, F. G., Leveno, K. J., Bloom, S. L., Spong, C. Y., Dashe, J. S., Hoffman, B. L., & Sheffield, J. S. (2014). *Williams obstetrics* (24th ed.). New York: McGraw-Hill.

Hall, J. E. (2015). *Textbook of medical physiology* (13th ed.). Philadelphia, PA: Elsevier.

Martin, J. A., Hamilton, B. E., Osterman, M. J. K., et al. (2015). Births: Final data for 2013. *National Vital Statistics Reports, 64*(1). Hyattsville, MD: National Center for Health Statistics.

Moore, K. L., Persaud, T. V. N., & Torchia, M. G. (2013). *Before we are born: Essentials of embryology and birth defects* (8th ed.). Philadelphia, PA: Saunders.

Moore, K. L., Persaud, T. V. N., & Torchia, M. G. (2016). *The developing human: Clinically oriented embryology* (10th ed.). Philadelphia, PA: Saunders.

Newman, R., & Unal, E. R. (2017). Multiple gestations. In S. G. Gabbe, J. R. Niebyl, J. L. Simpson, et al. (Eds.), *Obstetrics: Normal and problem pregnancies* (7th ed.) (pp. 706–736). Philadelphia, PA: Elsevier.

6

Maternal Adaptations to Pregnancy

Dawn Piacenza

OBJECTIVES

After studying this chapter, you should be able to:

1. Describe the physiologic changes that occur during pregnancy.
2. Differentiate presumptive, probable, and positive signs of pregnancy.
3. Describe the psychological responses of the expectant mother to pregnancy.
4. Identify the process of maternal role transition.
5. Explain the maternal tasks of pregnancy.
6. Describe the developmental processes of the transition to the role of father.
7. Describe the responses of prospective grandparents and siblings to pregnancy.
8. Discuss factors that influence psychosocial adaptation to pregnancy and explain how these factors affect nursing care.

From the moment of conception, changes occur in the pregnant woman's body. These changes are necessary to support and nourish the fetus, prepare the woman for childbirth and lactation, and maintain the woman's health. Pregnant women are often puzzled by the physical and psychological changes and unprepared for associated discomforts. Many women rely on nurses to provide accurate information and compassionate guidance throughout their pregnancy. To respond effectively, nurses should understand not only the physiologic and psychological changes but also how these changes affect the daily lives of expectant mothers and their families.

PHYSIOLOGIC ADAPTATIONS TO PREGNANCY

CHANGES IN BODY SYSTEMS

Although pregnancy challenges each body system to adapt to increasing demands of the fetus, the most obvious changes are in the reproductive system.

Reproductive System
Uterus

Growth. The most dramatic change during pregnancy occurs in the uterus, which before conception is a small, pear-shaped organ entirely contained in the pelvic cavity. The nonpregnant uterus weighs up to 70 g (2.5 oz) and has a capacity of approximately 10 mL (one-third of an ounce). By **term** (38 to 42 weeks of gestation) the uterus weighs 1100 to 1200 g (2.4 to 2.6 lb) and has a capacity of 5 L (Norwitz & Lye, 2014).

Uterine growth occurs as the result of hyperplasia and hypertrophy. Growth can be predicted for each **trimester** (one of three 13-week periods of pregnancy). Early in pregnancy, growth results from hyperplasia caused by estrogen and growth factors. In the latter half of pregnancy, uterine growth results mainly from hypertrophy as the muscle fibers stretch in all directions to accommodate the growing fetus. In addition to muscle growth, fibrous tissue accumulates in the outer muscle layer of the uterus and the amount of elastic tissue increases. These changes greatly increase the strength of the muscle wall (Cunningham et al., 2014).

Muscle fibers in the myometrium increase in both length and width. Although the uterine wall thickens during early pregnancy, the wall of the uterus thins to approximately 0.5 to 1 cm (0.2 to 0.4 inch) and the fetus can be palpated easily through the abdominal wall by term (Blackburn, 2013). As the uterus expands into the abdominal cavity, it displaces the intestines upward and laterally. The uterus gradually rotates to the right as a result of pressure from the rectosigmoid colon on the left side of the pelvis.

Pattern of Uterine Growth. The uterus grows in a predictable pattern that provides information about fetal growth (Fig. 6.1). This growth helps confirm the estimated date of delivery (EDD), sometimes called the estimated date of birth (EDB), or estimated date of confinement (EDC). By 12 weeks of gestation, the fundus can be palpated above the

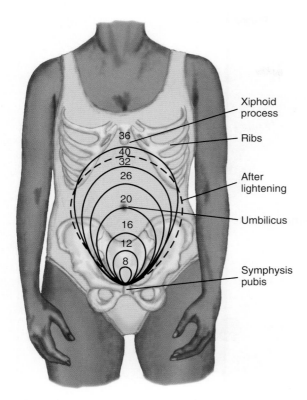

FIG. 6.1 Uterine growth pattern during pregnancy.

Labels on figure:
- Xiphoid process
- Ribs
- After lightening
- Umbilicus
- Symphysis pubis

symphysis pubis. At 16 weeks, the fundus reaches midway between the symphysis pubis and the umbilicus. It is located at the umbilicus at 20 weeks.

The fundus reaches its highest level at the xiphoid process at 36 weeks of gestation. It pushes against the diaphragm, and the expectant mother may experience shortness of breath, even during rest. By 40 weeks, the fetal head descends into the pelvic cavity and the uterus sinks to a lower level. This descent of the fetal head is called **lightening** because it reduces pressure on the diaphragm and makes breathing easier. Lightening is more pronounced in first pregnancies.

Contractility. Throughout pregnancy, the uterus undergoes irregular contractions called **Braxton Hicks contractions**. During the contractions, the uterus temporarily tightens and then returns to its original relaxed state. During the first two trimesters, the contractions are infrequent and usually not felt by the woman. Contractions occur more frequently during the third trimester and may cause some discomfort. They are called *false labor* when they are mistaken for the onset of early labor, and fail to result in cervical change.

Uterine Blood Flow. As the uterus enlarges, an increase in the size and number of blood vessels expands blood flow dramatically. As pregnancy progresses, the delivery of materials needed for fetal growth and the removal of metabolic wastes depends on adequate perfusion of the placental intervillous spaces. During late pregnancy, blood flow to the uterus and placenta reaches 1200 mL per minute and is 17% of maternal cardiac output (Koos, Kahn, & Equils, 2016). Almost 90% of the blood goes to the placenta

(Ross, Ervin, & Novak, 2017). Maternal blood carried by the myometrial arteries enters the intervillous spaces, where oxygen and nutrients are transferred to the chorionic villi and hence to the fetus. Metabolic wastes from the fetus diffuse into venous structures of the mother (see Chapter 5).

Cervix

The cervix also undergoes significant changes after conception. Water content and vascularity of the area increase. The most obvious changes occur in color and consistency. Increasing levels of estrogen cause **hyperemia** (congestion with blood) of the cervix, resulting in the characteristic bluish-purple that extends to include the vagina and labia. This discoloration, referred to as the **Chadwick's sign**, is one of the earliest signs of pregnancy.

The cervix is largely composed of connective tissue that softens when the collagen fibers decrease in concentration. Before pregnancy, the cervix has a consistency similar to that of the tip of the nose. After conception the cervix feels more like the lips or earlobe. The cervical softening is referred to as the **Goodell's sign**.

A less obvious change occurs as the cervical glands proliferate during pregnancy, and the glandular walls become thin and widely separated. As a result, the endocervical tissue resembles a honeycomb that fills with mucus secreted by the cervical glands. The mucus, which is rich in immunoglobulins, forms a plug in the cervical canal (Fig. 6.2). It blocks the ascent of bacteria from the vagina into the uterus during pregnancy to help protect the fetus and the uterine membranes from infection (Cunningham et al., 2014).

The mucous plug remains in place until term, when the cervix begins to thin and dilate, allowing the mucous plug to be expelled. One of the earliest signs of labor may be "bloody show," which consists of the mucous plug and a small amount of blood. Bleeding is produced by disruption of the cervical capillaries as the mucous plug is dislodged when the cervix begins to thin and dilate.

Vagina and Vulva

Increased vascularity causes the vaginal walls to appear bluish-purple. Softening of the abundant connective tissue allows the vagina to distend during childbirth. The vaginal mucosa thickens, and vaginal rugae (folds) become very prominent.

Vaginal cells contain increasing amounts of glycogen, which causes rapid sloughing and increased thick, white vaginal discharge. The pH of the vaginal discharge is acidic (3.5 to 6) because of the increased production of lactic acid that results from the action of *Lactobacillus acidophilus* on glycogen in the vaginal epithelium (Cunningham et al., 2014; Records & Tanaka, 2016). The acidic condition helps prevent growth of harmful bacteria in the vagina. However, the glycogen-rich environment favors the growth of *Candida albicans,* and persistent yeast infections (candidiasis) are common during pregnancy.

Increased vascularity, edema, and connective tissue changes make the tissues of the vulva and perineum more pliable. Pelvic congestion during pregnancy can lead to heightened sexual interest and increased orgasmic experiences.

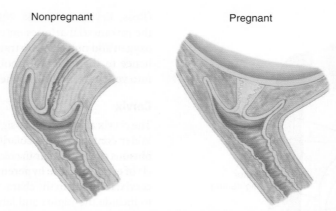

FIG. 6.2 Cervical Changes That Occur during Pregnancy. Note the thick mucous plug filling the cervical canal.

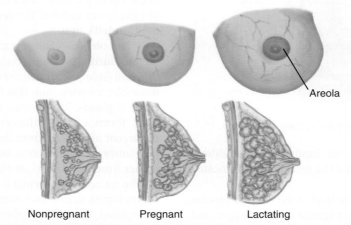

FIG. 6.3 Breast Changes That Occur during Pregnancy. The breasts increase in size and become more vascular, the areolae become darker, and the nipples become more erect.

Ovaries

Progesterone, called the "hormone of pregnancy," must be present in adequate amounts from the earliest stages to maintain pregnancy. Progesterone helps suppress contractions of the uterus and also may help prevent tissue rejection of the fetus (Blackburn, 2013). After conception, the corpus luteum of the ovaries secretes progesterone, mainly during the first 6 to 7 weeks of pregnancy (Cunningham et al., 2014). Between 6 and 10 weeks of gestation, the corpus luteum produces a smaller amount of progesterone as the placenta takes over production (Blackburn, 2013). The corpus luteum then regresses because it is no longer needed.

Ovulation ceases during pregnancy because the high circulating levels of estrogen and progesterone inhibit the release of follicle-stimulating hormone (FSH) and luteinizing hormone (LH), which are necessary for ovulation.

Breasts

During pregnancy the breasts change in both size and appearance (Fig. 6.3). Estrogen stimulates the growth of mammary ductal tissue, and progesterone promotes the growth of the lobes, lobules, and alveoli. The breasts become highly vascular, with a delicate network of veins often visible just beneath the surface of the skin. If the increase in breast size is extensive, striations ("stretch marks") similar to those that occur on the abdomen may develop.

Characteristic changes in the nipples and areola occur during pregnancy. The nipples increase in size and become darker and more erect, and the areola become larger and more pigmented. The degree of pigmentation varies with the complexion of the expectant mother. Women with very light skin tones exhibit less change in pigmentation than those with darker skin.

Sebaceous glands, called *tubercles of Montgomery*, become more prominent during pregnancy and secrete a substance that lubricates the nipples. In addition, a thick, yellowish fluid—**colostrum**—is secreted as early as 16 weeks of gestation (Records & Tanaka, 2016). Secretion of milk is suppressed during pregnancy by the high levels of estrogen and progesterone.

Cardiovascular System

During pregnancy, alterations occur in heart size and position, blood volume, blood flow, and blood components.

Heart

Heart Size and Position. Changes in the size and position of the heart are minor and reverse soon after childbirth. The muscles of the heart (myocardium) enlarge 10% to 15% during the first trimester (Blackburn, 2013). The heart is pushed upward and to the left as the uterus elevates the diaphragm during the third trimester. As a result of the change in position, the locations for auscultation of heart sounds may be shifted upward and laterally in late pregnancy.

Heart Sounds. Some heart sounds may be so altered during pregnancy that they would be considered abnormal in the nonpregnant state. The changes are first heard between 12 and 20 weeks and continue for 2 to 4 weeks after childbirth. The most common variations in heart sounds include splitting of the first heart sound and a systolic murmur that is found in more than 95% of pregnant women (Monga, 2014). The murmur is best heard at the left sternal border. Up to 90% of pregnant women have a third heart sound (Blackburn, 2013).

Blood Volume

Total blood volume increases significantly because of a combination of plasma and components such as red blood cells (RBCs, erythrocytes), white blood cells (WBCs, leukocytes), and platelets (thrombocytes). Total blood volume increase begins by 6 weeks of gestation and reaches an average of 30% to 45% during pregnancy (Blackburn, 2013).

The increased volume is needed to (1) transport nutrients and oxygen to the placenta, where they become available for the growing fetus; (2) meet the demands of the expanded maternal tissue in the uterus and breasts; and (3) provide a reserve to protect the pregnant woman from the adverse effects of blood loss that occurs during childbirth.

Plasma Volume. Plasma volume increases from 6 to 8 weeks until 32 weeks of gestation. The plasma volume is 40% to 60% (1200 to 1600 mL) greater than that in nonpregnant women (Blackburn, 2013). The increase is higher in multifetal pregnancies. The reason for the increase is unclear, but it may be related to vasodilation from nitric oxide and to estrogen, progesterone, and prostaglandin stimulation of the renin-angiotensin-aldosterone system, which causes sodium and water retention (Blackburn, 2013).

Red Blood Cell Volume. RBC volume increases by approximately 20% to 30% above prepregnancy values (Blackburn, 2013). Although both RBC volume and plasma volume expand, the increase in plasma volume is more pronounced and occurs earlier. The resulting dilution of RBC mass causes a decline in maternal hemoglobin and hematocrit. This condition is frequently called **physiologic anemia of pregnancy**, or *pseudoanemia of pregnancy,* because it reflects dilution of RBCs in the expanded plasma volume, rather than an actual decline in the number of RBCs, and does not indicate true anemia.

Physiologic anemia should not be dismissed as unimportant, however. Frequent laboratory examinations may be needed to distinguish between physiologic and true anemia. Generally, iron deficiency anemia occurs when the hemoglobin is less than 11 grams per deciliter (g/dL) in the first and third trimesters or less than 10.5 g/dL in the second trimester (Cunningham et al., 2014). Iron supplementation is often prescribed for all pregnant women by the second trimester to prevent anemia.

Dilution of RBCs by plasma may have a protective function. By decreasing blood viscosity, dilution may counter the tendency to form clots (thrombi) that could obstruct blood vessels and cause serious complications. Hemodilution may also increase placental perfusion (Monga, 2014).

Cardiac Output

The expanded blood volume of pregnancy results in an increase in cardiac output, the amount of blood ejected from the heart each minute. It is based on *stroke volume* (the amount of blood pumped from the heart with each contraction) and *heart rate* (the number of times the heart beats each minute). Cardiac output increases 30% to 50% with half of the rise occurring in the first 8 weeks of pregnancy and remains elevated throughout pregnancy (Beckmann, Ling, & Barzanski, 2014). The increase in cardiac output is the result of a gain in stroke volume and a heart rate acceleration that peaks at 15 to 20 beats per minute (bpm) by 32 weeks of gestation. Cardiac output is highest when the woman is lying on her side and is lower in the standing and supine positions (Antony, Racusin, Aagaard, & Dildy, 2017).

Systemic Vascular Resistance

Systemic vascular resistance falls during pregnancy. This change is likely because of (1) vasodilation resulting from the effects of progesterone and prostaglandins; (2) the addition of the uteroplacental unit, which provides a greater area for circulation and low resistance; (3) increased heat production from fetal, placental, and maternal metabolism, which produces vasodilation; (4) decreased sensitivity to angiotensin II; and (5) endothelial prostacyclin and endothelial-derived relaxant factors such as nitric oxide (Blackburn, 2013).

Blood Pressure

Blood pressure is an indirect measurement of the systemic vascular resistance. Due to the increased blood volume, the blood pressure changes during pregnancy are minimal (Blackburn, 2013). The diastolic pressure decreases slightly (about 10 to15 mm Hg) due to the influence of

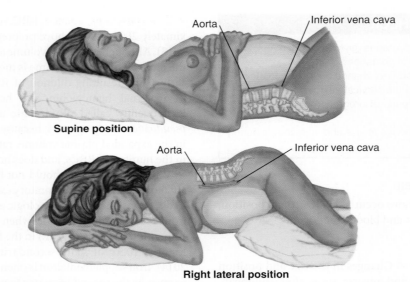

FIG. 6.4 Supine Hypotensive Syndrome. When the pregnant woman is in the supine position, the weight of the uterus partially occludes the vena cava and the aorta. The side-lying position corrects supine hypotension.

progesterone. This begins at six weeks of pregnancy and is most noticeable by the beginning of the third trimester.

Effect of Position and Other Variables. An accurate BP is affected by the maternal position. Systolic pressure remains largely unchanged or decreases slightly if it is measured when the woman is sitting or standing. Arterial pressures are approximately 10 mm Hg lower when the pregnant woman is in a side-lying or supine position than when she is sitting or standing (Antony et al., 2017). The most accurate and therefore preferred measurement is obtained with the woman in a sitting position. The position of the arm can make a difference in the reading. The arm should be at the level of the heart. If the arm is above the heart, the reading will be lower; if the arm is below the heart, the reading will be higher. The size of the cuff can affect the reading. A small cuff will show a higher reading and a large cuff will show a lower reading. It is important at every prenatal visit to measure the blood pressure with the woman in a seated position and using the appropriate cuff size. In addition, the same arm and position should be used consistently. These variables should be documented with the blood pressure reading.

Blood pressure can also be affected by age, activity, anxiety, chronic health conditions, pain, smoking, or use of alcohol or medications.

Supine Hypotension. When the pregnant woman is in the supine position, particularly in late pregnancy, the weight of the gravid (pregnant) uterus partially occludes the vena cava and the aorta (Fig. 6.4). The occlusion diminishes return of blood from the lower extremities and consequently reduces cardiac return. Cardiac output may be reduced 25% to 30% when the woman is in this position (Antony et al., 2017).

As many as 5% to 10% of women develop a drop in BP known as *supine hypotensive syndrome,* with symptoms of lightheadedness, dizziness, nausea, or *syncope* (a brief lapse in consciousness) when in the supine position (Antony et al., 2017). Blood flow through the placenta also decreases if the woman remains in the supine position for a prolonged time, which could result in fetal hypoxia.

Turning the woman to a lateral recumbent position alleviates the pressure on the blood vessels and quickly corrects supine hypotension. Women should be advised to rest in the side-lying position to prevent or correct the occurrence of supine hypotension. If they must lie in the supine position for any reason, a wedge or pillow under one hip may be effective in decreasing supine hypotension.

Blood Flow

Five major changes in blood flow occur during pregnancy:
- Blood flow is altered to include the uteroplacental unit.
- Renal plasma flow increases up to 30% to remove the increased metabolic wastes generated by the mother and the fetus (Koos et al., 2016).
- The woman's skin requires increased circulation to dissipate heat generated by increased metabolism during pregnancy.
- Blood flow to the breasts increases, resulting in engorgement and dilated veins.
- The weight of the expanding uterus on the inferior vena cava and iliac veins partially obstructs blood return from veins in the legs. Blood pools in the deep and superficial veins of the legs causing venous distention. Prolonged engorgement of the veins of the lower legs may lead to varicose veins of the legs, vulva, or rectum (hemorrhoids).

Blood Components

Although iron absorption is increased during pregnancy, sufficient iron is not always supplied by the diet. Iron supplementation is necessary to promote hemoglobin synthesis and ensure erythrocyte production adequate to prevent iron deficiency anemia.

Leukocytes increase during pregnancy, ranging from 5000 cells/mm^3 to 12,000 cells/mm^3 or as high as 15,000 cells/mm^3. Leukocytes increase further during labor and the early postpartum period, reaching levels of 25,000 cells/mm^3 to 30,000 cells/mm^3 (Blackburn, 2013).

Pregnancy is a hypercoagulable state because of an increase in factors that favor clotting and a decrease in factors that inhibit clotting. Fibrinogen (factor I), fibrin split products, and factors VII, VIII, IX, and X rise by 50% (Beckmann et al., 2014). These changes increase the ability to form clots. Fibrinolytic activity (to break down clots) decreases during pregnancy. The platelet count may decrease slightly but generally remains within the normal range (Blackburn, 2013). These changes offer some protection from hemorrhage during childbirth but also increase the risk for thrombus formation. The risk is a concern if the woman must stand or sit for prolonged periods with stasis of blood in the veins of the legs.

> ### KNOWLEDGE CHECK
>
> 6. Why is expanded blood volume important during pregnancy?
> 7. How does physiologic anemia or pseudoanemia differ from iron deficiency anemia?
> 8. Why might some pregnant women feel faint when they are in a supine position?
> 9. Why is circulation to the kidneys and skin increased during pregnancy?

Respiratory System

The major respiratory changes in pregnancy are the result of three factors: increased oxygen consumption, hormonal factors, and the physical effects of the enlarging uterus.

Oxygen Consumption

Oxygen consumption rises by 20% in pregnancy. Half the increase is used by the uterus, the fetus, and the placenta, 30% by the heart and kidneys, and the rest by the respiratory muscles and breast tissues (Beckmann et al., 2014). The tidal volume (the volume of gas moved into or out of the respiratory tract with each breath) increases by 30% to 40%. Although residual volume decreases by 20%, total lung capacity decreases by only 4%. To compensate for the increased need, progesterone causes the woman to hyperventilate slightly by breathing more deeply, although her respiratory rate remains unchanged. The partial pressure of carbon dioxide (Pco$_2$) decreases. Increased excretion of hydrogen ions from the kidneys partially compensates for the resulting mild respiratory alkalosis. The hyperventilation and respiratory alkalosis facilitate transfer of carbon dioxide from the fetus to the mother (Antony et al., 2017).

Hormonal Factors

Progesterone. Progesterone is considered a major factor in the respiratory changes of pregnancy. Progesterone, along with prostaglandins, helps decrease airway resistance by up to 50% by relaxing the smooth muscle in the respiratory tract. Progesterone is also believed to increase the sensitivity of the respiratory center in the medulla oblongata to carbon dioxide, thus stimulating the increase in minute ventilation. These two factors are responsible for the heightened awareness of the need to breathe, shortness of breath, and increased respirations experienced by many women during pregnancy (Blackburn, 2013).

Estrogen. Estrogen causes increased vascularity of the mucous membranes of the upper respiratory tract. As the capillaries become engorged, edema and hyperemia develop within the nose, pharynx, larynx, and trachea. This congestion may cause nasal and sinus stuffiness, epistaxis (nosebleed), and deepening of the voice. Increased vascularity also causes edema of the eardrum and eustachian tubes and may result in a sense of fullness in the ears.

Physical Effects of the Enlarging Uterus

During pregnancy, the enlarging uterus lifts the diaphragm approximately 4 cm (1.6 inches). The elevation of the diaphragm does not impede its movement which is increased by about 1 to 2 cm (0.4 to 0.8 inch) during respirations. The ribs flare, the substernal angle widens, and the transverse diameter of the chest expands by about 2 cm (0.8 inches) to compensate for the reduced space. These changes begin when the uterus is just beginning to enlarge. They result from the hormone relaxin, which causes relaxation of the ligaments around the ribs. Breathing becomes thoracic rather than abdominal, adding to the dyspnea that as many as 60% to 70% of women experience beginning in the first or second trimester (Blackburn, 2013).

Gastrointestinal System

The gastrointestinal system undergoes changes that are clinically significant because they may cause discomfort for the expectant mother.

Appetite

Unless the woman is nauseated, her appetite is often increased during pregnancy. This helps her consume the additional calories recommended. Food intake may increase by 15% to 20% beginning in early pregnancy (Blackburn, 2013).

Mouth

Elevated levels of estrogen cause hyperemia of the tissues of the mouth and gums and may lead to gingivitis and bleeding gums. Some women develop a highly vascular hypertrophy of the gums, called *epulis.* The condition regresses spontaneously after childbirth.

Although the amount of saliva does not usually change, some women experience *ptyalism,* or excessive salivation. The cause of ptyalism may be decreased swallowing, associated with nausea or stimulation of the salivary glands by the ingestion of starch (Records & Tanaka, 2016; Cunningham et al., 2014). Small, frequent meals and use of chewing gum and oral lozenges offer limited relief to some women.

Many women think that pregnancy causes loss of minerals from teeth to meet fetal needs. However, this is not true, and the tooth enamel is stable during pregnancy. Tooth decay may occur because of changes in saliva and the nausea and vomiting of pregnancy. Periodontal disease may result in infections that precipitate preterm labor (Blackburn, 2013).

Esophagus

The lower esophageal sphincter tone decreases during pregnancy, primarily because of the relaxant activity of progesterone on the smooth muscles. These changes, along with upward displacement of the stomach, allow gastroesophageal reflux of acidic stomach contents into the esophagus and produces heartburn (pyrosis).

Stomach

Elevated levels of progesterone relax all smooth muscle, decreasing tone and motility of the gastrointestinal tract. The effect on emptying time of the stomach is unclear, with some studies showing a decrease and others showing no change during pregnancy. Gastric acidity is decreased during the first two trimesters and increased during the third trimester. The risk for gastric ulcers decreases during pregnancy.

Large and Small Intestines

Emptying time of the intestines increases, allowing more time for nutrient absorption. It also may cause bloating and abdominal distention. Calcium, iron, some amino acids, glucose, sodium, and chloride are better absorbed during pregnancy, but absorption of some of the B vitamins is reduced (Blackburn, 2013). Decreased motility in the large intestine allows time for more water to be absorbed, leading to constipation. Constipation may cause or exacerbate hemorrhoids if the expectant mother must strain to have bowel movements. Flatulence also may be a problem.

Liver and Gallbladder

Although the size of the liver and gallbladder remains unchanged during pregnancy, estrogen and progesterone cause functional changes. The enlarging uterus pushes the liver upward and backward during the last trimester, and liver function is also altered. The serum alkaline phosphatase level rises two to four times that in nonpregnant women. Serum albumin and total protein fall, partly because of hemodilution (Williamson, Mackillop, & Heneghan, 2014).

The gallbladder becomes hypotonic, and emptying time is prolonged. The bile becomes thicker, predisposing to the development of gallstones. Reduced gallbladder tone also leads to a tendency to retain bile salts, which can cause itching (pruritus) (Records & Tanaka, 2016).

Urinary System

Bladder

The woman experiences frequency and urgency of urination throughout her pregnancy. Although uterine expansion within the pelvis is one cause of these urinary changes, frequency begins before the uterus is big enough to exert pressure on the bladder. Hormonal influences, increased blood volume, and changes in renal blood flow and glomerular filtration rate (GFR) may play a significant role in urinary frequency. Stress and urge incontinence begin at any time during pregnancy and continue until after delivery is experienced by 30% to 50% of pregnant women (Blackburn, 2013). Although frequency and urgency are normal during pregnancy, they are also signs of infection and, if accompanied by burning sensation or pain, may indicate urinary tract infection.

Bladder capacity doubles by term, and the tone is decreased in response to progesterone (Blackburn, 2013). Nocturia is common because sodium and water are retained during the day and excreted during the night when the woman is lying down. Pressure from the uterus pushes the base of the bladder forward and upward near the end of pregnancy. The bladder mucosa becomes congested with blood, and the bladder walls become hypertrophied as a result of stimulation from estrogen. Decreased drainage of blood from the base of the bladder results in edema of its tissues and renders the area susceptible to trauma and infection during childbirth.

Kidneys and Ureters

Changes in Size and Shape. During pregnancy, the kidneys change in both size and shape because of dilation of the renal pelves, calyces, and ureters above the pelvic brim. The dilation begins during the second month of pregnancy. The ureters become elongated and are compressed between the enlarging uterus and the bony pelvic brim.

The flow of urine through the ureters is partially obstructed, causing hydrostatic pressure against the renal pelvis. This occurs especially on the right side because the ureter turns toward the right during pregnancy and crosses the iliac and right ovarian veins. As much as 300 mL of urine may be present in the ureters (Blackburn, 2013). The resulting stasis of urine is important because it allows time for bacteria to multiply. The risk for bacteriuria, which may be asymptomatic, is increased, and pyelonephritis results in 30% of these women (Antony et al., 2017).

Functional Changes of the Kidneys. Renal plasma flow increases by 50% to 80% during pregnancy. This change results from increases in plasma volume and cardiac output. The flow is highest when the woman is in the left side-lying position. The GFR rises by as much as 50% because of the higher renal blood flow (Cunningham et al., 2014).

The increases in renal plasma flow and GFR are necessary for excretion of additional metabolic waste from the mother and the fetus. Glucose excretion increases, and glycosuria, or glucosuria, is common during pregnancy. Small quantities of amino acids, water-soluble vitamins, and electrolytes are also excreted because the filtered load of these substances exceeds the ability of the renal tubules to reabsorb them. Bacteria thrive in urine that is rich in nutrients, increasing the risk for urinary tract infections during pregnancy.

Urine output increases throughout pregnancy. Mild proteinuria is common and does not necessarily indicate abnormal kidney function or preeclampsia (Blackburn, 2013).

Protein level may be monitored throughout pregnancy to identify increases that would indicate a problem. Tests of renal function may be misleading during pregnancy. As a result of increased GFR, serum creatinine and blood urea nitrogen decrease and creatinine clearance levels increase (Antony et al., 2017).

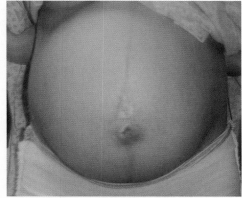

FIG. 6.5 Linea Nigra. A dark pigmented line from the fundus to the symphysis pubis.

> ### ❓ KNOWLEDGE CHECK
>
> 10. Why do some women experience dyspnea during pregnancy?
> 11. How does the respiratory system compensate for upward pressure exerted on the diaphragm by the enlarging uterus?
> 12. How does pregnancy affect the gastrointestinal system?
> 13. Why are pregnant women at increased risk for urinary tract infection?

Integumentary System
Skin

Circulation to the skin increases to help dissipate excess heat produced by increased metabolism. Pregnant women feel warmer and perspire more, particularly during the last trimester. Accelerated activity by the sebaceous glands fosters the development of acne. Additional changes include hyperpigmentation and vascular changes in the skin.

Hyperpigmentation. Increased pigmentation from elevated levels of estrogen, progesterone, and melanocyte-stimulating hormone occurs in 91% of pregnant women (Rapini, 2014). Women with dark hair or skin exhibit more hyperpigmentation than women with very light coloring.

Areas of pigmentation include brownish patches called **melasma**, chloasma, or the "mask of pregnancy." Melasma involves the forehead, cheeks, and bridge of the nose and occurs in approximately 70% of pregnant women. It also may occur in nonpregnant women taking oral contraceptives. Melasma increases with exposure to sunlight, but use of sunscreen may reduce the severity. Although melasma usually resolves after delivery when estrogen and progesterone levels decline, it continues for months or years in about 30% of women (Rapini, 2014).

The linea alba—the line that marks the longitudinal division of the midline of the abdomen—darkens to become the **linea nigra** (Fig. 6.5). This dark line of pigmentation may extend from the symphysis pubis to as high as the top of the fundus. Preexisting moles (nevi), freckles, and the areolae become darker as pregnancy progresses. Hyperpigmentation usually disappears after childbirth.

Cutaneous Vascular Changes. During pregnancy, blood vessels dilate and proliferate, which is an effect of estrogen. Changes in surface blood vessels are obvious during pregnancy, especially in women with fair skin. These include angiomas (vascular spiders, telangiectasia) that appear as tiny red elevations branching in all directions and occur most often on areas exposed to the sun. Redness of the palms of

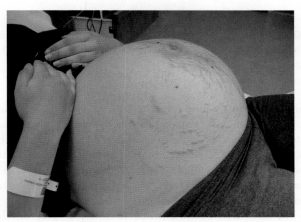

FIG. 6.6 Striae Gravidarum. Lineal tears that may occur in connective tissue.

the hands or soles of the feet, known as *palmar erythema,* also occurs in many White women and some African American women. Vascular changes may be emotionally distressing for the expectant mother, but they are clinically insignificant and usually disappear shortly after childbirth.

Connective Tissue

Linear tears may occur in the connective tissue, most often on the abdomen, breasts, and buttocks, appearing as slightly depressed, pink to purple streaks called **striae gravidarum,** or "stretch marks" (Fig. 6.6). They occur in 50% to 80% of pregnant women, and 10% have severe striae (Rapini, 2014). Women are concerned about striae because they do not disappear after childbirth, although the marks usually fade to silvery lines. Laser therapy is sometimes used after childbirth to reduce or eliminate severe striae. Many women believe that striae can be prevented by massaging with oil, vitamin E, or cocoa butter, but these substances have not been found effective. Antipruritic creams may be effective in controlling the itching that often occurs.

Hair and Nails

Because fewer follicles are in the resting phase, hair grows more rapidly and less hair falls out during pregnancy. After

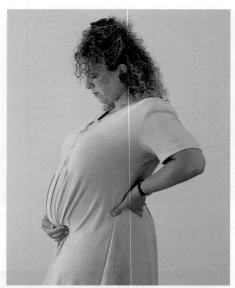

FIG. 6.7 Lordosis increases by the third trimester as the uterus grows larger, and the woman must lean backward to maintain her balance.

childbirth, hair follicles return to normal activity, and many women become concerned at the rate of hair loss that occurs 2 to 4 months after childbirth. They need reassurance that more follicles have returned to the normal resting phase and excessive hair loss will not continue. Hair growth returns to normal within 6 to 12 months after childbirth (Beckmann et al., 2014).

The nails may become brittle or softer or may develop transverse grooves. Some women's nails grow faster or split or break more easily during pregnancy. These changes end after childbirth and no treatment is needed.

Musculoskeletal System
Calcium Storage
During pregnancy, fetal demands for calcium increase, especially in the third trimester. Absorption of calcium from the intestine doubles during pregnancy. Calcium is stored for use during the third trimester, when fetal needs peak. Although 28 to 30 grams of calcium from maternal bone stores is transferred to the fetus, this amount is small compared with total maternal stores and does not deplete the maternal bone density (Blackburn, 2013).

Postural Changes
Musculoskeletal changes are progressive. They begin early in pregnancy when relaxin and progesterone initiate relaxation of the ligaments. At 28 to 30 weeks, the pelvic symphysis separates (Beckmann et al., 2014). The increased mobility of the pelvic joints causes the pregnant woman to assume a wide stance with the "waddling" gait of pregnancy.

During the third trimester, as the uterus increases in size, the expectant mother must lean backward to maintain her balance (Fig. 6.7). This posture creates a progressive lordosis or curvature of the lower spine and often leads to backache. Obesity or previous back problems increase the problem.

Abdominal Wall
The abdominal muscles may be stretched beyond their capacity during the third trimester, causing **diastasis recti**, separation of the rectus abdominis muscles (see Fig. 17.4). The extent of the separation varies from slight and clinically insignificant to severe, when a large portion of the uterine wall is covered only by the peritoneum, fascia, and skin.

Endocrine System
Numerous changes in hormones occur in pregnancy (Table 6.1).

Pituitary Gland
The anterior pituitary gland increases in size during pregnancy. Serum prolactin levels increase 10-fold by term to prepare the breasts for lactation (Blackburn, 2013). The hormones FSH and LH are not needed to stimulate ovulation during pregnancy and are suppressed by high levels of estrogen and progesterone.

The posterior pituitary releases oxytocin, which stimulates contractions of the uterus. This action is inhibited by progesterone, produced mainly by the placenta during pregnancy. In the second half of pregnancy, estrogen causes a gradual rise of oxytocin receptors in the uterus, increasing contractions near term (Boron & Boulpaep, 2017). After childbirth, oxytocin plays an important role in keeping the uterus contracted to prevent excessive bleeding. Oxytocin also stimulates the milk-ejection reflex after childbirth.

Thyroid Gland
Hyperplasia and increased vascularity cause the thyroid gland to enlarge during pregnancy (Cunningham et al., 2014). The availability of thyroid hormones increases by 40% to 100% (Cunningham et al., 2014).

Early in the first trimester, a rise in total thyroxine (T4) and thyroxine-binding globulin occurs. Levels of serum-unbound or free T4 rise early in pregnancy but return to normal nonpregnant levels by the end of the first trimester (Cunningham et al., 2014). Both T4 and triiodothyronine (T3) cross the placenta. Maternal thyroid hormones are important for fetal neurologic function because the fetus does not synthesize thyroid hormones until 10 to 12 weeks of gestation (Cunningham et al., 2014).

Parathyroid Glands
Parathyroid hormone, which is important in calcium homeostasis, is decreased by 10% to 30% in the first trimester and increases by term. However, it remains in the normal range throughout pregnancy (Blackburn, 2013). Calcium supplies for transfer to the fetus are adequate.

Pancreas
Significant changes in the pancreas during pregnancy are the result of alterations in maternal blood glucose levels and fluctuations in insulin production. Blood glucose levels are 10% to 20% lower than before pregnancy, and hypoglycemia may develop between meals and at night as the fetus continuously draws glucose from the mother (Blackburn, 2013).

TABLE 6.1   Hormones Related to Pregnancy

Hormone	Source	Major Effects
Prolactin	Anterior pituitary	Primary hormone of milk production, insulin antagonist
Follicle-stimulating hormone (FSH)	Anterior pituitary	Initiates maturation of ovum, suppressed during pregnancy
Luteinizing hormone (LH)	Anterior pituitary	Stimulates ovulation of mature ovum in nonpregnant state, suppressed in pregnancy
Oxytocin	Posterior pituitary	Stimulates uterine contractions, stimulates milk-ejection reflex after birth, inhibited during pregnancy
Thyroxine (T4)	Thyroid	Increased during pregnancy to stimulate basal metabolic rate, used by fetus in early pregnancy
Cortisol	Adrenals	Increased during pregnancy, insulin antagonist, active in metabolism of glucose, protein, and fats
Aldosterone	Adrenals	Increased during pregnancy to conserve sodium and maintain fluid balance
Human chorionic gonadotropin (hCG)	Trophoblast	Prevents involution of corpus luteum to maintain production of estrogen and progesterone until placenta is formed
Estrogen	Corpus luteum of ovary, placenta	Suppresses FSH and LH, stimulates development of uterus and breasts, causes vascular changes in skin, uterus, respiratory tract, and bladder, causes hyper-pigmentation, insulin antagonist, increases fat stores
Progesterone	Corpus luteum of ovary, placenta	Maintains uterine lining for implantation, relaxes smooth muscles, decreases uterine contractions, develops breasts for lactation, increases carbon dioxide sensitivity, increases resistance to insulin, inhibits FSH and LH, prevents fetal tissue rejection, retains sodium
Human chorionic somato-mammotropin (human placental lactogen)	Placenta	Stimulates metabolism of fat to provide maternal energy, antagonistic to insulin, promotes sodium retention, prepares breasts for lactation, acts as growth hormone
Relaxin	Corpus luteum, decidua, placenta	Inhibits uterine activity, softens connective tissue of cervix, relaxes cartilage and connective tissue

FSH, Follicle-stimulating hormone; *LH,* luteinizing hormone.

During the second half of pregnancy, maternal tissue sensitivity to insulin begins to decline because of the effects of human chorionic somatomammotropin (hCS), prolactin, estrogen, progesterone, and cortisol. The mother uses fatty acids to meet energy needs. Fasting blood glucose level is decreased as glucose passes to the fetus. Postprandial (after a meal) blood glucose level is higher than before pregnancy because of insulin resistance, making more glucose available for fetal energy needs. In healthy women, the pancreas produces additional insulin. In some women, however, insulin production cannot be increased and these women experience periodic hyperglycemia or gestational diabetes (see Chapter 10).

Adrenal Glands

Although the adrenal glands enlarge only slightly during pregnancy, significant changes occur in two adrenal hormones: cortisol and aldosterone. The concentrations of both serum cortisol and free (unbound) cortisol, the metabolically active form, are higher. The increase is the result of the elevated estrogen level and a decrease in metabolic clearance rate doubling the half-life of cortisol (Blackburn, 2013). Cortisol regulates carbohydrate and protein metabolism. It stimulates gluconeogenesis (formation of glycogen from noncarbohydrate sources such as amino and fatty acids) whenever the

supply of glucose is inadequate to meet the body's needs for energy.

Aldosterone regulates the absorption of sodium from the distal tubules of the kidneys. It increases very early in pregnancy to overcome the salt-wasting effects of progesterone. This helps maintain the necessary level of sodium in the greatly expanded blood volume to meet the needs of the fetus. Aldosterone level is closely related to water metabolism.

Changes Caused by Placental Hormones

Human Chorionic Gonadotropin. In early pregnancy, human chorionic gonadotropin (hCG) is produced by the trophoblastic cells surrounding the developing embryo. The primary function of hCG in early pregnancy is to prevent deterioration of the corpus luteum so it can continue producing estrogen and progesterone until the placenta is sufficiently developed. The presence of this hormone produces a positive pregnancy test result.

Estrogen. Early in pregnancy, estrogen is produced by the corpus luteum. The placenta produces estrogen for the remainder of pregnancy. The effects of estrogen during pregnancy include the following:

- Suppression of FSH and LH
- Stimulation of uterine growth
- Increased blood supply to uterine vessels

- Added deposit of maternal fat stores to provide a reserve of energy
- Increased uterine contractions near term
- Development of the glands and ductal system in the breasts in preparation for lactation
- Hyperpigmentation
- Stimulation of vascular changes in the skin, breasts, upper respiratory tract, and bladder
- Antagonist to insulin

Progesterone. Progesterone is produced first by the corpus luteum and then by the fully developed placenta. Progesterone is the most important hormone of pregnancy. Its major effects include:

- Suppression of FSH and LH
- Maintenance of the endometrial layer for implantation of the fertilized ovum and prevention of menstruation
- Decreased uterine contractility to prevent spontaneous abortion
- Increased fat deposits
- Stimulation of development of the lobes, lobules, and ducts in the breast for lactation
- Relaxation of smooth muscles of the uterus, gastric sphincter, bowel, ureters, bladder
- Increased respiratory sensitivity to carbon dioxide, stimulating ventilation
- Suppression of the immunologic response, preventing rejection of the fetus
- Antagonist to insulin
- Retention of sodium

Human Chorionic Somatomammotropin. Also called *human placental lactogen (hPL),* human chorionic somatomammotropin (hCS) is present early in pregnancy and increases steadily throughout pregnancy. Its primary function is to increase the availability of glucose for the fetus. A potent insulin antagonist, hCS reduces the sensitivity of maternal cells to insulin and decreases maternal metabolism of glucose. This frees glucose for transport to the fetus, who needs a constant supply. In addition, hCS encourages the quick metabolism of free fatty acids to provide energy for the pregnant woman. hCS also helps prepare the breasts for lactation and may act as a growth hormone.

Relaxin. Relaxin is produced by the corpus luteum, the decidua, and the placenta and is present by the first missed menstrual period. Relaxin inhibits uterine activity, softens connective tissue in the cervix, and relaxes cartilage and connective tissue to increase mobility of the pelvic joints (Blackburn, 2013).

Changes in Metabolism

During pregnancy, approximately 3.5 kg of fat and 30,000 kcal, are accumulated. In addition, the woman, fetus, and placenta synthesize 900 grams of new protein (Blackburn, 2013). The basal metabolic rate increases 10% to 20% by the third trimester (Cunningham et al., 2014).

Weight Gain. A correlation exists between inadequate weight gain in pregnancy and small-for-gestational age infants, as well as between excessive weight gain and increased risk for large-for-gestational age infants. Therefore women of normal prepregnancy weight are encouraged to gain an average of 11.5 to 16 kg (25 to 35 lb) during pregnancy (ACOG, 2013). The fetus, placenta, and amniotic fluid make up less than half the recommended weight gain. The remainder is found in the increased size of the uterus and breasts, increased blood volume, increased interstitial fluid, and maternal stores of subcutaneous fat.

Water Metabolism. The amount of water needed during pregnancy increases to meet the needs of the fetus, placenta, amniotic fluid, and increased blood volume. Total body water increases by 6.5 to 8.5 L by term (Antony et al., 2017). The kidneys must compensate for the many factors that influence fluid balance. Increased GFR, prostaglandins, decreased concentrations of plasma proteins, and increased progesterone level all result in an increase in sodium excretion. However, increased concentrations of estrogen, deoxycorticosterone, hCS, and aldosterone all tend to promote the reabsorption of sodium. The net effect of the combined hormonal action is the maintenance of the sodium and water balance (Blackburn, 2013).

Edema. Because of hemodilution, colloid osmotic pressure decreases slightly, which favors the development of edema during pregnancy. Edema further increases toward term when the weight of the uterus compresses the veins of the pelvis. This process delays venous return, causing the veins of the legs to become distended, and increases venous pressure, resulting in additional fluid shifts from the vascular compartment to interstitial spaces.

Up to 70% of women have dependent edema during pregnancy. Accumulation of 2 L or more of fluid occurs with edema of the feet. The edema is obvious at the end of the day (particularly if a pregnant woman stands for prolonged periods), and the force of gravity contributes to the pooling of blood in the veins of the legs. Generalized edema occurs if women retain 4 to 5 L of water (Blackburn, 2013). Dependent edema is clinically insignificant if no other abnormal signs are present.

Carbohydrate Metabolism. Carbohydrate metabolism changes markedly during pregnancy when more insulin is needed as pregnancy progresses as a result of increased insulin resistance (Cunningham et al., 2014). (See previous section, Pancreas, for more information.)

Sensory Organs
Eye

Corneal edema may cause women who wear contact lenses to have some discomfort. The problem resolves after childbirth, and women should not get new prescriptions for lenses for several weeks after delivery. Intraocular pressure decreases, which may cause improvement and a need for less medication in women with glaucoma (Blackburn, 2013).

Ear

Changes in the mucous membranes of the eustachian tube from increased levels of estrogen may cause women to have blocked ears and a mild, temporary hearing loss.

Immune System

Immune function is altered during pregnancy to allow the fetus, which is foreign tissue for the mother, to grow undisturbed without being rejected by the woman's body. This may cause some autoimmune conditions such as rheumatoid arthritis and multiple sclerosis to improve during pregnancy (Cunningham et al., 2014). Resistance to some infections is decreased, however, and some viral and fungal infections occur more often during pregnancy (Blackburn, 2013; Koos et al., 2016).

❓ KNOWLEDGE CHECK

14. What causes the progressive changes in posture and gait during pregnancy?
15. What are the reasons that women do not ovulate and have menstrual periods during pregnancy?
16. Why do maternal needs for insulin change during pregnancy?

CONFIRMATION OF PREGNANCY

Although many women undergo early ultrasonography to confirm the pregnancy, the diagnosis of pregnancy has traditionally been based on symptoms experienced by the woman as well as signs observed by a physician, nurse-midwife, or nurse practitioner. Fig. 6.8 summarizes maternal changes that occur throughout pregnancy. (See Chapter 5 for a discussion on fetal growth and development.)

The signs and symptoms of pregnancy are grouped into three classifications: presumptive, probable, and positive indications. A diagnosis of pregnancy cannot be made solely on the presumptive or probable signs because they may have other causes, listed in Table 6.2. A definitive diagnosis of pregnancy can be based only on positive signs.

Presumptive Indications of Pregnancy

Most, but not all, presumptive indications are subjective changes experienced and reported by the woman. These changes are the least reliable indicators of pregnancy because they can be caused by conditions other than pregnancy.

Amenorrhea

Absence of menstruation (**amenorrhea**) in a sexually active woman who menstruates regularly is one of the first changes noted and strongly suggests that conception has occurred. Menses cease after conception because progesterone and estrogen, secreted by the corpus luteum, maintain the endometrial lining in preparation for implantation of the fertilized ovum. A small amount of bleeding from implantation of the blastocyst may cause the woman to think she is having a period. This occurs in 30% to 40% of pregnant women (Hobel & Williams, 2016).

Nausea and Vomiting

Approximately 60% to 80% of women experience nausea and vomiting that begin at 4 to 8 weeks of pregnancy and resolve at 10 to 12 weeks, but some women experience it earlier and longer (Blackburn, 2013). Although the problem occurs most often in early pregnancy, a study of over 500 women found 45% experienced nausea and vomiting during the third trimester (Kramer et al., 2013). Nausea and vomiting are believed to be caused by the increased hormones (such as hCG and estrogen) and decreased gastric motility (an effect of progesterone).

Fatigue

Many pregnant women experience fatigue and drowsiness during the first trimester. The direct cause is unknown, but it may be from changes in hormones such as progesterone.

Urinary Frequency

Urinary frequency begins in the first few weeks of pregnancy and results from hormonal and fluid volume changes. It continues later as the expanding uterus exerts pressure on the bladder. Late in the third trimester, the fetus settles into the pelvic cavity and causes more frequency and urgency of urination as the uterus presses against the bladder.

Breast and Skin Changes

Breast changes begin by the 6th week of pregnancy. The expectant mother experiences breast tenderness, tingling, feelings of fullness, and increased size and pigmentation of the areolae.

Many women observe increased pigmentation of the skin (such as melasma, linea nigra, darkening of the areolae of the breasts) during pregnancy. These skin changes are the result of estrogen and progesterone on melanocytes (Blackburn, 2013).

Vaginal and Cervical Color Change

The cervix, vagina, and labia change from pink to a dark bluish purple. This color change, called the *Chadwick's sign,* is another presumptive sign of pregnancy (Blackburn, 2013; Cunningham et al., 2014; Gambone, 2016; Records & Tanaka, 2016). It results from increased vascularity of the pelvic organs and is present by 8 weeks of pregnancy.

Fetal Movement

Unlike other presumptive indications of pregnancy, fetal movement (quickening) is not perceived until the second trimester. Although some women become aware of fetal movement sooner, most expectant mothers notice subtle fetal movements, which gradually increase in intensity between 16 and 20 weeks of gestation.

Probable Indications of Pregnancy

Probable indications of pregnancy are objective findings that can be documented by an examiner. They are primarily related

Gestational age 5-8 weeks

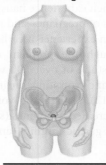

Woman misses menstrual period. Nausea; fatigue. Tingling of breasts. Uterus is size of a lemon; positive Chadwick, Goodell, and Hegar signs. Urinary frequency; increased vaginal discharge.

Gestational age 9-12 weeks

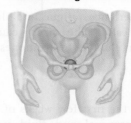

Nausea usually ends by 10 to 12 weeks. Uterus is size of an orange; palpable above symphysis pubis. Vulvar varicosities may appear. Fetal heartbeat may be heard with a Doppler.

Gestational age 13-16 weeks

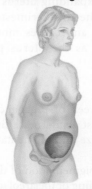

Fetal movements may be felt at about 16 weeks. Uterus has risen into the abdomen; fundus midway between symphysis pubis and umbilicus. Colostrum present; blood volume increases.

Gestational age 17-20 weeks

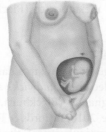

Fetal movements felt. Heartbeat can be heard with fetoscope. Skin pigmentation increases: areolae darken; melasma and linea nigra may be obvious. Braxton Hicks contractions palpable. Fundus at level of umbilicus at about 20 weeks.

Gestational age 21-24 weeks

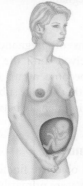

Relaxation of smooth muscles of veins and bladder increases the chance of varicose veins and urinary tract infections. Woman is more aware of fetal movements.

Gestational age 25-28 weeks

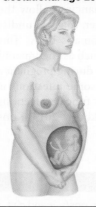

Period of greatest weight gain and lowest hemoglobin level begins. Lordosis may cause backache.

Gestational age 29-32 weeks

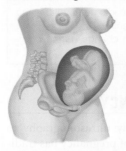

Heartburn common as uterus presses on diaphragm and displaces stomach. Braxton Hicks contractions more noticeable. Lordosis increases; waddling gait develops due to increased mobility of pelvic joints.

Gestational age 33-36 weeks

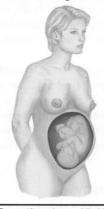

Shortness of breath caused by upward pressure on diaphragm; woman may have difficulty finding a comfortable position for sleep. Umbilicus protrudes. Varicosities more pronounced; pedal or ankle edema may be present. Urinary frequency noted following lightening when presenting part settles into pelvic cavity.

Gestational age 37-40 weeks

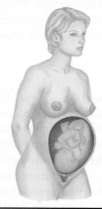

Woman is uncomfortable; looking forward to birth of baby. Cervix softens, begins to efface; mucous plug is often lost.

FIG. 6.8 Maternal responses based on the date of the last menstrual period.

TABLE 6.2 Indications of Pregnancy and Other Possible Causes

Sign	Other Possible Causes
Presumptive Indications	
Amenorrhea	Emotional stress, strenuous physical exercise, endocrine problems, chronic disease, early menopause, anovulation, low body weight
Nausea and vomiting	Gastrointestinal virus, food poisoning, emotional stress
Fatigue	Illness, stress, sudden changes in lifestyle
Urinary frequency	Urinary tract infection
Breast and skin changes	Premenstrual changes, use of oral contraceptives
Chadwick's sign	Infection or hormonal imbalance causing pelvic congestion
Quickening	Intestinal gas, peristalsis, or pseudocyesis (false pregnancy)
Probable Indications	
Abdominal enlargement	Abdominal or uterine tumors
Goodell's sign	Hormonal contraceptives or imbalance
Hegar's sign	Hormonal imbalance
Ballottement	Uterine or cervical polyps
Braxton Hicks contractions	Intestinal gas
Palpation of fetal outline	Large leiomyoma that feels like the fetal head, small soft leiomyoma that simulates fetal body parts
Uterine souffle	Confusion with the mother's pulse
Positive pregnancy test	Hematuria, proteinuria, some medications, tumors that produce human chorionic gonadotropin, some drugs
Positive Indications	
Auscultation of fetal heart sounds	
Fetal movements detected by an examiner	
Visualization of embryo or fetus	

to physical changes in the reproductive organs. Although these signs are stronger indicators of pregnancy, a positive diagnosis cannot be made because they may have other causes.

Abdominal Enlargement

Enlargement of the abdomen during the childbearing years is generally a reliable indication of pregnancy, particularly if it corresponds with a slow, gradual increase in uterine growth. Pregnancy is even more likely when abdominal enlargement is accompanied by amenorrhea.

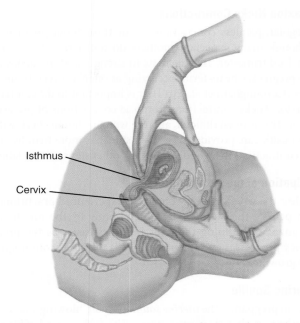

FIG. 6.9 Hegar's sign demonstrates softening of the isthmus of the cervix.

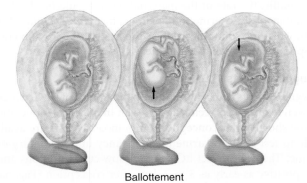

Ballottement

FIG. 6.10 When the cervix is tapped, the fetus floats upward in the amniotic fluid. A rebound is felt by the examiner when the fetus falls back.

Cervical Softening

In the early weeks of pregnancy, the cervix softens because of pelvic vasocongestion (Goodell's sign). Cervical softening is noted during pelvic examination (Records & Tanaka, 2016).

Changes in Uterine Consistency

About 6 to 8 weeks after the last menses, the lower uterine segment is so soft it can be compressed to the thinness of paper. This is called the **Hegar's sign** (Fig. 6.9). The body of the uterus can be easily flexed against the cervix.

Ballottement

Near midpregnancy, a sudden tap on the cervix during vaginal examination may cause the fetus to rise in the amniotic fluid and then rebound to its original position (Fig. 6.10). This movement, called *ballottement,* is a strong indication of pregnancy, but it may also be caused by other factors such as uterine or cervical polyps.

Braxton Hicks Contractions

Irregular, painless contractions occur throughout pregnancy, although many expectant mothers do not notice them until the third trimester. They increase in strength and frequency as the pregnancy nears term, occurring as often as every 10 minutes (Cunningham et al., 2014). It is important to differentiate Braxton Hicks contractions from the contractions of preterm labor. This is often difficult, and the woman should check with her health care provider if she is unsure, has more than five or six contractions in an hour, or has any other signs of early labor.

Palpation of the Fetal Outline

Unless the woman is very obese, an experienced practitioner can palpate the outlines of the fetal body by the middle of pregnancy. Outlining the fetus becomes easier as the pregnancy progresses and the uterine walls thin to accommodate the growing fetus.

Uterine Souffle

Late in pregnancy, the *uterine souffle*—a soft, blowing sound—may be auscultated over the uterus. This is the sound of blood circulating through the dilated uterine vessels, and it corresponds to the maternal pulse. Therefore to identify the uterine souffle, the rate of the maternal pulse should be checked simultaneously. Uterine souffle differs from *funic souffle*—the soft, whistling sound heard over the umbilical cord and corresponding to the fetal heart rate.

Pregnancy Tests

Pregnancy tests detect hCG or the beta subunit of hCG, which is secreted by the placenta and present in maternal blood and urine shortly after conception. Immunoassay tests are available to test blood or urine for pregnancy in a laboratory or home. They can detect hCG at very low concentrations and are positive as early as 3 to 7 days after conception (Pagana, Pagana, & Pagana, 2017). For home testing, the woman places her urine sample on a strip or wick and watches for a color or digital change. The first morning void is preferred because it is most concentrated. Instructions vary with different tests, and the woman should read the directions carefully when testing at home.

Inaccurate Pregnancy Test Results. When pregnancy test results are reported as negative and the woman is in fact pregnant, the results are called *false-negative*. False-negative results may occur when the instructions are not followed properly, it is too early in the pregnancy, the urine is too dilute, or the woman is taking drugs such as diuretics. Hematuria, proteinuria, or some tumors may cause *false-positive* results, in which the test indicates a pregnancy when the woman is not pregnant. Some anticonvulsants, antiparkinsonian drugs, tranquilizers, and hypnotics also may cause a false-positive result (Pagana et al., 2017).

Positive Indications of Pregnancy

Only three signs are accepted as positive confirmation of pregnancy: auscultation of fetal heart sounds, fetal movement detected by an examiner, and visualization of the embryo or fetus.

Auscultation of Fetal Heart Sounds

Fetal heart sounds can be heard with a fetoscope by 18 to 20 weeks of gestation (Beckmann et al., 2014). The electronic Doppler, which is used more often, detects heart motion and makes an audible sound by as early as 6 weeks of gestation (Gambone, 2016).

To distinguish the fetal heartbeat from the maternal pulse, the examiner palpates the maternal pulse while auscultating the fetal heartbeat. The normal fetal heart rate is 110 to 160 bpm. The fetal heart rate is muffled by the amniotic fluid, and the location changes because the fetus moves freely in the amniotic fluid.

Fetal Movements Detected by an Examiner

Fetal movements are considered a positive sign of pregnancy when felt or visualized by an experienced examiner who is not likely to be deceived by peristalsis in the large intestine.

Visualization of the Embryo or Fetus

Confirmation of pregnancy has become much simpler since the development of ultrasonography, which makes it possible to view the embryo or fetus and observe the fetal heartbeat very early in pregnancy. Positive confirmation of pregnancy is possible by transvaginal ultrasonography as early as 3 to 4 weeks of gestation (Beckmann et al., 2014).

? KNOWLEDGE CHECK

17. How do presumptive and probable indications of pregnancy differ?
18. Why is "fetal" movement felt by the pregnant woman not a positive sign of pregnancy?
19. What are the most common causes of inaccurate pregnancy test results?

PSYCHOSOCIAL ADAPTATIONS TO PREGNANCY

Becoming a parent who is capable of loving and caring for a totally dependent infant is more than a biologic event. The process begins before conception and involves major changes in the woman, her partner, and the entire family. Although each couple adapts to pregnancy in a unique way, the psychological responses of prospective parents change as the pregnancy progresses. Although the initial reaction may be uncertainty, by the time the infant is born the woman and her partner have completed **developmental tasks**, maturation steps that allow further development. These help them become parents in the true sense of the word. Both social and cultural factors influence their adjustment to the pregnancy.

MATERNAL PSYCHOLOGICAL RESPONSES

A woman's psychological response to pregnancy changes over time. Initially, she may be uncertain or ambivalent about the pregnancy and her primary focus is on herself. Gradually, her focus shifts, and she becomes increasingly concerned about protecting and providing for the fetus.

First Trimester

Uncertainty

During the early weeks, the woman is unsure if she is pregnant and tries to confirm it. She observes her body carefully for changes indicating pregnancy. She may confer with family and friends about the probability and often uses an over-the-counter pregnancy test kit for validation.

Reaction to the uncertainty of pregnancy depends on the individual. Usually, she seeks confirmation from a physician, nurse-midwife, or nurse practitioner during the first trimester of pregnancy.

Ambivalence

Whether or not the pregnancy was planned, once it is confirmed, many women have conflicting feelings, or **ambivalence**, about being pregnant (Link, 2016b). Pregnancy causes permanent life changes for the woman, and she often begins to examine expected changes and decide how she will cope with them. If it is her first pregnancy, the woman may worry about the added responsibility and feel unsure of her ability to be a good parent. A multipara may be apprehensive about how this pregnancy will affect her relationship with her other children and her partner. Ambivalence has usually changed to acceptance by the second trimester.

The Self as Primary Focus

Throughout the first trimester, the woman's primary focus is on herself, not on the fetus. Early physical responses to pregnancy, such as nausea and fatigue, confirm something is happening to her, but the fetus seems vague and unreal. Because she has not gained weight to confirm a growing, developing fetus, she often thinks more about being pregnant than about the coming baby.

Physical changes and increased hormone levels may cause emotional lability (unstable moods). Her mood can change quickly from contentment to irritation or from optimistic planning to an overwhelming sleepiness. These changes may be confusing to her partner and her family, who are accustomed to more stability.

Nurses should concentrate on the mother's physical and psychological needs during this period of maternal self-focus. Teaching should be aimed at the common early changes of pregnancy and their normality. Ways of coping with morning sickness, sexuality, and mood swings are important subjects to explore with the couple (Link, 2016a). The nurse should assess how the couple is managing these changes and explain that such changes are normal and generally do not indicate problems.

Second Trimester

Physical Evidence of Pregnancy

During the second trimester, physical changes occur in the expectant mother that make the fetus "real." The uterus grows rapidly and can be palpated in the abdomen, weight increases, and breast changes are obvious. Ultrasound examination allows the woman to see the fetus. During this time, she feels the fetus move (quickening). This experience is important because it confirms the presence of the fetus with each movement. As a result, she no longer thinks of the fetus as simply a part of her body but now perceives it as separate, although entirely dependent on her.

The Fetus as Primary Focus

The fetus becomes the woman's major focus during the second trimester. The discomforts of the first trimester have usually decreased, and her size does not affect her activity. She is now concerned about producing a healthy infant. She is often interested in information about diet and fetal development. A feeling of creative energy and satisfaction is common.

Narcissism and Introversion

At this time, many women become increasingly concerned about their ability to protect and provide for the fetus. This concern is often manifested as **narcissism** (undue preoccupation with oneself) and **introversion** (concentration on the self and body). Selecting exactly the right foods to eat or the right clothes to wear may assume more importance than earlier in the pregnancy. Some women lose interest in their jobs, which may seem alien compared with the events taking place inside them.

If this is her first pregnancy, the expectant mother wonders about the infant. She looks at baby pictures of herself and her partner and may want to hear stories about what they were like as infants. Although multiparas know more about infants in general, they are interested in this infant and concerned with this child's acceptance by siblings and grandparents. Expectant mothers also may examine their relationships with others and how these ties will change after the birth (Link, 2016a).

The woman often spends much time thinking about the fetus and daydreaming or fantasizing about what life will be like when it is born. She may call it by the name chosen and talk about the personality of the fetus. Some mothers enjoy reading about fetal development to see what changes are happening each week. This intense introspection may be confusing to her partner and family because it is so different from her usual behavior.

Body Image

Rapid and profound changes take place in the body during the second trimester. Changes in body size and contour are obvious with thickening of the waist, bulging of the abdomen, and enlargement of the breasts.

Changes may be welcomed because they signify growth of the fetus and give the woman and her partner a feeling of pride. They increase the woman's **body image** (subjective view of self). For some women, however, the change in body size and shape, coupled with hyperpigmentation of the skin and striae gravidarum, may contribute to a negative body image. Changes in body function such as altered balance, reduced physical endurance, and discomfort in the pelvis and lower back areas may also affect her body image.

NURSING CARE PLAN
Body Image during Pregnancy Assessment

Shannon is a 34-year-old primigravida in the 26th week of pregnancy. Both she and her husband have been runners for several years. With her physician's permission, she continued running until 6 weeks ago, when she began to find it uncomfortable. Shannon says she now walks "like other old ladies." She expresses concern about the brown discoloration on her face and her increasing size and says she feels "fat, awkward, and ugly." She states, "I hate the way I look! I can't wait to get back into shape." She also has questions about what sexual activity is allowed during pregnancy.

Identification of Patient Problem

Altered self-image because of changes in body size, contour, and function secondary to pregnancy

Planning: Expected Outcomes

By the end of her next prenatal visit Shannon will do the following:
1. Make statements that indicate acceptance of expected body changes during her pregnancy.
2. Express her feelings about body changes to her husband and the health care team.
3. Set realistic goals for weight loss and the resumption of a running program after childbirth.
4. Report continued mutually satisfactory sexual activity during pregnancy.

Interventions and Rationales

1. Acknowledge Shannon's feelings. "I can see you're disappointed about not being able to run and concerned about how pregnancy has changed your body." *Feelings should be acknowledged, reflected, and dealt with before the underlying cause can be addressed.*
2. Clarify her concerns. "You've always been an athlete. Women often wonder if changes in pregnancy will affect them permanently." *An underlying unvoiced concern may be that pregnancy will change the woman so that she will be unable to continue athletics. This altered perception of herself may cause fear, grief, or both.*
3. Suggest that she share her feelings with her husband and seek his support. Model this interaction, if necessary: "I feel awkward and left out of a big part of our lives. I need some reassurance from you." *Although the woman may assume her partner recognizes and understands her negative feelings, this may not be true.*
4. Discuss types of low-impact, moderate exercise, such as walking or swimming, that would be beneficial for Shannon. *Moderate daily exercise is encouraged during uncomplicated pregnancy.*

5. Describe the expected pattern of weight gain for the rest of the pregnancy and correlate this with the growth and development of the fetus. Explain that adipose tissue provides needed energy for birth and lactation. *Knowledge of the expected weight gain and understanding that weight gain shows the fetus is growing may allay unexpressed fears of excessive weight gain.*
6. Help Shannon make realistic plans to lose weight and recover her strength and endurance after childbirth.
   a. Explain the expected pattern of weight loss after childbirth.
   b. Demonstrate graduated exercises that increase muscle tone and strength.
   c. Discuss a diet that meets her needs for breastfeeding.
      Many women are relieved to know that the added weight will be lost gradually. Breastfeeding requires additional calories and nutrients.
7. Explain that the discoloration on her face (melasma) is normal and usually disappears after pregnancy. Suggest she limit exposure to the sun and use sunscreen. *Knowledge of what is normal is comforting. Limiting exposure to the sun and using sunscreen may help decrease the severity.*
8. Determine Shannon's specific concerns about sexuality and respond to those in particular. Concerns vary among couples. *Some couples worry about harming the fetus or causing discomfort for the mother.*
9. Reassure her that sexual activity poses no harm to either the mother or the fetus in a normal pregnancy. Explain the anatomy of the vagina, cervix, and uterus. Suggest she bring her partner to the next visit if he has concerns. *Knowledge of the separation between the vagina and the fetus may relieve concern about the safety of vaginal intercourse during pregnancy.*
10. Suggest that alternative positions such as side-lying, woman-superior, and vaginal entry from the back be used for intercourse during the third trimester. *The male-superior position becomes uncomfortable for the woman when the uterus is large and heavy, and it increases the risk for supine hypotension.*

Evaluation

At the next prenatal visit, Shannon speaks with pride about how big the baby is growing and makes other statements showing more acceptance of body changes. She reports that her husband has shown increased concern about her feelings and has been very supportive since she shared her feelings with him. Shannon has explored other types of exercises and has found several she will use during the rest of her pregnancy. She begins to plan a realistic schedule of diet and exercise that she will follow after the birth. She relates mutually satisfying sexual experiences.

Changes in Sexuality

The sexual interest and activity of pregnant women and their partners are unpredictable and may increase, decline, or remain unchanged. The woman's physical comfort and sense of well-being are closely linked to her interest in sexual activity. The culture of the couple is also important. Intercourse during pregnancy is allowed and encouraged in some cultures but strictly forbidden in others.

During the first trimester, freedom from worry about becoming pregnant or the need for contraception may provide a sense of freedom and enhance sexual interest in both partners. However, nausea, fatigue, and breast tenderness may interfere with erotic feelings. Fear of miscarriage may cause couples to avoid intercourse, particularly if the woman has previously lost a pregnancy or has had infertility therapy. Nurses can reassure the couple that no evidence shows intercourse to be related to early pregnancy loss when no complications are present.

In the second trimester, women experience increased sensitivity of the labia and clitoris and increased vaginal lubrication from pelvic vasocongestion. Nausea is no longer a concern by this time for most women. Many have a general feeling of well-being and energy that may increase sexual responsiveness. Orgasm may occur more frequently and with greater intensity during pregnancy because of these changes. Although orgasm causes temporary uterine contractions, they are not harmful if the pregnancy has been normal.

During the third trimester, the "missionary position" (male on top) may cause discomfort because of abdominal pressure. Heartburn, indigestion, and supine hypotensive syndrome also increase in this position. The pressure of the fetus low in the pelvis may add to the discomfort. Moreover, fatigue, ligament pain, urinary frequency, and shortness of breath may be problems.

The nurse can suggest alternative positions such as female-superior, side-to-side, or vaginal rear-entry for intercourse. The side-lying position may be the most comfortable and require the least amount of energy during the third trimester. Hugging, cuddling, kissing, and mutual massage or masturbation are other ways to express affection without vaginal intercourse.

As they become larger, some women believe their bodies are ugly and worry about their partner's reaction to their increased size. Sexual response varies widely among men. Some men report heightened feelings of sexual interest, but others perceive the woman's body in late pregnancy as unattractive, and erotic feelings decrease. In addition, fear of harming the fetus or causing discomfort to the woman may interfere with sexual activity.

Despite the need for information, many women are reluctant to initiate a discussion about sexual activity. Unfortunately, most health care professionals do not introduce the topic. They may fear offending the woman or may be uncomfortable with their own sexuality and embarrassed to begin a discussion. They often lack time for any but the most pressing assessments. The result may be that an important aspect of care is ignored.

A broad opening statement may help initiate discussion about sexual activity—for example, "Sometimes couples are concerned about having sex during pregnancy." Such statements introduce the subject in a way that lets the woman feel comfortable either pursuing it or ignoring it.

The couple should be made aware of the normal changes in sexual desire that occur during pregnancy and the importance of communicating their feelings openly with each other to find solutions to problems. The nurse can reassure the couple that their feelings are normal.

Intercourse is safe throughout pregnancy if there are no complications. Bleeding, an incompetent cervix, placenta previa, rupture of membranes, and history of preterm labor in the present pregnancy are contraindications for intercourse. In addition, blowing into the vagina should be avoided at any time because it can cause an air embolus (Cunningham et al., 2014; Link, 2016b).

Third Trimester
Vulnerability
The sense of well-being and contentment that dominates the second trimester gives way to increasing feelings of vulnerability that peak in the third trimester during the 7th month (Link, 2016b). The expectant mother may worry that the precious baby may be lost or harmed if not protected at all times. She often has fantasies or nightmares about having a deformed baby or harm coming to the infant and may become very cautious as a result. She may avoid crowds because she feels unable to protect the infant from infectious diseases or potential physical dangers. She needs reassurance that such dreams and fears are not unusual in pregnancy.

Increasing Dependence
The expectant mother often becomes increasingly dependent on her partner in the last weeks of pregnancy (Link, 2016a). She may insist that he be easy to reach at all times and may call his cell phone or place of work several times during the day. She may rely on her partner and others more at this time and seek their help in making decisions. This may be frustrating if it is a marked change for her.

Women often have fears about the safety of the partner and that something will happen to him. Her need for love and attention from her partner is even more pronounced in late pregnancy. When she is assured of his concern and willingness to provide assistance, she feels more secure and able to cope.

Although the woman may not be able to explain the increasing dependence, she expects her partner to understand the feeling and may become angry if he is not sympathetic. Irritability may increase because of her fatigue at this time as well. The nurse can encourage couples to discuss fears and feelings openly so that misunderstandings can be avoided.

Some pregnant women have difficulty with tasks that require direct, sustained attention, particularly in the third trimester. Women may feel they have trouble concentrating or focusing on learning new material or skills at this time. Teaching should be clear and concise to help women learn most easily.

Preparation for Birth
Gradually, the feelings of vulnerability decrease as the woman comes to terms with her situation. The fetus continues to grow, and fetal movements are no longer gentle. The woman's relationship with the fetus changes as she acknowledges that although she and the fetus are interrelated, the baby is a pervasive presence and not a part of herself. Although she may not consciously acknowledge the increasing feelings of separateness, she longs to see the baby and become acquainted with her child (Link, 2016a).

Most pregnant women are concerned about their ability to determine when they are in labor. Many couples are anxious about getting to the birth facility in time for the birth, and they may be worried about coping with labor.

During the last few weeks, the woman becomes increasingly concerned about her due date and the experience of

TABLE 6.3 Progressive Changes in Maternal Responses to Pregnancy

First Trimester	Second Trimester	Third Trimester
Emotional Responses		
Uncertainty, ambivalence, focus on self, emotional lability	Wonder, increased narcissism, introversion, concern about changes in her body and sexuality	Vulnerability, increased dependence, acceptance that fetus is separate but totally dependent
Physical Validation		
No obvious signs of fetal growth	Quickening, enlarging abdomen	Obvious fetal growth, discomfort, decreased maternal activity
Role		
May begin to seek safe passage for self and fetus	Seeks acceptance of fetus and her role as mother	Prepares for birth, sets up expectations of herself as a mother
"Self-Statement"		
"I am pregnant."	"I am going to have a baby."	"I am going to be a mother."

labor and delivery. They often say they are tired of being pregnant and want the pregnancy to be over (Link, 2016a).

Women pregnant for the first time are more likely to fear childbirth than multiparas. Many women fear the pain of childbirth or that something will go wrong during labor. Multiparas who had a previous negative pregnancy or birth experience have increased concerns during the current pregnancy. Worry may also increase if friends or relatives have had difficult pregnancies.

Women may seek help for their fears by talking to members of their support system or by seeking information from health care professionals, books, television, or the Internet. However, information from websites or TV may not always be scientifically based, show practices that are evidence based, or depict experiences that are most common.

During the third trimester an expectant mother prepares for the infant, if that is appropriate in her culture. "Nesting" behavior includes obtaining clothing and furniture and arranging a place for the infant to sleep. Negotiation of how the couple will share household tasks is among the plans made at this time. In addition, many couples complete childbirth education classes (see Chapter 7). Table 6.3 summarizes changes in maternal responses during pregnancy.

KNOWLEDGE CHECK

20. Why might an expectant mother say, "I am pregnant" during the first trimester and "I am going to be a mother" late in pregnancy?
21. How might pregnancy affect the sexual responses of the mother and the father?

MATERNAL ROLE TRANSITION

Becoming a mother involves intense feelings of love, tenderness, and devotion that endure over a lifetime. How does a woman learn to be a mother?

Role transition is changing from one pattern of behavior and self-image into another. The transition into the mother role begins during pregnancy and increases with gestational age. The woman must accept the pregnancy and the changes that will result. She develops a relationship with the unborn child, first as part of herself and then as a separate individual (Link, 2016a). Near the end of pregnancy, she must prepare herself for the birth and for parenting the new baby.

Transitions Experienced Throughout Pregnancy

The woman undergoes transitions in relationships that continue throughout the pregnancy. She becomes more aware of herself and the changes occurring in her life. Her relationship with the father changes as they both prepare for parenthood. Her relationship with her own mother is often examined and may change as the expectant mother develops a view of herself as a mother and what that role entails. The woman needs mentors to help her understand that her feelings and experiences during pregnancy are normal. She also needs support from other new mothers (Alden, 2014).

Steps in Maternal Role Taking

Rubin (1984), in her classic work, observed specific steps that provide a framework for understanding the process of maternal role taking: mimicry, role play, fantasy, the search for a role fit, and grief work.

Mimicry

Mimicry involves observing and copying the behaviors of other women who are pregnant or mothers to discover what the role is like. Mimicry often begins in the first trimester, when the woman may wear maternity clothes before they are needed to understand the feelings of women in more advanced pregnancy and see how others react to her. She may also mimic the waddling gait or posture of a woman who is close to delivery long before these changes occur for her.

Role Play

Role play consists of acting out some aspects of what mothers do. The pregnant woman searches for opportunities to hold or care for infants in the presence of another person. Role playing gives her an opportunity to "practice" the expected role and receive validation from an observer that she has functioned well. She is particularly sensitive to the responses of her partner and her own mother.

Fantasy

Fantasies (mental images formed to prepare for the birth of a child) allow the woman to consider a variety of possibilities and daydream or "try on" a variety of behaviors. Fantasies often revolve around how the infant will look and what characteristics he or she will have. The woman may daydream about taking her child to the park or reading or singing songs to the child. She may also have vivid dreams at night.

At times, fantasies are fearful. Fearful fantasies often provoke a pregnant woman to respond by seeking information or reassurance. For instance, she may ask her partner if he will love the baby even if he or she is not perfect, or she may strive to learn all she can about caring for a baby who is difficult to console.

Fantasies may change during each trimester and may be different for primigravidas and multigravidas. Fantasies are most frequent during the third trimester. The nurse shows acceptance and understanding by listening to women's fantasies. In addition, listening helps the nurse identify concerns that may need further discussion.

The Search for a Role Fit

The search for a role fit occurs once the woman has established a set of role expectations for herself and internalized a view of a "good" mother's behavior. She then observes the behaviors of various mothers and compares them with her own expectations of herself. She imagines herself acting in the same way and either rejects or accepts the behaviors, depending on how well they fit her idea of what is right. This process implies that the woman has explored the role of mother long enough to have developed a sense of herself in the role and to be able to select behaviors that reaffirm her view of how she will fulfill the role.

Grief Work

Although grief work seems incongruous with maternal role taking, women often experience a sense of sadness when they realize that they must give up certain aspects of their previous selves and can never go back. A primigravida will never again be a carefree woman who has not had a child. She must relinquish some of her old patterns of behavior to take on the new identity as a mother. Even simple things such as going shopping or to the movies will require planning to include the infant or find alternative care. The multipara will have one more child claiming her attention. Changes may be particularly difficult for the adolescent mother, who is not used to planning ahead and may have to give up or change school plans as well.

Maternal Tasks of Pregnancy

To become mothers, pregnant women spend a great deal of time and energy learning new behaviors. As the woman works to establish a relationship with the infant, she must also reorder her relationship with her partner and family.

This psychological work of pregnancy has been grouped into the following four maternal tasks of pregnancy (Rubin, 1984):

1. Seeking safe passage for herself and baby through pregnancy, labor, and childbirth
2. Gaining acceptance of the baby and herself from her partner and family
3. Learning to give of herself
4. Developing attachment and interconnection with the unknown child

Seeking Safe Passage

Seeking safe passage for herself and her baby is the woman's priority task. If she cannot be assured of that safety, she cannot move on to the other tasks. Behaviors that ensure safe passage include seeking the care of a physician or nurse-midwife and following recommendations about diet, vitamins, rest, and subsequent visits for care. In addition to following the advice of health care professionals, the pregnant woman must also adhere to cultural practices that ensure safety for herself and the infant.

Securing Acceptance

Securing acceptance is a process that continues throughout pregnancy. It involves reworking relationships so that the important persons in the family accept the woman in the role of mother and welcome the baby into the family constellation.

In her first pregnancy, the woman and the father of the baby must give up an exclusive relationship and make a place in their lives for a child. When her partner expresses pride and joy in each pregnancy, the woman feels valued and comforted. This feeling is so important that many women retain a memory of the partner's reaction to the announcement of pregnancy for many years.

Support and acceptance from her own mother are also important. The pregnant woman gains energy and contentment when her mother freely offers acceptance and support. Many expectant mothers gain a sense of increased closeness with their mothers during pregnancy (Fig. 6.11).

Problems may occur if the family strongly desires a child with particular characteristics and the woman thinks the family may reject an infant who does not meet the criteria.

Learning to Give of Herself

Giving is one of the most idealized components of motherhood, but one that is essential. Learning to give to the coming infant begins in pregnancy when the woman allows her body to give space and nurturing to the fetus. She tests her ability to derive pleasure from giving by providing food, care, and acts of thoughtfulness for her family. The acceptance and enjoyment of the "gift" enhance her pleasure and strengthen the role. She also may give small gifts to friends, especially those who are pregnant.

Pregnant women also learn to give by receiving. Gifts received at "baby showers" are more than needed items. They also confirm continued interest and commitment from friends and family and enhance the woman's ability to give. Intangible gifts from others, such as companionship,

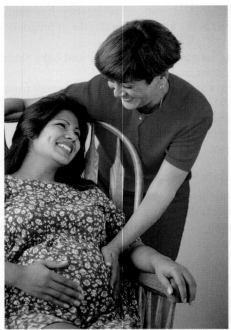

FIG. 6.11 The bond between a pregnant woman and her own mother is particularly important to the young mother.

attention, and support, help increase her energy and affirm the importance of giving.

Committing Herself to the Unknown Child

The process of **attachment** (development of strong affectional ties) begins in early pregnancy when the woman accepts or "binds in" to the idea that she is pregnant, even though the baby is not yet real to her. During the second trimester, the baby becomes real and feelings of love and attachment surge. This is especially true when quickening occurs or after an ultrasound shows recognizable parts of the baby.

Mothers report feedback from their unborn infants during the third trimester and describe unique characteristics of the fetus about sleep-wake cycles, temperament, and communication. Love of the infant becomes possessive and leads to feelings of vulnerability. The woman integrates the role of mother into her image of herself. She becomes comfortable with the idea of herself as mother and finds pleasure in contemplating the new role (Mercer & Ferketich, 1994).

Some women delay attachment to the fetus until they feel sure the pregnancy is normal and will continue. This is especially true for women who have lost a pregnancy previously. They may begin to have feelings of attachment after they have passed a critical time that correlates to the time they lost a previous pregnancy.

KNOWLEDGE CHECK

22. What does "looking for a fit" mean in role transition?
23. Why is grief work part of maternal role transition?
24. How does the pregnant woman seek safe passage for herself and the baby?

PATERNAL ADAPTATION

Expectant fathers do not experience the biologic processes of pregnancy, but they also must make major psychosocial changes to adapt to a new role. These changes may be more difficult because the male partner is often neglected by the health care team and his peer group, because attention is focused on the woman. His concerns and anxieties may remain unknown because of the lack of focus on him.

Variations in Paternal Adaptation

Wide variations exist in paternal responses to pregnancy. Some men are emotionally invested and comfortable as full partners exploring every aspect of pregnancy, childbirth, and parenting. Others are more task oriented and view themselves as managers. They may direct the woman's diet and rest periods and act as coaches during childbirth but remain detached from the emotional aspects of the experience. Some men are more comfortable as observers and prefer not to participate. In some cultures, men are conditioned to see pregnancy and childbirth as "women's work" and may not be able to express their true feelings about pregnancy and fatherhood.

Readiness for fatherhood is more likely if a stable relationship between the partners, financial security, and a desire for parenthood are present. Additional factors include the man's relationship with his own father, his previous experience with children, and his confidence in his ability to care for the infant.

Fathers have many concerns during a pregnancy. Coping with the expectant mother's emotional lability can be confusing and difficult. Common concerns include anxiety about the health of the mother and baby, financial concerns, and apprehension about his role during the birth and about the changes that will result when the baby arrives.

Financial concerns may be especially acute in a two-income family if the mother develops complications that prevent her from working as long as expected. Men may seek a second job or work overtime to prepare for the increased financial needs.

Developmental Processes

The responses of the expectant father are dynamic, progressing through phases that are subject to individual variation. Jordan (1990) describes the following three developmental processes that an expectant father must address:
- Grappling with the reality of pregnancy and the new child
- Struggling for recognition as a parent from his family and social network
- Making an effort to be seen as relevant to childbearing

The Reality of Pregnancy and the Child

The pregnancy and the child must become real before a man can assume the identity of father. The process requires time and may be incomplete until the birth. Initially, the pregnancy is a diagnosis only, and changes in the expectant woman's behavior, such as nausea and fatigue, are perceived as symptoms of illness that have little to do with having a baby.

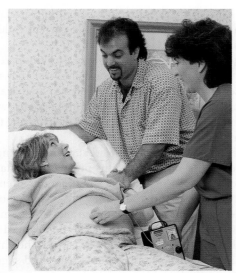

FIG. 6.12 Reality boosters such as hearing the sounds of the fetal heart make the fetus more real for the father.

A man's initial reaction to the announcement of pregnancy may be pride and joy, but he often experiences the same ambivalence as his partner. Various experiences act as catalysts or "reality boosters" that make the child more real (Fig. 6.12). The most frequently mentioned experiences are seeing the fetus on an ultrasound, hearing the baby's heartbeat, and feeling the infant move.

Preparing room for the baby and accumulating supplies also reinforce the reality of the coming child. These tasks often represent the first time the expectant father has the opportunity to do something directly for the baby. The birth itself is the most powerful reality booster, and the infant becomes real to the father when he has an opportunity to see and hold the baby.

The Struggle for Recognition as a Parent

Men are often perceived by others as helpmates but not parents in their own right. Some men may be upset that their feelings are not validated and that they may not be recognized as parents as well as helpers. Many men accept that the focus should be on their partners, but others are frustrated by the lack of understanding of their own experiences.

Support groups or classes for expectant fathers are sometimes available. These groups allow them to talk with other men about changes resulting from the pregnancy and how these changes have affected them. Knowing his experiences and feelings are shared by other men in the same situation is very helpful.

Expectant mothers play an important role in helping their partners gain recognition as parents. Women who openly share their physical sensations and emotions help expectant fathers feel they are part of the process. These women often say "we" are pregnant and include their partners in all discussions and decisions.

Nurses should learn to view the mother, the father, and the infant as one patient and not focus exclusively on the mother and the fetus. The nurse should encourage men to ask questions about their partners' pregnancies. These men are entitled to as much advice and reassurance as expectant women. Men who have sufficient information about pregnancy, birth, and newborn care are less likely to be as psychologically stressed as men who do not feel they have enough information. Internet resources such as that of the American College of Obstetricians & Gynecologists also provide valuable information for partners at www.acog.org.

The nurse can guide the couple in discussion of the role the father will play during and after the birth. How actively will he participate during labor? Will he be involved in infant care from the start or wait until the baby is older? The expectant parents may be surprised to learn each other's views and will need to negotiate, taking the beliefs of each partner into consideration to determine the roles each will play.

Creating the Role of the Involved Father

Men use various means to create a parenting role that is comfortable for them. They may seek closer ties with their fathers to reminisce about their own childhoods. They may fantasize about their relationships with their children as they progress through the stages of childhood.

Expectant fathers also observe men who are already fathers and "try on" fathering behaviors to determine whether they are comfortable and fit their own concepts of the father role. Some men change their self-images and even their appearances to fit their new images (Link, 2016b). In addition, many men assertively seek information about infant care and growth and development so they will be prepared.

Parenting Information. Expectant fathers need information about infant care and parenting. Although adequate information may be given to them, fathers may not be ready to learn at the time it is provided. As a result, they may have unrealistic expectations and be unprepared to care for the newborn. Nurses should review information about infant care and growth and development after the infant is born when the knowledge is immediately relevant.

Couvade. The term **couvade** refers to pregnancy-related symptoms and behavior in expectant fathers. In primitive cultures, couvade took the form of rituals involving special dress, confinement, limitations of physical work, avoidance of certain foods, sexual restraint, and, in some instances, performance of "mock labor."

In modern practice, expectant fathers sometimes experience physical symptoms similar to those of pregnant women, such as loss of appetite, nausea, headache, fatigue, and weight gain. Symptoms are more likely to occur in early pregnancy and lessen as the pregnancy progresses. They may be caused by stress, anxiety, or empathy for the pregnant partner. They are usually harmless but may persist and result in nervousness, insomnia, restlessness, and irritability. Although the symptoms are almost always unobserved by the health care team, anticipatory guidance is beneficial for both partners.

ADAPTATION OF GRANDPARENTS

The initial reaction of grandparents depends on factors such as their ages, the number and spacing of other grandchildren, and their perceptions of the role of grandparents.

Age

Age is a major determining factor in the emotional responses of prospective grandparents. Older grandparents have often already dealt with their feelings about aging and react with joy when they find they are to become grandparents. They look forward to being able to love grandchildren, who signify the continuity of life and family.

Younger grandparents may not be happy with the stereotype of grandparents as old persons. They may experience conflict when they must resolve their self-image with the stereotype. They often have career responsibilities and may not be accessible because of the continuing demands of their own lives.

Number and Spacing of Other Grandchildren

The number and spacing of other grandchildren also determine grandparents' reactions. A first grandchild may be an exciting event that creates great joy. If the grandparents have other grandchildren, another may be welcomed, but with less excitement. The subdued reaction may be disappointing to the couple, who may desire the same reaction as that expressed for the first grandchild.

Perceptions of the Role of Grandparents

Grandparents' beliefs about their importance to grandchildren vary widely. Many grandparents see their relationships with grandchildren as second in importance only to the parent-child relationship. They want to be involved in the pregnancy, and grandmothers often engage in rituals such as shopping and gift-giving showers that confirm their role as important participants. Many grandparents are intimately involved in child care and offer unconditional love to the child. They offer to care for older children while the mother gives birth, and they assist during the first weeks after childbirth.

In the past, grandparents were often asked for advice about childbearing and child-rearing. Health care personnel have now become the "experts," and many grandparents have difficulty adjusting to this change. Some grandparents may withdraw, sensing that their participation is no longer valued. Other grandparents worry about their lack of familiarity with modern ways of childbearing and parenting. Special classes are often available to teach them about current childbearing practices.

On the other hand, some contemporary grandparents plan little participation in pregnancy or child care. They may say, "I've raised my children, and I don't plan to do it again." This attitude often results in conflict with the parents, who may feel hurt and wish for the grandparents' help during the third trimester and after the birth.

Nurses can assist families to verbalize their feelings about the grandparents' responses to the pregnancy by statements such as, "It may seem that the grandparents aren't interested in the baby, but perhaps they are uneasy about what their role should be." Parents and grandparents may need to negotiate how the grandparents can be involved without feeling that they must assume more care of the child than they desire. For instance, the couple may need suggestions to help the grandparents participate in family gatherings that do not involve babysitting or child care. Letting grandparents know that the parents want them to share in the joy the child brings without other expectations may ease the situation.

ADAPTATION OF SIBLINGS

Sibling adaptation to the birth of an infant depends largely on age and developmental level.

Toddlers

Children 2 years old or younger are unaware of the maternal changes occurring during pregnancy and are unable to understand that a new brother or sister is going to be born. Because toddlers have little perception of time, many parents delay telling them that a baby is expected until shortly before the birth.

Although preparing very young children for the birth of a baby is difficult, the nurse can make suggestions that may prove helpful. Any changes in sleeping arrangements should be made several weeks before the birth so the child does not feel displaced by the new baby. Family members should be prepared that toddlers may show feelings of jealousy or resentment. Toddlers need frequent reassurance that they are loved.

Older Children

Children from 3 to 12 years are more aware of changes in the mother's body and may realize a baby is to be born. They may enjoy observing the mother's abdomen, feeling the fetus move, and listening to the heartbeat. They may have questions about how the fetus will develop, how it was created, and how it will get out of the abdomen. Although they look forward to the baby's arrival, preschool children may expect the infant to be a full-fledged playmate and may be shocked and disappointed when the infant is small and helpless. They also need preparation for the fact the mother will go away for several days when the baby is born.

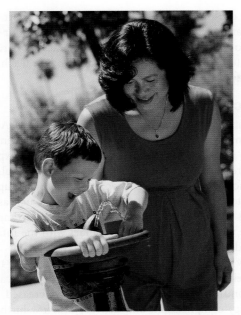

FIG. 6.13 A pregnant woman who spends time with an older child can provide affection and a sense of security.

School-age children are often told about the pregnancy during the second trimester and benefit from being included in preparations for the new baby. They are interested in following the development of the fetus, preparing space for the infant to sleep, and helping accumulate supplies the infant will need. They should be encouraged to feel the fetus move, and many come close to the mother's abdomen and talk to the fetus.

School-age children may wonder how the birth will affect their role in the family. Parents should address these concerns and reassure the children about their continued importance. Providing time alone with the parents may help them gain a sense of security (Fig. 6.13). Reading books about other children's experiences after the birth of a sibling may be helpful.

Children as young as 3 years can benefit from sibling classes. The classes provide an opportunity for them to discuss what newborns are like and what changes the new baby will bring to the family. They are encouraged to bring a doll to these classes to simulate caring for the infant.

In some settings, siblings are permitted to be with the mother during childbirth. They should attend a class that prepares them for the event. During the birth, a familiar person who has no other role but to support and care for younger siblings should be available to explain what is taking place and to comfort or remove them if events become overwhelming.

Adolescents

The response of adolescents also depends on their developmental level. Some are embarrassed because the pregnancy confirms the continued sexuality of their parents. Many adolescents are immersed in their own developmental tasks involving loosening ties to their parents and coming to terms with their own sexuality. They may be indifferent to the pregnancy unless it directly affects them or their activities. Other adolescents become very involved and want to help with preparations for the baby.

FACTORS INFLUENCING PSYCHOSOCIAL ADAPTATIONS

Age

Pregnancy presents a challenge for teenagers, who must cope with the conflicting developmental tasks of pregnancy and adolescence at the same time. The major developmental task of adolescence is to form and become comfortable with a sense of self. On the other hand, one of the major tasks of pregnancy involves learning to "give of self," a process that includes sacrificing personal desires for the benefit of the fetus.

Nurses who work with pregnant teenagers should help them adjust to their changing bodies and the increasing presence of the developing fetus. Adolescents also need prompting to follow a lifestyle that promotes the best outcomes for them and their infants.

The pregnant woman over 35 years of age also may have some concerns. Pregnancy may mean a major change in her life. She may have medical conditions that have an impact on the pregnancy, as well. Concerns relating to the pregnant adolescent and the older woman are discussed further in Chapter 11.

Multiparity

The assumption that a multipara needs less help than a first-time mother is inaccurate. Pregnancy tasks are often more complex for the multipara than for the primigravida. The multipara does not have as much time to take special care of herself as she did during the first pregnancy. She is more likely to experience fatigue and may have serious concerns about her other children accepting the infant. She may worry about finding time and energy for additional responsibilities. When seeking acceptance of the new baby, the multipara may find the family less excited than they were for the first child. The couple's celebration is also more subdued.

The woman spends a great deal of time developing a new relationship with the first child, who may become demanding. This behavior may foster feelings of guilt as the mother tries to expand her love to include the second child. Developing attachment for the coming baby is hampered by feelings of loss between herself and the first child. She senses that the child is growing up and away from her, and she may grieve for the loss of their special relationship.

Nurses cannot assume that the process is "old hat" and that information about labor, breastfeeding, and infant care is not needed. The parents also may need special assistance in integrating an additional infant into the family structure.

Social Support

Social support has been found to be a significant predictor of health-related quality of life during the perinatal period (Alden, 2014). Social support comes from the woman's partner, family, friends, and coworkers. Generally, support from the woman's partner and her mother is particularly important.

Depression may occur in women who have little support during pregnancy, and they are more likely to begin prenatal care late. The nurse should assess for signs of depression in all women and refer them for help when necessary. (See Chapter 11 for a discussion of peripartum depression.) When social support is inadequate the nurse can help the woman explore potential sources such as support groups, childbearing education classes, church, work, or school. Some community programs employ nurses or paraprofessionals to visit expectant mothers to provide teaching and social support.

Absence of a Partner

Pregnant single women may have special concerns. Although some unmarried women have the financial and emotional support of a partner, others do not. They may experience more stress about telling their family and friends about the pregnancy. They may have to enlist more social support to substitute for that of a partner. Legal issues such as whom to list as the father on birth records and what arrangements must be made to allow paternal contact with the infant may be added concerns.

Many single women without partners live below the poverty level. They are more likely to delay prenatal care until the second or third trimester and are at increased risk for pregnancy complications and delivery of a low-birth-weight infant.

Nurses should recognize the single mother's needs for accessible and affordable prenatal care. In addition, nurses should be prepared to offer specialized supportive care for single mothers. Necessary social services may include Medicaid; the Special Supplemental Nutrition Program for Women, Infants, and Children (WIC) for food vouchers; and transportation to prenatal appointments.

Some women are single by choice. They may have been inseminated to achieve pregnancy or choose not to continue the relationship with the father. If the pregnancy was planned, these women may have fewer financial concerns.

Abnormal Situations

Other factors that influence psychosocial adaptation during pregnancy include abnormal situations such as intimate partner violence, substance abuse (see Chapters 2 and 11), or the death of a partner. The nurse should assess all women for both of these risk factors during pregnancy so that appropriate referrals for help can be given.

SUMMARY CONCEPTS

- Pregnancy causes a predictable pattern of uterine growth. In general, the uterus can be palpated halfway between the symphysis pubis and the umbilicus at 16 weeks of gestation, at the level of the umbilicus at 20 weeks, and at the xiphoid process by 36 weeks.
- Thick mucus fills the cervical canal and protects the fetus from infection caused by bacteria ascending from the vagina.
- Plasma volume expands faster and to a greater extent than red blood cells, resulting in a dilution of hemoglobin concentration. This physiologic anemia (pseudoanemia) does not reflect an inadequate number of red blood cells.
- Although blood volume increases, blood pressure is not elevated during normal pregnancy.

- The gravid uterus partially occludes the vena cava and aorta when the mother is supine, causing supine hypotensive syndrome. This can be prevented or corrected if she assumes a lateral position.
- During the last trimester, the uterus pushes the diaphragm upward. To compensate, the ribs flare, the substernal angle widens, and the circumference of the chest increases.
- Slight hyperventilation and decreased airway resistance allow increased oxygen needs to be met.
- Increased progesterone level is associated with relaxation of smooth muscles, resulting in stasis of urine and increasing the risk for urinary tract infections and constipation.
- Increased renal plasma flow causes increased glomerular filtration rate and effectively removes additional metabolic

- wastes produced by the mother and the fetus but often results in "spilling" of glucose and other nutrients into urine.
- Increased blood flow to the skin reduces heat generated by the increased metabolic rate.
- Forms of hyperpigmentation during pregnancy include melasma and linea nigra.
- Striae gravidarum occur from separation of connective tissue fibers.
- Increased estrogen and human chorionic gonadotropin and decreased gastric motility are associated with nausea in early pregnancy. Morning sickness will not harm the fetus and usually ends by 10 to 12 weeks.
- The expanding uterus causes progressive changes that can lead to muscle strain and backache during the last trimester.
- Progesterone maintains the uterine lining for implantation, prevents uterine contractions during pregnancy, and helps prepare the breasts for lactation.
- Presumptive and probable signs of pregnancy may be caused by conditions other than pregnancy and cannot be considered positive or diagnostic signs. Positive signs can have no other cause.
- Maternal psychological responses progress during pregnancy from uncertainty and ambivalence to feelings of vulnerability and preparation for the birth of the infant.
- As the fetus becomes real, usually in the second trimester, maternal focus shifts from the self to the fetus and the woman turns inward to concentrate on the processes taking place in her body.
- Sexual activity varies among couples and may be culturally influenced. It is safe throughout pregnancy if no complications are present.

- Changes in the maternal body during pregnancy may result in a negative body image that affects sexual responses. This change may be especially troubling if the couple does not discuss emotions and concerns related to the changes in sexuality.
- Making the transition to the role of mother involves mimicking the behavior of other mothers, role play, fantasizing about the baby, developing a sense of self as mother, and grieving the loss of previous roles.
- To complete the maternal tasks of pregnancy the woman must seek safe passage for herself and the infant, gain acceptance from significant persons, and learn to be giving while forming an attachment to the unknown child.
- Paternal responses change throughout pregnancy and depend on the ability to perceive the fetus as real, gain recognition for the role of parent, and create a role as involved father.
- The most powerful reality boosters for the expectant father during pregnancy are hearing the fetal heartbeat, feeling the fetus move, and viewing the fetus on an ultrasound.
- In primitive cultures, *couvade* refers to pregnancy-related rituals performed by the father. Today, it refers to a cluster of pregnancy-related symptoms experienced by the father.
- The response of grandparents to pregnancy depends on their ages and beliefs about the role of grandparents as well as the number and ages of other grandchildren.
- The response of siblings to pregnancy depends on their ages and developmental levels.
- Completing the developmental tasks of pregnancy may be more difficult for multiparas because they have less time, experience more fatigue, and must negotiate a new relationship with the older child or children.

REFERENCES & READINGS

Alden, K. R. (2014). Nursing care of the family during pregnancy. In S. E. Perry, M. J. Hockenberry, D. L. Lowdermilk, & D. Wilson (Eds.), *Maternal child nursing care* (5th ed.) (pp. 186–226). S. Louis, MO: Mosby.

American College of Obstetricians and Gynecologists (ACOG). (2013). Weight gain during pregnancy, ACOG committee opinion #548. *ACOG: Obstetrics & Gynecology, 121*, 210–212.

Antony, K. M., Racusin, D. A., Aagaard, K., & Dildy, G. A. (2017). Maternal physiology. In S. G. Gabbe, J. R. Niebyl, J. L. Simpson, et al. (Eds.), *Obstetrics: Normal and problem pregnancies* (7th ed.) (pp. 38–63). Philadelphia, PA: Elsevier.

Beckmann, C. R. B., Ling, F. W., Barzansky, B. M., et al. (2014). *Obstetrics and gynecology* (7th ed.). Philadelphia, PA: Lippincott Williams & Wilkins.

Blackburn, S. T. (2013). *Maternal, fetal, and neonatal physiology: A clinical perspective* (4th ed.). St. Louis, MO: Saunders.

Boron, W. F., & Boulpaep, E. L. (2017). *Medical physiology* (3rd ed.). Philadelphia, PA: Saunders.

Cunningham, F. G., Leveno, K. J., Bloom, S. L., et al. (2014). *Williams obstetrics* (24th ed.). New York: McGraw-Hill.

Gambone, J. C. (2016). Clinical approach to the patient. In N. F. Hacker, J. C. Gambone, & C. J. Hobel (Eds.), *Essentials of obstetrics and gynecology* (6th ed.) (pp. 12–22). Philadelphia, PA: Saunders.

Hobel, C. J., & Williams, J. (2016). Antepartum care. In N. F. Hacker, J. C. Gambone, & C. J. Hobel (Eds.), *Essentials of obstetrics and gynecology* (6th ed.) (pp. 76–95). Philadelphia, PA: Saunders.

Jordan, P. L. (1990). Laboring for relevance: Expectant and new fatherhood. *Nursing Research, 39*(1), 11–16.

Koos, B. J., Kahn, D. A., & Equils, O. (2016). Maternal physiologic and immunologic adaptation to pregnancy. In N. F. Hacker, J. C. Gambone, & C. J. Hobel (Eds.), *Essentials of obstetrics and gynecology* (6th ed.) (pp. 61–75). Philadelphia, PA: Saunders.

Kramer, J., Bowen, A., Stewart, N., et al. (2013). Nausea and vomiting of pregnancy: Prevalence, severity and relation to psychosocial health. *MCN: The American Journal of Maternal/Child Nursing, 38*(1), 21–27.

Link, D. G. (2016a). Nursing care of the family during pregnancy. In D. L. Lowdermilk, S. E. Perry, K. Cashion, & K. R. Alden (Eds.), (11th ed.) (pp. 301–343). St. Louis, MO: Elsevier.

Link, D. G. (2016b). Psychology of pregnancy. In S. Mattson, & J. E. Smith (Eds.), *Core curriculum for maternal-newborn nursing* (5th ed.) (pp. 108–122). St. Louis, MO: Saunders.

Mercer, R. T., & Ferketich, S. L. (1994). Predictors of maternal role competence by risk status. *Nursing Research, 43*(1), 38–43.

Monga, M. (2014). Maternal cardiovascular, respiratory, and renal adaptation to pregnancy. In R. K. Creasy, R. Resnik, J. D. Iams, et al. (Eds.), *Maternal-fetal medicine: principles and practice* (7th ed.) (pp. 93–99). Philadelphia, PA: Saunders.

Norwitz, E. R., & Lye, S. J. (2014). Biology of parturition. In R. K. Creasy, R. Resnik, J. D. Iams, et al. (Eds.), *Maternal-fetal medicine: principles and practice* (7th ed.) (pp. 66–79). Philadelphia, PA: Saunders.

Pagana, K. D., Pagana, T. J., & Pagana, T. N. (2017). *Mosby's diagnostic and laboratory test reference* (13th ed.). St. Louis, MO: Mosby.

Rapini, R. P. (2014). The skin and pregnancy. In R. K. Creasy, R. Resnik, J. D. Iams, et al. (Eds.), *Maternal-fetal medicine: principles and practice* (7th ed.) (pp. 1146–1155). Philadelphia, PA: Saunders.

Records, K., & Tanaka, L. (2016). Physiology of pregnancy. In S. Mattson, & J. E. Smith (Eds.), *Core curriculum for maternal-newborn nursing* (5th ed.) (pp. 83–107). St. Louis, MO: Saunders.

Ross, M. G., Ervin, M. G., & Novak, D. (2017). Fetal development and physiology. In S. G. Gabbe, J. R. Niebyl, J. L. Simpson, et al. (Eds.), *Obstetrics: normal and problem pregnancies* (7th ed.) (pp. 26–37). Philadelphia, PA: Saunders.

Rubin, R. (1984). *Maternal identity and the maternal experience*. New York, NY: Springer.

Williamson, C., Mackillop, L., & Heneghan, M. A. (2014). Diseases of the liver, biliary system, and pancreas. In R. K. Creasy, R. Resnik, J. D. Iams, et al. (Eds.), *Maternal-fetal medicine: principles and practice* (7th ed.) (pp. 1075–1091). Philadelphia, PA: Saunders.

Antepartum Assessment, Care, and Education

Tania Lopez

OBJECTIVES

After studying this chapter, you should be able to:

1. Compute gravida, para, and estimated date of delivery.
2. Describe preconception, initial, and subsequent antepartum assessments in terms of history, physical examination, and risk assessment.
3. Describe the common discomforts of pregnancy in terms of causes and measures to prevent or relieve them.
4. Apply the nursing process to care of the antepartum patient.

5. List the goals of perinatal education.
6. Describe various types of education for childbearing families.
7. Explain the purposes of a birth plan.
8. Describe techniques for pain relief taught in childbirth classes.

ANTEPARTUM ASSESSMENT AND CARE

The objective of antepartum care is to promote optimum health of the mother and infant. Prenatal care involves early and continuing risk assessments, health education, counseling, and social support.

Ideally, antepartum care begins before conception and continues on a regular basis until birth. Although no prospective controlled trials have demonstrated the efficacy of prenatal care overall, inadequate antepartum care is associated with low birth weight and an increased incidence of prematurity. Prenatal visits provide clinicians with the opportunity to address primary health care concerns as well as assessing pregnancy risks and potential or existing complications (Gregory, Ramos, & Jauniaux, 2017).

In 2015, birth certificate data show 77% of women giving birth received early prenatal care in the first trimester, while 6.0% of women began prenatal care in the third trimester or did not receive any prenatal care (National Center for Health Statistics - NCHS, 2017). The *Healthy People 2020* goal is for at least 77.6% of women to begin antepartum care in the first trimester (DHHS, 2010).

Preconception and Interconception Care

Ideally, the first visit takes place before conception. Preconception care (the period of time prior to conception) and interconception care (the period of time between pregnancies) are important to identify problems or risk factors that might harm the mother or the infant once pregnancy

occurs and to provide education to help promote a healthy pregnancy. The early weeks of pregnancy are particularly important because the fetal organs are forming and are especially sensitive to harm. Many women do not begin prenatal care until after this sensitive period, and injury may already have transpired. Interconception care is especially important for women who have had previous pregnancy or birth complications. It also identifies and treats risk factors that have occurred since the last pregnancy.

Because many pregnancies are unintended, any visit to a health care provider by a woman of childbearing age should be seen as an opportunity for preconception or interconception care. This care can be part of developing a reproductive life plan that includes deciding the desired number and spacing of pregnancies. Such a plan helps women make changes to improve birth outcomes (Nypaver, Arbour, & Niederegger, 2016). Chronic conditions such as asthma, obesity, diabetes, or hypothyroidism should be addressed before pregnancy occurs. Previous reproductive problems and family history of possible genetic conditions are explored. Genetic testing may be indicated by the family history (see Chapter 4).

During a preconception visit, the health care provider obtains a complete history and performs a physical examination. The woman is assessed for health problems (e.g., diabetes, hypertension, sexually transmitted diseases [STDs], or psychological problems), harmful habits (such as use of alcohol or drugs), or social problems (such as intimate partner violence) that might adversely affect pregnancy. If problems are discovered, intervention may be started immediately to avoid complications or worsening of the woman's condition or situation because of pregnancy. Screening for rubella, varicella, and hepatitis B is performed, and the vaccines are given, if indicated. The woman should be instructed to wait at least 1 month after receiving rubella and varicella vaccines before conceiving to minimize risk to the fetus (CDC, 2016).

If the woman is taking prescription and over-the-counter (OTC) drugs, vitamins, or other supplements, their effect on pregnancy is evaluated and changes made, if necessary. Approximately 50% of women report taking at least one medication during pregnancy (Mitchell et al., 2011). Potentially teratogenic medications should be evaluated and changed to less harmful drugs, if possible, before attempting pregnancy.

Use of complementary or alternative therapies is addressed because some may be safe at other times but harmful during pregnancy. Avoidance of common teratogens or other harmful substances is discussed. Women who are obese can obtain help to lose weight before conceiving. Referral to smoking cessation programs may be indicated.

The woman is advised to consume 400 to 800 micrograms (mcg) (0.4 to 0.8 mg) of folic acid daily for at least 1 month before conception and 2 to 3 months after conception to decrease the risk for neural tube defects (U.S. Preventive Services Task Force, 2016). A daily intake of 600 mcg (0.6 mg) is recommended for the rest of pregnancy. Women who have previously given birth to an infant with a neural tube defect should consult with their provider about increasing the dosage to 4000 mcg (4 mg) of folic acid daily during the 4 weeks before pregnancy and throughout the first trimester. Women on antiepileptic medications are advised to take 1000 mcg of folic acid during this time frame as well (West, Hark, & Catalano, 2017).

Initial Prenatal Visit

If a preconception visit has occurred recently, many initial prenatal assessments will have been completed. If not, the nurse practitioner, nurse-midwife, or physician will complete a thorough history and physical examination. The obstetric nurse may play an essential role in this intake visit as well, verifying history, uncovering potential risk factors, and providing early pregnancy education. The following are the primary objectives of the first antepartum visit:

- Establish trust and rapport with the childbearing family.
- Verify or rule out pregnancy.
- Evaluate the pregnant woman's physical and psychological health relevant to childbearing.
- Assess the growth and health of the fetus.
- Establish baseline data for comparison with future observations.
- Evaluate the psychosocial needs of the woman and her family.
- Assess the need for counseling or teaching.
- Negotiate a plan of care to promote optimal health of the mother and baby.

History

Obstetric History. The obstetric history provides essential information about previous pregnancies and may alert the health care provider to possible problems in the present pregnancy. Components of this history include the following:

- Gravida, para, abortions (spontaneous or elective termination of pregnancies before the 20th week of gestation; spontaneous abortion is frequently called *miscarriage*), and living children
- Length of previous gestations
- Weight of infants at birth
- Labor experiences, type of deliveries, locations of births, and names of providers
- Types of anesthesia and any difficulties with anesthesia during childbirths or previous surgeries
- Maternal complications such as hypertension, diabetes, infection, bleeding, or psychologic complications
- Infant complications
- Methods of infant feeding used in the past and currently planned
- Special concerns

Gravida refers to a woman who is or has been pregnant, regardless of the length of the pregnancy. A **primigravida** is a woman pregnant for the first time. A **multigravida** has been pregnant more than once. **Para** refers to the number of pregnancies that have ended at 20 or more weeks, regardless of whether the infant was born alive or stillborn. A multiple gestation pregnancy, such as twins or triplets, is still one pregnancy and therefore one para. A **nullipara** is a woman who has never been pregnant or has not completed a pregnancy of 20 weeks or more. A **primipara** has delivered one pregnancy of at least 20 weeks. A **multipara** has delivered two or more pregnancies of at least 20 weeks.

There are two methods of summarizing a woman's obstetric history (gravida and para). The first uses two digits, gravida (the number of times she has been pregnant) and para (the number of completed pregnancies of 20 weeks or more). The second method, described by the acronym GTPAL, is more informative because it uses five digits: G = pregnancies or gravida, T = term pregnancies delivered, P = preterm pregnancies delivered, A = abortions (spontaneous and induced), and L = living children (Box 7.1).

Nurses should use caution when discussing gravida and para with the expectant mother in the presence of her family or significant other. Although the antepartum record may indicate a previous pregnancy or childbirth, she may not have shared this information with her family, and her right to privacy could be jeopardized by probing questions in their presence. The pregnancy may have terminated in elective or spontaneous abortion or in the birth of an infant who was placed for adoption. The confidentiality of the pregnant woman should always be protected. The nurse should wait until the woman is alone if it is necessary to clarify information about her gravida or para.

Menstrual History and Estimated Date of Delivery. A complete menstrual history is necessary to establish the estimated date of delivery (EDD) and therefore the gestational

BOX 7.1 Calculation of Gravida and Para

A method for calculating gravida and para is to separate pregnancies and their outcome using the acronym GTPAL: G = gravida, T = term, P = preterm, A = abortions, and L = living children.

The following examples illustrate the use of this method:

- Jennie is 6 months pregnant. She had one spontaneous and one elective abortion in the first trimester. She has a son who was born at 40 weeks of gestation and a daughter who was born at 34 weeks of gestation. Using the two-digit method, Jennie is gravida 5, para 2. The two abortions are counted in the gravida but not included in the para because they occurred before 20 weeks of gestation. Using the five-digit method, GTPAL is 5-1-1-2-2. (G = all pregnancies, including the current one; T = 1,the son born at 40 weeks; P = 1, the daughter born at 34 weeks; A = 2 , the spontaneous and elective abortions in the first trimester; and L = 2, the number of current living children).
- Lani gave birth to twins at 32 weeks of gestation and to a stillborn infant at 24 weeks of gestation. Approximately 2 years later, she experienced a spontaneous abortion at 12 weeks of gestation. If pregnant now, she is gravida 4, para 2 (the twins count as 1 parous experience and the stillborn infant counts as 1 parous experience because the pregnancy extended past 20 weeks gestation, the spontaneous abortion does not count as a parous experience because the pregnancy ended before 20 weeks gestation). If the GTPAL acronym is used, G = 4, T = 0 (no pregnancies went to term), P = 2 (the twins count as 1 and the stillborn infant counts as 1 pregnancy ending in preterm birth), A = 1 (the 12 weeks spontaneous abortion), L = 2 (the two living children).

age of the fetus and any given time. The EDD is important in deciding when to schedule certain tests or procedures commonly performed during pregnancy. Common practice is to estimate the EDD on the basis of the first day of the last normal menstrual period (LNMP), although ovulation and conception occur approximately 2 weeks after the beginning of menstruation in a regular 28-day cycle. The average duration of pregnancy from the first day of the LNMP is 40 weeks, or 280 days.

The Nägele's rule is often used to establish the EDD. This method involves subtracting 3 months from the date the LNMP began, adding 7 days, and then correcting the year, if appropriate. For example:

- LNMP: August 30, 2018
- Subtract 3 months: May 30, 2018
- Add 7 days and change the year: June 6, 2019

Calculations of EDD may be inaccurate in some situations. For example, the Nägele's rule is less accurate when the woman's menstrual cycle is very irregular. To determine EDD quickly, many health care providers also use a gestational wheel or an EDD calculator tool application designed for electronic medical records or smart phones (ACOG, 2016a, Cunningham et al., 2014).

Ultrasound measurements taken early in pregnancy (before 20 weeks of gestation) can more accurately determine the gestational age.

Gynecologic and Contraceptive History. Any previous gynecologic problems should be identified. STDs should be treated. Infertility problems with past or the current pregnancy should be discussed.

A detailed history of contraceptive methods is important. Studies have shown no increased risk for congenital malformations when women conceive while using hormonal contraceptives (Charlton et al., 2016). Any woman who becomes pregnant should stop taking hormonal contraceptives and consult with a health care provider.

Pregnancy with an intrauterine device (IUD) in place is unusual, but it can cause complications such as spontaneous abortion, infection, and preterm delivery. The patient should be evaluated for ectopic pregnancy. As soon as the pregnancy is confirmed, the IUD should be removed promptly by a provider. A woman who shows signs of infection with an IUD in place should receive intensive antibiotic treatment and have her uterus evacuated (Cunningham et al., 2014).

Medical and Surgical History. Chronic conditions can affect the outcome of the pregnancy and should be investigated. Infections, surgical procedures, and trauma may complicate the pregnancy or childbirth and should be documented. The history includes the following:

- Age, race, and ethnic background (risk for specific genetic problems such as sickle cell disease, thalassemia, cystic fibrosis, and Tay-Sachs disease)
- Childhood diseases and immunizations
- Chronic illnesses (onset and treatment) such as asthma, heart disease, hypertension, diabetes, renal disease, and lupus
- Previous illnesses, surgical procedures, and injuries (particularly of the pelvis and back)
- Previous infections such as hepatitis, STDs, tuberculosis, and presence of group B *Streptococcus*
- History of and treatment for anemia, including any previous blood transfusions
- Bladder and bowel function (problems or changes)
- Amount of caffeine and alcohol consumed each day
- Tobacco use in any form (number of years and daily amount)
- Prescription, OTC, and illicit drugs (name, dose, frequency)
- Complementary or alternative therapies used
- Appetite, general nutrition, history of eating disorders
- Contact with pets, particularly cats (increased risk for infections such as toxoplasmosis)
- Allergies and drug sensitivities
- Occupation and related risk factors

Family History. A family history provides valuable information about the general health of the family, including chronic diseases such as diabetes and heart disease and infections such as tuberculosis and hepatitis. In addition, it may reveal information about patterns of genetic or congenital anomalies.

Partner's Health History. The partner's history may include significant health problems such as genetic abnormalities, chronic diseases, and infections. Use of drugs such as cocaine and alcohol may affect the family's ability to cope with pregnancy and childbirth. Tobacco use by the partner increases the risk for upper respiratory tract infections for both the mother and the infant from exposure to passive smoke.

In addition, the father's blood type and Rh factor are important if the mother is Rh-negative or type O because blood incompatibility between the mother and fetus is possible.

Psychosocial History. The psychosocial history, including mental health, substance abuse, risk for violence or abuse, and coping abilities, should be elicited during the initial visit.

Physical Examination

Many women have not had a recent physical examination before becoming pregnant. Therefore a thorough evaluation of all body systems is necessary to detect previously undiagnosed physical problems that may affect the pregnancy outcome. It also establishes baseline levels to guide the treatment of the expectant mother and fetus throughout pregnancy.

Vital Signs

Blood Pressure. Position, anxiety, pain, and the use of alcohol or tobacco products can affect blood pressure (BP). BP should be obtained using an appropriate size cuff with the woman seated and her arm supported in a horizontal position at heart level. The same arm should be used for each assessment. There may be differences between BP values obtained manually and BP values obtained with automatic cuffs. Documentation should include the position, arm used, pressures obtained, and type of sphygmomanometer used. The nurse may notice a normal decrease in BP during first and second trimesters, which normalizes by the third trimester (see Chapter 6). A BP of 140/90 mm Hg or higher may indicate chronic hypertension or preeclampsia and requires additional evaluation (Chapter10).

Pulse. The normal adult pulse rate is 60 to 90 beats per minute (bpm). Tachycardia is associated with anxiety, hyperthyroidism, and infection and should be investigated. Apical pulse should be assessed for at least 1 minute to determine the amplitude and regularity of the heartbeat and presence of murmurs. Pedal pulses are assessed to determine the presence of circulatory problems in the legs. Pedal pulses should be strong, equal, and regular.

Respirations. Respiratory rate during pregnancy is in the range of 16 to 24 breaths per minute. Tachypnea may indicate respiratory tract infection or cardiac disease. Breath sounds should be equal bilaterally, chest expansion should be symmetric, and lung fields should be free of abnormal breath sounds.

Temperature. Normal temperature during pregnancy is 36.6°C to 37.6°C (97.8°F to 99.6°F). Fever suggests infection and may require medical management.

Cardiovascular System. Additional assessment of the cardiovascular system includes observation for venous congestion, which can develop into varicosities and edema. Venous congestion is most commonly noted in the legs, the vulva (as varicosities), or the rectum (as hemorrhoids). Edema of the legs may be a benign condition that reflects pooling of blood in the extremities caused by occlusion of the pelvic veins and inferior vena cava by the large uterus. This results in a shift of intravascular fluid into interstitial spaces. When pressure exerted by a finger leaves a persistent depression, pitting edema is present (see Fig. 17.6).

Musculoskeletal System. Body mechanics and changes in posture and gait should be addressed. Poor body mechanics during pregnancy may place strain on the muscles of the lower back and legs. Many joints have increased mobility during pregnancy which contributes to posture changes, potentially leading to lower back pain.

Height and Weight. An initial weight is recorded to establish a baseline for evaluation of weight gain throughout pregnancy. The body mass index should be calculated. Women who are underweight before pregnancy are at risk for having low-birth-weight infants (Hobel & Williams, 2016).

Obesity is a special concern during pregnancy (Chapter 10). Obesity increases the incidence of hypertensive disorders, gestational diabetes, postpartum hemorrhage, poor labor progression, cesarean delivery, anesthesia complications, wound infection, and birth of large-for-gestational age infants (Cunningham et al., 2014). Obese women often need closer observation and careful management of complications during pregnancy. Tests of fetal well-being may be important during the third trimester.

Abdomen. The contour, size, and muscle tone of the abdomen should be assessed. The fundal height should be measured if the fundus is palpable above the symphysis pubis (Fig. 7.1). The fetal heart rate should be auscultated, counted, and recorded if the pregnancy is advanced enough (10 to 12 weeks by Doppler; 18 to 20 weeks by fetoscope).

Neurologic System. A complete neurologic assessment is not necessary for women who have a negative history and are free of signs or symptoms indicating a problem. However, deep tendon reflexes should be evaluated because hyperreflexia is associated with complications of pregnancy (Chapter 10).

Carpal Tunnel Syndrome. Carpal tunnel syndrome is believed to result when edema compresses the median nerve

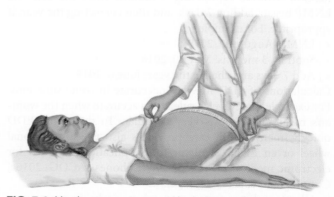

FIG. 7.1 Uterine measurements include the distance between the upper border of the symphysis pubis and the top of the fundus.

at the point where it passes through the carpal tunnel of the wrist. Symptoms include pain, burning, numbness, or tingling of the hand and wrist. Splinting of the wrist at night may provide improvement. It resolves by 3 months after childbirth for most women (Blackburn, 2013).

Integumentary System. Skin color should be consistent with racial background. Pallor may result from anemia, and jaundice may indicate hepatic disease. Lesions, bruising, rashes, areas of hyperpigmentation related to pregnancy (melasma, linea nigra), and stretch marks (striae) should be noted. Nail beds should be pink with instant capillary return.

Endocrine System. The thyroid enlarges moderately during the second trimester. However, gross enlargement, nodules, or tenderness may indicate thyroid disease and requires further medical evaluation.

Gastrointestinal System

Mouth. Mucous membranes should be pink, smooth, glistening, and uniform. Lips should be free of ulcerations. Gums may be red, tender, and edematous and may bleed more easily. Teeth should be in good repair. Dental plaque may increase, and a temporary increase in tooth mobility may occur (Blackburn, 2013).

The woman should be referred for regular dental care. The second trimester may be the most comfortable time for dental care. However, if necessary, dental care can be performed during the third trimester if the woman is positioned to avoid supine hypotensive syndrome.

Intestine. A warm stethoscope for assessing bowel sounds is most comfortable for the pregnant woman. Bowel sounds may be diminished because of the effects of progesterone on smooth muscle. Bowel sounds are often increased if a meal is overdue or diarrhea is present. Problems with constipation can be discussed during abdominal examination.

Urinary System. A clean-catch midstream urine sample is tested for urinary tract infection (UTI) and indicators of other complications. Although a trace amount of protein may be present in the urine, the amount should not increase. Its presence may indicate kidney disease, preeclampsia, or contamination by vaginal secretions. Small amounts of glucose may indicate physiologic "spilling" that occurs during normal pregnancy. Ketones may be found in the urine after heavy exercise or as a result of inadequate intake of food and fluid. Increased bacteria in urine is associated with UTI, which is common during pregnancy. A baseline urinalysis or culture may detect any underlying bacterial infections that warrant treatment to prevent more serious UTIs such as pyelonephritis (Cunningham et al., 2014).

Reproductive System

Breasts. Breast size and symmetry, condition of the nipples (erect, flat, inverted), and presence of colostrum should be noted. Any lumps, dimpling of the skin, or asymmetry of the nipples requires further evaluation. Breast tissue changes during pregnancy frequently cause increased tenderness and sensitivity during breast examination.

External Reproductive Organs. The skin and mucous membranes of the perineum, vulva, and anus are inspected for excoriations, growths, ulcerations, lesions, varicosities,

warts, chancres, and perineal scars. Enlargement, tenderness, redness, or discharge from the Bartholin or Skene gland may indicate gonorrheal or chlamydial infection. The examiner should obtain a specimen for culture from any discharge from lesions or inflamed glands to determine the causative organisms and to provide effective care.

Internal Reproductive Organs. A speculum inserted into the vagina permits the examiner to see the walls of the vagina and the cervix. The cervix should be pink in a nonpregnant woman and bluish purple in a pregnant woman (Chadwick's sign). The external cervical os is closed in primigravidas, but one fingertip may be admitted in multiparas. The cervix feels relatively firm except during pregnancy, when marked softening is noted (Goodell's sign). Routine cervical cultures for gonorrhea and chlamydial infection are generally obtained during the initial pregnancy examination. The examiner also collects a specimen for a Papanicolaou (Pap) test to screen for cervical cancer if indicated.

A bimanual examination involves the use of both hands, one on the abdomen and the other in the vagina, to palpate the internal genitalia. The examiner palpates the uterus for size, contour, tenderness, and position. The uterus should be movable between the two examining hands and should feel smooth and enlarged according to gestational age. The ovaries, if palpable, should be about the size and shape of almonds and nontender.

Pelvic Measurements. Pelvic measurements may be assessed at this time to determine whether the shape and size of the bony pelvis are adequate for a normal vaginal birth (see Fig. 12.4).

Laboratory Data

Table 7.1 lists laboratory tests commonly performed during pregnancy and describes the purpose and significance of each test. Table 7.2 shows laboratory values for pregnant and nonpregnant women.

Risk Assessment

Risk assessment begins at the initial visit when the health care provider identifies factors that put the expectant mother or fetus at risk for complications and determines the need for specialized care. Women with identified risk factors may require closer surveillance to monitor maternal and fetal well-being. Furthermore, risk factors change as pregnancy progresses, and risk assessment should be updated throughout pregnancy. Table 7.3 lists major risk factors and their implications.

❓ KNOWLEDGE CHECK

1. Why is a preconception visit important?
2. Why are medical, surgical, psychological and obstetric histories necessary?
3. Why is it important for all caregivers to be consistent when measuring BP?
4. What are major risk factors during pregnancy?

TABLE 7.1   Common Laboratory Tests

Test	Purpose	Significance
Complete blood count (CBC)	To detect infection, anemia, or cell abnormalities	More than 15,000/mm³ white blood cells or decreased platelets require follow-up.
Hemoglobin (Hgb) or hematocrit (Hct)	To detect anemia; often checked several times during pregnancy	Low Hgb or Hct may indicate need for added iron supplementation.
Blood grouping, Rh factor, and antibody screen	To determine blood type to screen for maternal-fetal blood incompatibility	Identifies possible causes of incompatibility that may result in jaundice in neonate. If father is Rh-positive and mother is Rh-negative and unsensitized, Rho (D) immune globulin will be given to the mother at 28 wk.
Venereal Disease Research Laboratory (VDRL) test or rapid plasma reagin (RPR)	To screen for syphilis	Treat, if results are positive. Retest, as indicated.
Rubella titer	To determine immunity	If titer is ≤1:8, the woman is not immune. Immunize postpartum if not immune.
Tuberculin skin test	To screen for tuberculosis	If positive, refer for additional testing or therapy.
Genetic testing (for sickle cell anemia, cystic fibrosis, Tay-Sachs disease, and other genetic conditions)	Offered if an increased risk for certain genetic conditions exists	If mother is positive, check partner. Counsel as appropriate for test results.
Hepatitis B screen	To detect presence of antigens in maternal blood	If antigens are present, infants should be given hepatitis immune globulin and vaccine soon after birth.
Human immunodeficiency virus (HIV) screen	Encouraged at first visit to detect HIV antibodies	Positive results require retesting, counseling, and treatment to lower risk for infant infection.
Urinalysis	To detect renal disease or infection	Requires further assessment if positive for more than trace protein (renal damage, preeclampsia, or normal), ketones (fasting or dehydration), or bacteria (infection).
Papanicolaou (Pap) test	To screen for cervical neoplasia	Refer for treatment if abnormal cells are present.
Vaginal-rectal culture	To detect chlamydia and gonorrhea (in early pregnancy) and group B streptococci (in late pregnancy)	Treat and retest as necessary; treat chlamydia and gonorrhea when discovered and group B streptococci during labor.
Multiple marker screen: Maternal serum alpha-fetoprotein, human chorionic gonadotropin (hCG), and estriol. Inhibin A and nuchal lucency may also be measured	To screen for fetal anomalies	Abnormal results may indicate increased risk for chromosomal abnormality (e.g., trisomy 13, 18, or 21) or structural defects (e.g., neural tube defects or gastroschisis).
Glucose challenge test	To screen for gestational diabetes	If elevated, 3-hr glucose tolerance test is recommended.

Subsequent Visits

Ongoing antepartum care is important to the successful outcome of pregnancy. Although the recommended number of visits can be reduced for women without complications, the usual schedule for prenatal assessment in normal pregnancy is as follows (American Association of Pediatrics [AAP] & ACOG, 2012; Cunningham et al., 2014):

- Conception to 28 weeks—every 4 weeks
- 29 to 36 weeks—every 2 weeks
- 37 weeks to birth—weekly

Although the preceding schedule is the traditional model of prenatal care, other options do exist. "CenteringPregnancy" is an example of an evidence-based alternative method of care. The method involves 10 sessions of 1.5 to 2 hours with groups of 8 to 12 women meeting with a facilitator, who may be a nurse and a health care provider, beginning at 12 to 16 weeks of pregnancy and ending soon after childbirth. Women assess their own BP and weight during the first 30 minutes of the session, promoting personal ownership and responsibility. Each visit includes an individual assessment with time alone with the health care provider, typically a nurse-midwife or nurse-practitioner. They then participate in a group educational discussion with peers who are of similar gestational ages (Barger, Faucher, & Murphy, 2015). The social support provided by the group is an important benefit. Women participating in this form of care have been satisfied with their care, reported a greater positive influence on stress, and had favorable pregnancy outcomes (Heberlein et al., 2016). More information is available at www.centeringhealthcare.org.

Merging CenteringPregnancy & Individual Care during Pregnancy

CenteringPregnancy is a program that emerged in the 1990s as a model for prenatal care that is provided to groups of women rather than individual visits with a provider. CenteringPregnancy provides women with 10 sessions of 1.5 to 2 hours. During the first part of the visit, the women assess and document their own blood pressure and weight and are seen by a provider, usually a nurse midwife or nurse practitioner, for assessment of fetal heart rate and fetal growth. The last part of the visit (60–75 min) is spent in interactive group discussion and education led by a facilitator. The group is composed of 8–12 women with similar due dates; the members of the group are consistent. The group forms a powerful support network. Assessment, education and support are the components of CenteringPregnancy.

Current research indicates that women who participate CenteringPregnancy are more knowledgeable and feel better prepared for labor than women in traditional care models. The women are highly satisfied with the format for prenatal visits, they have higher breastfeeding initiation rates, and may have decreased preterm birth rates. Limitations of CenteringPregnancy include the substantial initial implementation costs, typical limitation of the program to low-risk women and the time commitment required of the women.

Because of these limitations, Lathrop and Pritham (2015) conducted a pilot study of Healthy Pregnancy, Healthy Childbirth, Healthy Parenting (HPCP), a blended prenatal care model that combines individual visits with group education. In HPCP, one group visit replaces one routine individual visit each trimester. Each group visit lasts approximately 2 hours, with a 30-min assessment and documentation of blood pressure and weight by a medical assistant and a private visit with the woman's provider (a nurse practitioner in this study). The last 90 min of the group visit is spent in the group setting for discussion and education. In HPCP, the peer group doesn't necessarily stay the same – women are free to attend any group visit that fits their schedule.

The purpose of the pilot study was to evaluate education-focused group prenatal care visits to determine: (1) if the woman's knowledge of self-care, childbirth and infant care improved, (2) if the woman's self-efficacy (belief in one's ability to be successful) improved and (3) if the woman perceived the prenatal care experience as positive. The researchers found that maternal knowledge increased in each trimester after attending the group visit, there was an increase in the women's self-efficacy scores, although in some cases it was too small to be statistically significant, and more than 85% of the women perceived the experience as positive and said they would recommend HCHP to other mothers.

The authors identified the strengths of the program as increased time for patient education and the opportunity for the women to learn from each other, individualized experience (the women still get individual prenatal care) which allows for inclusion of high-risk women, flexibility in the group discussion and education to allow the leader to address specific needs of the women attending the group and a lower implementation cost than CenteringPregnancy. The weaknesses were fewer contact hours per patient compared to CenteringPregnancy; the times for group sessions weren't convenient for all women; the peer cohort changed, so opportunities for friendship and powerful peer support are limited compared to CenteringPregnancy and education topics aren't covered as fully as in CenteringPregnancy. Other than the small sample size, the primary limitation of the study was that data collection was limited to 5 months. Therefore, they were not able to compare results between women who attended all group visits and those who attended only one or two visits. In addition, they were not able to collect pregnancy outcome data such as preterm birth rate.

Questions

1. Do you think HPCP will have similar rates of preterm birth and initiation of breastfeeding compared to CenteringPregnancy? Why or why not?
2. What would be the advantages and disadvantages of HPCP compared to traditional prenatal care combined with prepared childbirth classes?

Reference

Lathrop, B., & Pritham, U. A. (2014). A pilot study of blended group and individual prenatal care visits for women with low income. *Nursing For Women's Health, 18*(6), 462–474.

TABLE 7.2 Laboratory Values in Nonpregnant and Pregnant Women

Value	Nonpregnant	Pregnant
Red blood cell count (million/mm³)	4.0-5.2	2.71-4.55 Decreases slightly because of hemodilution
Hemoglobin (g/dL)	12-16	10.5- 11 (consider anemia if <11.0 in 1st or 3rd trimester; < 10.5 in 2nd trimester)
Hematocrit, packed cell volume (%)	35.4-44.4	28-41
White blood cell (mm³)	5000-10,000	5000-15,000
Platelets (mm3)	165,000-415,000	146,000-429,000
Prothrombin time (seconds)	12.7-15.4	9.5-13.5
Activated partial thromboplastin time (seconds)	26.3-39.4	22.6-38.9
D-dimer (µg/mL)	0.22-0.74	0.05-1.7
Blood glucose, fasting (mg/dL)	70-100	95 or lower
Creatinine (mg/dL)	0.5-0.9	0.4-0.9
Creatinine clearance, 24 hour urine (mL/min)	91-130	50-166
Fibrinogen (mg/dL)	233-496	244-696

Data from Cunningham, F. G., Leveno, K. J., Bloom, S. L., Spong CY, Dashe JS, Hoffman BL, Sheffield JS. (2014). *Williams' obstetrics* (24th ed.). New York, NY: McGraw-Hill; and Pagana, K. D., & Pagana, T. J. (2014).
Uptodate, 2017. Normal reference ranges in pregnant women. Retrieved from www.uptodate.com.

TABLE 7.3 Summary of Major Risk Factors in Pregnancy

Factors	Associated Problems
Demographic Factors	
<16 yr of age	Preterm birth, low birth weight, perinatal mortality, anemia, human immunodeficiency virus (HIV), sexually transmitted diseases (STDs), insufficient prenatal care, and substance abuse.
>35 yr of age	Gestational diabetes, hypertension, prolonged labor, cesarean birth, congenital anomalies, infant mortality, placenta previa.
Low socioeconomic status or dependence on public assistance	Preterm labor, maternal perinatal mortality, low birth weight, chromosomal disorders, fetal growth disorders, insufficient prenatal care.
Nonwhite race	Low birth weight, preterm birth, infant mortality for some groups.
Multiparity	Abnormal fetal presentation, antepartum or postpartum hemorrhage, cesarean birth.
Social and Personal Factors	
Low prepregnancy weight	Low birth weight.
Obesity	Preterm birth, hypertension, gestational diabetes, stillbirth, failure to progress in labor, macrosomia, cesarean birth, wound infections, anesthesia complications, postpartum hemorrhage, thromboembolism.
Height <152 cm (5 feet)	Cesarean birth because of cephalopelvic disproportion.
Smoking	Spontaneous abortion, low birth weight, placental abruption, placenta previa, preterm birth, perinatal mortality, sudden infant death syndrome (SIDS).
Use of alcohol or illicit drugs	Congenital anomalies, neonatal withdrawal syndrome, fetal alcohol spectrum disorder, risky lifestyle behaviors.
Domestic violence	Poor pregnancy weight gain, infection, anemia, tobacco use, stillbirth, pelvic fracture, placental abruption, fetal injury, preterm delivery and low birth weight. Violence may escalate, causing severe maternal injury or death.
Obstetric Factors	
Birth of previous infant >4000 g (8.8 lb)	Maternal gestational diabetes, cesarean birth; birth injury, neonatal hypoglycemia.
Previous fetal or neonatal death	Maternal psychological distress.
Rh sensitization	Jaundice, fetal anemia, erythroblastosis fetalis, kernicterus.
Previous preterm birth	Repeated preterm birth.
Existing Medical Conditions	
Diabetes mellitus	Preeclampsia, cesarean birth, preterm birth, infant either small or large for gestational age, neonatal hypoglycemia, congenital anomalies
Hypothyroidism	Gestational hypertension, low birth weight, mental and motor developmental delay, placental abruption, postpartum hemorrhage.
Hyperthyroidism	Spontaneous abortion, heart failure, thyroid storm, preeclampsia, growth restriction, fetal or neonatal thyrotoxicosis, stillbirth.
Cardiac disease	Congestive heart failure, arrhythmias, stroke, maternal mortality, growth restriction, preterm birth.
Renal disease	Maternal renal failure, preeclampsia, preterm delivery, perinatal mortality, growth restriction.
Concurrent infections	Severe fetal implications (heart disease, blindness, deafness, bone lesions) if maternal disease occurred in first trimester, increased incidence of spontaneous abortion or congenital anomalies associated with some infections. If occurring after 20 weeks, preterm delivery and increased fetal and maternal morbidity and mortality.
Psychological conditions	Perinatal mood disorders (anxiety, depression)

Vital Signs

Significant deviations from baseline values for vital signs indicate the need for further assessment. BP should be measured in the same arm, with the mother in the same position each time.

Weight

Weight should be recorded and evaluated for expected progress. Inadequate weight gain may indicate the pregnancy is not as advanced as was thought or the fetus is not growing as expected. A sudden, rapid weight gain may indicate excessive fluid retention.

Urine

Urine may be tested at each visit for protein, glucose, and ketones. Urine is also checked for nitrates to identify UTI and the need for a urine culture.

Fundal Height

Measuring fundal height is an inexpensive and noninvasive method of evaluating fetal growth and confirming gestational age. It is performed at each visit once the fundus is high enough to be palpated in the abdomen. The bladder should be empty to avoid elevation of the uterus. The woman lies on her back with her knees slightly flexed. The top of the fundus is palpated, and a tape measure is stretched from the top of the symphysis pubis, over the abdominal curve, to the top of the fundus (see Fig. 7.1).

From 20 weeks until 32 weeks of gestation, the fundal height, measured in centimeters, is approximately equal to the gestational age of the fetus in weeks. If a discrepancy between fundal height and weeks of gestation is present, additional assessment is necessary. The EDD may be incorrect and the pregnancy more or less advanced than thought. The number of fetuses present, fetal growth, the amount of amniotic fluid, presence of leiomyomata (fibroids), or gestational trophoblastic disease (hydatidiform mole) will affect the fundal height. Ultrasonography may be performed to obtain further information.

Leopold Maneuvers

Leopold maneuvers provide a systematic method for palpating the fetus through the abdominal wall during the latter part of pregnancy. These maneuvers provide valuable information about the location and presentation of the fetus (see Procedure 15.1).

Fetal Heart Rate

The fetal heart rate should be between 110 and 160 bpm. The location of the fetal heart sounds helps determine the position in which the fetus is entering the pelvis. For example, fetal heart sounds heard in an upper quadrant of the abdomen suggest the fetus is in breech presentation.

Fetal Activity

Fetal movements (**quickening**) are usually first noticed by the expectant mother at 16 to 20 weeks of gestation and gradually increase in frequency and strength. In the last trimester, the woman may be asked to count fetal movements, commonly called *kick counts*. In general, fetal activity is a reassuring sign of a physically healthy fetus. Obese women may have decreased perception of fetal movements.

Signs of Labor

The woman should be asked about signs of labor at each visit. A discussion of contractions, bleeding, and rupture of membranes will help the woman learn to identify preterm labor. She should be cautioned to call the health care provider or go to the hospital if she thinks she might be in labor. During the third trimester, a discussion of the normal course of labor is important to prepare the woman.

Ultrasonographic Screening

Ultrasonography is a commonly used prenatal diagnostic procedure (Chapter 9). During early pregnancy, ultrasonography helps determine gestational age, fetal number, and cardiac activity. Ultrasound during the second and third trimesters can be useful when there is a discrepancy between the woman's last menstrual period and uterine size, to detect fetal anatomic defects, to observe for abnormal fetal growth, to check placental location and amniotic fluid volume estimates, and to determine fetal gender. Ultrasound also may be used to measure cervical length in women at risk for preterm delivery (Barron, 2014).

Glucose Screening

Initial screening for diabetes in pregnant women may be by medical history, clinical risk factors, and/or laboratory tests (ACOG, 2015a). For women with significant history or risk factors, the blood glucose level is assessed at 24 to 28 weeks of gestation with a 1-hour oral glucose challenge test. If the result is 140 milligrams per deciliter (mg/dL) or higher, the woman receives a 3-hour oral glucose tolerance test to determine whether she has gestational diabetes. In high-risk women or high-risk populations, laboratory screening at the initial visit is also indicated and includes a fasting glucose test and a hemoglobin A1C (Barron, 2014) (Chapter 10).

Isoimmunization

Antibody tests may be repeated in the third trimester in women who are Rh-negative if the father of the baby is Rh-positive. If unsensitized, the woman should receive Rho (D) immune globulin (RhoGAM) prophylactically at 28 weeks of gestation, after any invasive procedure, such as amniocentesis, or abdominal trauma, and again within 3 days after birth. The woman should be counseled to notify her provider of any episodes of vaginal bleeding or abdominal trauma during the pregnancy.

Pelvic Examination

During the last month of pregnancy, the obstetric provider may perform a pelvic examination to determine cervical changes. The descent of the fetus and the presenting part are also assessed at this time.

Psychosocial Assessments

The woman's psychosocial adaptation should be assessed at each visit (Table 7.4). The nurse should ask the patient about mood swings, body image, dreams, and concerns. In addition to assessment for normal psychosocial changes in pregnancy, ACOG (2015d) recommends all women be screened at least once during the perinatal period for depression and anxiety.

Multifetal Pregnancy

A multifetal pregnancy is a pregnancy in which two or more embryos or fetuses are present simultaneously.

Diagnosis

Multifetal pregnancies are more likely in women who are over 35 years of age or in those who have a personal or family history of multifetal pregnancies. Advances in reproductive technology has contributed to an increased incidence of multifetal gestation (Hobel, 2016).

Women with multifetal pregnancies are larger than expected for the weeks of gestation, report increased fetal movements, and gain more weight. The fundal height is often 4 cm larger than expected on the basis of gestational age computed from the last menstrual period (Beckmann, Ling, Herbert, Laube, & Smith, 2014). When more than one fetus is

TABLE 7.4   Psychosocial Assessment

Normal Findings (Findings of Concern)	Sample Questions	Nursing Implications
Psychological Response		
First trimester: Uncertainty, ambivalence, mood changes, self as primary focus	"How do you and your partner feel about being pregnant?"	Use active listening and reflection to establish a sense of trust.
Second trimester: Wonder, joy, focus on fetus	"How will the pregnancy change your lives?"	Reevaluate negative responses (fear, apathy, anger) in subsequent assessments.
Third trimester: Vulnerability, preparing for birth (fear, anger, apathy, ambivalence, lack of preparation)	"How do you feel about the changes in your body?" "How are you getting ready for the baby?"	
Availability of Resources		
Financial concerns (lack of funds or insurance)	"What are your plans for prenatal care and birth?"	Determine adequacy of financial means. Refer to resources such as a public clinic for care, Program for Women, Infants, and Children (WIC) for food.
Availability of grandparents, friends, family (family geographically or emotionally unavailable)	"How do your parents feel about being grandparents?" "Who else can you depend on besides your family?" "Who helps you when there is a problem?"	Help the couple discover alternative resources if family is unavailable. Identify family conflicts early to allow time for resolution.
Changes in Sexual Practices		
Mutual satisfaction with changes (excessive concern with comfort or safety, excessive conflict)	"How has your sexual relationship changed during this pregnancy?" "How do you cope with the changes?" "What concerns you most?"	Offer reassurance that intercourse is safe if pregnancy is normal. Suggest alternative positions and open communication.
Educational Needs		
Many questions about pregnancy, childbirth, and infant care (no questions, absence of interest in educational programs)	"How do you feel about caring for an infant?" "What are your major concerns?" "Where do you get information about pregnancy?"	Respond to needs that are expressed. Refer couple to appropriate child and parenting classes, reliable Internet sources of information.
Cultural Influences		
Ability of either the woman or her family to speak English or availability of fluent interpreters	"What foods and practices are recommended during pregnancy?" "What is forbidden?"	Locate fluent interpreters, if needed. Avoid labeling beliefs as "superstition."
Cultural influences that support a healthy pregnancy and infant (harmful cultural beliefs or health practices)	"What is most important to you in your care?" "How do your religious beliefs affect pregnancy?"	Reinforce beliefs that promote a good pregnancy outcome. Elicit help from accepted sources of information to overcome harmful practices.

suspected, diagnosis should be confirmed with ultrasonography. Separate fetuses and heart activities may be seen as early as 6 weeks of gestation (Hobel, 2016).

Maternal Adaptation to Multifetal Pregnancy

The degree of maternal physiologic changes is greater with multiple fetuses than with a single fetus. For example, with twins, blood volume increases 500 mL more than the amount needed for a single fetus. This increases the workload of the heart and may contribute to fatigue and activity intolerance. The additional size of the uterus intensifies the mechanical effects of pregnancy. The uterus may achieve a volume of 10 L or more and weigh more than 9 kg (20 lb) (Cunningham et al., 2014). Respiratory difficulty increases because the overdistended uterus causes greater elevation of the diaphragm.

The uterus may also cause more compression of the large vessels, resulting in more pronounced and earlier supine hypotension. Greater compression of the ureters can occur, and maternal edema and slight proteinuria are common. Compression of the

bowel makes constipation and hemorrhoids persistent problems. Nausea and vomiting occur three times as often as in single-fetus pregnancies because of the increased hormones (Cunningham et al., 2014). Fatigue and backache are also increased.

Antepartum Care in Multifetal Pregnancy

Early diagnosis of multifetal pregnancy allows time for the family to be educated about the many ways in which the pregnancy will differ from those involving a single fetus. Special antepartum classes can explain the need for increased nutrition, rest, and fetal monitoring. Instruction about signs of preterm labor, a common complication, should begin early. Discussions of the possible need to reduce activity and take frequent rest periods as well as the potential family stress caused by a high-risk pregnancy should be included.

Women with multifetal pregnancies have more frequent antepartum visits to allow early detection of common complications. These include preeclampsia, preterm labor, placental abruption, congenital anomalies, low birth weight, and postpartum hemorrhage (Beckman et al., 2014; Cunningham et al., 2014). Ultrasound scanning may be performed every 4 to 6 weeks beginning at 24 weeks of gestation to assess the growth of each fetus. Assessment of cervical lengths using ultrasound may help determine increased risk for preterm delivery (Hobel, 2016).

Nutritional education is essential. Adequate calories, iron, calcium, folic acid, and vitamins are important. Women with a normal prepregnancy weight are advised to gain 37 to 54 pounds (lb) during a twin pregnancy (Luke, 2015).

The woman may have many concerns and may need more support than women with only one fetus. Discomforts of pregnancy, which are merely annoying to other women, are increased during multifetal pregnancies. Because preterm birth is the most frequent complication in multifetal pregnancies, teaching about signs of labor and how to respond should begin early in pregnancy.

In addition, the financial burden of medical and hospital care during and after pregnancy is increased. Concerns about the effect of more than one newborn on the family should be discussed. The woman may need referral for assistance in these areas.

❓ KNOWLEDGE CHECK

5. What is the recommended schedule for antepartum visits?
6. How does fundal height relate to gestational age?
7. How does maternal adaptation differ in multifetal pregnancies?

Common Discomforts of Pregnancy

Many women experience discomforts of pregnancy that are not serious but detract from their feeling of comfort and well-being (see Patient Teaching: Discomforts of Pregnancy).

PATIENT TEACHING

Discomforts of Pregnancy

Nausea and Vomiting
- Eat crackers, dry toast, or dry cereal before arising in the morning; then get out of bed slowly.
- Eat small amounts of high-carbohydrate, low-fat foods every 2 hours and a total of five to six small meals per day to prevent an empty stomach.
- Eat a protein snack before bedtime.
- Suck on hard candy.
- Drink fluids frequently but separately from meals. Try small amounts of ice chips, water, and clear liquids like gelatin or frozen juice bars. Avoid coffee.
- Avoid fried, high-fat, greasy, or spicy foods and those with strong odors such as onion and cabbage. Instead, try bland foods that may be more easily tolerated.
- If cooking odors are bothersome, open a window to help disperse them.
- Experiment with different foods that may be helpful, such as ginger (tea, cookies, soda), peppermint (tea or candy), tart and salty combinations such as potato chips and lemonade or green apples, or sweet and salty combinations.
- Take prenatal vitamins at bedtime because they may increase nausea if taken in the morning.
- Use an acupressure band over a point approximately three fingerwidths above the wrist crease on the inner arm.
- Nap and rest more frequently, if possible, because fatigue may increase nausea.
- Check with your health care provider before taking any herbal remedies.
- Notify your health care provider for severe nausea and vomiting or signs of dehydration (dry, cracked lips, elevated pulse, fever, concentrated urine).

Heartburn
- Eat small meals every 2 to 3 hours and avoid fatty, acidic, or spicy foods.
- Eliminate or curtail smoking and drinking coffee and carbonated beverages, which stimulate acid formation in the stomach.
- Avoid citrus fruits and juices, tomato-based products, chocolate, and peppermint if they increase symptoms.
- Try chewing gum.
- Avoid bending over or lying flat.

- Wear loose-fitting clothes.
- Take deep breaths and sip water to help relieve the burning sensation.
- Use antacids, but avoid those that are high in sodium and cause fluid retention (such as Alka-Seltzer, baking soda). Antacids high in calcium (such as Tums, Alka-Mints) are effective but may cause rebound hyperacidity. Take calcium-magnesium based antacids after meals and at bedtime. Avoid antacids containing phosphorus, sodium, or aluminum. Liquid antacids may be more effective, as they coat the esophagus.
- Remain upright for 1 to 2 hours after eating to reduce reflux and relieve symptoms.
- Avoid eating or drinking for 2 to 3 hours before bedtime and sleep with an extra pillow to elevate your head.

Backache
- Maintain correct posture with the head up and the shoulders back.
- Avoid high-heeled shoes because they increase lordosis and back strain.
- Do not gain excess weight.
- Do not lift heavy objects.
- To pick up objects, squat rather than bend from the waist.
- When sitting, use foot supports, arm rests, and pillows behind the back.
- Exercise: Tailor sitting, shoulder circling, and pelvic rocking strengthen the back and help prepare for labor.
- Application of heat or acupuncture may help.
- Standing with one foot in front of the other and rocking back and forth may help.

Round Ligament Pain
- Use good body mechanics, and avoid very strenuous exercise.
- Do not make sudden movements or position changes.
- Do not stretch and twist at the same time. When getting out of bed, turn to the side first without twisting, and then get up slowly.
- Bend toward the pain, squat, or bring the knees up to the chest to relieve pain by relaxing the ligament.
- Apply heat and lie on the right side if discomfort persists.

Continued

PATIENT TEACHING—cont'd

Discomforts of Pregnancy

Urinary Frequency and Loss of Urine

- Restrict fluids in the evening but take adequate amounts during the day.
- Limit intake of natural diuretics such as coffee, tea, and other sources of caffeine.
- Perform Kegel exercises to help maintain bladder control:
  - Identify the muscles to be exercised by stopping the flow of urine midstream. Do not routinely perform the exercise while urinating, however, because it might cause urinary retention and increase the risk of urinary tract infection.
  - Slowly contract the muscles around the vagina and hold for 10 seconds. Relax for at least 10 seconds.
  - Repeat the contraction-relaxation cycle 30 or more times each day.

Varicosities

- Avoid constricting clothing and crossing the legs at the knees, which impede blood return from the legs.
- Rest frequently with the legs elevated above the level of the hips and supported with pillows.
- Apply support hose or elastic stockings that reach above the varicosities before getting out of bed each morning. Putting them on later makes them less effective because pooling begins on rising.
- If working in one position for prolonged periods, walk around for a few minutes at least every 2 hours to stimulate blood flow and relieve discomfort.
- Walk frequently to stimulate circulation in the legs.
- Do foot circles and flex your feet toward your head frequently if sitting for long periods.

Constipation

- Self-care measures generally are as effective as laxatives but do not interfere with absorption of nutrients or lead to laxative dependency.
- Drink at least eight glasses of liquids including water, juice, or milk each day. These should not include coffee, tea, or carbonated drinks because of their diuretic effect. After drinking diuretic beverages, drink a glass of water to counteract its effect.
- Add foods high in fiber to help maintain bowel elimination. Include unpeeled fresh fruits and vegetables, whole-grain breads and cereals, bran muffins, oatmeal, potatoes with skins,

dried beans, and fruit juices. Four pieces of fruit and a large salad provide enough fiber requirements for 1 day.
- Restrict consumption of cheese, which causes constipation.
- Curtail the intake of sweets, which increases bacterial growth in the intestine and can lead to flatulence.
- Do not discontinue taking iron supplements if they have been prescribed. If constipation persists, consult your health care provider about use of stool softeners.
- Exercise stimulates peristalsis and improves muscle tone. Walking briskly for at least 1 mile per day, swimming, or riding a stationary bicycle may be helpful.
- Establish a regular pattern by allowing a consistent time each day for elimination. One hour after meals is ideal to take advantage of the gastrocolic reflex (the peristaltic wave in the colon that is induced by taking food into the fasting stomach).
- Use a footrest during elimination to provide comfort and decrease straining.

Hemorrhoids

- Avoid constipation to prevent straining that causes or worsens hemorrhoids. Drink plenty of water, eat foods rich in fiber, and exercise regularly.
- To relieve existing hemorrhoids, take frequent tepid baths. Apply cool witch hazel compresses or anesthetic ointments.
- Lie on your side with the hips elevated on a pillow.
- If pain or bleeding persists, call your health care provider.

Leg Cramps

- To prevent cramps, elevate the legs frequently to improve circulation.
- To relieve cramps, extend the affected leg, keeping the knee straight. Bend the foot toward the body, or ask someone to assist. If alone, stand and apply pressure on the affected leg with the knee straight. These measures lengthen the affected muscles and relieve cramping.
- Avoid excessive foods high in phosphorus, such as soft drinks.
- Check with your health care provider regarding the need for supplemental calcium, magnesium, or sodium chloride.

Dependent Edema

- Apply support stockings before getting out of bed.
- Sit or lie with the legs elevated often.

Nausea and Vomiting

The nausea and vomiting of pregnancy are frequently called *morning sickness* because these symptoms are more acute on arising. However, they may occur at any time and may continue throughout the day. Symptoms may be aggravated by odors (such as from cooking), fatigue, and emotional stress. Women need reassurance that although morning sickness is distressing, it is common, temporary, and will not harm the fetus. Morning sickness should be distinguished from *hyperemesis gravidarum*—severe vomiting accompanied by weight loss, dehydration, electrolyte imbalance, and ketosis (see Chapter 10).

Nausea and vomiting that significantly interfere with the woman's intake of nutrients may decrease the nutrients available to the fetus. Eating small, frequent meals and high-protein

snacks may help alleviate symptoms. Vitamin B_6 (pyridoxine), doxylamine, and phenothiazines may be prescribed by the health care provider, if necessary (Cunningham et al., 2014). Many nonpharmacologic alternative therapies may be helpful, including ginger, peppermint tea, and acupressure. Although these therapies may be helpful in some women, the efficacy of many of these alternative remedies is not significant (Boelig et al., 2016; Matthews et al., 2015). The health care provider should be consulted before complementary and alternative methods are used.

Heartburn

Heartburn, an acute burning sensation in the epigastric and sternal regions, occurs in up to 80% of pregnant women

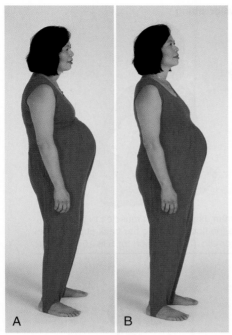

FIG. 7.2 Posture during pregnancy may cause or alleviate backache. **A,** Incorrect posture. The neck is jutting forward, the shoulders are slumping, and the back is sharply curved, creating back pain and discomfort. **B,** Correct posture. The neck and shoulders are straight, the back is flattened, and the pelvis is tucked under and slightly upward.

(Blackburn, 2013). It is caused by reverse peristaltic waves that produce regurgitation of stomach contents into the esophagus. The underlying causes are diminished gastric motility, displacement of the stomach by the enlarging uterus, relaxation of the lower esophageal and gastric sphincters, and increased intraabdominal and intragastric pressure as pregnancy progresses. If common remedies and dietary changes are not effective, the provider may prescribe histamine-2 receptor inhibitors (Blackburn, 2013).

Backache

Backache occurs in 45% to 59% of pregnant women (Blackburn, 2013). Increased joint mobility, lumbar lordosis, and relaxed ligaments contribute to the problem. Teaching correct posture and body mechanics can help prevent back pain (Fig. 7.2). Stooping or bending puts a great deal of strain on the muscles of the lower back. Instruction should include correct and incorrect methods of lifting (Fig. 7.3) and exercises to relax the shoulders and help prevent backache (Fig. 7.4).

Round Ligament Pain

Round ligament pain is a sharp pain in the inguinal area or on the side, usually on the right. It results from softening and stretching of the ligament from hormones and uterine growth. In some instances, it may be difficult for the woman to distinguish from uterine contractions. Careful assessment to rule out contractions followed by reassurance are appropriate measures.

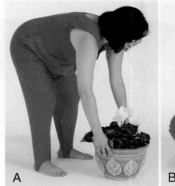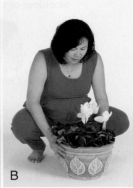

FIG. 7.3 **Techniques for Lifting.** Squatting places less strain on the back. **A,** Incorrect technique. Stooping or bending places a great deal of strain on muscles of the lower back. **B,** Correct technique. Squatting close to the object permits the stronger muscles of the legs to do the lifting.

Urinary Frequency

Although urinary frequency is a common complaint during pregnancy, the condition is temporary and is managed by most women without undue distress. Urinary incontinence, especially in the third trimester, may occur. Kegel exercises may be helpful in maintaining bladder control.

Varicosities

Varicosities occur in 40% of pregnancies (Blackburn, 2013). They are seen more often in women who are obese, are multiparas, or have a family history of varicose veins. During pregnancy, the weight of the uterus partially compresses the veins returning blood from the legs, and estrogen causes elastic tissue to become more fragile. As blood pools, the vessels dilate and become engorged, inflamed, and painful. Varicose veins are exacerbated by prolonged standing, during which the force of gravity makes blood return more difficult.

Varicosities are usually confined to the legs but may involve the veins of the vulva or rectum (hemorrhoids). Varicosities may range from barely noticeable blemishes with minimal discomfort at the end of the day to large, tortuous veins that produce severe discomfort with any activity. They usually improve after childbirth but do not go away completely.

Hemorrhoids

Hemorrhoids are varicosities of the rectum and may be external (outside the anus) or internal (above the sphincter). Some common causes are vascular engorgement of the pelvis, constipation, straining at stool, and prolonged sitting or standing. Pushing during the second stage of labor aggravates the problem, which may continue into the postpartum period. Hemorrhoids often shrink and become less troublesome postpartum.

Constipation

Occasional constipation is not harmful, although it can cause feelings of abdominal fullness and flatulence and aggravate

Shoulder circling

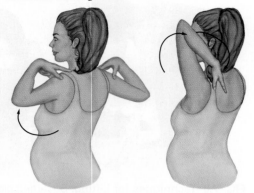

The fingertips are placed on the shoulders, then the elbows are brought forward and up during inhalation, back and down during exhalation. Repeat five times.

Tailor sitting

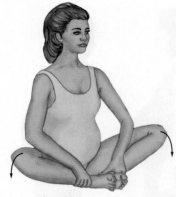

The woman uses her thigh muscles to press her knees to the floor. Keeping her back straight, she should remain in the position for 5 to 15 minutes.

Pelvic tilt or pelvic rocking

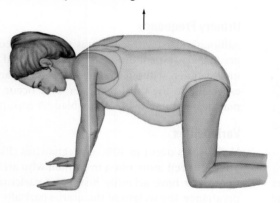

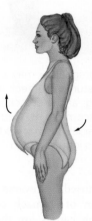

This exercise can be performed on hands and knees, with the hands directly under the shoulders and the knees under the hips. The back should be in a neutral position, not hollowed. The head and neck should be aligned with the straight back. The woman then presses up with the lower back and holds this position for a few seconds, then relaxes to a neutral position. Repeat 5 times. The exercise may also be performed in a standing position when the pelvis is rotated forward to flatten the lower back.

FIG. 7.4 Exercises to prevent backache.

painful hemorrhoids. Intestinal motility is reduced during pregnancy as a result of progesterone, pressure from the enlarged uterus, and decreased activity. The result may be hard, dry stools and decreased frequency of bowel movements. Iron supplementation often increases constipation. Increasing fluid and fiber intake may help to decrease this condition.

Leg Cramps

Painful contractions of the muscles of the legs occur in 25% to 50% of pregnant women (Blackburn, 2013). Cramps often occur during sleep when the muscles are relaxed or when the woman stretches and extends her feet with the toes pointed. Magnesium and vitamin D supplementation may be used (Hobel, 2016). Venous congestion in the legs during the third trimester also contributes to leg cramps. Dorsiflexion of the foot may relieve the cramp.

KNOWLEDGE CHECK

8. What are some relief methods for morning sickness?
9. How can backache be decreased during pregnancy?

◆ APPLICATION OF THE NURSING PROCESS: FAMILY RESPONSES TO PHYSICAL CHANGES OF PREGNANCY

The nursing process focuses on identifying each family's unique responses to the physiologic changes of pregnancy, determining factors that might interfere with their ability to adapt to changes, and finding solutions to identified problems.

◆ Assessment

Assess the woman's responses to the physiologic processes of pregnancy and explore the family's preparation for the birth.

Use structured interviews and planned teaching sessions, as well as more informal spontaneous discussions during assessments. Review the history and physical examination to obtain important data. Gather information from the expectant mother as well as from her partner and significant family members, if appropriate.

◆ Identification of Patient Problems

When analyzing data, nurses should use all their critical thinking skills before reaching a conclusion about the most significant patient problems or opportunities.

Much of the time, the nurse will work with the family to enhance their opportunity for health improvement during the antepartum period. Most families express an intense desire to protect the health of the unborn child and the well-being of the mother.

◆ Planning: Expected Outcomes

If the expected outcomes have been achieved, the woman will:
- Explain self care practices that promote safety and well being for herself and the fetus.
- Describe relief measures for common discomforts of pregnancy.
- Identify personal habits or behaviors that could adversely affect her health or the health of the fetus and develop a plan to modify these behaviors.

◆ Interventions

Teaching Health Behaviors

Teaching should be addressed at each visit and should focus on the mother's immediate questions and concerns. Common concerns are discussed here.

Bathing. Bathing protects pregnant women from infections and promotes comfort by dissipating heat produced by the increased metabolism. During the last trimester, when her balance is altered by a changing center of gravity, the woman is prone to falls. Advise her to use nonskid pads in the tub or shower.

Tubs and Saunas. Although warm baths and showers help relax tense and tired muscles, pregnant women should avoid activities that may cause hyperthermia. Maternal hyperthermia, particularly during the first trimester, may be associated with fetal anomalies. Caution the woman not to be in a sauna for more than 15 minutes or a hot tub for more than 10 minutes and to keep her head, chest, shoulders, and arms out of the water (Beckmann et al., 2014).

Douching. Some women douche because they believe it increases cleanliness and prevents infection. However, despite increased vaginal discharge during pregnancy, douching is unnecessary at any time. Douching increases the risk for ectopic pregnancy, cervical cancer, STDs, pelvic inflammatory disease, and endometritis. Bacterial vaginosis occurs more often in women who douche. In pregnancy, bacterial vaginosis has been associated with spontaneous abortion, preterm birth, premature rupture of membranes, and chorioamnionitis (Cunningham et al.,

2014). Discuss women's reasons for douching and explain it is unnecessary.

Breast Care. Instruct the expectant mother to avoid using soap on her nipples because it removes the natural lubricant secreted by Montgomery glands in the areola. Advise her to wear a well-fitting supportive bra to help prevent loss of tone as the breasts become heavier during pregnancy. Wide bra straps distribute the weight evenly across the shoulders and provide greater comfort.

Inform the couple that breast stimulation increases oxytocin secretion and may cause uterine contractions. Therefore it is unsafe if the woman has a history of preterm labor or existing signs of preterm labor such as rhythmic pelvic pressure or regular uterine contractions. No breast or nipple preparation is necessary during pregnancy for breastfeeding (Wright, 2015). Nurses and providers should promote and discuss the benefits of breastfeeding early in pregnancy and throughout prenatal care.

Clothing. Recommend practical, comfortable, and nonconstricting clothing. Tight jeans or pantyhose, which may impede venous circulation, should be avoided or worn only for short periods. Suggest the woman wear low heels because they do not interfere with balance. High heels increase the curvature of the lower spine (lordosis) increasing backache and making her more likely to fall.

Exercise. Exercise during pregnancy is generally beneficial and can strengthen muscles, reduce backache and stress, and provide a feeling of well-being. The amount and type of exercise recommended depend on the physical condition of the woman and the stage of pregnancy. Exercise tolerance is often decreased, but mild to moderate exercise is generally not a problem.

Teach women who have no medical or obstetric complications to exercise in moderation for at least 20 to 30 minutes or more on most if not all days of the week (ACOG, 2015b; Beckmann et al., 2014). Recreational sports can be continued if no risk for falling or abdominal trauma is present. Joint and ligament laxity and lumbar lordosis increase the risk for injury, especially in the third trimester. Contact sports and exercise with a high risk for falling such as rock climbing or skiing should be avoided. Exercise in the supine position should be discontinued after the first trimester to avoid supine hypotensive syndrome.

Walking is an ideal exercise because it stimulates muscular activity, gently increases respiratory and cardiovascular effort, and does not result in fatigue or strain. Swimming and water exercises are excellent during pregnancy because the buoyancy of the water helps prevent injuries. Riding a stationary bike and yoga are also helpful. Exercise classes especially for pregnant women are often available and offer companionship with other women having similar experiences.

Instruct the woman not to begin strenuous exercise programs or intensify training during pregnancy. Those who have been exercising strenuously before pregnancy should consult the health care provider but may be able to continue

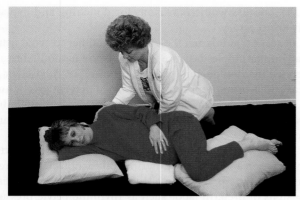

FIG. 7.5 During the third trimester, pillows supporting the abdomen and back provide a comfortable position for rest.

some of their usual routine. As pregnancy progresses, the exercise program may need modification because the change in the woman's center of gravity makes her more prone to falls. Therefore an activity may be safe in the first trimester but not in the third trimester.

Pregnant women should avoid becoming overheated during exercise because heat is transmitted to the fetus, causing an increase in fetal oxygen needs. Women should allow a cool-down period of mild activity after exercising. To prevent dehydration, it is important to take liquids frequently while exercising.

Exercise should be tailored to the way the woman feels to avoid becoming overly fatigued. Generally, if a woman cannot carry on a conversation while exercising, she is doing too much. The woman should stop exercising and seek medical advice if she has chest pain, dizziness, headache, vaginal bleeding, decreased fetal movement, or signs of labor while exercising.

Sleep and Rest. Problems sleeping may begin as early as the first trimester and continue throughout pregnancy (Gordon, 2017). Finding a comfortable position for rest may be difficult by the third trimester. Backache, abdominal discomfort and contractions, leg cramps, fetal movement, and urinary frequency may interfere with sleep.

Suggest the woman use pillows to support the abdomen and back to enhance sleep (Fig. 7.5). Emphasize that frequent rest periods are beneficial, even if the woman does not fall asleep. Suggest relaxation exercises to use during the day and before bed. In addition, avoiding caffeine and limiting fluids at night may be helpful.

Sexual Activity. Sexual intercourse is generally safe for the healthy pregnant woman.

Nutrition. A discussion of nutrition should be part of each visit. The nurse should assess the woman's diet and use of prenatal vitamins and answer any questions she may have (see Chapter 8).

Employment. Most women of childbearing age in the United States are employed outside the home, and most continue to work during pregnancy. Women with uncomplicated pregnancies can usually continue working until they begin labor, if they wish (AAP & ACOG, 2012). However, the level of physical activity involved and the risk

for exposure to environmental toxins and industrial hazards should be considered.

Maternal Safety. Work should not lead to undue fatigue. Frequent rest periods with the feet elevated are essential. Women with jobs that require constant standing or sitting should change positions often or walk briefly to stimulate circulation and reduce fatigue. Tasks that require balance may be hazardous as the center of gravity shifts. Heavy lifting should be avoided.

Working women have many home responsibilities. The fatigue and stress of both the home and employment workloads may be difficult during pregnancy. If possible, the expectant mother should adapt her home and employment workloads during pregnancy to reduce fatigue and stress (Gregory et al., 2017).

Exposure to Teratogens. Intrauterine exposure to toxic substances is of particular concern during the first trimester, the period of organogenesis. Advise women to investigate their own occupational hazards. For example, nurses and hospital personnel may be exposed to chemotherapy drugs, radiation, anesthetic gases, and infectious diseases such as cytomegalovirus infection; hair and nail salon workers may be exposed to hair spray and nail products; laundry and dry-cleaning workers may be exposed to fetotoxic compounds; and farm workers may be exposed to pesticides. In addition, some women are exposed to passive smoking in the work place, which is harmful to both mother and fetus.

Travel. Car travel is safe during normal pregnancies. Generally, no more than 6 hours of car travel is recommended a day during pregnancy (Gregory et al., 2017). Suggest the woman stop to walk every 2 hours to increase venous return from the legs and consider compression stockings. Hydration is also important.

Instruct the woman to fasten the seat belt snugly with the lap belt under her abdomen and across her thighs and the shoulder belt in a diagonal position across her chest and above the bulge of her uterus. This position is uncomfortable for some women, and it causes concern about internal injuries if a collision occurs. However, it is safer to wear the belt than to leave it off and risk ejection from the vehicle during an accident.

Travel by plane is generally safe for up to 36 weeks in the absence of complications of pregnancy. Support stockings, periodic movement of the legs and ambulation, avoidance of restrictive clothing, and adequate hydration may help avoid venous thrombosis. The seat belt should be worn at all times because air turbulence is unpredictable (ACOG, 2016b). The belt should be buckled below the abdomen (AAP & ACOG, 2012). Advise the woman to walk at least every hour to maintain adequate peripheral circulation and avoid thromboembolism. The woman should not travel to remote locations where medical care is unavailable. Suggest she take a copy of her medical records if traveling a long distance.

Immunizations. In general, immunizations with live virus vaccines (such as measles, mumps, rubella, and varicella) are contraindicated during pregnancy because they may have teratogenic effects on the fetus. Inactivated vaccines are safe and can be used in women who have a risk for developing diseases such as tetanus and influenza. Inactivated influenza vaccine is especially important for women who are pregnant during flu season because they can have serious complications from the disease. It can be given at any point in pregnancy (AAP & ACOG, 2012; ACOG, 2014; CDC, 2016). The Centers for Disease Control and Prevention (CDC) recommends administration of the Tdap vaccination between 27 and 36 weeks of each pregnancy (CDC, 2016). (See the CDC website at www.cdc.gov/vaccines for current information.)

Teaching Necessary Lifestyle Changes

Many expectant parents are willing to make changes in lifestyle to avoid adversely affecting the fetus.

Prescription and Over-the-Counter Drugs. Advise pregnant women to consult with their health care providers before taking any drugs. This applies to OTC drugs as well as prescription drugs. Some nonsteroidal antiinflammatory drugs such as aspirin should be avoided because they may increase bleeding. When prescription drugs are necessary, the health care provider weighs the risks against the benefits to decide if a drug can be used safely or if changes are necessary. Drugs taken during the first trimester are of particular concern because of the risk to developing fetal organs.

Complementary and Alternative Therapies. Some complementary and alternative therapies are very safe and helpful during pregnancy. It is estimated that over one third of pregnant women in the United States use some type of alternative therapies during pregnancy, and many of these are seeking treatment for back pain (Holden, Gardiner, Birdee, Davis, & Yeh, 2015). Many have not been studied adequately. Ask about any complementary or alternative therapies used and advise the woman to discuss them with her health care provider.

Tobacco. An important aspect of prenatal care is assessment of and intervention for smoking. Approximately 10% of women smoked during the 3 months before pregnancy, and 8.4% of women in the United States smoke at some time during their pregnancy (Curtain & Mathews, 2016). A *Healthy People 2020* objective is that the number of women who stop smoking during the first trimester and do not restart for the entire pregnancy increase to 30% from a baseline of 11.3% (DHHS, 2010).

Identify women who smoke, and explain the effects of smoking during pregnancy. Every nurse should screen for tobacco use and refer women to smoking cessation programs as needed. Make every effort to motivate expectant mothers to stop smoking and to avoid contact with others who smoke. Secondhand smoke during pregnancy increases the risk for miscarriage, preterm birth, low birth weight, sudden infant death syndrome (SIDS), and other complications (AAP, 2015). The "5A" approach to smoking cessation is often effective:

1. *Ask* the woman at each visit if she smokes, if the amount of smoking has changed, and if she would like to quit. Pregnancy is a time when women are motivated to make changes to benefit their health and the health of the fetus.
2. *Advise* the woman about the importance of not smoking.
3. *Assess* the woman's willingness to try to stop smoking. Discuss motivational information if the woman is not willing to quit at this time. Refer the woman to a smoking cessation program if she is willing to try to stop smoking.
4. *Assist* the woman in making a plan to stop smoking, and provide practical counseling on how to solve the problems she may encounter—for example, avoiding others who smoke and being aware of activities she associates with smoking may be helpful. Advise her that total abstinence is essential to success.
5. *Arrange* follow-up visits or phone calls to discuss the woman's progress and any problems she may have experienced and to offer encouragement. Telephone support may be beneficial in preventing smoking relapse in women who have stopped smoking (ACOG, 2015c; Dennis & Kingston, 2008).

Include the woman's partner in discussions of smoking cessation and the effects of smoking on the fetus. The partner's support is especially important in helping the pregnant woman quit smoking. The partner who smokes may be interested in joining a cessation program, too.

Approximately 50% to 60% of women who stop smoking during pregnancy begin smoking again within 1 year after they give birth (ACOG, 2015c). Explain the effects of smoking on infants and provide continued support for smoking cessation during the postpartum period.

Although nonpharmacologic methods of smoking cessation are best, nicotine replacement therapy may be used if other methods are unsuccessful (Cunningham et al., 2014). Use of nicotine replacement therapy during pregnancy should occur only under the close supervision of the health care provider (AAP & ACOG, 2012; ACOG, 2015c).

Alcohol. Alcohol is a known teratogen, and maternal alcohol use is a leading cause of intellectual disability in the United States. Alcohol may produce a characteristic cluster of developmental anomalies known as fetal alcohol spectrum disorders. Conclusive data about fetal effects of social or moderate drinking are not available, but no amount of alcohol consumed during pregnancy is known to be safe. Therefore the best advice for women who are pregnant or who plan to become pregnant is to abstain from all alcohol.

Illicit Drugs. Use of so-called street or recreational drugs such as cocaine, heroin, and methamphetamines is harmful to the fetus. Advise the pregnant woman to seek help to discontinue all illicit drug use.

Teaching about Signs of Possible Complications

Instruct the pregnant woman and her family about signs and symptoms that should be reported immediately because they indicate a serious danger (see "Critical to Remember: Signs of Possible Pregnancy Complications"). The woman should be instructed to call her health care provider or go to the hospital immediately if she thinks she is experiencing complications.

Although making the expectant mother aware of signs of complications during pregnancy is crucial, the nurse should take care not to overly worry her. Avoid the term *danger signs* when talking to the woman and her family, because it may be frightening. It is less alarming to say, "The signs I am about to explain to

CRITICAL TO REMEMBER

Signs of Possible Pregnancy Complications

Signs	Possible Causes
Vaginal bleeding with or without discomfort	Spontaneous abortion, placenta previa, placental abruption, lesions of the cervix or vagina, "bloody show"
Escape of fluid from the vagina	Rupture of membranes
Swelling of the fingers (rings become tight) or puffiness of the face or around the eyes	Excessive edema, preeclampsia
Continuous pounding headache	Chronic hypertension or preeclampsia
Visual disturbances (such as blurred vision, dimness, flashing lights, spots before the eyes)	Worsening preeclampsia
Seizures	Eclampsia
Persistent or severe abdominal or epigastric pain	Ectopic pregnancy (if early), worsening preeclampsia, placental abruption
Chills or fever	Infection
Painful urination	Urinary tract infection
Persistent vomiting	Hyperemesis gravidarum
Change in frequency or strength of fetal movements	Fetal compromise or death
Signs or symptoms of preterm labor: Uterine contractions, cramps, constant or irregular low backache, pelvic pressure, watery vaginal discharge	Labor onset

you are unusual, but if you notice them, notify your health care provider at once because they require immediate attention."

Providing Resources

Provide the woman with sources for more information. These may include Internet websites such as the March of Dimes at www.marchofdimes.com for information about pregnancy and infants. The Association of Women's Health, Obstetric, and Neonatal Nurses (AWHONN), American College of Nurse-Midwives (ACNM), and ACOG provide information websites for all women's health topics, including pregnancy, at www.health4mom.org, www.ourmomentoftruth.com/Your-Health, and www.acog.org/Patients.

A free service providing information about pregnancy and infants through 1 year is available by text to mobile phones. The service can be accessed by going to the website at www.text4baby.org. The service is supported by both private and governmental agencies and provides three text messages weekly with health tips appropriate to the week of pregnancy or age of the infant.

◆ Evaluation

Interventions can be considered to effectively meet the established outcomes if the mother and her family (1) discuss and practice self-care measures to promote safety and health of the mother and fetus, (2) explain methods to help relieve common discomforts of pregnancy, and (3) identify a plan early in pregnancy to modify habits or behaviors that could adversely affect health. If interventions are ineffective, the nurse collaborates with the family to define new plans and work out additional interventions.

◆ APPLICATION OF THE NURSING PROCESS: PSYCHOSOCIAL CONCERNS

◆ Assessment

The purpose of a psychosocial assessment is to monitor the adaptation of the family to pregnancy, which may require a major transition in role function and relationships. For some families, pregnancy offers the potential for growth. For others, an alteration in family processes requires guidance and information. Specific needs can be discovered during a thorough psychosocial assessment. Table 7.4 identifies areas for assessment, provides sample questions, and indicates nursing implications.

◆ Identification of Patient Problems

Most families strive to maintain the health of the expectant mother and fetus and to complete developmental tasks that help the couple to take on the parent role. Perhaps the most encompassing patient issue is the opportunity for improved family coping, because of the desire to meet added family needs and assume parenting roles.

◆ Planning: Expected Outcomes

Expected outcomes include:

- The expectant parents will verbalize emotional responses that are appropriate to each trimester.
- The family will describe methods to help the expectant parents complete the developmental processes of pregnancy.
- The family will identify cultural factors that may produce conflicts and collaborate to reduce those conflicts.

◆ Interventions

Providing Information

Provide the prospective parents with information and anticipatory guidance to prepare them for the progressive changes that occur during pregnancy, and reassure them that their feelings and behaviors are normal. Guidance also gives them an opportunity to ask questions and explore their feelings. Common subjects include the following:

- The emotional changes that occur during pregnancy
- The developmental tasks of the mother
- Role transition
- The developmental processes of the prospective father

Adapting Nursing Care to Pregnancy Progress

Adapt nursing care to the changes that occur in each trimester of pregnancy. During the first trimester, focus on the woman's acceptance of the pregnancy. Tailor teaching to her feelings (physical and psychological), as this is a period of self-focus. The second trimester is a time to concentrate more on the fetus and how the woman and her family will adapt to the changes resulting from the birth. Ask about her fantasies about the baby and her relationships with significant others. The focus is on the woman's discomforts and readiness to give birth during the third trimester. Observe for signs the mother is having difficulty with any of the tasks or steps throughout pregnancy.

Discussing Resources

Initiate a discussion of the adequacy of the financial situation and support systems, and help couples without financial resources or insurance coverage find a convenient location to obtain prenatal care. This is particularly important for the new poor, who have little knowledge about how to gain access to government-sponsored care. Emotional resources include those that help the new family adjust to the demands of pregnancy and parenting.

Discuss the responses and participation of the grandparents. Although emotional responses vary, the family unit is strengthened and the attachment of the grandparents to the child is enhanced when grandparents actively participate in the pregnancy.

If family members who traditionally offer help in times of stress are unavailable, refer the prospective parents to community resources such as support groups and childbirth education, sibling, breastfeeding, and new parenting classes.

Helping the Family Prepare for Birth

During the last trimester, discuss lifestyle changes that will occur when the infant is born. Unanticipated changes that accompany this dramatic life event may add stress and disrupt family processes. Help the prospective parents make practical plans for the infant, such as obtaining clothing and needed equipment and choosing the method of feeding.

Assist the parents in planning sibling preparation. Older siblings should be prepared several weeks or even months before the birth. They often benefit from participating in planning for the baby. Younger children have a poor concept of time and can be prepared shortly before the birth.

Suggest the expectant parents consider how they will divide household chores, parenting tasks, and child care especially if the mother will return to work after childbirth. If these issues are not resolved, the couple can experience frustration and anger when one parent, usually the mother, assumes total care of the infant and attempts to complete all household tasks. Exhaustion and frustration can overwhelm the joys of parenting when one parent must provide all care.

Modeling Communication Technique

When disagreements are evident, discuss and model therapeutic communication techniques that include all significant family members. Techniques to clarify, summarize, and reflect feelings can defuse negative feelings that might result in family disruption.

Identifying Conflicting Cultural Factors

Explore possible areas of conflict related to cultural beliefs and health practices that affect pregnancy.

Expectant mothers are reassured when nurses support beneficial health beliefs before confronting them with concerns about health care practices. For example, "The foods you are choosing are very good for you and the baby. I am worried, though, because you missed your last appointment."

If a conflict occurs because of differences in time orientation, acknowledge the problem, convey understanding of the differences, and emphasize the importance of calling when appointments cannot be kept. Many families do not realize that when they miss an appointment, another family misses the opportunity for health care.

◆ Evaluation

When the family verbalizes concerns and emotions at each visit, the initial goal is met. Continued interest and involvement of the partner and significant family members are evidence that the family has completed the developmental tasks of pregnancy. Participation with health care workers to find a compromise if differing cultural beliefs cause conflict confirms that the family will identify and initiate measures to reduce conflicts.

PERINATAL EDUCATION CLASSES

The goals of perinatal education are to help parents become knowledgeable consumers, take an active role in maintaining health during pregnancy and birth, and learn coping techniques for pregnancy, childbirth, and parenting. Meeting these goals helps reduce parents' fear of the unknown and increases their abilities to make informed decisions regarding childbirth and parenting with confidence and satisfaction. Although much perinatal education is accomplished during the prenatal visits, many classes are available and valuable.

Perinatal education classes are strongly recommended by the AAP and the ACOG because they can have a beneficial effect on patients' experience (AAP & ACOG, 2012). A *Healthy People 2020* goal is to increase the proportion of women who attend a series of prepared childbirth classes (DHHS, 2010).

Expectant families have many choices for prenatal education classes. Their decisions are based on the classes available in the area, costs, and types of information they need. Small classes of a few women and their partners are ideal but may be too expensive or unavailable. The teacher is usually an RN who has experience in maternity nursing and is certified by a nationally known organization such as Lamaze International or the International Childbirth Education Association (ICEA).

Although most people think of perinatal education primarily as preparation for the birth experience, classes are available for all areas of pregnancy, childbirth, and parenting.

Nurses help the woman and her partner find classes suited to their educational needs, provide a list and description of classes in the community, and suggest they talk with others who have taken various classes. The couple may wish to interview teachers to learn about their preparation and philosophies. Some couples want classes that consider avoidance of medication a primary goal of childbirth. Many prefer those that consider a variety of tools, including medication, for coping with pain.

Preconception Classes

Classes for couples who are thinking about having a baby are designed to help them have a healthy pregnancy from the beginning. Information about nutrition before conception, healthy lifestyle, signs of pregnancy, and choosing a caregiver is presented. The effects of pregnancy and childbirth on a woman's relationships and career are discussed. Preconception classes emphasize early and regular prenatal care beginning before pregnancy and ways to reduce risk factors for poor pregnancy outcome.

Education in First Trimester

First-trimester classes cover information on adapting to pregnancy and understanding what to expect in the months ahead (Box 7.2). Emphasis is placed on how to have a healthy pregnancy by obtaining prenatal care and avoiding hazards to the fetus.

One important task for expecting women during early pregnancy is to choose the provider and setting that is most appropriate (see Chapter 1). Some women may wish to prepare a birth plan (Box 7.3).

Education in Second Trimester

Second-trimester classes focus on changes occurring during middle pregnancy and what to expect during the third trimester. Teachers discuss childbirth choices and information to help students become more knowledgeable consumers. With a CenteringPregnancy model of care, much of the perinatal education is incorporated into the regular prenatal visit. Exercise classes help women keep fit and healthy during pregnancy. Written consent from the primary caregiver may be required to ensure that the woman can participate safely. The instructor should understand the special needs of pregnancy and teach low-impact exercises preceded by warm-up routines. Women should avoid excessive heart rate elevation to prevent diversion of blood away from the uterus.

The woman with a high-risk pregnancy may have activity restrictions and may be unable to attend regular perinatal classes.

BOX 7.2 Topics Covered in Early Pregnancy Classes

Pregnancy changes
  Anatomy and physiology
  Physiologic and psychological changes
  Fetal development
  Hazards to the mother and fetus (e.g., drugs, alcohol, smoking, environmental hazards)
  Prenatal care (e.g., what to expect at each visit)
  Communication with the provider
  Prenatal screening tests
Self-care
  Hygiene
  Nutrition
  Exercise and body mechanics
  Discomforts of pregnancy
  Warning signs and actions to take
  Sexuality
  Work and pregnancy
Infant care
  Selection of a pediatric provider
  Infant development
  Infant feeding
Birth
  Birth options (such as birth plan, costs)
  Preterm labor

BOX 7.3 Birth Plan

Help couples prepare a plan for their birth experience if they wish. The birth plan, sometimes called a *family preference plan*, describes the couple's desires as they consider their choices in childbirth. The plan may be unwritten and very simple or a list of very specific items to be included in the childbirth experience. Cultural wishes can be incorporated into the birth plan.

The birth plan is a tool for expanding communication with health care professionals. It helps couples learn about their options and make informed choices and ensures their wishes are known before labor begins. It may help the couple choose the provider, setting, and classes most conducive to meeting specific needs. The couple should discuss the plan with the health care provider during pregnancy and with the nurse in the labor and delivery unit when they are admitted. This may result in a more satisfying birth experience even if not everything goes according to the expectations.

Help the couple learn about locally available choices and explain any restrictions. For example, insurance coverage may dictate which facility a woman must use. Those without insurance are concerned about the cost of various options. In addition, the health care provider or birth agency may have set policies on certain issues. Complications during labor and birth may necessitate changes in the plan.

If the couple has not chosen a health care provider, suggest they interview several physicians or nurse-midwives to learn about the provider's usual practices and possible exceptions. If they have a provider, emphasize the importance of discussing their plan with him or her. With discussion, the couple and provider can create a plan that is satisfactory to all.

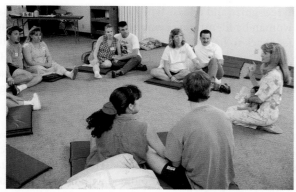

FIG. 7.6 The nurse teaching this class discusses movement of the fetus through the pelvis.

If possible, help her arrange for individual instruction. Online courses, CDs, written materials, and phone or e-mail contact with an instructor are ways she can learn and practice techniques without attending classes.

Education in Third Trimester

During the third trimester, women may enroll in prenatal classes to cope with vulnerabilities and fears regarding the upcoming birth.

In childbirth preparation classes during the third trimester, women and their support persons learn self-help measures, what to expect during labor and birth (Fig. 7.6), and how to prepare for the big day (Boxes 7.4 and 7.5). Although once referred to as "natural childbirth classes," they are now called *prepared childbirth classes* to denote the woman's preparation for all aspects of childbirth.

Couples learn coping methods to help them approach childbirth in a positive manner. Teachers do not promise prevention of all pain in labor. However, the increased confidence and the techniques learned in prepared childbirth classes may help increase tolerance of pain during labor and increase maternal satisfaction with their birth experience. Class series range from a 1-day class to 3 to 12 meetings, depending on the content included. Supervised practice of relaxation, breathing techniques, and coping strategies in "labor rehearsals" may be part of every class (Fig. 7.7).

Most classes cover information about both pharmacologic and nonpharmacologic methods of coping with labor pain. Although many women plan to have epidural anesthesia during childbirth, nonpharmacologic pain relief measures may be very helpful until the woman can obtain pharmacologic pain relief or in case the anesthesia does not provide complete relief.

By learning what to expect during labor and birth, women and their support persons are able to rehearse the experience in their minds in preparation for the actual event. They practice coping techniques during simulated contractions. Realistic, valid class information and discussion of possible variations are essential so couples are adequately prepared.

Prepared childbirth classes based in birth facilities include detailed information on what to expect in that particular setting but may not cover unavailable options. A tour of the maternity areas may be offered as part of the class or as a separate class.

? CRITICAL THINKING EXERCISE 7.1

Liz, gravida 2, para 1, tells you that she does not plan to attend prepared childbirth classes because she took classes before her son, Danny, was born 5 years ago.

Question
1. What should you discuss with her?

BOX 7.4   Topics Included in Prepared Childbirth Classes

Some topics may be presented in separate classes.
Physical and psychological changes of the last trimester
   Common discomforts and concerns
   Nutrition
   Exercise and body mechanics
   Sexuality
   Danger signs and actions to take
Labor and birth
   Anatomy and physiology of labor
   Plans for the birth (e.g., options, birth plan)
   Signs of labor and when to go to the hospital
   Hospital admission, procedures, and policies
   Physical and emotional aspects of labor
   Labor variations (e.g., back labor)
   Medical procedures (e.g., induction, augmentation, amniotomy, episiotomy, vacuum extraction)
   Birthing process
   Recovery
   Tour of maternity unit
   Role of the labor partner
   Techniques for support
Coping techniques for labor
   Relaxation and breathing techniques
   Comfort measures
   Labor rehearsals
   Pain relief (pharmacologic and nonpharmacologic)
Complications
   Fetal testing
   Preterm labor
   Hypertension
   Cesarean birth
High-risk pregnancy

BOX 7.5   What to Take to the Hospital

Items to Be Included in the Labor Bag
Focal point
Lotion, oil, or powder to make massage more comfortable
Warm socks for cold feet
Colored washcloths for washing face (white ones might be lost)
Hand-held fan
Elastic bands and clips for hair
Tennis balls in a sock for sacral pressure
Sugar-free sour lollipop for dry mouth
Mouthwash
Lip balm, unflavored

Continued

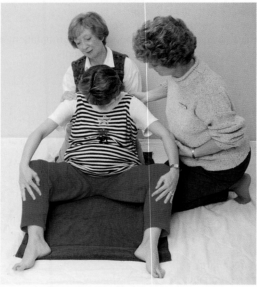

FIG. 7.7 The teacher helps each couple, individually and together, practice pushing during a labor rehearsal.

Coping Techniques

Relaxation. Tension and anxiety during labor cause tightening of abdominal muscles, impeding contractions and increasing pain by stimulation of nerve endings that heighten awareness of pain. Prolonged muscle tension causes fatigue and increased pain perception. When anxiety and tension are high, uterine contractions are less effective and the length of labor increases. The ability to relax during labor is an important component of coping effectively with childbirth. Relaxation conserves energy, decreases oxygen use, and enhances other pain relief techniques. Most childbirth preparation classes teach women exercises to help them recognize and release tension. The labor partner assists the woman by identifying symptoms of tension and providing feedback to help her relax. For example, she may tighten her shoulders, frown, or jiggle her foot when stressed. Her partner helps her focus on areas she finds difficult to relax. Positive feedback from the partner and teacher encourages increased relaxation.

Relaxation exercises should be practiced frequently to be useful during labor. Couples begin practice sessions in a quiet, comfortable setting. Later, they practice in other places to simulate the noise and unfamiliar setting of the hospital. Relaxation exercises may be combined with other techniques such as imagery and massage.

Breathing. Historically, specific breathing techniques were taught in childbirth preparations classes. Today, breathing is taught in conjunction with relaxation techniques. Many classes teach a variety of techniques to allow the woman to pick and choose those that work best for her. The cleansing breath, a deep inhalation followed by complete exhalation is used at the beginning and end of each contraction. This bookmarks the contraction and oxygenates the mother and fetus. With slow abdominal breathing, the patient is told to relax in a comfortable position, breathe in through the nose until she cannot comfortably take in any more air, then breathe out through her mouth, forcing out as much air as she can. Breathing techniques maintain oxygenation and provide a distraction for the mother. Breathing techniques include slow paced, modified paced, and pant-blow. With slow-paced breathing, the woman is told to breath at about half of her normal rate (in-2-3-4; out-2-3-4). Modified-paced breathing is slightly faster than normal but no more than twice the normal rate (in-2, out-2). Pant-blow is also at about twice the normal respiratory rate. With this technique, the woman is taught to take short, shallow breaths in and out with an occasional long exhale, like a sigh. The woman may be taught to "say" a quiet "he" with each of the pants and "ho" with the exhale, or blow. The ratio of pants to blows can be varied to provide additional distraction. For example: pant-2-3-4-5, blow; pant-2-3-blow.

Conditioning. Many techniques for prepared childbirth are based partially on theories of conditioned response, in which certain responses to stimuli become automatic through frequent association. Women learn to associate uterine contractions with relaxation by practicing relaxation techniques with mental images of contractions. Because effective conditioning requires a great deal of practice, women are encouraged to practice their techniques daily. For some women, the intensity of real uterine contractions is surprisingly different from their experiences during practice sessions. They may have difficulty with relaxation as a result and may need to use other methods along with conditioning.

Labor Partner. Almost all types of childbirth preparation encourage the participation of someone who remains with the woman throughout labor. This person may be called a *labor partner, support person, coach,* or *labor companion.* The presence of a labor partner may help the woman cope more effectively, decrease her distress during labor, and result in greater satisfaction with the childbirth experience. This support person shares the experience and helps the woman remain focused and calm during labor.

The person who takes on this role may be the baby's father, a relative, a friend and/or a doula. The labor partner generally attends classes with the mother to learn about labor, birth, and techniques to assist during labor. By practicing together, the woman and her partner learn to work smoothly as a team during labor. Classes may increase confidence for support persons, who learn specific techniques to use during labor. When the labor partner is the father, communication and a sense of closeness between the expectant parents may be enhanced. Many women hire a doula to assist with labor support. The doula may attend or teach the childbirth class. Encourage couples to think about the support person's labor role before labor begins and then encourage the partner in whatever role is chosen. Labor partners should not feel responsible for more than is included in the role. Teachers should discuss the duties of the labor nurse and encourage labor partners to seek assistance when they are uncertain. The labor nurse may have helpful suggestions and adaptations of techniques.

Class discussion of complications should include the role of the support person in these situations.

Methods of Childbirth Education

Although all methods of prepared childbirth education use some combination of pain management techniques, each method has unique aspects. Many classes have a holistic approach, providing a variety of techniques from which couples can choose those that work best for them. The nurse should give the family a list and description of classes in their community and the philosophies of each class.

Dick-Read Childbirth Education. Grantly Dick-Read was an English physician who was one of the first to use education and relaxation techniques to help women through childbirth. According to Dick-Read, fear of childbirth results in tension and pain. To prevent the fear-tension-pain cycle, he developed a method of slow abdominal breathing in early labor and rapid chest breathing in advanced labor. His methods were the first to be called *natural childbirth.*

Bradley Childbirth Education. The Bradley method was the first to include the father as a support person for "husband-coached childbirth." Abdominal breathing to increase relaxation and breath control are taught in these classes. The Bradley method also emphasizes avoidance of medications and other interventions. In addition, classes include general information included in most other childbirth preparation classes.

Lamaze Childbirth Education. The Lamaze method is often called **psychoprophylaxis** because it uses the mind to prevent pain. It involves concentration and conditioning to help the woman respond to contractions with relaxation and various techniques to decrease pain. The Lamaze method is the most popular method used today. A variety of techniques are taught, and women should feel free to choose among them (Table 7.5). Women should not be taught that there is only one right way of responding to labor.

KNOWLEDGE CHECK

10. What are the goals of perinatal education?
11. What information is typically covered in preconception classes? Early pregnancy classes? Second-trimester classes?
12. What techniques are commonly taught in childbirth preparation classes during the third trimester?
13. How is the woman in labor helped by having a labor partner?
14. What are the various roles the support person might take?

Breastfeeding Classes

Prenatal breastfeeding education is important because of the short time available after birth to help breastfeeding mothers in the birth facility. Classes help increase a woman's confidence in her ability to breastfeed successfully and provide her with resources if she encounters difficulties. Teachers are often certified lactation consultants who have special education and advanced knowledge about breastfeeding.

Breastfeeding classes include information about the various aspects of lactation and help support persons attending learn methods of providing assistance during breastfeeding (Box 7.6). Resources for additional help are provided in case the woman encounters difficulties. Some teachers hold additional sessions after the birth to provide ongoing counseling at a time when mothers may experience unexpected problems. These sessions allow discussion of problems as they occur.

Classes for Partners

Classes for partners often focus on the male perspective of pregnancy, birth, and parenting. They provide an opportunity for men to meet other expectant partners and ask questions they might not ask in classes that include expectant mothers. Some involve practicing infant care techniques with dolls. Classes are often taught by nurses who are experienced partners, or new partners are invited to come and share their experiences.

Classes for Siblings

Sibling classes are usually for children aged 3 to 12 years. The classes teach them about newborn characteristics and help decrease anxiety about the approaching birth (Fig. 7.8).

Many young children have never seen a newborn and are expecting a child near their own age who can be a playmate. A visit with a newborn infant allows them to see newborns at close range and learn to be safe helpers. Videos and stories promote discussion about normal feelings of jealousy and anger. Emphasis is placed on the important role of big brothers and sisters and that a baby could not replace them in their parents' affection.

A separate parent discussion may provide suggestions for further preparation and ways to cope with the transition after birth. Concerns about sibling rivalry and meeting the needs of more than one child are common topics.

Special sibling classes may be held for children who will be present at the birth. These help prepare the child for the sights and sounds of birth. The child's support person also attends the class.

TABLE 7.5 Methods of Pain Management Taught in Childbirth Classes

Method	Examples and Techniques	Descriptions	Effect on Pain	Notes
Positioning	Ambulation Position changes	Ambulation, sitting on exercise ball, rocking in rocking chair, squatting, kneeling, all four's, side-lying.	Increase comfort and decrease muscle fatigue; upright position makes contractions more efficient and less painful. Frequent position changes promote labor progress.	Position should be changed at least every 30–60 min during labor. Classes focus on teaching different positions, the need for frequent position changes and the benefits of ambulation in early labor.
Hydrotherapy	Shower Submersion in water	Shower with or without hand-held spray; tub, whirlpool.	Supplements relaxation and thermal techniques. Buoyancy supports the body, equalizes pressure and aids muscle relaxation. Spray provides cutaneous stimulation.	Check with provider and facility protocol before submersion if membranes are ruptured.
Relaxation	Progressive relaxation	Contracting/consciously releasing muscle groups. Repeated throughout the body until all voluntary muscles are relaxed. The woman learns to differentiate between feelings of tense and relaxed muscles, enabling her to systematically assess and release muscle tension throughout her body.	Reduces tension that increases pain perception and decreases pain tolerance. Conserves energy, decreases oxygen use and enhances other pain relief methods.	Learning multiple techniques provides options during labor. Techniques should be practiced frequently during pregnancy to be useful for labor.
	Neuromuscular disassociation	Learn to relax body during uterine contractions. The woman contracts an area such as an arm or leg, then concentrates on releasing tension from the rest of her body.		
	Touch relaxation	Learn to loosen taut muscles when touched by partner. The woman tenses an area (or multiple areas) and relaxes the area as her partner strokes and massages it.		
	Relaxation against pain	Practice using techniques against discomfort to simulate labor pain. Partner applies pressure against a tendon or large muscle of the arm or leg while the woman uses relaxation techniques. Alternately, ice may be applied as the source of discomfort.		

Category	Technique	Description	Rationale	Notes
Cutaneous stimulation	Pressure/counter pressure	Firm pressure applied to palms, fingertips, soles of the feet or sacral area of the back. (Tennis balls may be used to apply pressure to the back)	Pressure receptors travel more rapidly than pain receptors, closing "gate" on pain receptors.	
	Effleurage	Slow, light massage of abdomen during contraction using light touch in circular or other patterns.	Touch stimulates sensory fibers and interferes with transmission of pain impulses. Use of variety of patterns may provide source of concentration and increased input to the brain.	
	Thermal stimulation (heat and cold)	Cool cloths to the face, neck; ice chips eaten by the woman, ice pack to lower back. Warm blanket, moist towel, cloth bags or socks filled with rice and warmed in a microwave.	Application of heat and cold may stimulate thermoreceptors and reduce pain sensation. Heat increases local blood flow, skin and muscle temperature, tissue metabolism, relaxation; decreases muscle spasms. Cold decreases muscle temperature, relieves muscles spasms	Place a barrier (cloth or towel) between the woman's skin and source of heat or cold.
	Massage	Rub back, shoulders, legs; any area the woman finds helpful.	Increases circulation and reduces muscle tension.	Use lotion or powder to decrease friction. (Avoid inhalation of powder; keep powder away from newborn.)
Mental stimulation	Focal point	Attention centered on an object during contractions to direct thoughts away from contractions. Thoughts should focus on the object – shape, size, gradations of colors, etc.	Occupies the woman's mind and competes with pain stimuli. Helps woman dissociate from painful aspects. Also promotes relaxation by providing a tranquil imaginary atmosphere.	
	Imagery	Imagine self in a pleasant scene or setting, promoting feeling of peacefulness during the contraction. Partner or nurse describes the scene, using all senses applicable – the sights, sounds, smells, feeling on skin (such as warmth of sun, or splashing waves)		
	Sounds	Sounds of rainfall or waves; favorite playlist of various types of music to promote relaxation, energy, or sense of well-being.		
Breathing	Focused or controlled techniques	Cleansing breath, Slow-Paced Breathing, Modified-Paced Breathing, Patterned Breathing. (See Figs. 13.5, 13.6, 13.7, 13.9)	Provides a different focus during contractions, interfering with pain sensory transmission.	Once major focus of many classes, now considered one of many coping strategies. Selected techniques should be practiced before labor for best results. Should be used only when needed, usually when the woman can no longer walk or talk during the contractions.
Support	Labor partner, husband or partner Labor nurse, Doula	Advocate and speak for mother during labor, support with techniques practiced before labor, provide comfort measures, and emotional support – encouragement, reassurance.	Helps the woman use coping strategies, decreases fear, promotes relaxation	Some cultures may discourage men from participating. Support person may be another relative or friend.

BOX 7.6   Topics Included in Breastfeeding Classes

Anatomy and physiology
Preparation for breastfeeding
First feedings
Positioning and latch-on
Establishment of milk supply
Prevention and solutions for problems: Engorgement, sore nipples, nipple confusion, insufficient milk supply, mastitis
Nutrition
Use of bottles and storage of breast milk
Breast pumps
Role of support person(s)
Work and breastfeeding
Weaning

BOX 7.7   Topics Included in Parenting and Infant Care Classes

Normal newborn appearance: Marks, rashes, normal behavior
General care: Diapering, cord care, circumcision care, bathing
Behavior cues
Feeding methods and problems, schedules, colic
Other concerns: Crying, comforting techniques, sleeping through the night
Safety: Car seats, positioning for sleep, "baby-proofing" the home
Baby equipment
Early growth and development: Expectations, infant stimulation, immunization
Illness: Signs of common conditions, taking a temperature, calling the physician
Infant cardiopulmonary resuscitation
Family and relationship changes

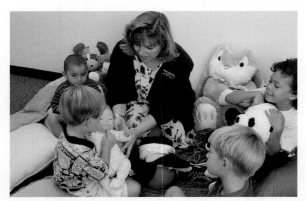

FIG. 7.8 During sibling classes, children learn about the new babies coming into their lives.

Parenting and Infant Care Classes

Content for parenting classes typically includes information parents need during the early weeks after the birth (Box 7.7).

Baby equipment such as infant car seats is often displayed. Practice with dolls may be included. Classes may continue after the birth of the infant.

Postpartum Classes

Although the postpartum period is discussed briefly in prepared childbirth classes, in some areas, the mother also can attend classes after birth. Content frequently focuses on exercise and nutrition, but may also include the physiologic and psychological changes of the postpartum period, role transition, and sexuality. Signs of postpartum depression may be discussed, with emphasis on when the woman should seek help. Some classes are informal support groups led by a knowledgeable professional.

SUMMARY CONCEPTS

- The preconception, interconception, or initial prenatal visit includes a complete history and physical examination to determine potential risks to the mother and fetus and obtain baseline data for a plan of care.
- Assessment of risk for problems is performed at each prenatal visit because pregnancies considered low risk in early pregnancy may later become high risk.
- Multifetal pregnancies impose greater physiologic changes than a single-fetus pregnancy and require extra vigilance to detect possible complications.
- Families need information related to self-care, health promotion, and coping with the common discomforts of pregnancy.
- Nurses use the nursing process and critical-thinking skills to assist the parents to make necessary changes in lifestyle.

- Education for childbearing helps couples become knowledgeable consumers and active participants in pregnancy and childbirth.
- Many classes are available for pregnant women and their support persons. Preconception and early pregnancy classes emphasize ways to have a healthy pregnancy. Classes conducted in later pregnancy focus on preparation for childbirth, breastfeeding, and early parenting.
- Classes for partners and siblings help all family members prepare for the birth.
- Education, relaxation, breathing, and conditioning are used to increase coping ability for childbirth.
- Having a labor partner or support person increases a woman's satisfaction with childbirth.

REFERENCES & READINGS

American Academy of Pediatrics (AAP). (2015). *The dangers of second hand smoke*. Retrieved from www.healthychildren.org.

American Academy of Pediatrics (AAP) & American College of Obstetricians and Gynecologists (ACOG). (2012). *Guidelines for perinatal care* (7th ed.). Elk Grove Village, IL: Author.

American College of Obstetricians and Gynecologists (ACOG). (2014). Influenza vaccination during pregnancy, Committee Opinion No. 608. *American College of Obstetrics and Gynecologists. Obstetrics & Gynecology.*

American College of Obstetricians and Gynecologists (ACOG). (2015a). *Gestational diabetes mellitus. Practice Bulletin* 137, 2013. reaffirmed, 2015. Author.

American College of Obstetricians and Gynecologists (ACOG). (2015b). *Physical activity and exercise during pregnancy and the postpartum period, ACOG Committee Opinion No. 650*. Online at www.acog.org.

American College of Obstetricians and Gynecologists (ACOG). (2015bc). *Smoking cessation during pregnancy, ACOG Committee Opinion No. 471*. ACOG: Obstetrics & Gynecology.

American College of Obstetricians and Gynecologists (ACOG). (2015d). *Screening for perinatal depression, ACOG Committee Opinion No 630*. ACOG: Obstetrics & Gynecology.

American College of Obstetricians and Gynecologists (ACOG). (2016a). *ACOG reinvents the pregnancy wheel*. ACOG: Obstetrics & Gynecology.

American College of Obstetricians and Gynecologists (ACOG). (2016b). *Air travel during pregnancy, ACOG Committee Opinion No 443*. ACOG: Obstetrics & Gynecology.

Barger, M., Faucher, M. A., & Murphy, P. A. (2015). Part II: The Centering Pregnancy Model of Group Prenatal Care. *Journal of Midwifery & Women's Health, 60*(2), 211–213.

Barron, M. L. (2014). Antenatal care. In K. R. Simpson, & P. A. Creehan (Eds.), *AWHONN perinatal nursing* (4th ed.) (pp. 89–122). Philadelphia, PA: Lippincott Williams & Wilkins.

Beckmann, C. R. B., Ling, F. W., Herbert, W. N. P., Laube, D. W., & Smith, R. P. (2014). *Obstetrics and gynecology* (7th ed.). Philadelphia, PA: Lippincott Williams & Wilkins.

Blackburn, S. T. (2013). *Maternal, fetal, and neonatal physiology: A clinical perspective* (4th ed.). St. Louis, MO: Saunders.

Boelig, R. C., Barton, S. J., Saccone, G., Kelly, A. J., Edwards, S. J., & Berghella, V. (2016). Interventions for treating hyperemesis gravidarum. *Cochrane Database of Systematic Reviews, 2016*(5).

Centers for Disease Control and Prevention (CDC). (2016). *Guidelines for vaccinating pregnant women*. Retrieved from www.cdc.gov.

Charlton, B. M., Mølgaard-Nielsen, D., Svanström, H., Wohlfahrt, J., Pasternak, B., & Melbye, M. (2016). Maternal use of oral contraceptives and risk of birth defects in Denmark: prospective, nationwide cohort study. *BMJ 2016*, 352.

Cunningham, F. G., Leveno, K. J., Bloom, S. L., Spong, C. Y., Dashe, J. S., Hoffman, B. L., & Sheffield, J. S. (2014). *Williams' obstetrics* (24th ed.). New York, NY: McGraw-Hill.

Curtain, S. A., & Mathews, T. J. (2016). Smoking prevalence and cessation before and during pregnancy: data from the birth certificate, 2014. *National Vital Statistics Report, 65*(1). Hyattsville, MD: National Center for Health Statistics .

Dennis, C. L., & Kingston, D. (2008). A systematic review of telephone support for women during pregnancy and the early postpartum period. *Journal of Obstetric, Gynecologic, and Neonatal Nursing, 37*(3), 301–314.

Gordon, M. C. (2017). Maternal physiology. In S. G. Gabbe, J. R. Niebyl, J. L. Simpson, et al. (Eds.), *Obstetrics: normal and problem pregnancies* (6th ed.) (pp. 42–65). Philadelphia, PA: Saunders.

Gregory, K. D., Ramos, D. E., & Jauniaux, E. R. M. (2017). Preconception and prenatal care. In S. G. Gabbe, J. R. Niebyl, J. L. Simpson, et al. (Eds.), *Obstetrics: normal and problem pregnancies* (6th ed.) (pp. 102–121). Philadelphia, PA: Saunders.

Heberlein, E. C., Picklesimer, A. H., Billings, D. L., Covington-Kolb, S., Farber, N., & Frongillo, E. A. (2016). Qualitative comparison of women's perspectives on the functions and benefits of group and individual prenatal care. *Journal of Midwifery & Women's Health, 61*(2), 224–234.

Hobel, C. J. (2016). Multifetal gestation and malpresentation. In N. F. Hacker, J. C. Gambone, & C. J. Hobel (Eds.), *Hacker & Moore's essentials of obstetrics and gynecology* (6th ed.) (pp. 170–182). Philadelphia, PA: Elsevier.

Hobel, C. J., & Williams, J. (2016). Antepartum care. In N. F. Hacker, J. C. Gambone, & C. J. Hobel (Eds.), *Hacker & Moore's essentials of obstetrics and gynecology* (6th ed.) (pp. 76–95). Philadelphia, PA: Elsevier.

Holden, S. C., Gardiner, P., Birdee, G., Davis, R. B., & Yeh, G. Y. (2015). Complementary and alternative medicine use among women during pregnancy and childbearing years. *Birth, 42*(3), 261–269.

Luke, B. (2015). Nutrition for multiples. *Clinical Obstetrics and Gynecology, 58*(3), 585–610.

Matthews, A., Haas, D. M., O'Mathúna, D. P., & Dowswell, T. (2015). Interventions for nausea and vomiting in early pregnancy. *Cochrane Database of Systematic Reviews* (3) CD007575.

Mitchell, A. A., Gilboa, S. M., Werler, M. M., Kelley, K. E., Louik, C., Hernández-Díaz, S., & National Birth Defects Prevention Study. (2011). Medication use during pregnancy, with particular focus on prescription drugs: 1976–2008. *American Journal of Obstetrics & Gynecology, 205*(1), 51.e1–51.e8.

National Center for Health Statistics. (2017). *Data File Documentations, Natality, 2015*. Hyattsville, MD: Author.

Nypaver, C., Arbour, M., & Niederegger, E. (2016). Preconception care of women and families. *Journal of Midwifery and Women's Health, 61*(3), 356–364.

U.S. Department of Health and Human Services. (2010). *Healthy people 2020*. Washington, DC: Author.

U.S. Preventive Services Task Force. (2016). *Folic acid for the prevention of neural tube Defects: U.S. Preventive Services Task Force Draft Recommendation Statement*. Retrieved from https://www.uspreventiveservicestaskforce.org/.

West, E. H., Hark, L., & Catalano, P. M. (2017). Nutrition during pregnancy. In S. G. Gabbe, J. R. Niebyl, J. L. Simpson, M. B. Landon, H. L. Galan, E. R. M. Jauniaux, et al. (Eds.), *Obstetrics: Normal and Problem Pregnancies* (7th ed.) (pp. 122–135). Philadelphia, PA: Elsevier.

Wright, E. M. (2015). Breastfeeding and the mother-newborn dyad. In T. L. King, M. C. Brucker, J. M. Kriebs, J. O. Fahey, C. L. Gegor, & H. Varney (Eds.), *Varney's Midwifery* (5th ed.) (pp. 704–705). Burlington, MA: Jones & Bartlett Learning.

Nutrition for Childbearing

Kari Mau

At no other point in a woman's life is nutrition as important as it is during pregnancy and lactation. At this time, she must nourish not only herself but also her baby. Nutrition may affect the size of the fetus and determine whether it has adequate stores of some nutrients after birth. If the woman fails to consume sufficient nutrients during pregnancy, her own stores of some nutrients may be depleted to meet the needs of the fetus, who also may be deprived of essential nutrients.

Nurses have ongoing contact with pregnant women and can provide education about nutrition on a continuing basis. This is especially important because many women do not understand the nutritional needs of pregnancy. Nurses are often able to offer nutrition counseling before conception to women who are considering becoming pregnant. Such counseling increases the chances that a woman will be nutritionally healthy at the time of conception and will continue to practice good nutrition throughout pregnancy. It also may increase the level of nutrition the woman provides for her entire family. Therefore nutritional education is an essential part of nursing care.

WEIGHT GAIN DURING PREGNANCY

Weight gain during pregnancy is an important determinant of fetal growth. Insufficient weight gain during pregnancy has been associated with low birth weight (less than 2500 grams [g], or 5.5 pounds [lb]), small-for-gestational age (SGA) infants, preterm birth, and failure to initiate breastfeeding (Agency for Healthcare Research and Quality, 2014).

Low weight gain in the second trimester is especially associated with poor infant birth weight, even if overall gain is within the recommended range (Grodner, Escott-Stump, & Dorner, 2016). Lower caloric intake and decreased intake of important nutrients are present when poor maternal weight gain occurs.

Excessive weight gain is also a problem. It is associated with gestational hypertension, preeclampsia, gestational diabetes, prolonged labor, cesarean birth, macrosomia, stillbirth, and congenital anomalies, including neural tube defects (American Dietetic Association [ADA], 2016). Approximately 20% of women gain more than 18 kg (40 lb) during pregnancy (American College of Obstetricians and Gynecologists [ACOG], 2013b; Centers for Disease Control and Prevention [CDC], 2015a). The nutrient intake is even more important than the weight gain itself. Weight gain from a diet lacking in essential nutrients is not as beneficial as weight gain from a balanced diet. It could be inadequate in nutrients such as protein, iron, or folic acid, which could cause anemia, neural tube defects, or inadequate fetal nutrient stores.

Recommendations for Total Weight Gain

Recommendations for weight gain during pregnancy have changed considerably over the years. In the late nineteenth century, rickets, a disease of the bones resulting from deficiencies of calcium and vitamin D, caused some women to have small, distorted pelves. Restricted weight gain kept the fetus small and facilitated delivery. Later, weight gain was limited because of the inaccurate understanding that large gains caused preeclampsia.

❓ CRITICAL THINKING EXERCISE 8.1

Cheryl, age 22 years, has gained 4.5 kg (10 lb) more than recommended at 31 weeks of pregnancy. She asks the nurse for help because she is very worried about her weight gain and thinking of starting a severe weight loss diet. She started pregnancy at the upper end of the normal body mass index (BMI) and should gain 25 to 35 lb during the pregnancy. She has no apparent edema or other complications of pregnancy.

Questions

1. Why is Cheryl's weight gain a problem?
2. What suggestions should the nurse make to help Cheryl with her diet?

TABLE 8.1 Recommended Weight Gain during Pregnancy

Weight before Pregnancy	Total Gain	Range and Mean of Weekly Gain (Second and Third Trimesters)
Underweight (BMI <18.5)	12.5-18 kg (28-40 lb)	Range: 0.44-0.58 kg (1-1.3 lb) Mean: 0.51 kg (1 lb)
Normal weight (BMI 18.5-24.9)	11.5-16 kg (25-35 lb)	Range: 0.35-0.5 kg (0.8-1 lb) Mean: 0.42 kg (1 lb)
Overweight (BMI 25-29.9)	7-11.5 kg (15-25 lb)	Range: 0.23-0.33 kg (0.5-0.7 lb) Mean: 0.28 kg (0.6 lb)
Obese (BMI ≥30)	5-9 kg (11-20 lb)	Range: 0.17-0.27 kg (0.4-0.6 lb) Mean: 0.22 kg (0.5 lb)

BMI, Body mass index.
Note: Weight gain during the first trimester should be 0.5 to 2 kg (1.1 to 4.4 lb).
Data from Rasmussen, K.M., & Yaktine, A.L. (Eds.), (2009). *Weight gain during pregnancy: Reexamining the guidelines.* Washington, DC: National Academies Press.

Weight gain recommendations are based on the woman's prepregnancy body mass index (BMI). BMI is calculated by dividing the weight in kilograms by the height in meters squared. Another method is to divide the weight in pounds by the height in inches squared and multiply the result by 703 (CDC, 2015a). For example, if a woman weighs 56 kg (124 lb) before pregnancy and is 163 cm (64 inches) tall, her BMI is 21, which shows normal weight for height. A calculator to measure BMI is available at www.nhlbi.nih.gov/health/educational/lose_wt/BMI/bmicalc.htm.

Recommended gains vary according to the woman's BMI before pregnancy (Table 8.1). The recommended weight gain during pregnancy is 11.5 to 16 kg (25 to 35 lb) for women who begin pregnancy at normal BMI. (IOM, 2009). The range allows for individual differences because no precise weight gain is appropriate for every woman. It provides a target and allows for variations in individual needs.

Low prepregnancy weight is associated with preterm labor, SGA, and increased perinatal mortality (Cunningham, Leveno, Bloom, Spong, & Dash, 2014). Women who are underweight should gain more to meet the needs of pregnancy as well as their own need to gain weight. They should gain 12.5 to 18 kg (28 to 40 lb).

Obesity is an increasing problem. When obese women become pregnant, they are at higher risk for spontaneous abortion, gestational diabetes, gestational hypertension, preeclampsia, prolonged labor, cesarean birth, congenital anomalies, macrosomia, postpartum hemorrhage, wound complications, thromboembolic disorders, and other postpartum complications (Cunningham et al., 2014). Their children have an increased risk for childhood obesity. Overweight and obese women should be advised to lose weight before conception to achieve the best pregnancy outcomes.

The current recommended gain for overweight women is 7 to 11.5 kg (15 to 25 lb) to provide sufficient nutrients for the fetus. The weight gain for obese women is 5 to 9 kg (11 to 20 lb). Lower weight gain or weight loss for obese women during pregnancy is not recommended at this time because evidence on the effect on neurologic development of the infant is insufficient. More research is needed in this area. Inadequate gain may cause catabolism of fat stores producing ketones, which may lead to preterm labor (ACOG, 2013b; Cunningham et al., 2014; Grieger, Grzeskowiak, & Clifton, 2014).

In the past, it was recommended that shorter women should gain only the lowest amount of the recommended range. However, evidence to support these guidelines has not been identified. These women should gain according to recommendations for their BMI (CDC, 2015a).

Adolescents should gain weight according to their prepregnancy BMI using adult rather than pediatric BMI categories. Using adult BMI categories may place adolescents in a lighter group who are advised to gain more weight, but additional weight gain in younger adolescents often improves birth outcomes (ACOG, 2013b; CDC, 2015a).

Another consideration is the woman who is pregnant with more than one fetus. Infants of a multifetal pregnancy are often born before term and tend to weigh less than those born of single pregnancies. A greater weight gain in the mother may help prevent low birth weight. The recommended gain for women of normal prepregnancy weight who are carrying twins is 17 to 25 kg (37 to 54 lb) (Luke, 2015).

Pattern of Weight Gain

The pattern of weight gain is as important as the total increase in weight. Early and adequate prenatal care allows assessment of weight gain on a regular basis throughout pregnancy. The general recommendation is approximately 0.5 to 2 kg (1.1 to 4.4 lb) during the first trimester, when the mother may be nauseated and the fetus needs few nutrients for growth. During the rest of the pregnancy, the weekly expected weight gain ranges and means for various prepregnancy weights are shown in Table 8.1.

Maternal and Fetal Weight Distribution

Women often wonder why they should gain so much weight when the fetus weighs only 3.2 to 3.6 kg (7 to 8 lb). The nurse should explain the distribution of weight to help them understand this need (Fig. 8.1).

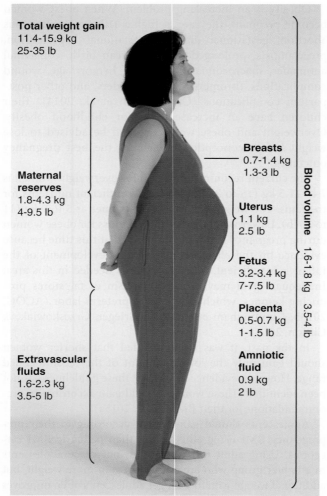

Total weight gain
11.4-15.9 kg
25-35 lb

Maternal reserves
1.8-4.3 kg
4-9.5 lb

Extravascular fluids
1.6-2.3 kg
3.5-5 lb

Breasts
0.7-1.4 kg
1.3-3 lb

Uterus
1.1 kg
2.5 lb

Fetus
3.2-3.4 kg
7-7.5 lb

Placenta
0.5-0.7 kg
1-1.5 lb

Amniotic fluid
0.9 kg
2 lb

Blood volume 1.6-1.8 kg   3.5-4 lb

FIG. 8.1 Distribution of Weight Gain in Pregnancy for Women of Normal Prepregnancy Weight. The numbers represent a general distribution because variation among women is great. The component with the greatest fluctuation is the weight increase attributed to extravascular fluids (edema) and maternal reserves of fat.

Factors That Influence Weight Gain

The nurse can positively influence the expectant mother's weight gain by teaching her the importance of her diet for fetal growth. A discussion of the effects of maternal intake on fetal growth and storage of nutrients often motivates women to improve their nutrition. Knowledge of factors that may negatively influence nutrient intake and weight gain helps the nurse devise plans for improving nutrition.

❓ KNOWLEDGE CHECK

1. How does weight gain in the mother relate to the birth weight of the infant?
2. How much weight should the average woman gain during pregnancy? What factors might change this?
3. What pattern of weight gain is recommended for the average woman?

NUTRITIONAL REQUIREMENTS

Nutrient needs increase during pregnancy to meet the demands of the mother and fetus. The amount of increase for each nutrient varies. In most cases, the increases are not large and are relatively easy to obtain through the diet.

Dietary Reference Intakes

In the United States, **dietary reference intakes** (DRIs) are used to estimate nutrient needs. DRIs include the following four categories:

- **Recommended dietary allowance (RDA)**—The amount of a nutrient sufficient to meet the needs of almost all (97% to 98%) healthy people in an age group. The actual needs of individuals (particularly for calories and protein) may vary according to body size, previous nutritional status, and usual activity level.
- Adequate intake (AI)—The nutrient intake assumed to be adequate when an RDA cannot be determined.
- Tolerable upper intake level (UL)—The highest amount of a nutrient that can be taken by most people without probable adverse health effects.
- Estimated average requirement (EAR)—The amount of a nutrient estimated to meet the needs of half the healthy people in an age group.

Tables of recommendations are based on a reference individual, a hypothetical person of medium size. These tables are used to calculate nutrient needs based on age, gender, and size. Recommendations for energy, carbohydrate, and protein intakes are shown in Table 8.2. Recommendations for vitamin and mineral intake and food sources are shown in Table 8.3.

Energy

The energy provided by foods for body processes is calculated in kilocalories. **Kilocalories** (commonly called *calories* [the term used in this book]) refers to a unit of heat and is used to show the energy value in foods. Calories are obtained from carbohydrates and proteins, which provide 4 calories in each gram, and fats, which provide 9 calories in each gram.

Carbohydrates

Carbohydrates may be simple or complex. The most common simple carbohydrate is sucrose (table sugar), which is a source of energy but provides no other nutrients. Fruits and vegetables contain simple sugars along with other nutrients. Complex carbohydrates are present in starches such as cereal, pasta, and potatoes. They supply vitamins, minerals, and fiber. They should be the major source of carbohydrates in the diet because of their value in providing other nutrients.

Another type of carbohydrate is fiber, the nondigestible product of plant foods and an important source of bulk in the diet. Fiber absorbs water and stimulates peristalsis, causing food to pass more quickly through the intestines. Fiber helps prevent constipation and also slows gastric emptying, causing a sensation of fullness.

TABLE 8.2 Recommendations for Daily Energy, Carbohydrate, and Protein Intakes for Women Aged 15 to 50 Years

Nonpregnant Adult Female	Pregnancy	Lactation
Energy		
Varies greatly according to body size, age, and physical activity level	First trimester: No change from nonpregnant needs	First 6 months: 330 kcal above nonpregnant needs (with an additional 170 kcal drawn from maternal stores)
Example:	Second trimester: 340 kcal above nonpregnant needs	
Woman, 30 years, active, height 1.65 m (65 inches), weight 50.4 kg (111 lb), body mass index (BMI) 18.5 needs 2267 kcal	Third trimester: 452 kcal above nonpregnant needs	Second 6 months: 400 kcal above nonpregnant needs
Same woman, weight 68 kg (150 lb), BMI 24.99 needs 2477 kcal		
Carbohydrate		
130 g	175 g	210 g
Protein		
46 g	71 g	71 g

Data from Institute of Medicine, Food, Nutrition Board. (2005). *Dietary reference intakes for energy, carbohydrates, fiber, fat, fatty acids, cholesterol, protein and amino acids (macronutrients).* Washington, DC: National Academies Press.

TABLE 8.3 Recommendations for Vitamins and Minerals

Adult Females: Nonpregnant	Pregnancy and Lactation	Sources	Importance in Pregnancy
Vitamins			
Vitamin A			
Ages 14-50: 700 mcg (RDA)*	*Pregnancy:* Ages 14-18: 750 mcg Ages 19-50: 770 mcg *Lactation:* Ages 14-18: 1200 mcg Ages 19-50: 1300 mcg	Dark green, yellow, or orange vegetables; whole or fortified low-fat or nonfat milk; egg yolk; butter and fortified margarine	Fetal growth and cell differentiation. Excessive intake causes spontaneous abortions or serious fetal defects. Isotretinoin (Accutane), a vitamin A derivative for acne, should not be taken during pregnancy because it causes fetal defects.
Vitamin D			
Ages 14-50: 600 IU (15 mcg) (RDA)	*Pregnancy and lactation:* Ages 14-50: 600 IU (15 mcg) (RDA)	Fortified milk, margarine, and soy products; butter; egg yolks Synthesized in skin exposed to sunlight Vegans and those who are not exposed to sun and who do not eat fortified foods need supplements.	Necessary for metabolism of calcium. Inadequate amounts may cause neonatal hypocalcemia and hypoplasia of tooth enamel. Excessive intake causes hypercalcemia and possible fetal deformities. Supplements should be taken with caution.
Vitamin E			
Ages 14-50: 15 mg (RDA)	*Pregnancy:* Ages 14-50: 15 mg *Lactation:* Ages 14-50: 19 mg (RDA)	Vegetable oils, whole grains, nuts, dark green leafy vegetables	Rarely deficient in pregnant women, but deficiency can cause anemia in mother and fetus.
Vitamin K			
Ages 14-18: 75 mcg Ages 19-50: 90 mcg (AI)	*Pregnancy and lactation:* Ages 14-18: 75 mcg Ages 19-50: 90 mcg (AI)	Dark green leafy vegetables Also produced by normal bacterial flora in small intestine	Newborns are temporarily deficient and receive one dose by injection at birth to prevent hemorrhage.

Continued

TABLE 8.3 Recommendations for Vitamins and Minerals—cont'd

Adult Females: Nonpregnant	Pregnancy and Lactation	Sources	Importance in Pregnancy
Vitamin B₆ (Pyridoxine) Ages 14-18: 1.2 mg Ages 19-50: 1.3 mg (RDA)	*Pregnancy:* Ages 14-50: 1.9 mg *Lactation:* Ages 14-50: 2 mg (RDA)	Chicken, fish, pork, eggs, peanuts, whole grains, cereals	Increased metabolism of amino acids during pregnancy.
Vitamin B₁₂ Ages 14-50: 2.4 mcg (RDA)	*Pregnancy:* Ages 14-50: 2.6 mcg *Lactation:* Ages 14-50: 2.8 mcg (RDA)	Meat, fish, eggs, milk, fortified soy and cereal products	Cell division, increased formation of red blood cells, and protein synthesis.
Folic Acid Ages 14-50: 400 mcg (RDA)	*Pregnancy:* Ages 14-50: 600 mcg *Lactation:* Ages 14-50: 500 mcg (RDA)	Dark green leafy vegetables, legumes (beans, peanuts), orange juice, asparagus, spinach, and fortified cereal and pasta May be lost in cooking	Increased maternal red blood cell (RBC) formation, tissue growth. Deficiency in first weeks of pregnancy may cause spontaneous abortion and neural tube defects.
Thiamin Ages 14-18: 1 mg Ages 19-50: 1.1 mg (RDA)	*Pregnancy and lactation:* Ages 14-50: 1.4 mg (RDA)	Lean pork, whole or enriched grain products, legumes, organ meats, seeds, nuts	Forms coenzymes necessary to release energy, aids in nerve and muscle functioning. Increased need because of greater intake of calories.
Riboflavin Ages 14-18: 1 mg Ages 19-50: 1.1 mg (RDA)	*Pregnancy:* Ages 14-50: 1.4 mg *Lactation:* Ages 14-50: 1.6 mg (RDA)	Milk, meat, fish, poultry, eggs, enriched grain products, dark green vegetables	Forms coenzymes necessary to release energy, aids in nerve and muscle functioning. Increased need because of greater intake of calories.
Niacin Ages 14-50: 14 mg (RDA)	*Pregnancy:* Ages 14-50: 18 mg *Lactation:* Ages 14-50: 17 mg (RDA)	Meats, fish, poultry, legumes, enriched grains, milk	Forms coenzymes necessary to release energy, aids in nerve and muscle functioning. Increased need because of greater intake of calories.
Vitamin C Ages 14-18: 65 mg Ages 19-50: 75 mg (RDA)	*Pregnancy:* Ages 14-18: 80 mg Ages 19-50: 85 mg *Lactation:* Ages 14-18: 115 mg Ages 19-50: 120 mg (RDA)	Citrus fruit, peppers, strawberries, cantaloupe, green leafy vegetables, tomatoes, potatoes Destroyed by heat and oxidation	Formation of fetal tissue, collagen formation, tissue integrity, healing, immune response, and metabolism.
Minerals **Iron** Ages 14-18: 15 mg Ages 19-50: 18 mg (RDA)	*Pregnancy:* Ages 14-50: 27 mg *Lactation:* Ages 14-18: 10 mg Ages 19-50: 9 mg (RDA)	Meats, dark green leafy vegetables, enriched bread and cereal, dried fruits, tofu, legumes, nuts, blackstrap molasses	Expanded maternal blood volume, formation of fetal red blood cells, and storage in fetal liver for use after birth.

TABLE 8.3 Recommendations for Vitamins and Minerals—cont'd

Adult Females: Nonpregnant	Pregnancy and Lactation	Sources	Importance in Pregnancy
Calcium Ages 14-18: 1300 mg Ages 19-50: 1000 mg (AI)	*Pregnancy and lactation:* Ages 14-18: 1300 mg Ages 19-50: 1000 mg (AI)	Dairy products, salmon, sardines with bones, legumes, fortified juice, tofu, broccoli	Mineralization of fetal bones and teeth.
Phosphorus Ages 14-18: 1250 mg Ages 19-50: 700 mg (RDA)	*Pregnancy and lactation:* Ages 14-18: 1250 mg Ages 19-50: 700 mg	Dairy products, lean meat, fish, poultry, cereals; high in processed foods, snacks, carbonated drinks	Mineralization of fetal bones and teeth; excessive intake causes binding of calcium in intestines and prevents calcium absorption.
Zinc Ages 14-18: 9 mg Ages 19-50: 8 mg (RDA)	*Pregnancy:* Ages 14-18: 12 mg Ages 19-50: 11 mg *Lactation:* Ages 14-18: 13 mg Ages 19-50: 12 mg (RDA)	Meat, poultry, seafood, eggs, nuts, seeds, legumes, wheat germ, whole grains, yogurt	Fetal and maternal tissue growth, cell differentiation and reproduction, DNA and RNA synthesis, metabolism, acid-base balance.
Magnesium Ages 14-18: 360 mg Ages 19-30: 310 mg Ages 31-50: 320 mg (RDA)	*Pregnancy:* Ages 14-18: 400 mg Ages 19-30: 350 mg Ages 31-50: 360 mg *Lactation:* Ages 14-18: 360 mg Ages 19-30: 310 mg Ages 31-50: 320 mg (RDA)	Whole grains, nuts, legumes, dark green vegetables, small amounts in many foods	Cell growth and neuromuscular function; activates enzymes for metabolism of protein and energy.
Iodine Ages 14-50: 150 mcg (RDA)	*Pregnancy:* Ages 14-50: 220 mcg *Lactation:* Ages 14-50: 290 mcg (RDA)	Seafood, iodized salt	Important in thyroid function. Deficiency may cause abortion, stillbirth, congenital hypothyroidism, neurologic conditions.

DNA, Deoxyribonucleic acid; *RNA*, ribonucleic acid.
*Dietary reference intakes are listed as recommended daily allowance (RDA) or adequate intake (AI).
Data from Institute of Medicine (IOM), Food and Nutrition Board (FNB). (1997). *Dietary reference intakes for calcium, phosphorus, magnesium, vitamin D, and fluoride.* Washington, DC: National Academies Press; IOM, FNB. (1998). *Dietary reference intakes for thiamin, riboflavin, niacin, vitamin B6, folate, vitamin B12, pantothenic acid, biotin, and choline.* Washington, DC: National Academies Press; IOM, FNB. (2000). *Dietary reference intakes for vitamin C, vitamin E, selenium, and carotenoids.* Washington, DC: National Academies Press; IOM, FNB. (2001). *Dietary reference intakes for vitamin A, vitamin K, arsenic, boron, chromium, copper, iodine, iron, manganese, molybdenum, nickel, silicon, vanadium, and zinc.* Washington, DC: National Academies Press; IOM (2011). *Dietary reference intakes for calcium and vitamin D.* Washington, DC: The National Academies Press.

Fats

Fats provide energy and fat-soluble vitamins. When decreasing calories is necessary, a reduction, but not elimination, of carbohydrates and fats is important. If carbohydrate and fat intake provides insufficient calories, the body uses protein to meet energy needs. This use decreases the amount of protein available for building and repairing tissue.

Women often restrict fat to prevent weight gain. However, essential fatty acids such as alpha-linolenic acid and linoleic acid help in fetal neurologic and visual development. Docosahexaenoic acid (DHA) is also important for fetal visual and cognitive development. These fatty acids are found in canola, soybean, and walnut oils, as well as some seafood such as bass or salmon.

Calories

Approximately 75,000 additional calories are needed during pregnancy. These extra calories furnish energy for production and maintenance of the fetus, placenta, added maternal tissues, and increased basal metabolic rate. Most pregnant women need a daily caloric intake of 2200 to 2900 calories, depending on their age, activity level, and prepregnancy BMI (ACOG, 2013b; CDC, 2015a).

TABLE 8.4 Extra Foods Needed to Meet Pregnancy Requirements*

Energy (kcal)	1 slice whole wheat bread, 1 T peanut butter, ½ banana, *and* 1/2 c low-fat milk in second trimester; add 1 oz cheddar cheese and 1-2 carrots in third trimester
Protein	3 oz meat or poultry *or* 3 c milk *or* 3½ oz cheddar cheese *or* 1 c cottage cheese *or* 3¾ oz peanuts *or* 1⅔ c pinto or kidney beans
Iron	1 c raisin bran, *or* 1 c beef chuck + 1 c pinto beans, + 3 eggs
Thiamin	1½ oz pork *or* 2½ oz peanuts *or* 1⅔ c brown rice *or* 1½ c orange juice
Riboflavin	¾ c low-fat milk *or* ¾ c low-fat cottage cheese *or* ¾ c cooked spinach *or* 2 chicken drumsticks *or* 4 oz lean beef
Niacin	2 T peanut butter *or* 3 oz ground beef *or* 1½ oz salmon; also made by body from tryptophan
Vitamin C	2 T orange juice *or* 1½ peaches *or* 1 banana *or* 1½ pear *or* 1 c watermelon *or* ¼ c tomato juice

c, Cup; *kcal*, calories; *T*, tablespoon.
Data from U.S. Department of Agriculture, Agricultural Research Service (2016). U.S. Department of Agriculture, Agricultural Research Service, Nutrient Data Laboratory. USDA National Nutrient Database for Standard Reference, Release 28. Version Current: September 2015, slightly revised May 2016. Internet: /nea/bhnrc/ndl
*Examples of foods that would meet the additional requirements of pregnancy for women between the ages of 19 and 50 years.

During the first trimester of pregnancy, no added calories are needed. However, the daily caloric intake for pregnant women should increase by 340 calories during the second trimester and 452 calories during the third trimester (Cunningham et al., 2014; IOM, 2006). This increase can be achieved relatively easily with a variety of foods and only a small increase in food (Table 8.4).

Nutrient Density. The quantity and quality of the various nutrients in each 100 calories of food is the **nutrient density**. Foods of high nutrient density have large amounts of quality nutrients per serving. During pregnancy, the increased need for most nutrients may not be met unless calories are selected carefully. The term *empty calories* refers to foods high in calories but low in other nutrients. Many snack foods contain excessive calories and low nutrient density and are high in fat and sodium. Increased calories should be "spent" on foods that provide the nutrients needed in increased amounts during pregnancy.

Women often use sugar substitutes to reduce their caloric intake. Saccharin (Sweet'N Low), sucralose (Splenda), aspartame (Equal or NutraSweet) and steviol glycosides from stevia leaves (Stevia) are considered safe for use in moderation (Cox & Carney, 2017). Use of aspartame by women with phenylketonuria can result in fetal brain damage because these women lack the enzyme to metabolize aspartame (Pope, Koren, & Bozzo, 2014).

Protein

Protein is necessary for metabolism, tissue synthesis, and tissue repair. The daily protein from Recommended Dietary Allowances (RDA) is 46 g for females, depending on age and size. A protein intake of approximately 71 g each day is recommended during the second half of pregnancy because of expansion of blood volume and growth of maternal and fetal tissues (Grodner et al., 2016). This is an increase of 25 g of protein daily.

Protein is generally abundant in diets in most industrialized nations. Diets low in caloric intake also may be low in protein, however. If calories are low and protein is used to provide energy, fetal growth may be impaired.

The nurse should teach women at risk for poor protein diets how to determine intake and increase food sources of protein. When a woman needs to increase intake, she should eat more protein-rich foods rather than use high-protein powders or drinks. Protein substitutes increase protein intake but do not have the other nutrients provided by foods.

Vitamins

Although most people do not eat as much of every vitamin and mineral each day as recommended, true deficiency states for most nutrients are uncommon in North America.

Fat-Soluble Vitamins

Fat-soluble vitamins (A, D, E, and K) are stored in the liver. Deficiency states are not as likely to occur, but excessive intake of these vitamins can be toxic. For example, too much vitamin A can cause fetal defects. The nurse should ask about vitamins and medications taken by pregnant women and counsel them about the dangers of excess vitamins (see Table 8.3).

Water-Soluble Vitamins

Water-soluble vitamins (B_6, B_{12}, and C; folic acid; thiamin; riboflavin; and niacin) are not stored in the body as easily as fat-soluble vitamins. Therefore they should be included in the daily diet. Because excess amounts are excreted in urine, the chances of toxicity from excessive intake are lower, but toxicity can occur with megadoses.

Water-soluble vitamins are easily transferred from food to water during cooking. Foods should be steamed, microwaved, or prepared in only small amounts of water. The remaining water can be used in other dishes such as soups.

Folic Acid

Folic acid (also called *folate*) can decrease the occurrence of neural tube defects such as spina bifida and anencephaly in newborns. It also may help prevent cleft lip, cleft palate, and some heart defects (CDC, 2015b). Adequate intake of folic acid is especially important before conception and during the first trimester because the neural tube closes before many women realize they are pregnant. Because approximately half of pregnancies are unplanned, all women of childbearing age should consume at least 400 micrograms (mcg) (0.4 milligram [mg]) of folic acid every day. Once pregnancy occurs, daily intake of 600 mcg (0.6 mg) of folic acid is recommended.

Although the CDC recommends a daily folic acid intake of 400 mcg (0.4 mg) for women capable of childbearing (CDC, 2015b), the U.S. Preventive Services Task Force (USPSTF) recommends 400 to 800 mcg (0.4 to 0.8 mg) each day. The dose should be taken for at least 1 month before conception and for 2 to 3 months after conception (USPSTF, 2017). No change has been made in USPSTF's recommendation of 600 mcg (0.6 mg) of folic acid daily for the rest of pregnancy. For women who have previously had a child with a neural tube defect, the recommended dose is 4 mg (4000 mcg) daily during the months before conception (CDC, 2015b).

Women often do not realize the importance of folic acid in their diet before pregnancy begins, and many do not meet the recommended level in spite of a national campaign to make the public aware of this problem. Inadequate intake of folic acid is the most prevalent vitamin deficiency during pregnancy. One third of births occur in women ages 18 to 24 years, but women in this group have lower intake of supplements containing folic acid than older women (CDC, 2015b). More education is necessary to increase folic acid use in women of childbearing age. Fortunately, since food fortification with folic acid was begun, folic acid deficiency has decreased.

A *Healthy People 2020* goal is for women of childbearing potential to take in at least 400 mcg of folic acid each day (U.S. Department of Health and Human Services [DHHS], 2010). To help achieve adequate intake in the United States and Canada, folic acid is added to breads, cereals, and other products containing enriched flour.

KNOWLEDGE CHECK

4. How many additional calories should a woman consume each day during pregnancy?
5. How much protein is recommended during pregnancy?
6. Which vitamins are in the fat-soluble and water-soluble groups? What is the difference in the way the body stores them?
7. Why should all women of childbearing age consume 400 mcg of folic acid daily?

Minerals

Although most minerals are supplied in sufficient amounts in normal diets, the intake of iron and calcium may not be adequate before pregnancy (Lumish et al., 2014).

Iron

Iron helps form some enzymes necessary for metabolism and is important in the formation of hemoglobin (Hgb). The pregnant woman needs 27 mg of iron daily (an increase from 18 mg for a nonpregnant woman). The additional iron is needed for increased production of RBCs and for transfer to the fetus. Fetal stores of iron, which double during the last weeks of pregnancy, are important because the infant's intake of iron is low for the first 4 to 6 months after birth. Iron will be transferred to the fetus even if the mother is anemic, but infants will have less stored iron and an increased risk for anemia during the first year (Blackburn, 2013; Cantor, Bougatsos, Dana, Blazina, & McDonagh, 2015).

TABLE 8.5   Foods High in Iron Content*

Food and Amount	Average Amounts of Iron Supplied (mg)
Meats and Poultry (3-oz serving)	
Beef (average)	2
Chicken	1
Turkey	2
Legumes	
Kidney beans (1 cup [c])	3
Lentils (1 c)	6.6
Chickpeas (garbanzo beans) (1 c)	4.7
Lima beans (1 c)	4.5
Peas, green (1 c)	2.4
Peanuts, dry roasted (4 oz)	1.8
Sunflower seeds (¼ c)	1.2
Grains	
Rice, white enriched cooked (1 c)	2.8
Bread, wheat (slice)	1
Bagel, plain enriched, medium	3.8
Enriched cereals	7-18
Fruits	
Raisins (1 c)	2.7
Apricots, dried (10 halves)	0.9
Prune juice (1 c)	3
Vegetables (1 c)	
Broccoli	1
Collards	2.2
Tomatoes, stewed	3.4
Other	
Tofu, hard, 3.5 oz.	2.75

*The recommended daily allowance for iron during pregnancy is 27 mg. Although many women take supplements because they do not eat enough iron-containing foods in their daily diet to meet this need, iron in foods is often better absorbed. Therefore the nurse should suggest ways a woman can increase her dietary iron.
Data from U.S. Department of Agriculture, Agricultural Research Service. (2016). *USDA national nutrient database for standard reference, release 28.* Retrieved from www.ars.usda.gov/northeast-area/beltsville-md/beltsville-human-nutrition-research-center/nutrient-data-laboratory/docs/usda-national-nutrient-database-for-standard-reference/.

Even though iron is better absorbed during pregnancy, it is probably the only nutrient that cannot be supplied completely and easily by the diet. Iron is present in many foods but in small amounts (Table 8.5). The average woman's daily diet contains approximately 6 mg of iron for each 1000 calories. In addition, some women restrict their intake of meats and grains in an effort to cut down on fat, carbohydrates, and calories. Menstrual bleeding causes loss of iron. Therefore women frequently enter pregnancy with low iron stores (Cunningham et al., 2014). A *Healthy People 2020* goal is to reduce iron deficiency in pregnant women to 14.5% from a baseline of 16.2% (DHHS, 2010).

Approximately 25% of iron from animal sources (called **heme iron**) is absorbed. Only approximately 5% of **nonheme** iron (from plants and fortified foods) is absorbed (Grodner et al., 2016). Absorption of iron is affected by intake of other substances. Calcium and phosphorus in milk and tannin in tea and red wine decrease iron absorption if they are consumed during the same meal. Coffee binds iron, preventing it from being fully absorbed. Antacids, phytates (in grains and vegetables), oxalic acid (in spinach), and ethylenediaminetetraacetic acid (EDTA; a food additive) also decrease absorption. Foods cooked in iron pans contain more iron. Foods containing ascorbic acid and meat, fish, or poultry eaten with non-heme iron–containing foods increase absorption (Grodner et al., 2016).

Because of the difficulty of obtaining enough iron in the diet, health care providers often prescribe iron supplements of 30 mg/day. Women who are anemic, have more than one fetus, or begin supplementation late may need 60 to 100 mg daily (Cunningham et al., 2014). Supplementation may begin during the second trimester when the need increases and morning sickness has usually ended. Women who take high doses of iron also need zinc supplements because iron interferes with the absorption and use of this mineral (Cantor et al., 2015).

Iron taken between meals is absorbed more completely, but many women find it difficult to tolerate iron without some food. Iron taken at bedtime may be easier to tolerate. For best results, it should be taken with water or a source of vitamin C such as orange juice, but not with coffee, tea, or milk. Side effects occur more often with higher doses and include nausea, vomiting, heartburn, epigastric pain, constipation, diarrhea, and black stools.

Women should be reminded to keep iron and all other medicines out of the reach of children. Accidental iron overdose is a significant cause of childhood poisoning.

Calcium

Calcium is necessary for bone formation, maintenance of cell membrane permeability, coagulation, and neuromuscular function. It is transferred to the fetus, especially in the last trimester, and is important for mineralization of fetal bones and teeth. Calcium absorption and retention increase during pregnancy, and it is stored for use in the third trimester when fetal needs are highest.

Although a small amount of calcium is removed from the mother's bones, it is insignificant and mineralization of the woman's bones is usually not affected. A common myth is that calcium is removed from teeth during pregnancy. In reality, the calcium in teeth is stable and not affected by pregnancy.

Dairy products are the best source of calcium. Whole, low-fat, and nonfat milk all contain the same amount of calcium and may be used interchangeably to increase or reduce calorie intake. Women with **lactose intolerance** (lactase deficiency resulting in gastrointestinal problems when dairy products are consumed) need other sources of calcium (Box 8.1).

Calcium is also present in legumes, nuts, dried fruits, broccoli, and dark green leafy vegetables. Although spinach and chard contain calcium, they also contain oxalates that decrease calcium availability, making them poor sources. Caffeine increases excretion of calcium. Large amounts of fiber interfere with calcium absorption. More calcium is needed by women younger than 18 years because their bone density is incomplete. The recommendations for calcium intake during pregnancy and lactation are the same as those for nonpregnant women.

BOX 8.1 Calcium Sources Approximately Equivalent to 1 Cup of Milk*

¾ cup (c) yogurt
1½ ounces (oz) hard cheese
1½ c low-fat cottage cheese
1 c calcium-fortified orange juice
1¾ c ice cream
3 c sherbet
3½ c pinto beans
½ block tofu
4½ c broccoli
1 c cooked collard greens (frozen)
6 oz canned salmon with bones
3 oz canned sardines with bones

*This list can be used to counsel women who are vegans or lactose intolerant. Lactose-intolerant women often can manage small amounts of yogurt and cheese without distress. Although the amounts of some foods listed are more than would be likely to be eaten within 1 day, they serve for comparison.
Data from U.S. Department of Agriculture, Agricultural Research Service. (2016). U.S. Department of Agriculture, Agricultural Research Service, Nutrient Data Laboratory. USDA National Nutrient Database for Standard Reference, Release 28. Version Current: September 2015, slightly revised May 2016. Internet: /nea/bhnrc/ndl

---

BOX 8.2 High-Sodium Foods*

Products containing the words *salt*, *soda*, or *sodium*, such as table salt, garlic salt, monosodium glutamate, bicarbonate of soda (baking soda)
Salty tasting foods, including sauerkraut and snack foods such as popcorn, potato chips, pretzels, crackers
Condiments and relishes such as catsup, chili sauce, horseradish, mustard, soy sauce, bouillon, pickles, green and black olives
Smoked, dried, and processed foods such as ham, bacon, lunch meats, corned beef
Canned soups, meats, and vegetables unless the label states the contents are low in sodium
Canned tomato and vegetable juices
Packaged mixes for sauces, gravies, cakes, and other baked foods

*During pregnancy, foods high in sodium should be consumed in moderation. Expectant mothers should be taught to read labels and avoid or limit products in which sodium is listed among the first ingredients.

Women who do not eat dairy products because of lactose intolerance, to avoid eating animal products, or for other reasons should take supplements unless they can meet their needs with other calcium-rich foods. Calcium should be taken with vitamin D, which increases its absorption. It is better absorbed when taken with meals, separately from iron supplements.

Sodium

Sodium needs are increased during pregnancy to provide for an expanded blood volume and the needs of the fetus. Although sodium is not restricted during pregnancy, excessive amounts should be avoided. Women are advised that a moderate intake of salt or the salting of foods to taste is acceptable, but intake of high-sodium foods (Box 8.2) should be limited.

Nutritional Supplementation

Purpose

Food is the best source of nutrients. Health care providers usually prescribe prenatal vitamin-mineral supplements, and they are seen as an important part of pregnancy by many women. However, women with adequate diets may not need supplements except for iron and folic acid, which are often not obtained in adequate amounts through normal food intake. Expectant mothers who are vegetarians, are lactose intolerant, or have special problems in obtaining nutrients through diet alone may need supplements. Assessment of each woman's individualized needs determines whether supplementation is appropriate.

Disadvantages and Dangers

Because they believe supplements are a harmless way to improve their diets, some women take large amounts without consulting a health care provider. No standardization or regulation of the amounts of ingredients contained in supplements is available at this time. Label information for some supplements may not be accurate and the supplement may not fulfill the health claims made for it.

The use of supplements may increase the intake of some nutrients to doses much higher than recommended. Excessive amounts of some vitamins and minerals may be toxic to the fetus. Excessive levels of vitamin A can cause fetal anomalies of the bones, urinary tract, and central nervous system. High doses of some vitamins or minerals may interfere with the ability to use others. If women understand this, they are less likely to exceed recommended doses.

Some women believe their nutrient needs can be met by vitamin-mineral supplements and are less concerned about their food intake. Supplements do not generally contain protein and calories and may lack many necessary nutrients. Nurses should emphasize that supplements are not food substitutes and do not contain all the nutrients needed during pregnancy. In fact, some nutrients important to pregnancy and provided by foods may be unknown at this time.

Water

Water is important during pregnancy for the expanded blood volume and as part of the increased maternal and fetal tissues. Women should drink approximately 8 to 10 cups (1920 to 2400 mL) of fluids that are mostly water each day (Cox & Carney, 2017). Fluids low in nutrients (e.g., carbonated beverages, coffee, tea, or juice drinks with high amounts of sugar and little real juice) should be limited because they are filling and replace other more nutritional foods and drinks.

MyPlate

The U.S. Department of Agriculture (USDA) MyPlate provides a guide for healthy eating for adults and children. Guidelines for pregnancy and lactation are discussed later and summarized in Table 8.6. Pregnant women can go to the website www.choosemyplate.gov to get an individualized diet plan specifically adapted for them and their needs during pregnancy.

TABLE 8.6 Food Plan for Pregnancy and Lactation

Food and Amounts per Serving	Recommended Intake for Pregnancy*	Recommended Intake for Lactation[†]
Whole grains (1 oz = 1 slice bread, ½ c rice or pasta)	6-8 oz	7 oz
Vegetables	2½-3 c	3 c
Fruits	1½-2 c	2 c
Dairy group (1 c milk or yogurt, 1½ oz hard cheese, 2 c cottage cheese)	3 c	3 c
Protein group (1 oz meat/poultry/fish, 1 egg, ¼ c cooked beans, ¼ c tofu, 1 tbsp peanut butter)	5-6½ oz	6 oz

c, Cup; *oz*, ounce; *tbsp*, tablespoon.
*Example for a woman 5 feet, 4 inches tall weighing 125 lb before pregnancy. Specific individualized food plans can be found at www.choosemyplate.gov.
[†]Amounts are for exclusive breastfeeding.
Data from www.choosemyplate.gov.

Whole Grains

Breads, cereals, rice, and pastas provide complex carbohydrates, fiber, vitamins, and minerals. At least half of the daily servings should be whole grains because they provide more nutrients than processed grain products. Although foods can be enriched to replace some nutrients lost during processing, not all nutrients are restored by enrichment. MyPlate recommendations are for 6 oz each day for adult women. Pregnant women should have 7 to 9 oz, and lactating women should have 9 oz daily.

Vegetables and Fruits

Vegetables and fruits are important sources of vitamins, minerals, and fiber. The daily recommendation for vegetables for nonpregnant adult women is 2.5 cups, 3 to 3.5 cups for pregnancy, and 3 cups for lactation. Adult women should have 2 cups of fruit daily. Pregnant and lactating women should also have 2 cups of fruit daily. A wide range of vegetables and fruits provides the best nutrition. Dark green and orange or dark yellow vegetables are especially nutritious.

Dairy Group

The dairy group includes foods such as milk, yogurt, and cheese. They contain approximately the same nutrient values whether they are whole (4% fat), low fat (2% fat), or nonfat/skim (0% fat), but calories and fat are reduced in the latter two. The dairy group has especially good sources of calcium. Adult women and those who are pregnant or lactating need 3 cups or the equivalent from this group.

Protein Group

Many adults think of meat, poultry, fish, and eggs as the only sources of protein. However, legumes (e.g., beans, peas, lentils), nuts, and soybean products such as tofu are also good sources. Adult women should consume 5 to 5.5 oz or the equivalent each day. Pregnant women need 6 to 6.5 oz and lactating women need 6 oz of protein foods daily. A typical portion of meat, fish, and poultry varies in size. A 3-oz portion is about the size of a deck of playing cards.

Other Elements

Concentrated sugars, fats, and oils should be eaten sparingly. They provide calories for energy but few other nutrients. An adequate allowance for oils for adult women is 5 to 6 teaspoons of unsaturated oils. Pregnant women need 6 to 8 teaspoons and lactating women need 6 teaspoons of unsaturated fats daily. Foods containing saturated fats and *trans*–fatty acids should be avoided.

Food Precautions

Although fish are an excellent source of nutrients, certain precautions should be taken. Large fish often have high levels of mercury, which can damage the fetal central nervous system. Pregnant and lactating women should avoid those fish. Other types of fish have smaller amounts of mercury and can be eaten weekly (American Academy of Pediatrics & American College of Obstetricians and Gynecologists [AAP & ACOG], 2014). Raw fish may contain parasites or bacteria and should be avoided.

> **! SAFETY CHECK**
>
> ### *Food Safety during Pregnancy and Lactation*
>
> Do not eat shark, swordfish, king mackerel, and tilefish.
> Eat up to 12 oz of shrimp, salmon, pollack, catfish, and canned light tuna (but only 6 oz of white albacore tuna) each week.
> Do not eat raw or undercooked fish, meat, poultry, or eggs.
> Avoid luncheon meats and hot dogs unless reheated until steaming hot.
> Avoid soft cheeses unless made with pasteurized milk.
> Do not consume refrigerated pâté, meat spreads, or smoked seafood.
> Do not consume raw (unpasteurized) milk or milk products.

Some foods may be contaminated with *Listeria monocytogenes,* which may cause listeriosis. If contracted during pregnancy, listeriosis may result in abortion, stillbirth, or severe illness of the newborn. More information about food safety during pregnancy can be obtained from the FDA website at www.fda.gov.

Eggs can be contaminated with harmful bacteria and should not be eaten unless fully cooked. Only eggs pasteurized in the shell are safe to eat raw or partially cooked. Unpasteurized juices, cold deli salads, and raw sprouts should also be avoided. Eating raw or undercooked meat or unwashed fruits or vegetables may cause toxoplasmosis with severe consequences to the fetus. Toxoplasmosis also can be contracted by contact with cat feces.

> **? KNOWLEDGE CHECK**
>
> 8. Which minerals are often below the recommended amounts in the diets of pregnant women?
> 9. Why is excessive use of vitamin-mineral supplements unnecessary and possibly dangerous?
> 10. How much fluid should a woman drink each day during pregnancy?
> 11. How much of each food group is recommended during pregnancy?

FACTORS THAT INFLUENCE NUTRITION

Age, knowledge about nutrition, exercise, and cultural background influence the food choices women make and their nutritional status. The nurse should consider these factors when counseling women about their diets.

Age

Age is an important consideration. The adolescent who is not fully mature needs nutritional support for her own growth. Older women who are in good health have the same nutritional requirements as younger pregnant women. They may have more knowledge about nutrition through life experiences or need as much teaching as younger women. Older women are more likely to be financially secure than very young women.

Nutritional Knowledge

Once pregnancy is confirmed, even women who have not previously been attentive to their diets often want to learn about the relationship between what they eat and the effect on the fetus. Although women know they should "eat well" during pregnancy, they may have little idea of what "eating well" means. Some lack basic understanding of nutrition and have misconceptions based on common food myths that interfere with good nutritional choices. They may seek information about nutrition from books, magazine articles, TV, and the Internet. They benefit by receiving nutritional education from nurses.

Exercise

Moderate exercise during pregnancy is encouraged. Women who exercise more strenuously or are athletes may need modifications of their diet to meet additional nutritional needs. Extra calories may be needed to restore the energy used during exercise. A serving of fruit, yogurt, or pasta before and after exercise may be sufficient. Additional fluids should be taken during and after exercise as well.

Culture

Food is important in all cultures and often has special meaning during pregnancy and childbirth when certain foods may be favored or discouraged. Nurses need to know about the habits of a variety of cultures so they can provide culturally appropriate nutritional counseling. Before making assumptions about the influence of a woman's culture on her diet, the nurse should assess each woman individually. Not all women follow food practices considered typical for their cultures.

The nurse should assess the woman's age, how long she has lived in North America, and whether she has adopted any common American eating habits. Greater exposure to the North American diet may cause younger members of a group to make more dietary changes compared with their older relatives. Some women who usually follow an American diet may return to some aspects of their traditional cultural diet during pregnancy to "make sure" they do not harm the fetus.

Nurses often give women pamphlets in the appropriate language during nutritional teaching.

Before giving a woman printed materials, the nurse should determine whether the woman prefers to read English or her native language. People who cannot read may not readily admit it to others. In addition, the reading level may be too complicated for a woman with little education. Having an interpreter discuss the material with the woman helps determine how well she can read and aids in other teaching.

People of many cultures believe certain foods, conditions, and medicines are "hot" or "cold" and should be balanced to preserve health. Foods considered hot in one culture may not fit in that category in another culture, and the designation does not necessarily match the temperature or spiciness of the food. In the Chinese culture, this belief is expressed with terms such as *yin* for cold and *yang* for hot and may influence what the mother eats during pregnancy and the postpartum period.

Food taboos may determine what some women eat during the childbearing period. For example, Samoan women avoid eating octopus or raw fish during pregnancy. Haitian women believe they should eat for two and eat a hearty diet with lots of red fruits and vegetables. They also believe eating white foods such as milk, white beans, and lobster after birth will increase the lochia. Some Asians believe vitamin preparations that contain iron harden the bones, making birth more difficult. Chinese women may avoid spicy foods such as chili peppers but eat bird's nests, considered a delicacy (Callister, 2013).

Special foods may be customary during pregnancy or after birth. Punjabi women may drink milk to prevent melasma. A Korean family may bring the new mother a hot beef and seaweed soup to cleanse her body and increase breast milk production (Callister, 2013).

Cultural preferences for foods are extremely varied. For example, some African-Americans follow a diet similar to that of people living in the southeastern United States. Common foods include okra, collard greens, mustard greens, ham hocks, black-eyed peas, and hominy or grits. The diet of other African-Americans, however, varies according to the geographic area in which they live. Lactose intolerance is common and results in a lack of calcium if other sources are not present in the diet. Intake of high-sodium and fried foods may present health problems.

Some Jewish women follow a strictly kosher diet. They avoid meat from animals without cloven hooves or do not chew their cud, which excludes pork and pork products. The meat must be processed to remove all blood and cannot be eaten in the same meal as milk. Muslim women also do not eat pork and may fast on certain days. Although the religion exempts pregnant and nursing women from obligatory fasting, the woman must make up the fasting days at another time. Some choose to fast, regardless, for spiritual reasons or so they do not have to make up the days later.

The diet of Native American women may contain blue cornbread, potatoes, wild greens, legumes, nuts, tomatoes, and squash. Lactose intolerance is common, and milk and cheese are avoided. Meats may include wild game and poultry. Fried dough ("fry bread") is frequently served. Low-income Native Americans may receive food vouchers from the Special Supplemental Nutrition Program for Women, Infants, and Children (WIC).

Food preferences for two cultures, Southeast Asian and Hispanic, are explored further here to show the influence of culture on diet. Immigrants from Southeast Asia are likely to follow diets similar to those in their homelands. Hispanics are a large minority group in the United States. Nurses throughout the United States need information about food preferences prevalent in these groups (Callister, 2013).

Southeast Asian Dietary Practices

Southeast Asians include those from Cambodia, Laos, and Vietnam. Traditional cooking methods in these countries include searing fresh vegetables quickly with small portions of meat, poultry, or fish in a little oil over high heat. Meals cooked in this manner are low in fat and retain vitamins. Most meals are accompanied by rice, which increases the intake of complex carbohydrates, and soup. White rice is usually preferred over brown rice. A salty fish sauce called *nuoc mam* is also part of most meals (Appel, 2013). Tofu and fresh fruits are frequent additions.

Many Southeast Asians eat American foods along with their traditional diet. Such foods as eggs, beef, pork, and bread add nutrients but also fat to the diet. Candy, soft drinks, coffee, butter or margarine, and fast foods have been less favorable influences because they are low in nutrients but high in sugar or fat.

Effect of Culture on Diet during Childbearing. In Southeast Asian cultures, pregnancy (especially the third trimester) is considered "hot," and women eat "cold" foods to maintain a balance. The diet includes sour foods, fruits, noodles, spinach, and mung beans and avoids fish, excessively salty or spicy foods, alcohol, and rice. Unfamiliar foods are avoided for fear they may harm the mother or her fetus.

The postpartum period is considered "cold," partly because of the loss of blood, which is "hot." Mothers avoid losing more heat, which would negatively affect their health. They stay warm physically and choose to eat "hot" foods, including rice with fish sauce, broth, salty meats, fish, chicken, and eggs. They may refuse cold drinks but welcome hot fluids, requesting tea or plain hot water. The family frequently brings food to the mother while she is in the hospital because hospital food may not meet her preferences (Callister, 2013).

Increasing Nutrients with Traditional Foods. Milk products are not part of the traditional Southeast Asian diet, and lactose intolerance is common. Soy milk may be used instead. Increasing the intake of commonly used dark green leafy vegetables such as mustard greens, bok choy, and broccoli increases calcium, iron, magnesium, and folic acid intake. Tofu is a good source of calcium and iron. A broth made from pork or chicken bones soaked in vinegar, which removes calcium from the bones, is frequently served. If the mother avoids fortified milk, she may need vitamin D supplementation. Increasing the intake of meats and poultry elevates levels of protein, iron, vitamin B_6, and zinc.

Hispanic Dietary Practices

Spanish-speaking people such as Mexican Americans, Puerto Ricans, and Cuban Americans are often referred to as *Hispanics* or *Latinos*. Like Asians, many Hispanics follow the theories of "hot" and "cold" foods and conditions. They also consider pregnancy to be "hot" and the postpartum period to be "cold" and adjust the diet accordingly. During pregnancy, Hispanic women may not take prenatal vitamins or iron because they are considered "hot" or may take a "cold" food such as fruit juice to neutralize the effect (Callister, 2013).

Dried beans (especially pinto beans) are a staple of the Mexican American diet and are part of most meals, served alone, as refried beans, or mixed with other foods such as rice. The major grain is corn, which is ground and made into a dough called *masa* to make corn tortillas. The corn is treated with lime and is a good source of calcium. Corn or flour tortillas are eaten with most meals. Rice is also an important grain. Many Hispanics are lactose intolerant, and milk is not commonly used. However, cheese is used in many dishes. Chili peppers and tomatoes are the most common vegetables. Green leafy and yellow vegetables are seldom included.

Hispanic foods are often hot, spicy, and fried. The diet is high in fiber and complex carbohydrates. However, it also tends to be high in calories and fat, leading many Mexican Americans to become overweight.

Puerto Rican and Cuban diets are similar to the Mexican American diet, with the addition of tropical fruits and vegetables from the homeland, when available. *Viandas* (starchy fruits and vegetables such as plantains, green bananas, white and sweet potatoes, and chayote squash) are common. They may be cooked with codfish and onion. Guava, papaya, mango, and eggplant also are used when available.

NUTRITIONAL RISK FACTORS

The nurse should identify factors that may interfere with a woman's ability to meet the nutritional needs of pregnancy.

Socioeconomic Status
Poverty

Low-income women may have deficient diets because of lack of financial resources and nutritional education. Carbohydrate foods are often less expensive than meats, dairy products, fresh fruits, and vegetables. Therefore the diet may be high in calories but low in vitamins and minerals. A referral to Temporary Assistance for Needy Families (TANF) or WIC may be helpful if a woman's food intake is inadequate because of lack of money. Vitamin-mineral supplementation may be important, especially if her diet is likely to be inconsistent. Low-income families may experience food shortages at the end of the month when resources are depleted or when food is shared with a large number of people.

Food Supplement Programs

The WIC program is administered by the USDA to provide nutritional assessment, counseling, and education to low-income women and children up to age 5 years who are at nutritional risk. The program also provides vouchers for foods such as milk, cheese, tofu, eggs, whole wheat bread, brown rice, tortillas, fruits and vegetables, iron-fortified cereal, juice, legumes, peanut butter, and formula to qualified women and their children. Eligibility is based on an income at or below 185% of the federal poverty level. Women are eligible throughout pregnancy and for 6 months after birth if formula feeding or 1 year if breastfeeding. Children at risk for poor nutrition may be eligible until 5 years of age. Further information is available at www.fns.usda.gov/wic.

<table>
<tr><td>❓ KNOWLEDGE CHECK</td></tr>
<tr><td>12. When the nurse assesses cultural influences on nutrition during pregnancy, what factors should be considered?
13. For what nutritional problems should the nurse assess when caring for low-income women?</td></tr>
</table>

Vegetarianism

A **vegetarian** is a person who eats only or mostly plant foods. It occurs in a variety of forms. **Vegans** avoid all animal products and may have the most difficulty meeting their nutrient needs. Their diet may be lacking in adequate calcium, iron, zinc, riboflavin, and vitamins D, B_6, and B_{12}. Vegans should pay particular attention to obtaining these nutrients in food or supplement form. It is easier for **lactovegetarians** (those whose diet includes milk products), **ovovegetarians** (those who include eggs), and **lacto-ovovegetarians** (those who include milk products and eggs) to meet their nutrient needs (Piccoli et al., 2015).

Although not true vegetarianism, a diet without red meats to decrease intake of saturated fats and cholesterol is a growing trend. Women who follow this type of diet usually eat small amounts of chicken, fish, and dairy products.

Although the knowledgeable vegetarian may eat a very nutritious diet, she is at higher risk during pregnancy. If she is new to vegetarian food practices, uninformed about pregnancy needs, or careless with her diet, she could fail to meet her nutrient needs (Piccoli et al., 2015).

Meeting the Nutritional Requirements of the Pregnant Vegetarian

Energy. Vegetarian diets may be low in calories and fat, and some do not meet the energy needs of pregnancy. The diets are high in fiber and may cause a feeling of fullness before enough calories are eaten. A pregnant woman can increase caloric intake by eating snacks and higher calorie foods. If carbohydrate and fat intakes are too low, her body may use protein for energy, making it unavailable for other purposes.

Protein. Although most vegetarians get enough protein, this area needs consideration, especially in vegan diets. **Complete proteins** contain all the **essential amino acids** (amino acids the body cannot synthesize from other sources). Animal proteins are complete, but plant proteins (with the exception of soybeans) are **incomplete proteins**, lacking one or more of the essential amino acids.

However, even a diet with only plant proteins can meet the needs of pregnancy. Combining incomplete plant proteins with other plant foods with complementary amino acids allows intake of all essential amino acids. Dishes with grains (e.g., wheat, rice, corn) and legumes (e.g., garbanzo, navy, kidney, or pinto beans; peas; peanuts) are combinations that provide complete proteins. Complementary proteins do not have to be eaten at the same meal if they are consumed in a single day.

Incomplete proteins also can be combined with small amounts of complete protein foods such as cheese or milk to provide all amino acids. Therefore women who include even small amounts of animal products meet their protein needs more easily.

Many vegetarians use tofu, made from soybeans, which provides protein as well as calcium and iron. Meat analogs with a texture similar to meat but made from vegetable protein are available. Some look and taste like hamburgers, bacon, lunch meats, chicken patties, and other commonly eaten foods. Meat analogs may be fortified with nutrients that are often low in vegan diets (Piccoli et al., 2015).

Calcium. Vegetarians who include milk products in their diet may meet the pregnancy needs for calcium. Vegans obtain calcium from dark green vegetables and legumes, but their high-fiber diet may interfere with calcium absorption. Calcium-fortified juices or soy products such as soy milk or tofu may meet the requirements. Calcium supplements may be necessary. Vitamin D supplementation is especially important if the woman drinks no milk and has little exposure to sunlight. Soy milks may be enriched with vitamin D.

Iron. Iron from plants in the vegetarian diet is poorly absorbed. Absorption is enhanced by eating a source of vitamin C in the same meal in which nonheme iron is consumed or by preparing food in iron pans. Iron supplements are particularly important for vegetarian women during pregnancy.

Zinc. Because the best sources of zinc are meat and fish, vegetarians may be deficient in this mineral. Fortified cereals, nuts, and dried beans increase zinc intake. Vegans may need zinc supplements to meet their needs.

Vitamin B_{12}. Vitamin B_{12} is obtained only from animal products. Because vegetarian diets contain large amounts of folic acid, anemia from inadequate intake of vitamin B_{12} may not be apparent at first. Vegans may eat fortified foods such as cereal and soy products or take B_{12} supplements.

Vitamin A. Vitamin A is generally abundant in vegetarian diets. If a pregnant vegetarian takes a multiple vitamin-mineral supplement, her intake of vitamin A may be excessive. Toxic effects include anorexia, irritability, hair loss, dry skin, and damage to the fetus. Supplementation should be individualized for each woman on the basis of her diet and needs.

Lactose Intolerance

Lactose intolerance is caused by a deficiency of the small intestine enzyme lactase, which is necessary for absorption of lactose, a milk sugar. Some degree of lactose intolerance is normal for most of the world's population after early childhood. This includes many African-American, Hispanic, Asian, Pacific Islander, Native American, and Middle-Eastern people. Although those with lactose intolerance may tolerate cultured and fermented milk products such as aged cheese, buttermilk, and some brands of yogurt, symptoms may occur after drinking as little as 1 cup of milk. Symptoms include nausea, bloating, flatulence, diarrhea, and intestinal cramping.

Although the ability to tolerate lactose may increase during pregnancy, women who avoid dairy foods may not get the recommended amounts of calcium. Most women can tolerate small amounts (½ cup) of milk with meals, and they should increase their intake of other food sources of calcium. Soy milk, low-lactose milk, and milk treated with lactase are available. The enzyme lactase can be purchased to be added to milk or taken as a tablet. Nondairy sources of calcium should be increased (see Box 8.1). Calcium supplements may be necessary for some lactose-intolerant women.

Nausea and Vomiting of Pregnancy

Morning sickness usually disappears soon after the first trimester, although some women experience nausea at other times of the day and for a longer time. Most women can consume enough food to maintain nutrition sufficiently. They are often able to manage frequent small meals better than three large meals. Protein and complex carbohydrates are often tolerated best, but fatty foods increase nausea. Drinking liquids between meals instead of with meals often helps. Eating a bedtime protein snack helps maintain glucose levels through the night. A carbohydrate food such as dry toast or crackers eaten before getting out of bed in the morning helps prevent nausea. Peppermint or ginger tea may relieve nausea in some women.

Anemia

Anemia is a common concern during pregnancy. Hgb values decrease during the second trimester of pregnancy as a result of plasma increases diluting the blood. This physiologic anemia is normal (see Chapter 6). During the third trimester, Hgb levels generally rise to near prepregnant levels because of increased absorption of iron from the gastrointestinal tract, even though iron is transferred to the fetus primarily during this time.

A woman may begin pregnancy with anemia or develop it during pregnancy. She is considered anemic if her Hgb is less than 11 grams per deciliter (g/dL) or her hematocrit (Hct) is less than 33% during the first and third trimesters, her Hgb is less than 10.5 g/dL, or her Hct is less than 32% in the second trimester (Cunningham et al., 2014).

If fetal iron stores during the third trimester are sufficient, anemia will not develop in the newborn for the first 4 to 6 months after birth. However, if the woman's intake of iron is insufficient, her Hgb levels may not rise during the third trimester, iron deficiency anemia may develop, and transfer of iron to the fetus may be decreased. Anemic women need iron supplements and help choosing foods high in iron (see Table 8.5).

Abnormal Prepregnancy Weight

In addition to teaching about dietary changes, the nurse should be alert for problems associated with abnormal prepregnancy weight. The woman who is below normal weight may not have enough money for food or may have an eating disorder. Obese women may have other health problems such as hypertension that may affect the nurse's nutritional counseling plan.

Eating Disorders

Eating disorders include **anorexia nervosa** (refusal to eat because of a distorted body image and feelings of obesity) and **bulimia** (overeating followed by induced vomiting, fasting, or use of laxatives or diuretics). These conditions can be a threat to pregnancy and fetal development and require close supervision during pregnancy. They are associated with miscarriage, low birth weight, preterm birth, congenital anomalies, and postpartum depression. Women with anorexia often have amenorrhea and have difficulty conceiving. Women with bulimia or subclinical anorexia are more likely to become pregnant. All women should be asked about eating disorders, and nurses should assess for behaviors of disordered eating (Cardwell, 2013).

Some women with these disorders eat normally during pregnancy for the sake of the fetus. For others, the normal weight gain of pregnancy may be very stressful as old fears about obesity are reactivated. They may return to their previous eating patterns during pregnancy or in the early postpartum period when they do not lose weight immediately. Explaining that women often lose weight during breastfeeding may encourage them to breastfeed and eat a good diet during lactation. Women with eating disorders need a great deal of individual counseling to ensure they meet the increased nutrient needs of pregnancy and understand normal postpartum weight loss. Assessment of weight gain at each prenatal visit is especially important (Cardwell, 2013).

Food Cravings and Aversions

Women may have a strong preference or a strong dislike for certain foods only during pregnancy. Cravings for pickles, ice cream (not necessarily together), pizza, chocolate, cake, candy, spicy foods, and dairy products are common. Food aversions often include those to coffee, alcoholic beverages, highly seasoned or fried foods, and meat. The cause of cravings and aversions is not known, but they may be a result of changes in the sense of taste and smell. They are generally not harmful, and some, like aversion to alcohol, may be beneficial.

Satisfying food cravings during pregnancy is thought important in many cultures. For example, women from India may believe cravings during pregnancy should be satisfied because they come from the fetus (Callister, 2013). Ethiopian women may believe that unfulfilled food cravings during pregnancy may cause miscarriage.

Pica

Some women have cravings for nonnutritive substances. The practice of eating substances not usually considered part of a normal diet is called **pica**. Ice, clay or dirt, and laundry starch or cornstarch are the most common materials, but other items such as chalk, baking soda, antacid tablets, coffee grounds, freezer frost, toothpaste, burnt matches, or ashes may be included (Lumish et al., 2014; Miao, Young, & Golden, 2015).

Pica is practiced by approximately 20% of pregnant women. It is more common in women from inner cities, rural areas, and the southeastern United States; African-Americans; women who live in poverty and have poor nutrition; and those with a childhood or family history of the practice. However, pica is not limited to any one socioeconomic group or geographic area. Pica may be present before pregnancy occurs (Lumish et al., 2014; Miao et al., 2015).

The cause of pica is unknown, although cultural values may make pica a common practice. Pica may be related to beliefs regarding the effects of the substance on labor or the baby. Iron deficiency is often associated with pica, and the woman should be tested to see if she needs additional iron supplementation (Rabel, Leitman, & Miller, 2015). Clay and dirt are not sources of iron and may decrease the absorption of iron and other minerals (Lumish et al., 2014; Miao et al., 2015).

Substances eaten may be contaminated with parasites, other organisms, or toxins such as lead. Clay and dirt may cause constipation or intestinal blockage. Eating large amounts of ice may cause dental problems. Pica also may decrease the intake of foods and essential nutrients. Some women fear that their eating habits are harmful but are unable to ignore the cravings. They often hide their eating practices from caregivers who might disapprove.

Multiparity and Multifetal Pregnancy

The number and spacing of pregnancies and the presence of more than one fetus influence nutritional requirements. The woman who has had previous pregnancies may begin a pregnancy with a nutritional deficit. In addition, she may be too busy meeting the needs of her family to be attentive to her own nutritional needs.

Pregnancies spaced at least 18 to 23 months apart are healthier for the mother and the fetus. An interval of less than 6 months between pregnancies increases the risk for preterm and low-birth-weight infants, as well as maternal morbidity and mortality (Cunningham et al., 2014; Luke, 2015).

Closely spaced pregnancies may not allow a woman to remedy any nutritional deficits originating during a previous pregnancy. If she has inadequate nutrient stores, she must meet nutritional needs from her daily diet and supplementation alone. Morning sickness from a new pregnancy soon after delivery may further interfere with an expectant mother's ability to eat an adequate diet.

The woman with a multifetal pregnancy must provide enough nutrients to meet the needs of each fetus without depleting her own stores. She needs more calories to meet her weight gain and energy needs. A woman of normal prepregnancy weight should gain 17 to 25 kg (37 to 54 lb) if she is pregnant with twins, a gain of 5.5 to 9 kg (12 to 19 lb) more than for women with a single fetus. When these women meet the recommended weight gain, they are less likely to deliver their twins before 32 weeks of gestation and the infants are more likely to weigh more than 2500 g (5.5 lb) (Luke, 2015).

Women carrying triplets should gain a total of 23 to 27 kg (50 to 60 lb). Women pregnant with more than one fetus should consume an additional 300 calories per day for each fetus (Luke, 2015). Additional vitamin-mineral supplementation may also be necessary.

Substance Abuse

Substance abuse often accompanies a lifestyle that is unlikely to promote healthy eating habits. The expense of supporting a substance abuse habit decreases money available to purchase food. Therefore nutrition in pregnant women who abuse substances should be explored fully. Usually, more than one substance is involved, and the effects of various combinations of substances on nutrition are not fully understood. The damaging effects of smoking, alcohol, and illicit drug use on the fetus are discussed further in Chapter 11.

Smoking

Cigarette smoking increases maternal metabolic rate and decreases appetite, which may result in a lower weight gain. As the amount of smoking increases, infant birth weight decreases in spite of an adequate diet. Smoking decreases the availability of some vitamins and minerals, and vitamin-mineral supplements are important during pregnancy. Counseling to help the woman stop smoking or at least decrease the number of cigarettes smoked during pregnancy is essential.

Caffeine

The evidence regarding the effect of caffeine on nutrition during pregnancy is conflicting, and more research is needed. At this time, it appears that caffeine intake less than 200 mg/day is not a major contributing cause of miscarriage or preterm birth. Until more is known about its effects on nutrition and the fetus, caffeine intake should be limited during pregnancy to less than 200 mg/day (ACOG, 2015). An 8-oz cup of brewed coffee contains approximately 137 mg, brewed tea contains 48 mg/8 oz, cola beverages contain 37 mg/12 oz, and cocoa mix contains 8 to 12 mg/packet or 3 teaspoons (March of Dimes, 2015). The nurse should discuss other sources of caffeine, including some over-the-counter medications.

Alcohol

Because of the association between drinking and fetal alcohol spectrum disorders, women should avoid alcohol completely during pregnancy. Alcohol affects the absorption of vitamin B_{12}, folic acid, and magnesium, and often takes the place of food in the diet. Vitamin-mineral supplementation may be necessary for women who had large intakes of alcohol before pregnancy, even if they stop drinking after conception because their nutrient stores may be depleted.

Drugs

The use of drugs other than those prescribed during pregnancy increases danger to the fetus and may interfere with nutrition. Even some prescribed drugs have risks during pregnancy that should be weighed against their benefits. The interaction of various drugs with nutrients is not fully understood.

Marijuana increases appetite, but women may not satisfy their hunger with foods of good nutrient quality. Heroin alters metabolism and may cause a woman to become malnourished. Cocaine acts as an appetite suppressant, interfering with nutrient intake. Vasoconstriction from cocaine use decreases nutrient flow to the fetus. Cocaine users also tend to drink more caffeine and alcoholic beverages. Amphetamines and methamphetamines depress appetite. Women who use amphetamines for dieting should be warned that these drugs should be discontinued during pregnancy.

Adolescence

Adolescent pregnancies are associated with higher risk for complications for both the expectant mother and the fetus. Pregnant adolescents who are younger than 4 years **gynecologic age** (number of years since menarche) and those who are undernourished at the time of conception have the greatest nutritional needs (Robinson, Baird, & Godfrey, 2014; Larson, Stang & Leak, 2017). Maternal growth may interfere with placental blood flow and transfer of nutrients to the fetus. As a result, the adolescent mother may add weight and fat to her own body rather than use it for support of the fetus. This leads to a tendency to have smaller infants even with good weight gain in the mother.

Nutrient Needs

The DRIs for nutrients needed by pregnant adolescents are the same as those for older women for most nutrients. Adolescents need more calcium, phosphorus, magnesium, and zinc to meet their own growth needs. Individualized assessment of gynecologic age, nutritional status, and daily diet may indicate the need for increases in other areas as well.

Common Problems

The diets of teenagers before pregnancy are often low in vitamin A, folic acid, calcium, iron, and zinc. Although they may get 3 or 4 servings of vegetables daily, 1 or 2 may be potatoes and often are French fries. Girls average only 1.5 servings of fruits and dairy a day. Foods high in sugar and fat are common (Robinson et al., 2014; Larson, Stang & Leak, 2017). These habits often lead to inadequate stores of nutrients for pregnancy. Supplements may be prescribed, but the adolescent may not take them regularly. This combination of poor intake and unreliable supplementation may further deplete nutrient stores and general nutritional status.

Adolescents are often concerned about body image. If weight is a major focus for a teenager and her peers, she is more likely to restrict calories to prevent weight gain during pregnancy. Teenagers tend to skip meals, especially breakfast. The fetus requires a steady supply of nutrients, and the expectant mother's stores may be used if intake is not sufficient to meet fetal needs.

Teenagers are often in a hurry and want fast and convenient foods. Meals may be irregular and often eaten away from home. A significant part of the adolescent diet may consist of fast foods from restaurants or snack machines. These foods are often high in fat, sweeteners, and sodium and low in vitamins, minerals, and fiber. Peer pressure is an important influence on nutritional status. Choosing fast foods that do not make her appear different from her peers yet meet her added nutrient needs is important for the pregnant adolescent.

Teaching the Adolescent

Teaching the adolescent about nutrition can be a challenge for nurses. It is essential to establish an accepting, relaxed atmosphere and show willingness to listen to the teenager's concerns. Her lifestyle, pattern of eating, and food likes and dislikes should be explored to determine whether changes are needed in her diet.

The adolescent's home life may affect her nutritional status. She may live at home where the whole family may eat together. Or she may eat with the family only occasionally because she is often away at mealtimes. Some pregnant adolescents are homeless or in unstable situations. The number of other people in the home and the sufficiency of the food available also affect the dietary intake.

The nurse should keep suggestions to a minimum and focus on only the most important changes. If an adolescent believes she must eliminate all her favorite foods, she is likely to rebel. Asking for the adolescent's input increases the likelihood she will follow suggestions. When changes are necessary the nurse should explain why they are important for both the fetus and the expectant mother. A teenager, like other pregnant women, often makes changes for the sake of her unborn baby that she would not consider for herself alone.

The teenager's likes and dislikes should be considered, and snacks should be included in the meal plan. The need to be like her peers is of major importance to the adolescent, especially when she is going through the changes of pregnancy. With education about appropriate choices, she can eat fast foods with her friends and still maintain a nourishing diet. Giving her plenty of examples of alternatives from which she can choose should be very helpful (Table 8.7 and "Patient Teaching: Fast Foods and Nutrition").

TABLE 8.7	**Nutritious Choices from Snack Machines***
Food	**Nutrients Provided**
Yogurt, white or chocolate milk	Protein, calcium
Fruit juices, fresh fruits (usually apples or oranges), dried fruit	Vitamins, fiber
Vegetables such as baby carrots	Vitamins, fiber
Popcorn (best without butter or salt)	Fiber
Peanuts, almonds (roasted)	Protein, vitamins, calcium, iron
Granola or granola bars, trail mix, sunflower seeds	Fiber, protein
Crackers and cheese	Protein, calcium
Crackers and peanut butter	Protein

*Snack machines generally dispense foods high in calories, fats, and sodium and low in nutrients. Some of the foods listed here are somewhat high in calories, but all provide other worthwhile nutrients.

PATIENT TEACHING

Fast Foods and Nutrition

Add cheese to hamburgers to increase calcium and protein. Include lettuce and tomato for vitamins A and C.

Avoid dressings on hamburgers because they tend to be high in calories and fat.

To reduce fat and calories, choose broiled, roasted, and barbecued foods (e.g., chicken breast, roast beef). Avoid fried foods (e.g., French fries, fried zucchini, onion rings, fried cheese) because they are high in fat and the high heat may destroy some vitamins. Breaded foods such as chicken nuggets and breaded clams are high in calories and absorb more oil if they are fried.

Try wraps instead of sandwiches to decrease calories.

Baked potatoes with broccoli, cheese, and meat fillings provide better nutrition than French fries or baked potatoes with sour cream and butter.

Pizza is high in calories, but the cheese provides protein and calcium. Ask for vegetable toppings or add a salad to increase vitamins.

Salad bars are often available at fast food restaurants and provide vitamins and minerals without adding too many calories. Use only a small amount of salad dressing, which is high in fat.

Milk, milkshakes, and orange juice provide more nutrients than carbonated beverages, which are high in sodium and calories.

Avoid pickles, olives, and other salty foods. Too much sodium may increase swelling of the ankles. Add only small amounts of salt to foods to prevent or decrease swelling.

Other Risk Factors

Women who follow food fads may not meet the nutritional requirements for pregnancy. Those who have followed a severely restricted diet for a long time may have depleted nutrient stores. Nurses can help them understand the necessary changes to help ensure successful pregnancies.

Women with complications of pregnancy such as diabetes, heart disease, and preeclampsia may need dietary alterations. Those with other medical conditions such as extreme obesity, history of bariatric surgery, cystic fibrosis, and celiac disease may need nutritional counseling from a dietitian. Women with phenylketonuria should follow a low-phenylalanine diet before conception and during pregnancy to prevent cognitive impairment and other defects in the infant. This is true even if the woman has not usually followed the diet during adulthood (American Academy of Pediatrics & American College of Obstetricians & Gynecologists [AAP & ACOG], 2012).

KNOWLEDGE CHECK

14. What suggestions can the nurse give the vegan about diet during pregnancy?
15. How can lactose-intolerant women increase their intake of calcium?
16. What other conditions present nutritional risk factors during pregnancy?
17. What nutritional problems may the adolescent have during pregnancy?

NUTRITION AFTER BIRTH

Nutritional requirements after birth depend on whether the mother breastfeeds or formula feeds her infant. The nurse should review the woman's nutritional knowledge as she returns to her prepregnancy diet and teach the breastfeeding mother how to adapt her diet to meet the needs of lactation.

Nutrition for the Lactating Mother

The lactating mother must nourish both herself and her baby as she did during pregnancy. Therefore she continues to need a highly nutritious diet. Some DRIs for lactation are higher than those for nonpregnant adult women. Lactating women with poor diets may have reduced milk levels of fatty acids, selenium, iodine, vitamin A, and some B vitamins (Bronner, 2014).

Energy

During the first 6 months of lactation, the estimated energy requirement (EER) is 330 calories each day in addition to normal needs for women according to age, weight, and height. In addition to the calories consumed, approximately 170 calories per day are drawn from the woman's fat stores. This provides a total of 500 calories each day above prepregnancy requirements to meet the needs of lactation. The use of calories from fat stores aids in postpartum weight loss.

The EER for the second 6 months of lactation is 400 calories more than prepregnancy needs. Although the infant takes solids after 6 months and decreases the milk intake, it is assumed that maternal energy stores have been used and the calories should come from the woman's daily intake (IOM, 2002). Milk volume is usually adequate even when a mother's diet is less than optimal, but volume may be reduced and maternal nutrient stores will be depleted with very low caloric intake.

Protein

The DRI for protein during lactation is 71 g each day. Although there is no change from the pregnancy DRI, it is important for the woman to maintain her protein intake throughout the breastfeeding period.

Fats

The long-chain polyunsaturated omega-3 and omega-6 fatty acids are present in human milk. Therefore they should be included in the mother's diet during lactation.

Vitamins and Minerals

The DRIs for lactating women are higher than for pregnancy for vitamins A, B_6, B_{12}, C, and E and riboflavin, zinc, iodine, potassium, copper, and selenium. Lactating women who eat a well-balanced diet generally consume adequate amounts of essential nutrients to meet the infant's and their own needs. Although the quality of the milk is not affected by the mother's intake of most minerals, the vitamin content may be decreased if her diet is consistently low in vitamins.

Vitamin D is low in breast milk and supplements are recommended for infants (AAP & ACOG, 2012). Milk levels of some nutrients such as calcium remain constant because some nutrients are drawn from the mother's stores if her intake is poor. Many health providers recommend women continue to take their prenatal vitamin-mineral supplements during lactation.

Specific Nutritional Concerns

Some women have difficulty consuming all required nutrients and need special counseling. This group includes women who are dieting, adolescents, vegans, women who avoid dairy products, and those whose diet is inadequate for other reasons.

Dieting. Women who are concerned about losing weight after pregnancy need special consideration. After the initial losses in the first month, weight gradually decreases as maternal fat is used to meet a portion of the energy needs of lactation. However, breastfeeding does not necessarily result in weight loss, and some women maintain or even gain weight during lactation. This is more likely when weight gain during pregnancy was excessive.

Dieting should be postponed for at least 3 weeks after birth to allow the woman to recover fully from childbirth and establish her milk supply if she is breastfeeding. Gradual weight loss is preferable and should be accomplished by a combination of moderate exercise and a diet high in nutrients with at least 1800 calories per day (Bronner, 2014). Weight loss of approximately 0.45 to 0.68 kg (1 to 1.5 lb) a week is generally considered safe and will not compromise milk supply. Nursing mothers should avoid appetite suppressants, which may pass into the milk and harm the infant. They should not use liquid diet drinks or diets that severely restrict any nutrient because they will not meet the infant's needs.

Adolescence. The problems of the adolescent diet continue to be of concern during lactation. The adolescent may be deficient in the same nutrients as other mothers during lactation and may have a low iron intake. If she dislikes or cannot afford fruits and vegetables, her intake of vitamins A and C may be inadequate.

Vegan Diet. The milk of vegan mothers may contain inadequate amounts of vitamin B_{12}, and they may need supplements. Vegans can meet their need for other nutrients during lactation by diet alone with careful planning. Those who are not knowledgeable about nutrition should take supplements.

Avoidance of Dairy Products. The recommendation for calcium is the same for pregnancy and lactation, and the calcium content of breast milk is not affected by maternal intake. Less calcium is excreted in urine during lactation. Although calcium is removed from the mother's bones during lactation, it is replaced when she is no longer breastfeeding (Bronner, 2014). Women who do not eat dairy products should obtain calcium from other sources or take a calcium supplement. Unless they consume foods fortified with vitamin D or are exposed to sunlight, they may require vitamin D supplementation, which is necessary for calcium absorption.

Inadequate Diet. Women with cultural or other food prohibitions may need help choosing a diet adequate for lactation. Low-income women may need referral to agencies such as WIC. If the mother must take medications that interfere with absorption of certain nutrients, her diet should be high in foods containing those nutrients.

Alcohol. Although the relaxing effect of alcohol was once thought to be helpful to the nursing mother, the deleterious effects of alcohol are too important to consider this suggestion appropriate today. Alcohol may interfere with the milk-ejection reflex and may be harmful to the infant. Alcohol level in the milk peaks at 30 to 60 minutes after drinking if it is taken alone and 60 to 90 minutes if taken with food. When mothers drink alcohol they should not breastfeed for at least 2 hours (ACOG, 2013a).

Caffeine. Foods high in caffeine should be limited. Infants of mothers who drink more than 2 to 3 cups of caffeinated coffee or the equivalent each day may be irritable or have trouble sleeping.

Fluids. Nursing mothers should drink fluids sufficient to relieve thirst, which often increases in the early breastfeeding period. Eight to ten cups of non-caffeinated fluids is adequate. Drinking large quantities of fluids, as was once recommended, is not necessary.

Nutrition for the Nonlactating Mother

The postpartum woman who is not breastfeeding can return to her prepregnancy diet, provided it meets recommendations for adult women. Her diet should contain enough protein and vitamin C to promote healing. Many health care providers suggest that the woman continue to take her prenatal vitamin-mineral supplements until her supply is finished. This ensures adequate intake during the time of involution and helps renew nutrient stores.

The nurse should assess the mother's understanding of the amount of food she needs from each food group. A review of important nutrient sources for calcium and iron may be relevant. If the woman was anemic during pregnancy, she should continue to take an iron supplement until her Hgb level returns to normal.

Weight Loss

When her baby is born, a woman can expect to lose about 4.5 to 5.8 kg (10 to 13 lb) immediately. She loses approximately another 3.2 to 5 kg (7 to 11 lb) during the first week. Weight loss continues with the greatest loss during the first 3 months. If her weight gain during pregnancy has not been excessive, she will probably lose all but about 1 kg (2.2 lb) within a year if she follows a well-balanced diet (Blackburn, 2013). She should decrease her caloric intake to her normal nonpregnant levels to avoid retaining weight. Suggestions for sensible calorie reduction combined with exercise are appropriate.

Women who gain excess weight during pregnancy may have difficulty losing it after birth and may need help from a dietitian to plan a weight loss program. Those who do not lose the weight gained during pregnancy may begin the next pregnancy overweight, and this may lead to further retention of weight after birth.

Mothers are sometimes so involved with the needs of the infant that they fail to eat properly. They may snack instead of planning meals for themselves, especially if they are home alone with the baby during the early weeks. The nurse should remind them that snacking often involves high caloric intake without meeting nutritional needs. During the postpartum period the mother needs to ensure her own good health so that she is able to care for her baby. Therefore meals and snacks should be high in nutrient content.

◆ APPLICATION OF THE NURSING PROCESS: NUTRITION FOR CHILDBEARING

The nursing process focuses on determining any factors that might interfere with the woman's ability to meet the nutrient needs of pregnancy, the postpartum period, and lactation and finding solutions to any problems identified. This process primarily involves education of the woman.

◆ Assessment
Interview

The interview provides an opportunity to develop rapport and identify any specific problems affecting dietary intake.

Appetite. Begin the interview by discussing the woman's appetite. Has it changed during the pregnancy? How does it compare with her appetite before pregnancy? Morning sickness may decrease food intake during the first trimester. Determine the severity and duration of nausea and vomiting. Hyperemesis gravidarum is the most serious form of this problem and may require intravenous correction of fluid and electrolyte imbalance and parenteral nutrition (see Chapter 10).

Eating Habits. Assess the usual pattern of meals to discover poor food habits such as skipping breakfast, eating only snack foods for lunch, or eating fast foods for most meals. Determine who cooks for the family. If someone else does the cooking, discuss nutritional needs during pregnancy with that person. If the woman does the cooking herself, the likes and dislikes of other family members may influence what she serves, especially if she has little understanding of her own needs during pregnancy.

Food Preferences. Ask the woman about her food preferences and dislikes. Some women experience aversions to certain foods such as meats only during pregnancy. Careful counseling helps work around dislikes and aversions to find ways of obtaining the nutrients needed. For example, if she dislikes most vegetables, fruits may often be substituted.

Discussing likes and dislikes provides an opening to ask about food cravings and pica. Cravings may be for nutritional foods or foods low in nutrient density or eaten in amounts that interfere with intake of other foods. Ask about pica in a matter-of-fact manner to avoid giving an impression of disapproval. Food items such as ice are included in pica, and the nurse should ask about it as well. Also determine whether the mother eats large amounts of a particular food or group of foods.

When assessing for pica the nurse might say, "Have you had any cravings for special things to eat during your pregnancy?" This can be followed with, "Women sometimes eat things like ice, clay, dirt and laundry starch during pregnancy. Have you tried these?"

Potential Problems. Identify any obvious areas of potential deficiency. For example, the woman might eat little meat, avoid vegetables, be lactose intolerant, or follow a fad diet. Assess the woman's knowledge about nutritional needs during pregnancy. Inquire how long the vegetarian has followed her diet, determine which foods she includes, and question her awareness of changes necessary during pregnancy.

Psychosocial Influences

Psychosocial factors should be assessed because they can affect dietary intake. Women who are fatigued, stressed, and anxious during pregnancy may consume more high-calorie foods but have lower intake of some important nutrients. The diets of postpartum women are also affected by psychosocial factors. Those with stress, weight-related concerns, negative body image, and depressive symptoms are less likely to eat healthful diets.

Identify cultural or religious considerations that affect the diet. Do these apply only during pregnancy or at all times? Assess whether the woman follows all or only certain restrictions, and determine the effect on her nutrient intake.

Identify other factors that affect nutrition. Women with low incomes may not know about sources of assistance. A woman's smoking habits, alcohol intake, and other substance abuse may become obvious during the interview. Determine whether she takes medications that interfere with nutrient absorption. Other questions include the amount of time she has for food preparation and the frequency of fast food intake.

Provide an opportunity for the woman to ask about special concerns regarding her diet. This may bring out fears about weight gain, worry that specific foods could hurt the fetus, or other issues that have not yet been addressed.

Diet History

Diet histories provide information about a woman's usual intake of nutrients. Food intake records, 24-hour diet histories, and food frequency questionnaires can form a basis for counseling about any changes required to meet pregnancy needs. They also help the woman become more aware of her eating habits.

Food Intake Records. Food intake records are used to report foods eaten over 1 or more days. Instruct the woman to list everything she eats throughout the day. The list is more accurate if she writes down each food immediately after eating. Some women eat more nutritious foods during the recording period when they are concentrating on good diet and then return to a less wholesome diet later.

24-Hour Diet History. Ask the woman to recall what she ate at each meal and snack during the previous 24 hours. Use specific questions about the size of portions, ingredients, and food preparation for each meal. Models of food items and measuring utensils may be helpful to determine portion sizes. Inquire about beverages and snacks between meals and at bedtime. Ask if this sample is typical of her usual daily food intake. If it is not, ask what foods are more representative of her usual intake. Analyze her diet to determine whether the woman has met the recommendations for specific food groups, calories, and protein. Detailed analysis for individual nutrients is unnecessary because it is time consuming and because daily variation in intake occurs.

The food history may be inaccurate if the woman cannot remember what she ate or is mistaken about amounts of food. The expectant mother may alter her reported intake to make it appear she is eating better. She may be embarrassed about her inability to follow the diet prescribed because of lack of money or cooking facilities. The atmosphere created by the nurse is important in helping mothers feel free to be honest.

Food Frequency Questionnaires. Food frequency questionnaires, which contain lists of common foods, may provide information about diet over a longer period. Review the questionnaire with the woman, and ask her how often she eats each food. Foods consumed daily and weekly are her most common source of nutrients. Analyze the list to determine whether foods from each food group are eaten in adequate amounts to meet pregnancy needs and determine whether any major groups are omitted.

Physical Assessment

Information about nutritional status can be obtained during the physical assessment. This assessment includes measurement of weight and examination for signs of nutritional deficiency.

Weight and Height at Initial Visit. Weigh the woman at the first prenatal visit to provide a baseline value for future comparison. Ask if she has gained or lost weight. Measure her height without shoes because she may not have had a recent accurate measurement. Determine her BMI from her prepregnancy weight and height to draw conclusions about her nutritional condition. If her weight is low for height, nutritional reserves are marginal.

Weight at Subsequent Visits. Assessment of weight gain at each prenatal visit provides an easy method of estimating whether nutrition is adequate and serves as a basis for counseling. Weigh the woman at each visit on the same scale with approximately the same amount of clothing.

Record the weight on a weight grid at each visit throughout the pregnancy (Fig. 8.2). This grid allows examination of the pattern of weight gain as well as the total gain to date. It also helps keep track of the amount of gain between individual visits.

Be careful not to overemphasize weight gain. In some instances, a woman may be afraid caregivers will be disapproving if she gains weight and consequently may diet or fast a day or two before her prenatal visit.

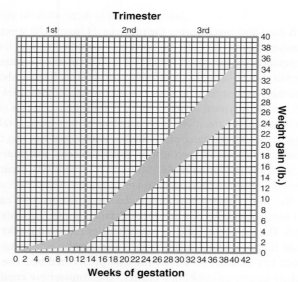

Trimester

FIG. 8.2 Weight Gain Grid for Pregnancy. The normal range for weight gain is 11.5 to 16 kg (25 to 35 lb).

Signs of Nutrient Deficiency. Observe for indications of nutritional status or any signs of deficiency. For example, bleeding gums may indicate inadequate intake of vitamin C. Actual deficiency states, however, are not likely to occur in women in most industrialized countries. The exception is iron deficiency anemia, which is common in a mild form. Signs and symptoms include pallor, low Hgb level, fatigue, and increased susceptibility to infection.

Laboratory Tests

Laboratory tests for in-depth analysis of nutrient intake are generally impractical. Analysis of specific nutrients is expensive, and normal laboratory values during pregnancy have not been determined for all laboratory tests. Hgb, Hct, and, in some cases, serum ferritin tests are most often used to determine anemia.

Ongoing Nutritional Status

At each prenatal visit (1) reassess the woman's dietary status; (2) ask if she has any questions about her diet or has had any difficulty; (3) check her weight gain to see whether she is within the expected pattern; (4) evaluate her Hgb and Hct levels to detect anemia, if appropriate; and (5) explain what assessments are being made and why.

◆ Identification of Patient Problems

Although some women consume more calories than necessary during pregnancy and risk obesity as a result, other women are likely to eat fewer nutrients than recommended. The problem may be related to many factors, the most common of which is general lack of knowledge of nutrition. Analysis of the data collected enables the nurse to identify actual and potential patient problems and develop an individualized plan of care.

◆ Planning: Expected Outcomes

The expected outcomes for an actual or potential nutritional problem in pregnancy include the following:
- The woman's daily diet will include the recommended amount of food from each food group for pregnancy.
- The woman with a normal BMI before pregnancy will gain approximately 0.5 to 2 kg (1.1 to 4.4 lb) during the first trimester and 0.35 to 0.5 kg (0.8 to 1 lb) per week during the second and third trimesters for a total gain of 11.5 to 16 kg (25 to 35 lb).

◆ Interventions
Identifying Problems

After analyzing food likes and dislikes and taking a 24-hour diet history, identify any obvious areas that are lacking and determine the woman's knowledge about the nutrient needs of pregnancy. If the woman is experiencing pica, try to find foods to replace the substances she is eating. Crunchy foods may replace some ice ingestion. Other women are willing to make substitutions such as nonfat dry milk powder for laundry starch (Lumish et al., 2014; Miao et al., 2015).

Explaining Nutrient Needs

Use the woman's diet history as a basis to introduce information about nutrition during pregnancy. Explain the recommended servings from each food group, help her analyze her own diet so she understands the process, and determine whether she meets the number of servings recommended for each food group. Explain which important nutrients are provided in each food group and why they are necessary for her and the fetus.

Calculate a rough estimate of calories, protein, iron, folic acid, and calcium in the diet to help her identify whether she eats enough of these foods on a regular basis. Compare the usual sources of these nutrients with her diet history and favorite foods. Suggest ways she can increase nutrients that are lacking by increasing foods that are good sources. Advise the woman that adequate nutrition, especially intake of iron and folic acid, may help reduce fatigue during pregnancy and after birth.

Providing Reinforcement

Give frequent positive reinforcement when the woman is eating appropriately. Assist her in evaluating weaknesses in her diet and planning ways to remedy them (Fig. 8.3). Ask her what problems she foresees in obtaining the nutrients she needs. Explore a variety of options to overcome expected problems, and ask about how these changes will affect the rest of her family. Perhaps the changes she needs to make for her own needs would be beneficial to the entire family.

If the woman can read, give her printed materials in her preferred language on nutrition during pregnancy and review them with her. If she can take the information home, she can review it to ensure she is eating properly. A small pamphlet with pictures might be placed on the refrigerator to help her remember what foods she needs each day.

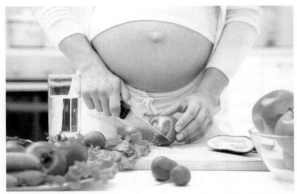

FIG. 8.3 Women often make changes in their diets for the sake of their unborn children that they would not consider for themselves alone. (YanLev, Photographer. © 2012 Photos. com, a division of Getty Images. All rights reserved.)

Demonstrate portion sizes by showing her plastic models of frequently eaten foods. These are available for various ethnic foods, as well, and help women understand how to incorporate cultural foods into the pregnancy food plan.

Evaluating Weight Gain

Compare the woman's weight with a weight gain chart to ascertain whether she has gained the appropriate amount of weight for this point in her pregnancy. Discuss the importance and expected pattern of weight gain and explain the need to eat foods high in nutrient density when she is increasing calories. If she is greatly outside of normal ranges, discuss necessary diet modifications with her primary health care provider. For example, an obese woman is expected to gain some weight, but the amount should be individualized according to her particular needs.

Although slight variations from the recommended weight gain have little significance, possible reasons for larger differences should be examined carefully. For women of normal weight, a monthly gain of less than 1 kg (2.2 lb) should lead to a discussion of diet and possible problems in food intake. A gain of more than 2.9 kg (6.5 lb) per month may signify edema. However, errors in calculation of gestation may reflect a pattern of weight gain different from that expected.

Encouraging Supplement Intake

If vitamin-mineral supplements have been prescribed, determine whether she takes them regularly and, if not, explore

---

BOX 8.3 Common Sources of Dietary Fiber

Fruits and vegetables (with skins, when possible): Apples, strawberries, pears, carrots, corn, potatoes with skins, and broccoli

Whole grains and whole grain products: Whole wheat bread, bran muffins, bran cereals, oatmeal, brown rice, and whole wheat pasta

Legumes: Peas, lentils, kidney beans, lima beans, baked beans, and nuts

---

reasons and possible solutions. Iron supplements often cause constipation, but dietary changes such as increased intake of fluids and fiber can help prevent this problem (Box 8.3). If she forgets, suggest she take vitamin-mineral supplements with meals or iron tablets with orange juice at bedtime just before brushing her teeth. If she avoids iron supplements because of side effects such as nausea, she can take them with meals or snacks. Even though taking iron supplements with food decreases the absorption of the iron, it is preferred to not using the supplements at all. Let her know that black stools are a harmless side effect of iron supplements.

Making Referrals

The nurse can provide adequate nutritional counseling for most women, but some situations warrant referral to other sources. Refer women with health problems that affect nutrition (such as diabetes, celiac disease, extreme weight problems) to a dietician with follow-up by the nurse. Women with inadequate financial resources to buy food can be referred to public assistance programs such as WIC. At the next visit, determine whether the woman obtained the help needed and whether other assistance is necessary.

◆ Evaluation

Ongoing evaluation of diet and pattern of weight gain throughout the pregnancy determines whether the goals have been met. The woman should eat the recommended amount of foods from each food group daily. She should gain approximately 0.5 to 2 kg (1.1 to 4.4 lb) during the first trimester and 0.35 to 0.5 kg (0.8 to 1 lb) per week during the rest of her pregnancy. Total weight gain should be about 11.5 to 16 kg (25 to 35 lb).

SUMMARY CONCEPTS

- Nutritional education during the childbearing period may have long-term positive effects on the mother, the infant, and the entire family.
- Weight gain during pregnancy is an important determinant of fetal growth. Poor weight gain in pregnant women is associated with low-birth-weight and small-for-gestational age infants. Excessive weight gain may lead to increased birth weight, gestational diabetes, labor complications, and postpartum weight retention.

- The recommended weight gain during pregnancy for women of normal prepregnancy weight is 11.5 to 16 kg (25 to 35 lb). The amount is greater for women who are underweight or who carry more than one fetus, and it is less for overweight and obese women.
- The pattern of weight gain is also important. The woman should gain 0.5 to 2 kg (1.1 to 4.4 lb) during the first trimester and 0.35 to 0.5 kg (0.8 to 1 lb) per week thereafter.

- The recommended increase in daily energy intake during pregnancy is 340 calories in the second trimester and 452 calories in the third trimester. Calorie increases should be attained by choosing foods high in nutrient density to meet the other needs of pregnancy.
- Protein should be increased to 71 g daily during pregnancy, which is 25 g more than nonpregnancy needs.
- Women may not eat enough foods high in vitamins and minerals to meet recommendations.
- Fat-soluble vitamins (A, D, E, K) are stored in the liver. Excess consumption may result in toxic effects.
- Daily intake of water-soluble vitamins and folic acid is necessary because excesses are not stored but excreted.
- Minerals that may not be consumed at recommended amounts during pregnancy are iron and calcium. Iron is often added as a supplement and calcium is added for women with low intake.
- Vitamin-mineral supplements should be used carefully to prevent excessive intake and toxicity. Increased intake of some nutrients interferes with use of others.
- Pregnant women should drink approximately 8 to 10 cups of fluids each day. They should eat 7 to 9 oz of whole grains, 3 to 3.5 cups of vegetables, 2 cups of fruits, 3 cups of the dairy group, and 6 to 6.5 oz of protein foods daily.
- Culture can influence diet during pregnancy. The nurse should learn whether a woman follows traditional dietary practices and whether her food practices are consistent with good nutrition.
- Both Asian and Hispanic dietary practices include the importance of *yin* and *yang* (cold and hot) foods. The nurse should know which foods are acceptable at what times.
- Low-income women may not have enough money or knowledge to meet the nutrient needs of pregnancy. Nurses should refer them for financial assistance and nutritional counseling.
- Pregnant vegetarians may need help choosing a diet with adequate nonanimal sources of nutrients.
- Lactose-intolerant women should increase calcium intake from foods other than milk, such as calcium-rich vegetables.
- Abnormal prepregnancy weight, anemia, eating disorders, pica, multiparity, substance abuse, closely spaced pregnancies, and multifetal pregnancies are all nutritional risk factors that warrant adaptations of diet during pregnancy.
- Adolescents may skip meals and eat snacks and fast foods of low nutrient density. They are subject to peer pressure that may decrease their nutritional intake.
- Lactating women need an additional daily intake of 330 calories during the first 6 months, with the remaining 170 calories drawn from maternal stores. During the second 6 months of breastfeeding, an added daily intake of 400 calories is needed.
- Lactating women should avoid alcohol and excess caffeine.
- The postpartum woman who does not breastfeed should resume her prepregnant caloric intake and eat a well-balanced diet to enhance recovery from childbirth. Weight loss should be accomplished slowly and sensibly.

REFERENCES & READINGS

Agency for Healthcare Research and Quality. (2014). *Maternal Weight Gain, Outcomes*. Retrieved from www.ahrq.gov/research/findings/evidence-based-reports/er168-abstract.html.

American Academy of Pediatrics & American College of Obstetricians and Gynecologists (AAP & ACOG). (2012). *Guidelines for perinatal care* (8th ed.). Elk Grove Village, IL: Author.

American Academy of Pediatrics & American College of Obstetricians and Gynecologists (AAP & ACOG). (2014). *Practice advisory: seafood consumption during pregnancy*. Washington DC: Author.

American College of Obstetricians and Gynecologists (ACOG). (2013a). *Committee Opinion: At risk: Drinking and Alcohol Dependence: Obstetric and Gynecologic Implications, 2011, reaffirmed 2013*. Washington DC: Author.

American College of Obstetricians and Gynecologists (ACOG). (2013b). Committee Opinion: Weight gain during pregnancy. *Obstetrics & Gynecology, 121*(1), 210–212.

American College of Obstetricians and Gynecologists (ACOG). (2015). *Committee opinion: moderate caffeine consumption during pregnancy, 2010, reaffirmed 2015*. Washington DC: Author.

American Dietetic Association (ADA). (2016). Position of the Academy of Nutrition and Dietetics: Obesity, Reproduction, and Pregnancy Outcomes. *Journal of the Academy of Dietetics and Nutrition, 116*(4), 677–691.

Appel, S. J. (2013). Vietnamese Americans. In J. N. Giger (Ed.), *Transcultural nursing: assessment and intervention* (6th ed.) (pp. 426–455). St. Louis, MO: Mosby.

Blackburn, S. T. (2013). *Maternal, fetal, and neonatal physiology: a clinical perspective* (4th ed.). St. Louis, MO: Saunders.

Bronner, Y. L. (2014). Maternal nutrition during lactation. In J. Riordan & K. Wambach (Eds.), *Breastfeeding and human lactation* (5th ed.). Sudbury, MA: Jones & Bartlett.

Callister, L. C. (2013). Integrating cultural beliefs and practices into the care of childbearing women. In K. R. Simpson & P. A. Creehan (Eds.), *AWHONN perinatal nursing* (4th ed.). Philadelphia, PA: Lippincott Williams & Wilkins.

Cantor, A., Bougatsos, C., Dana, T., Blazina, I., & McDonagh, M. (2015). Routine iron supplementation and screening for iron deficiency anemia in pregnancy: a systematic review for the U.S. Preventive Services Task Force. *Annals of Internal Medicine, 162*(8), 566–576.

Cardwell, M. S. (2013). Eating disorders during pregnancy. *Obstetrics and Gynecology Survey, 68*(4), 312–323.

Centers for Disease Control and Prevention [CDC]. (2015a). *About BMI for adults*. Retrieved from www.cdc.gov/healthyweight/assessing/bmi/adult_bmi/index.html#Interpreted.

Centers for Disease Control and Prevention [CDC]. (2015b). *Folic acid: Questions and answers*. Retrieved from www.cdc.gov/ncbddd/folicacid/faqs.html.

Cox, J. T. & Carney, V. H. (2017). Nutrition for reproductive health and lactation in. In L. K. Mahan & J. L. Raymond (Eds.),

Krause's food & the nutrition care process (14th ed.) (pp. 239–299). St. Louis, MO: Elsevier.

Cunningham, F., Leveno, K., Bloom, S., Spong, C., & Dash, L. (2014). *Williams obstetrics* (24th ed.). New York, NY: Mc-Graw-Hill.

Grieger, J. A., Grzeskowiak, L. E., & Clifton, V. L. (2014). Preconception dietary patterns in human pregnancies are associated with preterm delivery. *Journal of Nutrition, 144*(7), 1075–1080.

Grodner, M., Escott-Stump, S., & Dorner, S. (2016). *Nutritional foundations & clinical applications: a nursing approach* (6th ed.) (pp. 187–226). St. Louis, MO: Mosby.

Institute of Medicine. (2006). *Dietary Reference Intakes: The Essential Guide to Nutrient Requirements*. Washington, DC: The National Academies Press.

Institute of Medicine. (2009). *Weight gain during pregnancy: Reexamining the guidelines*. Retrieved from http://iom.edu/Reports/2009/Weight-Gain-During-Pregnancy-Reexamining-the-Guidelines.aspx.

Institute of Medicine, Food and Nutrition Board. (2002). *Dietary reference intakes for energy, carbohydrates, fiber, protein and amino acids (macronutrients)*. Washington, DC: National Academies Press.

Larson, N., Stang, J., & Leak, T. (2017). Nutrition in adolescence. In L. K. Mahan, & J. L. Raymond (Eds.), *Krause's food & the nutrition care process* (14th ed.) (pp. 331–351). St. Louis, MO: Elsevier.

Luke, B. (2015). Nutrition for multiples. *Clinical Obstetrics and Gynecology, 58*(3), 585–610.

Lumish, R., Young, S., Lee, S., Cooper, E., Pressman, E., Guillet, R., & O'Brien, K. (2014). Gestational iron deficiency is associated with pica behaviors in adolescents. *Journal of Nutrition, 144*(10), 1533–1539.

March of Dimes. (2015). *Caffeine in pregnancy*. Retrieved from www.marchofdimes.org/pregnancy/caffeine-in-pregnancy.aspx.

Miao, D., Young, S., & Golden, C. (2015). A meta-analysis of pica and micronutrient status. *American Journal of Human Biology, 27*(1), 84–93.

Piccoli, G.B., Clari, R., Vigotti, F.N., Leone, F., Attini, R., Cabiddu, G.,... Avagnina, P. (2015). Vegan-vegetarian diets in pregnancy: danger or panacea? A systemic narrative review. *British Journal of Obstetrics and Gynecology, 122*(5), 623–333.

Pope, E., Koren, G., & Bozzo, P. (2014). Sugar substitutes during pregnancy. *Canadian Family Physician, 60*(11), 1003–1005.

Rabel, A., Leitman, S., & Miller, J. (2015). Ask about ice, then consider iron. *Journal of the American Association of Nurse Practitioners*. Retrieved from www.onlinelibrary.wiley.com/journal/10.1002/%28ISSN%292327-6924/earlyview?start=21&resultsPerPage=20.

Robinson, S., Baird, J., & Godfrey, K. (2014). Eating for two? The unresolved question of optimal diet in pregnancy. *American Journal of Clinical Nutrition, 100*(5), 1220–1221.

U.S. Department of Health and Human Services. (2010). *Healthy People 2020*. Washington DC: Author.

U.S. Preventive Services Task Force. (2017). Folic Acid Supplementation for the Prevention of Neural Tube Defects US Preventive Services Task Force Recommendation Statement. *JAMA: The Journal of the American Medical Association, 317*(2), 183–189.

Assessing the Fetus

Becky Cypher

Prenatal and antepartum fetal testing are cornerstones in providing contemporary obstetric care. Expansion in fetal development and pathophysiology research, innovative technologic advances, and an evolution of novel testing methods have transformed how health care teams diagnose fetal abnormalities, determine fetal growth and development, and establish fetal well-being.

Historically, fundamental approaches were used to verify fetal life; assess fetal size, growth, and position; and quantify amniotic fluid volume. These methods, which are still used in modern obstetrics, include maternal perception of fetal movement using fetal movement counting (FMC), fundal height measurement, abdominal palpation, and fetal heart rate (FHR) assessment.

Prenatal screening and diagnosis, once associated with specific high-risk conditions and invasive procedures, now incorporates analysis of the family pedigree, population screening tests, fetal genetic risk assessment, and genetic counseling (Wapner, 2014). Advancements in chromosomal and biochemical markers, ultrasound, fetal monitoring, and fetal therapy have revolutionized how fetal abnormalities are identified and allow for greater accuracy in monitoring fetal condition.

PRENATAL SCREENING AND DIAGNOSIS

Women are often concerned about fetal health and well-being. Fortunately, twenty-first-century pregnancy care has brought a variety of new and updated prenatal screening and diagnostic testing options that provide women with previously unavailable pregnancy information (Table 9.1). The primary objective of prenatal screening and diagnosis is to detect genetic disorders or abnormalities that could affect the woman, fetus, and newborn (American College of Obstetricians and Gynecologists [ACOG], 2016a, b).

Screening versus Diagnostic Testing

There are two categories of testing: screening and diagnostic. Screening detects or identifies individuals who are at risk for an abnormality or disease. The test is performed by drawing blood at certain timeframes within the pregnancy. Single screening tests described in Table 9.1 include first-trimester screening (FTS), triple screen, quadruplet ("quad") screen, and cell-free DNA (cfDNA). Some screening tests combine portions of single screening tests. These are referred to as *integrated* and *sequential screening*. Along with drawing blood, the use of ultrasound may be used to assist in calculating the results of the screening test. Most prenatal screening tests look for only a few specific conditions. One limitation of screening tests is the risk of false-negative and false-positive results, because no screening test is 100% accurate. A false-negative is when the result is normal but a chromosomal problem such as trisomy 21 is present. A false-positive occurs when there is a positive result but the fetus is completely unaffected.

Diagnostic testing is the most precise test for a given condition. These tests are typically performed after a screening test in order to provide a diagnosis. Diagnostic testing options offered during pregnancy include chorionic villus sampling (CVS), amniocentesis, and preimplantation genetic diagnosis (PGD). Amniocentesis and CVS are more precise and usually provide "yes or no" answers about a condition or chromosomal abnormality.

TABLE 9.1   Prenatal Screening Tests

Name of Test	When	Description	What It Tells You
Nuchal translucency (NT) ultrasound	10 + 0 to 13 + 6 wk	Ultrasound measurement of small space behind fetal neck	Screens for chromosomal abnormalities, cardiac anomalies, and genetic disorders
Combined test	10 + 0 to 13 + 6 wk	1st-trimester test based on NT and maternal serum marker levels (hCG, PAPP-A)	Screens for trisomies 21 and 18
Multiple-marker triple screen	15-22 wk	2nd-trimester test based on maternal serum markers (AFP, estriol, and beta-hCG) with maternal age	Screens for trisomies 21 and 18, NTDs
Multiple-marker quadruplet screen	15-22 wk	2nd-trimester test based on maternal serum markers (AFP, estriol, beta-hCG, and inhibin-A) with maternal age	Screens for trisomies 21 and 18, NTDs
Integrated screen (full)	10 + 0 to 13 + 6 wk *then* 15-22 wk	Integration of measurements completed in 1st/2nd trimester (NT/PAPP-A with quad screen results) for a single test result with maternal age Screens for trisomies 21 and 28, NTDs	Screens for trisomies 21 and 28, NTDs
Serum integrated screen	10 + 0 to 13 + 6 wk *then* 15-22 wk	Integration of maternal serum markers only completed in 1st/2nd trimester (PAPP-A and quad screen)	
Cell-free DNA (cfDNA)	After 9 + 6 wk until delivery	Fetal cfDNA from maternal blood	Most target trisomy 21, but is expanding to include trisomy 18, trisomy 13, sex chromosome aneuploidies, and selected microdeletions and microduplications for numerous other conditions

AFP, Alpha-fetoprotein; *hCG,* human chorionic gonadotropin; *PAPP-A,* pregnancy-associated plasma protein-A.
Modified from American College of Obstetricians and Gynecologists (ACOG). (2016). Prenatal screening for fetal aneuploidy (Practice Bulletin 163). *Obstetrics and Gynecology, 127*(5), E123–E127; Driscoll, D. A., Simpson, J. L., Holzgreve, W., & Otano, L. (2017). Genetic screening and prenatal diagnosis. In S. G. Gabbe, J. R. Niebyl, J. L. Simpson, M. B. Landon, H. L. Galan, E. R. M. Jauniaux, . . . W. A. Grobman. (Eds), *Obstetrics: Normal and problem pregnancies* (7th ed., pp. 193–217). Philadelphia, PA: Elsevier; and Evans, M. I., Andriole, S., & Evans, S. M. (2015). Genetics: Update on prenatal screening and diagnosis. *Obstetrics and Gynecology Clinics of North America, 42*(2), 193–208.

ULTRASOUND

Obstetric ultrasound is a procedure in which high-frequency sound waves obtain real-time images of maternal structures, placenta, amniotic fluid, and fetus during the first, second, and third trimesters. Ultrasound is also used to assist in obstetric procedures such as amniocentesis. Sound waves from an ultrasound transducer penetrate to the level of the structure being evaluated. The sound waves bounce back to a computer screen with images that are then displayed as a type of video. Ultrasound may be paused at different points so measurements can be taken or closer imaging of specific structures can be acquired.

Ultrasound results are now considered to be one of the most valuable diagnostic tools in the field of obstetrics and should be readily available for members of the health care team (Richards, 2017). Results of ultrasound imaging is documented for each examination and placed in the woman's medical record. Ultrasound still images and those obtained with other types of media, such as video, are then uploaded into a secure clinic or hospital system connection for storage and review for future evaluations. Patients are sometimes provided still images of the fetus depending on each facility's policy.

Ultrasound images may appear as two- (2D), three- (3D), or four-dimensional (4D). 2D provides a flat picture of the image because sound waves are sent straight down and reflected back (Fig. 9.1). 3D ultrasound provides a more advanced imaging technology so the width, height, and depth of a structure can be visualized. This type of ultrasound also provides greater detail of typical features and assists in identifying abnormalities. Although 3D ultrasound is not considered a requirement in routine obstetrics at this time, some facilities use 3D as an adjunct to 2D ultrasound, particularly when identifying fetal facial anomalies such as cleft lips (ACOG 2014b; Richards, 2017) (Fig. 9.2). 4D ultrasound is similar to 3D ultrasound but has the capability of live streaming video images.

Obstetric ultrasound can be done transabdominally or transvaginally. The maternal bladder may need to be full when either approach is used in the first trimester to allow for better visualization. In the transabdominal approach, a water-soluble transmission gel or lotion is applied to the maternal abdomen as a lubricant to increase transmission of sound waves. After the gel is applied, a transducer is maneuvered back and forth across the maternal abdomen to allow visualization of multiple structures or to view a single structure from different angles (Fig. 9.3). Transvaginal ultrasound requires a specially shaped transducer with a disposable probe cover containing ultrasound gel. The transducer is inserted into the vagina to

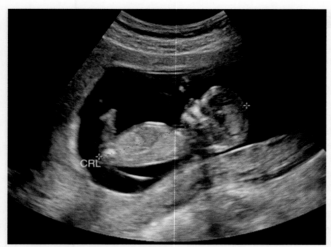

FIG. 9.1 Measurement of first-trimester crown–rump length (CRL) (From S. G. Gabbe, J. R. Niebyl, J. L. Simpson, et al. (Eds), *Obstetrics: Normal and problem pregnancies* (7th ed., p.177). Philadelphia: Elsevier.)

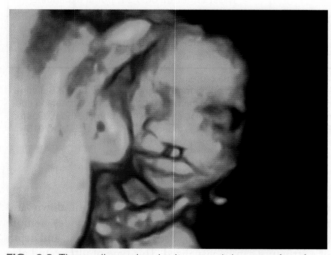

FIG. 9.2 Three dimensional ultrasound image of a fetus with a bilateral cleft lip (From Richards, D. S. (2017). In S. G. Gabbe, J. R. Niebyl, J. L. Simpson, et al. (Eds), *Obstetrics: Normal and problem pregnancies* (7th ed., pp. 160-192). Philadelphia: Elsevier.)

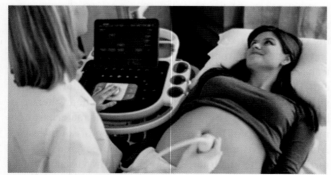

FIG. 9.3 A sonographer uses an abdominal transducer to perform an ultrasound on a pregnant woman (From http://www.usa.philips.com/healthcare/medical-specialties/mother-and-child-care)

create sharper images. Transvaginal ultrasound is commonly used in the first trimester for determining gestational age but is sometimes used later for cervical length measurements and to produce clearer images of placental location.

The three categories of obstetric ultrasound are standard (or basic), limited, and specialized (detailed or target). Basic obstetric ultrasound provides the following information (ACOG, 2014b; Salomon et al., 2011; Wax et al., 2014):

- Maternal anatomy (cervix, uterus, adnexa)
- Number of fetuses
- Biometry (fetal measurements of specific structures) that estimate gestational age and fetal weight or determines whether a structure is a normal or abnormal size
- Survey of fetal anatomy
- Fetal presentation
- Presence of fetal cardiac activity
- Placental location
- Amniotic fluid volume

Limited obstetric ultrasound provides information about a specific problem or concern that requires further evaluation (ACOG, 2014b). These are usually done in women who have already completed a basic obstetric ultrasound. An example of a limited ultrasound is confirmation of the presence of a fetal four-chamber heart when a woman is morbidly obese. The basic examination may have had inadequate views of the fetal heart because excess adipose tissue decreases the ability of sound waves to penetrate to the structure's level. The patient is asked to come back in 2 to 4 weeks for a limited ultrasound to ensure four chambers are visualized (Richards, 2017).

Specialized obstetric ultrasounds are performed when a specific fetal structure or organ system requires more detailed imaging than the basic examination (ACOG, 2014b; Salomon et al., 2011; Wax et al., 2014). This type of targeted ultrasound is performed by specially trained staff, such as maternal-fetal medicine physicians. Examples of indications for detailed obstetric ultrasound include the following:

- Suspected or known fetal structural anomaly (e.g., gastroschisis)
- Suspected or known fetal genetic or chromosomal abnormality (e.g., trisomy 13)
- History of previous pregnancy with anatomic, genetic, or chromosomal abnormality
- Fetal growth abnormalities (growth restriction or macrosomia)
- Maternal-fetal complications that affect the fetus (e.g., Rh sensitization)

Nonmedical Obstetric Ultrasound

In recent years, 3D and 4D ultrasound have been used in nonmedical locations for patient entertainment pictures and videos, especially in the identification of fetal gender. Although ultrasound has been used for many years and has been part of numerous research studies, ultrasound technology involves the delivery of sound waves that cannot be assumed to be harmless. There is a possibility, though small, that effects from these sound waves may have a biologic impact on the fetus (Richards, 2017). Ultrasound for nondiagnostic purposes by noncredentialed personnel has been criticized by multiple professional organizations. Concerns about these ultrasounds include theoretical adverse bioeffects of ultrasound, false reassurance to women because subtle abnormalities may be missed, and identification of abnormalities in a location where staff is not knowledgeable enough to discuss the abnormality or provide follow-up appointments (ACOG, 2014b; Richards, 2017). Nonmedical use of ultrasound is considered inappropriate and should not be used in obstetric practice. Obstetric ultrasound, while considered safe, should be used for medical and obstetric reasons only.

Patient Reactions to Obstetric Ultrasound

Most women in the United States have at least one ultrasound examination during pregnancy. Many women expect and often look forward to an ultrasound at some time during pregnancy. Ultrasound is often done with the first prenatal visit to confirm the pregnancy and the EDD determined by the women's last menstrual period (LMP).

Parental responses to ultrasonography vary widely. Some women are excited and report feelings of love and protectiveness when the fetus is visualized. Ultrasound may help women establish an early relationship with the pregnancy that will assist with maternal-newborn bonding in the postpartum period. Others report anxiety, fear, or concern that something will be wrong. Sometimes, an unexpected occurrence of an abnormality fails to give women the reassurance they were expecting. Women may not be sure how to manage an abnormal result. Some respond by gathering more information from the health care team before making pregnancy management decisions that may be difficult (Chard & Norton, 2016).

Fetal genitalia are differentiated as male or female by the 12th week of gestation. The gender may be determined during an ultrasound after this time. Many couples expect to know the gender of their fetus, others do not want to know, even if it is obvious, and prefer to wait and "be surprised." The parents' desires should be respected in this matter. The sonographer often provides the parents with still images as keepsakes.

KNOWLEDGE CHECK

1. What is the primary objective of prenatal screening and diagnosis?
2. What are three categories of obstetric ultrasound? What are the two routes used for obstetric ultrasound?
3. What information is obtained with a basic ultrasound?
4. Why is ultrasound transmission gel used during obstetric ultrasounds?

First-Trimester Ultrasonography

During the first trimester, transvaginal ultrasonography allows clear visualization of the uterus, gestational sac, embryo, and pelvic structures such as the ovaries and fallopian tubes.

Purposes

During the first trimester, ultrasonography is most frequently used to do the following:

- Confirm pregnancy
- Verify the location of the pregnancy (e.g., uterine, ectopic)
- Identify multifetal gestations
- Determine gestational age with measures such as crown–rump length (CRL) and head measurements
- Confirm number and viability of fetuses
- Identify markers such as nuchal translucency (NT), which suggest chromosome abnormalities
- Determine the locations of the uterus, cervix, and placenta

An embryo can be seen approximately 5 to 6 weeks after the LMP. At this time, the CRL of the embryo is the most reliable measure of gestational age. Fetal viability is confirmed by observation of fetal heartbeat, which is visible when the CRL of the embryo is 5 mm.

Procedure

The woman is placed in a lithotomy position for transvaginal ultrasound. A transvaginal probe encased in a disposable cover and coated with a gel that provides lubrication and promotes conductivity is inserted into the vagina. The procedure takes approximately 10 to 15 minutes to complete.

Second-Trimester and Third-Trimester Ultrasonography

Transabdominal ultrasonography is most often used during the second and third trimesters because the uterus extends out of the pelvis, allowing clear views of the fetus and placenta.

Purposes

Ultrasonography is used throughout the second and third trimesters for the following:

- Confirm fetal viability
- Evaluate fetal anatomy, including the umbilical cord, its vessels, and the insertion site
- Determine gestational age
- Assess serial fetal growth over several scans
- Evaluate quantity of fluid
- Compare fetal growth and amniotic fluid volumes in multifetal gestations
- Evaluate four or five markers in a biophysical profile (BPP)
- Locate the placenta when placenta previa (abnormal implantation of the placenta in the lower uterus) is suspected
- Determine fetal presentation

Gestational age determination with ultrasonography is increasingly less accurate after the first trimester because the combination of individual growth potential and intrauterine environment causes greater variations among fetuses. The following two methods improve the accuracy of gestational age determination in later pregnancy:

- Multiple measurements are calculated from measurements of the fetal head biparietal diameter, head circumference, abdominal circumference, and length of bones in the extremities.

- If the woman is between 24 and 32 weeks of gestation, two or three ultrasound measurements may be taken 2 weeks apart to compare against standard fetal growth curves. If measurements are done after 32 weeks of gestation, fetal age is subject to error.

Procedure

For transabdominal ultrasound, the woman is positioned on her back, with head and knees supported. Her hip may be wedged to either the left or right side with a pillow to prevent aortocaval syndrome from the gravid uterus. Warm transmission gel is spread over the abdomen, and the sonographer slowly moves the transducer over the abdomen to obtain the picture (see Fig. 9.3). The procedure takes 10 to 30 minutes.

PRENATAL SCREENING TESTS

First-Trimester Screening

In the first trimester, screening tests incorporate maternal serum results with ultrasound examinations. Fetal ultrasound is a valuable tool in the first trimester in identifying aneuploidies and structural abnormalities. First-Trimester Screening (FTS) includes nuchal translucency (NT) measurement (via ultrasound) with maternal serum analyte quantification of pregnancy-associated plasma protein-A (PAPP-A) and human chorionic gonadotropin (hCG). FTS screens for trisomy 21 and trisomy 18. NT is a first-trimester ultrasound measurement of the fluid-filled space measured at the back of the fetal neck (Fig. 9.4). This measurement can be obtained when a fetal crown–rump length is performed for gestational age dating. An enlarged NT, often defined as 3.0 mm or greater or above the 99th percentile for gestational age is associated with trisomy 21 as well as structural abnormalities such as congenital heart defects (ACOG, 2016b; Driscoll, Simpson, Holzgreve, & Otano, 2017).

Human chorionic gonadotropin (hCG) is a hormone produced by the embryo. The level in the mother's blood usually doubles every 2 days for the first 4 weeks of pregnancy, peaking at 8 to 10 weeks, and then declines for the remainder of the pregnancy. Increased levels of maternal serum hCG have been associated with trisomy 21, whereas trisomy 13 and 18 demonstrate decreased levels (Blackburn, 2013; Malone, 2008). PAPP-A is a glycoprotein made by the placenta and is released directly into the maternal bloodstream. This protein is detectable in maternal serum at approximately 6 weeks of gestation and peaks at 14 weeks of gestation. Low first-trimester PAPP-A maternal serum levels are linked to trisomy 21 (Blackburn, 2013).

An independent ultrasound marker that is sometimes used in addition to FTS is nasal bone assessment. Assessment of the fetal nasal bone is sometimes used in first-trimester detection of trisomy 21. One characteristic feature that is often found in individuals with trisomy 21 is midface hypoplasia and a flattened nose. In obstetric ultrasound at 11 to 14 weeks, the nasal bone may not be visible; the presence or absence of a visible nasal bone is an important ultrasound finding. Unfortunately, this type of imaging is technically

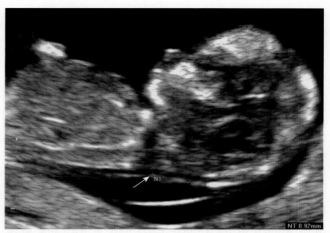

FIG. 9.4 Nuchal Translucency. (From Malone, F. D. (2008). First trimester screening for aneuploidy. In P. W. Callen (Ed.), *Ultrasonography in Obstetrics and Gynecology* (5th ed., pp. 60-69). Philadelphia: Saunders Elsevier.)

difficult and has not been shown to improve trisomy 21 prediction when combined with FTS or NT (Driscoll et al., 2017; Richards, 2017; Wapner, 2014).

Cell-Free Fetal DNA

Advances in genomics have resulted in the development of cell-free DNA (cfDNA) screening in obstetrics, as well as other fields such as oncology. In obstetrics, small fragments of cfDNA originating from maternal and fetal cell breakdown at the placental level mix freely in maternal circulation (Driscoll et al., 2017). cfDNA is found in maternal serum as early as 5 to 7 weeks of gestation, becomes a more suitable source of fetal genetic material after 10 weeks of gestation, and then dissipates shortly after delivery (ACOG, 2015a; Norton & Rink, 2016). This type of screening, sometimes referred to as *noninvasive prenatal screening*, is a maternal serum screening test that targets trisomy 21, trisomy 18, trisomy 13, sex chromosome composition, and selected microdeletions and microduplications (Gregg et al., 2013; Dar, Shani, & Evans, 2016). However, approximately 10% of cfDNA disseminated in maternal circulation is of fetal origin, with the remainder being of maternal origin (Gregg et al., 2013; Rink & Norton, 2016). This makes analysis of cfDNA challenging because the test cannot distinguish between fetal and maternal DNA, leading to false results (ACOG, 2015a; Wapner, 2014). Neural tube defects (NTDs) cannot be identified with cfDNA. At this time, cfDNA is just one of many screening options for aneuploidies and is not a primary prenatal screening test (ACOG, 2015a; Driscoll et al., 2017).

Initially, cfDNA screening in the obstetric population was designed for high-risk patients, including maternal age 35 years or older at delivery or ultrasound findings indicating an increased risk for an aneuploidy. The screening test was found to have high sensitivity and specificity for trisomy 21 in this population. Sensitivity means that if the test result is negative, trisomy 21 is unlikely in the pregnancy. If cfDNA screening is positive and the test is highly specific, trisomy 21 is probably present. Subsequently, cfDNA screening is now offered to women at both low and high risk. Unfortunately, there does appear to be a larger proportion of false-positive tests among low-risk patients compared with high-risk women. The test can be performed at approximately 10 weeks and has no gestational age cutoff. Results are returned within 1 week.

All women with a positive screening result should have diagnostic testing such as CVS or amniocentesis offered for diagnosis confirmation (ACOG, 2015a; Evans, Andriole, & Evans, 2015; Gregg et al., 2013).

Second-Trimester Multiple-Marker Screening

Second-trimester multiple-marker screening reports a woman's risk for trisomy 21, trisomy 18, and open NTDs (e.g., spina bifida and anencephaly). This screening method requires maternal serum to be drawn so specific maternal serum analytes can be measured. Screening is performed between 15 $^{0/7}$ and 22 $^{6/7}$ weeks of gestation but is optimal between 16 and 18 weeks to improve screening for open NTDs. Maternal analytes include: (1) hCG, (2) alpha-fetoprotein (AFP), (3) inhibin A, and (4) unconjugated estriol (uE3) (ACOG, 2016b). These hormones and proteins are produced by the fetus or the placenta and cross over into maternal circulation. Triple screens measure hCG, AFP, and uE3 levels. Quad screens determine the level of all four analytes. Results are based on computer risk calculations of the serum analyte levels, gestational age, maternal weight, ethnicity, presence of diabetes, and number of fetuses. Incorrect information, such as gestational age, entered into the computer will decrease result accuracy, which can delay future testing options. Accurate maternal weight is obtained at the time of the blood sample. The obese woman may have an inaccurate low AFP with serum dilution, whereas thin women may have inaccurate elevation. Women with type 1 diabetes have a greater risk for a fetus with an NTD, but have a lower AFP level. Black women have a lower risk for a fetus with an NTD, but have a higher AFP level than other ethnic groups. All results are reported as negative or positive.

AFP is a glycoprotein that is produced early in the first trimester in the yolk sac and eventually from the fetal gastrointestinal system. This protein is transported from fetal plasma into fetal urine, which is then excreted into amniotic fluid. Although a portion of AFP is swallowed and digested by the fetus, the remainder crosses fetal membranes through diffusion into maternal circulation. Levels increase until 10 to 14 weeks and then decline (Blackburn, 2013). Low levels of AFP suggest:

- chromosomal trisomies such as trisomy 21,
- gestational trophoblastic disease,
- a normal fetus with overestimation of gestational age or increased maternal weight.

Levels that remain elevated are most commonly associated with NTDs. Other circumstances associated with elevated AFP include the following (Driscoll et al., 2017):

- Underestimation of gestational age
- Undiagnosed multiple gestation
- Fetal demise

- Conditions associated with fetal edema such as cystic hygroma
- Other anomalies, specifically abdominal wall defects such as gastroschisis

NTDs are congenital anomalies affecting the brain and spinal cord. Different types of NTDs can occur, and each has a different level of severity. Two of the more common types of NTDs are anencephaly and spina bifida. Anencephaly is abnormal development of the brain and skull affecting brain function and is severe enough to result in fetal or neonatal death. In spina bifida, including meningocele and myelomeningocele, extensive nerve damage may be expected; in meningocele the meninges protrude from the spinal canal, and in myelomeningocele the spinal cord and meninges protrude through the defect. Complications of spina bifida include a range of minor physical disabilities with little functional impairment to severe physical and intellectual disabilities requiring specialized care and equipment (National Institute of Neurological Disorders and Stroke, 2015). Spina bifida occulta is not an open NTD and may cause no problems. Open NTDs are fairly common. However, since the introduction of folic acid to food products and additional supplementation in prenatal vitamins, the rate of NTDs has decreased.

uE3 is made by the fetal liver and placenta. Levels of this protein rise throughout the pregnancy. Trisomies 18 and 21 are associated with lower levels of uE3. Inhibin-A is another glycoprotein that originates in the placenta. Levels of this protein gradually rise through pregnancy. Levels of inhibin-A that are two times higher than normal are associated with trisomy 21 (Rink & Norton, 2016; Wapner, 2014).

Combined first- and second-trimester screening tests allow for a higher detection rate than FTS alone. This means that second-trimester screening tests can be joined with components of FTS. *Integrated screening* combines NT measurement and PAPP-A with a quad screen. The first portion of this test is done between 11 and 13 $^{6/7}$ weeks, followed by the second portion between 15 and 22 weeks of gestation. The *sequential stepwise screening* combines NT measurement, hCG, and PAPP-A with results from the quad screen. *Serum integrated screening* combines PAPP-A results with the quad screen, but NT measurement is omitted. Results for integrated, sequential stepwise, and serum integrated screening are not available until the second trimester (ACOG, 2016b).

❓ KNOWLEDGE CHECK

5. What is an NT measurement? What aneuploidy is associated with an increased NT measurement?
6. What conditions are associated with elevated AFP levels?
7. What is multiple-marker screening? Why is it performed?

PRENATAL DIAGNOSTIC TESTS

Chorionic Villus Sampling

A disadvantage of second-trimester screening and diagnostic testing is the delay in obtaining results. This can lead to a

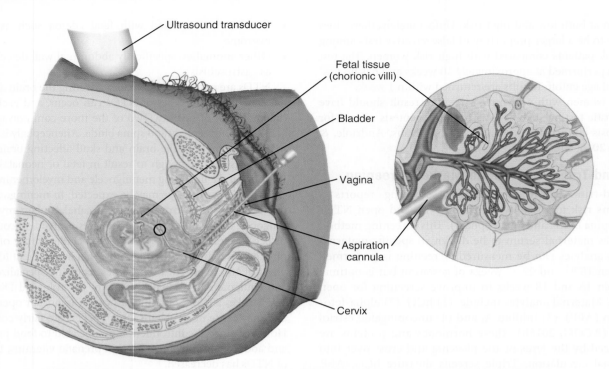

FIG. 9.5 Transcervical Chorionic Villus Sampling. Tissue is aspirated from placental tissue to detect fetal chromosomal, metabolic, and genetic material makeup, A transabdominal approach may be used as an alternative route.

prolonged interval between screening and diagnosis, which may have an impact on the pregnancy decision-making process (Wapner, 2014). Additionally, delaying diagnostic procedures until the second trimester, when maternal perception of fetal movement is more pronounced, may cause increased emotional stress for the woman (Malone, 2008; Wapner, 2014). As a result, first-trimester CVS allows for more immediate results early in pregnancy compared with other diagnostic testing options such as amniocentesis.

Chorionic villi are microscopic projections that develop from the chorion and burrow into endometrial tissue during placental formation. Chorionic villi are located in the placenta's intervillous space. These finger-like projections maximize contact with surface area that is exposed to maternal circulation for nutrient and gas exchange. Additionally, chorionic villi typically contain the chromosomal, metabolic, and genetic material makeup of the fetus (Blackburn, 2013).

CVS is normally performed between 10 and 13 weeks of gestation to diagnose fetal chromosomal, metabolic or deoxyribonucleic acid (DNA) abnormalities. Two approaches for aspiration of placental tissue can be used: transcervical or transabdominal. Both require ultrasound examination to confirm FHR, gestational age, and location of the uterus, cervix, and placenta. Either approach is acceptable. However, patient choice and technical difficulty based on a variety of situations are often considered when deciding between either approach (Driscoll et al., 2017; Wapner, 2014). For example, the transabdominal approach may be used in women who have active herpes to avoid transmission to the fetus. Final CVS results can be reported in 5 to 7 days (ACOG, 2016a; Wapner, 2014).

Patients can be provided reassurance when results are normal. If abnormal results are detected, the health care provider will discuss pregnancy management options with the woman that may include continuing the pregnancy or pregnancy termination. If chosen, pregnancy termination is generally safer for women at an early gestational age (Norton & Rink, 2016). When time is a factor, a technique called fluorescence in-situ hybridization (FISH) may be used for chromosome analysis. FISH offers an opportunity for rapid screening of aneuploidies resulting in turnaround time of 24 to 48 hours. Unfortunately, FISH is not diagnostic because the test is unable to detect other chromosomal abnormalities such as structural rearrangements. Women should wait for final CVS results before making decisions about pregnancy management (ACOG, 2016a).

Procedure

As with all diagnostic procedures, the woman should receive counseling about the procedure itself as well as genetic counseling about the specific defect for which CVS sampling is being performed. The risks and benefits of the procedure should be carefully explained, and a signed informed consent should be obtained.

Transcervical villus sampling is performed by inserting a flexible catheter through the cervix (Fig. 9.5). The transabdominal approach is performed using an 18- or 20-gauge spinal needle with a stylet attached. Both procedures require the insertion site be aseptically prepared.

Ultrasound is used to guide the catheter or needle placement. A sample of chorionic villi, usually between 10 and 30 ml, is aspirated into a syringe containing culture medium. If an insufficient sample is obtained, a second aspiration may be needed (Malone, 2008; Wapner, 2014). RhoGAM is administered to Rh-negative women after CVS to prevent alloimmunization, formerly referred to as isoimmunization. Alloimmunization is a maternal immune system response to foreign red blood cell surface antigens produced by the fetus. RhoGAM can assist in suppressing the immune system to avoid fetal risks for hemolytic diseases such as hydrops fetalis (Moise, 2017).

Women are often concerned about CVS procedure safety and pregnancy loss risk. There are varying opinions and research studies about pregnancy loss rates with CVS. In general, if CVS is accomplished by experienced specially trained physicians who perform a large volume of CVS procedures, the pregnancy loss rate is less than 1% (ACOG, 2016a; Evans et al., 2015; Norton & Rink, 2016). Limb reduction defects were once associated with CVS when the procedure was performed at less than 10 weeks gestation. Improvements in technique and timing of procedure shows no increased risk for this type of defect when CVS is performed at 10 weeks or greater, minimal risk between 8 and 9 weeks of gestation, and approximately 1% at less than 8 weeks (ACOG, 2016a; Evans et al., 2015). Other CVS complications include culture failure rate in growing chromosomes, subchorionic hematomas, infection, and spontaneous rupture of membranes (ACOG, 2016a; Wapner, 2014).

The most common patient complaint after CVS is post procedure spotting that appears red in the first 2 days and transitions to brown. Spotting occurs in up to 32% of women who had transcervical CVS procedures and less frequently with transabdominal approaches (ACOG, 2016a). Spotting generally resolves without intervention. Uterine cramping is normal the day of the procedure. Postprocedure recommendation includes resting for 24 hours and avoiding exercise, heavy lifting, and sexual intercourse for several days. All women should receive written and verbal instruction to report signs of heavy bleeding, clot or tissue passage, leaking of amniotic fluid, or temperature greater than 100.4°F.

KNOWLEDGE CHECK

8. What is the major advantage of CVS compared with amniocentesis?
9. What risk is associated with CVS when the procedure is performed at less than 10 weeks?

Amniocentesis

Amniocentesis is an invasive procedure that has been the foundation of prenatal diagnosis for many years (Evans et al., 2015). The procedure involves aspiration of amniotic fluid from the uterus (Fig. 9.6). Amniocentesis is performed for a variety of indications and at different gestational ages. Common indications for amniocentesis include identifying chromosomal, metabolic, or genetic abnormalities. Amniocentesis can assist in determining fetal lung maturity (FLM) status. Less common indications

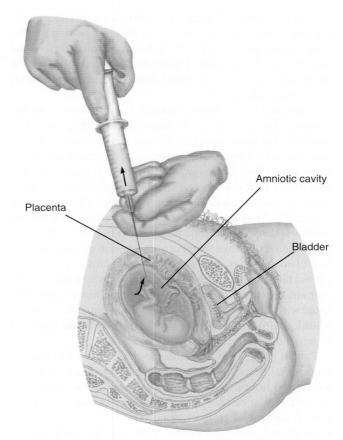

FIG. 9.6 Amniocentesis. Amniocentesis is a procedure that involves aspirating amniotic fluid (represented by arrows) from the uterus. Amniocentesis is performed for a variety of indications and at different gestational ages.

for amniocentesis include identification of fetal infection and therapeutic amniocentesis for amniotic fluid volume disorders such as hydramnios and oligohydramnios. Amniocentesis for severe hemolytic disease is no longer part of clinical practice. This has been replaced by less invasive techniques such as Doppler flow studies (Moise, 2017).

Procedure

Ultrasound is used to locate the fetus, placenta, and pockets of amniotic fluid. These pockets of fluid should be large enough to allow a needle to be advanced and generally should be free of fetal body parts and umbilical cord. The abdomen is prepared aseptically. A small amount of local anesthetic is sometimes injected subcutaneously into the skin for patient comfort, but women will still feel pressure and cramping as the needle enters the myometrium. A 20- to 22-gauge spinal needle with stylet is inserted into the fluid pocket. A syringe is then attached to the needle to allow for aspiration of 1 to 2 mL of amniotic fluid; the syringe is immediately discarded to prevent maternal cell contamination when fluid is sent for analysis. Another syringe is then connected, and approximately 20 mL or more of fluid is removed for examination. The amount removed is determined by the number of required diagnostic tests. Fetal cardiac activity and fetal movement is documented post procedure in midtrimester amniocentesis. For later gestational ages, electronic fetal monitoring may be implemented to monitor FHR and contraction pattern if the fetus is considered viable. RhoGAM is also administered to Rh-negative women to prevent hemolytic disease in the fetus or newborn (Moise, 2017).

Pregnancy loss is another concern for women after amniocentesis. Like CVS, accurate data reflecting pregnancy loss rates vary but most agree that the rate has decreased over the years because of better ultrasound equipment and procedure technique. Presently, pregnancy loss rate is quoted as less than 1% in facilities where experienced physicians perform frequent amniocentesis procedures (ACOG, 2016a; Driscoll et al., 2017). Women may experience vaginal spotting or continuous leakage of amniotic fluid, which occurs in 1% to 2% of procedures. Unlike spontaneous preterm premature rupture of membranes, which can occur because of infection, vaginal bleeding or uterine distention, rupture of membranes after amniocentesis is often short lived and not usually associated with adverse perinatal and neonatal outcomes (Norton & Rink, 2016). Incidences of needle injuries to the fetus and maternal infection are extremely rare.

Patient complaints are similar to those with CVS. Women may verbalize postprocedure uterine cramping that may last several hours. Some women experience low abdominal discomfort that can last 24 to 48 hours. Women may notice a small amount of amniotic fluid leakage the first day. This is associated with the needle puncture site between the uterus and amniotic membrane that usually reseals quickly. Postprocedure patient instructions include resting the day of the amniocentesis and resumption of normal activities the next day. Women should be instructed to report signs of bleeding, amniotic fluid that continues to leak after 24 hours, severe cramping that lasts several hours, or a temperature greater than 100.4°F.

Amniocentesis for Prenatal Diagnosis

Amniocentesis for prenatal diagnosis is usually performed midtrimester, between 15 and 20 weeks of gestation, when an adequate amount of amniotic fluid and viable fetal cells are available for chromosomal, genetic, and metabolic evaluation (ACOG, 2016a). The biggest disadvantage of performing amniocentesis for prenatal diagnosis is that final test results are not available for a minimum of 10 to 14 days. Longer periods of time are required than with CVS for fluid analysis and cell growth (Driscoll et al., 2017; Wapner, 2014). FISH testing also may be used, but, similar to CVS, results are interpreted only as preliminary findings. Another disadvantage of amniocentesis is the procedure takes place in the second trimester, when the pregnancy is more apparent and fetal movement has been perceived. The maternal bonding process has started, making decisions about pregnancy continuation versus termination more emotionally and physically difficult (Evans et al., 2015).

Early amniocentesis, before 15 weeks of gestation, has mostly been abandoned in clinical practice for a variety of reasons (Chard & Norton, 2016; Evans et al., 2015; Wapner, 2014). These include the following:

1. Increased degree of difficulty because of incomplete fusion of the amnion and chorion early in pregnancy. This results in membrane tenting, causing the needle to be unable to penetrate the membranes and resulting in a higher failed procedure rate.
2. Problems obtaining an adequate amount of fluid for sampling because the amount of amniotic fluid is less at early gestational ages.
3. Increased rates of pregnancy loss and amniotic fluid leakage has been linked to talipes equinovarus (clubfoot). The incidence of this deformity is approximately 1.3% compared with 0.1% midtrimester and is believed to occur as a result of disrupted amniotic membranes and amniotic fluid leakage.

Amniocentesis to Determine Fetal Lung Maturity

One of the last systems to mature structurally and physiologically in the fetus is the pulmonary system. One complex substance, surfactant, plays an important role in fetal lung maturation (FLM). Surfactant is primarily composed of phospholipids. Surfactant has many functions but primarily reduces surface tension on the inner walls of the alveoli, allowing them to stay slightly open during exhalation. Additionally, surfactant stabilizes lung volume, alters lung mechanics, and maintains gas exchange in the lung. Without adequate surfactant, lung walls adhere to one another, making alveoli inflation during inhalation difficult, which in turn increases the amount of pressure required to keep alveoli open (Blackburn, 2013). If this situation is not corrected, impaired oxygenation eventually leads to respiratory distress syndrome (RDS) and other neonatal complications, increasing the rates of neonatal morbidity and mortality.

Consequently, evaluation of FLM may be indicated to reduce neonatal complications (Greenberg & Druzin, 2017). Primary laboratory methods of evaluating FLM are using the lecithin-to-sphingomyelin (L/S) ratio, presence or absence of phosphatidylglycerol (PG), and lamellar body counting. Visual inspection of amniotic fluid can provide preliminary results. Amniocentesis for FLM is often performed to prevent iatrogenic preterm birth. For instance, a woman may present to an obstetric clinic with no prior prenatal care, a fundal height of 36 cm, and a history of two prior classic cesarean births. Ultrasound biometry to determine gestational age and weight at term can be off as much as 3 to 4 weeks (ACOG, 2014b). If FLM testing is performed in this situation and the results demonstrate mature fetal lungs, this decreases the concern for neonatal respiratory complications. Repeat cesarean birth then can be scheduled.

Amniocentesis is required to prevent iatrogenic preterm birth in women who request to deliver before 39 weeks for nonmedical indications (ACOG, 2015b). For example, a grand multiparous patient lives 45 minutes from the nearest hospital and is due in January during peak blizzard season. She requests to be delivered at 38 weeks for logistic reasons because the three preceding labors were less than 1 hour, the last delivery required aggressive postpartum hemorrhage management including blood transfusions, and she is able to arrange for childcare during that time. Although nonmedically indicated induction is seriously discouraged by professional organizations because of adverse neonatal outcomes in the early term period, amniocentesis may be performed to ensure FLM before scheduling an induction date. Finally, amniocentesis can guide clinical decision management about maternal-fetal risks for pregnancy continuation over maternal-fetal risks associated with preterm birth are being considered. This may be the case for a person with type 1 diabetes at 37 weeks who is experiencing new-onset extreme fluctuations in blood sugar results. If the FLM is mature, early delivery may decrease the risk for stillbirth.

Nurses should have a clear understanding of what each FLM test is evaluating. Lecithin is a phospholipid component of fetal lung fluid and surfactant. Concentrations of lecithin gradually increase throughout pregnancy and peak at 34 to 35 weeks of gestation. Sphingomyelin is an amniotic membrane lipid with a relatively stable concentration in amniotic fluid during the entire pregnancy (Blackburn, 2013). By 35 weeks, lecithin concentration over sphingomyelin increases markedly, with the L/S ratio changing from 1:1 to 2:1. A ratio of 2:1 or greater of lecithin to sphingomyelin generally indicates adequate surfactant and mature fetal lungs. In some situations, such as maternal diabetes, a L/S ratio of 2:1 may not indicate fetal lung maturity and additional testing is necessary.

Another component of surfactant that can be evaluated for FLM is establishing the presence of PG. Presence of PG supports the likelihood that fetal lungs are mature (Blackburn, 2013; Greenberg & Druzin, 2017). PG testing may be useful in preterm premature rupture of membranes when amniotic fluid can be collected from vaginal pooling, although fluid obtained this way may be contaminated by mucus, blood, and bacteria, which may interfere with the accuracy of the test. L/S ratio and PG testing can be affected by the presence of maternal or fetal blood and meconium in amniotic fluid that has been obtained by amniocentesis (Greenberg & Druzin, 2017; Miller, Miller, & Cypher, 2016).

Lamellar bodies are the storage form of surfactant produced by type II pneumocytes (Fig. 9.7). Counting lamellar bodies is another method of evaluating FLM. This test uses a hematology analyzer, which is used for platelet counting to evaluate 1 mL of amniotic fluid and takes approximately 15 minutes to complete. This test is more objective, is less labor intensive, does not require a special technique to perform, and is less expensive than other testing options (Neerhoff et al., 2001). A count greater than 30,000 to 55,000/µL is highly predictive of FLM. Counts below 10,000 to 15,000/µL suggests fetal lung immaturity, putting the neonate at significant risk for RDS (Greenberg & Druzin, 2017).

Visual inspection of amniotic fluid for color and particles can offer information about surfactant levels before amniotic fluid is sent to the laboratory for analysis. Amniotic fluid is yellow and clear in the first and second trimesters. In the third trimester, amniotic fluid becomes colorless. By 35 weeks of gestation, amniotic fluid is cloudy with particles of vernix appearing by 36 to 37 weeks of gestation (Verpoest, Seelen,

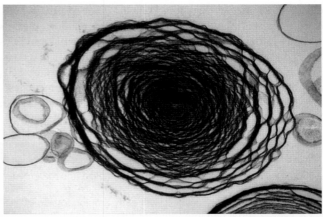

FIG. 9.7 Lamellar Body. (From Lu, J., Gronowski, A. M., & Eby, C. (2008). Lamellar body counts performed on automated hematology analyzers to assess fetal lung maturity. *Laboratory Medicine. 39*(7), 419.)

& Westerman,1976). Generally, amniotic fluid with obvious vernix or cloudy fluid that does not permit the reading of newsprint through the specimen tube is considered a mature L/S ratio. The foam stability test is another visual aid, which is not used as frequently. This test is based on surfactant's capacity to generate a foam ring around the inside of a glass tube when ethanol is added (Clements et al., 1972). Ethanol eliminates the effect of nonsurfactant factors on foam formation. After the mixture is shaken for approximately 15 seconds, a stable foam ring will form if surfactant is present (Miller et al., 2016).

Percutaneous Umbilical Blood Sampling

Percutaneous umbilical blood sampling (PUBS), also referred to as *cordocentesis,* is a diagnostic procedure typically performed after 18 weeks of gestation. This procedure is similar to amniocentesis, but requires fetal blood to be drawn from the umbilical cord through the maternal abdomen. A spinal needle, usually 21 or 22 gauge, is inserted via ultrasound guidance into the umbilical vein. The umbilical vein is preferred over other locations because this vessel is larger and less likely to cause complications such as fetal bradycardia or bleeding. Other complications include umbilical cord laceration, umbilical cord hematoma, thrombosis, infection, preterm labor resulting in an emergent preterm delivery of a compromised fetus, preterm premature rupture of membranes, and pregnancy loss. PUBS has been used to obtain fetal chromosomes, manage fetal hemolytic disease, and confirm congenital infection such as cytomegalovirus. Although PUBS is used in some high risk centers on a case-by-case basis, there may be alternatives, such as CVS, amniocentesis, or Doppler flow studies, that are safer, easier, and faster (Driscoll et al., 2017; Wapner, 2014).

Preimplantation Genetic Diagnosis

Preimplantation genetic diagnosis (PGD) is a testing option that is available only to patients undergoing in vitro fertilization. PGD analyzes one or more cells from an embryo between days 3 and 7 after fertilization. PGD looks for specific genetic conditions that may be inherited from one or both parents who are known carriers, such as sickle cell anemia and Tay-Sachs disease. Results are usually received within 1 to 2 days. PGD is not as reliable as CVS or amniocentesis because cells are obtained from an early embryo, so further diagnostic testing is recommended to validate a diagnosis (ACOG 2016a; Wapner, 2014).

> **❓ KNOWLEDGE CHECK**
>
> 10. What are second- and third-trimester indications for amniocentesis?
> 11. What risks are associated with early amniocentesis?
> 12. Why is surfactant important for fetal lung maturity?

WHO SHOULD BE OFFERED PRENATAL SCREENING AND DIAGNOSIS?

Prenatal screening and/or diagnosis is offered to all women who desire to be tested in pregnancy regardless of maternal age, family history, or obstetric history (ACOG, 2016b). Testing for underlying maternal medical conditions (e.g., diabetes) or exposure to environmental toxins may be suggested to patients. All prenatal tests are voluntary, but not all women choose to participate in prenatal testing options. Each woman has a choice on whether testing will be pursued. Unbiased, nondirective counseling about benefits and limitations of each test as well as informed patient consent should be provided before testing (Driscoll et al., 2017). Women who receive well-informed counseling about prenatal testing options are more likely to decline prenatal testing. This is a reflection that women feel enabled to make informed prenatal decisions (Kupperman et al., 2014).

Women are advised that there is no right or wrong answer when making decisions to pursue prenatal screening and diagnosis. Many women make decisions based on personal beliefs, values, traditions, and culture. Decisions also may be made with assistance from a spouse or significant other, family members, friends, religious affiliations, establishments, or trusted health care providers. Several questions are often asked during the education and counseling process.

1. *Why do you want this information?* Prenatal screening and diagnostic testing can offer vital information to women and health care providers on pregnancy options through shared decision-making process. For some patients, a normal result can provide reassurance. On the other hand, waiting for results can impart fear, anxiety, and concern.
2. *What will you do with the results?* If a screening test is positive, the patient has options to pursue more testing or decline anything further until after delivery. This can heighten anxiety for the remainder of the pregnancy. If diagnostic testing shows an abnormal result, this knowledge may give women and their families time to learn about the disorder, allow for referrals to specialists of the identified disorder, and seek information about the infant's future medical care. Alternatively, woman can choose to terminate the pregnancy.
3. *Will test results influence prenatal management?* Some prenatal tests detect structural anomalies such as a myelomeningocele (spina bifida) that may be surgically repaired in utero. Screening and diagnosis may identify a condition, such as a congenital heart defect that will require delivery at a specialized facility with immediate evaluation and treatment at the time of birth.

Nursing Role in Prenatal Screening and Diagnosis

In addition to physicians and genetic counselors, nurses play an important role in prenatal testing. Nurses are one of the patient's main resources of electronic and written information. Nurses often assist women in understanding available testing options and answer questions (Chard & Norton, 2016; Driscoll et al., 2017). Nurses sometimes help schedule tests and assist physicians with the more invasive procedures. Finally, nurses are a key source of emotional support to women and their families.

ANTEPARTUM FETAL TESTING

Fetal well-being may need to be assessed more frequently during the antepartum period, especially with a viable gestational age in a high-risk pregnancy (Table 9.2). The primary goal of antepartum fetal testing is identification of fetuses at risk for permanent neurologic injury or stillbirth so timely intervention can be done to decrease perinatal morbidity and mortality rates (ACOG, 2014a; Signore, Freeman, & Spong, 2009). Nevertheless, despite widespread use of antepartum fetal testing, there continues to be inadequate evidence to demonstrate an improvement in perinatal outcome except for fetal Doppler flow ultrasound (ACOG, 2014a; O'Neil & Thorp, 2012).

Antepartum surveillance methods are selected based on maternal-fetal risk factors, gestational age, and available technology. Common methods of fetal surveillance include the following:

1. Fetal movement counting (FMC)
2. Nonstress test (NST)
3. Contraction stress test (CST)
4. Biophysical profile (BPP)
5. Modified biophysical profile (MBPP)
6. Doppler flow studies

All of these methods are considered screening tests, and none are considered better than the other. Each one offers a different end point that is considered in the clinical decision-making process. Nevertheless, like all screening tests a false-negative rate or false-positive rate is possible. In most situations, normal antepartum fetal-testing results are encouraging, as reflected in the low false-negative rate for surveillance tests. False-negative in antepartum fetal testing is defined as a stillbirth occurring within 1 week of a *normal* antepartal fetal test result (Kaimal, 2014). In some cases, when an abnormal test result is obtained, the test is more likely to indicate a false-positive, which means the antepartum test is abnormal but an unaffected fetus is delivered (Miller et al., 2016).

TABLE 9.2 Indications for Antepartum Fetal Assessment

Maternal	Fetal	Other
Hypertensive disorders Gestational Preeclampsia Chronic	Decreased fetal movement	Previous stillbirth
Diabetes Type 1 Type 2 requiring medication Gestational on medication	Growth restriction	Advanced maternal age
Chronic renal disease	Post term	Obesity
Cyanotic heart disease	Fetal anomalies	Abnormal maternal serum markers PAPPA-A Two or more 2nd-trimester markers
Thrombophilia Antiphospholipid antibody syndrome	Multiple gestation	Substance abuse
Systemic lupus erythematosus	Amniotic fluid abnormalities Oligohydramnios Polyhydramnios	Poor education and low socioeconomic status
Cholestasis	Preterm premature rupture of membranes	Black race

PAPP-A, Pregnancy-associated plasma protein-A.
Modified from American College of Obstetricians and Gynecologists (ACOG). (2014). *Antepartum fetal surveillance* (Practice Bulletin No. 145). Washington, DC: Author; Signore, C., Freeman, R. K., & Spong, C. Y. (2009). Antenatal testing: a reevaluation—executive summary of a Eunice Kennedy Shriver National Institute of Child Health and Human Development workshop. *Obstetrics and Gynecology, 113*(3), 687–701.

True-positives occur when an abnormal result corresponds with a compromised fetus at delivery (ACOG, 2014a; O'Neil & Thorp, 2012). No test can predict stillbirths related to acute unpreventable circumstances such as an umbilical cord prolapse (ACOG, 2014a). Similar to prenatal screening and diagnostic tests, the nurse provides an appropriate level of patient education based on the obstetric situation (Chard & Norton, 2016). Tools such as educational pamphlets covering antepartum surveillance can reinforce key points on the maternal-fetal indication and method of assessment.

Risk Identification

Several risk factors have an obvious connection to fetal compromise or stillbirth because there is a presumed alteration in the maternal-fetal oxygenation pathway. Briefly, oxygen is carried from the environment to the fetus along a pathway

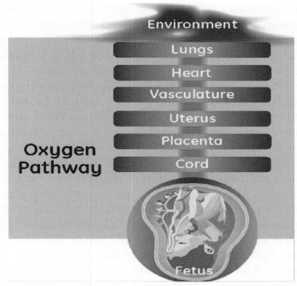

FIG. 9.8 Fetal Oxygenation Pathway. (From Miller, L. A., Miller, D. A., & Cypher, R. L. (2016). *Mosby's pocket guide to fetal monitoring: A multidisciplinary approach.* Elsevier Health Sciences.)

that includes the maternal lungs, heart, vasculature, uterus, placenta, and umbilical cord (Fig. 9.8). Interruptions can occur anywhere along this pathway (Miller et al., 2016). For example, severe hypertension in pregnancy can cause an oxygenation interruption at the level of the maternal vasculature, uterus, and placenta. Elevated blood pressures reduce maternal intravascular volume and cause vasoconstriction in both maternal and placental vasculature. Insufficient exchange in oxygen, carbon dioxide, nutrients, and waste products between maternal and fetal circulations may consequently lead to a fetal physiologic response such as an elevated FHR baseline or decelerations. In some clinical situations, antepartum fetal testing may identify fetal hypoxia early enough so treatment can begin before fetal oxygenation reaches a critical level. Using the example of blood pressures in the severe range, if administration of an antihypertensive agent lowers maternal blood pressure, the process may be reversed enough to allow improved blood flow to the fetus so adequate oxygen and nutrition exchange occurs. Otherwise if recurrent interruptions in the oxygenation pathway continue, decreased oxygen content in the blood (hypoxemia) progresses to hypoxia or decreased oxygen in fetal tissues. Anaerobic metabolism is then activated and lactic acid is produced, which can result in metabolic acidosis, metabolic acidemia, and finally potential neurologic injury or death (Miller et al., 2016). Other risk factors, such as maternal age and weight, are more complicated to understand because the link to neurologic injury or stillbirth is not as obvious as an interruption in the oxygenation pathway and cannot be modified.

Gestational Age and Frequency of Assessment

The gestational age to start antepartum fetal testing has not been defined (Greenberg & Druzin, 2017). Several factors go into decisions as to when to begin testing. Antepartum fetal surveillance is traditionally initiated at 24 to 32 weeks of gestation for high-risk pregnancies. Earlier testing may be recommended for a number of reasons, including risk factors, maternal comorbidities that existed before pregnancy, and previous testing results in the current pregnancy. Experts agree that antepartum testing, especially methods using electronic fetal heart monitoring (EFM), should not be initiated until the gestational age is sufficient to expect infant survival if intervention and delivery becomes necessary (Freeman, Garite, Nageotte, & Miller, 2012; Raju, Mercer, Burchfield, & Joseph, 2014). Frequency of testing is individualized to the patient and fetus, current clinical situation, and the health care team's judgment. Normally, antepartum testing is conducted weekly or biweekly. More frequent intervals of antepartum testing may be warranted if the clinical status of the woman or fetus deteriorates (ACOG, 2014a; Signore et al., 2009). For example, a woman may have biweekly NSTs and amniotic fluid index (AFI) measured for preterm gestational hypertension but is admitted to an inpatient antepartum unit for further evaluation of worsening blood pressures. NST frequency may be increased to daily while the woman is hospitalized. Sometimes, an isolated situation warrants antepartum testing but continued surveillance is not necessary. For example, an NST may be performed because of a patient complaint of decreased fetal movement. If the NST is reactive and the woman is reassured, no further testing is indicated.

Fetal Movement Counting

For women, maternal perception of fetal movement has been an indicator of fetal life, and absence of movement signaled death. As a fetus becomes more hypoxic because of potential interruptions in the oxygenation pathway, activity is reduced to conserve oxygen consumption. Eventually stillbirth may occur (Blackburn, 2013; Signore et al., 2009). Fetal movement counting (FMC) is considered a method to evaluate fetal well-being. Various counting methods for fetal movement have been suggested, but an optimal number of fetal movements or duration for counting has not been proposed (ACOG, 2014a; Greenberg & Druzin, 2017).

One approach to FMC is the "count to 10" method. Women are instructed to rest in a quiet location and count distinct fetal movements, such as kicks or rolls. Maternal perception of 10 distinct movements in a 1- to 2-hour period is reflective of a nonhypoxic fetus at that point in time. The count is discontinued once 10 movements are perceived (ACOG, 2014a; Freeman et al., 2012). Fetal movement is then recorded on paper or a cell phone application. Maternal perception of decreased fetal movement should alert a woman to seek further evaluation.

Some women have difficulty recognizing fetal movement related to fetal position, obesity, amniotic fluid volume abnormalities, and placental location (O'Neil & Thorp, 2012). For example, an anterior placenta or a breech position may alter a woman's perception of movement. In these situations, it is sometimes useful for nurses to assist women in abdominal palpation. Rarely, women may require ultrasound to assist in distinguishing fetal movement. The time of the day can potentially influence fetal kick count results. Fetal movement generally peaks between 9:00 PM and 1:00 AM, which is attributed to a fall in maternal glucose level. In this scenario, women may need to select a different time of day to perform counting (Greenburg & Druzin, 2017).

 KNOWLEDGE CHECK

13. What is the primary goal of antepartal fetal testing?
14. Describe one method of fetal movement counting as if you are explaining the procedure to a patient.

Nonstress Test

NSTs involve placement of an EFM for FHR and uterine activity observation. The NST is the primary means of fetal surveillance in pregnancies at risk for uteroplacental insufficiency (inability of placenta to exchange oxygen, carbon dioxide, nutrients, and waste products properly between maternal and fetal circulations) with consequent fetal hypoxia and acidosis. The NST identifies whether an increase in the FHR occurs when the fetus moves, indicating adequate oxygenation, a healthy neural pathway from the fetal central nervous system (CNS) to the fetal heart, and the ability of the fetal heart to respond to stimuli. FHR accelerations without fetal movement are also considered a reassuring sign of adequate fetal oxygenation. If the fetal heart does not accelerate with movement, however, fetal hypoxemia and acidosis are concerns.

NSTs are a result of early observations demonstrating that when normal oscillations and fluctuations in baseline FHR were present (now called *variability*), fetal well-being could be established. The presence of accelerations indicates intact CNS and normal autonomic regulation of the FHR, and it is predictive of the absence of fetal metabolic acidemia at the time of observation (Macones, Hankins, Spong, Hauth, & Moore, 2008; Miller et al., 2016). Accelerations are defined as visually apparent increases in the FHR that reach a peak of 15 beats per minute (bpm) above the baseline, with the entire acceleration lasting a minimum of 15 seconds but less than 2 minutes ("15 × 15"). Before 32 weeks of gestation, accelerations are defined as visually apparent increases in the FHR that reach a peak of 10 bpm above the baseline with the entire acceleration lasting at least 10 seconds ("10 × 10") (Macones et al., 2008). This is because preterm fetuses may not have the physiologic maturity to generate accelerations of 15 × 15. Accelerations can either be spontaneous or stimulated with fetal scalp stimulation or acoustic stimulation.

Procedure

NSTs are noninvasive and can be performed in a hospital or clinic setting. Women are placed in a comfortable position, such as semi-Fowler's with a lateral tilt, to reduce the risk for aortocaval compression, which may cause maternal hypotension and abnormal FHR changes. Fetal position is assessed with Leopold's maneuvers to allow correct EFM placement and maximize the ability to obtain a continuous tracing. The ultrasound transducer and tocotransducer are applied and secured to the woman's abdomen to detect FHR and presence or absence of uterine contractions. (Fig. 9.9).

Although *nonstress test* contains the word *"stress,"* the fetus is not physically challenged by factors such as increased maternal activity or contractions to obtain necessary data. Patients remain on continuous fetal monitoring for a minimum of 20 minutes. NSTs can be extended another 20 minutes for a total of 40 minutes to take into account normal fetal sleep-wake cycles (ACOG, 2014a).

Maternal ingestion of medications such as narcotics, barbiturates, benzodiazepines, or methadone, as well as alcohol, beta-blockers, tobacco, and corticosteroids for FLM have also been associated with altered fetal movement (Greenberg & Druzin, 2017). In these situations, fetal stimulation may be required to provoke a fetal response. One simple method uses an artificial larynx to provide vibroacoustic stimulation. The artificial larynx is placed on the maternal abdomen near the fetal head. Stimulation is applied for 1 to 2 seconds and can be repeated up to three times for progressively longer durations (3 seconds) if no response is elicited (ACOG, 2014a). Fetuses will respond to externally applied sound and vibration by displaying more FHR accelerations that have increased amplitude and duration (Read & Miller, 1977; Walker, Grimwade,

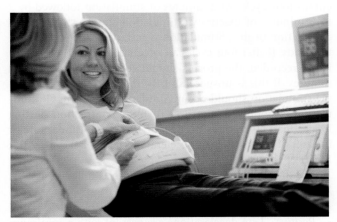

FIG. 9.9 Antepartum fetal testing typically involves use of an electronic fetal monitor in which fetal heart rate and uterine activity can be observed. (From http://images.philips.com/is/image/PhilipsConsumer/HC865132-UPL-global-001?wid=960&hei=500)

& Wood, 1971). Cell phones placed on the maternal abdomen and loud noises or vibration near the woman (e.g., vacuum cleaner) also may elicit a similar response. An event marker on the EFM may be pressed by the patient recording a symbol on the FHR tracing each time movement is perceived.

FHR and uterine activity is recorded on a paper tracing that comes from the EFM or an electronic tracing stored in computerized systems. Contractions not perceived by women may be identified during an NST depending on gestational age. These contractions, which are often mild on palpation and irregular, reflect normal structural and functional changes in the myometrium during pregnancy (Blackburn, 2013). However, if contraction frequency increases, appears to be more coordinated or changes intensity, women should be assessed for labor, especially in preterm gestations.

Interpretation

NSTs are interpreted as reactive or nonreactive. Reactive NSTs contain two or more FHR accelerations previously described within a 20-minute period (Fig. 9.10). Documentation of accelerations in relationship to fetal movement is not required for a reactive NST. Nonreactive NSTs are defined as fewer than two accelerations during a 40-minute period (Fig. 9.11). Variable decelerations are sometimes observed in NSTs and are typically associated with umbilical cord compression. As long as these decelerations are not recurrent and last less than 30 seconds, no further intervention or monitoring is required. However, if variable decelerations become more recurrent, defined as three or more in 20 minutes, the patient should be monitored for an extended period because this type of pattern has been associated with indeterminate and abnormal FHR patterns requiring further intervention. Decelerations that persist for 1 minute or longer during an NST have been associated with increased cesarean birth rates and stillbirth (ACOG, 2014a). Nurses may interpret NST results if facility educational and competency requirements have been met.

Contraction Stress Test

Contraction stress tests (CSTs) determine fetal well-being by monitoring FHR responses to contractions. A CST may be done if the NST findings are nonreactive. Usually a BPP

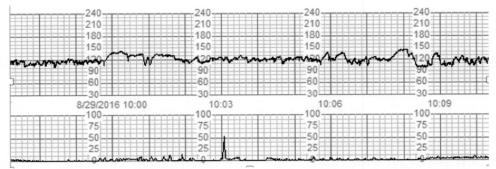

FIG. 9.10 Reactive nonstress tests contains two or more fetal heart rate accelerations within a 20-minute period. (Courtesy PeriGen, Princeton, New Jersey)

is performed in place of the CST. The physiologic premise behind CST is that between the uterus and placenta are a number of vessels, including uterine spiral arteries. These arteries carry oxygenated blood to the intervillous space, which contains chorionic villi. When the uterus contracts, uteroplacental blood flow is temporarily interrupted as a result of blood vessel compression. In response to contractions, healthy oxygenated fetuses can physiologically tolerate contractions and maintain FHR with normal characteristics such as a stable baseline rate and accelerations. In compromised fetuses, brief interruptions of oxygen transfer during contractions can result in late decelerations because the fetus is assumed to be in a state of hypoxemia. Late decelerations are defined as a gradual FHR decrease (≥30 seconds) from FHR baseline with a nadir (lowest part of the deceleration) occurring after a contraction peaks, followed by a gradual recovery to baseline after a contraction ends (Macones et al., 2008). If the contraction pattern continues, the fetus could progressively deteriorate down a pathway of hypoxia, metabolic acidosis, metabolic academia, and potential neurologic injury (Miller et al., 2016).

Other names for CSTs include the oxytocin challenge test (OCT), in which intravenous oxytocin is used to elicit contractions, and the nipple stimulation test, in which maternal manipulation of the nipple produces contractions. Regardless of which method is used, success rates for achieving an adequate contraction pattern to interpret test results are similar (Greenberg & Druzin, 2017).

Procedure

CSTs are typically performed in a hospital environment where interventions such as administration of intravenous medication or an immediate delivery can occur in the event of an emergency. Relative contraindications for performing the test include patients in whom vaginal delivery is not recommended at the time of the test. Examples include placenta previa, preterm premature rupture of membranes, preterm labor, history of preterm delivery, previous classic cesarean section, or multiple gestations (Freeman et al., 2012). Procedure steps are exactly the same as for an NST. Initial monitoring will determine whether at least three spontaneous contractions within a 10-minute timeframe are present. The duration of each contraction should be 40 seconds or longer and palpable

to the nurse. Contractions do not need to be painful to patients for test interpretation. If spontaneous contractions are sufficient, additional uterine stimulation is not needed. When adequate contractions are not present, oxytocin or nipple stimulation is required. An adequate contraction pattern with continuous FHR data on a tracing must be present to interpret CST results.

OCTs require an intravenous infusion of dilute exogenous oxytocin to stimulate contractions. Oxytocin is administered by a continuous infusion pump per hospital policy. One sample protocol starts oxytocin at 0.5 mU/min to 2 mU/min, with increases every 15 minutes until sufficient contractions are recorded. Oxytocin is discontinued once an adequate contraction pattern with interpretable data is recorded. If there is evidence of tachysystole (more than 5 contractions in a 10-minute segment averaged over a 30-minute period), prolonged decelerations, recurrent variable decelerations, or recurrent late decelerations, oxytocin also should be discontinued (Miller et al., 2016).

The alternative to oxytocin infusion is nipple stimulation. When breasts are stimulated, endogenous oxytocin is released from the posterior pituitary gland (Blackburn, 2013). In turn, contractions will occur. Women are asked to brush the nipple surface. One method of nipple stimulation entails four cycles of 2 minutes of stimulation followed by 2 to 5 minutes of inactivity. Stimulation should stop when a contraction begins. Stimulation is restarted when a contraction ends. If after four cycles an adequate contraction pattern is not recorded, the process should continue for another 10 minutes. If this is unsuccessful, 10 minutes of bilateral nipple stimulation should occur. Similar to OCTs, nipple stimulation is stopped when three or more contractions lasting longer than 40 seconds occur in a 10-minute time frame or in cases of tachysystole or decelerations (Freeman et al., 2012; Miller et al., 2016).

The interpretation criteria for CST are as follows (ACOG, 2014a):
- *Negative*—No late decelerations (Fig. 9.12)
- *Positive*—Late decelerations are present with a minimum of 50% of the contractions, even when fewer than three contractions occur in 10 minutes (Fig. 9.13)
- *Equivocal-suspicious*—Intermittent late decelerations or significant variable decelerations (sudden decreases in the FHR that quickly return to the baseline) (Fig. 9.14)

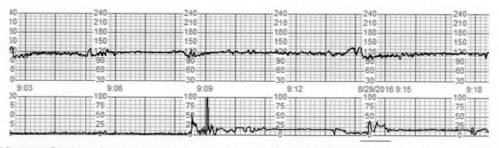

FIG. 9.11 Portion of a nonreactive nonstress test reflecting the absence of two or more fetal heart rate (FHR) accelerations despite a normal range FHR baseline. (Courtesy PeriGen, Princeton, New Jersey)

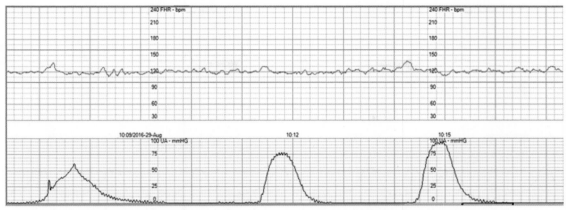

FIG. 9.12 Negative Contraction Stress Test. (Courtesy PeriGen, Princeton, New Jersey)

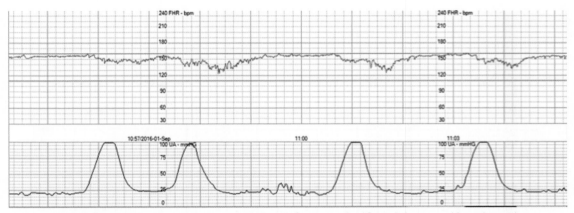

FIG. 9.13 Positive Contraction Stress Test. (Courtesy PeriGen, Princeton, New Jersey)

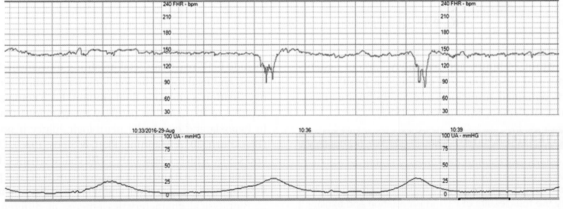

FIG. 9.14 Equivocal Suspicious. (Courtesy PeriGen, Princeton, New Jersey)

- *Equivocal*—FHR decelerations in the presence of contractions that are more frequent than every 2 minutes or last longer than 90 seconds (Fig. 9.15)
- *Unsatisfactory*—Fewer than three contractions in 10 minutes or a tracing that cannot be interpreted (Fig. 9.16)

A negative CST has been consistently associated with fetal well-being, meaning the stillbirth rate is less than 1 per 1000 as long as an acute event does not occur. Negative CSTs can be repeated in 1 week. Positive CSTs are linked to an increased incidence of fetal growth restriction, late decelerations in

labor, meconium-stained fluid, low 5-minute Apgar scores, and stillbirth. The likelihood of stillbirth varies between 7% and 15%. In the event of a positive CST result, the health care team will discuss management options with the patient that may include further testing or an expedited delivery. An equivocal, equivocal suspicious, or unsatisfactory CST result prompts further evaluation, including repeat testing within 24 hours, prolonged continuous monitoring, or using adjunct methods of testing unless there are other clinical indications for prompt delivery (Greenberg & Druzin, 2017). If a CST

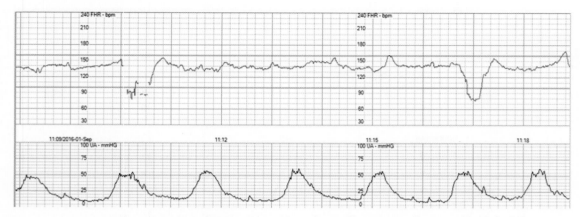

FIG. 9.15 Equivocal. (Courtesy PeriGen, Princeton, New Jersey)

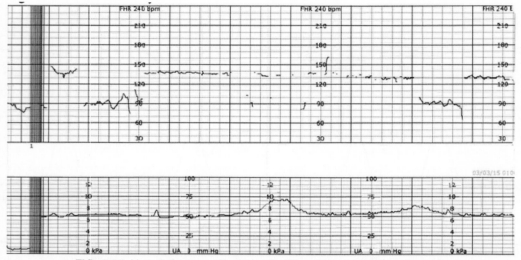

FIG. 9.16 Unsatisfactory. (Courtesy PeriGen, Princeton, New Jersey)

is repeated within 24 hours, approximately 7.5% of patients with an equivocal suspicious test exhibited a positive CST result, 38.8% remained suspicious, and 53.7% became negative (Freeman, Anderson, & Dorchester, 1982).

Biophysical Profile

Biophysical profiles (BPPs) combine EFM with ultrasound assessment of specific fetal biophysical characteristics. These include fetal movement, fetal tone, fetal breathing movement, and amniotic fluid amount. Biophysical characteristics are a reflection of the CNS and provide an indirect means of evaluating fetal oxygenation. Individual BPP components are a combination of short-term and long-term indicators of fetal well-being and sufficient oxygenation. Short-term indicators include FHR reactivity, fetal breathing movement, fetal movement, and fetal tone. The sole long-term indicator of adequate oxygenation is amniotic fluid amount. Each component is susceptible to oxygenation pathway interruptions that may lead to hypoxia and eventually neurologic injury if not corrected (Blackburn, 2013; Manning, Platt, & Sipos, 1980). Unlike NSTs and CSTs, which assess only FHR characteristics, biophysical scoring allows a more complete assessment of fetal growth and development, oxygenation, and uterine environment.

Biophysical characteristics emerge at different stages of fetal development. Fetal tone is established at approximately 7 to 8 weeks of gestation. Spontaneous fetal movement can be observed on ultrasound at 9 weeks of gestation starting with flexion-extension of the vertebral column. Fetal breathing can be detected at 10 weeks of gestation and becomes more apparent by 19 to 20 weeks of gestation. Sometimes referred to as "practice breathing," this biophysical characteristic is often rhythmic and is a reflection of diaphragmatic, laryngeal, and intercostal muscle contractions (Fig. 9.17). Amniotic fluid production by the fetal renal system is present at approximately 10 weeks of gestation. Finally, FHR reactivity is established by the end of the second trimester (Blackburn, 2013).

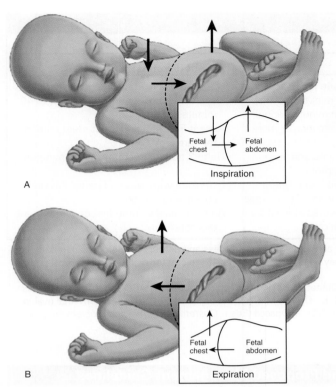

A

B

FIG. 9.17 Fetal Breathing. (From Fetal assessment (2014). In F. Cunningham, K. J. Leveno, S. L. Bloom, et al. (Eds), *William's Obstetrics* (24th ed., pp 335-349). New York: McGraw-Hill; 2013.)

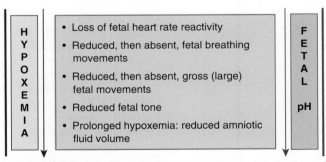

H Y P O X E M I A

- Loss of fetal heart rate reactivity
- Reduced, then absent, fetal breathing movements
- Reduced, then absent, gross (large) fetal movements
- Reduced fetal tone
- Prolonged hypoxemia: reduced amniotic fluid volume

F E T A L pH

FIG. 9.18 Effects of gradual hypoxemia and worsening of fetal acidosis.

Oxygenation disruption that leads to acute or chronic periods of hypoxia prompts the fetus to decrease biophysical activities in reverse order of pregnancy development to preserve energy and oxygen consumption. FHR reactivity disappears first, followed by fetal breathing movement. If hypoxia continues, decreased fetal movement and loss of fetal tone will occur. During this process, levels of amniotic fluid reach critical levels defined as oligohydramnios, because uteroplacental circulation is not adequate to oxygenate fetal kidneys (Fig. 9.18). Shunting occurs because fetuses redirect blood from areas not critical to fetal life, such as the kidneys, gastrointestinal tract, and extremities to the vital organs, which include the heart, brain, and adrenal gland. If changes

in oxygenation are prolonged, blood flow to the fetal kidneys ceases. Therefore oligohydramnios in fetuses with normal renal structures and intact amniotic membranes suggests prolonged fetal hypoxia and is a strong indication of fetal compromise (Manning, 1995; Vintzileos & Knuppel, 1994).

Procedure and Interpretation

NSTs are the EFM portion of BPPs. NSTs may be performed first to determine whether FHR is reactive or nonreactive. Sometimes, the NST is not performed if ultrasound is done first and all four biophysical characteristics are observed. If any of the biophysical characteristics are not met, an NST will follow.

Biophysical characteristics are evaluated simultaneously over a 30-minute period. This type of ultrasound is performed by sonographers, advanced practice nurses, or physicians. In some states, nurses may perform BPPs but must attend specialized training and successfully complete competency verification. A scoring technique is used to interpret data, with each parameter receiving a score of 2 which is normal or 0 which is abnormal (Table 9.3). Scores for all five BPP components are totaled together for interpretation and management (Table 9.4). BPP scores of 8 or 10 correlate with normal fetal oxygenation. A BPP score of 6 is interpreted as equivocal if there is normal fluid and suspicious for fetal asphyxia if there is abnormal fluid. In equivocal or suspicious cases, extending the testing period, retesting within 24 hours, or adding adjunct testing such as a CST may be done before making pregnancy management decisions (Greenberg & Druzin, 2017; Kaimal, 2014). Scores of 0 to 4 in situations in which previously APFT results were normal may justify delivery of a fetus depending on the clinical scenario. Abnormal scores of 0 to 4 are usually associated with acidemia or perinatal asphyxia, which leads to poor perinatal and neonatal outcomes including stillbirth.

Modified Biophysical Profile

Modified biophysical profile (MBPP) is a variation of a BPP. MBPPs combine NST with ultrasound measurement of amniotic fluid. Remember, NSTs are a short-term indicator of how well a fetus is oxygenated, and amniotic fluid amount is a long-term reflection of adequate oxygenation in which shunting has not taken place. This method can be done weekly or biweekly depending on maternal-fetal indication. Unlike the BPP, this test is not as time consuming and does not require more advanced ultrasound skill (O'Neill & Thorp, 2012).

NSTs are either reactive or nonreactive. Amniotic fluid amount is assessed by measuring the largest pocket of amniotic fluid in four maternal abdominal quadrants. The four measurements are totaled together to report the AFI. Oligohydramnios is considered an AFI of less than 5 cm in this procedure. Volume sums greater than 10 cm are considered reassuring. Some health care providers use measurement of one single deepest pocket instead of measuring four pockets. If a single deepest pocket is 2 cm or less, oligohydramnios is identified (ACOG, 2014a; Kaimal, 2014). An AFI higher than 18 to 20 cm suggests excess amniotic fluid volume or hydramnios. Results are interpreted as normal if the NST

TABLE 9.3   Biophysical Profile Scoring

Criterion	POINTS	
	Present (2 Points)	Absent (0 Points)
Nonstress test (NST) (if used)	Reactive NST (at least 2 fetal heart rate (FHR) accelerations peaking at least 15 beats per minute (bpm) above baseline for 15 seconds within a 20-minute period)	Nonreactive NST (absence of required characteristics for reactive test after 40 minutes of testing)
Fetal breathing movements (FBMs)	≥1 episode of rhythmic FBMs of 30 seconds or more within 30 minutes	Absent FBMs or none that meet criterion for "present"
Gross body movements	≥3 trunk movements in 30 minutes; limb and trunk movement is considered one movement	Up to 2 trunk movements in 30 minutes
Fetal tone	≥1 episode of fetal extremity extension with return to flexion; opening or closing of hand within 30 minutes	Extension with return to partial flexion; absence of flexion
Amniotic fluid volume	At least one pocket of fluid that measures at least 2 cm in two planes perpendicular to each other	Amniotic fluid volume that does not meet this criterion

Interpretation: Normal (reassuring) = 8 to 10 points; equivocal = 6 points; abnormal = 4 points or less and delivery may be considered. If oligohydramnios is present, more frequent testing is warranted, and delivery may be considered. If the NST is omitted from the biophysical profile (BPP), the maximum score of the four remaining ultrasound criteria is 8.
Data from American Academy of Pediatrics (AAP) & American College of Obstetricians and Gynecologists (AAP & ACOG). (2012). *Guidelines for perinatal care* (7th ed.). Elk Grove Village, IL: Author; and Greenberg, M. B., Druzin, M. L., & Gabbe, S. G. (2012). Antepartum fetal evaluation. In S. G. Gabbe, J. R., Niebyl, J. L. Simpson, M. B. Landon, H. L. Galan, & D. A. Driscoll (Eds.), *Obstetrics: Normal and problem pregnancies* (6th ed., pp. 237–263). Philadelphia, PA: Saunders.

TABLE 9.4   Biophysical Profile Interpretation and Proposed Management Guidelines

Score	Interpretation	Risk for Stillbirth Within 1 Week Without Intervention	Management
10 of 10 8 of 10 (normal fluid) 8 of 8 (NST not done)	Risk of fetal asphyxia extremely rare	1 per 1000	Intervene for obstetric and maternal factors only No indication for intervention for fetal disease
8 of 10 (abnormal fluid)	Probable chronic fetal compromise	89 per 1000	Determine that there is functioning renal tissue and intact membranes; deliver for fetal indications
6 of 10 (normal fluid)	Equivocal test, possible fetal asphyxia	Variable	If fetus is mature, deliver If fetus is immature, repeat BPP within 24 hr If < 6 of 10, deliver
6 of 10 (abnormal fluid)	Probable fetal asphyxia	89 per 1000	Deliver for fetal indications
4 of 10	High probability of fetal asphyxia	91 per 1000	Deliver for fetal indications
2 of 10	Fetal asphyxia almost certain	125 per 1000	Deliver for fetal indications
0 of 10	Fetal asphyxia certain	600 per 1000	Deliver for fetal indications

is reactive and oligohydramnios is not observed. Abnormal MBPPs are either a nonreactive NST, oligohydramnios, or if both are present (ACOG, 2014a). Further testing is indicated if test results are abnormal.

Fetal Doppler Flow Ultrasound

Fetal Doppler flow ultrasound is an assessment of placental condition. This noninvasive procedure assesses hemodynamic components of vascular resistance in high-risk pregnancies with fetal growth restriction (ACOG, 2014a). Doppler flow is also used as an alternative to detect fetal anemia when Rh alloimmunization is suspected (Moise, 2017). This method of

fetal assessment measures cardiac cycle differences between peak-systolic and end-diastolic blood flow velocity, referred to as the *S/D ratio*, amount of blood flow resistance, and pulsatility index in various fetal vessels (ACOG, 2014a; O'Neil & Thorp, 2012). Color may be added to assist in assessing blood flow velocity (Fig. 9.19). The most common vessels are umbilical arteries, which allow for assessment of blood flow from the fetus to the placenta. Measurements also can be taken of the middle cerebral artery, umbilical veins, and ductus venosus (Kaimal, 2014; O'Neil & Thorp, 2012). More attention is being paid to middle cerebral artery measurements because of the shunting phenomenon. Again, hypoxic fetuses shunt

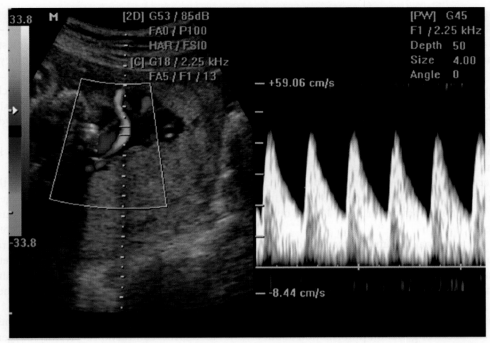

FIG. 9.19 Fetal Doppler flow ultrasound showing the umbilical artery with color. *Red* indicates that blood flow is going toward the transducer, and *blue* indicates blood flow going away from the transducer. The *white* peaks and valleys show a normal Doppler flow velocity. (From S. G. Gabbe, J. R. Niebyl, J. L. Simpson, et al. (Eds), *Obstetrics: Normal and Problem Pregnancies* (7th ed., p. 165). Philadelphia, PA: Elsevier.)

blood flow to the brain by reducing the amount of resistance in fetal cerebrovascular vessels. This allows for an increase in blood flow to the fetal brain.

Fetal Doppler flow ultrasound results are reported as normal, decreased, absent, or reversed. Fetuses that are not growth restricted will have normal high-velocity diastolic flow, whereas compromised fetuses may have decreased, absent, or reversed end-diastolic flow when deterioration occurs from an interruption in the oxygenation pathway. The sequence of events for abnormal Doppler flow starts with increased resistance in placental vasculature and is indicative of poor placental function. This leads to decreased diastolic velocities that eventually become absent. Once absent diastolic flow occurs, blood flow resistance continues to increase and an elastic component to fetal vasculature is added to this sequence of events. This causes reversed end-diastolic flow, and the placental circulation starts to recoil or "reverse" after being distended (Kaimal, 2014). Increased resistance occurs when approximately 30% of the fetal vasculature is abnormal (Morrow, Adamson, Bull, & Ritchie, 1989). Absent and reversed end-diastolic Doppler images are abnormal and have been linked to altered fetal acid-base status and poor perinatal outcomes including stillbirth (Kaimal, 2014; Miller et al., 2016; O'Neil & Thorp, 2012).

Patients with normal Doppler flow results are typically evaluated weekly. In the same week, an NST or MBPP may be requested. Increased frequency of Doppler examination and other adjuncts of fetal assessment occur when decreased, absent, or reversed flow is identified. As with other methods of APFT, Doppler results are interpreted in the context of the entire clinical scenario, including results of other surveillance methods to make pregnancy management decisions.

KNOWLEDGE CHECK

18. What are the four biophysical characteristics evaluated with ultrasound during a BPP and what do they reflect?
19. Why is amniotic fluid volume an important parameter in BPPs and MBPPs?
20. Describe the process of shunting in relationship to fetal oxygenation.

SUMMARY CONCEPTS

- There are two categories of prenatal testing. Screening detects or identifies individuals who are at risk for an abnormality or disease. Diagnostic testing identifies or confirms a diagnosis and is the most accurate test.
- First-trimester screenings incorporate maternal serum results of human chorionic gonadotropin and pregnancy-associated plasma protein-A with ultrasound nuchal translucency measurement to identify chromosomal anomalies. Nuchal translucency greater than 3.0 to 3.5 mm is associated with trisomy 21.
- Second-trimester multiple-marker screening is performed between 15 and 22 [67] weeks of gestation and is used to report a woman's risk for trisomy 21, trisomy 18, and open neural tube defects.
- Measurements of maternal serum human chorionic gonadotropin, alpha-fetoprotein, inhibin A, and unconjugated estriol 3 are calculated with gestational age, maternal weight, ethnicity, presence of diabetes, and number of fetuses.
- Chorionic villus sampling is an invasive procedure performed at 10 to 13 weeks of gestation. Information about chromosomal, metabolic, and genetic disorders is obtained from chorionic villus samples.
- Amniocentesis is an invasive procedure in which amniotic fluid is removed for prenatal diagnosis, fetal lung maturity status, and as a therapeutic measure for abnormal amniotic fluid volume.
- Amniocentesis is performed at 15 weeks of gestation and above.
- Ultrasound is widely used during pregnancy for a variety of indications to determine various fetal and placental conditions and as an adjunct to other fetal surveillance tests and procedures, such as amniocentesis.

- The primary goal of antepartum fetal testing is to decrease risk for permanent neurologic injury or stillbirth in high-risk pregnancies.
- Types of antepartum fetal testing include fetal movement counting, nonstress test, biophysical profile, modified biophysical profile, and fetal Doppler flow ultrasound.
- A simple evaluation tool for fetal well-being is maternal perception of fetal movement.
- Fetal activity becomes reduced when the fetus becomes hypoxic, to conserve energy and oxygen. If this occurs, women are advised to seek further evaluation.
- Accelerations in the fetal heart rate are a reflection of normal autonomic regulation and an intact central nervous system and is predictive of the absence of fetal metabolic acidemia.
- Nonstress tests are a form of antepartum fetal testing in which the presence or absence of fetal heart rate accelerations is assessed.
- Contraction stress tests evaluate fetal heart rate response to uterine contractions. Healthy oxygenated fetuses are able to tolerate temporary disruptions in oxygenation, whereas compromised fetuses will demonstrate fetal heart rate decelerations.
- Biophysical profiles assess fetal heart rate reactivity and four biophysical characteristics: fetal breathing movements, gross fetal movements, muscle tone, and amniotic fluid amount.
- A modified biophysical profile consists of a nonstress test and measurement of amniotic fluid volume.
- Fetal Doppler flow ultrasound is a method of measuring blood flow patterns in fetal circulation. Flow that is normal is associated with adequate fetal oxygenation. Absent or reversed flow is abnormal and is associated with a poor fetal prognosis.

REFERENCES & READINGS

American College of Obstetricians and Gynecologists (ACOG). (2014a). *Antepartum fetal surveillance (Practice Bulletin No.145)*. Washington, DC: Author.

American College of Obstetricians and Gynecologists (ACOG). (2014b). *Ultrasonography in pregnancy (Practice Bulletin No. 101)*. Washington, DC: Author.

American College of Obstetricians and Gynecologists (ACOG). (2015a). *Cell-free DNA screening for fetal aneuploidy*. Committee Opinion No. 640. Washington, DC: Author.

American College of Obstetricians and Gynecologists (ACOG). (2015b). *Induction of labor (Practice Bulletin No. 107)*. Washington, DC: Author.

American College of Obstetricians and Gynecologists (ACOG). (2016a). *Prenatal diagnostic testing for genetic disorders (Practice Bulletin 162)*. Washington, DC: Author.

American College of Obstetricians and Gynecologists (ACOG). (2016b). *Screening for fetal aneuploidy (Practice Bulletin 163)*. Washington, DC: Author.

Blackburn, S. T. (2013). *Maternal, fetal & neonatal physiology* (4th ed.). St. Louis, MO: Saunders.

Chard, R. L., & Norton, M. E. (2016). Genetic counseling for patients considering screening and diagnosis for chromosomal abnormalities. *Clinics in Laboratory Medicine, 36*(2), 227–236.

Clements, J. A., Platzker, A. C., Tierney, D. F., Hobel, C. J., Creasy, R. K., Margolis, A. J., & Oh, W. (1972). Assessment of the risk of the respiratory-distress syndrome by a rapid test for surfactant in amniotic fluid. *New England Journal of Medicine, 286*(20), 1077–1081.

Dar, P., Shani, H., & Evans, M. I. (2016). Cell-free DNA: comparison of technologies. *Clinics in Laboratory Medicine, 36*(2), 199.

Driscoll, D. A., Simpson, J. L., Holzgreve, W., & Otano, L. (2017). Genetic screening and prenatal diagnosis. In S. G. Gabbe, J. R. Niebyl, J. L. Simpson, M. B. Landon, H. L. Galan, E. R. M. Jauniaux, & W. A. Grobman (Eds.), *Obstetrics: normal and problem pregnancies* (7th ed.) (pp. 193–217). Philadelphia, PA: Elsevier.

Evans, M. I., Andriole, S., & Evans, S. M. (2015). Genetics: update on prenatal screening and diagnosis. *Obstetrics and Gynecology Clinics of North America, 42*(2), 193–208.

Freeman, R., Anderson, G., & Dorchester, W. (1982). A prospective multi-institutional study of antepartum fetal heart rate monitoring. II. CST vs NST for primary surveillance. *American Journal of Obstetrics and Gynecology, 143*(7), 771–777.

Freeman, R. K., Garite, T. J., Nageotte, M. P., & Miller, L. A. (2012). *Fetal heart rate monitoring*. Philadelphia, PA: Lippincott Williams & Wilkins.

Greenberg, M. B., & Druzin, M. L. (2017). Antepartum fetal evaluation. In S. G. Gabbe, J. R. Niebyl, J. L. Simpson, M. B. Landon, H. L. Galan, E. R. M. Jauniaux, & W. A. Grobman (Eds.), *Obstetrics: normal and problem pregnancies* (7th ed.) (pp. 219–243). Philadelphia, PA: Elsevier.

Gregg, A. R., Gross, S. J., Best, R. G., Monaghan, K. G., Bajaj, K., Skotko, B. G., Watson, M. S., et al. (2013). ACMG statement on noninvasive prenatal screening for fetal aneuploidy. *Genetics in Medicine, 15*(5), 395–398.

Kaimal, A. J. (2014). Assessment of fetal health. In R. K. Creasy, R. Resnik, J. D. Iams, et al. (Eds.), *Maternal-fetal medicine principles and practice* (7th ed.) (pp. 473–487). Philadelphia: Elsevier.

Kuppermann, M., Pena, S., Bishop, J. T., Nakagawa, S., Gregorich, S. E., Sit, A., & Norton, M. E. (2014). Effect of enhanced information, values clarification, and removal of financial barriers on use of prenatal genetic testing: a randomized clinical trial. *Journal of the American Medical Association, AMA, 312*(12), 1210–1217.

Macones, G. A., Hankins, G. D., Spong, C. Y., Hauth, J., & Moore, T. (2008). The 2008 National Institute of Child Health and Human Development workshop report on electronic fetal monitoring: update on definitions, interpretation, and research guidelines. *Journal of Obstetric, Gynecologic, & Neonatal Nursing, 37*(5), 510–515.

Malone, F. D. (2008). First trimester screening for aneuploidy. In P. W. Callen (Ed.), *Ultrasonography in obstetrics and gynecology* (5th ed.) (pp. 60–69). Philadelphia, PA: Saunders.

Manning, F. A. (1995). Dynamic ultrasound-based fetal assessment: the fetal biophysical profile score. *Clinical Obstetrics and Gynecology, 38*(1), 26–44.

Manning, F. A., Platt, L. D., & Sipos, L. (1980). Antepartum fetal evaluation: development of a fetal biophysical profile. *American Journal of Obstetrics and Gynecology, 136*(6), 787–795.

Miller, L. A., Miller, D. A., & Cypher, R. L. (2016). *Mosby's pocket guide to fetal monitoring: a multidisciplinary approach*. St Louis, MO: Elsevier.

Moise, K. J. (2017). Red cell alloimmunization. In S. G. Gabbe, J. R. Niebyl, J. L. Simpson, M. B. Landon, H. L. Galan, E. R. M. Jauniaux, & W. A. Grobman (Eds.), *Obstetrics: normal and problem pregnancies* (7th ed.) (pp. 770–785). Philadelphia, PA: Elsevier.

Morrow, R. J., Adamson, S. L., Bull, S. B., & Ritchie, J. K. (1989). Effect of placental embolization on the umbilical arterial velocity waveform in fetal sheep. *American Journal of Obstetrics and Gynecology, 161*(4), 1055–1060.

National Institute of Neurological Disorders and Stroke, National Institute of Health. (2015). *Spina Bifida Fact Sheet (NIH Publication No. 13-309)*. Retrieved from www.ninds.nih.gov/disorders/spina_bifida/detail_spina_bifida.htm#3258_10.

Neerhof, M. G., Haney, E. I., Silver, R. K., Ashwood, E. R., Lee, I. S., & Piazze, J. J. (2001). Lamellar body counts compared with traditional phospholipid analysis as an assay for evaluating fetal lung maturity. *Obstetrics & Gynecology, 97*(2), 305–309.

Norton, M. E., & Rink, B. D. (2016). Changing indications for invasive testing in an era of improved screening. *Seminars in Perinatology, 40*(1), 56–66.

O'Neill, E. R., & Thorp, J. (2012). Antepartum evaluation of the fetus and fetal well-being. *Clinical Obstetrics and Gynecology, 55*(3), 722–730.

Raju, T. N., Mercer, B. M., Burchfield, D. J., & Joseph, G. F. (2014). Periviable birth: Executive summary of a joint workshop by the Eunice Kennedy Shriver National Institute of Child Health and Human Development, Society for Maternal-Fetal Medicine, American Academy of Pediatrics, and American College of Obstetricians and Gynecologists. *American Journal of Obstetrics and Gynecology, 210*(5), 406–417.

Read, J. A., & Miller, F. C. (1977). Fetal heart rate acceleration in response to acoustic stimulation as a measure of fetal well-being. *American Journal of Obstetrics and Gynecology, 129*(5), 512–517.

Richards, D. S. (2017). In S. G. Gabbe, J. R. Niebyl, J. L. Simpson, M. B. Landon, H. L. Galan, E. R. M. Jauniaux, & W. A. Grobman (Eds.), *Obstetrics: normal and problem pregnancies* (7th ed.) (pp. 160–192). Philadelphia, PA: Elsevier.

Salomon, L. J., Alfirevic, Z., Berghella, V., Bilardo, C., Hernandez-Andrade, E., Johnsen, S. L., & Prefumo, F. (2011). Practice guidelines for performance of the routine mid-trimester fetal ultrasound scan. *Ultrasound in Obstetrics & Gynecology, 37*(1), 116–126.

Signore, C., Freeman, R. K., & Spong, C. Y. (2009). Antenatal testing: a reevaluation: executive summary of a Eunice Kennedy Shriver National Institute of Child Health and Human Development workshop. *Obstetrics and Gynecology, 113*(3), 687–701.

Verpoest, M. J., Seelen, J. C., & Westerman, C. F. (1976). Changes in appearance of amniotic fluid during pregnancy: the macroscore. *Journal of Perinatal Medicine-Official Journal of the WAPM, 4*(1), 12–25.

Vintzileos, A. M., & Knuppel, R. A. (1994). Multiple parameter biophysical testing in the prediction of fetal acid-base status. *Clinics in Perinatology, 21*(4), 823–848.

Walker, D., Grimwade, J., & Wood, C. (1971). Intrauterine noise: a component of the fetal environment. *American Journal of Obstetrics and Gynecology, 109*(1), 92–95.

Wapner, R. J. (2014). Prenatal diagnosis of congenital disorders. In R. K. Creasy, R. Resnik, J. D. Iams, et al. (Eds.), *Maternal-fetal medicine: principles and practice* (7th ed.) (pp. 417–464). Philadelphia, PA: Saunders.

Wax, J., Minkoff, H., Johnson, A., Coleman, B., Levine, D., Helfgott, A., & Benson, C. (2014). Consensus report on the detailed fetal anatomic ultrasound examination indications, components, and qualifications. *Journal of Ultrasound in Medicine, 33*(2), 189–195.

10

Complications of Pregnancy

Kristin L. Scheffer, Renee Jones, Karen S. Holub, Jessica L. McNeil

OBJECTIVES

After studying this chapter, you should be able to:

1. Describe the development and management of hemorrhagic conditions of early pregnancy, including spontaneous abortion, ectopic pregnancy, and gestational trophoblastic disease.
2. Explain physiology and management of placenta previa and placental abruption.
3. Discuss the effects and management of hyperemesis gravidarum.
4. Describe the development and management of hypertensive disorders of pregnancy.
5. Compare Rh and ABO incompatibility in terms of etiology, fetal and neonatal complications, and management.
6. Describe the effects of pregnancy on glucose metabolism.
7. Discuss the effects and management of preexisting diabetes mellitus during pregnancy.
8. Explain the physiology and management of gestational diabetes mellitus.
9. Describe the major effects of pregnancy on the woman who has heart disease and identify the goals of therapy.
10. Describe the effects of obesity during pregnancy.
11. Explain the maternal and fetal effects of specific anemias and the required management during pregnancy.
12. Identify the effects, management, and nursing considerations of specific preexisting immune complex and neurologic conditions discussed in this chapter.
13. Discuss the maternal, fetal, and neonatal effects of the most common infections that may occur during pregnancy.
14. Explain nursing considerations for each complication of pregnancy.

Although childbearing is usually a normal process, complications may arise threatening the well-being of the woman, the fetus, or both. Conditions that complicate pregnancy are divided into two broad categories: (1) those related to pregnancy and not seen at other times and (2) those that could occur at any time, but when they occur concurrently with pregnancy may complicate its course.

The most common pregnancy-related complications are hemorrhagic conditions that occur in early pregnancy, hemorrhagic complications of the placenta in late pregnancy, hyperemesis gravidarum (HEG), hypertensive disorders of pregnancy, and blood incompatibilities. Concurrent conditions include diabetes mellitus, cardiac disease, obesity, anemias, immune complex disorders, neurologic disorders, and infections.

PREGNANCY COMPLICATIONS

HEMORRHAGIC CONDITIONS OF EARLY PREGNANCY

The three most common causes of hemorrhage during the first half of pregnancy are abortion, ectopic pregnancy, and gestational trophoblastic disease.

Abortion

Abortion is the loss of pregnancy before the fetus is viable, or capable of living outside the uterus. The medical consensus today is that a fetus of less than 20 weeks of gestation or one weighing less than 500 grams (g) is not viable (Cunningham et al., 2014). Ending of pregnancy before this time is considered an abortion. Abortion may be either spontaneous or induced. *Abortion* is an accepted medical term for either a spontaneous or an induced ending of pregnancy, although the lay term *miscarriage* is sometimes used to denote spontaneous abortion. Elective termination of pregnancy, or induced abortion, is described in Chapter 27.

Spontaneous Abortion

Spontaneous abortion is a termination of pregnancy without action taken by the woman or another person.

Incidence and Etiology. Determining the exact incidence of spontaneous abortion is difficult because many unrecognized losses occur in early pregnancy, but it averages approximately 18% to 31% with any pregnancy (Blackburn, 2013). Most pregnancies (50% to 70%) are lost during the first trimester; many of these may occur before implantation or during the first month after the last menstrual period (Blackburn,

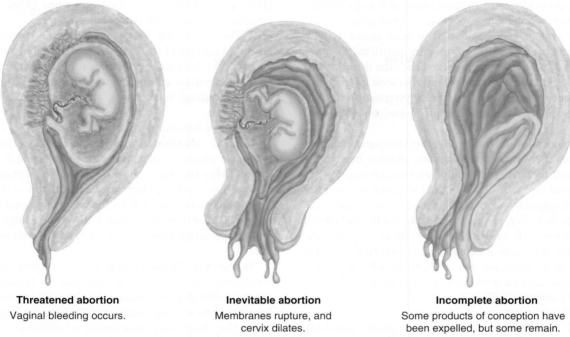

Threatened abortion	**Inevitable abortion**	**Incomplete abortion**
Vaginal bleeding occurs.	Membranes rupture, and cervix dilates.	Some products of conception have been expelled, but some remain.

FIG. 10.1 Three types of spontaneous abortion, also called *miscarriage*.

2013). The incidence of spontaneous abortion increases with parental age. The incidence is 12% for women younger than 20 years, rising to 26% for women older than 40 years. At a maternal age of 45 years, abortion risk is greater than 50%, about double the risk at 40 years. Paternal age younger than 20 years is associated with a spontaneous abortion rate of 12%, rising to 20% for fathers older than 40 years (Blackburn, 2013). About 80% of spontaneous abortions occur in the first 12 weeks of pregnancy, with the rate declining rapidly thereafter (Blackburn, 2013; Cunningham et al., 2014; Simpson & Jauniaux, 2017).

The most common cause of spontaneous abortion is severe congenital abnormalities that are often incompatible with life. Chromosomal abnormalities account for approximately 50% to 60% of spontaneous abortions within the first 12 weeks. Embryonic causes such as monosomy X (45,X) or autosomal trisomy contribute to chromosomal abnormalities. Another chromosomal abnormality is anembryonic (no embryo) or a "blighted ovum" causing a spontaneous abortion.

Additional causes include maternal infections such as syphilis, listeriosis, toxoplasmosis, brucellosis, rubella, cytomegalic virus, and periodontal disease and maternal endocrine disorders such as hypothyroidism, diabetes, and decreased progesterone. Other causes are related to inherited thrombophilias (factor V Leiden). Anatomic defects of the uterus, uterine septum, or cervical incompetence may contribute to pregnancy loss at any gestational age (Berghella & Iams, 2014). Finally, heavy alcohol consumption and heavy smoking may play a role in spontaneous abortion (Cunningham et al., 2014; Simpson & Jauniaux, 2017).

Spontaneous abortion is divided into six subgroups: threatened, inevitable, incomplete, complete, missed, and recurrent. Fig. 10.1 illustrates threatened, inevitable, and incomplete abortions.

Threatened Abortion

Clinical Manifestations. The first sign of threatened abortion is vaginal bleeding, which is rather common during early pregnancy. Approximately 25% of pregnant women experience "spotting" or bleeding in early pregnancy, and up to 50% of these pregnancies end in spontaneous abortion (Blackburn, 2013). Vaginal bleeding, which may be brief or last for weeks, may be accompanied by uterine cramping, persistent backache, or feelings of pelvic pressure. These added symptoms are more likely to be associated with loss of pregnancy.

Therapeutic Management. Bleeding during the first half of pregnancy should be considered a threatened abortion, and women should be advised to notify their physician or nurse-midwife if brownish or red vaginal bleeding is noted. When a woman reports bleeding in early pregnancy, the nurse obtains a detailed history that includes length of gestation (or first day of her last menstrual period) and the onset, duration, amount and color of vaginal bleeding. Any accompanying discomfort such as cramping, backache, or abdominal pain also is noted.

Ultrasound examination is performed to determine whether an embryo or fetus is present and alive, and if so, the approximate gestational age. Maternal serum beta-hCG and progesterone levels provide added information about the viability of the pregnancy (i.e., whether the levels are appropriate for gestation period and increase with fetal growth).

There is no evidence to support physical activity restrictions to stop spontaneous abortion (Cunningham et al., 2014). The woman may be advised to limit sexual activity until bleeding has ceased. The woman is instructed to count the number of perineal pads used and note the quantity and color of blood on the pads. She should also look for evidence of tissue passage, which would indicate progression beyond a threatened abortion. Drainage with a foul odor suggests infection.

Bleeding episodes are frightening, so psychological support is important. The woman often wonders whether her actions may have contributed to the situation and is anxious about her own condition and that of the fetus. The nurse should offer accurate information and avoid false reassurance because the woman may lose her pregnancy despite every precaution. Later problems such as prematurity, a small-for-gestational-age infant, abnormal presentation, or perinatal asphyxia may occur in pregnancies that do not end with a spontaneous abortion after early bleeding (Cunningham et al., 2014; Simpson & Jauniaux, 2017).

Inevitable Abortion

Clinical Manifestations. Abortion is usually inevitable (i.e., it cannot be stopped) when membranes rupture and the cervix dilates. Rupture of membranes generally is experienced as a loss of fluid from the vagina and subsequent uterine contractions and active bleeding. Incomplete evacuation of the products of conception can result in excessive bleeding or infection.

Therapeutic Management. Natural expulsion of uterine contents is common in inevitable abortion. **Vacuum curettage** (removal of uterine contents with a vacuum curet) is used to clear the uterus if the natural process is ineffective or incomplete. If the pregnancy is more advanced or if bleeding is excessive, a **dilation and curettage (D&C)** (stretching the cervical os to permit scraping the uterine walls) may be needed. Intravenous (IV) sedation or other anesthesia provides pain management for the procedure.

Incomplete Abortion

Clinical Manifestations. Incomplete abortion occurs when some but not all of the products of conception are expelled from the uterus. The major manifestations are active uterine bleeding and severe abdominal cramping. The cervix is open, and some fetal and/or placental tissues are passed.

Therapeutic Management. Retained tissue prevents the uterus from contracting firmly, thereby allowing excessive bleeding from uterine blood vessels. Initial treatment should focus on stabilizing the woman's cardiovascular state. A blood specimen is drawn for blood type and screen or crossmatch, and an IV line is inserted for fluid replacement and drug administration. When the woman's condition is stable, a D&C usually is performed to remove the remaining tissue. If the bleeding is later in pregnancy when the fetal tissue is larger, a greater cervical **dilation and evacuation (D&E)**, followed by vacuum or surgical curettage, is required. This procedure may be followed by IV administration of oxytocin (Pitocin) or intramuscular (IM) administration of methylergonovine (Methergine) to contract the uterus and control bleeding.

A D&C may not be performed if the pregnancy has advanced beyond 14 weeks because of the danger of excessive bleeding. In this case, oxytocin or prostaglandin is administered to stimulate uterine contractions until all products of conception (fetus, membranes, placenta, and amniotic fluid) are expelled.

Complete Abortion

Clinical Manifestations. Complete abortion occurs when all products of conception are expelled from the uterus. After passage of all products of conception, uterine contractions and bleeding subside and the cervix closes. The uterus feels smaller than the length of gestation would suggest. The symptoms of pregnancy are no longer present, and the pregnancy test becomes negative as hormone levels fall.

Therapeutic Management. Once complete abortion is confirmed, no additional intervention is required unless excessive bleeding or infection develops. The woman should be advised to rest and watch for further bleeding, pain, or fever. She should not have sexual intercourse until after a follow-up visit with her health care provider. Contraception is discussed at the follow-up visit if she wishes to prevent pregnancy.

Missed Abortion

Clinical Manifestations. Missed abortion occurs when the fetus dies during the first half of pregnancy but is retained in the uterus. When the fetus dies, the early symptoms of pregnancy (nausea, breast tenderness, urinary frequency) disappear. The uterus stops growing and decreases in size, reflecting the absorption of amniotic fluid and **maceration** (discoloration, softening, and eventual tissue degeneration) of the fetus. Vaginal bleeding of a red or brownish color may or may not occur.

Therapeutic Management. An ultrasound examination confirms fetal death by identifying a gestational sac or fetus that is too small for the presumed gestational age. No fetal heart activity can be found. Pregnancy tests for hCG show a decline in placental hormone production.

In most cases, the contents of the uterus would be expelled spontaneously, but this is emotionally difficult once the woman knows her fetus is not alive. Therefore her uterus usually is emptied by the most appropriate method for the size when the diagnosis of missed abortion is made. For a first-trimester missed abortion, a D&C usually can be done. If the missed abortion occurs during the second trimester, when the fetus is larger, a D&E may be done, or vaginal prostaglandin E_2 (PGE$_2$) or misoprostol (Cytotec) may be needed to induce uterine contractions that expel the fetus. A D&C may be needed to remove the placenta.

Two major complications of missed abortion are infection and disseminated intravascular coagulation (DIC). Signs such as elevation in temperature, vaginal discharge with a foul odor, and abdominal pain indicate uterine infection. Cultures are obtained, antimicrobial therapy is initiated, and the uterus is evacuated.

Recurrent Spontaneous Abortion

Clinical Manifestations. *Recurrent spontaneous abortion* usually is defined as three or more spontaneous abortions, although some authorities now use two or more pregnancy losses as the definition. The primary causes of recurrent abortion are believed to be genetic or chromosomal abnormalities and anomalies of the reproductive tract, such as **bicornuate** uterus (uterus with two horns) or incompetent cervix. Additional causes include an inadequate luteal phase with insufficient secretion of progesterone and immunologic factors that involve increased sharing of human leukocyte antigens by the sperm of the man and the ovum of the woman who conceived. The theory is that because of this sharing, the woman's immunologic system is not stimulated to produce blocking antibodies that protect the embryo from maternal immune cells or other damaging antibodies. Systemic diseases such as systemic lupus erythematosus and diabetes mellitus have been implicated in recurrent abortions. Reproductive infections and some sexually transmitted diseases (STDs) are also associated with recurrent abortions (Cunningham et al., 2014)

Therapeutic Management. The first step in management of recurrent spontaneous abortion is examination of the reproductive system to determine whether anatomic defects are the cause. If the cervix and uterus are normal, the woman and her partner are usually referred for genetic screening to identify chromosomal factors that would increase the possibility of recurrent abortions.

Additional therapeutic management of recurrent pregnancy loss depends on the cause. For instance, treatment may involve assisting the woman to develop a regimen to maintain normal blood glucose level if diabetes mellitus is a factor. Supplemental hormones may be given if her progesterone or other hormone levels are lower than normal. Antimicrobials are prescribed for the woman with infection, or hormone-related drugs may be prescribed if imbalance preventing normal fetal implantation and support is found.

Recurrent spontaneous abortion may be caused by **cervical incompetence**, also called **cervical insufficiency**, an anatomic defect that results in painless dilation of the cervix in the second trimester. In this situation, a **cerclage** procedure—suturing of the cervix to prevent early dilation—may be performed. The cerclage is most likely to be successful if done before much cervical dilation or bulging of the membranes through the cervix has occurred. Sutures may be removed near term in preparation for vaginal delivery, or they may be left in place if a cesarean birth is planned. Prophylactic antibiotics are ordered if the woman is at increased risk for infection. Preterm labor may still occur after the fetus is viable.

Rh immune globulin (RhoGAM) is given to the unsensitized Rho(D)-negative woman to prevent development of anti-Rh antibodies. A microdose (50 mcg) is given to the woman whose fetus is less than 13 weeks of gestational age at the time of the abortion.

Nursing Considerations. Nurses should consider the psychological needs of the woman experiencing spontaneous abortion. Vaginal bleeding is frightening, and waiting and watching are often difficult (although possibly the only treatment recommended). Many women and their families feel an acute sense of loss and grief with spontaneous abortion. Grief often includes feelings of guilt and speculation about whether the woman could have done something to prevent the loss. Nurses may help by emphasizing that abortions usually occur as the result of factors or abnormalities that cannot be avoided.

Anger, disappointment, and sadness are commonly experienced emotions, although the intensity of these feelings may vary. For many people, the fetus has not yet taken on specific physical characteristics, but they grieve for their fantasies of the unseen, unborn child. Recognizing the meaning of the loss to each woman and her significant others is important. Nurses should listen carefully to what the woman says and observe how she behaves. The woman or the couple may want to express their sadness but may think that family, friends, and often health care personnel are uncomfortable or diminish their loss. Nurses should convey their acceptance of the feelings expressed or demonstrated by the couple. Providing information and simple brief explanations of what has occurred and what will be done facilitates the family's ability to grieve.

The family should realize that grief may last up to 18 months. Many hospitals have grief support programs that families may attend for 12 weeks or as needed to assist with the grief process. Family support, knowledge of the grief process, spiritual counselors, and support from other bereaved couples may provide needed assistance during this time.

> **? KNOWLEDGE CHECK**
> 1. What are the signs of threatened abortion, and how do they differ from those of inevitable abortion?
> 2. What are the major causes of recurrent spontaneous abortion?
> 3. What interventions can nurses provide for families experiencing grief as a result of early pregnancy loss?

Ectopic Pregnancy

Ectopic pregnancy is an implantation of a fertilized ovum in an area outside the uterine cavity. Although implantation can occur in the abdomen or cervix, 97% of ectopic pregnancies occur in the fallopian tube (Cunningham et al., 2014). Fig. 10.2 shows the common sites of ectopic implantation.

Ectopic pregnancy has been called "a disaster of reproduction" despite our greater ability to recognize its occurrence. Ectopic pregnancy remains a significant cause of maternal death from hemorrhage. Tubal damage caused by an ectopic pregnancy reduces the woman's chances of subsequent pregnancies.

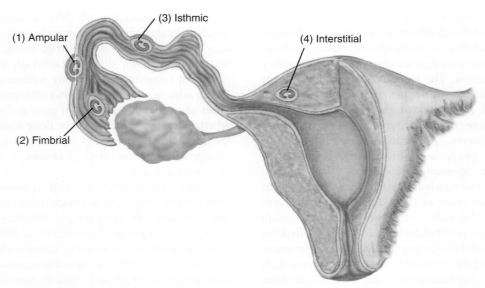

(3) Isthmic

(1) Ampular

(4) Interstitial

(2) Fimbrial

FIG 10.2 **Sites of Tubal Ectopic Pregnancy.** Numbers indicate the order of prevalence.

Incidence and Etiology

A common factor for the development of ectopic pregnancy in the fallopian tube is scarring of the fallopian tubes because of pelvic infection, inflammation, or surgery. Pelvic infection often is caused by *Chlamydia* or *Neisseria gonorrhoeae*. A failed tubal ligation, even if performed many years ago, and a history of previous ectopic pregnancy also increase the risk for an ectopic pregnancy in the fallopian tube. Greater incidences of ectopic pregnancies occur in women who conceived with assisted reproduction, most likely related to the tubal factors that contributed to infertility. Contraception such as intrauterine contraceptive devices or low-dose progesterone agents are associated with increased risk for ectopic pregnancy. (Cunningham et al., 2014).

Additional causes of ectopic pregnancy are delayed or premature ovulation, with the tendency of the fertilized ovum to implant before arrival in the uterus, and altered tubal motility in response to changes in estrogen and progesterone levels that occur with conception. Multiple induced abortions increase the risk for tubal pregnancy, possibly because of salpingitis (infection of the fallopian tube) that occurred after induced abortion (Box 10.1). Regardless of the cause of tubal pregnancy, the effect is that transport of the fertilized ovum through the fallopian tube is hampered.

Clinical Manifestations

The classic signs of ectopic pregnancy include the following:
- Missed menstrual period
- Positive pregnancy test
- Abdominal pain
- Vaginal "spotting"

More subtle signs and symptoms depend on the site of implantation. If implantation occurs in the distal end of the fallopian tube, which can contain the growing embryo longer, the woman may at first exhibit the usual early signs of pregnancy and consider herself to be normally pregnant. Several

| BOX 10.1 | **Risk Factors for Ectopic Pregnancy** |

History of previous ectopic pregnancies
Peak age-specific incidence 25 to 34 years
History of sexually transmitted diseases (gonorrhea, chlamydia)
Multiple sexual partners
Tubal sterilization and tubal reconstruction
Infertility
Assisted reproductive techniques such as gamete intrafallopian transfer
Intrauterine device
Multiple induced abortions

weeks into the pregnancy, intermittent abdominal pain and small amounts of vaginal bleeding occur, and initially this could be mistaken for threatened abortion. Because routine ultrasound examination in early pregnancy is common, however, it is not unusual to diagnose an ectopic pregnancy before onset of symptoms.

If implantation has occurred in the proximal end of the fallopian tube, rupture of the tube may occur within 2 to 3 weeks of the missed period because the tube is narrow in this area. Symptoms include sudden severe pain in one of the lower quadrants of the abdomen as the tube tears open and the embryo is expelled into the pelvic cavity, often with profuse abdominal hemorrhage. Radiating pain under the scapula may indicate bleeding into the abdomen caused by phrenic nerve irritation. **Hypovolemic shock** (acute peripheral circulatory failure from loss of circulating blood) is a major concern because systemic signs of shock may be rapid and extensive without external bleeding.

Diagnosis

The combined use of transvaginal ultrasound examination and determination of beta-hCG usually results in early detection of ectopic pregnancy. An abnormal pregnancy is suspected if beta-hCG is present but at lower levels than expected. If a gestational sac cannot be visualized when beta-hCG is present, a diagnosis of ectopic pregnancy may be made with great accuracy. Visualization of an intra-uterine pregnancy, however, does not absolutely rule out an ectopic pregnancy. A woman may have an intrauterine pregnancy and concurrently have an ectopic pregnancy. **Laparoscopy** (examination of the peritoneal cavity by means of a laparoscope) occasionally may be necessary to diagnose rupture of an ectopic pregnancy. A character-istic bluish swelling within the tube is the most common finding.

Therapeutic Management

Management of tubal pregnancy depends on whether the tube is intact or ruptured.

Medical management with methotrexate may be an option to surgery in the woman with an early ectopic preg-nancy if the tube is unruptured (Cunningham et al., 2014; Nelson & Gambone, 2016). The goal of medical manage-ment is to preserve the tube and improve the chance of future fertility. Methotrexate, a chemotherapeutic agent, is a folic acid antagonist that inhibits cell replication and therefore targets rapidly dividing cells, such as the tropho-blastic cells in early pregnancy. It is approximately 90% effective in treating ectopic tubal pregnancy (Cunningham et al., 2014). Successful medical management is associated with small ectopic size, low initial serum beta-hCG levels, and absent fetal cardiac activity (Cunningham et al., 2014; Nelson & Gambone, 2016). It may be given in a single dose or multiple dose protocol (Cunningham et al., 2014; Nelson & Gambone, 2016). The multiple dose protocol may be more successful, but the single dose protocol is less complex, is less expensive, and does not require as much follow-up as the multiple dose protocol (Cunningham et al., 2014). The single dose protocol calls for 50 mg/m^2 of body surface area. Follow-up hCG levels are required on days 4 and 7 and then weekly until hCG is not detectable in the woman's blood (Nelson & Gambone, 2016).

Surgical management of a tubal pregnancy that is unrup-tured may involve a **linear salpingostomy**, removal of the ectopic pregnancy from the tube in an effort to salvage the tube or a **salpingectomy**—removal of the tube. Salvaging the tube is particularly important to women concerned about future fertility, although the same cause may affect both tubes.

When ectopic pregnancy results in rupture of the fallopian tube, the goal of therapeutic management is to control the bleeding and prevent hypovolemic shock. Ruptured ectopic pregnancy is a major emergency (Blackburn, 2013). When the woman's cardiovascular status is stable, salpingectomy with ligation of bleeding vessels may be required.

Nursing Considerations

Nursing care focuses on prevention or early identification of hypovolemic shock, pain control, and psychological support for the woman who experiences ectopic pregnancy. Nurses monitor the woman for signs and symptoms that suggest tubal rupture or bleeding (e.g., pelvic, shoulder, or neck pain; dizziness or faintness; increased vaginal bleeding). Nurses administer ordered analgesics and evaluate their effectiveness so pain can be adequately controlled. The nurse administers Rh immune globulin to Rho(D)-negative women.

If the plan of care includes methotrexate, the nurse should be aware that methotrexate is a chemotherapeutic agent. Facility protocols for chemotherapy should be followed, including appropriate personal protective equipment (dou-ble glove) and verification of patient name, medication, and dosage by another nurse. Air should not be expelled from the syringe, because it could aerosolize the medication. The woman should be taught that her urine is considered toxic for 72 hours. She should be careful to avoid getting urine on the toilet seat. The toilet should be flushed twice with the lid closed when she voids. Additional patient teaching includes adverse side effects such as nausea and vomiting and the importance of informing the health care team of any physical changes. Transient abdominal pain occurs during methotrex-ate therapy, probably because of expulsion of the products of conception from the tube. The woman also should be instructed to refrain from drinking alcohol (which decreases the effectiveness of methotrexate), taking vitamins that con-tain folic acid, using nonsteroidal antiinflammatory drugs, and having sexual intercourse until beta-hCG is not detect-able in her blood. If the treatment is successful, this hormone disappears from plasma within 2 to 3 weeks. Maintaining fol-low-up appointments is essential to identify whether the hCG titer becomes negative and remains negative (Cunningham et al., 2014). Continued presence of hCG in the serum requires follow-up to identify whether the ectopic pregnancy is still present (Cunningham et al., 2014).

The woman and her family will need psychological sup-port to deal with intense emotions that may include anger, grief, guilt, and self-blame. The woman also may be anxious about her ability to become pregnant in the future. Because ectopic pregnancy may occur when a woman has undergone an assisted reproductive procedure, she may be more anx-ious about when she might become pregnant again and if similar risks exist for another pregnancy. The nurse should clarify the physician's explanation and use therapeutic com-munication techniques that assist the woman to deal with her anxiety.

Gestational Trophoblastic Disease (Hydatidiform Mole)

Hydatidiform mole is one form of **gestational trophoblastic disease**, which occurs when trophoblasts (peripheral cells that attach the fertilized ovum to the uterine wall) develop abnor-mally (Cohn, Ramaswamy, & Blum, 2014; Cunningham, 2014; DiGiuglio, Weidaseck & Monchek, 2012). The placenta does not develop normally and, if a fetus is present, there will be a fatal chromosome defect. Gestational trophoblastic disease is char-acterized by proliferation and edema of the chorionic villi. The fluid-filled villi form grapelike clusters of tissue that can rapidly grow large enough to fill the uterus to the size of an advanced pregnancy. The mole may be complete, with no fetus present, or partial, in which fetal tissue or membranes are present.

Incidence and Etiology

In the United States and Europe, the incidence of hydatidiform mole is 1 in every 1000 to 1500 pregnancies (Cohn et al., 2014; DiGiuglio et al., 2012). Age is a factor, with the frequency of molar pregnancies highest at both ends of reproductive life. The incidence is higher among Asian women. Women who have had one molar pregnancy have a greater risk to have another in a subsequent pregnancy (Cunningham et al., 2014; Salani & Copeland, 2017). Persistent gestational trophoblastic disease may undergo malignant change (choriocarcinoma) and may metastasize to sites such as the lung, vagina, liver, and brain.

Complete mole is thought to occur when the ovum is fertilized by a sperm that duplicates its own chromosomes and the maternal chromosomes in the ovum are inactivated. In a partial mole, the maternal contribution is usually present, but the paternal contribution is doubled, and therefore the karyotype is triploid (69,XXY or 69,XYY). If a fetus is identified with the partial mole, it is grossly abnormal because of the abnormal chromosomal composition.

Clinical Manifestations

Routine use of ultrasound allows earlier diagnosis of hydatidiform mole, usually before the more severe manifestations of the disorder develop. Possible signs and symptoms of molar pregnancy include the following:

- Higher levels of beta-hCG than expected for gestation
- Characteristic "snowstorm" ultrasound pattern that shows the vesicles and the absence of a fetal sac or fetal heart activity in a complete molar pregnancy
- A uterus that is larger than expected for gestational age
- Vaginal bleeding, which varies from dark-brown spotting to profuse hemorrhage
- Excessive nausea and vomiting or hyperemesis gravidarum (HEG) may be related to high levels of beta-hCG from the proliferating trophoblasts
- Early development of preeclampsia before 24 weeks gestation in an otherwise normal pregnancy

Diagnosis

Measurement of beta-hCG levels detects the abnormally high levels of the hormone before treatment. After treatment, beta-hCG levels are measured to determine whether they fall and then disappear.

In addition to the characteristic pattern showing the vesicles, ultrasound examination allows a differential diagnosis to be made between two types of molar pregnancies: (1) a partial mole that includes some fetal tissue and membranes and (2) a complete mole that is composed only of enlarged villi but contains no fetal tissue or membranes.

Therapeutic Management

Medical management includes two phases: (1) evacuation of the trophoblastic tissue of the mole and (2) continuous follow-up of the woman to detect malignant changes of any remaining trophoblastic tissue. At the same time, the woman is treated for any other problems such as preeclampsia or hyperemesis gravidarum (HEG).

Before evacuation, chest radiography, computed tomography (CT), or magnetic resonance imaging (MRI) may be performed to detect metastatic disease. A complete blood count, laboratory assessment of coagulation status, and blood type screening or crossmatching are also necessary in case a transfusion is needed. Blood chemistry examinations are done to evaluate renal, hepatic, and thyroid function.

The mole usually is removed by vacuum aspiration followed by curettage. After tissue removal, IV oxytocin is given to contract the uterus. Avoiding uterine stimulation with oxytocin before evacuation is important. Uterine contractions can cause trophoblastic tissue to be pulled into the large venous sinusoids in the uterus, resulting in embolization of the tissue and respiratory distress (Salani & Copeland., 2017). The tissue obtained is sent for laboratory evaluation. Although a hydatidiform mole is usually a benign process, choriocarcinoma may occur (Cohn et al., 2014).

Follow-up is critical to detect changes suggestive of trophoblastic malignancy (Cohn et al., 2014). Beta-hCG is repeated at 6 weeks postpartum. Follow-up protocol involves evaluation of serum beta-hCG levels monthly for 6 months, then every 2 to 3 months for 6 months until normal for three values. A persistent or rising beta-hCG level suggests continued gestational trophoblastic disease. Pregnancy must be avoided during the follow-up because the normal rise of beta-hCG level in pregnancy would obscure evidence of choriocarcinoma (Cohn et al., 2014).

Nursing Considerations

Bleeding is a possible complication with a molar pregnancy, but emotional care of the woman is also essential. Women who have had a hydatidiform mole experience emotions similar to those of women who have experienced any other type of pregnancy loss. In addition, they may be anxious about follow-up evaluations, the possibility of malignant change, and the need to delay pregnancy for at least 1 year (DiGiuglio et al., 2012).

❓ KNOWLEDGE CHECK

4. Why is ectopic pregnancy sometimes called a "disaster of reproduction"?
5. Why is the incidence of ectopic pregnancy increasing in the United States? How is ectopic pregnancy treated?
6. What is a hydatidiform mole, and why are two phases of treatment necessary?

◆ APPLICATION OF THE NURSING PROCESS: HEMORRHAGIC CONDITIONS OF EARLY PREGNANCY

Regardless of the cause of early antepartum bleeding, nurses play a vital role in its management. Nurses are responsible for monitoring the condition of the pregnant woman and for collaborating with the physician to provide treatment.

◆ Assessment

Confirmation of pregnancy and length of gestation are important initial data to obtain. Physical assessment focuses on determining the amount of bleeding and the description, location, and severity of pain. Estimate the amount of vaginal bleeding by examining the linen and peripads. If necessary, accurately assess the bleeding by weighing the linen and peripads (1 g weight equals 1 mL volume).

When asking a woman how much blood she lost at home, ask her to compare the amount lost with a common liquid measure such as a tablespoon or a cup. Ask also how long the bleeding episode lasted and what was done to control the bleeding.

🔆 CRITICAL THINKING EXERCISE 10.1

All women who have experienced prenatal bleeding and invasive procedures are at increased risk for infection.

Question

1. What common assumptions do nurses make about those who are at risk for developing infections?

Bleeding may be accompanied by pain. Uterine cramping usually accompanies spontaneous abortion; deep, severe pelvic pain is associated with ruptured ectopic pregnancy. In ruptured ectopic pregnancy, bleeding may be concealed and pain could be the only symptom.

The woman's vital signs and urine output give a clue to her cardiovascular status. A rising pulse rate and respiratory rate and falling urine output are associated with hypovolemia. The blood pressure usually falls late in hypovolemic shock. Check laboratory values for hemoglobin (Hgb) and hematocrit (Hct) and report abnormal values to the health care provider. Check laboratory values for coagulation factors to identify added risks for hemorrhage. Administer Rh immune globulin to appropriate Rho(D)-negative women.

Because vaginal bleeding and necessary medical interventions may be associated with infections, assess the woman for fever, elevated pulse rate, malaise, and prolonged or malodorous vaginal discharge. Determine the family's knowledge of needed follow-up care and how to prevent complications such as infection.

◆ Identification of Patient Problems

A variety of collaborative problems or nursing diagnoses should be considered in the woman who has a bleeding disorder of early pregnancy. Collaborative problems such as bleeding and potential for infection are present. Current diagnostic techniques often permit early diagnosis before hemorrhage occurs. An applicable patient problem for women with these early pregnancy disorders is "Need for Patient Teaching about diagnostic and therapeutic procedures, signs and symptoms of additional complications, measures to prevent infection and importance of follow-up care."

◆ Planning: Expected Outcomes

Goals and expected outcomes for this nursing diagnosis are that the woman will do the following:

- Verbalize understanding of diagnostic and therapeutic procedures
- Verbalize measures to prevent infection
- Verbalize signs of infection to report to the health care provider
- Maintain follow-up care

◆ Interventions

Provide Information about Tests and Procedures

Women and their families experience less anxiety if they understand what is happening. Explain planned diagnostic procedures such as transvaginal or transabdominal ultrasonography. Include the purpose of the tests, how long they will take, and whether the procedures cause discomfort. Briefly describe the reasons for blood tests, such as evaluation of hCG, Hgb, Hct, or coagulation factors (Moise, 2014). Explain that diagnostic and therapeutic measures sometimes must be performed quickly to prevent excessive blood loss. If surgical intervention is necessary, reinforce the explanations from the anesthesia professional about planned anesthesia. Obtain needed consents before procedures.

Teach Measures to Prevent Infection

The risk for infection is greatest during the first 72 hours after spontaneous abortion or operative procedures. Personal hygiene should include daily showers and careful handwashing before and after changing perineal pads. Perineal pads, applied in a front-to-back direction, should be used instead of tampons until bleeding has subsided. The woman should consult with the health care provider about safe timing for resuming intercourse.

Provide Dietary Information

Nutrition and adequate fluid intake help maintain the body's defense against infection, and the nurse should promote an adequate and culturally sensitive diet. The woman who has a hemorrhagic complication is also at risk for infection. She needs foods that are high in iron to increase Hgb and Hct values. These foods include liver, red meat, dried fruits, dried peas and beans, and dark green leafy vegetables. (Stopler & Weiner, 2017). Foods high in vitamin C include citrus fruits, broccoli, strawberries, cantaloupe, cabbage, and green peppers. Adequate fluid intake (2500 mL/day) promotes hydration after bleeding episodes and maintains digestive processes.

Iron supplementation is often prescribed, and the woman may require information on how to lessen the gastrointestinal upset that many people experience when iron is administered (Kilpatrick, 2014). Less gastric upset is experienced when iron is taken with meals. Iron supplements having a slow release may be better tolerated. A diet high in fiber and fluid helps reduce the commonly associated constipation.

Teach Signs of Infection to Report

Ensure that the woman has a thermometer at home and knows how to use it. Tell her to take her temperature every 8 hours for the first 3 days at home. Teach the woman to seek medical help if her temperature rises above 100.4°F (38°C) or as her physician instructs. She also should report other signs of infection, even if she does not have a fever, such as vaginal discharge with foul odor, pelvic tenderness, or persistent general malaise.

Reinforce Follow-Up Care

The woman with gestational trophoblastic disease, such as hydatidform mole, requires follow up every 1 to 2 weeks for evaluation of serum beta-hCG levels (Cunningham, 2014). Immunologic or genetic testing and counseling may be

---

❓ CRITICAL THINKING EXERCISE 10.2

Alice, a 24-year-old primigravida, had an incomplete abortion at 12 weeks of gestation. When she was admitted to the hospital, intravenous fluids were administered and blood was taken for blood typing and screening. A vacuum extraction with curettage was performed to remove retained placental tissue. She was discharged home after the bleeding subsided. The nurse providing discharge instructions comments to the woman, "These things happen for the best, and you are so lucky it happened early. You can have other children."

Questions

1. What assumptions has the nurse made? How might these comments affect the woman who suffered the spontaneous abortion or miscarriage?
2. Is the comment that the woman can have other children comforting? Why or why not?
3. If the nurse's response was not helpful, what responses from the nurse would be most helpful to Alice?

---

advised for couples having recurrent abortions. All couples who have had a pregnancy loss should be seen by health care professionals and counseled.

At this time, acknowledge their grief, which often manifests as anger. Many women have guilty feelings, which should be recognized. They often need repeated reassurance that the loss was not a result of anything they did or anything they neglected to do.

Women who do not desire pregnancy right away will need contraception. Reliable contraception for at least 1 year will be essential for women who have had a molar pregnancy. Teach the woman how to use the prescribed contraceptive method correctly to enhance effectiveness.

◆ Evaluation

Interventions are deemed successful and the goals and expected outcomes are met if the woman does the following:

- Verbalizes understanding of diagnostic and therapeutic procedures
- Verbalizes measures to prevent infection

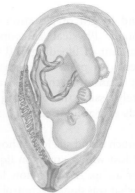

Marginal
Placenta is implanted in lower uterus but its lower border is >3 cm from internal cervical os.

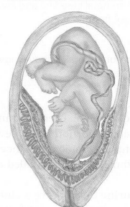

Partial
Lower border of placenta is within 3 cm of internal cervical os but does not fully cover it.

Total
Placenta completely covers internal cervical os.

FIG. 10.3 Examples of Three Classifications of Placenta Previa.

- Verbalizes signs of infection that should be reported to a health care professional
- Helps develop and participate in a plan of longer term follow-up care

HEMORRHAGIC CONDITIONS OF LATE PREGNANCY

After 20 weeks of pregnancy, the two major causes of hemorrhage are the disorders of the placenta called *placenta previa* and **placental abruption**. Placental abruption may be further complicated by disseminated intravascular coagulation (DIC).

Placenta Previa

Placenta previa is an implantation of the placenta in the lower uterus. As a result, the placenta is closer to the internal cervical os than to the presenting part (usually the head) of the fetus. The three classifications of placenta previa (total, partial, and marginal) depend on how much of the internal cervical os is covered by the placenta (Fig. 10.3). High-resolution ultrasound allows more accurate measurement of the distance between the internal cervical os and the lower border of the placenta, as follows:

- Marginal (sometimes called low-lying)—The placenta is implanted in the lower uterus, but its lower border is more than 3 cm from the internal cervical os.
- Partial—The lower border of the placenta is within 3 cm of the internal cervical os but does not completely cover the os.
- Total—The placenta completely covers the internal cervical os.

Marginal placenta previa is common in early ultrasound examinations and often appears to move upward and away from the internal cervical os (placental migration) as the fetus grows and the upper uterus develops more than the lower uterus. (Cunningham et al., 2014; Francois & Foley, 2017).

Incidence and Etiology

The average incidence of placenta previa is 1 in 200 births (Francois & Foley, 2017), and evidence indicates that the rate of placenta previa is increasing. It is more common in older women, multiparas, previous cesarean births, and prior uterine surgery. It is more likely to recur if a woman has had a placenta previa. Other risk factors include Asian ethnicity, current use of cocaine or cigarette smoking, and male fetus (Cunningham et al., 2014; Francois & Foley, 2017).

Clinical Manifestations

The classic sign of placenta previa is the sudden onset of painless uterine bleeding in the last half of pregnancy (Francois & Foley, 2017; Hull & Resnick, 2014). Many cases of placenta previa are diagnosed by ultrasound examination before any bleeding occurs. Bleeding results from tearing of the placental villi from the uterine wall as the lower uterine segment thins and the internal os begins to dilate near term. Bleeding is painless because it does not occur in a closed cavity and does not cause pressure on adjacent tissue. It may be scanty or profuse, and it may cease spontaneously, only to recur later.

Bleeding may not occur until labor starts, when cervical changes disrupt placental attachment. The admitting nurse may be unsure whether the bleeding is just heavy "bloody show" or a sign of a placenta previa, particularly if the woman had no prenatal care.

Digital examination of the cervical os or stimulation of contractions when a placenta previa is present can cause additional placental separation or tear the placenta itself, causing severe hemorrhage and extreme risk to the fetus. *Until the location and position of the placenta are verified by ultrasonography, no manual vaginal examinations should be performed, and administration of oxytocin should be postponed to prevent strong contractions that could result in sudden placental separation and rapid hemorrhage.*

Therapeutic Management

When the diagnosis of placenta previa is confirmed, medical interventions are based on the condition of the expectant mother and the fetus. The woman is evaluated to determine the amount of hemorrhage, and electronic fetal monitoring (EFM) is initiated to evaluate the fetus. Fetal gestational age is a third consideration.

Options for management include conservative management if the mother's cardiovascular status is stable and the fetus is immature and has a reassuring status by ultrasound examination and monitoring. Delaying birth may increase birth weight and maturity, and administration of corticosteroids to the mother speeds maturation of the fetal lungs, if needed. Conservative management may take place in the home or the hospital. Antepartum units are often designed to consider the woman's needs for physical and occupational therapy and for diversion as well as care for her pregnancy complication.

Home Care. Making a medical decision on home care versus inpatient care is difficult. General criteria for home care include the following (Francois & Foley, 2017):
- No evidence of active bleeding is present.
- The woman is able to maintain bed rest at home.
- Home is located within a short distance from the hospital.
- Emergency systems are available for immediate transport to the hospital 24 hours a day.
- The woman can verbalize her understanding of the risks associated with placenta previa and how to manage her care.

Nursing Considerations

Home Care. Nurses are often responsible for helping the woman and family understand the physician's plan of care. Nurses help the woman and family develop a workable plan for home care that may include strict bed rest except for elimination and shower, the presence of another adult to manage the home and be present if an emergency arises, and a procedure to follow if heavy bleeding begins. Teaching includes emphasizing the importance of (1) assessing color and amount of vaginal discharge or bleeding, especially after each urination or bowel movement; (2) assessing fetal activity (kick counts) daily; (3) assessing uterine activity at prescribed intervals; and (4) refraining from sexual intercourse to prevent disruption of the placenta. Home care nurses may be responsible for making daily phone contact to assess the woman's perception of uterine activity (cramping, regular or sporadic contractions), bleeding, fetal activity, and adherence to the prescribed treatment plan. In addition, they may make home visits for comprehensive maternal-fetal assessments with portable equipment, such as nonstress tests (NSTs). The woman and her family are instructed to report a decrease in fetal movement or an increase in uterine contractions or vaginal bleeding.

Nurses should provide specific, accurate information about the condition of the fetus. For example, parents are reassured when they hear that the fetal heart rate (FHR) is within the expected range and daily kick counts are normal. Nurses may need to help the family understand the physician's plan of care. For instance, the nurse may explain why a cesarean birth is necessary and why blood transfusion may be required.

Inpatient Care. Women with placenta previa are admitted to the antepartum unit if they do not meet the criteria for home care or if they require additional care to meet the goal of greater fetal maturity. When the expectant mother is confined to the hospital, nursing assessments focus on determining whether she experiences bleeding episodes or signs of preterm labor. Periodic electronic fetal monitoring (EFM) is necessary to determine whether there are fetal heart activity changes associated with fetal compromise. A significant change in fetal heart activity, an episode of vaginal bleeding, or signs of preterm labor should be reported immediately to the physician.

At times, conservative management is not an option. For instance, delivery may be scheduled if the fetus is older than 36 weeks of gestation and the lungs are mature. Immediate delivery may be necessary regardless of fetal immaturity if bleeding is excessive, the woman demonstrates signs of hypovolemia, or signs of fetal compromise are present. If cesarean birth is necessary, nurses should prepare the expectant mother for surgery. The preoperative procedures are often performed quickly if the woman is hemorrhaging, and the family may be anxious about the condition of the fetus and the expectant mother. Nurses should use whatever time is available to keep the family informed. Additional personnel will be needed to prepare the woman for cesarean birth. Preparations include one or more IV line starts, administration of preoperative antibiotics, anesthesia, Foley catheter insertion, and fetal monitoring. Neonatology or a team from the neonatal intensive care are usually notified and are present in the operating room for neonatal resuscitation.

Abruptio Placentae

Separation of a normally implanted placenta before the fetus is born (called *abruptio placentae, placental abruption,* or *premature separation of the placenta*) occurs in cases of bleeding and formation of a hematoma (clot) on the maternal side of the placenta. As the clot expands, further separation occurs. Hemorrhage may be apparent (vaginal bleeding) or concealed (Francois & Foley, 2017; Hull & Resnick, 2014). The severity of the complication depends on the amount of bleeding and the size of the hematoma. If bleeding continues, the hematoma expands and obliterates intervillous spaces. Fetal vessels are disrupted as placental separation occurs, resulting in fetal and maternal bleeding.

Placental abruption is a dangerous condition for both the pregnant woman and the fetus. The major dangers for the woman are hemorrhage and consequent hypovolemic shock and clotting abnormalities. The major dangers for the fetus are asphyxia, excessive blood loss, and prematurity.

Incidence and Etiology

The incidence of placental abruption varies but is approximately 0.5% to 1% of pregnancies (Hull & Resnick, 2014). Placental abruption accounts for 10% to 15% of perinatal deaths (Hull & Resnick, 2014).

The cause is not always known, but several factors that increase the risk have been identified. Maternal use of cocaine, which causes vasoconstriction in the endometrial arteries, is a leading cause of placental abruption. Other risk factors include maternal hypertension, maternal cigarette smoking, multigravida status, short umbilical cord, abdominal trauma, premature rupture of the membranes, and history of previous premature separation of the placenta (Cunningham et al., 2014; Francois & Foley, 2017).

Clinical Manifestations

Although verification of placental abruption may be quickly evident, it is not always a dramatic or acute event. Classic signs and symptoms of placental abruption include the following:

- Bleeding, which may be evident vaginally or concealed behind the placenta
- Uterine tenderness that may be localized at the site of the abruption
- Uterine irritability with frequent low-intensity contractions and poor relaxation between contractions
- Abdominal or low back pain that may be described as aching or dull
- High uterine resting tone identified with use of an intrauterine pressure catheter
- "Board-like" abdomen—the abdomen feels firm to touch because of the blood that can be concealed.
- "Port wine" colored amniotic fluid
- Nonreassuring FHR patterns or fetal death
- Signs of hypovolemic shock

Cases of placental abruption are divided into two main types: (1) those in which hemorrhage is concealed and (2) those in which hemorrhage is apparent. In either type, the placental abruption may be complete or partial. In cases of concealed hemorrhage, the bleeding occurs behind the placenta but the margins remain intact, causing formation of a hematoma. The hemorrhage is apparent when bleeding separates or dissects the membranes from the endometrium and blood flows out through the vagina. Amniotic fluid often has a classic "port wine" color. Fig. 10.4 illustrates placental abruption with external and concealed bleeding. Apparent bleeding does not always correspond to the actual amount of blood lost, and signs of shock (tachycardia, hypotension, pale color, and cold, clammy skin) may be present when little or no external bleeding occurs. Also, the woman may have an undiagnosed hypertensive disorder that masks hypovolemia until late hypotension occurs.

Abdominal pain is also related to the type of separation. It may be sudden and severe when bleeding occurs into the myometrium (uterine muscle) or intermittent and difficult to distinguish from labor contractions. The uterus may become exceedingly firm (board-like) and tender, making palpation of the fetus difficult. Ultrasound examination is helpful to rule out placenta previa as the cause of bleeding, but it cannot be used to diagnose placental abruption reliably because the separation and bleeding may not be obvious on ultrasonography.

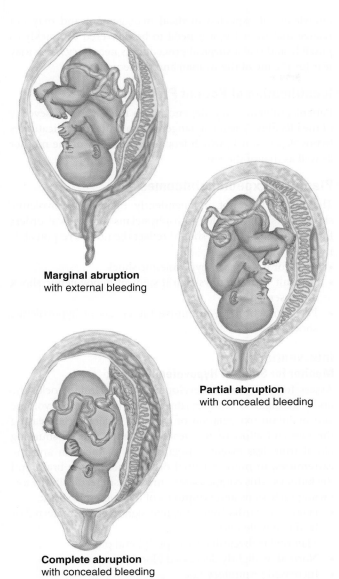

Marginal abruption
with external bleeding

Partial abruption
with concealed bleeding

Complete abruption
with concealed bleeding

FIG. 10.4 Types of placental abruption.

Therapeutic Management

Any woman who exhibits signs of placental abruption should be hospitalized and evaluated at once. Evaluation focuses on the cardiovascular status of the expectant mother and the condition of the fetus.

If the condition is mild and the fetus is under 34 weeks and shows no signs of distress, conservative management may be initiated. This includes bed rest and possible administration of tocolytic medications to reduce uterine activity and steroids to accelerate fetal lung maturity. Conservative management is rare and contraversial, however, because of the risks for fetal death and maternal hemorrhage associated with placental abruption (Cunningham et al., 2014; Francois & Foley, 2017).

Immediate delivery of the fetus is necessary if signs of fetal compromise exist or if the mother exhibits signs of excessive bleeding, either obvious or concealed. Intensive monitoring

of both the woman and the fetus is essential because rapid deterioration of either can occur. Blood products for replacement should be available, and two large-bore IV lines should be started for replacement of fluid and blood.

Women who have experienced abdominal trauma are at increased risk for placental abruption. They may be observed for up to 24 hours after significant trauma such as a motor vehicle accident, even if they are not having any signs of bleeding, because it may take this long for a placental abruption to develop. Serial Kleihauer-Betke (K-B) tests determine whether fetal bleeding is worsening (Cunningham et al, 2014; Hull & Resnick, 2014). For the Rh-negative woman, Rh immune globulin is usually administered to prevent possible maternal Rh sensitization.

Nursing Considerations

Placental abruption is frightening for a woman. She experiences severe pain and is aware of the danger to herself and to the fetus. She should be carefully assessed for signs of concealed hemorrhage.

If immediate cesarean delivery is necessary, the woman may feel powerless as the health care team hastily prepares her for surgery. If at all possible in the time available, nurses should explain the anticipated procedures to the woman and her family to reduce their fear and anxiety.

Excessive bleeding and fetal hypoxia are always major concerns with placental abruption, and nurses are responsible for continuous monitoring of both the mother and the fetus so that problems can be detected early before the condition of the woman or the fetus deteriorates.

> **! SAFETY CHECK**
>
> Signs of concealed hemorrhage in placental abruption include the following:
> - Increase in fundal height
> - Hard, board-like abdomen
> - High uterine baseline tone on electronic monitoring strip, especially when an intrauterine pressure catheter is used
> - Persistent abdominal pain
> - Systemic signs of early hemorrhage (tachycardia [maternal and fetal], tachypnea, falling blood pressure, falling urine output, restlessness)
> - Persistent late decelerations in fetal heart rate or decreasing baseline variability; absence of accelerations
> - Slight or absent vaginal bleeding

◆ APPLICATION OF THE NURSING PROCESS: HEMORRHAGIC CONDITIONS OF LATE PREGNANCY

◆ Assessment

For hemorrhagic conditions of late pregnancy, some nursing assessments should be performed immediately and others can be deferred until initial interventions have been taken to stabilize the cardiovascular status of the woman. Many nursing assessments are concurrent with medical assessments and include the following:

- Amount and nature of bleeding (time of onset, estimated blood loss before admission to hospital, and description of tissue or clots passed)—Peripads and underpads should be saved and weighed, as needed, to accurately assess blood loss.
- Pain (type [constant, intermittent, sharp, dull, severe]; onset [sudden, gradual]; and location [generalized over abdomen, localized in back])—Is uterine tenderness present with gentle palpation? Is the tenderness localized? Where?
- Maternal vital signs—Are these within normal limits, or is hypotension, tachycardia, or both present? A normal blood pressure may be misleading in a woman with placental abruption because she may have been hypertensive before the blood loss caused her blood pressure to fall to normal or hypotensive levels.
- Condition of the fetus—An electronic fetal monitor determines fetal heart rate, presence of accelerations, and fetal response to uterine activity. The presence of late decelerations or poor variability is of particular concern.
- Uterine contractions—Application of an external monitor determines frequency and duration of contractions. An intrauterine pressure catheter can identify hypertonic contractions and an increased resting tone associated with placental abruption if it is not contraindicated. Palpation can identify if the uterus does not relax fully between contractions. Thick abdominal adipose tissue reduces the ability to identify poor uterine relaxation by external means.
- Obstetric history (gravida, para, previous abortions, preterm infants, previous pregnancy outcomes)—Does the history include previous placental abruption?
- Length of gestation (date of last menstrual period, fundal height, correlation of fundal height with estimated gestation)—If bleeding occurs into the myometrium, the fundus enlarges as bleeding progresses. A piece of tape on the abdomen can mark the top of the fundus at a given time, and then the nurse can observe and report increasing fundal size, which suggests that bleeding into uterine muscles is occurring.
- Laboratory data—Laboratory studies include a complete blood count and blood typing and screening. Blood crossmatching is done if transfusion is likely. Type and Rh factor identify possible need for RhoGAM. Other tests may be done serially to identify whether the abruption is stable or worsening. The K-B test identifies fetal blood cells in the maternal circulation. Coagulation studies include fibrinogen, fibrin split products (FSPs), prothrombin and partial thromboplastin (PT/PTT) times, and D-dimer to identify fibrin degradation fragments. A drug screen is done if illegal drug use is suspected or if the woman had no prenatal care.

Despite the emphasis on physical assessment, the emotional response of the mother and her partner also should be addressed. They will most likely be anxious, fearful, confused, and overwhelmed by the activity. They may have little knowledge of expected medical management and may not realize that the fetus will need to be delivered as quickly as possible and that a surgical procedure is necessary. They may fear for the life of the woman and the fetus.

◆ Identification of Patient Problems

Patient problems vary, depending on the cause and severity of the bleeding. The most dangerous potential complication is hypovolemic shock, which jeopardizes the life of the mother as well as that of the fetus.

◆ Planning: Expected Outcomes

The nurse does not independently manage hypovolemic shock but should confer with physicians for medical orders for treatment. Planning should reflect the nurse's responsibility to:
- Monitor for signs of hypovolemic shock
- Consult with the physician if signs of hypovolemic shock are observed
- Perform actions to minimize the effects of hypovolemic shock

◆ Interventions
Monitor for Signs of Hypovolemic Shock

Assess for any sign of developing hypovolemic shock. The body attempts to compensate for decreased blood volume and maintain oxygenation of essential organs by increasing the rate and effort of the heart and lungs and by shunting blood from less essential organs, such as the skin and the extremities, to more essential organs such as the brain and the kidneys. This compensatory mechanism results in the following early signs and symptoms of hypovolemic shock:
- Fetal tachycardia (often the first sign of either maternal or fetal hypovolemia)
- Maternal tachycardia, weak peripheral pulses
- Normal or slightly decreased blood pressure
- Increased respiratory rate
- Low oxygen saturation
- Cool, pale skin and mucous membranes

The compensatory mechanism fails if hypovolemic shock progresses and insufficient blood exists to perfuse the brain, heart, and kidneys. Later signs of hypovolemic shock include the following:
- Falling blood pressure and oxygen saturation levels
- Pallor; skin becomes cold and clammy
- Urine output less than 30 mL/hr
- Restlessness, agitation, decreased mentation

Monitor the Fetus

Use continuous EFM so that signs of fetal compromise, such as tachycardia, decreasing baseline variability, or late decelerations, can be seen (see Chapter 14). If abnormal patterns are seen, contact the physician at once because the fetus often shows signs of compromise before maternal signs of hypovolemia are obvious. Give the physician a report on new laboratory data that suggest an increasing degree of placental abruption, such as rising K-B test levels after abdominal trauma.

Promote Tissue Oxygenation

The following should be done to promote oxygenation of tissues:

- Place the woman in a lateral position, with the head of the bed flat to increase cardiac return and thus to increase circulation and oxygenation of the placenta and other vital organs.
- Limit maternal activity to decrease the tissue demand for oxygen.
- Provide simple explanations, reassurance, and emotional support to the woman to reduce anxiety, which increases the metabolic demand for oxygen.
- Provide oxygen at 8 to 10 L/min via tight, non-rebreather face mask per hospital protocol and physician orders.

Collaborate with the Physician for Fluid Replacement

To replace fluids the following should be done:

- Insert IV lines according to hospital protocol. Two lines that use large-gauge catheters (16- to 18-gauge) are often recommended for rapid blood replacement, if needed.
- Administer fluids for replacement as directed by the physician to maintain a urinary output of at least 30 mL/hr.
- Obtain an order for blood typing and screening or cross-matching if not previously done.

Prepare the Woman for Surgery

Quick preparation of the woman for cesarean delivery may be necessary. The neonatal resuscitation team should be notified. See Chapter 15 for common preparations of a woman for cesarean.

Before and after birth assess bleeding from the vagina as well as from any surgical sites or puncture wounds (epidural or IV sites) to identify uncontrolled bleeding or bleeding from unexpected sites that may indicate DIC, requiring prompt medical management.

! SAFETY CHECK

Signs and symptoms of hypovolemic shock caused by blood loss include the following:

- Increased pulse rate, falling blood pressure, increased respiratory rate
- Weak, diminished, or "thready" peripheral pulses
- Cool, moist skin; pallor; or cyanosis (late sign)
- Decreased (<30 mL/hr) or absent urinary output
- Decreased Hgb, Hct levels
- Change in mental status (restlessness, agitation, difficulty concentrating)

Provide Emotional Support

Once the safety of the woman and the fetus is ensured, nursing interventions promote comfort and provide emotional support. Explain what is causing the discomfort, and reassure the woman that pain-relief measures that do not cause harm to the fetus will be initiated as soon as possible. Offering false reassurance about the condition of the fetus is unwise, but remain with the woman, and provide accurate and timely information. Explain your actions to the woman and her family. They can feel overwhelmed by all the activity. Visiting with the woman and her support person after birth helps clarify the problem and reasons for interventions to help put events in perspective.

◆ Evaluation

Patient-centered goals are not developed for collaborative problems, but the nurse collects and compares data with established norms and judges whether the data are within normal limits. For hypovolemic shock, the maternal vital signs remain within normal limits and the fetal heart demonstrates no signs of compromise such as abnormal rate, late decelerations, or decreasing baseline variability.

DISSEMINATED INTRAVASCULAR COAGULATION

Disseminated intravascular coagulation (DIC), also called *consumptive coagulopathy,* is a life-threatening defect in coagulation that may occur with several complications of pregnancy such as placental abruption or hypertension (Francois & Foley, 2017; Moise, 2014). DIC is not limited to obstetric conditions. At the same time anticoagulation is occurring, inappropriate coagulation also is taking place in the microcirculation. The results of DIC are excessive bleeding and the formation of tiny clots in tiny blood vessels, blocking blood flow to organs and causing ischemia.

In each of these disease processes, some factor initiates clotting mechanisms inappropriately. The first result is consumption of plasma factors, including platelets, fibrinogen, prothrombin, factor V, and factor VIII. When these plasma factors are consumed, the circulating blood then becomes deficient in clotting factors and is unable to clot. Fibrin degradation products accumulate and further interfere with coagulation.

Diseases that cause DIC fall into three major groups (Hull & Resnick, 2014; Moise, 2014):

1. Infusion of tissue thromboplastin into the circulation, which consumes, or "uses up," other clotting factors such as fibrinogen and platelets: Placental abruption (premature separation) and prolonged retention of a dead fetus cause this because the placenta is a rich source of thromboplastin.
2. Conditions characterized by endothelial damage: Severe preeclampsia and HELLP (*h*emolysis, *e*levated levels of *l*iver enzymes, and *low p*latelet levels) syndrome are characterized by endothelial damage.
3. Nonspecific effects of some diseases: Diseases such as maternal sepsis or amniotic fluid embolism are in this category.

DIC allows excess bleeding to occur from any vulnerable area such as IV sites, incisions, gums, or the nose and from expected sites such as the site of placental attachment during the postpartum period.

Laboratory studies help establish a diagnosis. Levels of fibrinogen and platelets usually are decreased, PT and activated PTT (aPTT) may be prolonged, and levels of fibrin degradation products, the most sensitive measurement, are increased. The D-dimer serum assay, which normally has negative results, confirms FSP and is presumptive for DIC when results are positive.

The priority in treatment of DIC is to correct the cause. In the case of a missed abortion, delivery of the fetus and the placenta ends the production of thromboplastin, which is fueling the process. Blood replacement products such as whole blood, packed red blood cells (RBCs), and cryoprecipitate are administered, as needed, to maintain the circulating volume and to transport oxygen to body cells.

Nursing Considerations

When caring for a woman who has any of the disorders that increase her risk for DIC, the nurse should observe for bleeding from unexpected sites including IV insertion and venipuncture sites for laboratory work. Nosebleeds or spontaneous bruising may be early indicators of DIC and should be reported. An additional IV line should be started to prepare for additional crystalloids, colloids, or blood products that may need to be administered. The nurse should apply oxygen at 10 liters per minute by face mask because of the blood loss. Monitoring of frequent vital signs includes temperature, blood pressure, pulse, and respirations to assess the cardiovascular status of the patient. An accurate record of intake and output should be obtained. Other nursing considerations include the weighing of all blood-soaked materials to obtain an accurate output. One gram is equal to 1 milliliter of blood (Association of Women's Health, Obstetrics, and Neonatal Nurses [AWHONN], 2012).

> ### KNOWLEDGE CHECK
>
> 7. What are the signs and symptoms of placenta previa? How is it managed in the home?
> 8. What are the signs and symptoms of placental abruption?
> 9. What are the major dangers to the mother and the fetus during the placental abruption?
> 10. What is DIC?

HYPEREMESIS GRAVIDARUM

Hyperemesis gravidarum (HEG) is persistent, uncontrollable vomiting that begins in the first weeks of pregnancy and may continue throughout pregnancy, although its severity usually lessens. Unlike morning sickness, which is self-limited and causes no serious complications, HEG can have serious consequences. Hyperemesis is associated with loss of 5% or more of prepregnancy weight, dehydration, acidosis from starvation, elevated levels of blood and urine ketones, alkalosis from loss of hydrochloric acid in the gastric fluids, and hypokalemia. Short-term hepatic dysfunction with elevated liver enzymes may occur. Deficiency of vitamin K may cause coagulation disorders, and deficiency of thiamine can cause encephalopathy (Cox & Carney, 2017).

Etiology

The cause of HEG is not known, but the condition is more common among unmarried White women, during first pregnancies, and in multifetal pregnancies. Other possible causes include allergy to fetal proteins, elevated levels of pregnancy-related hormones such as estrogen and beta-hCG, and maternal thyroid dysfunction. Association with the organism that causes peptic ulcer disease, *Helicobacter pylori,* is not conclusive. Psychological factors may interact with the nausea and vomiting that occurs during early pregnancy to worsen the condition (ACOG, 2015e; Cunningham et al., 2011; Gilbert, 2011; Kelly & Savides, 2014).

Therapeutic Management

Exclusion of other causes of persistent nausea and vomiting, such as cholecystitis, peptic ulcer disease, or gestational trophoblastic disease, should precede diagnosing hyperemesis. Laboratory studies include Hgb and Hct levels, which may be elevated because of dehydration, resulting in hemoconcentration. Electrolyte studies may reveal reduced sodium, potassium, and chloride levels. Elevated creatinine levels indicate renal dysfunction.

Treatment occurs primarily in the home, where the woman first attempts to control the nausea with methods that are used for morning sickness. In addition, some physicians prescribe vitamins such as pyridoxine (vitamin B_6), which may provide some relief. A daily vitamin and mineral supplement may be recommended.

Drug therapy may be required if the vomiting becomes severe. Drugs are evaluated for potential risks and benefits and may include the following:

- Diphenhydramine (Benadryl)
- Histamine-receptor antagonists such as famotidine (Pepcid) or ranitidine (Zantac)
- Gastric acid inhibitors such as esomeprazole (Nexium) or omeprazole (Prilosec)
- Metoclopramide (Reglan)
- Pyridoxine/doxylamine (Diclegis)

If simpler methods are unsuccessful and weight loss or electrolyte imbalance persists, IV fluid and electrolyte replacement or total parenteral nutrition (TPN) may be necessary. In some women, IV fluid replacement improves the nausea and vomiting quickly. The woman usually can be managed at home with periodic home nursing visits if she must have TPN. Periodic brief hospitalizations may be needed until the hyperemesis problem lessens. Enteral nutrition has also been used successfully (ACOG, 2015e; Cunningham et al., 2014).

Nursing Considerations

Nurses may be responsible for assessing and intervening for the woman with HEG in the hospital or the home. Physical assessment begins with determining the intake and output. Intake includes IV fluids and parenteral or enteral nutrition, as well as oral nutrition, which is resumed with control of vomiting. Output includes the amount and character of emesis and urinary output. As a rule of thumb, the normal urinary output is about 1 mL/kg/hr (1 mL/2.2 lb/hr). A record of bowel elimination also provides significant information about oral nutrition because a woman's intake may have been so minimal that many days have passed since her last normal bowel movement.

Laboratory data may be evaluated to determine fluid and metabolic status. Elevated levels of Hgb and Hct may occur as a result of dehydration, which results in hemoconcentration. Concentrations of sodium, potassium, and chloride may be reduced, resulting in hypokalemia and alkalosis.

Whether at home or at the hospital, the woman weighs herself daily, first thing in the morning, and in similar clothing each day. Weight loss and the presence of ketones in the urine suggest that fat stores and protein are being metabolized to meet energy needs.

Signs of dehydration include decreased fluid intake (less than 2000 mL/day), decreased urinary output, increased urine specific gravity (more than 1.025), dry skin or dry mucous membranes, and nonelastic skin turgor.

Nursing interventions focus on reducing nausea and vomiting, maintaining nutrition and fluid balance, and providing emotional support.

Reducing Nausea and Vomiting

When food is offered to the woman, portions should be small so that the amount does not appear overwhelming. Food should be attractively presented, and foods with strong odors should be eliminated from the diet because food smells often incite nausea. Low-fat foods and easily digested carbohydrates such as fruit, breads, cereals, rice, and pasta provide important nutrients and help prevent low blood glucose levels, which can cause nausea. Soups and other liquids should be taken between meals to avoid distending the stomach and triggering vomiting. Sitting upright after meals reduces gastric reflux. The use of ginger has been shown to help with reducing nausea and vomiting. Patients may be instructed to stop the use of iron supplements in the first trimester to assist with reduction of nausea and vomiting (ACOG, 2015e).

Maintaining Nutrition and Fluid Balance

Women with nausea and vomiting should eat every 1 to 2 hours. Salting the food helps replace the chloride lost when hydrochloric acid is vomited. Consuming potassium-rich and magnesium-rich foods and fluids should be encouraged when the woman can do so because stores of these nutrients are likely to be depleted and magnesium deficiency can exacerbate nausea. Potassium is found in fruits, vegetables, and meat. Sources of magnesium include seeds, nuts, legumes, and green vegetables. Many studies have shown that a high-protein diet may assist with nausea and vomiting (ACOG, 2015e).

IV fluids and TPN are administered as directed by the physician. IV fluid containing potassium is often ordered until the low serum level returns to normal. Small oral feedings of clear liquids are started when nausea and vomiting subside. When oral fluids and adequate food intake are tolerated, parenteral nutrition is gradually discontinued. Continued inability to tolerate oral feedings or continued episodes of vomiting should be reported to the physician.

Providing Emotional Support

The woman, and possibly her significant other, may have been surprised by the pregnancy and may not have accepted it. Helping the woman express reluctance to accept the pregnancy and identifying her sources of support may reduce nausea, although its intensity may remain higher than in most women. HEG can make early pregnancy unpleasant because of its unpredictability.

Although the woman with HEG needs the opportunity to express how it feels to be pregnant with constant nausea, she may experience a lack of sympathy and support from significant others. This attitude may stem from reports that the cause of HEG is always psychological. In addition, observation of the woman and her family may provide clues about family dynamics that may be contributing to her response to nausea of pregnancy. Nurses should use critical thinking to examine personal beliefs and biases so they can provide comfort and support.

> **? KNOWLEDGE CHECK**
>
> 11. How do "morning sickness" and HEG compare in terms of onset, duration, and effect on the woman?
> 12. What are the nursing goals in therapeutic management of HEG?
> 13. Why is critical thinking particularly important in the care of the woman with HEG?

HYPERTENSIVE DISORDERS OF PREGNANCY

Hypertension is one of the most common medical complications of pregnancy and a leading cause of maternal morbidity and mortality. Hypertension is defined as a systolic blood pressure of 140 mm Hg or greater or a diastolic blood pressure of 90 mm Hg or greater. The terminology used to describe hypertension in pregnancy is inconsistent and confusing. In an effort to standardize classifications of hypertension occurring during pregnancy and to clarify management, the National Heart, Lung, and Blood Institute (NHLBI) assembled a working group to update older recommendations. Four categories of hypertensive disorders that occur during pregnancy were identified by the group (Table 10.1; Cunningham et al., 2014; Druzin, Shields, Peterson, & Cape, 2013; Markham & Funai, 2014).

- Gestational hypertension: Onset of hypertension after 20 weeks of pregnancy *without* proteinuria. Gestational hypertension should be considered a working diagnosis because it may progress to preeclampsia. If gestational hypertension persists after 12 weeks postpartum, chronic hypertension is diagnosed.
- Preeclampsia-eclampsia: Onset of hypertension after 20 weeks of pregnancy that may be accompanied by proteinuria (≥300 mg in a 24-hour urine collection, which correlates with a random urine dipstick evaluation of ≥1+). ACOG's 2013 publication (ACOG, 2013a) defined preeclampsia both with and without proteinuria. Edema,

TABLE 10.1 Classification of Hypertension in Pregnancy

Classification	Characteristics
Chronic hypertension	BP ≥140 mm Hg systolic or 90 mm Hg diastolic predating conception Identified before 20 wk gestation Persists >12 wk postpartum Use of antihypertensive medications before pregnancy
Superimposed preeclampsia or eclampsia on chronic hypertension	New onset in a woman with hypertension before 20 wk Sudden increase in proteinuria if already present in early gestation Sudden increase in BP Development of HELLP syndrome Development of headache, scotomata, or epigastric pain
Gestational hypertension	Systolic pressure of 140 mm Hg or a diastolic pressure ≥90 mm Hg without proteinuria occurring after 20 wk gestation Transient diagnosis with normalization of BP by 12 wk postpartum May represent preproteinuric phase of preeclampsia or recurrence of chronic hypertension abated in midpregnancy May evolve to preeclampsia Retrospective diagnosis
Preeclampsia	Occurring after 20 wk of pregnancy BP ≥140 mm Hg systolic or ≥90 mm Hg diastolic or higher Proteinuria 0.3 g protein or higher in a 24-hour urine specimen *or* ≥ +1 per dipstick *or* P/C ratio ≥0.3 mg/dL
Eclampsia	Presence of new-onset grand mal seizures in a pregnant woman with preeclampsia (rule out idiopathic seizure disorder or other central nervous system pathologic processes such as intracranial hemorrhage, bleeding arteriovenous malformation, ruptured aneurysm) New-onset seizures 48 to 72 hours postpartum (other central nervous system pathologic process is the likely reason for the seizure after 7 days)
Severe preeclampsia	If one or more of the following criteria are present: 1. Blood pressure of ≥160 mm Hg systolic or ≥110 mm Hg diastolic or higher on two occasions at least 6 hr apart while the patient is on bed rest 2. Oliguria of <500 mL in 24 hr 3. Cerebral or visual disturbances 4. Pulmonary edema or cyanosis 5. Epigastric or right upper quadrant pain 6. Impaired liver function as indicated by abnormally elevated blood concentrations of liver enzymes (to twice normal concentration), severe persistent right upper quadrant or epigastric pain unresponsive to medication and not accounted for by alternative diagnoses, or both 7. Thrombocytopenia 8. Renal insufficiency
HELLP Syndrome (subset of severe preeclampsia)	**H**emolysis **E**levated **L**iver enzymes **L**ow **P**latelets

Data from Hypertension in Pregnancy: Report of the American College of Obstetricians and Gynecologists' Task Force on Hypertension in Pregnancy, November 2013.

although common in preeclampsia, is considered nonspecific because it occurs in many pregnancies not complicated by hypertension (Roberts, August, & Bakris, 2013).

- Eclampsia: Progression of preeclampsia to generalized seizures that cannot be attributed to other causes. Seizures may occur during antepartum, intrapartum, or postpartum periods.
- Chronic hypertension: Hypertension that is present before pregnancy, diagnosed before 20 weeks of gestation, or continuing beyond 12 weeks postpartum.
- Chronic hypertension with superimposed preeclampsia: Chronic hypertension as defined previously with one or more the following:
  - New-onset proteinuria after 20 weeks of gestation.

- Sudden increase in proteinuria in women with proteinuria present before 20 weeks.
- Sudden exacerbation of previously well-controlled hypertension.
- Change in laboratory values indicating multiorgan involvement (platelets less than 100,000, elevated liver enzymes, decreased kidney function, etc.).
- Development of headache, epigastric pain, or vision changes.

Preeclampsia

Preeclampsia is a condition in which hypertension develops after 20 weeks of gestation in a woman with previously normal blood pressure. In addition to hypertension, renal involvement may cause proteinuria. Many women also experience

TABLE 10.2 Maternal and Fetal Complications Associated with Preeclampsia

System	Maternal Complications
Cardiovascular	Decreased intravascular volume
	Severe hypertension including hypertensive crisis
	Pulmonary edema
	Congestive heart failure
	Future cardiac disease and dysfunction
Pulmonary	Pulmonary edema
	Hypoxemia/academia
Renal	Oliguria
	Acute renal failure
	Impaired drug metabolism and excretion
Hematologic	Hemolysis
	Decreased oxygen-carrying capacity
	Thrombocytopenia
	Coagulation defects (disseminated intravascular coagulation)
	Anemia
Neurologic	Seizures
	Cerebral edema
	Intracerebral hemorrhage
	Stroke
	Visual disturbances, blindness
Hepatic	Hepatocellular dysfunction
	Hepatic rupture
	Hypoglycemia
	Coagulation defects
	Impaired drug metabolism and excretion
Uteroplacental	Abruption
	Decreased uteroplacental perfusion

Fetal Complications

Intrauterine growth restriction
Intrauterine fetal death
Fetal intolerance to labor
Preterm birth
Low birth weight
Decreased oxygenation

BOX 10.2 Risk Factors for Pregnancy-Related Hypertension

First pregnancy
Men who fathered preeclamptic pregnancies are more likely to father further preeclamptic pregnancies
Age older than 35 years
African-American descent
History of thrombophilia such as hyperhomocysteinemia (elevated levels of homocysteine that increase the risk for developing clots, heart attack, and stroke); factor V Leiden; or protein C and protein S deficiencies
In vitro fertilization
Family or personal history of preeclampsia
Chronic hypertension or preexisting vascular or renal disease
Obesity
Diabetes mellitus
Metabolic syndrome
Antiphospholipid syndrome
Systemic lupus erythematosus
Multifetal pregnancy

From Cunningham, F. G., Leveno, K. J., Bloom, S. L., Spong, C. Y., Dashe, J. S., Hoffman, B. L., & Sheffield, J. S. (2014). *Williams' obstetrics* (24th ed.). New York, NY: McGraw-Hill; Sibai, B. M. (2017). Preeclampsia and Hypertensive disorders. In S. G. Gabbe, J. R. Niebyl, J. L. Simpson, M.B. Landon, H.L. Galan, R. M. Jauniaux, D.A. Driscoll, et al. (Eds.), *Obstetrics: Normal and problem Pregnancies* (7th ed., pp. 662–705). Philadelphia, PA: Saunders; and Markham, K. B., & Funai, E. F. (2014). Pregnancy-related hypertension. In R. K. Creasy, R. Resnik, J. D. Iams, C. Lockwood, T. Moore, M. Greene (Eds.), *Creasy & Resnik's Maternal-fetal medicine: Principles and practice* (7th ed., pp. 756–781). Philadelphia, PA: Saunders.

is detected early and managed carefully (Cunningham et al., 2014; Markham & Funai, 2014; Roberts et al., 2013).

Incidence and Risk Factors

Preeclampsia affects 5% to 10% of all pregnancies. Efforts to prevent hypertension in pregnancy have not been successful. The implications of a preeclampsia diagnosis are significant for both maternal and fetal well-being. Many adverse outcomes are associated with preeclampsia as seen in Table 10.2 (Cunningham et al., 2014; Markham & Funai, 2014; Sibai, 2017).

Although the cause of preeclampsia is not understood, several factors are known to increase a woman's risk (Box 10.2). Some factors such as obesity and prepregnancy diabetes may be interrelated. Although risk factors have been identified, the individual predictive value of these factors for screening and risk stratification has not been verified (Cunningham et al., 2014; Markham & Funai, 2014; Poole, 2014; Sibai, 2017).

generalized edema. Two categories of preeclampsia were defined in past literature: mild and severe. The characterization of "mild" can be misleading because maternal morbidity and mortality are significantly increased even in the absence of severe disease. Therefore, in 2013, the ACOG recommended the term *"mild preeclampsia"* be replaced with *"preeclampsia without severe features"* (ACOG, 2013a). The only known cure for preeclampsia is birth of the fetus and delivery of the placenta. Maternal and fetal morbidity can be minimized if preeclampsia

EVIDENCE-BASED PRACTICE

Racial Disparities in Comorbidities, Complications, and Maternal and Fetal Outcomes in Women with Preeclampsia/Eclampsia

Preeclampsia refers to a condition characterized by the new onset of hypertension and proteinuria after 20 weeks of gestation.

African American (AA) women experience a three-fold higher risk of mortality from complications related to pregnancy when compared to White American women. The mortality rate for AA as compared to White women is 38.9 and 12.0 per 100,000 live births. These numbers have remained consistent for the last 50 years.

Continued

Racial Disparities in Comorbidities, Complications, and Maternal and Fetal Outcomes in Women with Preeclampsia/Eclampsia

A cohort analysis using data from the National Inpatient Sample (NIS) from 2004 to 2012 was performed. The study included all women in the NIS with a diagnosis of preeclampsia/eclampsia in the stated range of years. In the study of 1,175,046 women with the diagnosis of preeclampsia, the incidence was greatest among African-American women; 6%. The incidence of Hispanic women was 2.58% as compared to 3.75% in White women. The study noted that in comparison to White women, AA women diagnosed with preeclampsia had a higher rate of hypertension, obesity, acute renal failure, and diabetes.

The incidence of complications during the peripartum period among AA women as compared to White women demonstrated higher probability of maternal complications such as acute respiratory distress, cardiac arrest, pulmonary edema, and peripartum cardiomyopathy. In the study, researchers learned that AA women had an increased risk of intrauterine fetal demise as compared to White women.

In conclusion, hypertension is a major cause of many maternal complications in pregnant women. It is noted that AA women develop severe hypertension earlier in the gestational period than White women and have a higher rate of mortality from hypertensive related issues.

Questions

1. There are risk factors of pre-existing hypertension before pregnancy and developing preeclampsia during pregnancy. What are some modifiable risk factors in women regardless of race?
2. Appropriate access to prenatal care and patient compliance during pregnancy might decrease the incidence of preeclampsia. What are some barriers to women in accessing medical care during pregnancy, especially with preexisting hypertension?

Reference

Shahul, S., Tung, A., Minhaj, M., Nizamuddin, J., Wnger, J., Mahmood, E., & Mueller, A. (2015). Racial disparities in comorbidities, complications, and maternal and fetal outcomes in women with preeclampsia/eclampsia. *Hypertension in Pregnancy, 34*(4), 506–515.

Pathophysiology

Preeclampsia is a result of generalized vasoconstriction and vasospasm resulting in a multiple system organ failure disease in pregancy as summarized in Table 10.3. The primary pathologic process of hypertension is vasoconstriction, whereas the underlying cause of vasospasm remains unknown. Several hypotheses regarding the etiology of this multisystem disease exist. Evidence suggests that the pathologic process begins in early pregnancy during placenta formation and implantation. Placenta pathologic examination reveals abnormal development in the maternal spiral arteries leading to decreased perfusion and oxygenation (Fig. 10.5). This diminished perfusion leads to a release of placental microparticles that generates a systemic inflammatory response. Other hypotheses include a dysregulation of maternal immune response to fetal and placental antigens leading to inflammatory changes and decreased maternal adaptation to pregnancy changes (Cunningham et al., 2014; Markham & Funai, 2014; Poole, 2014). In normal pregnancy, vascular volume and cardiac output increase significantly. Despite these increases, blood pressure does not rise in normal pregnancy. Pregnant women develop resistance to the effects of vasoconstrictors such as angiotensin II. Peripheral vascular resistance decreases because of the effects of certain vasodilators such as prostacyclin (PGI_2) and endothelium-derived relaxing factor (EDRF).

In preeclampsia, however, peripheral vascular resistance increases because preeclamptic women are sensitive to angiotensin II. They also may have a decrease in vasodilation. For instance, the ratio of thromboxane (TXA_2) to PGI_2 (prostacyclin) increases. TXA_2, produced by kidney and trophoblastic tissue, causes vasoconstriction and platelet aggregation (clumping). PGI_2, produced by placental tissue and endothelial cells, causes vasodilation and inhibits platelet aggregation.

Vasospasm decreases the diameter of blood vessels, which results in endothelial cell damage, decreasing EDRF, and increasing capillary permeability. Vasoconstriction also results in impeded blood flow and elevated blood pressure. As a result, circulation to all body organs, including the kidneys, liver, brain, and placenta, is decreased. The following changes are most significant (Markham & Funai, 2014):

- Decreased renal perfusion reduces the glomerular filtration rate. Blood urea nitrogen, creatinine, and uric acid levels rise.
- Reduced renal blood flow results in glomerular damage, allowing protein to leak across the glomerular membrane, which is normally impermeable to large protein molecules.
- Loss of protein from the kidneys reduces colloid osmotic pressure and allows fluid to shift to interstitial spaces. This may result in edema and a reduction in intravascular volume, which causes increased viscosity of the blood and a rise in Hct level. Generalized edema often occurs.
- In preeclampsia, the normal response to reduced intravascular volume, releasing additional angiotensin II and aldosterone trigger the retention of both sodium and water, does not occur. The noted change is significant susceptibility in preeclamptic women to the effects of the renin-angiotensin-aldosterone system, creating a pathologic systemic vasoconstriction process: angiotensin II results in further vasospasm and hypertension, aldosterone increases fluid retention, and edema worsens.
- Reduced liver circulation impairs function and leads to hepatic edema and subcapsular hemorrhage, which can result in hemorrhagic necrosis. This is manifested by elevation of liver enzymes in maternal serum. Epigastric pain is a common symptom.

TABLE 10.3 Preeclampsia Pathophysiology as a Multiorgan System Disease

System	Effect of Preeclampsia	Clinical Implications
Vascular bed 1. Endothelial dysfunction 2. Altered coagulation 3. Altered response to vasoactive substances	Increased release of cellular fibronectin, growth factors, VCAM-1, factor VIII antigen, and peptides Endothelial cell injury initiates coagulation either by intrinsic pathway (contact adhesion) or extrinsic pathway (tissue factor) Decreased production of prostacyclin and alteration in prostacyclin/thromboxane ratio	Endothelial dysfunction presents before clinical signs of the disease Increased thrombus formation, including pulmonary and cerebral emboli Vasoconstriction and vasospasm Increased sensitivity to vasoactive substance Capillary permeability, which contributes to edema formation
Cardiovascular and pulmonary 1. ↑ Vascular resistance 2. ↑ Cardiac output and stroke volume 3. ↓ Colloid osmotic pressure	Arteriolar narrowing ↑ Sympathetic activity ↑ Levels of endothelin-1, a vasoconstrictor ↑ Sensitivity to endogenous pressors, including vasopressin, epinephrine, and norepinephrine ↑ Capillary permeability Further depletion of intravascular colloids through capillary permeability and renal excretion of proteins	Increased blood pressure Hyperdynamic cardiac activity Epidurals can be used safely, but should be cautious if ephedrine is used to correct hypotension Subendocardial hemorrhages are present in >50% of women who die of eclampsia At risk for pulmonary edema, myocardial ischemia, left ventricular dysfunction
Renal 1. Proteinuria 2. Altered function	Slight decrease in glomerular size Diameter of glomerular capillary lumen decreased Glomerular endothelial cells are greatly enlarged and may occlude the capillary lumen Glomerular capillary endotheliosis Thickening of renal arterioles	Proteinuria plus hypertension is the most reliable indicator of fetal jeopardy, indicative of glomerular dysfunction ↑ Serum uric acid secondary to a ↓ urate clearance (uric acid better predictor of outcome than blood pressure) ↓ Creatinine clearance with an elevation of serum creatinine levels ↑ BUN mirrors changes in creatine clearance and also a function of protein intake and liver function Urine sediment analysis may not be beneficial At risk for oliguria, ATN, renal failure
Hepatic 1. Hepatic dysfunction 2. Hepatic rupture	Changes consistent with hemorrhage into hepatic tissue Later changes consistent with hepatic infarction ↑ Hepatic artery resistance Fibrin deposition Hepatocellular necrosis	Elevations of liver function tests; association of microangiopathic anemia and elevations of AST/ALT carries ominous prognosis for mother and fetus HELLP syndrome Possible elevations in bilirubin Signs of liver failure; malaise, nausea, epigastric pain, hypoglycemia, hemolysis, anemia
Hematologic 1. Thrombocytopenia 2. Altered platelet function 3. Hemolysis	↑ Platelet destruction ↑ Platelet aggregation ↓ Platelet life span Hemolytic anemia Destruction of RBCs in microvasculature	Platelets <100,000 increased risk for coagulopathy Platelets <50,000 increased risk for hemorrhage Platelets <20,000 increased risk for spontaneous bleeding Decreased oxygen-carrying capacity and organ oxygenation
Central nervous system (CNS) 1. Hyperreflexia	May indicate increasing CNS involvement, but not diagnostic of disease Alteration of cerebral autoregulation with seizures ↑ Intracranial pressures	Cerebral edema with severe disease Signs of CNS alterations: Headache, dizziness, changes in vital signs, diplopia, scotomata, blurred vision, amaurosis, tachycardia, alteration in level of consciousness
Fetal/neonatal 1. Fetal intolerance to labor 2. Preterm birth 3. Oligohydramnios 4. IUGR 5. IUFD 6. Abruptio placentae	Alteration in placental function At risk for indicated preterm birth secondary to maternal disease process	Must monitor signs for fetal compromise Monitoring for IUGR and IUFD At risk for abruptio placentae, oligohydramnios, indeterminate or abnormal fetal heart rate patterns
Uteroplacental 1. Spiral arteries 2. Changes consistent with hypoxia	Abnormal invasion Retain nonpregnant characteristics Limited vasodilatation Vessel necrosis	Decreases in uteroplacental perfusion Increased risk for fetal compromise and IUGR

AST/ALT, Aspartate aminotransferase/alanine aminotransferase; *ATN,* acute tubular necrosis; *BUN,* blood urea nitrogen; *HELLP,* hemolysis, elevated levels of liver enzymes, and low platelet levels; *IUFD,* intrauterine fetal death; *IUGR,* intrauterine growth restriction; *VCAM-1,* vascular cell adhesion protein 1.

From Simpson, K. R., & Creehan, P. A. (2014). *AWHONN's perinatal nursing* (4th ed.). Philadelphia, PA: Lippincott Williams & Wilkins. Copyright © 2014, 2008 by the Association of Women's Health, Obstetrics and Neonatal Nurses (AWHONN). p. 128.

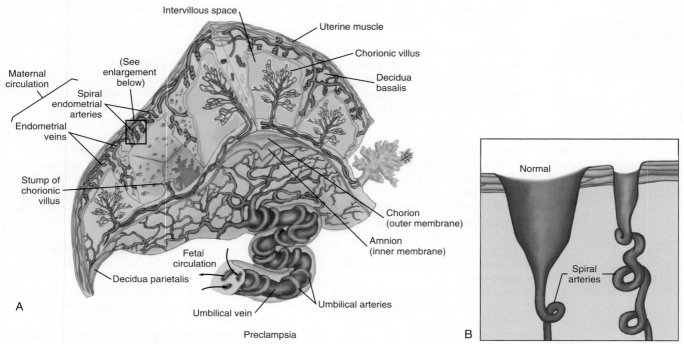

Preclampsia

FIG. 10.5 Abnormal development of the maternal spiral arteries in preeclampsia leads to decreased perfusion and oxygenation.

- Vasoconstriction of cerebral vessels leads to pressure-induced rupture of thin-walled capillaries, resulting in small cerebral hemorrhages. Symptoms of arterial vasospasm include headache and visual disturbances such as blurred vision, "spots" before the eyes, and hyperactive deep tendon reflexes (DTRs).
- Decreased colloid oncotic pressure can lead to pulmonary capillary leakage that results in pulmonary edema. Dyspnea is the primary symptom.
- Decreased placental circulation results in infarctions that increase the risk for placental abruption and HELLP syndrome. In addition, the fetus is likely to experience intrauterine growth restriction, persistent hypoxemia, and acidosis when maternal blood flow through the placenta is reduced.

Preventive Measures

Prenatal Care. Early and regular prenatal care with attention to weight gain patterns and close monitoring of blood pressure and urinary protein level may minimize maternal and fetal morbidity and mortality by allowing early detection of preeclampsia.

Attempts at prevention in women at high risk for recurrence have included low-dose aspirin, calcium and magnesium supplements, salt-restricted diet, and fish oil supplements. Low-dose aspirin of 81 mg/day appears to have minimum benefit in high-risk women. Calcium supplementation also appears to reduce the risk for preeclampsia in high-risk women with low calcium intake. Both salt restriction and fish oil supplements have failed to show an impact on the incidence or severity of preeclampsia. No

consensus on measures to reliably prevent preeclampsia in high-risk women exists at this time (Cunningham et al., 2014; Markham & Funai, 2014; Roberts et al., 2013, U.S. Preventive Services, 2014).

Clinical Manifestations of Preeclampsia

Diagnostic Criteria. Preeclampsia is hypertension (systolic blood pressure ≥14 mm Hg or diastolic ≥90 mm Hg) occurring after 20 weeks of pregnancy in women with previously normal blood pressure usually accompanied by proteinuria. Blood pressure measurements should be measured uniformly at each office visit. Blood pressure should be measured with the woman seated, feet flat on the floor, and arm supported, with the appropriate-size cuff placed on her arm at the level of her heart. After a 10-minute rest period, blood pressure should be assessed with a sphygmomanometer and a stethoscope to provide best audible identification of Korotkoff sounds. The diastolic pressure should be recorded at Korotkoff phase V, disappearance of sound. Hospitalizing the woman for serial observations of blood pressure may identify true elevations from those induced by anxiety.

Proteinuria can be identified using a clean-catch specimen or a 24-hour urine collection. Clean-catch urine specimens are used to prevent contamination of the specimen by vaginal secretions or blood. Women with urinary tract infections (UTIs) often have erythrocytes and leukocytes in their urine, which would elevate urine protein level in the absence of preeclampsia. Diagnostic values of 1+ or greater dipstick reading or 300 mg or greater in a 24-hour urine sample indicate developing preeclampsia. A protein-to-creatinine ratio of 0.3 mg or greater is also diagnostic.

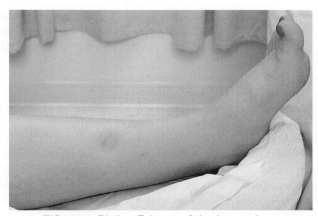

FIG. 10.6 Pitting Edema of the Lower Leg.

According to ACOG's 2013 publication *Task Force on Hypertension in Pregnancy* (ACOG, 2013a), diagnosis can occur in the absence of proteinuria. Therefore, if the following criteria are present in the absence of proteinuria, a diagnosis of preeclampsia is given (Roberts et al., 2013):

- Thrombocytopenia—platelets less than 100,000/μL
- Renal insufficiency—serum creatinine greater than 1.1 mg/dL or a doubling of the serum creatinine concentration in the absence of other renal disease
- Impaired liver function—elevated blood concentrations of liver transaminases to twice normal concentration
- Pulmonary edema
- Cerebral or visual symptoms

When the retina is examined, vascular constriction and narrowing of the small arteries are obvious in most women with preeclampsia. The vasoconstriction that can be seen in the retina is occurring throughout the body. DTRs may be very brisk (hyperreflexia), suggesting cerebral irritability secondary to decreased brain perfusion and edema.

Laboratory studies may identify liver, renal, and hepatic dysfunction if preeclampsia is severe. Coagulation may be impaired, as evidenced by a decrease in the number of platelets, which are often in the high-normal range in a woman without preeclampsia. See also the earlier discussion of DIC.

Although it is a nonspecific sign that may have many causes, generalized edema often occurs with preeclampsia and may be severe. Edema may first manifest as a rapid weight gain caused by fluid retention. It may present in the lower legs, which is common in pregnancy, and in the hands and face (Fig. 10.6). Substantial edema may alter the woman's appearance. Edema may not, however, be present in all women who develop preeclampsia, and it may be severe in women who do not have the disorder. Pulmonary edema is also more common in women with substantial edema from any cause

Symptoms. Preeclampsia is dangerous for the woman and the fetus for two reasons: (1) It can develop and worsen rapidly, and (2) the earliest symptoms are often not noticed by the woman. By the time she notices the symptoms, the disease may have progressed to an advanced state and valuable treatment time lost.

Certain symptoms such as continuous headache, drowsiness, or mental confusion indicate poor cerebral perfusion and may be precursors of seizures. Visual disturbances such as blurred or double vision or spots before the eyes indicate arterial spasms and edema in the retina. In rare instances, blindness can occur. Pathologic lesions present on the retina are caused by ischemia, infarction, or detachment. Numbness or tingling of the hands or feet occurs when nerves are compressed by retained fluid. Some symptoms such as epigastric pain or "upset stomach" are particularly ominous because they indicate distention of the hepatic capsule and increase the risk for liver rupture. Decreased urinary output indicates poor perfusion of the kidneys and may precede acute renal failure (Cunningham et al., 2104).

Therapeutic Management of Preeclampsia

The only cure for preeclampsia is delivery of the baby and placenta. However, the decision about delivery will be based on the severity of the hypertensive disorder and the degree of fetal maturity. Delivery is indicated in the woman with preeclampsia without severe features at 37 weeks of gestation. If the fetus is less than 34 weeks of gestation, steroids to accelerate fetal lung maturity may be given and an attempt made to delay birth for 48 hours. However, if the maternal or fetal condition deteriorates, the infant should be delivered, regardless of gestational age or administration of steroids. Vaginal birth is the preferred delivery method, reserving cesarean section for the usual obstetric implications (Cunningham et al., 2014; Roberts et al., 2013).

Home Care. Management in the home may be possible for select women without severe features and without evidence of worsening fetal or maternal status. The woman should be willing to adhere to a prescribed treatment plan that includes reduced activity (sedentary activity most of the day), home blood pressure monitoring, and follow-up visits to the provider every 3 to 4 days. The woman who is prescribed home care should be taught how to check her blood pressure and report symptoms that suggest worsening preeclampsia, such as visual disturbance, severe headache, or epigastric pain. Symptoms that suggest fetal compromise, such as reduced fetal movement, also should be taught. If the woman is hospitalized with preeclampsia, the assessments for home care in the following section are adapted for her inpatient care (Cunningham et al., 2014; Poole, 2014).

Activity Restrictions. The mother should rest frequently, although full bed rest is not required for preeclampsia. The lateral position decreases pressure on the vena cava, thereby increasing cardiac return and circulatory volume and improving perfusion of the woman's vital organs and the placenta. Although the efficacy of bed rest is not clearly established, it remains a usual and reasonable recommendation for preeclampsia management (Markham & Funai, 2014).

Blood Pressure. If blood pressure monitoring is prescribed, the family should be taught to use electronic blood pressure equipment, readily available in retail stores. Blood pressure should be checked in the same arm and in the same position two to four times each day. An appropriate-size cuff should be used. Although electronic equipment may underestimate blood pressure readings, not providing the precision of manual assessment, they are usually sufficient for home care.

Weight. Daily weight should be obtained each morning, preferably on the same scale and in clothing of similar weight. Increasing weight is an indicator of the degree of fluid retention occurring.

Urinalysis. A provider may order urine dipstick testing for protein. Typically the first voided midstream specimen of the day is used. A 24-hour urine specimens collected at home or in the hospital may be ordered for the most accurate urine protein levels.

Fetal Assessment. Because vasoconstriction can reduce placental flow, the woman will have increased fetal assessments to observe for evidence of fetal compromise. Fetal compromise can be evidenced by reduced fetal movement noted by the mother ("kick counts"). Additional surveillance includes ultrasonography for fetal growth and quantity of amniotic fluid or as part of a biophysical profile (BPP), as well as assessment of umbilical artery blood flow and resistance (Doppler velocimetry). A diminishing amount of amniotic fluid suggests placental impairment. If the pregnancy is less than 34 completed weeks and delivery is being considered but is not yet urgent, amniocentesis is often done to evaluate fetal lung maturity. See Chapter 9 for discussion of fetal surveillance methods (Cunningham et al, 2014; Markham & Funai, 2014).

Diet. The diet should have ample protein and calories. A regular diet without salt or fluid restriction is usually prescribed. Women who also have chronic hypertension or diabetes should have diet management appropriate for these disorders.

A nurse should reevaluate the woman's compliance with prescribed care and her understanding of signs or symptoms to promptly report at each contact, whether by phone or home care visit. The woman should go to the hospital for evaluation promptly if unable to contact her caregiver about signs or symptoms of concern.

Severe Preeclampsia

Diagnostic Criteria. Some clinical findings suggest an increased risk for morbidity and mortality resulting in a diagnosis of severe preeclampsia. Features of severe preeclampsia include one or more of the following (Cunningham et al., 2014; Druzin et al., 2013):

- Systolic blood pressure of 160 mm Hg or greater or a diastolic blood pressure of 110 mm Hg or greater on at least 2 occasions at least 4 to 6 hours apart while the patient is on bed rest
- Thrombocytopenia (platelet count less than 100,000)
- Impaired liver function as indicated by abnormally elevated liver enzymes (to twice normal concentration), severe persistent right upper quadrant, or epigastric pain unresponsive to medication and not accounted for by alternative diagnoses, or both

- Progressive renal insufficiency (serum creatinine concentration greater than 1.1 mg/dL or a doubling of the serum creatinine concentration in the absence of other renal disease)
- Pulmonary edema
- Cerebral or visual disturbances
- Oliguria of less than 500 mL in 24 hours

Nursing assessments focus on identification of disease progression and timely notification of the provider of such findings.

Management of Severe Preeclampsia. Severe preeclampsia requires inpatient hospitalization. Current recommendations for management depend on disease severity and include progression toward delivery, even if the gestation is less than 34 weeks.

Antepartum Management. Goals of management are to improve placental blood flow and fetal oxygenation and prevent seizures and other maternal complications, such as stroke, as the woman's condition is stabilized before birth. A decreased volume of amniotic fluid is considered significant because it suggests reduced placental blood flow, even if blood pressures are not high. Ultrasound may be done to evaluate fetal blood flow through the umbilical cord and placenta.

Bed Rest and Fetal Monitoring. The woman is prescribed bed rest in the lateral position, and her environment is kept quiet. External stimuli (e.g., lights, noise) that might precipitate a seizure should be reduced. EFM is indicated during hospitalization. The frequency of monitoring is individualized based on the patient's status (e.g., twice a day, three times per day, or continuously).

Antihypertensive Medications. Antihypertensive therapies are reserved for women with systolic blood pressure 160 mm Hg or greater or diastolic blood pressure 110 mm Hg or greater to decrease the risk for stroke or congestive heart failure (CHF). Antihypertensive medications are recommended to slowly reduce the woman's blood pressure. The following medications are considered first line because of their efficacy and preservation of uteroplacental blood flow:

- Labetalol—Has less maternal tachycardia and fewer adverse effects; contraindicated in patients with asthma, heart disease, or CHF; associated with hypoglycemia and small for gestational age infants.
- Hydralazine (Apresoline)—Higher doses are associated with maternal hypotension, headaches, and fetal distress
- Nifedipine—May be associated with reflex tachycardia and headaches; because of mechanism of action, a synergistic effect with magnesium sulfate may result in hypotension and neuromuscular blockade.

Caution is essential when antihypertensive medications are given to the woman receiving magnesium sulfate because hypotension may result, reducing placental perfusion (Cunningham et al., 2014; Poole, 2014).

Anticonvulsant Medications. Magnesium sulfate is the drug most often used to prevent seizures. Phenytoin (Dilantin) and diazepam (Valium) are not recommended as first-line agents because of their decreased efficacy compared with magnesium. However, phenytoin may be used in cases in which magnesium sulfate is inappropriate, such as in cases of myasthenia gravis, compromised renal function, or significant pulmonary concerns (Cunningham et al., 2014; Poole, 2014). Current recommendations are to administer magnesium sulfate for seizure prophylaxis in the patient with severe preeclampsia. Use of magnesium in the patient with preeclampsia without severe features remains controversial (Druzin et al., 2013). Magnesium acts as a central nervous system (CNS) depressant by blocking neuromuscular

transmission and decreasing the amount of acetylcholine liberated. Magnesium is not an antihypertensive medication, but it relaxes smooth muscle, including the uterus, and thus reduces vasoconstriction, possibly resulting in modest blood pressure reduction. Decreased vasoconstriction promotes circulation to the vital organs of the expectant mother and increases placental circulation. Increased circulation to the maternal kidneys leads to diuresis as interstitial fluid is shifted into the vascular compartment and excreted.

DRUG GUIDE

Magnesium Sulfate
Classification
Anticonvulsant

Action
Decreases acetylcholine released by motor nerve impulses, thereby blocking neuromuscular transmission. Depresses central nervous system irritability and relaxes smooth muscle, decreasing frequency and intensity of uterine contractions. Slows cardiac conduction. Produces flushing, hypotension, and vasodilation.

Indications
Prevention and control of seizures in severe preeclampsia, prevention of uterine contractions in preterm labor, and neuroprotection of preterm fetus.

Dosage and Route
A common intravenous (IV) administration protocol for preeclampsia includes a loading dose and a continuous infusion using a controlled infusion pump. The IV loading dose is 4 to 6 g of magnesium sulfate administered over 15 to 20 minutes. The continuing infusion to maintain control is 1 to 2 g/hr. Doses are individualized as needed. Deep intramuscular (IM) injection is acceptable but is painful, and the rate of absorption cannot be controlled. Dosing for IM injection is 10 g (5 g in each buttock), followed by 5 g every 4 hours. A mainline IV infusion with no medication is maintained, and the magnesium sulfate is piggy-backed into the port closest to the IV site.

Onset of Action
IV: Immediate. IM: 1 hour.

Excretion
Renal clearance. In women with normal kidney function, magnesium is excreted in approximately 4 hours.

Contraindications and Precautions
Contraindicated in persons with myocardial damage, heart block, myasthenia gravis, or impaired renal function. Magnesium toxicity, possibly related to incomplete renal drug excretion, may be evidenced by respiratory difficulty, lethargy, mental confusion, slurred speech, visual disturbances, or a decrease in reflexes.

Reactions
Result from magnesium overdose and include flushing, sweating, hypotension, depressed DTRs, and central nervous system depression, including respiratory depression.

Nursing Implications
Monitor blood pressure closely during administration. Assess the woman for respiratory rate above 12 breaths per minute, presence of DTRs, and urinary output greater than 30 mL/hr before administering magnesium. Place resuscitation equipment (suction and oxygen) in the room. Ensure calcium gluconate, which acts as an antidote to magnesium, is readily available, along with syringes and needles (Cunningham et al., 2014; Magnesium Sulfate Drug Information, 2016; Markham & Funai, 2014; Poole, 2014; Zeng et al., 2016).

Magnesium is administered by IV infusion, which allows for immediate onset of action and does not cause the discomfort associated with intramuscular administration. Magnesium is administered via a secondary line so the medication can be discontinued at any time while the primary line remains functional. The Institute for Safe Medication Practices (ISMP, 2014) lists 12 individual medications considered high risk. Magnesium sulfate is on that list. Therefore two qualified nurses check the orders and pump settings to ensure that the ordered grams per hour of magnesium is infused and the total IV fluid volume is correct.

Although magnesium sulfate is not risk-free, the major advantage of magnesium is its long record of safety for mother and baby while preventing maternal seizures (American Association of Pediatrics [AAP] & ACOG, 2012). Fetal magnesium levels are

nearly identical with those of the expectant mother. As a result, the fetal monitor tracing may show decreased FHR variability and reactivity. No cumulative effect occurs, however, because the fetal kidneys excrete magnesium effectively.

The therapeutic serum level for magnesium is 5 to 8 mg/dL, although it is elevated in terms of normal laboratory values. Adverse reactions to magnesium sulfate usually occur if the serum level becomes too high. The most significant adverse reaction is CNS depression, including depression of the respiratory center. Magnesium is excreted solely by the kidneys, and the reduced urine output that often occurs in preeclampsia allows magnesium to accumulate to toxic levels in the woman. Frequent assessment of serum magnesium levels, DTRs respiratory rate, and oxygen saturation can identify CNS depression before it progresses to respiratory depression or cardiac dysfunction. Monitoring urine output identifies oliguria that could allow magnesium to accumulate and reach excessive levels.

Intrapartum Management. Half of eclamptic seizures occur during labor or in the first 48 hours after birth. The other half occur antenatally (Cunningham et al., 2014; Poole, 2014).The fetus and the mother should be monitored continuously to detect signs of decreased fetal oxygenation and imminent seizures. The woman should be kept in a lateral position to promote circulation through the placenta, and efforts should focus on controlling pain that may cause agitation and precipitate seizures.

Oxytocin to stimulate uterine contractions and magnesium sulfate to prevent seizures are often administered simultaneously during labor when a woman has preeclampsia. The woman will have two secondary infusions in addition to her primary infusion line, one for oxytocin and one for magnesium. Antibiotics or other drugs may require additional lines. Multiple infusion pumps ensure that different medications and fluids are administered at the prescribed volume and dose. Equipment, IV lines, and IV sites should be checked carefully for correct placement and function.

Opiate analgesics or epidural analgesia may be administered to provide comfort and reduce painful stimuli that could precipitate a seizure. However, some women with severe preeclampsia have coagulation abnormalities that may contraindicate use of epidural analgesia.

Continuous EFM identifies changes in FHR patterns that suggest fetal compromise (see Chapter 14). Late decelerations and decreased variability are associated with reduced placental perfusion. The nurse continuously assesses the FHR pattern for any indeterminate or abnormal pattern. Interventions implemented are tailored to the fetal heart pattern identified, such as repositioning the mother, stopping the oxytocin infusion, altering other IV infusion rates, or administering oxygen to the mother. A neonatal resuscitation team is often called to the birth.

Postpartum Management. After birth, careful assessment of the mother's blood loss and signs of shock are essential because the hypovolemia caused by preeclampsia may be aggravated by blood loss during the delivery. Assessments for signs and symptoms of preeclampsia should be continued for at least 48 hours, and administration of magnesium along with its associated care usually is continued to prevent seizures for 24 hours.

Signs that the woman is recovering from preeclampsia include the following:
- Diuresis—Increased urinary output, which causes a rapid reduction in edema and rapid weight loss
- Decreased protein in the urine
- Return of blood pressure to normal
- Resolution of abnormal laboratory values

Therapeutic Management of Eclampsia. Eclampsia is a potentially preventable extension of severe preeclampsia marked by one or more generalized seizures, at times occurring before the woman goes to the hospital (Cunningham et al., 2014; Poole, 2014). Early identification

of preeclampsia in a pregnant woman allows intervention before the condition reaches the seizure stage in most cases. Generalized seizures are characterized by muscles alternately contracting and relaxing. These tonic-clonic movements last for about 1 minute. Breathing stops during a generalized seizure but resumes with a long, noisy inhalation. Gradually the muscle movements decrease until they finally stop and the woman lies motionless. The woman enters in an unresponsive state and is unlikely to remember the seizure when she resumes consciousness. This unresponsive state may be transient, or she may be in a coma for an unspecified time depending on the severity of the insult (Markham & Funai, 2014). Transient FHR patterns such as bradycardia, loss of variability, or late decelerations are anticipated. Fetal tachycardia may occur as the fetus compensates for the period of maternal apnea during the seizures.

The woman's blood volume is often severely reduced in eclampsia, increasing the risk for poor placental perfusion. Fluid shifts from her intravascular space to the interstitial space, including the lungs, causing pulmonary edema and possibly heart failure as forward blood flow from the maternal heart is impeded. Renal blood flow is severely reduced, resulting in oliguria (less than 30 mL/hr urine output) and possibly renal failure. Cerebral hemorrhage may accompany eclampsia because of the high blood pressure and coagulation deficits. The woman's lungs should be auscultated at regular intervals assessing for adventitious breath sounds. A pulse oximeter provides continuous readings of oxygen saturation. Furosemide (Lasix) may be administered if pulmonary edema develops. Administration of oxygen via a nonrebreather face mask at 10 L/min improves maternal and fetal oxygenation. Digitalis may be needed to strengthen contraction of the heart if circulatory failure results. Frequent assessments, usually at least hourly, of the previously mentioned parameters are indicated after an eclamptic seizure.

Because eclampsia stimulates uterine irritability, the woman should be monitored carefully for ruptured membranes, signs of labor, or placental abruption. While the woman is **postictal** (the unresponsive state after a seizure), she should be kept on her side to prevent aspiration and improve placental circulation. Aspiration of gastric contents is a leading cause of maternal morbidity after an eclamptic seizure (Roberts et al., 2013). Equipment to suction the woman's airway should be immediately available. The side rails should be raised to prevent a fall and possible injury. After initial stabilization, the nurse should anticipate orders for chest radiography and arterial blood gas determination to identify aspiration and possibly an order for head computed tomography (CT) to identify any cerebral hemorrhage (Markham & Funai, 2014; Poole, 2014). HELLP syndrome is associated with severe preeclampsia. DIC is an added complication of unexpected bleeding that may occur with coagulation abnormalities of severe preeclampsia or eclampsia. Laboratory studies are performed at frequent intervals to identify both falling and recovering coagulation values, as well as to identify hemolysis and elevated levels of liver enzymes. After maternal and fetal conditions have been stabilized, the fetus usually is delivered, either by induction of labor if the woman's cervix is favorable or by cesarean birth if she is remote from term.

KNOWLEDGE CHECK

14. What are the effects of maternal vasospasm on the fetus?
15. What are the signs and symptoms of preeclampsia? Why is reduced activity a part of management?
16. What is the effect of vasospasm on the brain?
17. What are the effects of magnesium sulfate, including the primary adverse effect?
18. What are the major complications of eclampsia?

◆ APPLICATION OF THE NURSING PROCESS: PREECLAMPSIA

◆ Assessment

Nursing assessment is one of the most important components of successful management of preeclampsia. Careful assessment is the only way to determine whether the condition is responding to medical management or whether the disease is worsening. A 1:1 nurse-to-patient ratio is needed for the unstable woman with severe preeclampsia.

Weigh the woman on admission and daily. Check vital signs, and auscultate the chest at least every 4 hours for crackles, adventitious breath sounds that indicate pulmonary edema. Assess the location and severity of edema at least every 4 hours. Table 10.4 provides a guideline to describe edema. Maintain strict intake and output monitoring. Insert an indwelling catheter to measure hourly urine output. Check the urine for protein as ordered. Apply an external electronic fetal monitor to identify changes in FHR resulting in indeterminate or abnormal patterns. Consider maternal medications and their relationship to the FHR pattern.

Check reflexes such as brachial, radial, and patellar reflexes for hyperreflexia, which indicates cerebral irritability. Determine whether clonus is present with hyperactive reflexes by dorsiflexing the woman's foot sharply and then releasing it while her knee is held in a flexed position. Clonus (rapidly alternating muscle contraction and relaxation) may occur when reflexes are hyperactive. If clonus is present, it should be reported to the provider (Kee-Hak, Steinberg, & Ramus, 2016). Procedure 10.1 illustrates how to assess and rate DTRs and clonus.

Question the woman carefully about symptoms she may be experiencing, such as headache, visual disturbances, epigastric pain, nausea or vomiting, or a sudden increase in edema.

Detailed questions are needed to identify important symptoms. Ask targeted questions such as "Do you have a headache? Describe it for me." "Do you have any pain in the abdomen? Show me where it hurts, and describe it." "Do you see spots before your eyes? Flashes of light?" "Do you have double vision?" "Is your vision blurred?" "Does the light bother you?" "Are you still able to wear your rings? Did you remove them because your hands were swollen? When did that happen?"

TABLE 10.4   Assessment of Edema

Characteristics	Grade
Minimal edema of lower extremities	+1
Marked edema of lower extremities	+2
Edema of lower extremities, face, hands, and sacral area	+3
Generalized massive edema that includes ascites (accumulation of fluid in peritoneal cavity)	+4

Retrieved from www.gbhn.ca/ebc/documents/ASSESSMENTOFPITTINGEDEMA.pdf

Assessments for Magnesium Toxicity

Obstetric units have protocols that address routine assessments and their frequency when magnesium is being administered. Reflexes may be slightly hypotonic but should not be absent at therapeutic levels of magnesium. Absent reflexes suggest CNS depression that precedes respiratory depression if magnesium levels are too high. Determining the respiratory rate and oxygen saturations by pulse oximetry identifies the adequacy of maternal respirations. Checking urine output identifies oliguria (below 30 mL/hr), which may result in magnesium toxicity as the drug accumulates. Assess the woman's level of consciousness (alert, drowsy [expected], confused, oriented, disoriented). Table 10.5 summarizes nursing assessments and their implications.

Psychosocial Assessment

The development of preeclampsia places added stress on the childbearing family. If the condition is not severe and the gestation period is early, the woman may be instructed to reduce her activity at home. She may be hospitalized, complicating care for other children. This creates anxiety about the condition of the fetus and that of the mother. Many families do not understand the seriousness of the disease. The possibility that a preterm birth may be necessary to reduce harm to mother and infant adds to the family's concerns about the outcome.

Explore how the family will function while the expectant mother is hospitalized. Determine how the woman is adapting to the "sick role" and the need of being dependent on others instead of functioning in her primary role. Ask how much support is available and who is willing to participate. Determine whether referrals to manage loss of income are needed. Finally, determine the priority concerns of the family.

◆ Identification of Patient Problems

Analysis of the data collected can lead to both nursing diagnoses and collaborative problems for potential complications. Both physician-prescribed and nurse-prescribed interventions are used to minimize the complications. Potential complications for the woman with preeclampsia are listed in Table 10.2.

◆ Planning: Expected Outcomes

Patient-centered nursing goals are inappropriate for the potential complications of eclamptic seizures and magnesium toxicity because the nurse cannot independently

NURSING PROCEDURE 10.1 Assessing Deep Tendon Reflexes

Purpose

To identify exaggerated reflexes (hyperreflexia) or diminished reflexes (hyporeflexia).

1. You will need a reflex hammer to best assess the brachial and the patellar reflexes. The patellar reflex is less reliable if the woman has had epidural analgesia. Upper extremity reflexes should be assessed.

2. Support the woman's arm, and instruct her to let it go limp while it is being held so that the arm is totally relaxed and slightly flexed as you assess the brachial reflex. If you have difficulty identifying the correct tendon to tap, have the woman flex and extend her arm until you can feel it moving beneath your thumb. Have her fully relax her arm after you identify the tendon.

3. Place your thumb over the woman's tendon, as illustrated, to allow you to feel as well as see the tendon response when it is tapped. Strike your thumb with the small end of the reflex hammer. The normal response is slight flexion of the forearm.

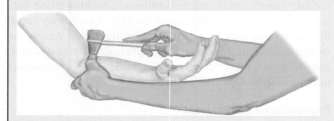

4. The patellar, or "knee-jerk," reflex can be assessed with the woman in two positions, sitting or lying. When the woman is sitting, allow her lower legs to dangle freely to flex the knee and stretch the tendons. If her patellar tendon is difficult to identify, have her flex and extend her lower legs slightly until you palpate the tendon. Strike the tendon directly with the reflex hammer just below the patella.

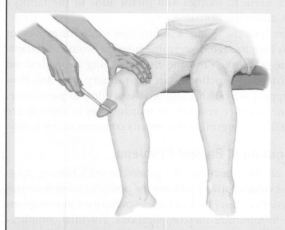

5. When the woman is supine, the weight of her leg should be supported to flex the knee and stretch the tendons. An accurate response requires that the limb be relaxed and the tendon partially stretched. Strike the partially stretched tendons just below the patella. Slight extension of the leg or a brief twitch of the quadriceps muscle of the thigh is the expected response.

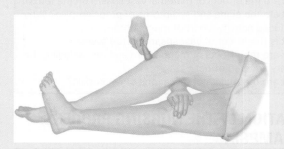

6. To assess for clonus, the woman's lower leg should be supported, as illustrated, and the foot well dorsiflexed to stretch the tendon. Hold the flexion. If no clonus is present, no movement will be felt. When clonus (indicating hyperreflexia) is present, rapid rhythmic tapping motions of the foot are present.

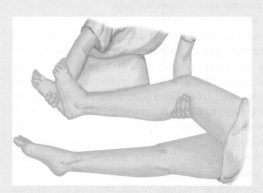

Deep Tendon Reflex Rating Scale

0	Reflex absent
+ 1	Reflex present, hypoactive
+ 2	Normal reflex
+ 3	Brisker than average reflex
+ 4	Hyperactive reflex; clonus may also be present

TABLE 10.5	Nursing Assessments for Preeclampsia and Magnesium Toxicity
Assessment	**Implications**
Daily weight	Provides estimate of fluid retention.
Blood pressure	Determines worsening condition, response to treatment, or both.
Respiratory rate, pulse oximeter readings	Drug therapy (magnesium sulfate) causes respiratory depression, and drug should be decreased or withheld and physician notified if respiratory rate is <12 breaths per minute or as specified by hospital policy. Pulse oximeter readings should be ≥95% in the pregnant patient and 92% in the nonpregnant patient.
Breath sounds	Identifies sounds of excess moisture in lungs associated with pulmonary edema.
Deep tendon reflexes and clonus	Hyperreflexia and clonus indicate increased cerebral irritability and edema; hyporeflexia is associated with magnesium excess.
Edema	Provides estimation of interstitial fluid.
Urinary output	Output of at least 30 mL/hr indicates adequate perfusion of the kidneys. Magnesium levels may become toxic if urinary output is inadequate.
Urine protein	Normal protein in random dipstick urine sample is negative or trace. Higher protein levels suggest greater leaking of protein secondary to glomerular damage with worsening preeclampsia. A 24-hr urine sample is most accurate for quantitative urine protein level.
Level of consciousness	Drowsiness or dulled sensorium indicates therapeutic effects of magnesium; no responsive behavior or muscle weakness is associated with magnesium excess.
Headache, epigastric pain, visual problems	These symptoms indicate increasing severity of condition caused by cerebral edema, vasospasm of cerebral vessels, and liver edema. Eclampsia may develop quickly.
Fetal heart rate and baseline variability	Rate should be between 110 and 160 bpm. Decreasing baseline variability may be caused by therapeutic magnesium level or by inadequate placental perfusion.
Laboratory data	Significant signs of increasing severity of disease are elevated serum creatinine level, elevated uric acid, elevated levels of liver enzymes, or decreased number of platelets (thrombocytopenia). Serum magnesium levels should be in therapeutic range designated by physician.

manage these conditions. The nurse should confer with physicians and use established protocols for treatment. Planning should reflect the nurse's responsibility to do the following:

- Perform actions that minimize the risk for seizures and prevent injury if seizures do occur.
- Monitor for signs of impending seizures.
- Consult with the physician if signs of impending seizures are observed.
- Support the family of the woman with eclampsia.
- Monitor for signs of magnesium toxicity.
- Consult with the physician if signs of magnesium toxicity are observed.
- Perform actions that reduce the possibility of magnesium toxicity.

◆ **Interventions**

Interventions for Seizures

Monitor for Signs of Impending Seizures. Assess for changes in the following:

- Hyperreflexia, possibly accompanied by clonus
- Increasing signs of cerebral irritability (headache, visual disturbances)
- Epigastric or right upper quadrant pain, nausea, or vomiting

Although none of these signs is a predictor of imminent seizure, nurses should be alert for subtle changes and be prepared for seizures in all women with preeclampsia.

Initiate Preventive Measures. In the presence of cerebral irritability, generalized seizures may be precipitated by excessive visual or auditory stimuli. Nurses should reduce external stimuli by doing the following:

- Keep the door to her room closed. Heightened surveillance of patient status is needed regardless of the specific room location that is available.
- Keep lights low and noise to a minimum. This may include blocking incoming telephone calls, instructing visitors to silence cell phones and electronic devices, and turning the noises of the electronic monitors (fetal monitor, pulse oximeter, IV pump) as low as possible.
- Group nursing assessments and care to allow the woman periods of undisturbed quiet.
- Move carefully and calmly around the room and avoid bumping into the bed or startling the woman.
- Collaborate with the woman and her family to restrict visitors.

Prevent Seizure-Related Injury. Hard side rails should be padded and the bed kept in the lowest position with the wheels locked to prevent trauma during a seizure.

Oxygen and suction equipment should be assembled and ready to use to suction secretions and to provide oxygen if it is not already being administered. Check equipment and connections at the beginning of each shift because sufficient time for setup will not exist if seizures occur.

The following equipment should be readily available: an Ambu bag with mask, reflex hammer, pulse oximeter, stethoscope, and syringes and needles. Medications that should be readily available include magnesium sulfate and calcium gluconate.

Protect the Woman and the Fetus during a Seizure. Nurses should protect the woman and the fetus during a seizure. The nurse's primary responsibilities are the following:

- Remain with the woman and press the emergency bell for assistance.
- If she is not on her side already, attempt to turn the woman onto her side when the tonic phase begins. A side-lying position permits greater circulation through the placenta and may prevent aspiration.
- Note the time and sequence of the seizure. Eclampsia is marked by a tonic-clonic seizure that may be preceded by facial twitching that lasts for a few seconds. A tonic contraction of the entire body is followed by the clonic phase, which may last about 1 minute.
- Maintain a patent airway after the seizure, and suction the woman's mouth and nose to prevent aspiration. Administer oxygen by nonrebreather facemask at 10 L/min to increase oxygenation of the placenta and all maternal body organs.
- Notify the physician that a seizure has occurred. This is an obstetric emergency that is associated with cerebral hemorrhage, placental abruption, severe fetal hypoxia, and death.
- Administer medications and prepare for additional medical interventions as directed by the physician.

These interventions are also relevant if the woman has a generalized seizure disorder that is unrelated to hypertension.

Provide Information and Support for the Family. Explain to the family what has happened without minimizing the seriousness of the situation. A generalized seizure is frightening for anyone who witnesses it. Explain that the woman will be unconscious and then may be drowsy for some time afterward. Acknowledge that the seizure indicates worsening of the condition and that it will be necessary for the physician to determine future management, which may include delivery of the infant as soon as possible.

Interventions for Magnesium Toxicity

Monitor for Signs of Magnesium Toxicity. Magnesium excess depresses the entire CNS, including the brainstem, which controls respirations and cardiac function, and the cerebrum, which controls memory, mental processes, and speech. Carbon dioxide accumulates if the respiratory rate is reduced, leading to respiratory acidosis and further CNS depression, which could culminate in respiratory arrest.

Signs of magnesium toxicity include the following (Cunningham et al., 2014):

- Respiratory depression, with a rate of fewer than 12 breaths per minute
- Chest pain
- Decreasing maternal pulse oximeter values:
  - Less than 95% during pregnancy
  - Less than 92% during postpartum phase
- Absence of DTRs
- Blurred vision

- Altered sensorium (confused, lethargic, slurred speech, drowsy, disoriented)
- Oliguria
- Hypotension
- Serum magnesium value greater than 8 mg/dL
- Respiratory/cardiac arrest

Respond to Signs of Magnesium Toxicity. Discontinue magnesium if the respiratory rate is below 12 breaths per minute, pulse oximeter rate is decreasing, or DTRs are absent. Additional magnesium will make the condition worse. Notify the provider of the woman's condition for additional orders. If the urinary output falls below 30 mL/hr, the provider may alter the drug dosage to maintain a therapeutic range.

Calcium opposes the effects of magnesium at the neuromuscular junction, and it should be readily available whenever magnesium is administered. Magnesium toxicity can be reversed by IV administration of 1 g (10 mL of 10% solution) of calcium gluconate over 3 minutes (Druzin, 2013).

◆ Evaluation

Collect and compare data with established norms and then determine whether the data are within normal limits. For seizures, interventions are deemed successful if the following occur:

- Reflexes remain within normal limits (+1 to +3).
- The woman is free of visual disturbances, headache, and epigastric or right upper quadrant pain.
- The woman remains free of seizures or free of preventable injury if a seizure occurs.

For magnesium toxicity, determine whether respiratory rates remain at least 12 breaths per minute, DTRs are present and not hyperactive, and maternal plasma levels of magnesium do not exceed the therapeutic range of 5 to 8 mg/dL.

❓ KNOWLEDGE CHECK

19. What nursing assessments should be made for the woman with preeclampsia? Why?
20. What measures may be initiated to prevent or manage seizures?
21. How can injury during seizure be prevented?
22. What are the signs of magnesium toxicity? How should it be managed?

HEMOLYSIS, ELEVATED LIVER ENZYMES, AND LOW PLATELETS SYNDROME

The syndrome of hemolysis, elevated liver enzymes, and low platelets (HELLP syndrome) is a life-threatening occurrence that complicates approximately 10% of pregnancies. Half of the women affected by HELLP also have severe preeclampsia, although hypertension may be absent. The normotensive woman should be considered to have preeclampsia if she has other signs of reduced organ perfusion. As in preeclampsia, HELLP syndrome may occur during the postpartum period (Cunningham et al., 2014; Williamson, Mackillop, & Heneghan, 2014).

Hemolysis is believed to occur as a result of the fragmentation and distortion of erythrocytes during passage through small damaged blood vessels. Liver enzyme levels increase when hepatic blood flow is obstructed by fibrin deposits. Hyperbilirubinemia and jaundice may occur as a result of liver impairment. Vasospasm causes vascular damage. Platelets aggregate at sites of damage resulting in low platelet levels (thrombocytopenia), which increases the risk for bleeding, frequently in the liver (Cunningham et al., 2014).

The prominent symptom of HELLP syndrome is pain in the right upper quadrant, the lower right chest, or the midepigastric area. This tenderness may result from liver distention. Additional signs and symptoms include nausea, vomiting, and severe edema. A sudden increase in intraabdominal pressure, including that caused by a seizure, could lead to rupture of a subcapsular hematoma, resulting in internal bleeding and hypovolemic shock. Hepatic rupture can lead to fetal and maternal mortality (Cunningham et al., 2014; Sibai, 2017; Williamson et al., 2014).

Women with HELLP syndrome should be managed in a setting with intensive care facilities. Treatment includes magnesium sulfate to control seizures and hydralazine or labetalol to control blood pressure. Fluid replacement is managed to avoid worsening the woman's reduced intravascular volume without giving her too much, because that could cause pulmonary edema or ascites. Cervical ripening with labor induction may be performed if the gestation is at least 34 weeks. Delivery may be delayed if the gestation is less than 34 weeks and the woman's condition is stable, to allow for steroid administration to stimulate fetal lung maturation (AAP & ACOG, 2012; Cunningham et al., 2014; Roberts et al., 2013; Sibai, 2017).

If the woman is near term and has a favorable cervix, induction of labor is preferred to avoid the bleeding and clotting complications that are more likely to occur with cesarean birth. Anesthesia choices are likely to be complicated by laryngeal edema (intubation difficulties), low platelet counts that may reduce safety of epidural block, and coagulation abnormalities that can have an impact on safety of pudendal blocks. Cesarean birth may be necessary if the woman is far from term or has an unfavorable cervix.

CHRONIC HYPERTENSION

A diagnosis of chronic hypertension is made if hypertension precedes pregnancy or is identified before 20 weeks of gestation. The diagnosis also can be based on blood pressure that remains elevated beyond postpartum week 12. Chronic hypertension is most often associated with advanced maternal age, obesity, and comorbidities such as diabetes. Heredity, including race, plays a role in the development of chronic hypertension, which is more common in African Americans at any age than in people of other races. Late childbearing and rising obesity rates add to the risks

for women. However, hypertension may be secondary to another problem, such as renal disease or an autoimmune disorder (Centers for Disease Control and Prevention [CDC], 2012; Cunningham et al., 2014).

Elevated circulating hormones, prostaglandins, and progesterone cause a decrease in blood pressure during early pregnancy; therefore the woman's blood pressure may appear normal when she enters prenatal care. Antihypertensive therapy is reserved for women with consistently elevated systolic pressures above 160 mm Hg or diastolic pressures above 90 to 100 mm Hg. If she already is taking an antihypertensive drug, she usually continues this drug unless her blood pressure becomes low because of vasodilation of pregnancy. Antihypertensive medications should be chosen carefully because they may reduce placental blood flow. Methyldopa (Aldomet) is the drug of choice because of its record of safety and effectiveness in pregnancy. Beta-blockers and calcium channel blockers also may be used if methyldopa is not effective, but their record of safety in pregnancy is less well established. Angiotensin-converting enzyme (ACE) inhibitors are not recommended in pregnancy but may be used in the postpartum period. Hydralazine is a vasodilator reserved for hypertensive crisis. Diuretics are avoided, if possible, because they may shrink the blood volume, which already may be reduced if preeclampsia exists with the chronic hypertension. In cases of pulmonary edema, diuretics may be necessary. (Cunningham et al., 2014; Markham & Funai, 2014).

The most common maternal complication is the development of preeclampsia, which occurs in approximately 25% of pregnant women with chronic hypertension. New-onset proteinuria or a significant rise in preexisting proteinuria identifies the development of superimposed preeclampsia. The rise in blood pressure with preeclampsia is likely to be greater in these women. Development of signs and symptoms indicating multiorgan development (headache, epigastric pain, or visual changes) are correlated to abnormal renal, hepatic, or hematologic laboratory values (Cunningham et al., 2014; Markham & Funai, 2014; NHLBI, 2000).

A dietitian should be consulted about the appropriate diet and weight gain because many of these women are obese and frequently have diabetes. Adequate intake of protein helps counteract the protein lost in urine. A reduced salt intake may be advised, unlike recommendations for the woman with preeclampsia alone. More frequent prenatal visits will be needed. Regular fetal surveillance by BPP and kick counts (see Chapter 9) is recommended to identify fetal compromise, such as poor growth patterns or decreasing amount of amniotic fluid.

❓ KNOWLEDGE CHECK

23. What does the acronym HELLP stand for? What are the prominent signs and symptoms of HELLP syndrome? Why should the liver not be palpated in a woman with HELLP syndrome?
24. Compare preeclampsia with chronic hypertension in terms of onset and treatment.

INCOMPATIBILITY BETWEEN MATERNAL AND FETAL BLOOD

Rh Incompatibility

Rhesus (Rh) factor incompatibility during pregnancy is possible only when two specific circumstances coexist: (1) the mother is Rh-negative (D-negative), and (2) the fetus is Rh-positive. For such a circumstance to occur, the father of the fetus must be Rh-positive. Rh incompatibility is a problem that affects the fetus; it causes no harm to the mother.

Rh-negative blood is an autosomal recessive trait, and a person must inherit the same gene from both parents to be Rh-negative. Approximately 15% of the White population in the United States is Rh-negative. The incidence is lower in the African-American and Asian populations (ACOG, 2016e).

Pathophysiology

People who are Rh-positive have the Rh antigen on their RBCs, whereas people who are Rh-negative do not have the antigen. When blood from a person who is Rh-positive enters the bloodstream of a person who is Rh-negative, the body reacts as it would to any foreign substance. It develops antibodies to destroy the invading antigen. To destroy the Rh antigen, which exists as part of the RBC, the entire RBC must be destroyed. The antibodies do not affect the Rh-negative RBCs because they do not have the Rh antigen. Exposure of the Rh-negative male or female to Rh-positive blood may occur unrelated to a pregnancy, such as during emergency blood transfusion. Destruction of Rh-positive cells occurs in the Rh-negative person after they have become sensitized (developed antibodies) to the Rh-positive antigens.

The Rh antigen does not cross an intact placenta; sensitization of the mother occurs when the Rh-positive blood of the fetus enters maternal circulation Theoretically, fetal and maternal blood do not mix during pregnancy. In reality, small placental accidents occur that allow a drop or two of fetal blood to enter the maternal circulation and initiate the production of antibodies to destroy the Rh-positive blood. Sensitization also can occur during a spontaneous or elective abortion or during antepartum procedures such as amniocentesis and chorionic villus sampling. A rapid immune response against Rh-positive blood occurs with an extensive fetal-maternal hemorrhage in complications such as placenta previa or placental abruption or with an uncomplicated birth.

Most exposure of maternal blood to fetal blood occurs during the third stage of labor, when active exchange of fetal and maternal blood may occur from damaged placental vessels. In this case the woman's first child is not usually affected because antibodies are formed after the birth of the infant. However, since the antibodies remain in the woman's body and cross an intact placenta, subsequent Rh-positive fetuses may be affected, unless the mother receives Rh immune globulin (RhoGAM) to prevent antibody formation after the birth of each Rh-positive infant.

Fetal and Neonatal Implications

If antibodies to the Rh factor are present in the pregnant mother's blood, they cross the placenta and destroy Rh-positive fetal erythrocytes. The fetus becomes deficient in RBCs, which are needed to transport oxygen to fetal tissue. As fetal RBCs are destroyed, fetal bilirubin levels increase (icterus gravis), which can lead to neurologic disease (**kernicterus** [staining of brain tissue], leading to bilirubin encephalopathy). This hemolytic process results in rapid production of erythroblasts (immature RBCs), which cannot carry oxygen. The entire syndrome is termed **erythroblastosis fetalis**. The fetus may become so anemic that generalized fetal edema (hydrops fetalis) results and can end in fetal CHF.

Prenatal Assessment and Management

Women should have a blood test to determine blood type and Rh factor at the initial prenatal visit. Rh-negative women should have an indirect Coombs' test to determine whether they are sensitized (have developed antibodies) as a result of previous exposure to Rh-positive blood. If the indirect Coombs' test is negative, it is repeated at 28 weeks of gestation to identify whether they have developed subsequent sensitization.

Rh immune globulin (RhoGAM) is administered to the unsensitized Rh-negative woman at 28 weeks of gestation to prevent sensitization, which may occur from small leaks of fetal blood across the placenta. RhoGAM is a commercial preparation of passive antibodies against Rh factor. It effectively prevents the formation of active antibodies against Rh-positive erythrocytes if a small amount of fetal Rh-positive blood enters the circulation of the Rh-negative mother during the remainder of the pregnancy. Administration of RhoGAM is repeated after birth if the woman delivers an Rh-positive infant.

> **! SAFETY CHECK**
>
> All unsensitized Rh-negative women should receive Rh immune globulin (RhoGAM) after abortion, ectopic pregnancy, chorionic villus sampling, amniocentesis, or birth of an Rh-positive infant. Rh immune globulin prevents the development of Rh antibodies that would result in destruction of fetal erythrocytes in subsequent pregnancies.

If the indirect Coombs' test result is positive, indicating maternal sensitization and the presence of antibodies, it is repeated at frequent intervals throughout the pregnancy to determine whether the antibody titer is rising. An increase in titer indicates that the process is continuing and that the fetus will be in jeopardy.

Ultrasound examination is used to noninvasively evaluate the condition of the fetus. Doppler studies allow evaluation of cardiac function and blood flow in fetal vessels. The systolic blood flow in the fetal middle cerebral artery is a noninvasive way to assess the degree of fetal anemia. An anemic fetus will increase blood flow to the brain in an effort to maintain oxygenation of the CNS. This increased blood flow is detected by Doppler sonography and can be quantified. Blood flow of 1.5 times the median for the fetal gestational age is predictive of moderate to severe fetal anemia (ACOG, 2016b). Generalized fetal edema, ascites, an enlarged heart, or hydramnios occurs when the fetus is very anemic. Percutaneous umbilical blood sampling (PUBS), or cordocentesis, allows invasive sampling of fetal blood from cord vessels to determine the degree of erythrocyte destruction. Because it is invasive, PUBS is reserved for the fetus thought to be significantly affected.

Intrauterine transfusion is the direct infusion of O-negative erythrocytes into the umbilical cord by percutaneous umbilical blood transfusion if the fetus is severely affected. The transfused erythrocytes must be compatible with maternal blood to avoid destruction by her antibodies. Whole blood is usually used to replace fetal serum proteins. Erythrocytes also may be transfused into the fetal abdominal cavity, where they are gradually absorbed into the circulation.

Postpartum Management

If the mother is Rh-negative, umbilical cord blood is taken at delivery to determine blood type, Rh factor, and antibody titer (direct Coombs' test) of the newborn. Rh-negative, unsensitized mothers who give birth to Rh-positive infants are given an intramuscular injection of RhoGAM within 72 hours after delivery. If RhoGAM is given to the mother within 72 hours after the birth of an Rh-positive infant, she does not form antibodies to the Rh antigen. If the infant is Rh-negative, Rh antibody formation does not occur and RhoGAM is not necessary.

⬮ DRUG GUIDE

Rho(D) Immune Globulin (RhoGAM, Hypro-D, Gamulin Rh)
Classification
Concentrated immunoglobulins directed toward the red blood cell (RBC) antigen Rho(D).

Action
Prevents production of anti-Rho(D) antibodies in Rh-negative women who have been exposed to Rh-positive blood by suppressing the immune reaction of the Rh-negative woman to the antigen in Rh-positive blood; prevents antibody response and thereby prevents hemolytic disease of the newborn in future Rh-positive pregnancies; used for both males and females who are Rh-negative but exposed to Rh-positive blood or for immune thrombocytopenic purpura (ITP).

Indications (Pregnancy Related)
Administered to Rh-negative women who have been exposed to Rh-positive blood by doing the following:
- Delivering an Rh-positive infant
- Aborting an Rh-positive fetus
- Undergoing chorionic villus sampling, amniocentesis, or intraabdominal trauma while carrying an Rh-positive fetus
- Receiving inadvertent transfusion of Rh-positive blood

Dosage and Route
One *standard* dose (300 mcg) administered intramuscularly:
1. At 28 weeks of pregnancy and within 72 hours of delivery of an Rh-positive infant, undergoing chorionic villus sampling, amniocentesis, or intraabdominal trauma.
2. Within 72 hours after termination of a pregnancy of 13 weeks or more of gestation.

One *microdose* (50 mcg) within 72 hours after the termination of a pregnancy of less than 13 weeks of gestation. The dose of

RhoGAM is calculated based on the volume of fetal-maternal hemorrhage or Rh-positive blood administered in transfusion accidents. A standard dose of 1500 international units or 300 mcg will protect against 30 mL of Rh-positive whole blood or 15 mL of packed RBCs (ACOG, 2016e; Cunningham et al., 2014).

Absorption
Well absorbed from intramuscular sites.

Excretion
Metabolism and excretion unknown.

Contraindications and Precautions
Women who are Rh-positive or women previously sensitized to Rho(D) should not receive Rho(D) immune globulin. It is used cautiously for women with previous hypersensitivity reactions to immune globulins.

Adverse Reactions
Local pain at intramuscular site, fever, or both.

Nursing Implications
Type and antibody screening of the mother's blood and cord blood type of the newborn should be performed to determine the need for the medication. The mother must be Rh-negative and negative for Rh antibodies. The newborn must be Rh-positive. If the fetal blood type after termination of pregnancy is uncertain, the medication should be administered. The newborn may have a weakly positive antibody test if the woman received Rho(D) immune globulin during pregnancy. The drug is administered to the mother, not the infant. The deltoid muscle is recommended for intramuscular administration.

Families often are concerned about the fetus, and nurses should be sensitive to cues that indicate that the family is anxious and should be able to offer honest reassurance. This is especially important if the woman is sensitized and fetal testing is necessary throughout pregnancy.

During labor, the nurse should carefully label the tube of cord blood obtained for analysis of the newborn's blood type and Rh factor. During the postpartum period, nurses are responsible for follow-up to determine whether RhoGAM is necessary and for administering the injection within the prescribed time.

ABO Incompatibility

ABO incompatibility occurs when the mother is blood type O and the fetus is blood type A, B, or AB. Types A, B, and AB blood contain an antigen that is not present in type O blood.

People with type O blood develop anti-A or anti-B antibodies naturally as a result of exposure to antigens in the foods they eat or to infection by gram-negative bacteria. As a result, some women with blood type O have developed high serum anti-A and anti-B antibody titers before pregnancy. The antibodies may be either immunoglobulin G (IgG) or IgM. When the woman becomes pregnant, the IgG antibodies cross the placenta and cause hemolysis of fetal RBCs. Although the first fetus can be affected, ABO incompatibility is less severe than Rh incompatibility because the primary antibodies of the ABO system are IgM, which do not readily cross the placenta.

No specific prenatal care is needed; however, the nurse should be aware of the possibility of ABO incompatibility. During the delivery, cord blood is taken to determine the blood type of the newborn and the antibody titer (direct Coombs' test). The newborn is carefully screened for jaundice, which indicates hyperbilirubinemia.

PATIENT TEACHING

Rh Incompatibility

What does it mean to be Rh-negative?
- Those who are Rh-negative lack a substance that is present in the red blood cells of those who are Rh-positive.

How can the expectant mother be Rh-negative and the fetus be Rh-positive?
- The fetus can inherit the Rh-positive factor from the father.

What does sensitization mean?
- *Sensitization* means that the Rh-negative person has been exposed to Rh-positive blood and has developed antibodies against the Rh factor.

Do the antibodies harm the woman?
- No, because she does not have the Rh factor.

Do Rh-positive men always father Rh-positive children?
- No. Rh-positive men who have an Rh-positive gene and an Rh-negative gene can father Rh-negative children. Two Rh-positive parents can conceive an Rh-negative fetus who inherits the Rh-negative gene from each parent.

Why is Rho(D) immune globulin (RhoGAM) necessary during pregnancy and after childbirth?
- RhoGAM prevents the development of Rh antibodies in the mother, which might be harmful to subsequent fetuses who are Rh-positive. Administering Rho(D) immune globulin during pregnancy to the mother who delivers an Rh-positive or Rh-negative infant is not harmful to the baby.

Why will the next fetus be jeopardized if RhoGAM is not administered?
- If RhoGAM is not administered when the newborn is Rh-positive, the woman may develop antibodies that cross the placental barrier and affect the next Rh-positive fetus.

❓ KNOWLEDGE CHECK

25. Why do unsensitized Rh-negative expectant mothers receive RhoGAM during pregnancy and after an abortion, amniocentesis, and childbirth?
26. What are the effects on the fetus of maternal Rh sensitization?
27. Why is the first fetus sometimes affected if ABO incompatibility occurs? Why are the effects of ABO incompatibility milder than those of Rh sensitization?

CONCURRENT CONDITIONS

Pregnancy affects the care of women with a medical condition in two ways. First, pregnancy may alter the course of the disease. Second, the disease or its treatment may have unwanted effects on the pregnancy. Antepartum care should be adapted to include increased surveillance of the mother and the fetus.

DIABETES MELLITUS

Etiology and Pathophysiology

Diabetes mellitus is a complex disorder of carbohydrate metabolism caused primarily by a partial or complete lack of insulin secretion by the beta cells of the pancreas. Some cells, such as those in skeletal and cardiac muscles and adipose tissue, rely on insulin to carry glucose across the cell membranes. Without insulin, glucose accumulates in blood, resulting in hyperglycemia. The body attempts to dilute the glucose load by any means possible. The first strategy is to increase thirst (**polydipsia**), a classic symptom of diabetes mellitus. Next, fluid from the intracellular spaces is drawn into the vascular bed, resulting in dehydration at the cellular level but fluid volume excess in the vascular compartment. The kidneys attempt to excrete large volumes of this fluid and the heavy solute load of glucose (**osmotic diuresis**). This excretion produces the second hallmark of diabetes, **polyuria**, with **glycosuria** (glucose in urine). Without glucose the cells starve, so weight loss occurs, even though the person ingests large amounts of food (**polyphagia**).

Because the body cannot metabolize glucose, it begins to metabolize protein and fat to meet energy needs. Metabolism of protein produces a negative nitrogen balance, and the metabolism of fat results in the buildup of ketone bodies (e.g., acetone, acetoacetic acid, or beta-hydroxybutyric acid) or **ketosis** (accumulation of acids in the body).

If the disease is not well controlled, serious complications may occur. Hypoglycemia or hyperglycemia can result if the amount of insulin does not match the diet. Fluctuating periods of hyperglycemia and hypoglycemia damage small blood vessels throughout the body. This damage can cause serious impairment, especially in the kidneys, eyes, and heart.

Effect of Pregnancy on Fuel Metabolism

To understand the relationship between diabetes mellitus and pregnancy, an understanding of the way pregnancy and diabetes alter the metabolism of food is necessary.

Early Pregnancy. Metabolic changes can be divided into those that occur early in pregnancy (from 1 to 20 weeks of gestation) and those that occur late in pregnancy (from 20 to 40 weeks of gestation). In early pregnancy, maternal metabolic rates and energy needs change little. During this time, however, insulin release in response to serum glucose levels accelerates. As a result, significant hypoglycemia may occur as more glucose is transported into the cells. The nausea, vomiting, and anorexia that often arise during the first weeks of pregnancy may increase the incidence of hypoglycemia

In an uncomplicated pregnancy, the availability of glucose and insulin, a **lipogenic** substance, favors the development and storage of fat during the first half of pregnancy. Accumulation of fat prepares the mother for the rise in energy use by the growing fetus during the second half of pregnancy.

Late Pregnancy. During the second half of pregnancy, levels of placental hormones rise sharply. These hormones, particularly estrogen, progesterone, and human placental lactogen (hPL), create resistance to insulin in maternal cells. This resistance allows an abundant supply of glucose to be available in the mother's blood for transport to the fetus. However, the hormones have a **diabetogenic effect** in that they may leave the woman with insufficient insulin and episodes of hyperglycemia.

For most women, insulin resistance is not a problem. The pancreas responds by simply increasing the production of insulin. If the pancreas is unable to respond adequately, the woman will have periods of hyperglycemia.

Birth. Maintenance of normal maternal glucose levels is essential during labor and birth to reduce neonatal hypoglycemia. Women with diabetes usually maintain their glucose testing and continue administration of doses of insulin the day before scheduled induction or cesarean birth. Women with an insulin pump continue using their pump through the night. After admission with nothing by mouth (NPO) after the prescribed time, their glucose level is checked and continuous infusion of insulin and glucose is started based on hourly glucose levels.

Postpartum Period. The need for additional insulin falls during the postpartum period. Breastfeeding is encouraged not only for the newborn's benefit but also because the added calorie used for lactation by the mother helps lower the amount of insulin needed in women with diabetes mellitus. The woman with gestational diabetes mellitus (GDM) usually needs no insulin after birth, but the greater risk for later development of type 2 diabetes should be emphasized with teaching before discharge.

Classification

Diabetes that exists before pregnancy is classified as type 1 (insulin deficient) or type 2 (insulin resistant, with a relative deficiency of insulin to metabolize carbohydrate. A third type is one in which any degree of glucose intolerance has its onset or first recognition during pregnancy. The term *gestational diabetes mellitus* refers to the onset of glucose intolerance during pregnancy.

> ### BOX 10.3   Classification of Diabetes Mellitus
>
> Type 1—Insulin dependence. Involves autoimmune destruction of pancreatic beta cells. Prone to ketosis.
> Type 2—May be diet controlled or require insulin related to increasing insulin resistance. Associated with obesity. Ketosis less likely to occur than in type 1 diabetes mellitus.
> Gestational (GDM)—Onset of glucose intolerance first diagnosed during pregnancy.

Data from American Diabetes Association (ADA). (2013). Diagnosis and classification of diabetes mellitus. *Diabetes Care, 36*(Suppl. 1), S67–S74; Landon, M. B., Catalano, P. M., & Gabbe, S. G. (2017). Diabetes mellitus complicating pregnancy. In S. G. Gabbe, J. R. Niebyl, J. L. Simpson, M.B. Landon, H.L. Galan, R. M. Jauniaux, D.A. Driscoll, et al. (Eds.), *Obstetrics: Normal and problem pregnancies* (7th ed., pp. 862–898). Philadelphia, PA: Saunders.

An additional classification of diabetes is sometimes used for descriptive purposes. The White classification describes the age at onset of diabetes, its duration based on the woman's current age, and vascular complications, such as retinopathy, that are present. GDM descriptions in White's classification include A-1 (diet controlled) and A-2 (diet and insulin controlled). Another classification for diabetes during pregnancy lists complications that may be found with type 1 or type 2 diabetes (retinopathy, nephropathy, coronary artery disease) and whether GDM is controlled by diet alone or also requires insulin to supplement diet control (Landon, Catalano, & Gabbe, 2017) (Box 10.3).

Incidence

Diabetes mellitus is a common medical condition that often affects pregnancy. Approximately 90% to 95% of diagnoses in the total population are of type 2, whereas type 1 accounts for about 5% of those diagnosed (CDC, 2014). The pregnant woman may have preexisting diabetes (type 1 or type 2), or she may develop GDM during the course of pregnancy. The pregnant woman may have had undiagnosed type 2 diabetes that is discovered during pregnancy screening for GDM and remains during the postpartum period (Landon et al., 2017).

Although the true incidence of gestational diabetes is unknown, one U.S. study found a prevalence rate of 9.2%, with a range of 16.3% to 6.8%, among different ethnic groups. The highest rates were found in Asian American or Pacific Islanders and Hispanics or Latinos, with the lowest rates in non-Hispanic whites (DeSisto, Kim, & Sharma, 2014). About half of women with GDM will develop type 2 diabetes later in life (ACOG, 2015c; American Diabetes Association [ADA], 2013; CDC, 2015a).

Preexisting Diabetes Mellitus

The course of pregnancy for women with diabetes mellitus has improved greatly as a result of treatments and more effective methods of fetal surveillance. However, the incidence of complications affecting the mother and fetus remains higher than that experienced by women who do not have diabetes.

TABLE 10.6   Major Effects of Diabetes Mellitus on Pregnancy

Effect	Probable Cause
Increased Maternal Risks	
Hypertension, preeclampsia	Unknown but increased even without renal or vascular impairment
Urinary tract infections	Increased bacterial growth in nutrient-rich urine
Ketoacidosis (risk for mother and fetus)	Uncontrolled hyperglycemia or infection; most common in women with type 1 diabetes
Labor dystocia, cesarean birth, uterine atony with hemorrhage after birth	Hydramnios secondary to fetal osmotic diuresis caused by hyperglycemia; uterus is overstretched
Birth injury to maternal tissues (hematoma, lacerations)	Fetal macrosomia causing difficult birth
Increased Fetal and Neonatal Risks	
Congenital anomalies	Maternal hyperglycemia during organ formation in first trimester
Perinatal death	Poor placental perfusion because of maternal vascular impairment, primarily in women with type 1 diabetes
Macrosomia (>4000 g)	Fetal hyperglycemia stimulating production of insulin to metabolize carbohydrates; excess nutrients transported to fetus
Intrauterine fetal growth restriction	Maternal vascular impairment
Preterm labor, premature rupture of membranes, preterm birth	Overdistention of uterus caused by hydramnios and large fetal size at preterm gestation
Birth injury	Large fetal size; shoulder dystocia or other difficult delivery
Hypoglycemia	Neonatal hyperinsulinemia after birth when maternal glucose is no longer available (but insulin production remains high)
Polycythemia	Fetal hypoxemia stimulating erythrocyte production
Hyperbilirubinemia	Breakdown of excessive red blood cells after birth
Hypocalcemia	Maternal relative hyperparathyroidism
Respiratory distress syndrome	Delayed maturation of fetal lungs; inadequate production of pulmonary surfactant; slowed absorption of fetal lung fluid

Maternal Effects

Diabetes can adversely affect a pregnant woman and her developing baby in several ways. During the first trimester, when major fetal organs are developing, the effects of the abnormal metabolic environment such as in hypoglycemia, hyperglycemia, and ketosis may lead to increased incidence of spontaneous abortion or major fetal malformations. Hypertension, especially preeclampsia, is more likely to develop if the woman has preexisting diabetes (Cunningham et al., 2014). The development of ketoacidosis is a threat to women with type 1 diabetes and is most often precipitated by infection or missed insulin doses. In addition, ketoacidosis may develop in these women at lower thresholds of hyperglycemia than those seen in nonpregnant individuals. Untreated ketoacidosis can progress to fetal and maternal death. UTIs are more common, possibly because of glucose in the urine, which provides a nutrient-rich medium for bacterial growth.

Other effects include **hydramnios**, which may result from fetal hyperglycemia and consequent fetal diuresis and premature rupture of membranes, which may be caused by overdistention of the uterus by hydramnios or a large fetus. Problems that arise during labor and childbirth if the fetus has **macrosomia** (weighs more than 8.8 lb [4000 g]) may include a difficult labor, shoulder **dystocia** (delayed or difficult birth of fetal shoulders after the head is born), and consequent injury to the birth canal or the infant. Large fetal size also increases the likelihood of a cesarean birth and the risk for postpartum hemorrhage (Table 10.6).

Fetal Effects

Fetal and neonatal effects of preexisting diabetes depend on the timing and severity of maternal hyperglycemia and the degree of vascular impairment that has occurred.

Congenital Malformation. Fewer malformations occur if the woman maintains a normal blood glucose level before conception and throughout pregnancy. The risk for a major congenital malformation is two to six times higher than for the general population of pregnant women if maternal hyperglycemia is not controlled during the first trimester. The most common major congenital malformations associated with preexisting diabetes are neural tube defects (NTDs), **caudal regression syndrome** (failure of sacrum, lumbar spine, and lower extremities to develop), and cardiac defects (Cunningham et al., 2014; Landon et al., 2017).

Variations in Fetal Size. Fetal growth is related to maternal vascular integrity. In women without vascular impairment, glucose and oxygen are easily transported to the fetus. If the mother is hyperglycemic, so is the fetus. Although maternal insulin does not cross the placental barrier, the fetus produces insulin by the tenth week of gestation. Fetal macrosomia results when elevated levels of blood glucose stimulate excessive production of fetal insulin, which acts as a powerful growth hormone. This is a major neonatal effect with consequent increase in the rate of cesarean birth or birth injury from shoulder dystocia.

Conversely, if vascular impairment is present in the mother, placental perfusion may be decreased. Vascular impairment may be caused by complications of the diabetes such as vasoconstriction, which occurs in preeclampsia or as a result of the disease process of diabetes. Impaired placental perfusion decreases supplies of glucose and oxygen delivered to the fetus. As a result, the infant is likely to be small for gestational age (SGA). This condition is called *intrauterine growth restriction* (IUGR). Amniotic fluid may be reduced (oligohydramnios) as the fetus conserves oxygen for the heart and brain rather than providing normal circulation to the kidneys.

Neonatal Effects

The four major neonatal complications of preexisting diabetes are hypoglycemia, hypocalcemia, hyperbilirubinemia, and respiratory distress syndrome. Maintaining normal maternal levels of glucose reduces the incidence and severity of neonatal complications.

Hypoglycemia. The neonate is at higher risk for hypoglycemia because fetal insulin production would have been accelerated during pregnancy to metabolize the excessive glucose received from the mother. The constant stimulation of hyperglycemia leads to hyperplasia and hypertrophy of the islets of Langerhans in the fetal pancreas. When the maternal glucose supply is abruptly withdrawn at birth, the level of neonatal insulin exceeds the available glucose, and hypoglycemia develops rapidly (Cunningham et al., 2014; Landon et al., 2017).

Hypocalcemia. Hypocalcemia is defined and a total serum calcium level of less than 7 mg/dL in a preterm infant or less than 8 mg/dL in a term infant (Blackburn, 2013). It is likely due to a relative hyperparathyroidism seen in many diabetic mothers (Blackburn, 2013, Rozance, McGowan, Price-Douglas, and Hay, 2016). Other possible causes include changes in the magnesium-calcium balance, asphyxia, or preterm birth (Cunningham et al., 2014).

Hyperbilirubinemia. The fetus experiencing recurrent hypoxia compensates by production of additional erythrocytes (polycythemia) to carry oxygen supplied by the mother. After birth, the excess erythrocytes are broken down, which releases large amounts of bilirubin into the neonate's circulation. Prematurity, more likely in the infant of a woman with poor glycemic control, further reduces the infant's ability to metabolize and excrete excess bilirubin (Cunningham et al., 2014; Landon et al., 2017).

Respiratory Distress Syndrome. Fetal hyperinsulinemia retards cortisol production, which is necessary for the synthesis of surfactant needed to keep the newborn's alveoli open after birth, thereby increasing the risk for respiratory distress syndrome. Reduced lung fluid clearance and delayed thinning of lung connective tissue also may be a factor. Respiratory distress syndrome is more likely to occur if the mother's glycemic control is poor, because wide fluctuations in her insulin and glucose levels have slowed lung maturation (Cunningham et al., 2014; Landon et al., 2017). Tests of fetal lung maturity will be done before elective delivery of the fetus by induction or scheduled cesarean birth if questions about maturity exist.

Complications in a mother and her fetus and then her newborn can be reduced if the mother maintains normal and stable blood glucose levels. The objective of the team providing treatment is to devise a plan that allows the woman to maintain a level as close to normal as possible.

? KNOWLEDGE CHECK

28. What effects do the hormones of pregnancy have on maternal glucose metabolism?
29. What are the maternal effects of type 1 diabetes mellitus? What are possible fetal and neonatal effects?
30. How do insulin needs vary from the first trimester through the postpartum period?

Maternal Assessment

Preconception care is ideal in a woman with preexisting diabetes. If the woman can have her body in the best condition before conception, including diabetes management, pregnancy is likely to have fewer or less severe complications than if she started care after conception. When the woman with preconception care or preexisting diabetes initiates care, a thorough evaluation of her health status should be completed. This evaluation includes history, physical examination, and laboratory tests.

History. A detailed history should include the onset and management of the diabetic condition. How long has she had the disease? How does she maintain a normal blood glucose level? Is she familiar with ways to monitor blood glucose level and administer insulin? The degree of glycemic control before pregnancy is of particular interest. Effective management depends on her adherence to a plan of care. Therefore her knowledge of how diabetes affects pregnancy and how pregnancy affects diabetes should be determined. The support person's knowledge also should be assessed, and specific learning needs should be identified. In addition, the woman's emotional status should be assessed to determine how she is coping with pregnancy superimposed on preexisting diabetes.

All women with diabetes should be seen by a qualified diabetes educator for an individualized assessment to ensure these women can monitor their blood glucose level accurately. Accurate readings depend on performing the test correctly and at the times recommended by the health care team. In addition to home monitoring of blood glucose level, the nurse should observe the woman's skill in mixing and self-administering insulin, using a sliding scale for added insulin or using an insulin pump if the drug will be given that way. Most pregnant women who need medication to reduce glucose levels take insulin via injection rather than as an oral agent, even if the oral agent had been effective in the woman with type 2 diabetes. The current ACOG (2016d) recommendation is limited on the individualized use of oral agents during pregnancy.

Physical Examination. In addition to routine prenatal examination, specific efforts should be made to assess the effects of diabetes. A baseline electrocardiogram (ECG) should be obtained to determine cardiovascular status. Evaluation for retinopathy should be performed, with referral to an ophthalmologist, if necessary. The woman's weight and blood pressure should be monitored because of the increased risk for hypertension, including preeclampsia. Fundal height should be measured, noting any abnormal increase in size that may indicate macrosomia or hydramnios, which may occur as a result of diuresis by the hyperglycemic fetus. Fundal height less than expected for the gestation may indicate fetal growth restriction or intrauterine death secondary to poor placental perfusion.

Laboratory Tests. In addition to routine prenatal laboratory examinations, baseline renal function should be assessed with a 24-hour urine collection for total protein excretion and creatinine clearance. A random urine sample should be checked at each prenatal visit for possible UTIs, which are common in women with diabetes. Urine also should be checked by using a dipstick for the presence of glucose, ketones, and protein. Thyroid function tests should be performed in the woman with preexisting diabetes because of her risk for coexisting thyroid disease.

Glycemic control should be evaluated on the basis of the level of glycosylated Hgb or hemoglobin A_{1c} (HbA_{1c}). The glycosylated Hgb assay is an accurate measurement of the average glucose concentrations during the preceding 2 to 3 months. Unlike tests that reflect the amount of glucose in the plasma at that moment, the HbA_{1c} measurement is not affected by recent intake or restriction of food.

Fetal Surveillance

Because of the increased risk for **congenital anomalies** or fetal death, surveillance should begin early for women with preexisting diabetes. Testing for anomalies includes multiple-marker screening to identify possible neural tube or other open defects and for possible chromosome abnormalities. Testing also includes performing ultrasonography at 18 to 20 weeks of gestation and fetal echocardiography at 20 to 22 weeks of gestation to determine the integrity of the fetal body and cardiac structure (ACOG, 2015c, 2016d; Cunningham et al., 2014; Landon et al., 2017).

During the third trimester, the goal of fetal surveillance is to identify markers that suggest a worsening intrauterine environment with an increased risk for fetal death. Surveillance may include maternal assessment of fetal movement ("kick counts"), BPPs, NSTs, and contraction stress tests (ACOG, 2016d; Landon et al., 2017). Serial sonograms are used to document fetal growth rates in an effort to identify fetuses at risk for macrosomia and shoulder dystocia (Landon et al., 2017). Doppler velocimetry of the umbilical artery may be used to assess vascular complications and poor fetal growth (ACOG, 2016d).

Therapeutic Management

The goals of therapeutic management for a pregnant woman with diabetes are to (1) maintain normal blood glucose levels, (2) facilitate the birth of a healthy baby, and (3) avoid accelerated impairment of blood vessels and other major organs. To achieve this outcome, an intensive, team approach to care is required.

Members of the team often include an endocrinologist or diabetologist, who assists in regulation of maternal blood glucose level; an obstetrician or a maternal-fetal medicine specialist (**perinatologist)** who monitors the mother and fetus and determines the optimal time for birth; a registered dietitian (RD) or registered dietary technician (RDT), who provides a balanced meal plan; and a diabetes educator, often a specialized nurse, who provides ongoing education and support as the therapy changes throughout pregnancy. The team is completed by a neonatologist, who will care for the newborn; the family physician and the pediatrician, who will provide ongoing care for the infant and the mother.

Preconception Care. Ideally, care should begin before conception. If diabetes exists before pregnancy, both prospective parents should participate in care sessions to learn more about the following measures that need to be taken by the health care team:

- Establishing the optimal time to undertake pregnancy, based on maintenance of normal maternal blood glucose levels, to reduce the risk for major fetal malformations
- Identifying whether diabetes complications exist in other organ systems
- Determining the degree of glycemic control based on client records or laboratory studies
- Instructing a woman about how to use a glucometer for blood glucose level measurement and having the woman demonstrate a correct technique
- Having the woman take a daily prenatal vitamin with folic acid A higher dose of folic acid is recommended for the woman who had a previous child with an NTD (Chapter 8)

Diet. Diet recommendations are individualized during pregnancy in a woman with diabetes. The average recommended caloric intake for the pregnant woman with diabetes who is of normal weight is 30 to 35 kilocalories per kilogram of body weight per day (kcal/kg/day). Approximately 40% to 50% of the calories should be from high-fiber complex carbohydrates, 20% from protein and up to 30% to 40% from fat (ACOG, 2016d; Landon et al., 2017). Caloric intake should be distributed among three meals and two or more snacks. The bedtime snack should include a complex carbohydrate and a protein. Women who are overweight or underweight usually have lower or higher caloric goals.

Self-Monitoring of Blood Glucose Level. The best frequency for self-monitoring of blood glucose (SMBG) level of capillary blood has not yet been established. One common testing regimen requires obtaining fasting and 2-hour postprandial levels. Another includes testing six times per day: a fasting capillary glucose level, 1 to 2 hours after breakfast, before and after lunch, before dinner, and at bedtime. Normal fasting and postprandial glucose levels have been associated with better outcomes, including a lower risk for macrosomia, neonatal hypoglycemia, and labor dystocia that results in cesarean birth. Preprandial glucose levels may be needed for smoother control if the glucose level is difficult to control. The target capillary blood glucose levels are as follows: fasting—95 mg/dL or less; premeal—100 mg/dL or less; 1-hour postprandial—140 mg/dL or less; and 2-hour postprandial—120 mg/dL or less (ACOG, 2016d). In addition to regular monitoring, the woman also should perform a glucose test whenever she experiences symptoms of hypoglycemia. The woman should record all test results on a log sheet or cell phone app for review by the health care provider at each visit.

Insulin Therapy. The need to maintain rigorous control of maternal metabolism during pregnancy requires more frequent doses of insulin than usual. Most treatment regimens rely on three daily injections, with a combination of short-acting (regular) insulin and intermediate-acting (neutral protamine Hagedorn [NPH]) insulin given before breakfast, regular insulin before dinner, and NPH insulin at bedtime. Lispro and aspart (Humalog and NovoLog, respectively) insulins act rapidly and should be injected just before a meal. Rapid-acting insulins have been shown to control postprandial hyperglycemia with less between-meal hypoglycemia (Landon et al., 2017). Because placental hormones cause insulin needs to change throughout pregnancy, insulin coverage will need to be adjusted as pregnancy progresses.

First Trimester. Insulin needs generally decline during the first trimester because the secretion of placental hormones antagonistic to insulin remains low. The woman also may experience nausea, vomiting, and anorexia, which result in decreased intake of food; therefore the woman requires less insulin. In addition, the fetus receives its share of glucose, which reduces maternal plasma glucose levels and decreases the need for maternal insulin.

Second and Third Trimesters. Insulin needs increase markedly during the second and third trimesters when placental hormones, which initiate maternal resistance to the effects of insulin, reach their peak. In addition, the nausea of early pregnancy usually resolves, and the diet includes additional calories per day to meet the increased metabolic demands of pregnancy.

During Labor. Maintenance of tight maternal glucose control during birth is desirable to reduce neonatal hypoglycemia. Continuous infusion of a regular insulin solution combined with a separate IV solution containing glucose, such as 5% dextrose in lactated Ringer's solution, allows titration to maintain blood glucose levels between 80 and 110 mg/dL or according to facility policy. The insulin solution is raised, lowered, or discontinued to maintain euglycemia based on hourly capillary blood glucose levels (ACOG, 2016d; Cunningham et al., 2014; Landon et al., 2017).

Postpartum Period. Insulin needs should decline rapidly after the delivery of the placenta and abrupt cessation of placental hormones. However, blood glucose levels should be monitored at least four times daily so that the insulin dose can be adjusted to meet individual needs. Women with type 1 diabetes usually return to their prepregnancy dosages. Women with type 2 diabetes are monitored, as ordered, and insulin is ordered only if needed.

EVIDENCE-BASED PRACTICE

Antenatal Corticosteroid Therapy in the Diabetic Patient

Women whose pregnancy is complicated by preexisting diabetes and those with new onset gestational diabetes are at higher risk of some obstetrical and medical complications. Some of these complications of pregnancy can put the mother and fetus at risk for preterm birth. Antenatal Corticosteroid (ACS) therapy is recommended to facilitate fetal lung maturity in women at risk for preterm birth within 7 days. Kalra, Kalra & Gupta (2014) conducted a literature review to examine the issues of (1) indications for ACS in gestational diabetes mellitus (GDM) complicated by threatened preterm birth, (2) effects of ACS on glycemia in previously euglycemic antenatal women, in women with GDM and in women with pre-existing diabetes, (3) glycemia monitoring in all women receiving ACS, in women with GDM receiving ACS, and in women with pre-existing or overt diabetes and (4) glycemic management after ACS administration.

They suggest that, while ACS therapy can cause hyperglycemia, diabetes is not considered a contraindication. It does, however, require close monitoring by the health care team and the mother to ensure tight glycemic control and avoid severe transient hyperglycemia. They recommend a blood glucose level prior to administration of ACS to evaluate for undiagnosed GDM and determine a baseline value. Because hyperglycemia starts approximately 12 hours after ACS and lasts up to five days, management should include more frequent blood glucose monitoring and strict management of nutritional intake. Typically there is a transient increase in insulin requirements. Since hyperglycemia can last for 5 days it is recommended that maternal-fetal surveillance be continued for at least 5 days; the type and frequency of the surveillance should be based on the character of the diabetes and the patient status.

Questions
1. How does this medical recommendation affect nursing care of the pregnant diabetic woman?
2. Based on this information, what patient teaching would you provide to the patient prior to administering ACS?
3. What symptoms should the nurse be looking for that might indicate hyperglycemia?
4. How would you counsel a woman who is having difficulty controlling her diet after receiving ACS? What recommendations would you give her?

Reference
Kalra, S., Kalra, B., & Gupta, Y. (2014). Glycemic Management after Antenatal Corticosteroid Therapy. *North American Journal of Medical Sciences, 6*(2), 71–76.

Timing of Delivery. If possible, the pregnancy is allowed to progress to 39 weeks or later to allow the fetal lungs to mature, reducing the risk for neonatal respiratory distress syndrome. With evidence of fetal compromise, such as a low BPP or reduced amniotic fluid, delivery may be required. If delivery before completion of 38 weeks is needed for nonemergency reasons, amniocentesis to determine fetal lung maturity is often performed because lung maturation may be slower than in nondiabetic pregnancies. Cesarean birth may be considered, to avoid traumatic birth injuries if the estimated fetal weight is more than 4500 g (ACOG, 2016d; Cunningham et al., 2014; Landon et al., 2017).

Gestational Diabetes Mellitus

Any degree of carbohydrate intolerance first diagnosed during pregnancy is classified as GDM (ACOG, 2015c). However, as the incidence of obesity and type 2 diabetes has increased, the number of women of childbearing age with undiagnosed preexisting diabetes also has increased (ACOG, 2015c, ADA, 2017a). Therefore the American Diabetes Association recommends a refinement of the definition to "diabetes diagnosed in the second or third trimester of pregnancy that was not clearly overt diabetes before gestation" (ADA, 2017a, p. S11). Women with risk factors should be tested for undiagnosed diabetes at their first prenatal visit. Diabetes identified during the first trimester should be classified as preexisting pregestational diabetes rather than gestational diabetes (ADA, 2017a). GDM is an added risk factor that a woman will develop type 2 diabetes later in life. Factors such as obesity, inactivity, abnormal cholesterol levels, vascular disease, or family members with type 2 diabetes further increase a woman's risk for developing type 2 diabetes (ACOG, 2015c; ADA, 2017a; CDC, 2014).

Risk Factors

Diagnosis of GDM begins with history-taking to identify the woman at risk. Factors known to increase the risk include the following (Cunningham et al., 2014; National Institutes of Health [NIH] & National Diabetes Information Clearinghouse [NDIC], 2013):

- Overweight (body mass index [BMI] ≥25 to 25.9), obesity (BMI ≥30), or morbidly obese (BMI ≥40 or higher)
- Maternal age older than 25 years
- Previous birth outcome often associated with GDM (neonatal macrosomia, maternal hypertension, infant with unexplained congenital anomalies, previous fetal death)
- Gestational diabetes in previous pregnancy
- History of abnormal glucose tolerance
- History of diabetes in a close (first-degree) relative
- Member of a high-risk ethnic group (African-American, Hispanic or Latino, American Indian, Asian American, or Pacific Islanders)
- History of prediabetes (elevated blood glucose that does not meet the criteria for diabetes)
- History of polycystic ovary syndrome (PCOS)

Women with any of these factors should be screened for type 2 or gestational diabetes at the first prenatal visit (ACOG, 2015c; ADA, 2017a).

Identifying Gestational Diabetes Mellitus

Screening. Women without any risk factors for gestational diabetes may be screened by history alone; blood glucose testing is not routinely required. For women with one or more risk factors, a two-step approach is the current recommendation for screening for GDM by the NIH and ACOG (ACOG, 2015c; Vandorsten et al., 2013).

Glucose Challenge Test. A glucose challenge test (GCT) is administered between 24 and 28 weeks of gestation. Fasting is not necessary for a GCT, and the woman is not required to follow any pretest dietary instructions. The woman should ingest 50 g of oral glucose solution. A blood sample is taken 1 hour later. If the blood glucose concentration is 140 mg/dL or greater, a 3-hour oral glucose tolerance test (OGTT) is recommended. Some practitioners use a lower cutoff of 130 or 135 mg/dL to identify more women at risk (ACOG, 2015c; Landon et al., 2017).

Oral Glucose Tolerance Test. The 3-hour OGTT is the gold standard for diagnosing diabetes, but it is a more complex test. The woman must fast from midnight on the day of the test. After a fasting plasma glucose level is determined, the woman should ingest 100 g of oral glucose solution. Plasma glucose levels are then determined at 1, 2, and 3 hours. A diagnosis of GDM is made if two or more of the values meet or exceed the threshold (ACOG, 2015c; ADA, 2017a; Landon et al., 2017):

- Fasting 95 mg/dL
- 1 hour, 180 mg/dL
- 2 hours, 155 mg/dL
- 3 hours, 140 mg/dL

Based on patient population, available resources, regional practice, and institutional policy, some providers may use thresholds of 105 for fasting, 190 for 1 hour, 165 for 2 hours, and 145 for 3 hours (ACOG, 2015c; ADA, 2017a; Landon et al., 2017).

Maternal, Fetal, and Neonatal Effects

With a few important exceptions, the effects of GDM are similar to those associated with preexisting diabetes. The exceptions are that GDM is not associated with an increased risk for maternal ketoacidosis or spontaneous abortion, and there is a decreased chance of preexisting maternal vascular and organ damage associated with diabetes. Because GDM develops after the first trimester, the critical period of major fetal organ development (organogenesis), it usually is not associated with an increase in major congenital malformations. Nevertheless, poorly controlled GDM, characterized by maternal hyperglycemia during the third trimester, is associated with increased neonatal morbidity and mortality. The major fetal complications are macrosomia, leading to birth injuries or cesarean birth, and neonatal hypoglycemia. Other problems such as hypocalcemia, hyperbilirubinemia, and respiratory distress also may occur (Cunningham et al., 2014; Landon et al., 2017). (See Table 10.6 for a summary of maternal, fetal, and neonatal effects of diabetes mellitus and their probable causes.)

Therapeutic Management

Diet. Ideally, an RD, RDT, or diabetes educator determines the dietary needs of the woman with GDM. The diet should provide the calories and nutrients needed for maternal and fetal health, result in euglycemia, avoid ketosis, and promote appropriate weight gain. Calories should be distributed in a way similar to that for preexisting diabetes. Simple sugars, found in concentrated sweets, should be eliminated from the diet. Based on a nonobese prepregnancy weight, an average of 30 to 35 kcal/kg per day is recommended. Calorie restriction to 25 kcal/kg each day may be recommended for women who are obese (Cunningham et al., 2014; Landon et al., 2017). These women may be prescribed a diet with a smaller percentage of carbohydrates than for women of normal weight to limit hyperglycemia. Carbohydrates at breakfast may be limited to 30 g during pregnancy because of increased levels of cortisol and growth hormones at that time of day. Protein foods at breakfast help satisfy early morning hunger. An evening snack is usually needed to prevent ketosis at night. Calories should be divided among three meals and two to four snacks (Franz & Evert, 2017).

Exercise. Research results have been mixed about whether exercise reduces the need for insulin in the woman with GDM. Nevertheless, exercise and an active lifestyle can improve cardiorespiratory fitness (Cunningham et al., 2014). A graduated physical exercise program should be recommended by a physician, taking into account each woman's risk factors as part of the treatment plan for women with GDM (ACOG, 2015c).

Blood Glucose Monitoring. Blood glucose levels should be evaluated to determine whether levels are normal. A common method is measurement of fasting blood glucose level (no food for the previous 4 hours) and postprandial blood glucose level (1 or 2 hours after each meal). Frequency of glucose monitoring may be modified once the glucose levels are well controlled by diet (ACOG, 2015c). If fasting capillary blood glucose levels repeatedly exceed 95 mg/dL or postprandial values exceed 140 mg/dL at 1 hour or 120 mg/dL at 2 hours, pharmacologic therapy may be added (ACOG, 2015c; Cunningham et al., 2014). Additional tests for glucose levels may be performed, as needed.

Pharmacologic Treatment. Pharmacologic treatment may be required for some women with GDM when diet and exercise do not achieve glycemic targets. Insulin is the preferred medication for treatment of hyperglycemia in GDM (ADA, 2017b). Insulin is typically started at 0.7 to 1 unit/kg/day given in divided doses (ACOG, 2015c; Cunningham et al., 2014). Intermediate-acting and short-acting insulin may be used alone or in combination. Dosage should be adjusted to the woman's blood glucose levels at particular times of the day (ACOG, 2015c; Cunningham et al., 2014).

Although insulin remains the only drug widely accepted for treatment of diabetes during pregnancy because it does not cross the placenta, oral agents are being studied more closely for GDM treatment (Landon et al., 2017). ACOG (2015c) recognizes that either insulin or oral agents may be used as an appropriate first-line pharmacologic therapy in GDM. Glyburide (Micronase) and metformin (Glucophage) have been studied for use with GDM and have demonstrated glucose control comparable to insulin without apparent maternal or neonatal complications (Landon et al., 2017). Because further research is needed on the long-term outcomes of oral diabetic therapy with GDM, ACOG (2015c) recommends patient counseling with this treatment plan.

Fetal Surveillance. Testing to identify fetal compromise may be of benefit for women with GDM and poor glycemic control, but there is no consensus regarding antepartum fetal testing for women with GDM and good glycemic control (ACOG, 2015c; Cunningham et al., 2014). Testing may begin as early as 28 weeks of gestation if the woman has poor glycemic control or by 32 to 34 weeks of gestation in lower risk women with GDM. The surveillance testing often includes "kick counts," ultrasonography for fetal growth and amniotic fluid volume, BPP, NSTs, contraction stress test, or amniocentesis for fetal lung maturity (Landon et al., 2017).

Nursing Considerations

The care of a pregnant woman with diabetes mellitus focuses primarily on maintaining normal blood glucose levels. As stated earlier, this maintenance involves a rather rigid schedule of controlling the diet, performing blood glucose tests, administering insulin, and performing regular fetal surveillance. Some women respond calmly to the intense medical supervision. Others respond with anxiety, fear, denial, or anger and may feel inadequate or unable to control the diabetes to the degree expected by the health care team. These feelings may not be shared spontaneously, but they may affect the woman's ability to achieve the desired outcomes. Also, nurses should remember to provide for normal pregnancy care in addition to monitoring the pregnant woman's diabetes.

Increasing Effective Communication. A woman often does not volunteer information about her feelings and concerns, especially if she has negative feelings about her care. In addition, the woman and the nurse both may be unaware of any misunderstanding or conflict regarding the plan of care. Nurses should ask specifically about the feelings and concerns the woman and her family have about the pregnancy.

❓ CRITICAL THINKING EXERCISE 10.3

A 28-year-old primigravida is diagnosed with gestational diabetes in her 30th week of pregnancy. The health care team provides her with a diet and exercise regimen and tells her that she will need weekly tests to monitor her condition and that of the fetus. Although she accepts the information without comment, she does not keep the next scheduled appointment.

Questions
1. What assumptions has the health care team made?
2. What could the team have done to improve the woman's compliance with the recommendations?

The woman is located and agrees to return to the clinic for follow-up care. She states she does not "see what all the fuss is about." She understands she may have a large baby but states that her mother had a 10-lb baby who did just fine. She wonders if the weekly tests are necessary and if they could harm the baby.

Questions
3. How can the nurse respond to the woman's comments about having a large baby without frightening her?
4. How can the nurse explain the need for weekly nonstress tests or biophysical profiles?

Broad opening questions such as "What are your major concerns?" and "How do you feel about the plan of care?" are helpful. These should be followed by more specific questions such as "How do you feel about the fetal testing?" and "What would you like to change about the diet?" The woman's responses may provide valuable information about her emotional response to the care plan. One woman remarked, "I can tell you one thing, I don't feel like a person. I feel like an incubator, a faulty incubator." Another woman who had a difficult time achieving the desired blood glucose level said, "I feel as though my whole life has been taken over by diabetes. I'm tired of feeling like a sick person."

The nurse should be an active listener and allow time for the woman and her family to express concerns and feelings. The nurse should convey acceptance of both negative feelings and positive feelings that are expressed. Many women are reassured to hear that their feelings of stress or anger are normal and learn that the health care team understands those feelings. Sharing of emotions will help her avoid or diminish unnecessary guilt, anxiety, and frustration and thus promotes positive feelings about her ability to participate successfully in her plan of care.

Most women benefit from praise when diabetes control is well maintained. They feel competent and trusted by the health care team and are motivated to continue their efforts.

Providing Opportunities for Control. Allowing the woman to make as many decisions as possible increases her sense of being in control. For instance, she can select foods from the exchange list that provide the necessary nutrients but still allow her some choice. A dietitian or dietary technician should be consulted if the list does not include foods she likes or that suit her ethnic or cultural preferences. A regular schedule of exercise and sleep that helps keep the blood glucose level under control is important. The woman can develop the schedule for rest and exercise that best suits her lifestyle. Nurses should allow as much flexibility as possible when scheduling stressful events such as fetal monitoring tests and amniocentesis.

Some women resent being "treated as though ill," even though their diabetes control is excellent. These women may be capable of making more decisions regarding their care during pregnancy, but they need the support of an understanding team to do this.

Providing Normal Pregnancy Care. Some women express a need for more attention to the normal aspects of their pregnancies. This can be overlooked because of the intense focus on preventing complications that can occur with diabetes. Women with diabetes also experience discomforts such as morning sickness, fatigue, backache, and difficulty sleeping that women without diabetes experience during pregnancy. The nurse caring for women with diabetes should therefore provide the usual education and counseling regarding pregnancy.

KNOWLEDGE CHECK

31. What is the importance of the glycosylated hemoglobin (Hb_{A1c}) measurement in monitoring diabetes mellitus?
32. How does GDM compare with type 1 and type 2 diabetes mellitus in terms of onset and treatment?
33. What is the difference between GCT and OGTT?
34. How do the maternal, fetal, and neonatal effects of gestational diabetes differ from those of preexisting diabetes?

◆ APPLICATION OF THE NURSING PROCESS: THE PREGNANT WOMAN WITH DIABETES MELLITUS

◆ Assessment

Determine how well the woman understands the prescribed management and how the family plans to carry out the recommended regimen. She may be newly diagnosed and have no experience in the necessary skills and procedures. The woman who had diabetes before becoming pregnant may be skilled in monitoring glucose level and administering insulin. However, the woman with preexisting diabetes may have no knowledge of how diabetes can affect pregnancy or how pregnancy can affect diabetes. She may have been using premixed insulin exclusively and now must begin mixing insulins of different types. A woman with type 2 diabetes may have taken only oral medication and now must learn to mix and inject insulin.

To determine whether the pregnant woman's techniques are accurate, ask her to demonstrate how she monitors blood glucose level and observe as she mixes and injects insulins if she has done that. Verify that she and her family are aware of the need to select appropriate sites and injection techniques that prevent insulin leakage.

Although diet is prescribed by a dietitian or diabetes educator, the nurse should assess how well the family understands the diet. Determine whether special problems with food preferences or availability of recommended foods exist. Diet recommendations include a target number of calories, plus targets for grams of carbohydrate, protein, and fat to meet calorie needs. Any of the several methods to count and exchange foods may be used. One method uses exchange lists, in which the listed foods all have about the same number of grams of carbohydrate, protein, and fat. Therefore one food from the list may be substituted, or exchanged, for another in the same list. Another method uses carbohydrate counting, in which foods on the starch, fruit, or milk list supply about 15 g of carbohydrate, or one carbohydrate choice. The diet plan would prescribe the number of carbohydrate choices for each meal and snack. Insulin is often adjusted according to the carbohydrate count for each meal or snack.

Identify special needs related to food preferences, culturally prescribed foods, or the availability of recommended foods. It may be necessary to review an exchange list and ask the woman how she plans to substitute and exchange foods to obtain the prescribed number of foods from each list.

Identify the woman's knowledge of potential complications such as hypoglycemia and hyperglycemia so that she and her family can be provided with pertinent information to avoid it or treat it.

Determine her knowledge of fetal surveillance techniques and her response to the need for frequent tests. Some women are highly motivated to continue the treatment regimen when test results indicate that the fetus is thriving. Other women find the frequent testing stressful and inconvenient.

◆ Identification of Patient Problems

A common patient problem for women with diabetes during pregnancy is "Need for Patient Teaching of (1) measures to maintain normal blood glucose levels, (2) measures to manage abnormal glucose levels, and (3) common fetal surveillance procedures."

◆ Planning: Expected Outcomes

Goals for this problem are that the woman and her family will do the following:

- Demonstrate competence in SMBG level and administration of insulin before home management is initiated.
- Describe a plan for meeting dietary recommendations that fits family lifestyle and food preferences.
- Identify signs and symptoms of hypoglycemia and hyperglycemia and the management required for each.
- Verbalize knowledge of fetal surveillance procedures and keep scheduled appointments for testing.

◆ Interventions

Management of diabetes mellitus during pregnancy is a team effort, and the nurse is responsible to provide or reinforce accurate information about the therapeutic regimen and offer consistent support for the woman's efforts to comply with the recommendations. It may be necessary to demonstrate specific skills that the woman and her support person should master and to review and reinforce information from other members of the health care team.

Teaching Self-Care Skills

Demonstrations and return demonstrations are effective ways to teach and evaluate psychomotor skills. The woman (and her family) should learn to (1) use a meter and obtain a small sample of blood, (2) test for glucose level, and (3) mix and inject insulin. The procedures are invasive and cause mild discomfort, which may make the woman reluctant to start. Mixing insulins accurately or using a sliding scale may be intimidating at first. Using food exchanges is often unfamiliar to the woman who is newly diagnosed, but it is critical to glucose control. Acknowledge these feelings before teaching begins.

Self-Monitoring of Blood Glucose Level. Spring-loaded lancets make home blood glucose monitoring easier. The side of the fingertip is less sensitive than the pad of the fingertip, so using the side reduces discomfort. Teach the woman to cleanse the area with warm water before obtaining a sample, to prevent infection. If alcohol is used to clean the area, let it dry thoroughly. The first drop of blood is wiped away, and the second drop is placed on the meter's strip. Each home monitoring kit contains specific instructions for use of the meter and the type of reagent strip or cartridge that should be used. Teach the woman how to record glucose values in a handwritten or other log. Teach her that current glucose monitors have a memory option to provide retrieval of previous glucose readings.

Insulin Administration. The woman is often prescribed a combination of short-acting and intermediate-acting insulins. Teach her about the difference in onset, peak, and duration of action of each type of insulin in her combination. She also needs to learn how to mix the two insulins in the same syringe. If she will use a sliding scale to keep glucose levels close to normal, she will need teaching about how to determine the additional dose of insulin if she has never used a sliding scale for insulin administration.

Insulin is administered subcutaneously. Common sites include the upper thighs, abdomen, and upper arms. Because the pregnant woman is injecting insulin frequently, emphasize the following precautions:

- To prevent hypoglycemia, a meal should be taken 30 minutes after regular insulin is injected. Because of its 10-minute onset of action, lispro (Humalog) insulin is injected just before eating.
- Unless the woman is very thin, insulin should be injected with the short needle inserted at a 90-degree angle so that the tip of the needle reaches the fatty tissue layer.
- The needle should be inserted quickly to minimize discomfort.
- The tissue pinch, if used, is released after inserting the needle and before injecting insulin because pressure from the pinch can promote insulin leakage from subcutaneous tissue.
- Aspirating is not necessary when injecting into subcutaneous tissue.
- Insulin is injected slowly (over 2 to 4 seconds) to allow tissue expansion and minimize pressure, which can cause insulin leakage.
- The needle is withdrawn quickly to minimize the formation of a track, which might cause insulin to leak out.

Emphasize the importance of administering the correct dosage at the correct time. Teach the woman and her family about the function of insulin and the importance of following the directions of her physician in regard to coordinating meals with the administration of insulin.

Continuous Subcutaneous Insulin Infusion. Many women who have preexisting diabetes use continuous subcutaneous insulin infusion and wish to continue with this method during pregnancy. The use of programmable insulin infusion pumps allows tailoring of insulin administration to the woman's individual lifestyle. Prompt emergency counseling and assistance should be available 24 hours a day to deal with unexpected problems such as pump malfunction.

Teaching Dietary Management

Although a dietitian prescribes the recommended diet, the nurse should be aware of the general requirements and be sensitive to the woman's dietary habits and preferences. Often, reviewing and clarifying how exchange lists are used to plan meals and snacks are necessary. Encourage the patient to avoid simple sugars (candy, cake, cookies), which raise the blood glucose levels quickly but may result in wide swings between high and low glucose levels.

It may be necessary to help the woman select foods that are high in nutrients but low in cost or meet cultural or religious constraints. Animal protein is especially expensive, and alternative sources of protein (beans, peas, corn, grains) can be substituted to meet some of the protein needs, as well as provide high-quality carbohydrate and fiber. A Nutrition and Dietetic Technician (NDTR) can help a pregnant woman who is a vegetarian meet her individual needs depending on what foods are acceptable to her.

Allow the expectant mother to verbalize her frustrations or problems with the diet, and collaborate with the dietitian if she has a particular problem.

Managing Hypoglycemia and Hyperglycemia

Every woman and her family should be aware of signs and symptoms that indicate abnormal glucose levels and how to correct the abnormal levels. Hypoglycemia and hyperglycemia pose a threat to the mother and the fetus if these problems are not identified and corrected quickly.

Hypoglycemia. Treat hypoglycemia at once to prevent damage to the fetal brain, which depends on glucose. The woman should take 15 g of carbohydrate if she can swallow food. Examples of foods that supply this are three glucose tablets or glucose gel, ½ cup of fruit juice or regular soft drink, 6 saltine crackers, or 1 tablespoon of syrup or honey. Large quantities of high-carbohydrate foods such as candy will increase the blood glucose excessively, making a sudden fall in the level more likely. The woman should retest 15 minutes after the carbohydrate intake and repeat the treatment if her blood glucose level remains below 70 mg/dL. If it is more than 1 hour until the next meal or snack, test again 60 minutes after treatment; additional carbohydrate may be required (Franz & Evert, 2017).

> **! SAFETY CHECK**
>
> Signs and symptoms of maternal hypoglycemia include the following:
> - Shakiness (tremors)
> - Sweating
> - Pallor; cold, clammy skin
> - Disorientation, irritability
> - Headache
> - Hunger
> - Blurred vision

Teach family members how to inject glucagon in the event that the woman cannot swallow or retain food. Notify the physician at once. IV glucose will be administered if she is hospitalized. If untreated, hypoglycemia can progress to seizures and death.

To prevent hypoglycemia, instruct the woman to have meals at a fixed time each day and to plan snacks at 10 AM, 3 PM, and bedtime. Suggest that she always carry glucose tablets or gel or some crackers with her.

Hyperglycemia. Because infection is the most common cause of hyperglycemia, pregnant women should be instructed to notify the physician whenever they have an infection of any type.

Untreated hyperglycemia can lead to ketoacidosis, coma, and maternal and fetal death. If signs and symptoms occur, notify the physician at once so treatment can be initiated. Hospitalization often is necessary to monitor blood glucose levels, for IV insulin administration to normalize glucose levels, and for treatment of any underlying infection.

> **! SAFETY CHECK**
>
> Signs and symptoms of maternal hyperglycemia include the following:
> - Fatigue
> - Flushed, hot skin
> - Dry mouth, excessive thirst
> - Frequent urination
> - Rapid, deep respirations; odor of acetone on the breath
> - Drowsiness, headache
> - Depressed reflexes

Explaining Procedures, Tests, and Plan of Care

Explain the schedule and the reasons for frequent checkups and necessary tests. Encourage the woman and her family to ask questions if any part of the schedule is confusing. This is particularly important for women who are aware that their prenatal care differs significantly from that of their friends who do not have diabetes. Knowing that the tests provide information about the condition of the mother and fetus reduces frustration and anxiety. Explain why more frequent antepartum surveillance testing is needed when diabetes complicates pregnancy. The woman needs to know her diabetic care will require more time and effort than it did before pregnancy but that this care greatly improves her likelihood of having a healthy infant.

◆ Evaluation

After procedures, tests, and plan of care have been explained, evaluation should ensure the following:

- The woman and at least one support person can demonstrate competence in home glucose monitoring and administration of insulin.
- The woman can describe a satisfactory plan for meeting her individual dietary requirements.
- The woman and at least one support person can list the signs and symptoms of hypoglycemia and hyperglycemia and describe the initial management of these conditions.
- The woman can verbalize knowledge of the reason for fetal surveillance procedures and keeps appointments for tests.

CARDIAC DISEASE

During pregnancy, significant hemodynamic adaptations occur to support maternal and fetal metabolic demands. These changes begin soon after conception and continue as gestation advances and are almost totally reversed within weeks to months after delivery. These cardiovascular adaptations can be problematic for the woman with cardiac disease. Such changes include increased blood volume, decreased systemic vascular resistance, increased clot formation, and increase in heart rate and cardiac output starting as early as 5 weeks of pregnancy (Arafeh, 2014; Blanchard & Daniels, 2014; Cunningham et al., 2014). Stroke volume is the primary reason cardiac output increases in early pregnancy, whereas in late pregnancy stroke volume decreases and heart rate increases, maintaining the elevation in cardiac output.

A normal heart can adapt to the changes so pregnancy and birth are tolerated without difficulty. For women with preexisting or underlying heart disease, however, the changes can impose an additional burden on an already compromised heart, which may result in cardiac decompensation leading to in ischemic events or **congestive heart failure** (CHF; failure of heart to maintain adequate circulation).

Incidence and Classification

Heart disease complicates 1% to 4% of pregnancies. The overall incidence of congenital heart disease (CHD) is increasing by 5% each year, which consequently increases the morbidity associated with cardiac disease in pregnant women (Arafeh, 2014; Elkayam, Goland, Pieper, & Silversides et al., 2016; Gaddipati & Troiano, 2013). Heart disease is now the leading cause of indirect maternal death—meaning death from a preexisting disease exacerbated by physiologic changes of pregnancy (Arafeh, 2014; Cunningham et al., 2014). Pregnancy may unmask a previously asymptomatic heart condition, or it may aggravate known heart disease. In some cases, pregnancy is contraindicated because of the severity of the mortality risk to the mother.

There are two major categories of heart disease: acquired and congenital. Acquired disease develops after birth and congenital disease is present at birth. Previously, acquired disease was the most prevalent form of heart disease because of increased incidence of rheumatic fever. Medical advances have made rheumatic fever uncommon, leaving CHD as the most common form in North America. Women with CHD are now likely to survive to reproductive age, adding cardiac risk to their pregnancy (Arafeh, 2014; Blanchard & Daniels, 2014; Cunningham et al., 2014). Cardiac disease effect on pregnancy depends on the woman's response to the hemodynamic changes and the severity of her disease.

Acquired Heart Disease
Rheumatic Heart Disease

Rheumatic heart disease is a complication that sometimes follows streptococcal pharyngitis ("strep throat"). Even one case of rheumatic fever may cause scarring of the heart valves, resulting in stenosis (narrowing) of the openings between the chambers of the heart. Early diagnosis and treatment of the streptococcal infection has resulted in a near-eradication of rheumatic fever in North America and Western Europe (Arafeh, 2014; Blanchard & Daniels, 2014).

The mitral valve is the most common site of stenosis. Mitral stenosis obstructs free blood flow from the left atrium to the left ventricle. The left atrium becomes dilated, and, as a result, pressure in the left atrium, pulmonary veins, and pulmonary capillaries is chronically elevated. This elevation may lead to pulmonary hypertension, pulmonary edema, aortic regurgitation, atrial fibrillation, or congestive heart failure (CHF). The first warnings of heart failure include persistent crackles at the base of the lungs, dyspnea on exertion, cough, and hemoptysis. Progressive edema and tachycardia are additional signs of heart failure (Blanchard & Daniels, 2014).

Valvular Stenosis

Valvular stenosis is most commonly caused by infection or blockage of the heart. Rheumatic fever and endocarditis are common infections that cause narrowing of heart valves. Some types of stenosis should be surgically repaired before pregnancy is attempted. Unrepaired stenotic valves may not tolerate the increased blood volume and cardiac output changes of pregnancy (Gaddipati & Troiano, 2013). Because of the increased risk for clot formation with valve replacement, anticoagulation is required (Arafeh, 2014). Bacterial endocarditis carries a high mortality risk for valvular heart disease and therefore should be treated in labor (ACOG, 2016f; Cunningham et al., 2014).

Myocardial Infarction

Myocardial infarction (MI) affects 1 in 10,000 pregnancies, with the highest incidence in the third trimester (Blanchard & Daniels, 2014; Gaddipati & Troiano, 2013). Maternal mortality rates at the time of the event are about 20%. Neonatal mortality is approximately 15% (Blanchard & Daniels, 2014; Gaddipati & Troiano, 2013). Risk factors associated with increased incidence of MI include (Arafeh, 2014):

- Smoking
- Hyperlipidemia—Increased total cholesterol, increased low-density lipoprotein (LDL), decreased high-density lipoprotein (HDL)
- Family history of MI
- Previously existing cardiovascular disease (hypertension, diabetes)
- Advanced maternal age

Common symptoms noted are radiating substernal chest pain, diaphoresis, nausea, and exertional dyspnea, although some women with coronary artery disease remain asymptomatic (Gaddipati & Troiano, 2013). In a study reviewing symptoms of different age groups of women, DeVon, Pettey, Vuckovic, Koenig, and McSweeney (2016) found that women 65 years old or older had less chest pain and more difficulty breathing compared with women younger than 65 years old. Delivery should be delayed, if possible, for 2 weeks after an event because mortality rates exponentially increase if delivery occurs in the following 14 days. Following an MI it is important to focus on supporting maternal heart function (Arafeh, 2014). Labor management should include:

- Lateral positioning (left or right) to maintain stable cardiac output during labor.
- Effective pain and anxiety management (epidural) to decrease maternal oxygen consumption.
- Second-stage labor management to include laboring down and avoiding the Valsalva maneuver through use of vacuum or forceps
- Antibiotic prophylaxis to decrease the risk for subacute bacterial endocarditis

Cardiomyopathy

Cardiomyopathy is a rare and often fatal disorder of the muscle structure of the heart and may be considered a diagnosis of exclusion. Although a number of cardiomyopathy forms exist, this chapter is focusing on peripartum cardiomyopathy (PPCM). This form occurs from late pregnancy to 5 months postpartum with no identifiable cause and no known previous heart disease. Left ventricular dysfunction is demonstrated by an ejection fraction less than 45%. PPCM is associated with advanced maternal age, African-American race, hypertension, multiple-fetus pregnancies, obesity, and tocolytic use and may have a familial genetic component (Arafeh, 2014; Blanchard & Daniels, 2014; Gaddipati & Troiano, 2013). The symptoms of PPCM are those of CHF: dyspnea on exertion, persistent basilar crackles, nocturnal cough, edema, weakness, chest pain, and heart palpitations (Cunningham et al., 2014). CHF is the primary sequela of PPCM and could be related to an underlying heart disease or a response to treatment.

Approximately 40% to 50% of women with cardiomyopathy may have a partial recovery with persistent CHF or other cardiac dysfunction. PPCM often recurs with subsequent pregnancies, particularly in women who did not have complete recovery of their left ventricular function. The woman should be informed of this risk (Blanchard & Daniels, 2014; Cunningham et al., 2014; Gaddipati & Troiano, 2013).

Anticoagulation with low-molecular-weight heparin (LMWH) to prevent clot formation is recommended when cardiac dysfunction is severe. Other medical therapy includes fluid restriction to reduce pulmonary edema, treatment of CHF and other pathologic processes associated with cardiomyopathy, and use of vasodilators (e.g., hydralazine) or dopamine agonists (e.g., bromocriptine) to support cardiac function (Blanchard & Daniels, 2014).

Congenital Heart Disease

Many congenital anomalies have no adverse effect on pregnancy. Malformations associated with high maternal and fetal morbidity and mortality may be surgically corrected before pregnancy. However, increased risk for miscarriage, cardiac complications, and premature delivery are noted in women with CHD despite advances in treatment and care. Congenital heart defects develop secondary to the following (Arafeh, 2014; Gaddipati & Troiano, 2013):

- Abnormal blood flow during organogenesis
- Maternal medical disorders (e.g., lupus, diabetes, phenylketonuria)
- Environmental exposure
  - Medications (e.g., anticonvulsants, street drugs, alcohol)
  - Infections (e.g., rubella, viruses, rheumatic fever)
- Genetics

Arafeh (2014) reports that congenital defects can be grouped into the following four structural defects:

- Holes (openings between structures of the heart)
- Stenosis (narrowing or stiffness resulting from obstruction)
- Hypoplasia or atresia (not developed or absent)
- Transposition, inversion, anomalous connections (wrong connection)

Defects that produce left-to-right shunting include atrial and ventricular septal defects and patent ductus arteriosus

(PDA). Shunting of extra blood to the right side of the heart leads to right-sided hypertrophy, which can lead to atrial arrhythmias and right-sided heart failure. In contrast, right-to-left shunting occurs when a cyanotic heart defect such as tetralogy of Fallot is present. Right-to-left shunting also may occur through a septal defect or PDA when pulmonary vascular resistance exceeds peripheral vascular resistance and pulmonary hypertension (Eisenmenger's syndrome) occurs. Fetal effects vary depending on the incidence and severity of the heart defect (Arafeh, 2014; Blanchard & Daniels, 2014).

Left-to-Right Shunt

Atrial Septal Defect. Atrial septal defect (ASD) often is first discovered in women of childbearing age because symptoms are absent or vague and include shortness of breath, syncope, palpitations, and inability to exercise without fatigue. This atrial septum opening produces a left-to-right shunt because of the increased pressure on the left side of the heart. Pregnancy is well tolerated by women with an uncomplicated ASD, and no specific treatment is recommended. Bacterial endocarditis is rare, and prophylactic antibiotics are not required. Occasionally, pulmonary hypertension develops as a result of the increased blood volume from the left side of the heart that is transported to the lungs through the pulmonary artery. ASD has the potential for causing CHF or atrial arrhythmias. If these complications are present, treatment would be indicated (Arafeh, 2014; Blanchard & Daniels, 2014; Cunningham et al., 2014; Gaddipati & Troiano, 2013).

Ventricular Septal Defect. Ventricular septal defects (VSDs) are more common than ASDs and are usually detected by auscultation at birth. Small defects often close with no surgical intervention; however, large defects will not spontaneously correct and therefore require surgery (Cunningham et al., 2014). Most women with VSD who become pregnant are asymptomatic, but fatigue or symptoms of pulmonary hypertension or congestion may occur (Arafeh, 2014; Cunningham et al., 2014).

Pregnancy is well tolerated with small to moderate left-to-right shunts. However, pregnancy occasionally precipitates heart failure or an arrhythmia. Antibiotic prophylaxis for bacterial endocarditis is no longer recommended unless recent surgical repair or a previous episode of endocarditis has occurred (Blanchard & Daniels, 2014).

Patent Ductus Arteriosus. The communicating shunt between the pulmonary artery and aorta typically closes from vasoconstriction after birth (Cunningham et al., 2014). If it doesn't, this shunt is usually discovered and treated in childhood because of the loud, continuous, machinery-like murmur (Blanchard & Daniels, 2014; Cunningham et al., 2014). If the condition is untreated, the physiologic effects are related to the size of the shunt. If this lesion is small, it may be well tolerated during pregnancy unless complicated by pulmonary hypertension. Bacterial endocarditis is common, and therefore antibiotic prophylaxis is recommended (Blanchard & Daniels, 2014; Cunningham et al., 2014).

Right-to-Left Shunt

Right-to-left shunting bypasses the pulmonary vasculature and therefore creates cyanosis. Cyanotic heart disease has relatively poor pregnancy outcomes, including miscarriage, preterm delivery, or fetal death (Cunningham et al., 2014). Surgical repair of the cyanotic defect decreases the maternal and fetal morbidity and mortality.

Tetralogy of Fallot. The most common cyanotic lesion noted is tetralogy of Fallot. The primary cause of right-to-left shunting is a combination of four defects (Arafeh, 2014; Blanchard & Daniels, 2014; Cunningham et al., 2014):

- VSD
- Pulmonary valve stenosis
- Right ventricular hypertrophy
- Overriding or displacement of the aorta toward the right ventricle

Patients with untreated tetralogy of Fallot have obvious symptoms of heart disease, including (1) cyanosis; (2) clubbing of the fingers and toes, (3) hypoxemia that creates reactive erythrocytosis causing elevated Hct; and (4) inability to tolerate activity (Blanchard & Daniels, 2014).

Women who have undergone repair and in whom cyanosis did not reappear may do well during pregnancy. With uncorrected tetralogy of Fallot, maternal and fetal mortality rates are high (Arafeh, 2014; Cunningham et al., 2014).

Eisenmenger's Syndrome. Eisenmenger's syndrome is a cyanotic heart condition that develops when pulmonary resistance equals or exceeds systemic resistance to blood flow and a right-to-left shunt develops. Several congenital defects may underlie the equalization of pressures within the ventricles, such as a large VSD or PDA. Operative closure of these defects should be done as soon as possible in defects that may cause Eisenmenger's syndrome. Deferring surgical intervention leads to irreversible pulmonary hypertension, creating an inoperable defect. Once Eisenmenger's syndrome is present surgical correction usually results in the woman's death (Blanchard & Daniels, 2014). Pregnancy carries a 50% maternal mortality risk for the patient with Eisenmenger's, usually from right ventricular failure or abnormal pulmonary blood flow as in pulmonary hypertension or pulmonary hemorrhage. Newborns carry the same mortality risk (50%) because of chronic hypoxemia (Arafeh, 2014; Blanchard & Daniels, 2014; Cunningham et al., 2014).

Other Congenital Lesions

Transposition of Great Vessels. Two varieties of transposition exist: levo-transposition (L-TGA) and dextro-transposition (D-TGA). L-TGA is congenitally corrected because the vessels along with the atria and ventricles are switched, which does not negatively affect oxygenation (Arafeh, 2014). In D-TGA the aorta arises from the right ventricle and the pulmonary artery from the left (Blanchard & Daniels, 2014). This transposition requires a shunt to allow oxygenating of the blood until completion of surgical repair. L-TGA may not be detected until adulthood, whereas D-TGA manifests with cyanosis shortly after birth (Arafeh, 2014).

Mitral Valve Prolapse. Mitral valve prolapse is one of the most common cardiac conditions among the general population. The incidence among otherwise normal young women is as high as 17%, but community-based studies have shown the incidence to be far lower, at 1% of the female population (Blanchard & Daniels, 2014). Although the condition appears to be inherited, it may be associated with a variety of other cardiac disorders such as ASDs and **Marfan syndrome**. In mitral valve prolapse, the leaflets of the mitral valve fall into the left atrium during ventricular contraction, which may allow blood to flow backward (regurgitation). Varying degrees of regurgitation are noted: absent, intermittent, or permanent (Blanchard & Daniels, 2014). Severe regurgitation can lead to left ventricular failure and pulmonary hypertension.

Mitral valve prolapse is considered a benign condition, and most women are asymptomatic and tolerate pregnancy well. Some women experience palpitations, syncope, fatigue, shortness of breath, chest pain, or anxiety (Cunningham et al., 2014). ACOG (2016f) does not recommend antibiotic prophylaxis for mitral valve prolapse. Beta-blockers may be given for chest pain or palpitations (Cunningham et al., 2014).

Coarctation of the Aorta. Coarctation of the aorta is a narrowing of the vessel, most commonly located distal to the subclavian artery (Blanchard & Daniels, 2014; Gaddipati & Troiano, 2013). Frequently coarctation is seen in conjunction with a bicuspid aortic valve, but is also associated with aortic stenosis, regurgitation, or long-standing arterial hypertension (Gaddipati & Troiano, 2013). Differentiation of complicated versus uncomplicated coarctation is important. Uncomplicated coarctations have no associated aneurysm or lesion that affects hemodynamics (Arafeh, 2014). Mortality associated with uncomplicated coarctation is 3% to 4%, whereas the mortality is up to 15% with complicated coarctation (Arafeh, 2014; Gaddipati & Troiano, 2013). Gaddipati and Troiano (2013) reported that measurement of the aortic gradient is useful in predicting pregnancy outcomes. Aortic gradients less than 20 mm Hg were associated with good outcomes (Gaddipati & Troiano, 2013). Therefore close monitoring of the lesion during pregnancy allows for timely intervention of worsening disease, creating optimal maternal and fetal outcomes.

Diagnosis and Classification

Early recognition of underlying heart disease is essential, and careful assessment for specific signs and symptoms of heart disease is part of every initial prenatal visit. Signs and symptoms include dyspnea, syncope (fainting) with exertion, hemoptysis, paroxysmal nocturnal dyspnea, progressive edema, tachypnea, tachycardia, and chest pain with exertion (Cunningham et al., 2014). Additional signs that confirm the diagnosis are (1) cyanosis; (2) clubbing; (3) diastolic, presystolic, or continuous heart murmur; (4) cardiac enlargement; (5) a loud, harsh systolic murmur associated with a thrill; and (6) serious arrhythmias (Blanchard & Daniels, 2014).

Class I—Uncompromised. No limitation of physical activity. Asymptomatic with ordinary activity.

Class II—Slightly compromised, requiring slight limitation of physical activity. Comfortable at rest, but ordinary physical activity causes fatigue, dyspnea, palpitations, or anginal pain.

Class III—Marked limitation of physical activity. Comfortable at rest, but less than ordinary activity causes excessive fatigue, palpitation, dyspnea, or anginal pain. Markedly compromised.

Class IV—Inability to perform any physical activity without discomfort. Symptoms of cardiac insufficiency even at rest.

*In general, maternal and fetal risks with classes I and II are small but are greatly increased with classes III and IV.

Diagnosis of heart disease may be made from clinical signs and symptoms and from findings on physical examination. It usually is confirmed by heart imaging studies such as transesophageal echocardiography.

Once the diagnosis is made, the severity of the disease is determined by the specific cardiac lesion, the functional status of the woman, and the development of complications (Gaddipati & Troiano, 2013). The New York Heart Association (NYHA) developed a clinical classification system to determine the effect of activity on the heart (Box 10.4) (American Heart Association, n.d.; Gaddipati & Troiano, 2013). Although this system helps determine the care needed for the pregnant woman with cardiac disease, it lacks the ability to predict the risk for adverse outcomes in pregnancy.

Therapeutic Management

Care of the pregnant woman with cardiac disease may include interventions not recommended in most pregnancies such as maintaining a low-sodium diet. Serial ultrasound scans to assess fetal growth and the presence of fetal congenital cardiac defects are recommended (Gaddipati & Troiano, 2013). Continual assessment of functional status and physical examination observing for signs and symptoms of cardiac compromise are essential during pregnancy.

Class I or II Heart Disease

Although pregnancy increases the demand placed on the woman's heart, women in New York Heart Association (NYHA) class I or II generally tolerate pregnancy changes well. The following are recommendations for women with heart disease (AHA, n.d.; Arafeh, 2014; Cunningham et al., 2014):

- Limit physical activity—This parameter is individualized to the patient's tolerance of activity. Demand should not exceed the functional capacity of the heart. In other words, the woman should remain free of symptoms of cardiac stress such as dyspnea, chest pain, and tachycardia during activity.

- Avoid excessive weight gain—Excessive weight increases demands on the heart. A diet adequate in protein, calories, and sodium is necessary. A low-sodium diet may be advised to avoid CHF.

- Prevent anemia—Anemia decreases the oxygen-carrying capacity of the blood and results in a compensatory increase in heart rate that a diseased heart may not be able to tolerate. Most anemia is prevented by administration of iron and folic acid.

- Prevent infection—Immunizations for influenza, pertussis, and pneumonia are available. Prevention may include administration of prophylactic antibiotics. As with other people, a pregnant woman with cardiac disease should be advised to avoid contact with those who may be ill during times when upper respiratory tract infections are prevalent, such as the winter months.

- Undergo careful assessment for the development of CHF, pulmonary edema, and cardiac arrhythmias—Characteristics of heart failure may include persistent basilar crackles, often accompanied by a cough during the night as the woman tries to sleep, sudden inability to carry out usual activities, dyspnea, cough, hemoptysis, increasing edema, altered level of consciousness, and tachycardia.

Class III or IV Heart Disease

NYHA class III or IV is associated with increased risk for morbidity and mortality in pregnancy (Cunningham et al., 2014; Gaddipati & Troiano, 2013). The primary goal of management is to prevent cardiac decompensation and development of CHF. Every effort is made to protect the fetus from hypoxia and IUGR, which can occur if placental perfusion is inadequate. In addition to the precautions listed for classes I and II heart disease, the woman may require bed rest, especially during the last trimester, because she has little reserve to tolerate rising metabolic demands. Reduced activity increases the maternal risk for thrombus formation and will require prophylaxis such as a sequential or boot compression device. Prophylactic anticoagulation may be needed.

Drug Therapy

Drug therapy for maternal cardiac disorders may extend from the prenatal period through the postpartum period. Medications that were part of a woman's treatment before pregnancy may be contraindicated during pregnancy. The medical team should consider risks and benefits when treating the pregnant woman with cardiac disease.

Anticoagulants. During pregnancy, clotting factors normally increase and thrombolytic activity decreases. These changes predispose the pregnant woman to thrombus formation. Superimposed cardiac problems such as mitral valve stenosis or atrial fibrillation may require anticoagulant therapy during pregnancy. Any patient requiring anticoagulation when not pregnant should be treated during pregnancy (Gaddipati & Troiano, 2013). Warfarin (Coumadin) is associated with fetal malformations and generally should be restricted throughout pregnancy. Certain conditions require warfarin for anticoagulation (e.g., mechanical heart valve replacement).

In such cases, the physician should discuss the risks and benefits of treatment options with the patient (ACOG, 2014b). Heparin, does not cross the placental barrier and is an effective alternative anticoagulant for most women. Careful monitoring of the partial thromboplastin time (PTT), activated partial thromboplastin time (aPTT), and platelet count is essential to achieve effective, safe anticoagulation. Enoxaparin (Lovenox), a LMWH, may be used instead of standard heparin because it requires less-frequent monitoring for bleeding complications. Enoxaparin and heparin are not interchangeable. Both are given subcutaneously, but only heparin may be given intravenously. Heparin is withheld during labor and resumed 6 hours after vaginal birth and 6 to 12 hours after cesarean birth (ACOG, 2014b; Gaddipati & Troiano, 2013). Postpartum anticoagulation is continued with warfarin (Cunningham et al., 2014; Gaddipati & Troiano, 2013).

Antiarrhythmics. Use of medications for heart disease during pregnancy should balance benefits to the mother against possible harm to the fetus. Another consideration is that maternal heart failure itself is harmful to the fetus. In addition to controlling arrhythmias, beta-blockers and calcium channel blockers may be used to control maternal hypertension. Digoxin, adenosine, and calcium channel blockers appear to be safe. Although beta-blockers have been associated with neonatal respiratory depression, sustained bradycardia, and hypoglycemia when administered late in pregnancy or just before delivery, they may be indicated in selected cases. The beta-blockers, atenolol and metoprolol, may be preferred because they do not cause the uterine stimulation or contractions that other drugs of this class may cause (Cunningham et al., 2014).

Antiinfectives. ACOG (2016f) set forth guidelines for use of antibiotic prophylaxis to prevent infective endocarditis in persons at high risk. The following cardiac conditions are considered high risk for development of endocarditis in the presence of bacteremia (ACOG, 2016f; Gaddipati & Troiano, 2013):

- Prosthetic heart valve or prosthetic material used for valve repair
- Previous infective endocarditis
- Congenital heart malformations, unrepaired or repaired using prosthetic material within 6 months of repair
- Residual heart defects at site of repair
- Surgically corrected systemic pulmonary shunts
- Dental procedures
- Cardiac transplantation recipients who develop disorders of heart valves

Antiinfective agents for endocarditis are chosen based on the infecting agent. Gram-positive *Staphylococcus* infections are common in IV drug users, and the mortality rate among them is high. Maternal gonorrhea infection may cause acute, rapidly developing endocarditis. A woman with an increased risk for bacterial endocarditis may receive prophylactic antibiotics such as amoxicillin, penicillin, ampicillin, and gentamicin at delivery. Ceftriaxone or vancomycin also may be given for acute endocarditis.

Drugs for Heart Failure. Myocardial response to CHF is ventricular wall thickening and dilation from fluid volume overload. This diminishes the contractile response of the cardiac muscle and decreases cardiac output (Blanchard & Daniels, 2014). Diuretics may be needed when CHF remains uncontrolled in spite of restriction of activity and sodium intake. Careful monitoring of electrolytes and fluid volume status through laboratory values and hemodynamic monitoring is necessary to avoid excessively reducing maternal blood volume with resulting adverse effects on the fetus. Furosemide has been associated with IUGR in the fetus. Additionally, thiazide diuretics are known to cause neonatal jaundice, thrombocytopenia, anemia, and hypoglycemia in the fetus (Blanchard & Daniels, 2014; Cunningham et al., 2014). ACE inhibitors or angiotensin receptor blockers are contraindicated in pregnancy. Therefore hydralazine is the preferred treatment in pregnancy (Blanchard & Daniels, 2014). Other medications approved for use in pregnancy include beta blockers and digoxin.

Intrapartum Management

Every effort is made to minimize the effects of labor on the cardiovascular system. With every contraction, 300 to 500 mL of blood is shifted from the uterus and placenta into the central circulation. This extra fluid causes a sharp rise in cardiac workload. Therefore careful management of IV fluid administration is essential to prevent fluid overload. The woman should be positioned on her side, with her head and shoulders elevated. Pulse oximetry is used to monitor oxygen saturation. The use of oxygen may be needed if oxygen saturation is below 95%. Pain increases oxygen consumption. The administration of pain medication or an epidural if not contraindicated should be given earlier in the pregnant intrapartum patient. The environment should be kept quiet and calm to prevent anxiety, which can cause a catecholamine release and further increase the workload of the heart (Gaddipati & Troiano, 2013). Maternal signs of cardiac decompensation (tachycardia, rapid respirations, moist crackles, and exhaustion) should be reported to the physician immediately. The fetus is monitored continuously for signs of compromise .

A vaginal birth is recommended for a woman with heart disease unless there are specific indications for a cesarean birth. Vacuum extraction or outlet forceps are used to minimize maternal pushing, which can add to the hemodynamic stress for the woman with cardiac disease. Cesarean birth may be chosen for obstetric indications. Although it is a common obstetric procedure, the woman and her physician should consider the added stress of major surgery on her heart. Expected blood loss is higher in cesarean birth than in vaginal birth. General anesthesia may be required if epidural anesthesia is not an option, leading to operative airway management by an anesthesiologist. Postoperative infection risk is greater with cesarean birth (Cunningham et al., 2014; Gaddipati & Troiano, 2013).

The fourth stage of labor is associated with risks. After delivery of the placenta, about 500 to 1000 mL of blood is returned to the intravascular volume creating an 80% increase in cardiac output within 10 to 15 minutes after delivery (Monga & Mastrobattista, 2014). To minimize the risks for overloading the heart, abrupt positional changes should be avoided. Repositioning the patient from lateral to supine can decrease cardiac output by 25% to 30% (Monga & Mastrobattista, 2014). Careful assessment for signs of circulatory overload, such as a bounding pulse, distended neck and peripheral veins, and moist crackles in the lungs, is performed throughout labor and the postpartum period.

Postpartum Management

Women who have shown no evidence of distress during pregnancy, labor, and childbirth may experience cardiac decompensation during the postpartum period. The relief of vena caval compression and autotransfusion of blood from the uterus after placental delivery abruptly increases the blood returning to the right side of the heart.

The woman should be observed for signs of infection, hemorrhage, and thromboembolism. These conditions can precipitate heart failure in women with underlying heart disease. The woman is vulnerable in the postpartum period, as interstitial fluid is mobilized into the vascular space for elimination. Astute management of intake and output is necessary to monitor for CHF and pulmonary edema. If the mother cannot assume care of her infant, nurses should make every effort to promote contact between the mother, her significant others, and the infant.

Breastfeeding imposes extra demands on the mother's heart and is advised on an individualized basis. Pumping may be initiated if the mother is in an ICU environment. Depending on the drugs the mother is given, her breastmilk may need to be be wasted. It is necessary to have the neonatologist and lactation consultant involved in the care.

> **! SAFETY CHECK**
>
> Signs and symptoms of congestive heart failure include the following:
> - Cough (frequent, productive, hemoptysis)
> - Progressive dyspnea with exertion
> - Orthopnea
> - Pitting edema of legs and feet or generalized edema of face, hands, or sacral area
> - Heart palpitations
> - Progressive fatigue or syncope with exertion
> - Moist crackles in lower lobes, indicating pulmonary edema
> - Altered level of consciousness

◆ APPLICATION OF THE NURSING PROCESS: THE PREGNANT WOMAN WITH HEART DISEASE

◆ Assessment

Begin with a review of the woman's medical record to determine the functional classification assigned (see Box 10.4). Assess the woman at each prenatal appointment to determine how pregnancy affects the functional capacity of the heart.

- Take vital signs and compare them with preconception levels. Note any changes such as tachycardia since the previous prenatal appointment.
- Assess the level of fatigue and any changes in fatigue since the previous prenatal appointment. This is especially important when fluid volume peaks and the chance of cardiac decompensation is greatest (18 to 32 weeks of gestation).
- Observe for signs or symptoms of CHF.
- Note additional factors that may increase the workload of the heart (anemia, infections, anxiety, lack of adequate support to manage the activities of daily living).
- Weigh the woman and compare the desired and actual patterns of weight gain to detect excessive weight gain or fluid retention.
- Assess the woman's knowledge of the prescribed regimen of care and her ability to comply with it.

◆ Identification of Patient Problems

The pregnant woman with a cardiac defect may be unable to tolerate activity to the same degree as before pregnancy because of the stress imposed on her cardiovascular system. Arriving at the patient problem, "Exhaustion because of insufficient knowledge of measures that reduce cardiac stress" is a priority.

◆ Planning: Expected Outcomes

Goals and outcomes are as follows:
- The woman (and her family) will identify factors that increase cardiac workload.
- The woman (and family) will describe measures that promote adaptation to activity restrictions.

◆ Interventions

Prenatal nursing care focuses on teaching the woman and her family about the possible effects of the disease on their lives. This teaching may include specific instructions about factors that increase the workload of the heart and measures to promote adaptation to activity restrictions during pregnancy and birth. Teaching also may reinforce or clarify the physician's instructions.

Teaching about Increased Cardiac Workload

Excessive Weight Gain and Anemia. Excessive weight gain and anemia increase the workload of the heart just as they do in the nonpregnant state and should be avoided. A well-balanced diet, with adequate high-quality protein and about 2200 calories is recommended. Emphasize the importance of taking any prescribed iron supplements to prevent anemia and reduce the risk for tachycardia. Folic acid should be taken prior to conception to prevent anemia and reduce the risk for NTDs in the fetus.

Exertion. Instruct the woman to modify her activity level to regulate energy expenditures and reduce cardiac workload. For example, she might take rest periods during the day and for an hour after meals. If possible, she should sit rather than stand when performing activities. She should rest every few minutes when performing an activity that increases heart rate to allow the heart time to recover. Emphasize that she should stop an activity if she experiences dyspnea, chest pain, or tachycardia.

Exposure. Instruct the woman to avoid unnecessary exposure to environmental extremes. She should dress warmly during cold weather and create a barrier to cold temperatures by wearing layers of clothing. Educate her that exertion in hot, humid weather or during extreme cold weather places additional demands on the heart and should be avoided.

Emotional Stress. Explain the effects of emotional stress on the cardiovascular system (increased blood pressure, heart rate, and respiratory rate). Help the woman identify areas of stress in her life. Discuss various methods for stress management such as meditation, progressive relaxation of muscles, and biofeedback. Teach that cigarette smoking and use of illicit drugs such as cocaine and amphetamines greatly increase stress on the heart and are associated with hypertension that further adds to cardiac workload and fetal compromise.

Helping Family Accept Restrictions on Activity

Assist family members to accept the need for activity restriction. The amount of activity that the woman can tolerate depends on the severity of the disease. However, all women with heart disease need 8 to 10 hours of sleep each night, with periods of morning and afternoon rest. For some women, bed rest with bathroom privileges is necessary during the last half of pregnancy, and this may create special problems for the family. Nurses often help family members plan ways to meet their needs while the mother continues bed rest.

Providing Postpartum Care

The woman is vulnerable in the postpartum period, as interstitial fluid is mobilized into the vascular space for elimination. Continue to observe for signs of CHF. Observe urine output because it is a direct indicator of renal blood flow. Inadequate urine output may reflect the heart's inability to circulate blood adequately to the kidneys.

After childbirth, the mother may be unable to assume care of the newborn, especially after a prolonged period of limited activity or bed rest. However, every effort should be made to promote contact between the mother and the baby. Many nurses assess the baby, perform the necessary newborn care at the bedside, and then allow the mother ample time to hold the infant. The father and other family members should be included in the care of the infant, whenever possible.

The decision about breastfeeding will be individualized according to the mother's condition and its demands on her energy. Regardless of feeding method, she should be encouraged to feed the infant whenever possible to promote maternal-infant attachment. Consult with physicians and make referrals as necessary for follow-up care, which may include home care by a nurse or nursing assistant. Be certain that the family understands the signs and symptoms of cardiac

Category	BMI
Underweight	<18.5
Normal weight	18.5-24.9
Overweight	25.0-29.9
Obesity class I	30.0-34.9
Obesity class II	35.0-39.9
Obesity class III	≥40

TABLE 10.7 World Health Organization Body Mass Categories

complications and when to notify the physician that problems have developed.

◆ Evaluation

The ability to identify the factors increasing cardiac workload offers reassurance that the woman and her family will initiate measures promoting adaptation to restricted activity.

KNOWLEDGE CHECK

35. How do the cardiovascular changes of pregnancy affect the condition of the woman who has a cardiac defect?
36. What are the two major categories of heart disease? What are the functional classifications of heart disease?
37. What are the primary goals for management of heart disease in terms of diet, activity, and weight gain?
38. Why should the administration of fluids, both oral and intravenous, be monitored closely during labor?
39. Why is the fourth stage of labor particularly dangerous for the woman with heart disease?

OBESITY

Obesity is determined by one's BMI defined as weight in kilograms divided by height in meters squared (kg/m^2). The World Health Organization (2006) organizes BMI into six categories: underweight, normal weight, overweight, and three classes of obesity (Table 10.7). Waist circumference and weight-to-hip ratios are used to determine central or abdominal obesity (Kriebs, 2014). An abdominal waist circumference of 35 inches or more is defined as central obesity.

Obesity is a public health epidemic in the United States. The rate of obesity among all adults from 2011 to 2014 was 36.5%; among young adults (20 to 39 years old), it was 32.3% (Ogden, Carroll, Fryar, & Flegal KM , 2015). Based on data from 2014, birth certificates from 47 states and the District of Columbia, 25.6% of the mothers were overweight (BMI is 25.0 to 29.9), and 24.8% were obese (BMI is greater than 29.9) before becoming pregnant. Increased rates of prepregnancy obesity were noted among non-Hispanic Black and non-Hispanic American Indian and Native Alaskan women. Increased maternal age, increased parity (3 or more), and low socioeconomic status are associated with higher rates of prepregnancy obesity (Branum A, Kirmeyer SE, Gregory ECW, 2016).

Risk

Pregnancy can exacerbate obesity-related comorbidities such as hypertension, diabetes, and asthma. Obese women are less fertile and have an increased risk for spontaneous abortions and stillbirth compared to women of appropriate weight. During pregnancy, obesity significantly increases risks to the mother, fetus and neonate.

Maternal risks associated with obesity in pregnancy include gestational diabetes, preeclampsia, venous thromboembolism, cesarean delivery, wound infection, respiratory complications, preterm birth, birth trauma, and postpartum anemia (ACOG, 2015f; 2016a; Kriebs, 2014). Infants of obese mothers have an increased risk for NTDs, hydrocephaly, and cardiovascular defect, as well as macrosomia, hypoglycemia, birth injury from shoulder dystocia, and neonatal intensive care admissions.

Antenatal Care

At the first prenatal visit, the woman's BMI should be determined. Obese pregnant women should be counseled on the risks associated with maternal obesity, and excessive weight gain during pregnancy is discussed at each prenatal visit (ACOG, 2013c). Proper nutrition to include a balanced diet, caloric intake, exercise, and behavior modification. The recommended weight gain in pregnancy is 11 to 20 lbs in obese women (BMI 30 or greater) and 15 to 25 lbs in overweight women (BMI 25 to 29.9) (ACOG, 2015f; Institute of Medicine [IOM], 2009). The recommended amount of exercise for pregnant women is 20 to 30 minutes preferably every day (ACOG, 2015a; Lindqvist et al., 2016). Referral to a Registered Dietician for development of a healthy eating plan may be appropriate. Because there is an association between obesity during pregnancy and psychological and emotional issues such as depression, anxiety and stress (Faria-Schützer, Surita, Nascimento, Vieira, & Turato, 2017; Wahedi, M., 2016), referral to a counselor or mental health provider may be reasonable.

Overweight and obese women have an increased risk for undiagnosed type 2 diabetes mellitus. They should be screened at the first prenatal visit and again at 24 to 28 weeks gestation. Additional laboratory tests may include a baseline metabolic or chemistry panel if hypertension is noted.

Obesity increases the risk for sleep apnea. If the obese pregnant patient has symptoms of snoring at night, sleepiness, or chronic fatigue or cannot concentrate, a referral for a sleep study may be appropriate. Finally, an ultrasound should be obtained between 18 and 22 weeks to review fetal anatomy. Serial growth scans may be needed because of difficulty assessing fetal growth by fundal height measurements.

Intrapartum Care

Special equipment for the obese gravida may be necessary during labor and delivery. These include a bariatric bed, commode or toilet seat, extra-large gowns, correct-size blood pressure cuff, correct-size sequential compression devices, bariatric wheelchairs, and a proper scale to weigh the patient. Should the patient require a cesarean section, a bariatric operating room table, as well as appropriate extra-long surgical instruments may be necessary.

Nursing care during labor involves frequent assessment of the FHR and uterine activity monitoring. It may be necessary for one-to-one nursing care or two-to-one nursing care in some cases. It can be difficult to monitor the FHR externally and may require the use of internal monitoring for the FHR as well as intrauterine pressure monitoring to assess uterine contractions.

Obese women are at an increased risk for dysfunctional labor leading to cesarean birth. Analgesia and anesthesia may be difficult to achieve. Regional anesthesia is difficult because of the decreased ability to identify landmarks and inability to correctly position the patient. In women who have a cesarean birth, risks for surgical site infection and endometritis are increased. Higher doses of preoperative antibiotics may need to be required. A vertical skin incision may be performed, and the physician may elect to involve a wound care nurse for follow up.

Postpartum

Obese mothers are at risk for pneumonia, infection, wound dehiscence, thromboembolism, and postpartum hemorrhage. Antibiotics may need to be continued during the postpartum period. Additionally, LMWH may be required to reduce the risk for thromboembolism. During the postpartum period, the nurse should encourage mothers to breastfeed their infants. Through breastfeeding, the obese will lose their pregnancy weight gain sooner than non-breastfeeding mothers. At the postpartum office appointment, gestational diabetes as well hypertension should be reassessed. Finally, obese postpartum women should be encouraged to optimize their health during the interconception period.

Pregnancy after Bariatric Surgery

Bariatric surgery is a common treatment for obesity. Although it is not appropriate during pregnancy, some obese women may elect to have weight reduction surgery before conceiving. In these women, the rates of obstetrical complications are lower than in the morbidly obese patient. The woman should postpone pregnancy for 12 to 24 months after bariatric surgery to allow her weight to stabilize. She should be assessed for vitamin and nutritional deficiency and be monitored for signs of intestinal obstruction (Cunningham et al., 2014).

Nursing Considerations

It is important to recognize one's own biases when caring for obese patients and remember that weight can be a very sensitive topic for the patient (ACOG, 2014a). Plans and discussions concerning weight loss and management with childbearing patients should be handled with the utmost respect and sensitivity and should take a team-based, patient-centered approach (ACOG, 2014a). Although the obese pregnant patient faces significant health risks, with proper and consistent education and treatment pregnant patients with obesity can experience healthy, successful pregnancies, lose weight, and improve their overall health and lifestyle.

> **? KNOWLEDGE CHECK**
>
> 40. How much should the pregnant obese patient gain during pregnancy?
> 41. What complications should the nurse assess during the intrapartum period?

ANEMIAS

Anemia is a condition in which a decline in circulating RBC mass reduces the capacity to carry oxygen to the vital organs of the mother or the fetus. Significant maternal anemia is associated with preterm birth and low birth weight. A pregnant woman is usually considered anemic if her Hgb level is less than 10.5 g/dL in the second trimester or less than 11 g/dL in the first and third trimesters (Blackburn, 2013; Cunningham et al., 2014; Kilpatrick, 2014; Samuels, 2017).

Anemia is one of the most common problems of pregnancy, affecting 15% to 25% of pregnant women. The incidence varies according to geographic location and socioeconomic group. Anemia may be caused by a variety of factors, including nutritional deficits, hemolysis, and blood loss. The most common type of anemia observed during pregnancy is iron-deficiency anemia; less common causes are folic acid deficiency, sickle cell disease, and thalassemia. The increase in bariatric surgery has increased the number of women with vitamin B_{12} deficiency (ACOG, 2015b; Samuels, 2017).

Iron-Deficiency Anemia

The total iron requirement for a typical pregnancy with a single fetus is approximately 1000 mg. Unfortunately, most women of reproductive age do not have this amount of iron stores because of menstrual blood loss. Furthermore, meeting pregnancy needs by diet alone is difficult, although iron is present in many foods. The primary sources of iron are meat, fish, chicken, liver, and green leafy vegetables.

Maternal Effects

Signs and symptoms of iron deficiency anemia include pallor, fatigue, lethargy, and headache. Clinical findings also may include inflammations of the lips and tongue. *Pica* (consuming nonfood substances such as clay, dirt, ice, and starch) may be a sign of iron-deficiency anemia. Laboratory findings for iron-deficiency anemia include RBCs that are microcytic (small) and hypochromic (pale). Plasma iron and serum ferritin levels are low, whereas the total iron-binding capacity is higher than normal. Women who have multifetal pregnancies or bleeding complications are more likely to be anemic during pregnancy (Kilpatrick, 2014).

Fetal and Neonatal Effects

All effects of maternal iron-deficiency anemia on the fetus and neonate are unclear. In general, even with significant maternal iron deficiency, the fetus will receive adequate stores at a cost to the mother. If the mother is severely anemic, the fetus may have reduced RBC volume, Hgb, and iron stores. Profound maternal anemia can reduce fetal oxygen supply (Kilpatrick, 2014).

Therapeutic Management

Routine supplemental iron therapy, rather than therapy based on an indication of anemia, is controversial. Ferrous sulfate 325 mg (which provides 60 to 65 mg of elemental iron), one to three times per day, is commonly prescribed. Many women experience less gastrointestinal discomfort if iron supplementation is taken with meals, although absorption is less. Taking iron supplementation with vitamin C may enhance absorption. Therapy is often continued for about 6 months after the anemia has been corrected. Parenteral therapy may be necessary for the woman who cannot or will not take oral iron supplementation and is significantly anemic, but does not require a transfusion (Samuels, 2017).

Folic Acid–Deficiency (Megaloblastic) Anemia

Folic acid, which functions as a coenzyme in the synthesis of DNA, is essential for cell duplication and fetal and placental growth. It also is an essential nutrient for the formation of RBCs.

Maternal Effects

Maternal needs for folic acid double during pregnancy in response to the demand for greater production of erythrocytes and fetal and placental growth. A deficiency in folic acid results in a reduction in the rate of DNA synthesis and mitotic activity of individual cells, resulting in the presence of large, immature erythrocytes (megaloblasts). Folate deficiency is the primary cause of megaloblastic anemia during pregnancy.

Nonfood factors that contribute to folic acid deficiency include hemolytic anemias with increased RBC turnover, multifetal pregnancies, some medications (such as anticonvulsants), and malabsorption entities. Folic acid deficiency often is present in association with iron-deficiency anemia.

Fetal and Neonatal Effects

Folate deficiency is associated with increased risk for spontaneous abortion, placental abruption, and fetal anomalies. A known association exists between folic acid deficiency and an increase in NTDs.

Therapeutic Management

The recommended daily allowance for folic acid doubles during pregnancy, and some women have difficulty ingesting the amount needed, even though it does occur widely in foods. The best sources of folic acid are fortified grains; beans such as black beans and lentils; peanuts; and fresh, dark-green leafy vegetables (see Table 8.3). Folic acid often is destroyed in cooking. As a result of the awareness of the association between folic acid deficiency and NTDs, it is now recommended that all women of childbearing age take 400 mcg (0.4 mg) of folic acid daily to reduce this risk. This supplementation should be increased to 600 mcg (0.6 mg) when pregnancy is confirmed. Women who have had a previous child with an NTD should take 4 mg of folic acid for 1 month before and during the first trimester of pregnancy (AAP & ACOG, 2012; U.S. Preventive Services Task Force, 2016).

Most prenatal vitamins contain 1 mg of folate to ensure sufficient intake. Higher doses of folate may be prescribed according to individual needs.

> **② KNOWLEDGE CHECK**
>
> 42. Why is supplemental iron needed by most women who are pregnant?
> 43. What are the neonatal effects of iron-deficiency anemia?
> 44. What are the fetal and neonatal effects of folic acid deficiency?

Sickle Cell Disease

Sickle cell disease is an autosomal recessive genetic disorder. It occurs when the gene for the production of Hgb S is inherited from both parents. The defect in the Hgb causes erythrocytes to become shaped like a sickle, or crescent, under certain conditions. Low oxygen concentration usually causes the sickling, with acidosis and dehydration worsening the process. At first the erythrocytes regain their normal shape, but eventually they remain permanently sickled. Because of their distorted shape, the erythrocytes cannot pass through small arteries and capillaries and tend to clump together and occlude the blood vessel.

The disease is characterized by chronic anemia because of the short life span of erythrocytes affected with Hgb S, increased susceptibility to infection, and periodic episodes of obstruction of blood vessels by the abnormally shaped erythrocytes. Sickle cell disease occurs most often in people who have ancestors from sub-Saharan Africa, Spanish-speaking countries in the Western hemisphere (South America, Caribbean, Central America), Saudi Arabia, India, and Mediterranean countries. In the United States approximately 1 in 500 births in the Black or African-American population and 1 in 36,000 births in the Hispanic population will result in an infant with sickle cell anemia. Sickle cell anemia affects 90,000 to 100,000 people in the United States. Of Blacks or African-Americans, 1 in 12 are carriers of the sickle cell trait and may pass the gene on to their children, even though they are not affected (ACOG, 2015d; NIH & NHLBI, 2012; Samuels, 2017).

Maternal Effects

Physiologic anemia, increased coagulation factors, and venous stasis, which are normal in pregnancy, may bring on sickle cell crisis, sometimes for the first time. This broad term includes several different conditions, particularly temporary cessation of bone marrow function, hemolytic crisis with massive erythrocyte destruction resulting in jaundice, and severe pain caused by infarctions located in the joints and the major organs. In addition, expectant mothers with sickle cell anemia are prone to pyelonephritis, bone infection, and heart disease. Preeclampsia occurs in approximately 14% of these women. Preterm birth and IUGR are common. Mothers with higher Hgb F (fetal Hgb) levels may have a lower perinatal mortality rate, but fetal safety has not been established for hydroxyurea that increases its production (ACOG, 2015d; NIH & NHLBI, 2012; Samuels, 2017).

Fetal and Neonatal Effects

In the absence of maternal sickle cell crisis, the fetus usually fares well, although complications such as prematurity and IUGR are more common. The incidence of fetal loss is high if sickle cell crisis occurs because of placental infarctions with loss of exchange surface on the placenta (ACOG, 2015d; NIH & NHLBI, 2012).

Therapeutic Management

Women with sickle cell disease should seek preconception care or early prenatal care and be informed of the maternal and fetal risks associated with the pregnancy. Folic acid supplementation of 4 mg (400 mcg) daily is prescribed, ideally before conception, because of frequent erythrocyte turnover. Frequent measurements of Hgb, complete blood cell count, serum iron, total iron-binding capacity, and serum folate are necessary to determine the degree of anemia and iron and folic acid stores. Testing is performed for infections such as hepatitis, human immunodeficiency virus (HIV) infection, tuberculosis, and STDs. Hepatitis B and varicella vaccines may be given to the noninfected woman who is not immune to these infections. Urinalysis, with culture and sensitivity, if indicated, identifies both clinical and subclinical UTIs that should be treated.

Fetal surveillance studies (ultrasonography, NSTs, and BPPs) assess fetal growth and development and placental function. Exchange transfusions or prophylactic transfusions may be used to increase the amount of normal Hgb in the mother's circulation and reduce severe anemia. Risks for prophylactic transfusions are comparable with risks in the woman without sickle cell disease. The woman with sickle cell disease may have a transfusion reaction and is likely to develop higher levels of antibodies to the cells in the transfused blood. Finding compatible blood for later transfusion might be more difficult. Prenatal supplementation of vitamins without iron may be prescribed for the woman who receives multiple transfusions but for whom additional folic acid is indicated (ACOG, 2015d; Cunningham et al., 2014; NIH & NHLBI, 2012; Samuels, 2017).

The goal of nursing management is to help the pregnant woman with sickle cell disease maintain a healthy state and avoid hospitalization. Women should be encouraged to keep all prenatal care appointments, usually every other week and more frequently, if needed. Topics in prenatal education include the need for (1) adequate hydration to prevent sickling, (2) adequate nutrition to meet metabolic needs, (3) folic acid supplementation for erythrocyte production, (4) rest periods throughout the day, (5) good hygiene practices and the avoidance of persons with infectious illnesses, and (6) prompt treatment for fever or other signs of infection.

Nurses should be alert for signs of a sickle cell crisis. The most common indications are pain in the abdomen, chest, vertebrae, joints, or extremities; pallor; and signs of cardiac failure. Nurses also should provide comfort measures such as repositioning and good skin care, assisting with ambulation and movement in bed, and assisting the woman to splint the abdomen with a pillow when she must cough or breathe deeply.

Nurses should remember that pain is not always related to the sickling crisis but could be related to a complication of pregnancy. Women with sickle cell disease also can have ectopic pregnancy, placental abruption, appendicitis, and other painful complications not related to their blood disorder.

Intrapartum care focuses on preventing the development of sickle cell crisis. Oxygen is administered continuously, and fluids should be administered to prevent dehydration because hypoxemia and dehydration, as well as exertion, infection, and acidosis, stimulate the sickling process. Prophylactic blood transfusions may be given in an attempt to reduce perinatal mortality (Cunningham et al., 2014).

Thalassemia

Like sickle cell anemia, thalassemia is a genetic disorder that involves the abnormal synthesis of alpha or beta chains of Hgb. This abnormal synthesis leads to alterations in the RBC membrane and decreased life span of RBCs. Thalassemia is named and classified by the type of chain that is abnormal. Beta-thalassemia is most frequently encountered in the United States, often in those of Mediterranean, Middle Eastern, and Asian descent.

Beta-thalassemia minor refers to the heterozygous form that results from the inheritance of one abnormal gene from either parent. *Beta-thalassemia major* refers to inheritance of the gene from both parents (homozygous form). Females with beta-thalassemia major (Cooley's anemia) usually die in young adulthood. Those females who survive are often sterile (ACOG, 2015d; Cunningham et al., 2014; Kilpatrick, 2014; Samuels, 2017).

Maternal Effects

Women with beta-thalassemia minor often are mildly anemic but otherwise healthy. Laboratory values normally associated with beta-thalassemia minor indicate a mild hypochromic and microcytic anemia. Large amounts of iron usually are not given despite the anemia because persons with beta-thalassemia absorb and store iron in their bodies excessively and must take a chelating agent to rid the excess. Chelation therapy to remove heavy metals such as iron is discontinued during pregnancy, if possible, because pregnancy safety has not been established (ACOG, 2015d; Samuels, 2017).

Fetal and Neonatal Effects

Whether the disorders are associated with increased fetal or neonatal morbidity remains unresolved because of the many variants of thalassemia. There appears to be no increase in the rate of prematurity, low-birth-weight infants, or abnormal size for gestation. Fetal anemia may be serious if inadequate fetal Hgb is produced. The fetus may inherit the serious problem of beta-thalassemia major if both parents have beta-thalassemia minor.

Therapeutic Management

No specific therapy for beta-thalassemia minor during pregnancy exists. Generally, the outcomes for the mother and fetus are satisfactory (ACOG, 2015d; Cunningham et al., 2014; Samuels, 2017). Infections that depress the production of RBCs and accelerate erythrocyte destruction should be identified and treated promptly.

> ### ❓ KNOWLEDGE CHECK
>
> 45. What are the maternal effects of sickle cell disease?
> 46. How is sickle cell disease treated during pregnancy?
> 47. Why is iron supplementation often not recommended for women with thalassemia?

OTHER MEDICAL CONDITIONS

Women with a preexisting medical condition should be aware of the effects that pregnancy will have on their conditions as well as the impact of their medical conditions on pregnancy outcome. Some conditions that complicate pregnancy are discussed in this section; others are described in Table 10.8.

Immune-Complex Diseases
Systemic Lupus Erythematosus

Systemic lupus erythematosus (SLE) is a chronic inflammatory autoimmune disease that can affect any organ or system in the body. The body attacks its own tissues as it would foreign antigens. Although the cause is unknown, an imbalance appears to exist between normal immune response to foreign antigens and an abnormal immune response of the body against its own cells. Signs and symptoms result from inflammation of multiple organ systems, especially the joints, skin, kidneys, and the CNS. The most common signs and symptoms of SLE are joint pain, photosensitivity, and a characteristic "butterfly rash" on the face, which may be less apparent during pregnancy because of the normal pigmentation changes. The disease is marked by episodes of *exacerbation* (flares), when the symptoms become worse, and *quiescence,* when the symptoms recede.

The disease tends to affect young women but may occur in any age group. Females are affected 6 to 10 times more often compared with males. There is sometimes a family aggregation, but it is usually sporadic. It is more common in women of African, Hispanic, Asian, and Native American descent (CDC, 2017b; Carpenter & Branch, 2017).

Women with a history of renal problems should be advised to seek the advice of a physician before becoming pregnant. Pregnancy is most likely to have a favorable outcome in the woman whose disease is well controlled at the beginning and who does not have renal involvement. However, flares

TABLE 10.8   Medical Conditions and Their Effects on Pregnancy

Condition	Maternal-Fetal Effects	Nursing Considerations
Appendicitis Inflammation of appendix, often with fever. Most common nongynecologic surgical emergency during pregnancy.	Is difficult to diagnose during pregnancy. Early symptoms mimic common conditions of pregnancy. Ultrasonography may help rule out other diagnoses such as ectopic pregnancy.	When reasonable doubt exists that patient has appendicitis, appendix should be removed to prevent rupture and consequent complications. Location of appendix often is altered by growing uterus. Fetal hyperthermia may be caused by maternal fever.
Asthma Obstructive lung disease caused by airway inflammation. Characterized by dyspnea, cough, wheezing. Course in pregnancy is variable.	Effective therapy and avoidance of severe attacks are associated with good pregnancy outcome. Medications used are well tolerated in pregnancy and appear to be safe for fetus. Breast-feeding is safe for newborn and may reduce risk for allergies.	Early use of antiinflammatory agents such as inhaled corticosteroids may prevent severe attacks. Inhaled cromolyn sodium and nedocromil sodium are effective but require more time to become effective than inhaled corticosteroids. Bronchodilators such as theophylline and inhaled beta-agonists may be required.
Glucose-6-Phosphate Dehydrogenase Deficiency Female-linked genetic disorder that predisposes to lysis of red blood cells when exposed to oxidizing drugs (salicylates, acetaminophen, phenacetin, and some sulfa drugs) and ingestion of fava beans in some people.	Is not affected by pregnancy unless complicated by anemia. Iron and folic acid supplementation is recommended. Newborn males have a higher incidence of severe jaundice.	Advise patient of risks and suggest she consult with her health care provider for recommended list of drugs for minor discomforts.
Hyperthyroidism An overactive, enlarged thyroid gland that is difficult to diagnose and manage during pregnancy because normal changes of pregnancy increase metabolic rate and mimic hyperthyroidism. Graves' disease is most common cause during pregnancy. Treatment ideally begins before pregnancy.	Increased incidence of hypertension such as preeclampsia and postpartum hemorrhage if not well controlled during pregnancy. Treatment is complicated by presence of fetus, which may be jeopardized by surgery or antithyroid medications. Propylthiouracil (PTU) has limited placental transfer and is widely used during pregnancy to control thyroid function. Additional drugs such as iodides and beta-blockers may be needed, particularly in a thyroid crisis.	Be aware of major signs that should be reported. These include resting pulse rate >100 bpm, loss of weight or failure to gain weight in spite of normal intake of food, heat intolerance, and abnormal protrusion of eyes (exophthalmos).
Hypothyroidism Characterized by inadequate thyroid secretion; confirmed by an elevated level of thyroid-stimulating hormone and low levels of triiodothyronine and thyroxine.	Women with hypothyroidism have a higher incidence of preeclampsia, abruptio placentae, and low-birth-weight, preterm, or stillborn infants. If woman is untreated, there is an increased risk for neonatal goiter and congenital hypothyroidism; severity of symptoms depends on time of onset and severity of hormonal deprivation but may include neurologic deficits. Treatment is with levothyroxine.	State screening for congenital hypothyroidism is required. Signs of congenital hypothyroidism may include skin mottling, a large tongue, hypotonia, depressed reflexes, and abdominal distention.
Maternal Phenylketonuria (PKU) Inherited autosomal recessive defect leading to inability to metabolize essential amino acid phenylalanine, resulting in high serum levels of phenylalanine. Irreparable intellectual disability occurs if pregnant woman is not treated early with a diet that provides adequate protein but restricts phenylalanine.	Woman must have low-phenylalanine diet before conception and pregnancy. If not, fetal risk for microcephaly, intellectual disability, heart defects, and intrauterine growth restriction increases.	Child either will be a carrier of the gene or will inherit the disease, depending on the presence of the gene in the father of the child. Special low-phenylalanine foods are expensive, but they may be obtained through the state's Supplemental Nutrition Program for Women, Infants, and Children (WIC) or Medicaid or may be covered by private insurance.

of SLE or disorders such as preeclampsia are more likely to occur during pregnancy and early postpartum (Carpenter & Branch, 2017).

SLE is associated with increased incidences of spontaneous abortion and fetal death during the first trimester. After the first trimester, the prognosis for a live birth is higher if no active disease exists. Newborn risks include preterm birth, often resulting from preterm rupture of the membranes, and growth restriction. The most serious potential complication for the neonate is a congenital heart block, which usually is permanent and will require a pacemaker (Carpenter & Branch, 2017).

Antiphospholipid Syndrome

Antiphospholipid syndrome (APS) is an autoimmune condition characterized by the production of antiphospholipid antibodies combined with certain clinical features. Specific clinical features include thrombosis confirmed by imaging or pathologic studies, abnormal and recurrent pregnancy outcomes, and elevated anticardiolipin antibody or presence of lupus anticoagulant. Pregnancy problems may include the following:

- One or more unexplained fetal deaths at or after 10 weeks of gestation
- One or more preterm births of a normal infant at or before 34 weeks of gestation that is related to severe preeclampsia or severe placental insufficiency
- Three or more unexplained recurrent spontaneous abortions before 10 weeks of gestation

Although the syndrome occurs most often in women with other underlying autoimmune diseases such as SLE, it also is diagnosed in women with no other recognizable autoimmune disease.

Women with APS should be informed about potential maternal and obstetric problems, including a possible risk for stroke. They should be assessed for evidence of anemia, thrombocytopenia, and underlying renal disease. Some physicians believe that treatment with heparin may be warranted on the basis of increased risk for thrombosis, even in women with no previous clotting problems. Combinations of low-dose aspirin and prophylactic heparin or enoxaparin are recommended for pregnant women with APS (Carpenter & Branch, 2017).

Hashimoto's Thyroiditis

Hashimoto's thyroiditis, characterized by antithyroid antibodies, causes most cases of hypothyroidism in women. Hypothyroidism in pregnancy increases risk for miscarriage, preterm birth, and preeclampsia. Maternal hypothyroidism during pregnancy can adversely affect the child's mental development. Thyroid-stimulating hormone (TSH) level should be tested before or in early pregnancy and hypothyroidism corrected with levothyroxine (ACOG, 2013b; Mestman, 2017).

Rheumatoid Arthritis

Rheumatoid arthritis (RA) is a chronic inflammatory disease that usually affects the synovial (hinged) joints. Although the cause is unknown, an autoimmune mechanism is suspected.

Marked improvement in symptoms of RA often occurs during pregnancy. The exact reason is unclear, but improvement is reported to parallel the rise in pregnancy-specific protein, which suppresses inflammatory reactions. Hormonal factors also have been suggested. For instance, increased levels of cortisol, estrogen, and progesterone may be beneficial in suppressing the immune response. Rheumatoid joints may become unstable in late pregnancy with the natural joint relaxation and changes in weight distribution. Unfortunately, a relapse (postpartum flare) occurs within 36 months after birth (Carpenter & Branch, 2017).

In contrast to SLE, the risk for abortion does not increase markedly in women with RA (Carpenter & Branch, 2017). Usually, obstetric problems do not occur at delivery unless the hips or cervical spine are significantly deteriorated.

Neurologic Disorders
Seizure Disorders

Seizures are the most common form of epilepsy, which is a recurrent disorder of cerebral function. Epilepsy occurs in about 1.8% of the general population (CDC, 2016a). Seizure control is the goal of treatment (Cunningham et al., 2014).

The effect of pregnancy on the course of epilepsy is variable and unpredictable. The frequency of seizures may increase, decrease, or remain the same. In general, the longer the woman has been seizure free before pregnancy, the less likely is the occurrence of seizures during pregnancy. Those with partial (focal) seizures are more likely to experience increased frequency. Vomiting, reduced gastric motility, use of gastrointestinal medications, and weight gain affect the absorption and distribution of anticonvulsant drugs. Serum levels of anticonvulsants may rise, fall, or remain the same during pregnancy.

Women with epilepsy have a higher than normal incidence of stillbirth, and some studies have shown a higher incidence of preterm labor. Maternal bleeding may occur because of a deficiency of clotting factors associated with anticonvulsant drugs such as hydantoins (Dilantin) and phenobarbital. Anticonvulsant drugs also compete with folate for absorption, which may result in folate deficiency. Most anticonvulsants are classified as pregnancy category C or D. Interactions between anticonvulsant drugs and other medications should be considered by the physician and pharmacist because dose changes or selection of valid alternative drugs may be needed. Effects of anticonvulsants and over-the-counter drugs should be considered as well.

A major concern is the teratogenic effects of anticonvulsant drugs. A specific syndrome known as *fetal hydantoin syndrome,* which includes craniofacial abnormalities, limb reduction defects, growth restriction, intellectual disability, and cardiac anomalies, has been described. Other anticonvulsants such as trimethadione, paramethadione, and carbamazepine also are associated with malformation syndromes. The teratogenic effects of phenobarbital are difficult to assess because it often is combined with other drugs. Newer anticonvulsants such as levetiracetam have fewer accumulated data related to fetal effects.

Health care professionals should recommend that the woman consult a neurologist before conception. The goal of treatment is to prevent generalized (formerly called *grand mal*) seizures and also reduce the adverse effects of anticonvulsant medications on the fetus. The family should be made aware of the risks involved when anticonvulsant drugs must be used. The woman and her family also should realize that treatment cannot be stopped during pregnancy unless the woman has been seizure free for a prolonged time and *stopped only at the directive of her physicians*. Generalized seizures result in fetal hypoxia and acidosis and therefore pose a serious problem for the fetus.

Bell's Palsy

Bell's palsy is a sudden unilateral neuropathy of the seventh cranial (facial) nerve that causes facial paralysis with weakness of the forehead and lower face. No cause for the neuropathy is often identified, although inflammation or viral infection of the facial nerve are possible causes. It is three times more common during pregnancy and generally occurs in the third trimester. Although the reason for the increase during pregnancy is unknown, one theory suggests that estrogen-induced edema causes pressure on the facial nerve, making the pregnant woman more vulnerable to the condition. The effect of pregnancy on the prognosis for Bell's palsy is unclear (Cunningham et al., 2014).

The face feels stiff and pulled to one side. Closing the eye on the affected side may be difficult or impossible. Difficulty with eating or fine facial movements may occur. The ability to taste also may be disturbed.

Treatment is controversial. Some physicians prescribe steroids within the first few days. Supportive care includes applying a patch over the eye and applying ointment or eye drops to prevent dryness or injury to the exposed cornea. Facial massage may be helpful, and the woman should be cautioned to chew carefully, because she could easily bite the inside of her mouth or her tongue. Psychological support is necessary to assist the woman and her family deal with the anxiety they naturally feel when sudden paralysis of the face occurs. They should be reassured that the condition is temporary in the majority of women who have Bell's palsy.

> **? KNOWLEDGE CHECK**
>
> 48. What are the maternal and fetal effects of SLE?
> 49. In what ways does pregnancy affect RA?
> 50. How can Hashimoto's thyroiditis affect the newborn?
> 51. What is the major concern about administering anticonvulsant drugs for the pregnant woman with epilepsy?
> 52. What is the recommended supportive care for pregnant women with Bell's palsy?

INFECTIONS DURING PREGNANCY

Some infections acquired during pregnancy can adversely affect the health of the fetus, the mother, or both. Some infections are mild or even subclinical in the mother and yet may cause severe birth defects or death of the fetus. Other infections may have adverse effects by increasing the risk for other pregnancy complications such as preterm labor. Some infections are transmitted primarily or exclusively by sexual means, whereas others may be transmitted not only in this way but also by other avenues.

The wide variety of infections affecting pregnancy care are divided into those caused by viruses and those caused by other organisms. Table 10.9 presents nursing considerations related to major STDs and vaginal infections. Table 10.9 also summarizes UTIs and their effects on pregnancy.

TABLE 10.9   Sexually Transmitted Diseases and Urinary Tract and Vaginal Infections
Impact on Pregnancy

Maternal, Fetal, and Neonatal Effects	Nursing Considerations
Sexually Transmitted Diseases (STDs)	
Syphilis (Causative Organism: Spirochete Treponema pallidum)	
If untreated, infection may cross placenta to fetus and result in spontaneous abortion, stillborn infant, premature labor and birth, or congenital syphilis. Major signs of congenital syphilis are enlarged liver and spleen, skin lesions, rashes, osteitis, pneumonia, and hepatitis.	Benzathine penicillin G is primary treatment to cure disease in both woman and fetus. Women who are allergic are desensitized and then treated.
Gonorrhea (Causative Organism: Bacterium Neisseria gonorrhoeae)	
Not transmitted via placenta; vertical transmission from mother to newborn during birth may cause ophthalmia neonatorum. Endocervicitis and weakness of fetal membranes increase risk for premature rupture of membranes and preterm labor. *Chlamydia* infection is likely to accompany gonorrhea infection.	Cephalosporins such as ceftriaxone (pregnancy category B) are recommended for gonorrhea during pregnancy. Because 20%-50% of women with gonorrhea also have chlamydial infection, azithromycin or amoxicillin (pregnancy category B) is recommended to accompany gonorrhea treatment. Partner also should be treated to prevent reinfection. Infants are treated with an ophthalmic antibiotic such as ceftriaxone at birth to prevent ophthalmia neonatorum. Tetracycline should not be used in a pregnant woman for chlamydial infection that often accompanies gonorrhea.

TABLE 10.9 Sexually Transmitted Diseases and Urinary Tract and Vaginal Infections—cont'd

Impact on Pregnancy

Maternal, Fetal, and Neonatal Effects	Nursing Considerations
Chlamydial Infection (Causative Organism: Bacterium Chlamydia trachomatis)	
Chlamydial infection is most common STDs in United States and often accompanies gonorrhea. Fetus may be infected during birth and suffer neonatal conjunctivitis or pneumonitis. Conjunctivitis is prevented by erythromycin ophthalmic ointment. *Chlamydia* may be responsible for premature rupture of membranes, premature labor, and chorioamnionitis.	Education is particularly important because infection is usually asymptomatic. Both partners should be treated to prevent recurrent infection. As with all STDs, use of condoms decreases risk for infection. Azithromycin or amoxicillin is recommended treatment during pregnancy. Tetracycline should not be used during pregnancy.
Trichomoniasis (Causative Organism: Protozoan Trichomonas vaginalis)	
Common cause of vaginitis in 10%-50% of pregnant women. Associated with premature rupture of membranes and postpartum endometritis.	Metronidazole (Flagyl), pregnancy category B, may be given to pregnant woman as 2-g single oral dose. Should withhold breastfeeding during treatment and 12-24 hr after last dose. Consistent association between fetal abnormalities or injury and metronidazole use has not been upheld.
Condyloma Acuminatum (Causative Organism: Human Papillomavirus [HPV])	
Transmission of condyloma acuminatum, also called venereal or genital warts, may occur during vaginal birth and is associated with development of epithelial tumors of mucous membranes of larynx in children. Pregnancy can cause proliferation of lesions, which are associated with cervical dysplasia and cancer.	Common choices for nonpregnant therapy (podophyllin, podofilox, imiquimod) are not recommended during pregnancy. Excision of maternal lesions by cryotherapy or cautery may be done. HPV vaccine is available in a three-dose series to protect against four strains of virus that are major causes of cervical cancer and genital warts. Routine immunization of girls should start at 11-12 yr but can start as young as 9 yr. Catch-up immunization is recommended for girls and women 13-26 yr to prevent infection with these four specific types of HPV. Immunization will not prevent disease if woman is already infected. Quadrivalent vaccine also can be used for males 9-26 yr. See www.cdc.gov/vaccines for current information.
Vaginal Infections	
Candidiasis (Causative Organism: Yeast Candida albicans)	
Oral candidiasis (thrush) may develop in newborns if maternal vaginal infection is present at birth. Thrush is treated with application of nystatin (Mycostatin) over surfaces of oral cavity four times a day for several days. Characteristic "cottage cheese" vaginal discharge with vulvar pruritus, burning, and dyspareunia. Vulva may be red, tender, and edematous.	*C. albicans* is part of the normal vaginal flora but may become pathogenic if the yeast becomes excessive. Candidiasis (sometimes called *Monilial vaginitis*) is a persistent problem for many women during pregnancy. Examples of maternal treatment choices include topical nystatin, miconazole, clotrimazole, butoconazole terconazole, and tioconazole.
Bacterial Vaginosis (Causative Organism: Gardnerella vaginalis)	
Adverse pregnancy outcomes include preterm rupture of membranes, preterm labor and birth, intraamniotic infection, and postpartum endometritis. Marked by a major shift in vaginal flora from normal predominance of lactobacilli to predominance of anaerobic bacteria. Causes profuse, malodorous, "fishy" vaginal discharge, itching, and burning. "Clue cells" may be seen microscopically in a wet mount preparation of vaginal secretions.	Metronidazole vaginal application or clindamycin oral therapy for 7 days is recommended during pregnancy. Clinical trials have shown that women at high risk for preterm birth may benefit from this medication regimen.
Urinary Tract Infections	
Asymptomatic Bacteriuria (Causative Organisms: Escherichia coli, Klebsiella, Proteus)	
Ascending bacterial infection can result in cystitis or pyelonephritis in later pregnancy if condition remains untreated.	Recovery of a urinary pathogen from a midstream, clean-catch urine specimen is defined as 100,000 colony-forming units (CFUs) per mL of urine. Rapid, less-expensive office tests to identify infection also may be used. Treatment for asymptomatic bacteriuria may include treatment for pathogens that also cause symptomatic cystitis.

Continued

TABLE 10.9   Sexually Transmitted Diseases and Urinary Tract and Vaginal Infections—cont'd

Impact on Pregnancy

Maternal, Fetal, and Neonatal Effects	Nursing Considerations
Cystitis (Causative Organisms: E. coli, Klebsiella, Proteus)	
Signs and symptoms include dysuria, frequency, urgency, and suprapubic tenderness. Ascending infection may lead to pyelonephritis.	Antibiotics used for both asymptomatic bacteriuria and cystitis may include amoxicillin, ampicillin, trimethoprim-sulfamethoxazole, nitrofurantoin, or a third-generation cephalosporin such as ceftriaxone. Emphasize importance of reporting signs of urinary tract infection. Stress importance of taking all medication prescribed in the 7-day course even if symptoms abate. Provide information about hygiene measures such as front-to-back perineal care after urination or bowel movements.
Acute Pyelonephritis (Causative Organisms: E. coli, Klebsiella, Proteus)	
Increased risk for preterm labor and premature delivery. Maternal complications include a high fever, flank pain, septic shock, and adult respiratory distress syndrome. Pregnant women often require hospitalization for acute care.	Inform women with asymptomatic bacteriuria or cystitis of signs and symptoms, such as sudden onset of fever (often higher than 102.2°F [39°C]), chills, flank pain or tenderness, nausea, and vomiting, so that treatment can begin promptly. Skin cooling equipment may be used to lower her temperature below 100.4°F (38°C), reducing possible compromise of fetal oxygen level. Woman may be hospitalized for intravenous administration of antibiotics. Common combinations include ampicillin or a cephalosporin plus an aminoglycoside. Serum levels of aminoglycosides are often measured to ensure an adequate dose without reaching a toxic level.

Data from Centers for Disease Control and Prevention. (2016). *MMWR Morbidity and Mortality Weekly Report, 59*(RR-12). Retrieved from www.cdc.gov/mmwr; and Duff, P. & Birsner, M (2017). Maternal and perinatal infection: Bacterial. In S. G. Gabbe, J. R. Niebyl, J. L. Simpson, M.B. Landon, H.L. Galan, R. M. Jauniaux, D.A. Driscoll, et al. (Eds.), *Obstetrics: Normal and problem pregnancies* (7th ed., pp. 1130–1146). Philadelphia, PA: Saunders.

Viral Infections

Pregnancy does not worsen the effects of most viral infections. Although viral infections may be mild or even asymptomatic in mothers, fetal and neonatal consequences can be catastrophic. Maternal infections with cytomegalovirus (CMV), rubella, varicella-zoster virus, herpes simplex, hepatitis B, and HIV have the greatest potential for causing harm to the fetus or newborn.

Cytomegalovirus

CMV, a member of the herpes virus group, is widespread and eventually infects most humans. CMV has been isolated from urine, saliva, blood, cervical mucus, semen, breast milk, and stool. Transmission may occur from contamination with any of these fluids, although close personal contact is required. CMV infection during pregnancy may be primary or recurrent. Symptoms of CMV infection are so vague that a woman is often unaware that she has an infection.

Daycare centers are a common place for transmission of CMV among children, especially toddlers, because they often share objects contaminated with saliva. Mothers and caregivers of young children who attend a daycare center should be aware that a child might acquire an infection in the center and transmit it to those who are at risk for a primary infection (Bernstein, 2017). As puberty approaches, behaviors such as kissing, sexual intercourse, and other close bodily contacts again increase the possibility that CMV infection will be transmitted to a female who may be pregnant (Cunningham et al., 2014).

After primary infection the virus becomes latent, but like other herpes virus infections, periodic reactivation and shedding of the virus may occur. Primary infection is more likely to cross the placenta, infecting the fetus, than is a reactivation infection. **Seroconversion** (change in blood test from negative to positive indicating development of antibodies in response to infection or immunization) and a rise in the specific IgM antibody titer may not differentiate a primary and recurrent infection. Specific CMV IgG avidity testing may be useful for this purpose (Cunningham et al., 2014). Most infections are asymptomatic, so they may not be suspected during pregnancy, and testing may not be done. Diagnosis of neonatal infection is by urine culture.

Fetal and Neonatal Effects. Approximately 5% to 10% of newborns infected with CMV show signs of congenital infection at birth, which may include intracranial calcifications, growth restriction, chorioretinitis, microcephaly, intellectual and physical disability, sensorineural deficits, hepatosplenomegaly, jaundice, hemolytic anemia, and thrombocytopenic purpura (Cunningham et al., 2014). Some infants who are asymptomatic at birth will develop late-onset signs such as neurologic deficits, learning disabilities, chorioretinitis, psychomotor disabilities, and hearing loss (Cunningham et al., 2014).

Therapeutic Management. No effective therapy is currently available for the treatment of congenital CMV infection. Ultrasound scanning may identify manifestations of the infection, such as cranial abnormalities or growth restriction. Antiviral agents such as ganciclovir and foscarnet may be used for severe infections, but these drugs are toxic and only temporarily suppress the shedding of the virus. Primary prevention—by emphasizing good hygiene and handwashing (especially to women who care for small children)—is the best way to prevent congenital CMV infections (Bernstein, 2017; Cunningham et al., 2014).

Rubella

Rubella is caused by a virus transmitted from person to person through droplets or through direct contact with articles contaminated by nasopharyngeal secretions. Rubella infection after birth is a mild disease, but congenital rubella could have severe consequences for the newborn. Common rubella signs and symptoms include fever, general malaise, and a characteristic maculopapular rash that begins on the face and migrates over the body. Fewer than 10% of pregnant women are not immune, because infection confers permanent immunity. The overall incidence of rubella has declined since the vaccine became available in 1969, although many young adults remain at risk. The decline in adult rubella has virtually eliminated congenital rubella. Most U.S. cases of congenital rubella occur in foreign-born mothers, although there have been periodic rubella outbreaks in the United States (Bernstein, 2017).

Fetal and Neonatal Effects. Rubella virus from the mother can cross the placental barrier and infect the fetus at any time during pregnancy. The greatest risk to the fetus is during the first trimester, when fetal organs are developing. If maternal infection occurs during this time, approximately one third of these cases will result in spontaneous abortions, and surviving fetuses may be seriously compromised. Deafness, developmental delay, cataracts, cardiac defects, IUGR, and microcephaly are the most common fetal complications. In addition, infants born to mothers who had rubella during pregnancy shed the virus for many months and therefore pose a threat to other infants and susceptible adults who come in contact with them. As pregnancy progresses, the risk for congenital rubella decreases (Bernstein, 2017; Duff, 2014).

Therapeutic Management. Prevention is the only effective protection for the fetus. Women who are immune do not become infected, so determining the immune status of all women of childbearing age is critical.

A rubella titer of 1:8 or greater provides evidence of immunity. Women who are not immune should be vaccinated before they become pregnant, and they should be advised not to become pregnant for 28 days after vaccination because of the possible risk to the fetus from the live-virus vaccine, although the actual risk appears to be low. Many nonimmune women are vaccinated during the postpartum period so they will be immune before becoming pregnant again. In most facilities, women of childbearing age must read and sign a document indicating they understand the risks to the fetus if they become pregnant within 28 days.

Varicella-Zoster Virus

Varicella infection (chickenpox) is caused by varicella-zoster virus (VZV), a herpes virus transmitted by direct contact or through the respiratory tract. Over 90% of people will have varicella infection before reaching reproductive age. After the primary varicella infection, the virus can become latent in the nerve ganglia. If VZV is reactivated, herpes zoster (shingles) results. Maternal complications of acute varicella infection may include preterm labor, encephalitis, and varicella pneumonia, which is the most serious complication associated with VZV. Varicella immunization has resulted in a marked decrease in children's varicella, well before they reach the reproductive age.

Fetal and Neonatal Effects. Fetal and neonatal effects depend on the time of maternal infection. If the infection occurs during the first trimester, the fetus has a small risk for congenital varicella syndrome (0.4%). The greatest risk for development of congenital varicella syndrome occurs during 13 to 20 weeks of gestation (2% of births). Clinical findings include limb hypoplasia, cutaneous scars, chorioretinitis, cataracts, microcephaly, and IUGR.

The infant who is infected during the perinatal period (5 days before through 2 days after birth) will not have the benefit of maternal antibodies. Four days before birth is not sufficient time for the mother to develop antibodies to VZV and pass them to the fetus. Varicella infection occurring in the fetus or infant just before or after birth would not be inactivated by antibodies, which leaves the infant at risk for life-threatening neonatal varicella infection. Varicella-zoster immune globulin (VZIG) is indicated for the infant infected perinatally. Infants born earlier than 28 weeks or who weigh 1000 g or less are given VZIG because maternal antibodies to VZV earlier in pregnancy have not yet crossed the placenta, reducing natural passive immunity (CDC, 2013).

Therapeutic Management. Immune testing may be recommended for pregnant women who are presumed to be susceptible. VZIG should be administered to women who have been exposed and whose fetuses are at high risk for congenital varicella syndrome, although this may not prevent primary infection. Women infected with varicella during pregnancy should be instructed to report pulmonary symptoms immediately. Hospitalization, fetal surveillance, full respiratory support, and hemodynamic monitoring should be available for women diagnosed with varicella-zoster pneumonia because it may become severe in a short time. Acyclovir is the primary drug used to treat varicella quickly.

For infants born to mothers infected with varicella during the perinatal period, immunization with VZIG as soon as possible but within 96 hours of birth provides passive immunity against varicella. Women and infants with varicella are highly contagious and should be placed in airborne and contact isolation. Only staff members known to be immune to varicella should come in contact with these clients.

Adult immunization with the live attenuated varicella vaccine (Varivax) is recommended for nonpregnant adults who have no evidence of having had varicella. A pregnant woman should not be immunized, but members of her household may be immunized because the vaccine is not transmissible from one person to another. A nonimmune postpartum woman should receive the vaccine before discharge and her second dose 4 to 8 weeks postpartum. She should be instructed to avoid pregnancy for 1 month after each of the two injections. Nonimmune health care workers should be immunized (Bernstein, 2017; CDC, 2016b).

Herpes Simplex Virus

Genital herpes is one of the most common STDs in the herpes simplex virus (HSV) group. It may be caused by HSV type 1 or 2. Most infections of genital herpes are caused by type 2. Type 1, which is more common in the mouth and upper body, also may infect the genital area. HSV infection occurs as a result of direct contact of the skin or mucous membrane with an active lesion. Lesions form at the site of contact and begin as a group of painful papules that progress rapidly to become vesicles, shallow ulcers, pustules, and crusts. The infected person sheds the virus until the lesions are healed. The virus then migrates along the sensory nerves to reside in the sensory ganglion, and the disease enters a latent phase. It can be reactivated later as a recurrent infection. Many women infected with HSV do not have signs and symptoms of infection and thus may shed the virus unknowingly (Bernstein, 2017).

Vertical transmission (from mother to infant) generally occurs in one of two ways: (1) after rupture of membranes, when the virus ascends from active lesions; or (2) during birth, when the fetus comes in contact with infectious genital secretions or when the fetal skin is punctured, such as with a fetal scalp electrode.

Diagnosis usually is based on clinical signs and symptoms. Definitive diagnosis requires culture of the virus from an active lesion, and results may take as long as 5 days. Newer tests based on genetic analysis (polymerase chain reaction [PCR]) are becoming common for detection of HSV and other infections.

Fetal and Neonatal Effects. Complications of pregnancy from a recurrent infection are rare. However, if primary infection occurs during pregnancy, the rates of spontaneous abortions, IUGR, and preterm labor increase. Neonatal herpes infection is uncommon but potentially devastating. The neonate may have infection limited to skin lesions or systemic (disseminated) infection. Symptoms usually appear within the first week, and the disease progresses rapidly. The likelihood of death or serious sequelae in infants who have systemic herpes infection is approximately 50%. The risk for neonatal infection is greatest if the mother has a primary (rather than recurrent) infection during the perinatal period. This is most likely because the amount of virus shed is higher during a primary infection than during subsequent ones (Bernstein, 2017).

Therapeutic Management. No known cure for herpes infection exists, although antiviral chemotherapy (acyclovir) is prescribed to reduce symptoms and shorten the duration of the lesions. Acyclovir may be given during late pregnancy to a woman with a recurrent outbreak to reduce the possibility of having active lesions at the time of birth.

For women with a history of genital herpes, vaginal birth is allowed if there are no genital lesions at the time of labor. Cesarean birth is recommended for women with active lesions in the genital area, whether recurrent or primary, at the time of labor. Use of fetal scalp electrodes, which cause a break in the skin, is acceptable when clinically indicated if there are no active lesions in the mother (ACOG, 2016c).

Expectant mothers need information about effective ways to deal with the emotional and physical effects of herpes. Many women are concerned about privacy and do not want family members to know why cesarean birth is necessary. These women should be assured that their wishes will be respected. Women may need an opportunity to discuss their feelings of shame, anger, or anxiety about the possible effects of the virus on their infant.

After delivery, isolation of the mother from her infant is not necessary if direct contact with lesions is avoided and mothers use careful handwashing techniques. Mothers may breastfeed if there are no lesions on the breasts. The infant is observed for signs of infection, including temperature instability, lethargy, poor sucking reflex, jaundice, seizures, and herpetic lesions. Acyclovir therapy is prescribed for neonatal infection (Pammi, Brand, & Weisman, 2016).

> ### ? KNOWLEDGE CHECK
>
> 53. What are the fetal and neonatal effects of CMV infection?
> 54. Why is rubella infection most dangerous in the first trimester?
> 55. How can rubella be prevented?
> 56. How are infants born to mothers with varicella treated?
> 57. How does vertical transmission of the herpesvirus occur?

Parvovirus B19

Erythema infectiosum (also called *fifth disease*), caused by human parvovirus B19, is an acute, communicable disease characterized by a highly distinctive rash. The rash starts on the face with a "slapped-cheeks" appearance, followed by a generalized maculopapular rash. Other symptoms include fever, malaise, and joint pain. Erythema infectiosum is most contagious before the rash is evident. The infection is more common among children and often occurs in community epidemics. The prognosis is usually excellent. However, if the disease occurs in pregnancy, potential fetal and neonatal effects exist. Parvovirus titers can be done if exposure during pregnancy is suspected to determine whether the mother is immune. PCR analysis of viral DNA is more sensitive than maternal antibodies, however (Bernstein, 2017).

Fetal and Neonatal Effects. When infection occurs during pregnancy, fetal death can result, usually from failure of fetal RBC production, followed by severe fetal anemia, hydrops (generalized edema), and heart failure. The level of maternal serum alpha-fetoprotein is sometimes elevated when fetal hydrops is present. Serial ultrasonography also can be performed to detect hydrops. Intrauterine transfusion is an option to treat severe fetal anemia if it does not resolve spontaneously. The risk to the fetus is greatest when the mother is infected in the first 20 weeks of pregnancy. The affected infant is examined for any defect, and the child is assessed regularly for several years to identify delayed complications such as persistent infection because of low levels of viral replication.

Therapeutic Management. No specific treatment exists. Starch baths may help reduce pruritus, and analgesics may be necessary to relieve mild joint pain.

Hepatitis B

Multiple serotypes of hepatitis are recognized, but three are common in the United States: A, B, and C. Other serotypes such as D, E, and G require the presence of other hepatitis viruses to exist. Hepatitis A is transmitted primarily by fecal-oral contamination and can be limited by simple hygiene. Hepatitis A is rarely transmitted perinatally, and supportive care is usually sufficient.

Hepatitis B is transmitted via blood, saliva, vaginal secretions, semen, or breast milk and readily crosses the placenta. Mortality associated with acute hepatitis B is about 1%, but about 85% to 90% of adults recover. Chronic hepatitis B develops in 10% of infected adults, who can continue to transmit the disease to others. Persons with chronic hepatitis B also are at greater risk for chronic liver disease, cirrhosis of the liver, and primary hepatocellular carcinoma (ACOG, 2016g; Bernstein, 2017). Hepatitis B is preventable with a vaccine, which is safe during pregnancy. Newborn vaccination against hepatitis B starts before discharge, with the second dose given 1 to 2 months later and the third dose given at 6 to 18 months.

The incidence of hepatitis B virus (HBV) has fallen significantly with screening and immunization of at-risk people, including health care providers. Goals to eliminate HBV in the United States include the following:

- Universal newborn vaccination
- Routine screening of all pregnant women and provision of immunoprophylaxis to infants born to infected mothers or women with unknown infection status
- Routine vaccination to unvaccinated children and adolescents

Vaccination of adults at increased risk for infection, including health care workers, those with STDs, household contacts or sexual partners of those having chronic HBV infection, multiple sex partners, recipients of certain blood products, and dialysis patients

Hepatitis C is acquired through blood products. Those at higher risk include IV drug users; those with recurrent STDs, including HIV; and persons needing recurrent blood products (such as hemophiliacs). Hepatitis C may remain undiagnosed until the woman develops chronic liver disease that often requires liver transplantation. The incidence of hepatitis C in pregnant women of childbearing age is approximately 1% (ACOG, 2016g; Bernstein, 2017).

Fetal and Neonatal Effects. The risk for prematurity, low birth weight, and neonatal death increases when the mother has HBV infection during pregnancy. Infection of the newborn whose mother is known to be HBsAg-positive usually can be prevented by administration of hepatitis B immune globulin (HBIG, Hep-B-Gammagee), followed by hepatitis B vaccine (Recombivax HB, Engerix-B) within 12 hours of birth. The newborn should be carefully bathed before any injections are given to prevent infections from skin surface contamination by the virus. The infant's vaccination should be repeated at 1 to 2 months and 6 to 18 months. Breastfeeding is considered safe as long as the newborn has received HBIG and the hepatitis B vaccine (ACOG, 2016g).

Therapeutic Management. Hepatitis B is a preventable infection. Simple hygiene measures such as safe sex and the use of standard precautions with bodily fluids provide primary prevention. Hepatitis B vaccines are available as a series of three intramuscular injections into the deltoid for adults, with the second and third doses given 1 and 6 months after the first. Vaccination is recommended for any population at risk, including nurses and other health care workers who frequently come in contact with body fluids.

All pregnant women should be screened for HBsAg. Women at high risk for hepatitis should be rescreened in the third trimester if the initial screen is negative. Household members and sexual contacts should be tested and offered vaccination if they are not immune. No specific treatment exists for acute HBV infection. Recommended supportive treatment includes bed rest and a high-protein, low-fat diet.

Human Immunodeficiency Virus

Acquired immunodeficiency syndrome (AIDS) is a failure in immune function caused by the retrovirus HIV. The infected person develops opportunistic infections or malignancies that ultimately are fatal. Transmission of HIV infection is predominantly through three modes: (1) sexual exposure to genital secretions of an infected person, (2) parenteral exposure to infected blood or tissue, and (3) perinatal exposure of an infant to infected maternal secretions through birth (vertical transmission). The continuing occurrence of HIV infections of infants demonstrates the importance of identifying and treating maternal infections during pregnancy to reduce the risks for infant infections. Breastfeeding is contraindicated for HIV positive women (AAP & ACOG, 2012: U.S. Department of Health and Human Services [DHHS], Panel on Treatment of HIV-Infected Pregnant Women and Prevention of Perinatal Transmission, 2013).

After rapid increase in the number of cases of HIV infections during the early years of the epidemic in the United States, deaths from AIDS have declined with improved antiretroviral therapies. New cases of HIV in heterosexual women in the United States in 2015 were estimated to be 4,524 among Black women, 1,131 among Hispanic women, and 1,431 among White women. (CDC, 2017a).

CRITICAL TO REMEMBER
Facts about Human Immunodeficiency Virus

- HIV is transmitted by sexual contact with an infected person, by contact with infected body fluids, and through the placenta from mother to fetus.
- During the initial phase of HIV, the person may be unaware of the infection, yet highly infectious.
- There is a latent period, averaging 10 years, from HIV infection to development of acquired immunodeficiency syndrome (AIDS), corresponding to the type of treatment received.
- A person infected by HIV can pass the virus to another person, even if he or she does not have symptoms.
- There is not yet a cure for the HIV infection or AIDS. Antiretroviral medications are available to slow the replication of the virus and delay the onset of opportunistic diseases.
- Antiretroviral treatment should be part of the medication regimen for a pregnant woman to reduce the risk for transmission to her fetus. The newborn also should receive antiretroviral treatment after birth.

Pathophysiology. Like other retroviruses, HIV integrates its viral genetic makeup into the genetic makeup of the cell when infecting it. This results in an abnormal cell that cannot perform its functions properly. At the same time, this cell replicates and produces more viruses that invade more cells. The disease worsens as more cells cease to function, and a greater number of viruses are produced. The principal mechanism by which HIV leads to immunodeficiency is through its destructive effect on cells that provide and regulate immunity. CD4 T lymphocytes, or helper T cells, play a key role in organizing the body's immune response to help immune functions. CD8 lymphocytes are T suppressor cells that limit excessive immune responses that might attack the person's own body tissues. When HIV infection invades body cells, the ratio of CD4 T lymphocytes to CD8 lymphocytes decreases. As the number of CD4 T lymphocytes declines, the immune response declines, and opportunistic infections can overwhelm the HIV-positive person. A CD4 T lymphocyte total count of less than 200 cells/ mm^3 or the development of opportunistic infections confirms the diagnosis of progression to AIDS (Bernstein, 2017; CDC, 2016h; Cunningham et al., 2014).

The clinical course of HIV infection follows fairly predictable stages:

- An early or acute stage occurs several weeks after HIV exposure (stage 1). Flulike symptoms may develop and last a few weeks.
- A middle or asymptomatic period of minor or no clinical problems follows (stage 2). This period is characterized by continuous low-level viral replication and CD4 cell loss.
- A late period of AIDS follows, which consists of opportunistic infections lasting months or years (stage 3).

During stages 1 and 2, the infected person is said to be HIV-positive. During stage 3 the immune system no longer offers adequate protection, and opportunistic diseases occur. The person is then said to have AIDS, regardless of the CD4 counts (Bernstein, 2017; CDC, 2016h).

Fetal and Neonatal Effects. Antiretroviral drugs have improved the prognosis for HIV-infected women and their infants. Mothers who receive no or minimal HIV care during the prenatal period may have higher rates of infected infants. Infant infection may occur during pregnancy, during labor and birth, or after birth if the infant is breastfed (Bernstein, 2017; DHHS Panel on Treatment of HIV-Infected Pregnant Women and Prevention of Perinatal Transmission, 2013).

Infant tests to diagnose HIV may include PCR for viral DNA and viral culture in addition to standard antibody tests. However, infant HIV tests can remain positive for up to 18 months after birth because of passive maternal antibodies. An infected newborn is typically asymptomatic at birth, but signs and symptoms may become obvious during the first year of life (Pammi et al., 2016). Early signs may include enlargement of the liver and spleen, lymphadenopathy, failure to thrive, persistent thrush, and chronic or recurrent diarrhea. Infected infants often have bacterial infections such as meningitis, pneumonia, osteomyelitis, and septic arthritis (Pammi et al., 2016).

Prompt treatment of the HIV-infected infant with appropriate antiretroviral medications and other prophylactic therapy may slow the infection's progress.

Prevention. Prevention remains the only way to control HIV infection. Sexual transmission can be avoided by several methods. Abstinence would render a person safe from all STDs, including HIV. However, for many people, sexual expression adds to their quality of life and many are not willing to practice abstinence. Transmission of HIV also can be prevented if infected persons do not have vaginal intercourse with susceptible persons. If intercourse does occur, barrier methods such as latex condoms reduce contact with infectious secretions. A condom also offers protection from transmission through oral sex.

Intravenous drug users who refuse rehabilitative treatment should be taught to wash the equipment with water, soap, and bleach before each use to reduce transmission of the virus through a soiled needle.

Therapeutic Management. Multiple antiretroviral drugs from different classes are beneficial in extending life after infection and reducing the transmission rate to the infant. Guidelines for the latest treatments from the National Institutes of Health for pregnant as well as nonpregnant patients may be found at www.aidsinfo.nih.gov/guidelines. Maternal zidovudine (ZDV) therapy to reduce infant HIV infection should consider many situations, such as the following:

- Whether the mother has had any antiretroviral therapy during pregnancy, including ZDV, and when it began
- Whether the mother had any prenatal care and when she started
- Fetal gestational age
- If the membranes have ruptured, how long they have been ruptured

Nursing Considerations. Learning of HIV infection during pregnancy can have a devastating and immobilizing effect on the entire family. A nurse should be careful not to allow personal attitudes to influence professional behavior or the care of the woman and family during pregnancy, birth, and the postpartum period. Care of the woman with HIV during pregnancy can present many challenges to the nurse. Issues that arise during the postpartum period may include the following:

- Whether to continue or stop antiretroviral therapy
- Support services needed after discharge
- Contraceptive counseling, including the information that condoms can reduce the risk for acquiring or transmitting STDs and HIV transmission but have a low rate of effectiveness for contraception
- Comprehensive follow-up for infection indicators and associated medical conditions, counseling for a new diagnosis, and evaluation of the need for continued antiretroviral therapy

A patient problem of "Emotional distress due to multiple losses that include the mother's shortened life expectancy and possible death of the infant" should be considered. Initially, crisis intervention may be necessary to help the family cope.

Nurses frequently must determine what the family perceives as the most pressing needs and worries. Some of the most common fears are loss of control, loss of support and love, social isolation, and loss of privacy. The nurse's response may involve finding ways for the woman to retain control while she is physically able and assisting her to select those in her family who will provide continued love and emotional support. Reassuring the woman that her right to privacy will not be violated is necessary.

Nurses should help the woman maintain the highest possible level of wellness. Adequate, high-quality nutrition decreases the risk for opportunistic infections and promotes vitality. A daily regimen should include sufficient rest and activity. Avoiding large crowds, travel to areas with poor sanitation, and exposure to infected individuals is important. Meticulous skin care is essential.

The nurse should also provide information on routine ongoing health care for women. Examples are cervical cancer screening, adult immunizations, and mental health or substance abuse treatment. Instruction in signs and symptoms of postpartum depression and providing sources of assistance should be offered before discharge, just as for any woman in the postpartum period.

The mother almost certainly will experience a great deal of anxiety about whether her infant will be HIV-positive. Nurses need to respond honestly that testing will be required but that most infants do not contract the virus if the medication regimen is followed carefully. In addition, nurses should reinforce information about medications that slow the progression of the disease in the mother as well as decrease the incidence of vertical transmission to the infant.

KNOWLEDGE CHECK

58. What are the fetal and neonatal effects of parvovirus B19 infection?
59. How is HBV transmitted? How are newborns treated?
60. How can HIV infection be prevented?
61. What is the medical management for a pregnant woman with HIV infection?

Nonviral Infections
Toxoplasmosis

Toxoplasmosis is a protozoan infection caused by *Toxoplasma gondii.* Infection is transmitted through organisms in raw and undercooked meat, through contact with infected cat feces or soil, and across the placental barrier to the fetus if the expectant mother acquires the infection during pregnancy. Toxoplasmosis is more common in Europe because of greater consumption of meats that are rare or undercooked (Duff & Birsner, 2017). Poor handwashing and sanitation of surfaces after food preparation increases the risk for toxoplasmosis in any country.

Toxoplasmosis often is subclinical. The woman may experience a few days of fatigue, muscle pains, and swollen glands, but she may be unaware of the disease. If the infection is suspected, diagnosis can be confirmed by positive results of serologic tests, which include indirect fluorescent antibody tests for IgG and IgM. Immune-compromised persons such as patients who received transplants or those infected with HIV are more likely to have severe toxoplasmosis infection.

Fetal and Neonatal Effects. Although toxoplasmosis may remain unnoticed in the pregnant woman, it may cause abortion or result in the birth of an infant with the disease. Approximately 40% of infants born to mothers who had an acute primary infection during pregnancy have congenital toxoplasmosis. About 50% of affected infants may be asymptomatic at birth, but others have serious effects such as low birth weight, enlarged liver and spleen, jaundice, and anemia or coagulation disorders. Severe complications may develop several years after birth. Symptoms of congenital toxoplasmosis include chorioretinitis that may lead to blindness, seizures, hepatosplenomegaly and mental retardation (Duff & Birsner, 2017).

Therapeutic Management. All pregnant women should be advised to do the following:

- Cook meat, particularly pork, beef, and lamb, thoroughly until the juices run clear.
- Avoid touching the mucous membranes of your mouth and eyes while handling raw meat.
- Wash all surfaces that come in contact with uncooked meat.
- Wash your hands thoroughly after handling raw meat.
- Avoid uncooked eggs and unpasteurized milk.
- Wash fruits and vegetables before consumption.
- Avoid contact with materials that are possibly contaminated with cat feces (such as cat litter boxes, sandboxes, garden soil).

Maternal treatment of toxoplasmosis during pregnancy is essential to reduce the risk for congenital infection. Sulfonamides can be used alone but are less effective than combination therapy. Spiramycin is successfully used in Europe for maternal toxoplasmosis and may be used according to specific guidelines within the United States (Duff & Birsner, 2017).

Group B *Streptococcus* Infection

Group B *Streptococcus* (GBS) is a leading cause of life-threatening perinatal infections in the United States. The gram-positive bacterium colonizes the rectum, vagina, cervix, and urethra of pregnant as well as nonpregnant women. Approximately 20% to 25% of pregnant women are colonized by GBS in the vaginal or rectal area (Duff & Birsner, 2017), but isolating the organism is often possible only intermittently. Often, these women are asymptomatic, although symptomatic maternal infections can occur. These infections include UTIs, intrauterine infections, and metritis. Most women respond quickly to antimicrobial therapy (AAP & ACOG, 2012; CDC, 2016e; Duff & Birsner, 2017)

Fetal and Neonatal Effects. Early-onset newborn GBS disease occurs during the first week after birth, often within 48 hours. Women who have GBS in the rectovaginal area at the time of birth have a 60% chance of transmitting the organism to the newborn, and about 1% to 2% of these infants will develop early-onset GBS disease. Sepsis, pneumonia, and meningitis are the primary infections in early-onset GBS disease (AAP & ACOG, 2012). Late-onset GBS disease occurs after the first week of life, and meningitis, pneumonia, and bacteremia are the most common clinical manifestations (Duff & Birsner, 2017).

Therapeutic Management. Health care providers have difficulty identifying pregnant women who are asymptomatic GBS carriers because the duration of carrier status is unpredictable. Optimal identification of the GBS carrier status is obtained by vaginal and rectal culture between 35 and 37 weeks of gestation. Women who have had a previous infant with GBS or a GBS in their urine in any trimester will be considered GBS-positive at delivery. A woman who delivers at or before 37 weeks, has ruptured membranes for 18 hours or more, or has a temperature of 100.4°F (≥38°C) or higher is also considered positive for GBS and should receive antibiotic therapy. Cesarean birth before membrane rupture does not require GBS antibiotic therapy.

Penicillin is the first-line agent for antibiotic treatment of the infected woman during birth. Cephazolin is the alternative for the patient with non–life-threatening penicillin allergy. Clindamycin is used for the woman at high risk for anaphylaxis.

Tuberculosis

Tuberculosis (TB) results from infection with *Mycobacterium tuberculosis*. It is transmitted by aerosolized droplets of liquid containing the bacterium, which are inhaled by a noninfected individual and taken into the lung. Initially, most individuals are asymptomatic. Women at risk should be screened for TB when obtaining prenatal care if they are not already known to be positive. This screening involves an intradermal injection of mycobacterial protein (purified protein derivative [PPD]). If the reaction is positive or the woman is already known to have a positive reaction, her abdomen should be protected by a lead shield while a chest radiograph is taken, preferably after the first trimester. Diagnosis is confirmed by isolating and identifying the bacterium in the sputum.

Signs and symptoms include general malaise, fatigue, loss of appetite, weight loss, and fever. Symptoms occur in the late afternoon and evening and are accompanied by night sweats. As the disease progresses, a chronic cough develops and mucopurulent sputum is produced.

TB increases with poverty, malnutrition, and HIV infection. Worldwide, it is responsible for more deaths than any other communicable disease. The incidence is increasing in inner-city areas and among homeless persons. It is also prevalent among immigrants from Southeast Asia and Central and South America.

Fetal and Neonatal Effects. Although perinatal infection is uncommon, it may be acquired as a result of the fetus swallowing or aspirating infected amniotic fluid. Diagnosis is made by finding the bacilli in the gastric aspirate of the neonate or in placental tissue. Signs of congenital TB include failure to thrive, lethargy, respiratory distress, fever, and enlargement of the spleen, liver, and lymph nodes. If the mother remains untreated, the newborn is at high risk for acquiring TB by inhalation of infectious respiratory droplets from the mother.

Therapeutic Management. Untreated TB poses a greater hazard to the fetus than its treatment (CDC, 2016i). Treatment of TB is based on two principles. First, more than one drug should be used to prevent the growth of resistant organisms. Second, treatment should continue for a prolonged period. The preferred treatment for pregnant women with active TB is isoniazid (INH), rifampin (RIF), and ethambutol (EMB) daily for 2 months, followed by INH and RIF daily or twice weekly for 7 months, for 9 months of total treatment duration. Pyridoxine (vitamin B_6) should be given with isoniazid to prevent fetal neurotoxicity and because pregnancy itself increases the demand for this vitamin. Drug resistance in the TB organism may require addition of other drugs, although the following drugs are not recommended in pregnancy: streptomycin, kanamycin, capreomycin, ethionamide, cycloserine, pyrazinamide, amikacin, and fluoroquinolones (CDC, 2016i; Whitty & Dombrowski, 2017).

Management of the infant born to a mother with TB involves preventing the disease and treating the infection early. If the mother's sputum is free of organisms, the infant does not need to be isolated from the mother. Breastfeeding is safe, and drugs may be secreted in breast milk. However, the maternal antituberculosis drugs in breast milk are not adequate for infant treatment. Drug serum levels in the infant can be measured to identify if levels are too high. Disease prevention focuses on teaching the mother and the family how the disease is transmitted so that they can protect the infant and other family members from airborne organisms. The infant should be skin-tested at birth and may be started on preventive isoniazid therapy immediately. Skin testing is repeated at 3 months. Isoniazid is usually continued for the infant until the mother's TB has been inactive for at least 3 months. Infant TB medication may be stopped if the mother and other family members have received full treatment and show no additional disease. If the skin test result shows conversion to positive, a full course of drug therapy should be given to the infant (AAP & ACOG, 2012; Whitty & Dombrowski, 2017).

? KNOWLEDGE CHECK

62. How can toxoplasmosis be prevented?
63. What are the risk factors for colonization of the newborn with GBS during the intrapartum period? How is colonization prevented?
64. How is TB treated in the mother? How is it diagnosed and treated in the newborn?

SUMMARY CONCEPTS

- Spontaneous abortion is a leading cause of pregnancy loss. Treatment is aimed at preventing complications such as hypovolemic shock and infection and providing emotional support for the grieving mother and her family.

- The incidence of ectopic pregnancy is increasing in the United States as a result of pelvic inflammation associated with sexually transmitted diseases. The goals of therapeutic management are to prevent severe hemorrhage and preserve the fallopian tube so that future fertility is retained.

- Management of gestational trophoblastic disease (hydatidiform mole) involves two phases: (1) evacuation of the molar pregnancy and (2) evaluation of serum beta-human chorionic gonadotropin levels monthly for 6 months, then every 2 to 3 months for 6 months until normal for three values. Pregnancy must be avoided during the follow-up because the normal rise of beta-human chorionic gonadotropin level in pregnancy would obscure evidence of choriocarcinoma.

- Disorders of the placenta (placenta previa and placental abruption) are responsible for hemorrhagic conditions of the last half of pregnancy. Either condition may result in maternal hemorrhage and fetal or maternal death.

- Disseminated intravascular coagulation is a life-threatening complication of missed abortion, placental abruption, and severe hypertension, in which procoagulation and anticoagulation factors are simultaneously activated. DIC may occur with problems unrelated to pregnancy.

- The cause of hyperemesis gravidarum remains unclear, but the goals of management are to prevent dehydration, malnutrition, excess weight loss, and electrolyte imbalance. Emotional support is an important responsibility of nurses, in addition to physical care.

- Classifications of hypertension during pregnancy include gestational hypertension, preeclampsia-eclampsia, chronic (preexisting or persistent) hypertension, and chronic hypertension with superimposed preeclampsia. The underlying pathologic process is vasoconstriction.

- Preeclampsia is caused by generalized vasospasm, which decreases circulation to all organs of the body, including the placenta. Major maternal organs affected include the liver, kidneys, heart, and brain.

- Treatment of preeclampsia includes reduced activity, reduction of environmental stimuli, and administration of medications to prevent generalized seizures.

- Magnesium sulfate, used to prevent preeclampsia from progressing to generalized eclamptic seizures, may have adverse effects. The most serious of these is central nervous system depression, which includes depression of the respiratory center. Adverse effects such as respiratory depression or absent deep tendon reflexes are more likely to occur if the blood level of magnesium rises over the therapeutic range.

- Nurses monitor the woman with preeclampsia to evaluate the effectiveness of medical therapy and identify signs that her condition is worsening, such as increasing hyperreflexia. Nurses also control external stimuli and initiate measures to protect her during eclamptic seizures.

- Pregnant women who have chronic hypertension are at increased risk for preeclampsia and should be monitored for worsening hypertension, proteinuria, change in laboratory values, or development of signs and symptoms of preeclampsia. Antihypertensive medication should be continued or initiated if blood pressure is consistently elevated above 160 mm Hg systolic and 90 to 100 mm Hg diastolic.

- Rh incompatibility can occur if an Rh-negative woman conceives a child who is Rh-positive. As a result of exposure to the Rh-positive antigen, maternal antibodies may develop that cause hemolysis of fetal Rh-positive RBCs in subsequent pregnancies.

- Administration of Rh immune globulin (RhoGAM) prevents production of anti-Rh antibodies, thereby preventing destruction of Rh-positive red blood cells in subsequent pregnancies.

- ABO incompatibility usually occurs when the mother has type O blood and naturally occurring anti-A and anti-B antibodies, which cause hemolysis if the fetus's blood is not type O. ABO incompatibility may result in hyperbilirubinemia of the infant, but it usually presents no serious threat to the health of the child.

- The release of insulin accelerates during early pregnancy, which may result in episodes of maternal hypoglycemia.

The availability of glucose and insulin favors the development and storage of fat that the mother will need later.

- Placental hormones, which reach their peak during the second and third trimesters, create resistance to insulin in maternal cells, resulting in increased insulin needs throughout the rest of pregnancy.

- Diabetes is classified according to onset (before or during pregnancy) and the pathology of the disease. Type 1 diabetes is due to beta cell destruction. There is usually absolute insulin deficiency and requires exogenous insulin for control. Type 2 diabetes is characterized by insulin resistance and may be diet controlled or may require both insulin and diet control.

- Type 1 diabetes adversely affects the mother in a variety of ways during pregnancy, including increasing her risk for hypertension, urinary tract infections, and ketosis.

- Because maternal hyperglycemia during the first trimester increases the risk for congenital anomalies in the fetus, a major goal of management is to establish normal blood glucose levels before conception.

- Fetal growth depends on the condition of maternal blood vessels. If no vascular impairment occurs, placental perfusion is adequate and the infant is likely to be large if maternal glucose levels remain too high (macrosomia). If vascular impairment does occur, placental perfusion may be reduced and the fetus may have intrauterine growth restriction.

- In addition to having an increased risk for congenital anomalies, the infant of a mother with preexisting diabetes has an increased risk for hypoglycemia, hypocalcemia, hyperbilirubinemia, and respiratory distress syndrome.

- Maternal adverse effects of gestational diabetes include increased urinary tract infections, hydramnios, premature rupture of membranes, and the development of preeclampsia.

- Gestational diabetes increases the risk for fetal macrosomia and neonatal hypoglycemia.

- In some cases, gestational diabetes usually can be treated by diet and exercise. However, insulin may be required if blood glucose levels remain high.

- Iron supplementation often is needed during pregnancy because most women do not have sufficient iron stores to meet the demands of pregnancy with diet alone.

- Folic acid deficiency is associated with increased risk for spontaneous abortion, placental abruption, and fetal anomalies such as neural tube defects. Folic acid supplementation of 400 mcg (0.4 mg) daily is recommended for all women of childbearing age to reduce the risk for neural tube defects.

- Sickle cell disease often is worsened by pregnancy, and a primary goal is to prevent sickle cell crisis during pregnancy.

- Laboratory values for thalassemia are similar to those for iron deficiency. However, administration of iron is risky because increased iron absorption and storage makes the woman susceptible to iron overload.

- Although the woman with systemic lupus erythematosus can have a normal pregnancy and give birth to a normal newborn, the pregnancy should be treated as high risk because of the increased incidence of abortion, fetal death during the first trimester, and possible exacerbation of the disease.

- Antiphospholipid syndrome is a cluster of clinical entities associated with an increased risk for thrombosis, fetal loss, and decreased platelets. Preeclampsia is more common in the woman with antiphospholipid syndrome.

- Marked improvement in rheumatoid arthritis often occurs during pregnancy, possibly as a result of pregnancy-specific hormone and hormonal factors. However, most women relapse soon after childbirth.

- Management of epilepsy is complex because of the teratogenic effects of anticonvulsant medications coupled with the importance of preventing seizures. Changes in anticonvulsant therapy that reduce the risks for adverse effects may be possible for the woman who wants to become pregnant.

- Although Bell's palsy usually is temporary, the woman may be anxious. Supportive care and emotional support are essential.

- Viral infections that occur during pregnancy can be transmitted to the fetus in two ways: across the placental barrier or by exposure to organisms during birth. Although they may be mild or even subclinical in the mother, viral infections can have serious effects on the fetus.

- The health care team is responsible for teaching how infectious diseases can be prevented and that early treatment may reduce fetal and neonatal exposure to infections.

- Human immunodeficiency virus is a retrovirus that gradually allows a decline in the effectiveness of the maternal immunity, often over many years in the treated woman. Maternal treatment with zidovudine, sometimes with other antiretroviral medications, can substantially reduce infection of the fetus with human immunodeficiency virus.

- Pregnant women who are HIV-positive experience anxiety, fear, and grief as they contemplate potential losses resulting from the disease. Nurses should provide emotional support, information, and counseling, which will help the woman cope with her emotions and retain control of her care for as long as possible.

- Specific pregnancy and postbirth treatment of nonviral infections such as toxoplasmosis, group B *Streptococcus* infection, and tuberculosis reduce long-term maternal and newborn complications.

REFERENCES & READINGS

American Academy of Pediatrics & American College of Obstetricians and Gynecologists (AAP & ACOG). (2012). *Guidelines for perinatal care* (7th ed.). Elk Grove Village, IL: Authors.

American College of Obstetricians and Gynecologists (ACOG). (2013a). *Task force on hyptertension in pregnancy*. Washington, DC: Author.

American College of Obstetricians and Gynecologists (ACOG). (2013b). *Thyroid disease in pregnancy (Practice Bulletin No. 37). Published 2002, reaffirmed 2013*. Washington DC: Author.

American College of Obstetricians and Gynecologists (ACOG). (2013c). *Weight Gain During Pregnancy*. Retrieved from http://www.acog.org/Resources-And-Publications/Committee-Opinions/Committee-on-Obstetric-Practice/Weight-Gain-During-Pregnancy.

American College of Obstetricians and Gynecologists (ACOG). (2014a). *Ethical Issues in the Care of Obese Women*. Retrieved from www.acog.org/-/media/Committee-Opinions/Committee-on-Ethics/co600.pdf?dmc=1&ts=20161006T2325227757.

American College of Obstetricians and Gynecologists (ACOG). (2014b). *Thromboembolism in Pregnancy. ACOG Practice Bulletin 123. Published 2011, reaffirmed 2014*. Washington DC: Author.

American College of Obstetricians and Gynecologists (ACOG). (2015a). *Physical Activity and Exercise During Pregnancy and The Postpartum Period*. Retrieved from www.acog.org/-/media/Committee-Opinions/Committee-on-Obstetric-practice/co650.pdf?dmc=1&ts=20161006T2248500684.

American College of Obstetricians and Gynecologists (ACOG). (2015b). *Anemia in pregnancy (Practice Bulletin No. 95)*. Washington, DC: Author.

American College of Obstetricians and Gynecologists (ACOG). (2015c). *Gestational diabetes (Practice Bulletin No. 137). Published 2013, reaffirmed 2015*. Washington, DC: Author.

American College of Obstetricians and Gynecologists (ACOG). (2015d). *Hemoglobinopathies in pregnancy (Practice Bulletin No. 78)*. Washington, DC: Author.

American College of Obstetricians & Gynecologists (ACOG). (2015e). *Nausea and vomiting of pregnancy (Practice Bulletin No. 153)*. Washington, DC: Author.

American College of Obstetricians and Gynecologists (ACOG). (2015f). *Obesity in Pregnancy Practice Bulletin (No. 156)*. Washington, DC: Author.

American College of Obstetricians and Gynecologist (ACOG). (2016a *FAQ Obesity and Pregnancy*. Retrieved from www.acog.org/Patients/FAQs/Obesity-and-Pregnancy.

American College of Obstetricians & Gynecologists (ACOG). (2016b). *Management of alloimmunization during pregnancy. (Practice Bulletin No. 75) published 2006, reaffirmed 2016*. Washington, DC: Author.

American College of Obstetricians and Gynecologists (ACOG). (2016c). *Management of herpes in pregnancy (Practice Bulletin No. 82)*. Washington, DC: Author.

American College of Obstetricians and Gynecologists (ACOG). (2016d). *Pregestational diabetes mellitus (Practice Bulletin No. 60) Published 2005, reaffirmed 2016*. Washington, DC: Author.

American College of Obstetricians & Gynecologists (ACOG). (2016e). *Prevention of Rh and Alloimmunization (Practice Bulletin, No. 4)*. Washington, DC: Author.

American College of Obstetricians and Gynecologists (ACOG). (2016f). *Use of prophylactic antibiotics in labor and delivery. ACOG Practice Bulletin 120. Published 2011, reaffirmed 2016*. Washington DC: Author.

American College of Obstetricians and Gynecologists (ACOG). (2016g). *Viral hepatitis in pregnancy (Practice Bulletin No. 86)*. Washington, DC: Author.

American Diabetes Association (ADA). (2013). Diagnosis and classification of diabetes mellitus. *Diabetes Care, 36*(Suppl. 1), S67–S74.

American Diabetes Association (ADA). (2017a). Classification and diagnosis of diabetes. *Diabetes Care, 40*(Suppl. 1), S11–S24.

American Diabetes Association (ADA). (2017b). Management of diabetes in pregnancy. *Diabetes Care, 40*(Suppl.1), S114–S119.

American Heart Association (AHA). (n.d.). Classes of Heart Failure. Retrieved from www.heart.org/HEARTORG/Conditions/HeartFailure/AboutHeartFailure/Classes-of-Heart-Failure_UCM_306328_Article.jsp#.V-hSTCErJD8.

Aminoff, M. J. (2014). Neurologic disorders. In R. K. Creasy, R. Resnik, J. D. Iams, C. J. Lockwood, & T. R. Moore (Eds.), *Creasy & Resnik's maternal-fetal medicine: principles and practice* (7th ed.) (pp. 1100–1121). Philadelphia, PA: Saunders.

Arafeh, J. (2014). Cardiac disease in pregnancy. In K. R. Simpson, & P. A. Creehan (Eds.), *Perinatal Nursing* (4th ed.) (pp. 224–229). Philadelphia: Lippincott Williams & Wilkins.

Association of Womens Health, Obstetric, and Neonatal Nurses (AWHONN). (2012). *Obstetric Hemorrhage Position Statement*. Washington, DC: Author.

Berghella, V., & Iams, J. D. (2014). Cervical insufficiency. In R. K. Creasy, R. Resnik, J. D. Iams, et al. (Eds.), *Creasy & Resnik's Maternal-fetal medicine: principles and practice* (7th ed.) (pp. 657–662). Philadelphia, PA: Saunders.

Bernstein, H. (2017). Maternal and perinatal infection: viral. In S. G. Gabbe, J. R. Niebyl, J. L. Simpson, M. B. Landon, H. L. Galan, R. M. Jauniaux, D. A. Driscoll, et al. (Eds.), *Obstetrics: normal and problem pregnancies* (7th ed.) (pp. 1099–1129). Philadelphia, PA: Saunders.

Blackburn, S. T. (2013). *Maternal, fetal, & neonatal physiology: a clinical perspective* (4th ed.). Philadelphia, PA: Saunders.

Blanchard, D. G., & Daniels, L. B. (2014). Cardiac diseases. In R. K. Creasy, R. Resnik, J. D. Iams, et al. (Eds.), *Creasy & Resnik's Maternal-fetal medicine: principles and practice* (7th ed.) (pp. 852–877). Philadelphia, PA: Saunders.

Branum, A., Kirmeyer, S. E., & Gregory, E. C. W. (2016). *Prepregnancy body mass index by maternal characteristics and state: data from the birth certificate, 2014. National vital statistics reports* (Vol. 65). Hyattsville, MD: National Center for Health Statistics. no 6.

Carpenter, J. R., & Branch, D. W. (2017). Collagen vascular diseases. In S. G. Gabbe, J. R. Niebyl, J. L. Simpson, M. B. Landon, H. L. Galan, R. M. Jauniaux, D. A. Driscoll, et al. (Eds.), *Obstetrics: Normal and Problem Pregnancies* (7th ed.) (pp. 981–997). Philadelphia, PA: Saunders.

Centers for Disease Control and Prevention (CDC). (2012). *Hypertension: high blood pressure facts*. Retrieved from www.cdc.gov.

Center for Disease Control and Prevention (CDC). (2013). Updated Recommendations for Use of VariZIG: United States, 2013. *MMR Morbidity and Mortality Weekly Report, 62*(28), 574–576.

Centers for Disease Control and Prevention (CDC). (2014). *National diabetes statistics report* (2014). Retrieved from www.cdc.gov/diabetes.

Centers for Disease Control and Prevention (CDC). (2015a). *Diabetes and Pregnancy*. Retrieved from www.cdc.gov/pregnancy/diabetes.

Centers for Disease Control and Prevention (CDC). (2015b). *Parvovirus and fifth disease*. Retrieved from www.cdc.gov.

Centers for Disease Control and Prevention (CDC). (2016a). *Epilepsy fast facts*. Retrieved from www.cdc.gov.

Centers for Disease Control and Prevention (CDC). (2016b). *Guidelines for vaccinating pregnant women*. Retrieved from www.cdc.gov.

Centers for Disease Control and Prevention (CDC). (2016c). *Immunization schedules for infants and children in easy-to-read formats*. Retrieved from www.cdc.gov/vaccines.

Centers for Disease Control and Prevention (CDC). (2016d). *Routine varicella vaccination. Vaccines and Preventable Diseases*. Retrieved from www.cdc.gov/vaccines/vpd/varicella/hcp/recommendations.html.

Centers for Disease Control and Prevention (CDC). (2016e). *Prevention of perinatal group B streptococcal disease: revised guidelines from CDC (2016)*. Retrieved from www.cdc.gov.

Centers for Disease Control and Prevention (CDC). (2016f). *Sexually transmitted diseases treatment guidelines*. Retrieved from www.cdc.gov/mmwr.

Centers for Disease Control and Prevention (CDC). (2016g). *Sexually transmitted diseases (STDs): Genital HPV infection fact sheet*. Retrieved from www.cdc.gov/std.

Center for Disease Control and Preventions (CDC). (2016h). *Stages of HIV infection*. Retrieved from www.aids.gov/hiv-aids-basics/just-diagnosed-with-hiv-aids/hiv-in-your-body/stages-of-hiv/index.html.

Centers for Disease Control and Prevention (CDC). (2016i). *TB treatment and pregnancy. Tuberculosis (TB)*. Retrieved from www.cdc.gov/tb/topic/treatment/pregnancy.htm.

Centers for Disease Control and Prevention (CDC). (2016j). *Viral hepatitis*. Retrieved from www.cdc.gov/hepatitis.

Centers for Disease Control and Prevention (CDC). (2017a). *HIV among African Americans*. Retrieved from www.cdc.gov/hiv/group/racialethnic/africanamericans/index.html.

Centers for Disease Control and Prevention (CDC). (2017b). *Lupus basic fact sheet. Systemic lupus erythematosus*. Retrieved from www.cdc.gov.

Centers for Disease Control and Prevention (CDC). (2017c). *Recommended adult immunization schedule. United States, 2016*. Retrieved from www.cdc.gov.

Cohn, D., Ramaswamy, B., & Blum, K. (2014). Malignancy and pregnancy. In R. K. Creasy, R. Resnik, J. D. Iams, et al. (Eds.), *Creasy & Resnik's Maternal-fetal medicine: principles and practice* (7th ed.) (pp. 932–948). Philadelphia, PA: Saunders.

Cox, J. T., & Carney, V. H. (2017). Nutrition for reproductive health and lactation. In L. K. Mahan, & J. L. Raymond (Eds.), *Krause's food and the nutrition care process* (14th ed.) (pp. 239–298). St. Louis, MO: Elsevier.

Cunningham, F. G., Leveno, K. J., Bloom, S. L., Spong, C. Y., Dashe, J. S., Hoffman, B. L., & Sheffield, J. S. (2014). *Williams' obstetrics* (24th ed.). New York: McGraw-Hill.

DeSisto, C. L., Kim, S. Y., & Sharma, A. J. (2014). Prevalence Estimates of Gestational Diabetes Mellitus in the United States, Pregnancy Risk Assessment Monitoring System (PRAMS), 2007–2010. *Preventing Chronic Disease, 11*, 130415.

DeVon, H. A., Pettey, C. M., Vuckovic, K. M., Koenig, M. D., & McSweeney, J. C. (2016). A Review of the Literature on Cardiac Symptoms in Older and Younger Women. *JOGNN: Journal of Obstetric Gynecologic and Neonatal Nurses, 45*, 426–437.

DiGiuglio, M., Weidaseck, S., & Monchek, R. (2012). Understanding hydatidiform mole. *MCN: American Journal of Maternal-Child Nursing, 37*(1), 30–34.

Druzin, M. L., Shields, L. E., Peterson, N. L., & Cape, V. (2013). *Preeclampsia Toolkit: Improving Health Care Response to Preeclampsia: A California Toolkit to Transform Maternity Care*. Developed under contract #11-10006 with the California Department of Public Health; Maternal, Child and Adolescent Health Division; Published by the California Maternal Quality Care Collaborative.

Duff, P. (2014). Maternal and fetal infections. In R. K. Creasy, R. Resnik, J. D. Iams, et al. (Eds.), *Creasy & Resnik's Maternal-fetal medicine: principles and practice* (7th ed.) (pp. 802–851). Philadelphia, PA: Saunders.

Duff, P., & Birsner, M. (2017). Maternal and perinatal infection: bacterial. In S. G. Gabbe, J. R. Niebyl, J. L. Simpson, M. B. Landon, H. L. Galan, R. M. Jauniaux, D. A. Driscoll, et al. (Eds.), *Obstetrics: normal and problem pregnancies* (7th ed.) (pp. 1130–1146). Philadelphia, PA: Saunders.

Elkayam, U., Goland, S., Pieper, P. G., & Silversides, C. K. (2016). High-Risk Cardiac Disease in Pregnancy. *Journal of the American College of Cardiology, 68*(4), 396–410.

Faria-Schützer, D. B., Surita, F. G., Nascimento, S. L., Vieira, C. M., Turato, E., & Faria-Schützer, D. B. (2017). Psychological issues facing obese pregnant women: a systematic review. *Journal Of Maternal-Fetal & Neonatal Medicine, 30*(1), 88–95.

Francois, K. E., & Foley, M. R. (2017). Antepartum and postpartum hemorrhage. In S. G. Gabbe, J. R. Niebyl, J. L. Simpson, M. B. Landon, H. L. Galan, R. M. Jauniaux, D. A. Driscoll, et al. (Eds.), *Obstetrics: normal and problem pregnancies* (7th ed.) (pp. 395–425). Philadelphia, PA: Saunders.

Franz, M. J., & Evert, A. B. (2017). Medical nutrition therapy for diabetes mellitus and hypoglycemia of nondiabetic origin. In L. K. Mahan, & J. L. Raymond (Eds.), *Krause's food and the nutrition care process* (14th ed.) (pp. 586–618). Philadelphia, PA: Saunders.

Gaddipati, S., & Troiano, N. H. (2013). Cardiac disorders in pregnancy. In N. H. Troiano, C. J. Harvey, & B. F. Chez (Eds.), *AWHONN High-risk & critical care obstetrics* (3rd ed.) (pp. 125–143). Philadelphia, PA: Lippincott Williams & Wilkins.

Gilbert, E. S. (2011). *Manual of high risk pregnancy & delivery* (5th ed.). St. Louis, MO: Mosby.

Hull, A. D., & Resnik, R. (2014). Placenta previa, placenta accreta, abruptio placentae, and vasa previa. In R. K. Creasy, R. Resnik, J. D. Iams, et al. (Eds.), *Creasy & Resnik's Maternal-fetal medicine: principles and practice* (7th ed.) (pp. 732–749). Philadelphia, PA: Saunders.

Institute of Medicine. (2009). *Weight gain during pregnancy: reexamining the guidelines*. Retrieved from http://iom.edu/Reports/2009/Weight-Gain-During-Pregnancy-Reexamining-the-Guidelines.aspx.

Institute for Safe Medication Practices. (2014). *ISMP list of high-alert medications in clinical practice*. Retrieved from www.ismp.org/tools/institutionalhighAlert.asp.

Kee-Hak, L., Steinberg, G., & Ramus, R. (2016). *Preeclampsia*. Retrieved from www.emedicine.medscape.com/article/1476919-overview.

Kelly, T. F., & Savides, T. J. (2014). Gastrointestinal disease in pregnancy. In R. K. Creasy, R. Resnik, J. D. Iams, et al. (Eds.), *Creasy & Resnik's Maternal-fetal medicine: principles and practice* (7th ed.) (pp. 1059–1074). Philadelphia, PA: Saunders.

Kilpatrick, S. J. (2014). Anemia and pregnancy. In R. K. Creasy, R. Resnik, J. D. Iams, et al. (Eds.), *Creasy & Resnik's Maternal-fetal medicine: principles and practice* (7th ed.) (pp. 918–931). Philadelphia, PA: Saunders.

Kreibs, J. M. (2014). Obesity in pregnancy: addressing risks to improve outcomes. *Journal of Perinatal and Neonatal Nursing, 28*(1), 32–40.

Kuklina, E. V., & Callaghan, W. M. (2011). Chronic heart disease and severe obstetric morbidity among hospitalizations for pregnancy in the USA: 1995-2006. *BJOG: An International Journal of Obstetrics and Gynecology, 118*(3), 345–352.

Landon, M. B., Catalano, P. M., & Gabbe, S. G. (2017). Diabetes mellitus complicating pregnancy. In S. G. Gabbe, J. R. Niebyl, J. L. Simpson, M. B. Landon, H. L. Galan, R. M. Jauniaux, D. A. Driscoll, et al. (Eds.), *Obstetrics: normal and problem pregnancies* (7th ed.) (pp. 862–898). Philadelphia, PA: Saunders.

Lindqvist, M., Lindkvist, M., Eurenius, E., Persson, M., Iversson, A., & Mogren, I. (2016). Leisure time physical activity among pregnant women and its associations with maternal characteristics and pregnancy outcomes. *Sexual and Reproductive Healthcare, 9*, 14–20.

Lockwood, C. J. (2014). Thromboembolic disease in pregnancy. In R. K. Creasy, R. Resnik, J. D. Iams, et al. (Eds.), *Creasy & Resnik's Maternal-fetal medicine: principles and practice* (7th ed.) (pp. 906–917). Philadelphia, PA: Saunders.

Magnesium Sulfate: Drug Information. (2016). Retrieved from www.uptodate.com/contents/magnesium-sulfate-drug-information?source=search_result&search=magnesium+sulfate&selectedTitle=1%7E147

Markham, K. B., & Funai, E. F. (2014). Pregnancy-related hypertension. In R. K. Creasy, R. Resnik, J. D. Iams, C. Lockwood, T. Moore, & M. Greene (Eds.), *Creasy & Resnik's Maternal-fetal medicine: principles and practice* (7th ed.) (pp. 756–781). Philadelphia, PA: Saunders.

Mestman, J. H. (2017). Thyroid and parathyroid diseases in pregnancy. In S. G. Gabbe, J. R. Niebyl, J. L. Simpson, M. B. Landon, H. L. Galan, R. M. Jauniaux, D. A. Driscoll, et al. (Eds.), *Obstetrics: normal and problem pregnancies* (7th ed.) (pp. 910–937). Philadelphia, PA: Saunders.

Moise, K. J. (2014). Hemolytic disease of the fetus and newborn. In R. K. Creasy, R. Resnik, J. D. Iams, et al. (Eds.), *Creasy & Resnik's Maternal-fetal medicine: principles and practice* (7th ed.) (pp. 558–568). Philadelphia, PA: Saunders.

Monga, M., & Mastrobattista, J. M. (2014). Maternal cardiovascular, respiratory, and renal adaptation to pregnancy. In R. K. Creasy, R. Resnik, J. D. Iams, et al. (Eds.), *Creasy & Resnik's Maternal-fetal medicine: principles and Practice* (7th ed.) (pp. 93–96). Philadelphia, PA: Saunders.

National Institutes of Health (NIH): National Diabetes Information Clearinghouse (NDIC). (2013). *What I need to know about gestational diabetes (NIH Publication No. 13–5129)*. Retrieved from www.diabetes.niddk.nih.gov.

National Institutes of Health (NIH), National Heart, Lung, and Blood Institute (NHLBI). (2000). *Report of the working group on research on hypertension during pregnancy*. Retrieved from www.nhlbi.nih.gov.

National Institutes of Health (NIH), National Heart, Lung, & Blood Institute (NHLBI). (2012). *What is sickle cell anemia?* Retrieved from www.nhlbi.nih.gov.

Nelson, A. L., & Gambone, J. C. (2016). Ectopic Pregnancy. In N. F. Hacker, J. C. Gambone, & C. J. Hobel (Eds.), *Hacker & Moore's Essentials of Obstetrics and Gynecology* (6th ed.) (pp. 304–313). Philadelpha, PA: Elsevier.

Ogden, C. L., Carroll, M. D., Fryar, C. D., & Flegal, K. M. (2015). *Prevalence of obesity among adults and youth: United States, 2011–2014. NCHS data brief, no 219*. Hyattsville, MD: National Center for Health Statistics.

Pammi, M., Brand, C. M., & Weisman, L. E. (2016). Infection in the neonate. In S. Gardner, B. Carter, M. Enzman-Hines, & J. Hernandez (Eds.), *Merenstein & Gardner's Handbook of Neonatal Intensive Care* (pp. 537–564). St. Louis, MO: Mosby.

Poole, J. H. (2014). Hypertensive Disorders of Pregnancy. In K. R. Simpson, & P. A. Creehan (Eds.), *Perinatal Nursing* (4th ed.) (pp. 122–142). Philadelphia. PA: Lippincott Williams & Wilkins.

Roberts, J. M., August, P. A., & Bakris, G. (2013). *Task Force on Hypertension in Pregnancy*. Washington D.C.: American College of Obstetricians and Gynecologists.

Rozance, P. J., McGowan, J. E., Price-Douglas, W., & Hay, W., Jr. (2016). In S. L. Gardner, B. S. Carter, M. E. Hines, & J. A. Hernandez (Eds.), *Merenstein & Gardner's Handbook of Neonatal Intensive Care* (8th ed.) (pp. 337–359). St. Louis, MO: Mosby.

Salani, R., & Copeland, L. J. (2017). Malignant diseases and pregnancy. In S. G. Gabbe, J. R. Niebyl, J. L. Simpson, M. B. Landon, H. L. Galan, R. M. Jauniaux, D. A. Driscoll, et al. (Eds.), *Obstetrics: Normal and problem pregnancies* (7th ed.) (pp. 1057–1074). Philadelphia, PA: Saunders.

Samuels, P. (2017). Hematologic complications of pregnancy. In S. G. Gabbe, J. R. Niebyl, J. L. Simpson, M. B. Landon, H. L. Galan, R. M. Jauniaux, D. A. Driscoll, et al. (Eds.), *Obstetrics: Normal and problem pregnancies* (7th ed.) (pp. 947–964). Philadelphia, PA: Elsevier.

Sibai, B. M. (2017). Preeclampsia and Hypertensive disorders. In S. G. Gabbe, J. R. Niebyl, J. L. Simpson, M. B. Landon, H. L. Galan, R. M. Jauniaux, D. A. Driscoll, et al. (Eds.), *Obstetrics: Normal and problem pregnancies* (7th ed.) (pp. 662–705). Philadelphia, PA: Saunders.

Simpson, J. L., & Jauniaux, E. R. M. (2017). Early pregnancy loss and stillbirth. In S. G. Gabbe, J. R. Niebyl, J. L. Simpson, M. B. Landon, H. L. Galan, R. M. Jauniaux, D. A. Driscoll, et al. (Eds.), *Obstetrics: Normal and problem pregnancies* (7th ed.) (pp. 578–594). Philadelphia, PA: Saunders.

Stopler, T., & Weiner, S. (2017). Medical nutrition for anemia. In L. K. Mahan, & J. L. Raymond (Eds.), *Krause's food and the nutrition care process* (14th ed.) (pp. 631–645). St. Louis, MO: Elsevier.

U.S. Department of Health and Human Services (USDHHS). Panel on Treatment of HIV-Infected Pregnant Women and Prevention of Perinatal Transmission. (2013). *Recommendations for Use of Antiretroviral Drugs in Pregnant HIV-1-Infected Women for Maternal Health and Interventions to Reduce Perinatal HIV Transmission in the United States*. Retrieved from https://aidsinfo.nih.gov/contentfiles/lvguidelines/PerinatalGL.pdf.

U.S. Preventive Services Task Force. (2014). *Low-Dose Aspirin Use for the Prevention of Morbidity and Mortality From Preeclampsia: Preventative Medication*. Retrieved from www.uspreventiveservicestaskforce.org/Page/Document/UpdateSummaryFinal/low-dose-aspirin-use-for-the-prevention-of-morbidity-and-mortality-from-preeclampsia-preventive-medication?ds=1&s=pregnancy.

U.S. Preventive Services Task Force. (2016). *Folic acid for the prevention of neural tube Defects: U.S. Preventive Services Task Force Draft Recommendation Statement*. Retrieved from https://www.uspreventiveservicestaskforce.org/.

Vandorsten, J. P., Dodson, W. C., Espeland, M. A., Grobman, W. A., Guise, W. A., Mercer, B. M., & Tital, A. T. (2013). NIH consensus development conference: diagnosis in gestational diabetes mellitus. *NIH Consensus and State-of-the-Science Statements, 29*(1), 1–31.

Wahedi, M. (2016). Should midwives consider associated psychological factors when caring for women who are obese? *British Journal of Midwifery, 24*(10), 724–735.

WHO. (2006). *BMI classification. Global database on body mass index.* Retrieved July 05, 2017, from http://apps.who.int/bmi/index.jsp?introPage=intro_3.html.

Whitty, J. E., & Dombrowski, M. P. (2014). Respiratory diseases in pregnancy. In R. K. Creasy, R. Resnik, J. D. Iams, C. J. Lockwood, & T. R. Moore (Eds.), *Creasy & Resnik's Maternal-fetal medicine: principles and practice* (7th ed.) (pp. 965–987). Philadelphia, PA: Saunders.

Whitty, J. E., & Dombrowski, M. P. (2017). Respiratory diseases in pregnancy. In S. G. Gabbe, J. R. Niebyl, J. L. Simpson, M. B. Landon, H. L. Galan, R. M. Jauniaux, D. A. Driscoll, et al. (Eds.), *Obstetrics: normal and problem pregnancies* (7th ed.) (pp. 828–849). Philadelphia, PA: Saunders.

Williamson, C., Mackillop, L., & Heneghan, M. A. (2014). Diseases of the Liver, Biliary System, and Pancreas. In R. K. Creasy, R. Resnik, J. D. Iams, et al. (Eds.), *Creasy & Resnik's Maternal-fetal medicine: principles and practice* (7th ed.) (pp. 1075–1091). Philadelphia, PA: Saunders.

Yakoob, M. Y., & Bhutta, Z. A. (2011). Effect of routine iron supplementation with or without folic acid on anemia during pregnancy. *BMC Public Health, 11*(11 Suppl. 21), 21.

Zeng, X., Xue, Y., Tian, Q., Sun, R., & An, R. (2016). Effects and Safety of Magnesium Sulfate on Neuroprotection: A Meta-analysis Based on PRISMA Guidelines. *Medicine, 95*(1):e2451. (1-12).

The Childbearing Family with Special Needs

Jessica L. McNeil, Karen S. Holub

All families must make major changes as they adapt to pregnancy and childbirth. For some families, however, the changes are particularly difficult. Such families have special needs related to parental age, substance abuse, birth of an infant with congenital abnormalities, perinatal loss, adoption, or mental health disorder. Perinatal nurses can make a difference in the lives of these families.

ADOLESCENT PREGNANCY

The 2015 birth rate to teenage mothers (age 15 to 19 years) in the United States was 22.3 per 1000 teenage women (229,715 babies were born to teenage mothers), decreasing 8% from 2014 (Centers for Disease Control [CDC], 2017). This continues to decline from 1991 when the rate was 61.8 per 1000 teenage women (United States Health and Human Services [DHHS], 2016). The reasons for the decline are not totally understood, however the evidence suggests abstinence rates are increasing among teenage women, and those who are sexually active are more likely to use contraceptives. (CDC, 2017). Although the decline is encouraging, teenage pregnancy rates in the U.S. are still substantially higher than in other western countries and there are significant racial disparities. The teenage birth rate was highest (34.9 per 1000) among Hispanic women, followed by non-Hispanic Black women (31.8 per 1000), American Indian/Alaska Native women (25.7 per 1000), non-Hispanic White women (16 per 1000) and Asian/Pacific Islander women (6.9 per 1000) (CDC, 2017).

Factors Associated with Teenage Pregnancy

Many factors may contribute to one becoming a teenage mother. The U.S. Department of Health and Human Services (DHHS) recognizes those teens who are homeless, in the juvenile justice system, and in the foster care system as most at risk for teenage pregnancy (Koh, 2014). Adolescents tend to engage in more frequent high-risk sexual behaviors because there may be a lack of consideration of the consequences that accompany their actions. Many adolescents believe teenage pregnancy will never happen to them. Increased abstinence, education, and more effective contraceptive practices have assisted in the recent decline of teenage pregnancies.

Some adolescents chance pregnancy and parenthood as a means of maintaining a relationship, and/or having someone to love them, whereas others see it as a means to gain independence. Factors that contribute to teenage pregnancy are listed in Box 11.1.

Sex Education

Sex education for teens should focus on helping them clarify their own values and beliefs regarding sexual behavior,

BOX 11.1   Factors That Contribute to Teenage Pregnancy

Peer pressure to begin sexual activity

High rate of sexual activity

Limited access to contraceptive devices

Lack of accurate information about how to use contraceptives correctly

Incorrect or lack of use of contraceptives

Fear of reporting sexual activity to parents

Ambivalence toward sexuality; intercourse not "planned"

Feelings of invincibility

Low self-esteem and consequent inability to set limits on sexual activity

Desire to attain love or escape present situation

Lack of appropriate role models

recognize consequences associated with risky sexual behaviors, understand how to set appropriate boundaries regarding their own sexual behaviors, and learn effective measures to prevent pregnancy and sexually transmitted disease (STD). It is especially important that teens learn the importance of setting limits on sexual behavior and are equipped with the tools to know how to say "not now," "not yet," and "not you." Many teenagers may find themselves feeling pressured by peers into engaging in sexual activities when they lack the emotional maturity to deal responsibly with intercourse, contraception, or an unplanned pregnancy.

When providing sex education, nurses should keep in mind that adolescent males and females mature at different rates and may be more comfortable learning and discussing topics in separate groups. In talking with teenagers, nurses should use simple but correct language such as, "uterus," "testicles," "penis," and "vagina."

Socioeconomic Implications

Teenage pregnancy can prove to be an economic burden because often the teen is still in school and unable to work and make enough money to sufficiently provide for the child. Often it is necessary for the teen to receive government assistance to have the basic resources needed to provide food and shelter. Categorically, teenage parents cost U.S. tax payers millions annually through government programs, the foster care system, and the legal system (Koh, 2014). Teenage parents are less likely than their childless peers to finish high school and go to college, more likely to live in poverty, and more likely to depend on government assistance (Koh, 2014).

Although the financial cost of teenage pregnancy is huge, there is also a psychosocial cost to the teen and a cost to society. The developmental tasks of adolescence such as achieving independence from parents and establishing a lifestyle that is personally satisfying may be interrupted when a pregnancy increases the need for financial and emotional support from parents (Table 11.1). Instead of becoming independent, they often become more dependent on their parents or

their boyfriends because of pregnancy. Education goals may be curtailed for some young mothers, limiting employment opportunities and resulting in reliance on the welfare system.

Positive outcomes from the pregnancy also may occur. For some adolescents, pregnancy provides them with a motivation to further their education and provide a better life for their child. Pregnancy and birth may have a stabilizing and maturing effect on adolescents who use the experience as an opportunity to change past poor lifestyle choices and become more goal-directed.

Implications for Maternal Health

Compared to older women, teenage mothers have an increased chance of perinatal complications including death, pregnancy-associated hypertension, anemia, preterm labor and birth, depression, substance abuse, intimate partner violence, poor nutrition and self-care, perineal lacerations, and striae gravidarum with itching. (ACOG, 2015; Asheer et al., 2014; Lee et al., 2016; Montgomery et al., 2014; Nove, Matthews, & Camacho, 2014) Teenage mothers may delay seeking prenatal care and delay finding and receiving postpartum care and care for their newborn (Lee, Tsui, & Wang, 2016). The lack of maturity and reasoning that often accompanies adolescence makes teenagers less likely to properly use reliable methods of birth control (Asheer, Berger, Meckstroth, Kisker, & Keating, 2014), increasing their risk for another pregnancy. (Fig. 11.1)

Statistics reveal that those who have had one teenage pregnancy have a 23% chance of having a second teenage pregnancy (Montgomery, Folken, & Seitz, 2014).

Some women may panic at the thought of an unplanned pregnancy and choose to have an abortion (Sedgh, Finer, Bankole, Eilers, & Singh, 2015). The decision to abort can bring conflicting feelings of sadness, guilt, and relief and be difficult for the teenager to process.

Implications for Fetal and Neonatal Health

Infants born to teenage mothers have a higher risk for preterm birth and low birthweight (Sedgh et al., 2015). Infants of teenage mothers tend to have lower Apgar scores at birth and experience higher rates of neonatal death (Lee et al., 2016).

The Teenage Expectant Father

The majority of teenage mothers have partners who are within 2 years of their age, but some may have partners who are older. These men may accept responsibility for the child, or they may become "phantom fathers" who are absent and rarely involved in raising the child.

Almost all adolescent expectant fathers indicate that they are not ready for fatherhood. Many are depressed as they grapple with the conflicting roles of adolescence and fatherhood. Although some express interest in learning about childbirth and child care, those who do not want to be fathers are less likely to be supportive. Some do not wish to be involved in the child's life, leaving the young pregnant woman to seek support elsewhere. Other fathers are involved to some degree during the pregnancy and early years of the

TABLE 11.1   Impact of Pregnancy on the Developmental Tasks of Adolescence

Developmental Task*	Impact of Pregnancy	Nursing Considerations
Achievement of a Stable Identity: How the person sees himself or herself and how the person perceives that others see and accept him or her. Peer group approval provides confirmation and is a major component of identity development.	The ability to adapt and respond to stress is a good indicator of identity development. Adolescents who become pregnant before a stable identity is developed may not be able to accept the responsibilities of parenthood and to plan for the future.	Explore the availability of a school-based mothers' program that will provide the peer support that is very important. Emphasize the importance of prenatal classes and the effect of prenatal care on pregnancy. Encourage both parents to attend parenting classes, and describe the expected growth and development of infants. Focus on the infant's need to develop trust and on the parenting behaviors that promote this.
Achievement of Comfort with Body Image: Requires internalization of mature body size, contour, and function.	The adolescent must learn to cope with body changes of pregnancy (increasing size, contour, pigmentation changes, and striae) before she has learned to accept the body changes of puberty. May deny pregnancy or severely restrict calories to avoid gaining weight. May be disgusted with the physical changes of pregnancy that make her look different from her peers.	Allow time for the teenager to verbalize her feelings about the body changes of pregnancy. Emphasize that dieting is harmful to the infant and will not stop the changes in body size and contour. Provide exercises that will help her regain her figure after the birth of the infant.
Acceptance of Sexual Role and Identity: Requires internalization of strong sexual urges and achievement of intimacy with others.	The adolescent may need to achieve an intimate relationship with another person and form an exclusive relationship before she is ready. The pregnant teenager will also need to cope with changes in relationships with friends. She often has difficulty seeing herself as a sexual being or as a mother.	Allow the teenager to express her feelings about sexuality and about motherhood. Initiate groups designed specifically for adolescents (e.g., childbirth education, parenting classes, groups focused on nutrition). This will help her deal with changing relationships with her peers and move toward a mothering role.
Development of a Personal Value System: Able to consider the rights and feelings of others.	Pregnancy may occur before the adolescent is able to move from following rules to considering the rights and feelings of others and developing ethical standards. She may experience conflict when she must adjust to the responsibilities of premature motherhood.	Initiate a discussion of the teenager's feelings of conflict about her role as mother versus her role as student. Explore her views about motherhood: How does she expect it to change her life? What are her future plans? Present options and assist her to explore her goals.
Preparation for Vocation or Career: Completing educational or vocational goals; youths living in poverty may not have the means or encouragement to accomplish this.	Pregnancy often interrupts school for both parents. This may be a major frustration, and it may result in permanent withdrawal from school and limited access to jobs that pay more than the minimum wage.	Discuss the importance of continued education, and elicit the teenager's feelings and plans to accomplish this. Determine the amount and availability of support from her parents. Refer her to social services for needed assistance.
Achievement of Independence from Parents: Competent in the social environment and able to function without parental guidance.	Must adjust to the need for continued financial assistance and dependence on parents at a time when achieving independence is a major priority.	Assist the teenager to verbalize her feelings about continued dependence on parents. Discuss the reality of the situation and her need for financial support and help with the care of the infant. Determine the reaction of her parents to the pregnancy and if she will continue to live at home. How much support will they provide? What are the conditions for her remaining in her parents' home with the infant?

Modified from Mercer, R. T. (1990). *Parents at risk*. New York, NY: Springer.

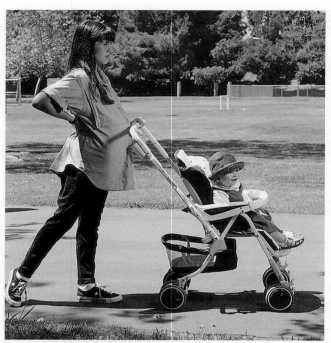

FIG. 11.1 Pregnant Adolescent. Approximately 23% of pregnant adolescents will have a second teenage pregnancy.

child's life but become less involved over time. Many adolescent mothers perceive that support from their partners is inadequate.

A disproportionate number of teenage expectant fathers are from environments of poverty and lack job skills or educational preparation. Many need job training before they can earn enough money to contribute to the support of their children. To help provide financial support, the father may have to interrupt his education to find a job.

Impact of Teenage Pregnancy on Parenting

Evidence shows that 82% of teenage pregnancies are unintended (Koh, 2014). This unexpected and unwanted life event can lead to difficulties in the mother establishing a bond with her child and embracing the new role as parent. Teenage parents are still growing and developing a sense of self and often do not possess the maturity or patience to parent well, and thus children born to teenage mothers are at greater risk for abuse and cognitive delays (Montgomery et al., 2014). Teenage parents often need substantial resources to adequately provide for their children. Community resources such as parenting classes, as well as self-help and career classes, are beneficial in preparing teenage parents to assume new roles and prepare to meet the physical and emotional needs of their child (Asheer et al., 2014).

> **KNOWLEDGE CHECK**
> 1. How does pregnancy affect the developmental tasks of adolescence?
> 2. What are the major problems associated with teenage pregnancy in terms of maternal and fetal health?

◆ APPLICATION OF THE NURSING PROCESS: THE PREGNANT TEENAGER

◆ Assessment

Physical Assessment

Assessment of pregnant teenagers is like that of older women in many respects. At the initial visit, obtain a thorough health and family history to determine whether conditions such as diabetes or infectious diseases increase the risk for the mother and the fetus. Monitor closely for signs of iron-deficiency anemia, preeclampsia, or STDs. Attempt to identify behavioral risk factors such as poor nutrition, smoking, alcohol or drug use, or unprotected sex, which could harm the mother or the fetus. Screen for physical or sexual abuse, which is more common in pregnant teenagers.

Teenagers are sometimes defensive and inconsistent in their responses. Because they may not volunteer information about nutrition, exercise, and the use of alcohol or other drugs, the nurse needs to press for details. The teenager's statement "I eat okay, and I'm pretty active" requires follow-up questions worded to obtain specific information: "What foods do you especially like? What did you eat yesterday?" "What kind of things do you like to do?"

Structure the interview so questions can be interspersed in a more general conversation that explores the teenager's likes and concerns. For example, a question such as "Will you be able to continue the swim team after the baby is born?" may help the nurse establish rapport, gain a better understanding of the teenager, and determine whether she is making plans for the future.

Cognitive Development

Determine the teenager's level of cognitive development and ability to absorb health counseling. The three most important areas of cognitive development are as follows:

1. Egocentrism (interest centered on the self), which involves the ability to defer personal satisfaction to respond to the needs of the infant: "What will you do when the baby gets sick?" "How will you help the baby get better?"
2. Present-future orientation, which involves the ability to make long-term plans: "What are your plans for finishing high school?" "What will you and the infant need in the first year of the infant's life?"
3. Abstract thinking, which involves identifying cause and effect: "Why is it important to keep clinic appointments?" "Why should condoms be used during sex even though you're pregnant?"

Knowledge of Infant Needs

Assess knowledge of infant needs and parenting skills. How does the teenager plan to feed the infant? (Nurses should encourage breast feeding. See Chapter 22.) What will she do when the infant cries? How will she know when the infant is ill and should be taken to a pediatrician? Does she know how much the infant should sleep? What plans have been made to provide for the safety needs of the infant?

Family Assessment

Begin assessment of the family unit by determining the degree of participation by the father of the infant. The father may deny responsibility for the pregnancy, be married to or plan to marry the expectant mother, participate in the pregnancy and rearing of the child without marriage, or be totally uninvolved.

Assessing the adolescent without the presence of her parents is important, yet it is crucial to determine the availability and amount of family support. Will the pregnant teenager live with her parents? How do her parents feel about the pregnancy? How will they incorporate the mother and her infant into the family?

Families generally respond in one of the following three ways:

1. A family member (often the adolescent's mother) assumes the mothering role, which the teenager may abdicate willingly.
2. All care and responsibilities are left to the adolescent mother, although shelter and food are provided.
3. The family shares care and responsibilities, which allows the teenager to grow in the mothering role while completing the developmental tasks of adolescence.

It is particularly important to assess the perceptions of the pregnant teenager's mother. How does she feel about becoming a grandmother? Many women feel embarrassed and disgraced. She may feel that she has "failed" as a mother, or she may resent the new cycle of child care in which the pregnancy involves her. Is communication with her daughter open? Is she aware of the difficult role conflict (as adolescent and mother) that her daughter will experience? Many pregnant adolescents live with their mothers, who provide various levels of support.

If the family is unable or unwilling to provide care for an adolescent with an infant, what other social support can be identified? In some situations, the family of the baby's father may be of assistance.

◆ Identification of Patient Problems

Many adolescents wait until the second or third trimester to seek prenatal care because they either do not realize they are pregnant, continue to deny they are pregnant, or want to hide the pregnancy. They may not know where to go for care and may fear the effects of pregnancy on their lives and relationships. In addition, many teenagers have little information about physiologic demands such as the increased need for nutrients that pregnancy imposes on their bodies. As a result, they may have a pattern of sporadic prenatal care and missed appointments. Many adolescents are unaware of ways to promote health during pregnancy and therefore need health teaching. Increased family stress as a result of inadequate coping strategies is another common problem.

◆ Planning: Expected Outcomes

The expected outcomes for the need for health teaching are as follows:

1. The expectant mother will keep prenatal appointments and follow health care instructions throughout pregnancy.

2. She will communicate her concerns throughout pregnancy and participate in learning about infant care.
3. The family will verbalize emotions and concerns and maintain functional support of the expectant mother and her infant.

◆ Interventions
Eliminating Barriers to Health Care

The two major barriers to health care are (1) scheduling conflicts and (2) negative attitudes of some health care workers. Help the adolescent locate the clinic closest to her that offers appointments when she (and her partner, if they wish) is available. Provide information about public transportation to that location, if necessary. Some clinics are open in the evening or on Saturday.

Communicating with adolescents requires special skills. Nurses should match their teaching with the teenager's cognitive development. Those who are 15 years old or younger need concrete explanations because their ability to understand abstract reasoning is not yet developed. Nurses should avoid seeming authoritarian because teens may see this behavior as interfering with their independence and may not return for care. When nurses work with adolescents as partners in care, adolescents are more likely to follow nursing recommendations.

Applying Teaching and Learning Principles

The lives of adolescents change greatly during pregnancy and even more after the infant is born. They often feel isolated from peers, who may not understand the responsibilities of parenthood. They no longer may be able to participate in activities with their friends because of child care obligations.

Teens often are hesitant to ask questions. Discuss concerns that are common to pregnant adolescents, and ask the pregnant teenager if she has other questions. Because peers are important to adolescents, arrange for them to participate in small groups with common concerns. Being with peers may make her feel more comfortable in asking questions and voicing concerns. Specific needs that might be addressed are the benefits of prenatal care or help in eliminating unhealthy habits such as smoking, drug use, or alcohol consumption. Find common goals that may be discussed in groups in which the teens can assist each other to have a healthier pregnancy. As pregnancy progresses, needs and group focus change and preparation for labor and delivery and infant care become priorities.

Repetition is an important method of teaching and clarifying misinformation. Allow ample time for discussions. Although teenagers often do not read or benefit from printed materials to the same degree that older parents do, material that is prepared with adolescents in mind may be helpful. Information regarding reliable Internet sites may be well received. Teens often respond well to audiovisual aids. Numerous well-made videos are available that deal with all aspects of prenatal and infant care.

It is particularly important that the nurse does not sound like a parent when working with adolescents. Avoid using the words "should" and "ought," offering unwanted advice, and making decisions for the teenagers. Maintain an open, friendly posture and convey empathy by using attending behaviors such as eye contact, frequent nodding, and leaning toward the speaker. Box 11.2 summarizes additional recommended methods for teaching adolescents.

Counseling

Allow time to counsel teenagers about their specific concerns such as nutrition, stress reduction, and infant care.

Nutrition. Nutrition counseling is one way to help reduce the incidence of low-birth-weight infants. Determine the adolescent's general nutritional status and assess for eating disorders that would reduce caloric intake and possibly affect fetal growth. Emphasize that she is still growing and her intake should be adequate for her own growth as well as that of the fetus. Ask if she prepares her own meals, if someone else prepares them, or if she eats away from home for most meals. Discuss nutrition during lactation, pointing out the advantages for both mother and baby.

Tailor information to suit the individual adolescent's likes and peer group habits. Teach her how to prepare simple meals and how to make the most nutritious selection from fast-food menus or select and plan for healthy snacks when she is away from home (see Chapter 8). Nutrition education should be socially and culturally appropriate.

Refer the teen to food stamp providers; the Special Supplemental Food Program for Women, Infants, and Children (WIC); surplus food distributors; and food banks, if necessary. Many teenagers have limited access to food and lack the ability to store or prepare it.

Self-Care. Provide the same teaching about self-care that would be given to an older woman. In addition, emphasize the importance of using a condom for prevention of STDs even though she is pregnant. Counsel the adolescent about lifestyle changes such as cessation of smoking or substance abuse, which will benefit her and the fetus, and refer her to resources that offer help with these problems.

Stress Reduction. Identify the stressors in the adolescent's life. Stress may be related to basic needs such as food, shelter, and health care. Fear of labor and delivery and fear of being single, alone, and unsupported all create stress. Meeting the

developmental tasks of adolescence while working on the tasks of pregnancy is another stressor.

A variety of measures may be used to reduce stress, depending on the teenager's age, situation, and available support. Refer adolescents with chronic life stress to a social worker for help to achieve stability. If the girl is very young or the pregnancy is a result of rape or incest, social services and law enforcement agencies should become involved to provide protection and assistance.

The pregnant teenager often experiences stress because she has not told her parents or the father of the infant about the pregnancy. Explore her reluctance to do this, and role-play the encounter with her to help her work out a plan for breaking the news. Although there is strain on the relationship when the teen first tells her parents, their relationship may improve over time if her parents are supportive. If appropriate, encourage her to tell the expectant father so that he can work out his role.

Teens who experience high levels of stress during pregnancy and the postpartum period may spend less time on infant care activities, feel less competent as parents, and have a more difficult time adjusting to being mothers compared with teens with lower levels of stress during pregnancy and postpartum. Therefore interventions to reduce stress in pregnant adolescents have an impact on the infant as well as the mother.

Help the teen think ahead to how her life will change because of the pregnancy and what may interfere with the mother role. Help her identify possible solutions to the problems presented. Assistance with resolving conflict with support persons and identifying new sources of support are other important interventions.

Attachment to the Fetus. Because attachment begins during pregnancy, helping the adolescent begin this process is important. Seeing the fetus move during an ultrasound often changes any pregnant woman's perceptions about the fetus. Hearing the fetal heartbeat and feeling the baby move may increase attachment. Looking at illustrations of the fetus at different gestational ages increases the mother's interest. A heightened awareness of the fetus may make her more likely to follow suggestions that will enhance fetal well-being. Discussion of the fetal changes month to month may lead to discussion of the capabilities and needs of the neonate.

Infant Care. The priorities for teaching gradually change from maternal needs to infant needs, with emphasis on infant care and normal growth and development. Discuss common early developmental changes to help the young mother understand the normal progression of infant abilities.

Explain and demonstrate infant cues (using behaviors of the infants in videos or in the group as examples) in terms of gaze, vocalization, facial expression, body position, and limb movement. Describe the way infants use these behaviors to "talk" without words and ways in which parents can use the behaviors to respond to their infants. Emphasize that eye contact, holding, cuddling, and verbal stimulation are important for the child's development.

Because adolescents tend to have a more rigid and punitive approach to child care, explain that infants develop a sense of trust when their needs are met promptly and gently. In addition, their future development depends on attaining a sense of trust during infancy. Emphasize that crying does not indicate that the infant is spoiled but simply that the infant has a need for food, warmth, or comfort and love.

If a support person will be involved in helping care for the infant, include that person in teaching, especially if the support person has limited experience with babies. Having a support person learn with her may help the teenager remember the information better.

Breastfeeding. Adolescents who decide to breastfeed their infants need support in their endeavor. They should be praised for their decision to do what is best for the baby. Adapt teaching to the mother's level of understanding. Encourage questions because the young mother may have much misinformation. Privacy is important to adolescents; they often feel embarrassed to breastfeed in front of others. Provide help with correct positioning and latching-on of the infant. Show her how to drape a blanket to cover her breast and the nursing infant.

Check on the mother frequently during feedings to identify any problems and intervene appropriately and in a timely manner. Discuss problems that may occur, so she has a realistic understanding of them and knows when and where to seek help, if necessary. Offer praise liberally. Success in the baby latching-on to the breast and seeing the infant gain weight may be very rewarding for the mother.

Promoting Family Support

The pregnant teenager needs encouragement to include her family in her decision making and problem solving. The involvement of her mother, older sister, or other close relative is particularly important in terms of future plans. Discuss topics such as who will care for the infant, whether the teenager will return to school, and what financial assistance is available from the family and the infant's father. Adolescent mothers who have adequate emotional support are more likely to learn appropriate parenting techniques.

However, if the family has multiple problems such as substance abuse or family violence, involving them may be inappropriate. In such situations, the teenager should be encouraged to communicate instead with a family friend or another trusted adult.

Providing Support during Labor

The needs of pregnant adolescents during labor are similar to those of the older woman. Nursing support at this time is especially important in helping them feel safe and cared for so they can have a successful childbirth experience.

Providing Referrals

Make referrals to conveniently located national and community resources for pregnant adolescents. Include well-baby clinics offered by the public health service and assistance programs offered by state social services agencies. Church and community organizations also may provide needed assistance. Childbirth education classes specifically for teenagers are often available.

Programs for school-age mothers are offered by many school districts and provide an opportunity to complete high school education and take the much-needed classes in childbearing and parenting. Some schools include pregnant adolescents in regular classes and add other classes to meet their special needs.

◆ Evaluation

Nursing care has been effective if the pregnant adolescent keeps prenatal appointments and participates actively in her plan of care, as demonstrated by asking questions, sharing concerns, and adhering to the recommended program of care. She should demonstrate basic knowledge of the infant's needs and care of the infant. Family support should be available, but if it is not, referrals to agencies that can provide assistance should be made.

> **KNOWLEDGE CHECK**
>
> 3. What methods are effective for teaching pregnant teenagers?
> 4. What should prospective teenage parents be taught about infant growth and development?

DELAYED PREGNANCY

It has become increasingly common for women to delay childbearing to further their careers, marry later, or establish financial security. However, delaying childbearing is not without risk. With advanced maternal age comes an increased risk for infertility (American College of Obstetricians and Gynecologist [ACOG], 2014). Although advances in contraception and fertility management have provided options to women who choose to delay childbearing and the ability to still conceive, there are physical and financial constraints they may face. A women's fertility begins to decline at 32 years of age, with the most significant decrease taking place at around 37 years of age (ACOG, 2014).

Maternal and Fetal Implications

Some of the risks associated with advanced maternal age aside from infertility include miscarriage, multiple gestations, and chromosome disorders such as Down's syndrome and aneuploidy (ACOG, 2014). Older mothers are also at an increased risk for preexisting chronic conditions such as hypertension, diabetes mellitus, and uterine myomas (fibroids). One should also consider the psychological implications that may come with infertility struggles. Women may experience a wide array of emotions such as depression, anxiety, and guilt for delaying childbearing (Kearney & White, 2016).

Advantages of Delayed Childbirth

Some significant advantages also are found with the delayed childbirth. Patients who have delayed childbirth tend to be

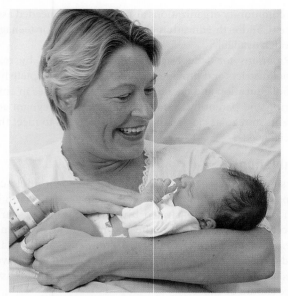

FIG. 11.2 Older primigravidas bring maturity and problem-solving skills to the maternal role, but they are at somewhat increased risk for physiologic problems related to pregnancy and birth.

more mature and of higher education and socioeconomic status. These traits result in them often being better equipped to deal with the emotional and financial demands of parenthood (Fig. 11.2)

Nursing Considerations

All women of advanced maternal age (older than 35 years at estimated day of birth) should receive honest and clear preconception education so a plan can be identified with their health care provider before trying to conceive. Chronic conditions should be treated before conception. Women should be counseled on all diagnostic tests available to detect chromosomal abnormalities early in the pregnancy so they can make educated decisions. For some women, these tests may result in the choice to terminate the pregnancy should an abnormality be detected. As a nurse it is important to recognize any bias regarding the patient's decision making, and remain nonjudgmental and respectful to the patient during this difficult time. Other women may choose to undergo genetic testing to make necessary arrangements should the child be affected with a disorder.

There are also emotional difficulties for the patient who has chosen to delay childbearing. The more mature patient may have had an imagined plan and picture of what pregnancy and parenthood should look like and may find it difficult to cope when things do not go exactly as planned. This new journey to motherhood may mean the patient has to give up or alter career plans. For the more accomplished patient this may be a difficult and unexpected transition. Nurses should be prepared to address both the physical and emotional needs of a patient experiencing delayed childbirth. Although these patients may have some unique needs throughout their

journey to motherhood, many go on to have healthy, enjoyable pregnancies.

Facilitating Expression of Emotions

Several days or weeks may pass between performance of some diagnostic studies and receipt of the results. This is a particularly difficult time for many expectant parents, and nurses often assist the couple to express their concerns and emotions.

A broad statement such as "Many couples find it difficult to wait for the results" will often elicit free expression of the parents' feelings. Follow-up questions such as "What concerns you most?" may reveal anxiety about the procedure itself or about the possible effects of the procedure on the fetus. Simply acknowledging that it is a stressful time helps the couple cope with their emotions.

Women who have undergone many tests and procedures for infertility may be especially anxious. Once pregnancy is achieved, they worry about their ability to carry the fetus to term and may see themselves as being at higher risk than they actually are. If they have had unsuccessful pregnancies in the past, the fear that the present pregnancy may also be lost makes it hard for them to be optimistic about success.

Mature gravidas also worry about complications that may affect the fetus or their own health. They are aware that they may not have another opportunity for pregnancy because of their age. They may be concerned about their ability to balance their careers with increased family responsibilities.

Providing Parenting Information

Nurses often help the mature mother prepare for effective parenting by pointing out her individual strengths and advantages. Anticipatory guidance about measures that will help conserve energy after childbirth is very useful. These include meal planning and setting realistic housekeeping goals. In addition, many older mothers need to mobilize all available support so they can reserve their energy for care of the infant.

When giving suggestions about conserving energy and obtaining support, avoid using terms like "elderly primipara" when referring to the expectant mother. It is important not to make her feel abnormal because of her age. Unless she has complications, she should know that her prenatal course will be the same as that for any other pregnant woman.

During the first weeks after childbirth the mother may experience feelings of social isolation, particularly if her friends have children who are much older. She may miss the mental stimulation of a job while staying at home. If she elects to return to work, she is likely to experience guilt and grief because she must leave her infant. Balancing the needs of the infant and the challenges of a career or occupation may be difficult.

Older mothers are likely to seek information they need from a variety of sources. They are particularly interested in learning how the infant grows and develops and what they can do to provide nurturing care for the infant. Meeting other older expectant parents in classes may provide friendships that can continue after the birth and help women provide support for each other. Play groups are another source of support where mothers can compare notes on parenting.

Older parents may interview care providers before choosing one. They may have special concerns and ask many questions. They often adopt health-promoting activities such as improving nutrition and eliminating harmful substances. Printed materials that can be used to reinforce teaching are often helpful.

> **❓ KNOWLEDGE CHECK**
>
> 5. What special resources do mature gravidas often have?
> 6. Why is it important to offer prenatal testing to the mature gravida?
> 7. What anticipatory guidance should the nurse provide the older mother for the first weeks at home after childbirth?

SUBSTANCE ABUSE

Chemical dependence is the physical and psychological dependence on a substance such as alcohol, tobacco, or drugs, either legal or illicit. When present during pregnancy, it can pose serious risk to both the mother and infant.

Incidence

Data have shown that approximately 5.9% of women use illicit drugs during pregnancy, 8.5% use alcohol, and 15.9% smoke cigarettes (DHHS, 2013). Over the last decade, the number of women abusing prescription opiates and heroin increased dramatically, thus necessitating that increased attention and resources be spent on this significant issue that affects a vulnerable population (Cleveland, 2016).

Maternal and Fetal Effects

When a pregnant woman uses a substance by drinking, smoking, snorting, or injecting it, the fetus experiences the same systemic effects as the expectant mother but often more severely and for a longer time. Because the fetus is unable to metabolize drugs efficiently, a drug that causes intoxication in the woman causes it for prolonged periods in the fetus. Therefore substances taken by the woman can have a great impact on the fetus and interfere with normal fetal development and health.

Maternal, fetal, and neonatal effects of commonly abused substances are summarized in Table 11.2.

Tobacco

Tobacco is one of the most common harmful substances used by women in pregnancy (Passey, Sanson-Fisher, D'Este,

TABLE 11.2   Maternal and Fetal or Neonatal Effects of Commonly Abused Substances

Substance	Maternal Effects	Fetal or Neonatal Effects
Caffeine (coffee, tea, cola, chocolate, cold remedies, analgesics)	Stimulates CNS and cardiac function, causes vasoconstriction and mild diuresis, half-life triples during pregnancy	Crosses placental barrier and stimulates fetus; teratogenic effects are undocumented
Tobacco	Decreased placental perfusion, abruptio placentae, anemia, PROM, preterm labor, spontaneous abortion	Prematurity, LBW, neurodevelopmental problems, increased incidence of SIDS, perinatal mortality
Alcohol (beer, wine, mixed drinks, after-dinner drinks)	Spontaneous abortion, abruptio placentae	Fetal demise, FGR, fetal alcohol spectrum disorders, FAS (facial and cranial anomalies, developmental delay, cognitive impairment, short attention span)
Marijuana ("pot" or "grass")	Often used with other drugs: tobacco, alcohol, cocaine; exact effects undetermined	Unclear; more study needed; may be related to problems in motor development; increased risk for anomalies or mortality unproven
Cocaine ("crack")	Hyperarousal state, euphoria, generalized vasoconstriction, hypertension, tachycardia, STDs, spontaneous abortion, abruptio placentae, preeclampsia, PROM, preterm labor, precipitous delivery	Fetal hypoxia, tachycardia, meconium staining, stillbirth, prematurity, irritability, sleep followed by agitation, poor response to comforting or interaction, possible attention and language problems
Amphetamines and methamphetamines ("speed," "crystal," "glass," "ice," "ecstasy")	Malnutrition, vasoconstriction, tachycardia, hypertension, spontaneous abortion, preterm labor, abruptio placentae, preeclampsia, retroplacental hemorrhage	Increased risk for FGR, prematurity, abnormal sleep patterns, agitation, poor feeding, vomiting
Opioids (heroin, methadone, morphine)	Malnutrition, anemia, increased incidence of STDs, HIV exposure, hepatitis, thrombosis, cardiac disease, spontaneous abortion, preterm labor	FGR, LBW, NAS, perinatal asphyxia, meconium aspiration syndrome, fetal or neonatal death, SIDS, child abuse and neglect; long-term developmental effects unclear
Antidepressants such as selective serotonin reuptake inhibitors	Relief of anxiety and depression, risk for anomalies with paroxetine, small risk for anomalies with other antidepressants	Transient respiratory problems, irritability, poor tone, persistent pulmonary hypertension

CNS, Central nervous system; *FAS,* fetal alcohol syndrome; *FGR,* fetal growth restriction; *HIV,* human immunodeficiency virus; *LBW,* low birth weight; *NAS,* neonatal abstinence syndrome; *PROM,* premature rupture of membranes; *SIDS,* sudden infant death syndrome; *STDs,* sexually transmitted diseases.

& Stirling, 2014). Tobacco is very addictive and harmful to the developing fetus in several ways. Nicotine causes vasoconstriction and reduces placental blood circulation. Carbon monoxide inactivates fetal and maternal hemoglobin. This combination significantly reduces the amount of oxygen that goes to the baby (ACOG, 2013).

Maternal and Fetal Effects. Some maternal effects of cigarette smoking include decreased appetite, poor weight gain, and poor nutritional status.

Neonatal Effects. Neonatal effects include risk for low birth weight, increased risk for sudden infant death syndrome (SIDS), and increased risk for colic, asthma, and childhood obesity (ACOG, 2013).

Alcohol

Alcohol is a teratogen known to have the potential to cause both mental delays and birth defects in the developing fetus. The amount and timing of alcohol ingested have a direct impact on the degree of impact to the fetus. Although alcohol intake during the first trimester appears to have the largest negative impact on cell growth and division, alcohol use during any point in the pregnancy can have harmful effects on the fetus. Studies have shown that compared with other harmful substances in pregnancy, alcohol causes the most significant harm and long-term impact (Bingham, 2015).

Maternal and Fetal Effects. The use of alcohol in pregnancy can increase the risk for miscarriage (Bingham, 2015) and the risk for preterm labor.

Neonatal Effects. Alcohol crosses the placenta and reaches the fetal liver; however, the fetal liver is unable to metabolize alcohol (ACOG, 2013). The teratogenic impacts of alcohol can lead to fetal alcohol spectrum disorders, the most severe of which is fetal alcohol syndrome (ACOG, 2013). Fetal alcohol syndrome is characterized by three distinct features: prenatal and postnatal growth restriction, central nervous system (CNS) impairment, and an identifiable grouping of facial features. Growth restriction is evident in length, weight, and head circumference. CNS deficits include intellectual incapacities, learning disabilities, attention deficit disorder, and reduced short-term memory. Facial features frequently associated with fetal alcohol syndrome include microcephaly, short palpebral fissures (the openings between the eyelids), epicanthal folds, flat midface with a low nasal bridge, indistinct philtrum (groove between the nose and upper lip), and a thin upper lip. Although not all infants exposed to alcohol during pregnancy will have signs or symptoms of fetal alcohol syndrome, it's important to educate patients that there is no safe level of alcohol during pregnancy.

Marijuana

Recent studies have shown that as many as 10% of women have used marijuana during pregnancy (Roth, Satran, & Smith, 2015).

Maternal and Fetal Effects. Consumed in large doses, marijuana can cause anxiety, tachycardia, confusion, panic, and hallucinations (Roth et al., 2015). When consumed in small amounts, marijuana increases sympathetic nervous system

stimulation and decreases parasympathetic stimulation, which in turn causes tachycardia and increased cardiac output (Roth et al., 2015).

Neonatal Effects. There is little definitive research to show the absolute impact of marijuana use to the fetus; however, preliminary studies show that marijuana use can lead to cognitive, behavioral, and emotional deficits in the infant as well as memory and problem-solving issues (Roth et al., 2015).

Cocaine

Cocaine is a powerful short-acting CNS stimulant. It blocks the reuptake of the neurotransmitters *norepinephrine* and *dopamine* at the nerve terminals, producing a hyperarousal state that results in euphoria, sexual excitement, increased alertness, and a heightened sense of well-being. Physical effects of cocaine use are related to cardiovascular stimulation and vasoconstriction. Hypertension, tachycardia, arrhythmias, tremors, anemia, anorexia, and even death to both the mother and/or fetus can occur.

When the initial euphoria wears off, a period of irritability, exhaustion, lethargy, depression, and anxiety occurs. This state elicits a strong desire for additional cocaine so that the initial feelings can be recaptured.

Maternal and Fetal Effects. Because many women who use cocaine also use other drugs, such as alcohol, tranquilizers, heroin, or marijuana, to "come down" from the hyperarousal state that cocaine produces, it is difficult to define the exact effects of cocaine on the fetus. Women who abuse cocaine are less likely to seek prenatal care or eat a diet that contains adequate nutrition. Sex may be exchanged for drugs, increasing the risk for STDs.

Because of the vasoconstriction of placental vessels caused by cocaine use, placental abruption is a known risk. Cocaine also stimulates uterine contractions, resulting in increased incidence of spontaneous abortion, premature rupture of membranes, preterm labor, and precipitous delivery.

Neonatal Effects. Maternal cocaine use puts the infant at risk for preterm birth, preterm rupture of the membranes, intrauterine growth restriction and low birth weight (Wisner, Sit, Bogen, Altemus, Pearlstein, Svikis, Misra, & Miller, 2017).

Bath Salts

A new class of drugs known as psychoactive bath salts have become increasing popular in recent years, and like other illegal drugs pose a significant threat to both mothers and babies. Bath salts are synthetic cathinones or methcathinones that come from the khat plant (Gray & Holland, 2014). Bath salts can come in their pure form or be mixed with other drugs and can be taken in pill form, smoked, or snorted (Gray & Holland, 2014). When ingested, bath salts induce feelings of euphoria, increased alertness, decreased need for sleep, hallucinations, agitation, and delusions (Gray & Holland, 2014). They have also been shown to cause tachycardia, hypertension, stroke, and acute myocardial infarction (Gray & Holland, 2014). Although little is known of their exact effect on pregnancy, the serious maternal impact can lead one to infer that they would be harmful to a developing fetus. There is also evidence that the khat plant increases blood pressure, gastric reflux, and constipation, which can all cause issues in pregnancy (Gray & Holland, 2014).

Amphetamines and Methamphetamines

Amphetamines and methamphetamines are CNS stimulants that when taken leave users with the feeling of immense pleasure.

Maternal and Fetal Effects. Amphetamine and methamphetamine use in pregnancy causes increases in blood pressure and an increased risk for placental abruption. It also has the potential to cause impaired brain development, delayed motor development, and delayed white matter maturation in the developing fetus (Chang, Oishi, & Skranes, 2016).

Neonatal Effects. Infants exposed to amphetamines or methamphetamines frequently exhibit signs of neonatal abstinence syndrome such as poor feeding and sucking reflexes, jitteriness, irritability and high-pitched cry (ACOG, 2016).

Antidepressants

Antidepressants such as selective serotonin reuptake inhibitors (SSRIs) are frequently prescribed during pregnancy for women with depression and anxiety. Although negative side effects and risk to the baby can occur when taking these medications, in many cases the benefits and safety to the mother outweigh the risk.

Maternal, Fetal, and Neonatal Effects. SSRIs can cause thrombocytopenia and persistent pulmonary hypertension in newborns (Roth, Hering, & Campos, 2015).

Opiates

Opiates include drugs such as morphine, methadone, meperidine (Demerol), oxycodone (OxyContin), hydromorphone hydrochloride (Dilaudid), and heroin. Many opiates are frequently used and prescribed by physicians to treat chronic pain; however, they are very addictive. Heroin is the most frequently abused drug in pregnancy because it is easy to obtain and is cheap (McKeever, Spaeth-Brayton, & Sheerin, 2014). Heroin rapidly crosses the placenta (within 1 hour), leading to quick exposure to baby (McKeever et al., 2014). Opiates are CNS depressants, and they generally leave individuals experiencing feelings of drowsiness, mental dullness, and stupor. Heroin acts as an appetite suppressant, and patients abusing it should be evaluated for poor nutritional intake and inadequate weight gain during pregnancy. These patients also should be tested for STDs, especially human immunodeficiency virus (HIV) infection because of the increased risk noted when sharing needles (McKeever et al., 2014). Pregnant women who abuse opiates have an increased risk for developing chorioamnionitis, cellulitis, and endocarditis (McKeever et al., 2014).

Maternal and Fetal Effects. With opiate use there is an increased incidence of placental abruption, intrauterine growth restriction, preterm labor, and fetal death (ACOG, 2016). Because of the addictive nature of opiates such as

heroin, patients will typically alternate between periods of overdose and periods of withdrawal. These episodes expose the neonate to intermittent hypoxia, which increases the risk for meconium aspiration syndrome. Heroin use can lead to maternal kidney and liver disease, heart and lung infections, and severe respiratory distress (March of Dimes, 2016). As a result of the highly addictive nature of heroin and other opiates, these medications cannot be immediately stopped. The sudden discontinuation of heroin can cause dangerous complications for both mother and baby, the most serious of which is death (March of Dimes, 2016).

Neonatal Effects. Opiates such as heroin frequently cause neonatal abstinence syndrome. These infants can experience seizures, birth defects, and dysfunctions in brain organization (Artigas, 2014).

Diagnosis and Management of Substance Abuse

It is not uncommon for women with substance abuse disorders to obtain prenatal care late in their pregnancy, if at all (ACOG, 2016). The woman may fear that the baby will be taken away if a health care provider finds out she has a substance abuse disorder. Statistics show that mental illness often accompanies substance abuse disorders in pregnancy (McKeever et al., 2014). For these reasons, it is important for nurses to carefully assess their patients for any signs or symptoms of substance abuse and/or mental illness and report their findings to the proper members of the health care team so the patient can get access to needed care and treatment. In recent years there has been an increased push to reduce the numbers of prescribed opiates for both pregnant and nonpregnant patients and replace these medications with something safer and less addicting (Hunt & Hellwig, 2015). Women with opiate abuse may need to be treated with methadone or buprenorphine under the watchful care of a medical provider to safely wean off the drugs (March of Dimes, 2016). Methadone can be taken orally and is long acting, providing consistent blood levels to decrease the adverse fetal effects of wide swings in blood level found with heroin use. The daily dose can be gradually decreased to wean the woman off the drug. However, if the baby is born before the drug is discontinued, the newborn must withdraw from methadone after birth. Buprenorphine may be used instead of methadone. Although neonatal withdrawal still occurs, it is shorter and less severe than with methadone.

Ensuring the patient has access to treatment resources is important because research has shown that the greatest risk for substance abuse relapse is in the immediate postpartum period because patients think they no longer run the risk for causing harm to the baby (McKeever et al., 2014). Women who are actively seeking or receiving treatment should be strongly encouraged to hold and bond with their baby, and those who are not currently using drugs but are receiving methadone or buprenorphine can and should be encouraged to breastfeed (Cleveland, 2016). To reduce the number of women abusing drugs in pregnancy, some states have moved to pressing criminal charges against women found to have a substance abuse disorder in pregnancy; however, the Association of Women's Health, Obstetric and Neonatal

Nurses (AWHONN, 2015) opposes this action because it can impede women coming forward and admitting that they are abusing drugs out of fear of incarceration. The AWHONN recommends universal substance abuse screening for all patients, as well as priority to substance abuse treatment centers for those who are pregnant (AWHONN, 2015). Nurses should be able to identify patients who need help in relation to substance use and abuse and ensure the appropriate care for both the women and their babies.

> **? KNOWLEDGE CHECK**
>
> 8. How does smoking affect the neonate? What are the long-term effects on the child?
> 9. What problems are associated with fetal alcohol syndrome?
> 10. What are the effects of maternal cocaine use on the infant?
> 11. Why are women who use heroin encouraged to use methadone during pregnancy?

◆ APPLICATION OF THE NURSING PROCESS: MATERNAL SUBSTANCE ABUSE

Nursing care related to substance abuse may occur during the antepartum, intrapartum, or postpartum period.

ANTEPARTUM PERIOD

◆ Assessment

Polydrug abuse appears to be the most common substance abuse problem among women, and all women should be screened at the first prenatal visit for tobacco, alcohol, and other drug use. Because substance abuse occurs in all populations, the nurse should not make assumptions based on class, race, or economic status.

Certain behaviors are strongly associated with substance abuse: seeking prenatal care late in the pregnancy, failing to keep appointments, and following recommended regimens inconsistently.

> **! SAFETY CHECK**
>
> ### Signs of Possible Drug Use
>
> Seeking prenatal care late in pregnancy
> Failure to keep prenatal appointments
> Inconsistent follow-through with recommended care
> Poor grooming, inadequate weight gain
> Needle punctures, thrombosed veins, cellulitis
> Defensive or hostile reactions
> Anger or apathy regarding pregnancy
> Severe mood swings

Women who use drugs have low self-esteem. They are dealing with conflicting issues: the physical and psychological need for the substance, the need to deny that the substance is harming the fetus, and guilt that they may be

responsible for harming the fetus. Fear of prosecution for use of illegal drugs may prevent the woman from seeking prenatal care, increasing risk for the woman and her fetus. In addition, many women with substance abuse problems face discrimination and resentment from health care professionals who direct their frustration at the woman rather than the problem.

Given the powerful deterrents to self-disclosure, extensive history taking provides the best opportunity to determine current and past substance use. The nurse taking the health history should maintain a nonjudgmental attitude, exhibit patience and empathy, and display an attitude of concern for the woman and her infant.

Medical History

Determine whether the woman has medical conditions that are prevalent among women who use drugs—for example, seizures, hepatitis, cellulitis, STDs, hypertension, depression, and suicide attempts. Current problems may include insomnia, panic attacks, exhaustion, heart palpitations, depression, and suicidal ideation.

Obstetric History

Evaluate for past and current complications of pregnancy. Spontaneous abortions, premature deliveries, placental abruption, and stillbirths are associated with substance abuse. Current complications may include STIs, vaginal bleeding, and an inactive or hyperactive fetus. Fundal height may be inconsistent with gestational age, suggesting fetal growth restriction.

Investigate emotional responses such as anger or apathy regarding the pregnancy. These feelings are particularly significant during the latter half of the pregnancy, when the normal feelings of ambivalence are usually resolved. Negative feelings toward the pregnancy may interfere with prenatal compliance with recommended care.

History of Substance Abuse

Obtaining an accurate history of substance abuse is difficult and depends in large part on the way the health care worker approaches the woman. A sincere, nonjudgmental, and empathic approach promotes open exchange of information. (Suggestions for interviewing are given in Box 11.3.)

Ask about all forms of drug use, including cigarettes, e-cigarettes, over-the-counter drugs, prescription medications, alcohol, and illicit drugs. Examine patterns of drug use, which can range from occasional recreational use to weekly binges to daily dependence on a particular drug or group of drugs.

◆ Identification of Patient Problems

Some women acknowledge the use of harmful substances but do not fully understand the adverse effects. Other women are aware of the risks but are unable to stop using these substances. Common patient problems include lack of knowledge of the effects of substance abuse on self and fetus and inability to manage stress without the use of drugs. Both of these problems can result in the need for health teaching.

BOX 11.3 Techniques for Interviewing a Woman about Substance Abuse

To determine whether the woman abuses substances:

- Display an accepting and nonjudgmental attitude.
- Explain why it is important to know about substance abuse: "We need to know about anything that might affect you or your baby during the pregnancy."
- Let her know that the questions are asked of all pregnant women.
- Acknowledge that women may be reluctant to disclose information: "I know it's difficult to talk to us about this, but we need to know so that we can give you and your baby the best care possible."
- Begin with questions about over-the-counter or prescription drugs and lead up to use of tobacco, alcohol, and, finally, illicit drugs.
- Demonstrate knowledge of types and forms of drugs commonly used in the community: "Do you have friends who are using ecstasy?"

When substance abuse is acknowledged, the important points in the drug history include the following:

- The type of drug used
- The amount of drug used
- The frequency of use
- The time of last dose

Ask specific questions:

- How often have you taken over-the-counter medications?
- What drugs did you take last month? Were they prescribed?
- How many cigarettes do you smoke on a daily basis? Are there times when you smoke more?
- How many times a week do you drink alcoholic beverages (beer, wine, mixed drinks)?
- How many in a day? Are there times when you have more drinks?
- How often did you use [drug used] before becoming pregnant? How often do you use it now? Do you snort? Smoke crack? Shoot cocaine? How many lines do you use? How long do you stay high?

◆ Planning: Expected Outcomes

Expected outcomes are that the woman will do the following:

1. Identify the harmful effects of substances on herself and her infant.
2. Verbalize feelings related to continued use of harmful substances.
3. Identify personal strengths and accept resources offered by the health care delivery system to stop using drugs.

◆ Interventions

Effective interventions for substance abuse require the combined efforts of nurses, physicians, social workers, and numerous community and federal agencies. Nurses should realize that progress is slow and frustrating. The major priority is to protect the fetus and the expectant mother from the harmful effects of drugs.

Examining Attitudes

When working with pregnant women with substance abuse problems, nurses should identify their own knowledge level, feelings, and prejudices. They may have limited knowledge about perinatal substance abuse and negative attitudes toward mothers who abuse substances. Nurses may be angry at the woman who not only engages in self-destructive behavior but also may be inflicting harm on her fetus. Maintaining feelings of empathy or concern without becoming judgmental or even unknowingly punitive to the pregnant woman may be difficult. Nurses also may feel helpless and discouraged when the pregnant woman continues to abuse drugs despite the best efforts of the health care team.

In-service education, professional consultation, and peer support are all helpful for professionals working with pregnant women who abuse drugs. These processes can allow opportunities for discussion and sharing of feelings, problems, and particularly troublesome treatment issues.

Preventing Substance Abuse

Participate in campaigns to prevent substance abuse throughout the community. Provide accurate information in terms that patients can easily understand. Use posters, diagrams, pamphlets, and other visual aids to describe the effects of tobacco, alcohol, and other drugs on the fetus. Post visual aids in schools, supermarkets, shopping centers, and other areas where women of childbearing age will be exposed to them.

Focus on the benefits of remaining drug free, which include a decrease in maternal and neonatal complications. For example, the effects of smoking tobacco are dose related and cumulative, and nurses should encourage and support cessation at any point during pregnancy.

Women who use alcohol during pregnancy may not realize the effect on the fetus. Social drinkers will often stop drinking once they know about the dangers. Those with heavy alcohol use need counseling and referral for further treatment.

Communicating with the Woman

Ask the expectant mother about stressors in her life that may be contributing to her substance abuse. Additional stressors may include inadequate housing, economic predicaments, intimate partner violence, and emotional or physical illness.

Be honest at all times, while displaying a patient, nonjudgmental attitude and genuine interest and concern. This is especially important when the woman relapses into substance-abusing patterns. Allow her to express guilt, and reassure her that abstinence is possible and that she can and must begin again.

Helping the Woman Identify Strengths

Assist the pregnant woman with substance abuse problems in identifying personal strengths because she generally has a poor self-image. Acknowledge her actions when she abstains from drugs or alcohol for even a short time. Praise for maintaining an adequate weight gain and attending prenatal classes may increase her confidence and compliance with the recommended regimen of care.

Providing Ongoing Care

At each antepartum visit, consider the current status of substance use, social service needs, education needs, and compliance with treatment referrals. Address current drug use because women may change their pattern of drug use during pregnancy. For example, they may stop using cocaine but may increase their use of heroin or alcohol.

Verify compliance with recommended treatment regimens such as antepartum clinics and chemical-dependence referral programs. Coordinate care among various service providers such as group therapy and prenatal classes. Establish communication with all agencies that provide care, and facilitate communication that helps the woman with a chaotic lifestyle meet treatment objectives.

Provide continuing prenatal education about the anatomy and physiology of pregnancy and consequences of prenatal substance abuse. Describe how the newborn benefits when the mother abstains from using drugs, including tobacco and alcohol. Drug screens will be performed periodically throughout the pregnancy. Praise any attempts at abstinence and encourage the expectant mother to try again if she relapses.

Assess signs of maternal attachment to the fetus, because it may help her reduce or eliminate her substance use. Fetal movement often increases the woman's awareness of the fetus and may lead to a discussion about her plans for the infant and changes in her life that have occurred and will occur. Help her make realistic plans for care of the baby. Include support persons if possible.

When the woman's partner abuses substances, she is more likely to continue to use them or to stop during the pregnancy but start again after birth. Explain to the partner the importance of avoiding use for both members of the couple to enhance the outcome of the pregnancy and avoid exposure of children to the adverse effects of substances.

When women use substances during pregnancy, child welfare services may be involved to ensure the safety of the infant after discharge. The infant may become a ward of the courts and be placed in foster care until the mother can show she is in rehabilitation. Use therapeutic communication techniques to help the mother express her feelings about this loss. Help her make plans for implementing changes that will allow her to be with her infant.

◆ Evaluation

Interventions have been successful if the expectant mother identifies the harmful effects of substance abuse on herself and on the fetus, discusses her strengths and her feelings about continued use of substances, and is receptive to assistance to stop using drugs.

INTRAPARTUM PERIOD

◆ Assessment

Nurses who work in labor and delivery units should become skilled at identifying drug-induced signs and symptoms.

Cocaine

Behaviors associated with frequent or recent use of cocaine include profuse sweating, hypertension, tachycardia, and irregular respirations combined with a lethargic response to labor and apparent lack of interest in the necessary interventions. Additional signs include dilated pupils, increased body temperature, and sudden onset of severely painful contractions. Fetal signs often include tachycardia and excessive fetal activity. Fetal bradycardia and late decelerations may occur.

Emotional signs of recent cocaine use may include angry, caustic, or abusive reactions to those attempting to provide care. Emotional lability and paranoia are signs of cocaine intoxication.

Heroin

Typically, the pregnant woman dependent on heroin comes to the labor and delivery unit intoxicated from recent drug use. When the effects of the drug begin to wear off, withdrawal symptoms may be observed. These include yawning, diaphoresis, rhinorrhea, restlessness, excessive tearing of the eyes, nausea, vomiting, and abdominal cramping.

◆ Identification of Patient Problems

One of the most immediate patient problems during the intrapartum period is potential injury of the mother, fetus, and newborn because of physiologic and psychological effects of recent drug use.

◆ Planning: Expected Outcomes

The major goal or expected outcome for this patient problem is that the woman and the fetus will remain free from injury during labor and childbirth.

◆ Interventions

Preventing Injury

When a laboring woman has recently used a substance, the nurse should intervene to meet the needs of the woman and the fetus for safety, oxygen, and comfort.

Admitting Procedure. Two nurses may be needed to admit the woman into the labor unit and to persuade her to assume a safe position. One nurse helps the woman into bed, initiates electronic fetal monitoring, and begins administration of oxygen, as needed. The other nurse acts as the communicator.

Because the woman who has recently used a drug may have difficulty following directions, she should hear only one voice telling her what to do. This nurse states firmly what is happening and exactly what the woman should do: "Lie on your left side." "This helps us watch how the baby is doing." "This gives you more oxygen." Maintain eye contact with the woman while giving her instructions.

Setting Limits. It is essential to set limits to protect the safety of the mother and the fetus. For instance, the mother cannot smoke. The nurse may say, "It's difficult not to smoke, but there is real danger to everyone if you smoke when oxygen is being used." The mother who must remain in bed may become agitated. The nurse may say, "I know it's hard to stay in bed, but we can't take good care of the baby when you walk." If walking is safe for the woman, the nurse should set limits about where she can walk (in the labor room, not to the cafeteria).

Initiating Seizure Precautions. The laboring woman who recently used cocaine is at risk for seizures. Take the following seizure precautions:

- Keep the bed in a low, locked position.
- Pad the side rails, and keep them up at all times.
- Check the oxygen and oxygen administration equipment.
- Make sure that the suction equipment functions properly to prevent aspiration.
- Reduce environmental stimuli (lights, noise) as much as possible.

Maintaining Effective Communication

Establishing a therapeutic pattern of communication is essential. Avoid confrontation. Instead, acknowledge feelings: "I know you hurt and are frightened. I'll do everything I can to make you comfortable." When the woman is abusive, be careful not to take the abuse personally or react in a defensive manner.

Examine your own feelings when women are abusive and acknowledge when anger is getting in the way of providing care. Another nurse may need to assume care of the woman for a time to allow some relief from being the target of unrelenting abusive comments or actions.

Providing Pain Control

Pain control for women who are substance abusers poses a difficult problem because it is often impossible to determine the type or combination of drugs that were used before admission. If pain medication can be administered safely, do not withhold it under the false assumption that the woman does not need it or that medication will contribute to her chemical dependence. Include nonpharmacologic comfort measures such as sacral pressure, back rubs, a cool cloth on the forehead, and continual support and encouragement as for any other woman in labor.

Preventing Heroin Withdrawal

To prevent heroin withdrawal during labor, give as ordered to the woman who usually receives it at a chemical-dependence center if she did not receive her daily dose. Administer it intramuscularly if the woman is nauseated or vomiting. It is important to avoid the use of opioid agonist-antagonist drugs such as butorphanol (Stadol) and nalbuphine (Nubain) in women who are opiate dependent because acute withdrawal signs and symptoms will occur in the woman and the fetus.

◆ Evaluation

Both the expectant mother and the fetus may have experienced the harmful effects of drugs throughout pregnancy. However, the interventions for this patient problem can be considered effective if neither the woman nor the fetus sustains additional injury during labor and childbirth.

POSTPARTUM PERIOD

During the postpartum period, nursing care is focused on helping the mother with bonding, providing infant care, and planning to provide care of herself and the infant after discharge. Observe for signs of recent drug use and continue to assess the vital signs and level of consciousness of the mother.

Observe the mother–infant interaction so that bonding and attachment can be promoted. This is a major concern at this time. Encourage the woman to continue her efforts to stop taking substances. Women who stop or reduce use during pregnancy may return to using at previous levels after pregnancy and need support to continue abstinence. Referral to social services and child protective agencies may be necessary for the follow-up care of the mother and the infant.

KNOWLEDGE CHECK

12. What prenatal behaviors may indicate substance abuse?
13. What signs and symptoms indicate recent cocaine use?
14. How does nursing care differ during the intrapartum period when the woman has recently taken illicit drugs?

BIRTH OF AN INFANT WITH CONGENITAL ANOMALIES

Even when everything goes according to plan, childbirth is a time of stress for parents. Their anxiety about the condition of the infant is obvious as they carefully trace the features and count the fingers and toes of their newborn. When the infant is not perfect but is born with anomalies, the parents are often overwhelmed with shock and grief. What may appear to be a minor defect to health care workers may seem a severe impairment to parents (Gardner & Carter, 2016). Nurses have an opportunity to help the family adjust and cope with their feelings.

Factors Influencing Emotional Responses of Parents

Timing and Manner of Being Told

At one time, common practice was to remove the infant from the delivery area before parents could see a congenital anomaly and to tell them about it later. This practice changed, however, when it was realized that parents experienced less stress if they were told at once and were permitted to hold their baby if the physical status of the infant allowed. The manner of presenting information also changed. Physicians and nurses became aware of the importance of helping the parents accept and bond with the newborn.

Prior Knowledge of the Defect

Although ultrasonography does not identify all fetal anomalies, many parents become aware of congenital anomalies during ultrasound examinations performed during pregnancy. These parents have time for anticipatory grieving before the birth. They may not demonstrate the shock and disbelief at the birth that are seen in parents who are unprepared. Their reactions should not be interpreted to mean that they do not experience grief but rather that they have completed some of the early phases of grieving before the birth. Their grief is real and profound, even though it is expressed differently.

One couple was aware from 18 weeks of gestation that the fetus had hydrocephalus and protrusion of brain tissue from the skull. The mother elected to carry the fetus to term so that the infant would have "every chance at life." When the infant died within minutes after birth, the parents calmly held their child and called the infant by the name they had selected several weeks previously. The only overt signs of grief were silent tears and a request to see their clergy.

Once the anomaly is discovered by ultrasound, the pregnancy is no longer seen as normal and the focus may be on specialized care for the mother in preparation for the birth. Parents may feel isolated from those with normal pregnancies. Some parents seek information from parents who have a child with a similar anomaly. The full extent of the problem may not be known until after the birth. There may be a long period of worry and fear between the ultrasound diagnosis and the birth.

Type of Defect

Although any defect in a newborn produces extreme concern and anxiety, certain defects are associated with long-term parenting problems. Accepting an infant with facial or genital anomalies is particularly difficult for the family and the community.

The face is visible to everyone, and parents are fearful about whether the child will be accepted. If the defect is cleft lip and palate, the parents are concerned about surgical repair. They are often anxious about how grandparents and siblings will accept the child. With time and support, parents often work out unique methods to help the family develop strong feelings of attachment.

Gender is at the core of a person's identity, and any defect of the genitals, however slight or correctable, arouses deep concern in both parents. Some anomalies such as hypospadias (opening of the urethra on the underside of the penis) are repaired in early childhood. Other genital anomalies such as ambiguous genitalia (when assignment of gender is in doubt) cause extreme concern in the family and affect such basic issues as what to name the infant, how to dress the infant, and how to respond to questions about the infant's gender.

Irreparable Defect

Although the initial impact of any defect is profound disappointment and concern, when the defect is irreparable, the parents must grapple with the knowledge that the infant will have a lifelong disability. Examples of irreparable defects include Down's syndrome, microcephaly, and amelia (absence of an entire limb).

Grief and Mourning

Grief describes the emotional response to loss. Mourning is the process of going through the phases of grief until the loss can be accepted and resolved. Birth of an infant with an anomaly evokes a grief response. The family must mourn the loss of the perfect infant they imagined during pregnancy. They must detach from and mourn the fantasy baby to be able to attach to the actual infant (Gardner & Carter, 2016). Early emotions include denial, anger, and guilt.

Denial and disbelief are the initial reactions of most parents to the birth of an infant with a congenital defect. "How could this happen?" Anger is often a pervasive response and may take the form of fault-finding or resentment. Anger may be directed toward the family, the medical personnel, or the self, but it is seldom directed toward the infant. Guilt may be expressed as a question of responsibility for the defect as many parents search for a cause: "I shouldn't have worked so much while I was pregnant."

Other emotions include fear, which may be expressed as concern about what must be done in the immediate or distant future (surgical procedures, complicated care, the infant's potential for a normal life). Sadness and depression, manifested by crying, withdrawal from relationships, lack of energy, inability to sleep, and decreased appetite, may precede acceptance and resolution. Gradually—often after a prolonged time—the feelings of sadness abate and the family is able to adapt to the loss and resolve its grief.

> ### ❓ KNOWLEDGE CHECK
>
> 15. When should parents be told that the infant has anomalies?
> 16. What types of defects most affect parenting?
> 17. How can the reaction of parents to birth anomalies be described?

Nursing Considerations
Assisting with the Grieving Process

Whenever possible, both parents should be present when they are told about the infant's condition. The nurse should use therapeutic communication techniques to help them discuss their feelings and fears. They should be given as much information as possible about the anomaly before the birth. If the infant will go to the neonatal intensive care unit (NICU), a tour before the birth may help them understand the type of care their infant will receive.

At birth, the parents continue to grieve the loss of the perfect infant they expected and form an attachment with this newborn. Whether the parents learned about the problem before or after the birth, it is helpful if the nurse remains with them as they go through the initial phase of shock and disbelief. The nurse maintains an atmosphere that encourages them to express their feelings by listening carefully to what the parents say and reflecting the content and feelings they express.

For example, the mother of an infant girl with cleft palate says, "How could this happen? I should have gone to the doctor earlier." A helpful response might be, "It sounds like you feel responsible for this problem. Actually, we don't know the exact causes of cleft palate, but let's talk about how you are feeling." This offers reassurance but keeps the interaction open to explore the underlying feelings of guilt the mother may be expressing.

Nurses should recognize that grief responses vary among individuals, and cultural and religious beliefs affect the expression of grief. Members of some groups express grief

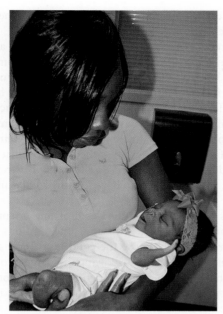

FIG. 11.3 Touching and cuddling by a mother whose infant has a congenital anomaly fosters attachment and helps them cope with the grieving process. This infant has anomalies of the hand and arm. (Courtesy Cheryl Briggs, RNC, Annapolis, MD).

openly by crying, becoming angry, or seeking comfort from a support group. Those in other cultures (e.g., Asian and Native American) may appear stoic and may not reveal the depths of their grief. In some cultures (such as Hispanic), it is acceptable for women, but not for men, to grieve publicly. The couple should be offered a private room, if possible. The infant should be examined in front of the parents so that they can ask questions. Information about normal needs of the newborn should be given at the same time as information about the anomaly.

Promoting Bonding and Attachment

A priority nursing intervention is to promote bonding and attachment, which may be disrupted when the infant is born with an abnormality. The process is facilitated when the nurse communicates acceptance of the infant.

To promote bonding, the nurse handles the newborn gently and presents the infant as someone precious. Parents are particularly sensitive to facial expressions of shock or distress. The infant should be called by name. Many nurses emphasize the normal aspects of the infant's body: "She's so alert, and she has beautiful eyes." Perhaps it is most important to help the parents hold their infant as soon as possible. Touching and cuddling are essential to caring (Fig. 11.3).

Providing Accurate Information

Nurses who work in perinatal settings should be aware of follow-up treatment and timing of surgical procedures for common anomalies so they can clarify and reinforce the information provided by the physician. This involves discussing the plan of care with the physician as well as researching the nursing care that will be required. Parents develop trust in the health care team when consistent information is presented clearly and explained fully.

If possible, one primary nurse or a team of nurses should work with the family throughout the hospital stay. The nurse should assess the parents' understanding of the condition and the treatment plan. Parents often need information repeated frequently because it is difficult for them to absorb all they are told at this time of intense emotions.

Facilitating Communication

Nurses are sometimes fearful of being asked questions they are unable to answer, or they fear they will say the wrong thing.

The most helpful course of action is to answer questions as honestly as possible. If uncertain about information, say so: "I'm not sure about that, but I'll find out for you." In addition to answers, parents need kindness, support, and genuine concern.

It is crucial that family members communicate with one another as well as with the health care professionals. Information and empathy should be offered consistently to both parents. Fathers should be included in all discussions, demonstrations, and care of the infant. Without this attention, the father cannot be expected to support his partner, explain the infant's condition to relatives and friends, or cope with his own shock and sadness.

The nurse should assess the mother for signs of postpartum depression. The support person should be made aware of the mother's increased risk for prolonged depression. The signs of depression and the differences among normal "baby blues," normal grieving, and postpartum depression should be explained.

Participating in Infant Care

Parents should be involved in giving care to the infant as soon as possible to increase bonding and help them feel they can be real parents to the infant. Providing care for the infant also helps reduce parental anxiety as they get to know their baby (Ballard, 2015).

Planning for Discharge

Teach parents the special feeding, holding, and positioning techniques that their infant needs. Early participation in infant care fosters feelings of attachment and responsibility for the infant as well as increasing feelings of confidence. They should also know what type of follow-up care with the health care provider is necessary and what other services may be needed.

Provide other anticipatory guidance that may help prevent problems when the infant is discharged. The reaction and behavior of siblings depend on their ages and abilities to understand the needs of the infant. Young children, who are often jealous of the attention and care the infant requires, may regress to infantile behaviors such as bedwetting and thumb sucking. Remind parents that this indicates a need for attention rather than naughtiness.

Although grandparents can be a great source of strength and support, they also may have difficulty adjusting to the infant with an abnormality. When appropriate and if the parents are willing, include grandparents when teaching the special care the infant will need.

Providing Referrals

Initiate referrals to national and community resources, as needed. In addition to a referral to the social worker or grief counselor in the hospital, parents may also benefit from information about the Easter Seal Disability Services, the March of Dimes, or the disabled children's services of the public health department. In addition, organizations such as the Shriners provide funds for the care of children. Support groups vary among communities, and perinatal nurses may wish to provide a list of the names, addresses, and telephone numbers of these organizations.

KNOWLEDGE CHECK

18. How do nurses promote bonding in families of an infant with congenital anomalies?
19. What should be included in discharge planning for the family of an infant with congenital anomalies?

PERINATAL LOSS

Perinatal death can occur at any time. Early spontaneous abortion, ectopic pregnancy, fetal demise at any point in pregnancy, stillbirth, or neonatal death when the infant survives for a few days or weeks can be equally devastating for the parents. The death may occur after a complicated pregnancy or one in which all seemed well until the baby died. Parents may have a short time with their baby while it still lives or none at all.

Parents experiencing perinatal death often feel alone in their grief. Friends and family members may be hesitant to discuss the loss for fear of saying the wrong thing. They may be uncomfortable with the topic and change the subject when parents want to talk.

Early Pregnancy Loss

Early pregnancy loss from spontaneous abortion or ectopic pregnancy may precipitate intense grief in the parents. The parents may not yet have told family and friends about the pregnancy. Those who do know may minimize the grief that occurs at this time. Comments such as "You shouldn't have any problems getting pregnant again" discount the intensity of the parents' feelings. Frequently, the health care of a woman experiencing early pregnancy loss focuses on her physical needs with little attention given to the emotional needs of the woman and her family. In a small study of such women, Johnson and Langford (2015) found that bereavement interventions provided immediately after the pregnancy loss enhanced women's ability to cope.

Concurrent Death and Survival in Multifetal Pregnancy

Parents experience conflicting and complex feelings of joy and grief when one or more infants in a multifetal pregnancy live and one or more infants in the same gestation die. Parents

do not grieve less for the dead infant because of the joy they experience in the surviving child.

For parents experiencing survival of one infant and death of another, the grieving process may be more complicated. They may have fears about the health of the surviving infant, especially if the infant is preterm or ill. They may be unable to grieve for the dead child because of their concerns and responsibilities for the surviving child. They also may experience problems with attachment to the surviving infant because of grieving and fear that they will lose that infant as well. In addition, they may receive less support from others compared with parents who have lost their child in a single gestation.

Parents who experience the death of one infant and the survival of another need the same interventions as those offered for parents who lose the child in a single gestation. These interventions include allowing the parents to hold the dead infant and gathering mementos. In addition, nurses should be prepared to confirm the cause of death, if known, and the health status of the surviving infant.

Perinatal Palliative or Hospice Care Services

Some parents learn that the fetus has a condition that is terminal. They may choose to continue the pregnancy and deliver at term, knowing that the infant will survive only a short time. Perinatal palliative or hospice care services provide care by nurses experienced in hospice or palliative care. These nurses assist the family through the processes of birth, death, and grief. The emphasis of care is on promoting quality of life, minimizing suffering, and supporting parents in their grief. It allows parents to plan for the birth and death of their baby. They make choices about care and make memories that make their parenting more meaningful, even though it lasts only a short time (Limbo & Wool, 2016).

Previous Pregnancy Loss

Women who have experienced previous pregnancy losses, regardless of the gestational age at the time of the loss, often have higher levels of anxiety, grief, depression, and posttraumatic stress than women who have not experienced such loss (Hutti, Armstrong, Myers, & Hall, 2015).

Having other, healthy children does not reduce the degree of anxiety during a pregnancy that follows a perinatal loss. Parents may delay telling family and friends about the pregnancy until they feel confident about the outcome. They may not tell those who do not already know about the loss of the previous pregnancy. Some do not prepare the baby's room at all during the pregnancy. Others wait until near the end of pregnancy to make preparations to bring an infant into the home. Conflicting emotions of excitement, fear, and doubt occur as the pregnancy progresses normally.

Early prenatal care is especially important during a pregnancy after a loss. Both parents may be more comfortable with more frequent contact with the health care provider. Women tend to be extra careful to do what is recommended in pregnancy and hypervigilant about signs that might indicate something is wrong. Less fetal activity than usual is very worrying, and feeling the baby move is reassuring. They need frequent reassurance about the status of the fetus and emotional support throughout the pregnancy.

Although mothers may request extra diagnostic testing to help relieve their anxiety, they may not always feel as reassured by normal test results as they had hoped. It is important for nurses to provide an opportunity for these mothers to express their distress and fears. Referrals to support groups or mental health providers may be appropriate.

◆ APPLICATION OF THE NURSING PROCESS: PREGNANCY LOSS

◆ Assessment

Nursing assessment of the family that has experienced the loss of a fetus or infant requires sensitivity. Collect as much information as possible before meeting the woman and her family for the first time so that hurtful mistakes can be avoided. Knowing the child's gender, weight, length, gestational age, and whether any abnormalities were noted will help the nurse communicate effectively.

Many perinatal units design a sticker or symbol to place on the door and chart so that all staff who encounter the family will be alerted that the infant has not survived. This visual symbol diminishes the chance that an uninformed person will make inadvertent comments that cause pain.

Nurses are often unsure about how to interact with a family that has experienced the loss of an infant. It is helpful to acknowledge the situation and clarify the nurse's role at once: "I'm Dawn, and I'll be your nurse today. I'm so sorry for your loss. What can I do today that would be most helpful to you?" This is not an appropriate time for self-disclosure or for false reassurance. Keep the focus on the family's response and their ability to support one another.

Initial grief responses are similar to those expressed by parents of infants with anomalies. Crying and expressions of anger often occur during the woman's stay in the birth facility. Guilt is often an underlying feeling as the parents search for a reason for their child's death.

Nurses who provide home care or make follow-up telephone calls should be aware of subtle cues of grief such as sighing, excessive sleeping, apathy, poor hygiene, and loss of appetite. These signs are especially important when assessing members of cultural groups who do not display grief publicly. In addition, nurses should observe for signs of postpartum depression, posttraumatic stress disorder, and panic disorder, which may occur after perinatal loss.

Evaluate the availability of a support system that includes family members or faith leaders. Ask whether the family would like a spiritual advisor called. The family may want the infant baptized or blessed.

Assess the father's needs as well because they are sometimes perceived as needing less support than the mother. Fathers grieve differently from mothers. An acceptance of the differences in their grieving style, tolerance, and respect for each other may enable couples to strengthen their relationship during this experience (Avelin, Rådestad, Säflund, Wredling, & Erlandsson, 2013).

◆ Identification of Patient Problems

Perinatal loss affects the entire family. Many families experience changes in their relationships and family processes because of grief.

◆ Planning: Expected Outcomes

Expected outcomes for changes in family processes are that the parents will do the following:
1. Acknowledge their grief and express the meaning of the loss.
2. Share their grief with significant others.
3. Provide support to each family member.

◆ Interventions

Allowing Expression of Feelings

Stay with the parents as they express their feelings. Allow them to cry or respond as they wish. Parents may want to have some time alone but may also appreciate having the nurse sit quietly nearby. When they are ready to talk, listen attentively.

Acknowledging the Infant

It was once believed that when an infant was stillborn or died shortly after birth, the less parents knew of the infant, the less they would grieve. The infant often was whisked away so that the parents never saw their newborn. Relatives disposed of the clothes and infant equipment before the mother returned home, and the parents were left with very few memories of the infant's birth.

The response to perinatal death changed as nurses discovered that the most helpful interventions for grieving parents were those that acknowledged the rights of the baby. These include the right to the following (Primeau & Lamb, 1995):
• Be recognized as a person who was born and died
• Be named
• Be seen, touched, and held by the family
• Have life ending acknowledged
• Be put to rest with dignity

Allow the parents to talk about the baby as much as they wish. Refer to the infant by name. If the infant lived for a time, talk about what happened during that time and answer any questions the parents have. If the infant is dying, allow parents to hold and care for their baby. Take pictures of the infant if the parents wish.

Presenting the Infant to the Parents

When the baby dies, the way in which the infant is presented to the parents is extremely important because these are the memories they will retain. Parents should be prepared for the appearance of the infant, especially if maceration (peeling) of the skin is present or there are disfigured areas. If necessary, wash the infant and apply baby lotion. The sense of smell is very powerful. Applying baby lotion provides olfactory stimulation. Wrap the infant in a soft, warm blanket. Some parents may wish to participate in bathing and dressing the baby.

If possible, bring the parents and the infant together while the infant is still warm and soft. Keeping the infant in a warmed incubator may be necessary if some time elapses before the parents have contact with the infant. If this is not possible, rewarm the infant under a radiant warmer. Wrap the infant in warmed blankets. Allow the parents to keep the infant as long as they wish, and tell them to feel free to unwrap the infant if they wish.

When the stillborn infant has severe deformities, explain the defect briefly and gently. Wrap the infant to expose the most normal aspects. When the infant has deformities of the head and face, wrap the infant with the blanket draped loosely over the most severely affected areas so that the parents do not see those areas first. Use diapers to cover genital defects and booties and mittens to cover abnormalities of the hands and feet.

It is not advisable to try to hide the defects completely. Allow parents to progress at their own speed in inspecting the infant. Parents may look at the abnormality or choose to leave the infant wrapped. They may quietly discuss positive features of the infant: "He has your ears." "Look at her long fingers."

Some parents may provide care before their baby dies. If death is near, ventilators and other equipment may be removed so that the parents can feel closer to the infant. They may hold the infant during the dying process. Many feel that this is very helpful to them, as it provides a chance to say goodbye and is the only opportunity they will have to parent their baby. Other family members also may be present at this time. Stay with the family, if they wish, to help them at this difficult time.

Allow as much privacy and time as the parents and other family members need to be together. Remain sensitive to cues that members of the family want to talk or prefer silence. A sympathetic smile or a promise to return at a certain time and then returning at that time are equally important. It is all right to say, "Do you want to talk?" Then all that is required is listening quietly and reflecting the mother's or father's feelings. Allow the parents to be alone if they wish, and check intermittently to see if they need assistance.

Although many parents want to spend time caring for or holding their baby before or after death, others may not. It is important not to make the parents feel guilty or that they should behave in a certain way. Nurses should accept that each family needs to go through this difficult experience in their own way.

Preparing a Memory Packet

Mourning requires memories. Nurses have explored measures that help the family create memories of the infant so the existence of the child is confirmed and the parents can complete the grieving process. Helping families create memories and providing support are part of a perinatal grief support nursing care quality measure under development by the AWHONN (2014).

Most parents treasure a memory packet. Prepare one that includes a photograph; a birth identification band with the date and time of birth; the crib card with the infant's name, weight, and length; a tape measure; and a blanket and cap used for the baby. If the baby has enough hair, ask the parents for permission to cut a lock of hair from the nape of the neck where it will not be noticeable. Some hospitals offer commercial remembrance materials to parents. The packets or boxes may contain clothing for the baby to wear and provide a place to keep baby items. Make paper handprints or soft modeling material impressions of the infant's hands and feet.

Take photographs of the infant to help parents remember the baby's features, and assist them through the grieving process. Take photographs of the infant dressed and undressed, wrapped and unwrapped, and of the parents and other family members with the infant. The infant should be positioned in natural newborn positions for the photos such as lying on the stomach with the knees tucked under and the head turned to one side. Professional photographers may be available from the Now I Lay Me Down To Sleep Foundation, a nonprofit organization that provides bereavement photos to families. A list of photographers and their locations is available at www.nowilaymedowntosleep.org. Keep the memory packet and photographs on file if the parents do not wish to take them home because they may want them at a later time. Many couples feel these concrete forms of remembrance are invaluable in helping them remember the baby as a person who really existed when they have no other signs of that life.

Respecting Cultural Practices

In some cultures, seeing or holding the baby after death is not acceptable. Cutting a lock of hair may not be permissible. It is culturally unacceptable in certain groups to take photographs of a person after death. Therefore ask permission before taking pictures. Pictures taken before death occurs may be more acceptable. Expression of grief may be loud and open, or parents may appear stoic, depending on cultural expectations. The nurse should be accepting of the family's method of coping with their loss.

Assisting with Other Needs

If the family includes other children, help the parents plan how to tell them about the death of the expected infant. Give them information about sibling responses and needs based on the ages of their other children. Provide the parents with written information about perinatal loss, grieving, and children's responses to death for later use. Other family members and close friends may be important in helping care for siblings as the parents cope with their own grief.

Offer to call clergy or other faith leaders, and discuss plans for a funeral or memorial service, if the family wishes. Parents may want to discuss this with their own faith leader, or a hospital chaplain may assist them. Discuss the normal grieving process, and explain that a considerable amount of time is involved. Describe common reactions that family members and friends might have. For example, some family members or friends may minimize the loss, whereas others, in a misguided attempt to offer comfort, may urge the couple to have another baby. Let them know that grandparents also go through grief because of the loss of their grandchild as well as the pain their children must endure.

Providing Follow-Up Care

Parents may find that friends and relatives expect them to recover quickly from perinatal loss and cannot understand their continued grief. Suggest that they allow the parents to "tell the story" of the infant as often as they want because this helps them in the grief process. Suggest that they help parents collect and talk about mementos to help establish memories of the infant.

Siblings are often expecting to be a "big brother" or "big sister" and need help understanding why that will not occur. Help the parents explore how they will tell their other children that the new baby will not be coming home. Explain that some young children think they have done something to cause the death and need reassurance. They may have questions (such as "Is the baby still dead?" or "Is the baby alive?") that should be answered simply but truthfully. Because the mother and the father experience grief in different ways, they may not understand each other's responses. Mothers who want to talk about the loss repeatedly may have partners who deal with their grief by being stoic and brooding or by focusing their energy on work. Emphasize the individuality of grief and that no single method or duration of grieving is right for everyone.

Couples usually want to know the cause of their infant's death. An autopsy may be recommended even if the cause of death is obvious. This gives parents the most accurate diagnosis for risk for recurrence in a future pregnancy. In some cases, the cause may never be found. Referral for genetic counseling may be appropriate for some parents who are concerned about the risk for a repeated tragedy. Future pregnancies will be stressful, and the woman will need closer follow-up than usual to identify any problems as soon as possible. The anxiety may continue in the neonatal period, and parents may need education and emotional support during this time.

Providing Referrals

Many birth agencies offer bereavement programs or counselors to provide ongoing help to parents. A social services referral is important. Telephone calls made during the first week, 1 to 2 weeks later, at the time of the postpartum checkup, and at the 1-year anniversary are helpful. Sympathy cards may be sent by agency staff with a list of resources that may be helpful. The greatest help often comes from contact with people who have experienced a similar loss, and a variety of support groups have been formed.

Refer parents to resources at the birth facility or in the community designed to help parents cope with loss. Many Internet resources are available. Examples are the MISS Foundation at www.misschildren.org and Helping After Neonatal Death (HAND) at www.handonline.org.

Some families join Internet perinatal loss support groups. Such groups may be particularly helpful after the immediate period surrounding the death. Extended family and friends may no longer be as supportive at this time and do not realize the length of time involved in grieving. Gaining a feeling of control over their lives and being able to make decisions gradually develop as the parents move toward healing.

◆ Evaluation

Nursing care has been successful if the family members share their feelings of loss and grief, communicate them to their significant others, and are supportive of one another.

? KNOWLEDGE CHECK

20. How should the stillborn infant be presented to the parents? Why?
21. What is a memory packet, and what should it include?

ADOPTION

Although pregnancy is a planned and exciting time for some, it can be a time of great strife and distress for others. For some women, pregnancy can be unexpected and for a variety of reasons they may find themselves choosing adoption for their child. Caring for a patient deciding on adoption can present interesting challenges for women's health nurses. Deciding for adoption can be one of the most difficult yet rewarding experiences for a birth mother (Clutter, 2014). Although the birth mother may find a great sense of joy in knowing she could give her child a better life through making a decision for adoption, she may also struggle with intense feelings of guilt, depression, and regret.

Adoption has changed greatly in recent years, and now offers birth parents the option of choosing how involved they would like to be in their child's life. The decision for adoption is a very personal one and will look different for each person. For some individuals, it is very important to them that they have a relationship with their child and that they have an opportunity to be a part of the child's life, whereas for others, having a relationship may prove too emotionally difficult and they choose to not maintain any relationship or communication with the child or adopted parents. For this reason, many adoption agencies now offer a variety of choices to birth mothers deciding on adoption, ranging from having an open adoption that permits the birth mother to have regular contact with the child and adoptive family, to partially open, or to closed adoptions. The relationship between birth mothers and adoptive parents may vary greatly among patients. Some birth mothers can interview and pick which family they would like to adopt their child. They may have had time to develop a close relationship throughout the pregnancy, with the adoptive family attending doctor appointments and in some cases even attending the birth. In other circumstances, the birth mother may choose to let an adoption agency make the decision on where to best place her child and not know or have any contact with the adoptive family at all.

It is important that health care providers are equipped to deal with both the physical and emotional needs of patients deciding on adoption, as well as the adopting family. Knowing if the patient has made a decision for adoption, as well as whether an adoptive family has been chosen, and who she would like to be a part of her delivery are vital pieces of information a nurse should have to best support the patient. Health care providers should be sensitive and nonjudgmental in their speech and care of the patient deciding on adoption. It is important that nurses withhold any personal biases they may have and remember that making a decision for adoption is a courageous act of love by the birth mother, not abandonment. Nurses should make every effort to respect and meet any special needs or requests the patient may have during the birth experience. Most birth mothers make a plan for how much contact they would like with the infant, how involved in the infant's care they would like to be, and how involved they would like the adoptive parents to be during the hospital stay. It is common for birth mothers to want as much information as possible about the infant and have some time alone with the infant. The birth mother should be encouraged to take as much time as she would like with the infant, and hospital mementos such as keep-sake footprints, baby bands, and infant blankets should be given to the birth mother if she wishes. Such actions provide memories of the infant and help the mother through the grieving process that accompanies deciding on adoption.

It is important that the nurse is able to form a rapport and trusting relationship with the birth mother. Therapeutic communication techniques are useful in helping the mother explore her feelings. Although the mother has made a choice for adoption, the grief she feels may be similar to that experienced when there is a death. Her grief may not be shared with family or friends, and those close to her may not understand her feelings. It is imperative that the nurse acknowledge any feelings the mother may have, while avoiding offering advice or coming across as judgmental. The ability for the patient to see the nurse as an advocate for her feelings and well-being will assist the patient in being able to successfully transition through a very emotional and difficult experience.

In the event that adoptive parents have been chosen, the nurse should acknowledge their needs and emotions as well. All efforts should be made to give adoptive parents a private room to process through emotions and adapt to their new role as parents. Nurses should teach adoptive parents how to care for their newborn and what to expect in growth and development. This family will need all teaching that is standard for new parents. Adoptive parents may be anxious, overwhelmed, and even experience postadoption depression (Foli, 2015). Demonstrations as well as return demonstrations may be helpful in assisting them in learning to care for their newborn.

? KNOWLEDGE CHECK

22. What is meant by the phrase "Adoption is an act of love"?
23. What are the nurse's responsibilities to the adoptive parents?

PERINATAL PSYCHOLOGICAL COMPLICATIONS

Although pregnancy and birth is a time of great joy and excitement for many women, for others it can be a time of great stress and sadness and bring to the forefront underlying psychological disorders. Psychological disorders can arise at the beginning of the pregnancy, or existing disorders can be intensified by the huge hormonal surges and shifts that occur during pregnancy (McKeever, Alderman, Luff, & Dejesus, 2016). Left untreated, perinatal psychological complications can result in serious harm to both the mother and infant. Historically, many obstetricians and women's health professionals have been ill prepared to address the needs of patients with psychological complications during the perinatal period (Schaar & Hall, 2013). Fortunately, in recent years increased attention has been given to the importance of appropriate screening and treatment for this vulnerable population of patients.

Perinatal Mood Disorder

Perinatal mood disorder, also known as a major depressive disorder, is generally characterized as unipolar depression or a major depressive disorder with associated psychotic features (McKeever et al., 2016). Signs and symptoms of a mood disorder include anxiety, agitation, a constant sad mood, feelings of worthlessness, difficulty thinking or concentrating, loss of energy, crying fits, fatigue, headache, and loss of appetite (McKeever et al., 2016). Psychosis-associated mood disorders include symptoms of delusions, auditory hallucinations, cognitive impairment, disorganized thinking, failure to distinguish delusions from reality, poor hygiene, and anger (McKeever et al., 2016). These types of disorders affect 3% to 6% of perinatal patients, with the disorder most frequently being seen in adolescent patients and those in their early 20s (McKeever et al., 2016). Although the disorders occur more often during the postpartum period, prenatal episodes are also possible.

EVIDENCE-BASED PRACTICE

Postpartum depression (PPD) is a common disorder that causes significant functional impairment and increases risk of poor mother-infant bonding and delays in infant development. Kayton et al. (2014) studied 3039 women receiving prenatal care and delivering at the University of Washington. Of these women, 1515 were excluded due to lack of postpartum assessment. The participants of this study were screened at 4 months or 8 months of pregnancy (or both) and then again at 6 weeks postpartum. This study found that younger age, unemployment, antenatal depressive symptoms, taking antidepressants, psychosocial stressors, prepregnancy chronic physical illnesses (diabetes, and neurologic conditions), and smoking were independent predictors of development of PPD.

Questions

1. With knowledge of risk factors for PPD, what can the maternity nurse do to initiate dialogue with new mothers and their families about postpartum mood disorders?
2. What screening tools are appropriate for use prior to discharge from the facility?
3. What should be included in discharge teaching about PPD? What resources are available?

Reference

Katon, W., Ruso, J., & Gavin, A. (2014). Predictors of Postpartum Depression, *Journal of Women's Health* (15409996), *23*(9), 753–759.

Postpartum Depression

Postpartum depression is defined as depression that takes place after childbirth and persists longer than 2 weeks. In contrast, postpartum blues (*baby blues, maternity blues*) is a mild, transient condition which resolves within 2 weeks (see Chapter 17). Postpartum depression typically presents within the first 3 months postpartum and has the potential to last up to a year (McKeever et al., 2016). Postpartum depression is the most common complication of childbirth, with up to 20% of mothers experiencing postpartum depression during one of their pregnancies (McKeever et al., 2016). Women who have a history of depression are at an increased risk for being affected by the disorder (McKeever et al., 2016). Although postpartum depression can affect anyone after giving birth, patients with a history of sexual abuse, patients experiencing an unexpected or unwanted pregnancy, those who smoke, and those who formula feed their baby are all at increased risk for this disorder (McKeever et al., 2016) (Box 11.4). Some women may be reluctant to care for their infants or continue to breastfeed because of the extreme feelings of depression; however, research has shown that breastfeeding can actually decrease the risk for developing postpartum depression and in some cases may even be beneficial to those experiencing postpartum depression because it allows them to bond and connect with their baby despite the depressive feelings they have (Olson & Bowen, 2014). As medical professionals, it is imperative to remember that each patient's experience is different and that care and treatment options should be individualized to the patient. It is also important to note that acknowledgment of depressive symptoms, screening, and treatment vary throughout different countries and regions and may be accepted differently based on the patient's culture (Norhayati, Nik-Hazlina, Asrenee, & Wan Emilin, 2015). A patient's family and support system should be a part of her care and treatment as much as possible, because social support has been shown to play a significant role in a patient's ability or lack thereof to overcome this disorder (Biaggi, Conroy, Pawlby, & Pariante, 2016).

> **! SAFETY CHECK**
>
> Signs and symptoms of postpartum depression include the following:
> Anxiety
> Feelings of guilt
> Agitation
> Fatigue, sleeplessness
> Feeling unwell
> Irritability
> Difficulty concentrating or making decisions, confusion
> Appetite changes
> Loss of pleasure in normal activities
> Lack of energy
> Crying
> Sadness
> Depression (may not be present at first)
> Suicidal thoughts
> Less responsive to infant

BOX 11.4 Risk Factors for Postpartum Depression

Depression during pregnancy or previous postpartum depression (strong predictors)
First pregnancy
Hormonal fluctuations that follow childbirth
Medical problems during pregnancy or after birth, such as preeclampsia, preexisting diabetes mellitus, anemia, or postpartum thyroid dysfunction
Personal or family history of depression, mental illness, or alcoholism
Personality characteristics, such as immaturity and low self-esteem
Marital dysfunction or difficult relationship with the significant other, resulting in lack of support
Anger or ambivalence about the pregnancy
Single status
Young maternal age
Feelings of isolation, lack of social support, or support that does not meet the mother's needs
Fatigue, lack of sleep
Financial worries
Child care stress (infant who is ill, has anomalies, or has a difficult temperament)
Multifetal pregnancy
Chronic stressors
Unwanted or unplanned pregnancy

Postpartum Psychosis

Postpartum psychosis is an intense type of deep depression or relapse of an underlying psychotic disorder such as schizophrenia (McKeever et al., 2016). Postpartum psychosis is characterized by serious mood instabilities that peak from 48 hours to 2 weeks postpartum. To truly be characterized as a postpartum psychosis episode, the following criteria are required: major depressive disorder with psychotic traits, bipolar I, bipolar II, unspecified functional psychosis, schizoaffective disorder, or short-term psychotic disorder (McKeever et al., 2016). Postpartum psychosis is a serious medical emergency that requires immediate intervention, usually hospitalization, psychotherapy and appropriate medication. There is an increased risk for development of postpartum psychosis in women of advanced maternal age, as well as with those with a lower socioeconomic status (McKeever et al., 2016). In addition to having symptoms similar to those seen with postpartum depression, symptoms of postpartum psychosis include the failure to be able to identify reality; confusion, auditory, and visual hallucinations; insomnia; hyperactivity; suicide, homicide, and infanticide (McKeever et al., 2016).

Bipolar II Disorder

Bipolar disorder is a combination of depressive and manic symptoms. There are three types of bipolar disorder with clinical manifestations that differ for each type: bipolar I, bipolar II, and cyclothymic. A diagnosis of bipolar I requires manic episodes and depressive episodes, a bipolar II diagnosis requires depressive episodes and hypomania, and a cyclothymic diagnosis requires recurrent mood changes of both depressive episodes and hypomania (McKeever et al., 2016). Pregnancy often intensifies symptoms for the patient with bipolar disorder and can send them into a depressive or manic episode; however, many patients stop taking their medications during pregnancy out of fear they will cause harm to the baby. It is imperative that medical professionals work with these patients to establish risk versus benefit regarding medications during pregnancy. This may mean that the patient may have to continue to take medications despite known risk to the baby, to ensure safety and well-being to the mother. It is also important that patients are educated on the increased risk for mood disorder relapse with each subsequent pregnancy, because this might play a significant role in the patient's family planning (Di Florio et al., 2014). Some signs and symptoms that accompany bipolar disorder are frequent mood swings, impulsiveness, loneliness, guilt, hopelessness, increased or decreased energy, irritability, euphoria, and excessive thoughts and speech (McKeever et al., 2016).

Postpartum Anxiety Disorders

Posttraumatic stress disorder, panic disorder, obsessive-compulsive disorder, phobias, and generalized anxiety disorder are all considered postpartum anxiety disorders (McKeever et al., 2016). The signs and symptoms of an anxiety disorder include inability to relax, restlessness, difficulty concentrating, irritability, insomnia, anguish about making decisions, irritable bowel syndrome, constant worrying, and the inability to stop worrying (McKeever et al., 2016). It is estimated that 4.5% to 15% of pregnant and postpartum women have an anxiety disorder (McKeever et al., 2016).

❓ CRITICAL THINKING EXERCISE 11.1

Aricella, a 23-year-old multipara, gave birth 10 days ago to her second baby. It is obvious to the nurse making a telephone follow-up call after discharge that Aricella is crying. She says, "I don't know what's wrong with me! I can barely get out of bed in the morning and I'm worn out just trying to take care of the kids." The nurse responds, "Oh, that's just the 'baby blues.' Just look at that beautiful baby and you'll feel better."

Questions
1. What assumptions has the nurse made?
2. Is the nurse's response helpful for Aricella? Why or why not?
3. What would be a more therapeutic response?
4. What additional action should the nurse take?

◆ APPLICATION OF THE NURSING PROCESS: PERINATAL PSYCHOLOGICAL COMPLICATIONS

◆ Assessment

Women should be assessed for depression during pregnancy, at the birth facility, and during follow-up visits after birth. Early identification is paramount. The woman should be reassessed at each contact with health care providers (including follow-up telephone calls). Women whose infants are in a NICU should be assessed for postpartum depression during visits to their infants.

Assessment tools such as the Postpartum Depression Predictors Inventory–Revised may be helpful. This inventory identifies prenatal depression, life stress, social support, prenatal anxiety, satisfaction with marital relationship, history of depression, self-esteem, unwanted or unplanned pregnancy, marital status, socioeconomic status, child care stress, infant temperament, and maternity blues as factors that may predict the likelihood of a woman developing postpartum depression (Beck, Records, & Rice, 2006). In addition, screening for excessive fatigue in the first 2 weeks after childbirth may help identify women who will later develop postpartum depression and enable them to get early treatment.

Some examples of other screening tools include the Edinburgh Postnatal Depression Scale and the Postpartum Depression Screening Scale. Ask the woman if she is often sad or depressed, or if she has felt a loss of pleasure or interest in things she once enjoyed. These questions may enable early identification and treatment of depression.

Observe for subjective symptoms, such as apathy, lack of interest or energy, anorexia, or sleeplessness. The mother's verbalizations of failure, sadness, loneliness, anxiety, or vague confusion are important cues. Focus on the frequency, duration, and intensity of the woman's feelings to determine their severity.

Assess for objective data, such as crying, sleeplessness, poor personal hygiene, or inability to follow directions or concentrate. Determine what, if any, support is available. Mothers with an absent or unavailable support system may feel increasingly isolated, leading to stress and a feeling that they are unable to manage. Inappropriate expressions of blame or anger toward the partner and unmet expectations of the baby or the parenting role are sometimes present.

◆ Identification of Patient Problem

Women with psychological disorders during the perinatal period lack effective coping techniques to manage the stressors associated with childbirth and parenting.

◆ Planning: Expected Outcomes

To achieve the expected outcomes for this patient problem, the new mother will do the following:

- Verbalize feelings with the health care provider and significant other throughout the postpartum period.

- Discuss her own strengths.
- Identify available resources for the postpartum period.

◆ Interventions

Providing Anticipatory Guidance

Because of short hospital stays for new mothers, and timing of the usual onset of affective disorders, most incidences of postpartum depression (and postpartum psychosis) occur after the woman has gone home. Anticipatory guidance of the mother and her family is the most critical nursing intervention. Success of treatment is largely affected by early diagnosis. During the prenatal period, initiate a discussion with all pregnant women and their partners to provide anticipatory guidance about the early weeks at home. Explain the signs of postpartum depression and the importance of seeking early help to decrease the length of time the condition lasts.

Discuss the need for frequent contact with other adults so the mother does not become isolated. Emphasize the importance of continued communication with the partner or a close friend who can provide support when loneliness or anxiety becomes a problem.

Explain that adequate rest and nutrition can help the mother maintain energy and a feeling of health and well-being. Teach mothers and their support persons the signs of postpartum depression and other postpartum psychological disorders, including when they should seek help.

Demonstrating Caring

Conveying a caring attitude is an important nursing strategy to help mothers decrease their emotional distress and guide them in regaining their well-being during the peripartum period. Acknowledge that something is wrong and that the woman seems depressed. Spend time with her and reassure her that the condition is not her fault.

Explain to the woman that what she is feeling is a common experience after childbirth. Encourage her to talk about her feelings and reassure her that help is available.

Helping the Mother Verbalize Feelings

Because women are expected to be happy after giving birth, many women do not discuss their negative feelings with others. They may feel ashamed and believe a social stigma is attached to admitting to depression at any time and especially after giving birth. They may fear that their infants may be taken away from them if they disclose their problem. If they do discuss their feelings, their friends or even health care workers may trivialize the problem by making comments such as, "You'll get over it. After all, you have a beautiful baby." Women and their families minimize depression because they cannot find the exact cause.

Recommend that although some of her feelings may seem "unreasonable" (anger, guilt, shame), the woman should acknowledge negative feelings to herself and insist that others recognize them too. Discuss the realities of parenting and the fact that it is often exhausting. It may be helpful to rehearse some of the situations that may occur, such as a fussy baby or being home alone and feeling lonely.

Enhancing Sensitivity to Infant Cues

Point out infant cues and explain their meaning. Model behavior to show the mother how to respond to the infant's cues. Suggest measures that may enhance her sensitivity to cues. Measures to help the mother relax may help improve her mood and her response to her infant.

Assess the infant's growth and development. Depressed mothers may not give the care and nurturing needed. Determine the infant's weight gain or loss and observe the mother's response to the infant's crying. If the mother is breastfeeding, make suggestions to help her continue because it may increase her feelings of closeness to the infant. If she is taking medication, be sure that it is recommended for use during lactation.

Helping Family Members

Include the father in discussions about depression, before and after the birth. Acknowledge his feelings and those of the mother. Stress his role in helping his partner and other family members. Offer practical suggestions of ways he can help manage the changes in their lives. Discuss ways to help, such as arranging for the mother to get more sleep and to eat better, which may help decrease her irritability and anxiety. Determine the father's need for additional support and explain the impact of postpartum depression on each family member. Emphasize the importance of the mother taking medications as ordered. Discuss signs that the mother's depression is worsening and when to call the health care provider.

Providing Help

Explore with the family practical suggestions on how to help the mother. Explain the importance of sleep and suggest that another family member care for the infant at night, if possible, to allow the mother to sleep. Because depressed mothers do not interact with their infants well, emphasize the importance of other family members holding and interacting with the infant.

Discussing Options and Resources

Ask the mother about stressors in her life that may be contributing to her depression. Help her plan ways to reduce common areas of stress. Assist the mother and her partner to identify people who are available to provide support. In addition, provide telephone numbers for local postpartum depression support groups. Internet sources are another place to find help. Examples are Postpartum Support International (www.postpartum.net), and the National Women's Health Information Center (www.womenshealth. gov).

◆ Evaluation

The interventions are successful if the mother does the following:

- Talks about her feelings to staff and family members.
- Identifies her personal strengths.
- Discusses community and family resources and makes plans to use them.

KNOWLEDGE CHECK

24. What are the symptoms of postpartum depression, and how does it differ from postpartum blues?
25. How can nurses intervene for postpartum depression?
26. What is the therapeutic management for postpartum psychosis?

SUMMARY CONCEPTS

- Teenage pregnancy is a major health problem in the United States. Adolescents need to receive accurate information about contraceptives and how to set limits on sexual behavior.
- Adolescent pregnancy imposes serious physiologic risks that result in a higher incidence of complications for the mother and the fetus.
- Teenage pregnancy interrupts the developmental tasks of adolescence and may result in childbirth before the parents are capable of providing a nurturing home for the infant without a great deal of assistance.
- The mature gravida often has financial and emotional resources that younger women do not have. She may experience anxiety, however, about recommended antepartum testing and her ability to parent effectively.
- Polydrug abuse is a widespread problem that can have devastating fetal and neonatal effects, which may persist and become long-term developmental problems for the child.
- The lifestyle associated with illicit drug abuse includes inadequate nutrition, inadequate prenatal care, and increased incidence of sexually transmitted diseases. It requires interdisciplinary interventions to prevent injury to the expectant mother and the fetus.

- The birth of an infant with congenital anomalies produces strong emotions of shock and grief in the family. It calls for a sensitive response from the health care team to help the family grieve for the loss of the perfect or "fantasy" infant and form an attachment to the newborn.
- Pregnancy loss at any stage produces grief that should be acknowledged and expressed before it can be resolved. Nurses realize that mourning requires memories, and they intervene to arrange unlimited contact between the family and the stillborn infant and gather a memento packet for the family.
- Nursing care for the mother who is placing her infant for adoption is based on the knowledge that adoption is an act of love, not abandonment.
- Mood disorders include postpartum blues, postpartum depression, and postpartum psychosis.
- Postpartum depression is a disabling affective disorder that has an impact on the entire family. Nurses help the woman acknowledge her feelings and assist her in identifying measures that will help her cope with the condition.
- Anxiety disorders include panic disorder, postpartum obsessive-compulsive disorder, and posttraumatic stress disorder.

REFERENCES & READINGS

American College of Obstetrics and Gynecology (ACOG). (2013). *FAQ: Tobacco, Alcohol, Drugs, & Pregnancy*. Retrieved from www.acog.org/Patients/FAQs/Tobacco-Alcohol-Drugs-and-Pregnancy.

American College of Obstetricians and Gynecologists (ACOG). (2014, March). *Female Age-Related Fertility Decline*. Retrieved from www.acog.org/-/media/Committee-Opinions/Committee-on-Gynecologic-Practice/co589.pdf?dmc=1&ts=2016100 9T0222301693.

American College of Obstetricians and Gynecologists (ACOG). (2015, April). *Frequently asked questions especially for teens: Having a baby. FAQ 103*. Retrieved from www.acog.org/Patients/FAQs/Having-a-Baby-Especially-for-Teens#risks.

American College of Obstetricians and Gynecologists (ACOG). (2016). *Committee Opinion: Opioid Abuse, Dependence, and Addiction in Pregnancy. Published 2012, reaffirmed 2016*. Retrieved from www.acog.org/-/media/Committee-Opinions/Committee-on-Health-Care-for-Underserved-Women/co524.pdf?dmc=1&ts=20161016T2008315728.

Artigas, V. (2014). Management of neonatal abstinence in the newborn nursery. *Nursing for Women's Health, 18*(5), 509–514.

Asheer, S., Berger, A., Meckstroth, A., Kisker, E., & Keating, B. (2014). Engaging pregnant and parenting teens: Early challenges and lessons learned from the evaluation of adolescent pregnancy prevention approaches. *Journal of Adolescent Health, 54*, S84–S91.

Association of Women's Health, Obstetric, and Neonatal Nurses (AWHONN). (2014). *Women's health and perinatal nursing care quality. Refined draft measures specifications*. Washington, DC: Author.

Association of Women's Health Obstetric and Neonatal Nurses (AWHONN). (2015). Criminalization of Pregnant Women With Substance Use Disorders. *Journal of Obstetric, Gynecologic, & Neonatal Nursing, 9*(1), 93–95.

Avelin, P., Rådestad, I., Säflund, K., Wredling, R., & Erlandsson, K. (2013). Parental grief and relationships after the loss of a stillborn baby. *Midwifery, 29*(2013), 668–673.

Ballard, R. A. (2015). Attachment challenges with premature or sick infants. In R. J. Martin, A. A. Fanaroff, & M. C. Walsh (Eds.), *Fanaroff and Martin's neonatal-perinatal medicine* (10th ed.) (pp. 636–638). St. Louis, MO: Saunders.

Beck, C. T., Records, K., & Rice, M. (2006). Further development of the postpartum depression predictors inventory-revised. *Journal of Obstetric, Gynecologic, and Neonatal Nursing, 35*(6), 735–745.

Biaggi, A., Conroy, S., Pawlby, S., & Pariante, C. (2016). Identifying the women at risk of antenatal anxiety and depression: a systematic review. *Journal of Affective Disorders, 19,* 162–177.

Bingham, R. J. (2015). Latest evidence on alchol and pregnancy. *Nursing for Women's Health, 19*(4), 338–344.

Centers for Disease Control (CDC). (2017). *Reproductive health: Teen pregnancy. About teen pregnancy: Teen pregnancy in the United States.* Retrieved from https://www.cdc.gov/teenpregnancy/about/index.htm.

Chang, L., Oishi, K., & Skranes, J. (2016). Sex-specific alterations of white matter developmental trajectories in infants with prenatal exposure to methamphetamine and tobacco. *JAMA Psychiatry, 73*(12), 1217–1227.

Cleveland, L. M. (2016). Breastfeeding recommendations for women who receive medication-assisted treatment for opioid use disorders: AWHONN practice brief number 4. *Journal of Obstetric, Gynecologic, & Neonatal Nursing, 20*(4), 432–434.

Clutter, L. B. (2014). Adult birth mothers who made open infant adoption placements after adolescent unplanned pregnancy. *Journal of Obstetric, Gynecologic, & Neonatal Nursing, 43*(2), 190–199.

Di Florio, A., Jones, L., Forty, L., Gordon-Smith, K., Robertson Blakemore, E., Heron, J., & Jones, I. (2014). Mood disorders and parity: a clue to the aetiology of the postpartum trigger. *Journal of Affective Disorders, 152–154,* 334–339.

Foli, K. J. (2015). Longitudinal course of risk for parental postadoption depression. *Journal of Obstetric, Gynecologic, & Neonatal Nursing, 45*(2), 210–226.

Gardner, S. L., & Carter, B. S. (2016). Grief and perinatal loss. In S. L. Gardner, B. S. Carter, M. Enzman-Hines, et al. (Eds.), *Merenstein & Gardner's handbook of neonatal intensive care* (8th ed.) (pp. 865–902). St. Louis, MO: Mosby.

Gray, B. A., & Holland, C. (2014). Implications of psychoactive "bath salts" use during pregnancy. *Nursing for Women's Health, 18*(3), 220–230.

Hunt, S., & Hellwig, J. (2015). Prescription opioid use in pregnancy. *Nursing for Women's Health, 19*(2), 123–127.

Hutti, M. H., Armstrong, D. S., Myers, J. A., & Hall, L. A. (2015). Grief intensity, psychological well-being, and the intimate partner relationship in the subsequent pregnancy after a perinatal loss. *Journal of Obstetric, Gynecologic, & Neonatal Nursing, 44*(1), 42–50.

Johnson, O. P., & Langford, R. W. (2015). A randomized trial of a bereavement intervention for pregnancy loss. *Journal of Obstetric, Gynecologic, & Neonatal Nursing, 44*(4), 492–499.

Kearney, A., & White, K. (2016). Examining the pyschosocial determinents of women's decisions to delay childbearing. *Human Reproduction, 31*(8), 1776–1787.

Koh, H. (2014). The teen pregnancy prevention program: An evidence-based public health program model. *Journal of Adolescent Health, 54*(3), S1–S2.

Lee, W.-L., Tsui, K.-H., & Wang, P.-H. (2016). Is nutrition deficiency a key factor of adverse outcomes for pregnant adolescents? *Journal of the Chinese Medical Association, 79*(6), 301–303.

Limbo, R., & Wool, C. W. (2016). Perinatal palliative care. *Journal of Obstetric, Gynecologic, & Neonatal Nursing, 45*(5), 611–613.

March of Dimes. (2016, July). *Heroin and Pregnancy.* Retrieved from http://www.marchofdimes.org/pregnancy/heroin-and-pregnancy.aspx.

McKeever, A. E., Spaeth-Brayton, S., & Sheerin, S. (2014). The role of nurses in comprehensive care management with drug addiction of pregnant women. *Nursing for Women's Health, 18*(4), 283–293.

McKeever, A., Alderman, S., Luff, S., & Dejesus, B. (2016). Assessment and care of childbearing women with severe and persistent mental illness. *Nursing for Women's Health, 20*(5), 484–499.

Montgomery, T., Folken, L., & Seitz, M. A. (2014). Addressing adolescent pregnancy with legislation. *Nursing for Women's Health, 18*(4), 277–283.

Norhayati, M., Nik-Hazlina, N., Asrenee, A., & Wan Emilin, W. (2015). Magnitude and risk factors for postpartum symptoms: a literature review. *Journal of Affective Disorders, 175*(1), 34–52.

Nove, A., Matthews, Z., & Camacho, V. A. (2014). Maternal mortality in adolescents compared with women of other ages: evidence from 144 countries. *The Lancet, 2*(3), e155–e164.

Olson, T., & Bowen, A. (2014). Dispelling myths to support breastfeeding in women with postpartum depression. *Nursing for Women's Health, 18*(4), 304–313.

Passey, M. E., Sanson-Fisher, R. W., D'Este, C. A., & Stirling, J. M. (2014). Tobacco, alcohol and cannabis use during pregnancy: clustering of risks. *Drug and Alcohol Dependence, 134*(1), 44–50.

Primeau, M. R., & Lamb, J. M. (1995). When a baby dies: Rights of the baby and parents. *Journal of Obstetric, Gynecologic, and Neonatal Nursing, 24*(3), 206–208.

Roth, C. K., Hering, S. L., & Campos, S. (2015). Serotonin syndrome in pregnancy. *Nursing for Women's Health, 19*(4), 345–349.

Roth, C. K., Satran, L. A., & Smith, S. M. (2015). Marijuana Use in Pregnancy. *Nursing for Women's Health, 19*(5), 431–437.

Schaar, G. L., & Hall, M. (2013). A nurse-led initiative to improve obstetricians' screening for postpartum depression. *Nursing for Women's Health, 17*(4), 306–316.

Sedgh, G., Finer, L. B., Bankole, A., Eilers, M. A., & Singh, S. (2015). Adolescent pregnancy, birth, and abortion rates across countries: levels and recent trends. *Journal of Adolescent Health, 56*(2), 223–230.

United States Department of Health and Human Services. (2013). *Substance A, Mental Health Services Administration. Center for Behavioral Health S Quality: National Survey on Drug Use and Health, 2012.* Interuniversity Consortium for Political and Social Research (ICPSR) [distributor]10.3886/ICPSR34933.v3.

United States Department of Health and Human Services. (2016). *Trends in teen pregnancy and childbearing: Teen births.* Retrieved from www.hhs.gov/ash/oah/adolescent-development/reproductive-health-and-teen-pregnancy/teen-pregnancy-and-childbearing/trends/index.html.

Wisner, K. L., Sit, D. K. Y., Bogen, D. L., Altemus, M., Pearlstein, T. B., Svikis, D. S., Misra, D., & Miller, E. S. (2017). Mental health and behavioral disorders in pregnancy. In S. G. Gabbe, J. R. Niebyl, J. L. Simpson, M. B. Landon, H. L. Galan, R. M. Jauniaux, D. A. Driscoll, et al. (Eds.), *Obstetrics: Normal and problem pregnancies* (7th ed.) (pp. 1147–1172). Philadelphia, PA: Saunders.

12

Processes of Birth

Kristine DeButy, Kristin L. Scheffer

Understanding the physiologic and psychological components of the birth process helps the nurse provide safe, effective care for the childbearing family. Awareness of expected changes allows the nurse to support the laboring woman when these occur and provides a basis for identifying abnormal occurrences. This chapter focuses on the physiology of birth.

PHYSIOLOGIC EFFECTS OF THE LABOR PROCESS

The birth process affects the physiologic systems of both the mother and fetus.

Maternal Response

The most obvious changes of pregnancy and birth occur in the woman's reproductive system, but significant changes also occur during labor in her cardiovascular, respiratory, gastrointestinal, urinary, and hematopoietic systems.

Reproductive System

Characteristics of Contractions. Normal labor contractions are coordinated, involuntary, and intermittent.

Coordinated. The uterus can contract and relax in a coordinated way like the heart and other smooth muscles.

Contractions during pregnancy are of low intensity and uncoordinated. As the woman approaches full term, contractions become organized and gradually assume a regular pattern of increasing **frequency** *(period from the beginning of one uterine contraction to the beginning of the next),* **duration** *(period from the beginning of a uterine contraction to the end of the same contraction),* and **intensity** *(strength of a contraction)* during labor. Coordinated labor contractions begin in the uterine fundus and spread downward toward the cervix to propel the fetus through the pelvis.

Involuntary. Uterine contractions are involuntary and are not under conscious control. The mother cannot cause labor to start and stop by conscious effort. However, walking and other activities may stimulate existing labor contractions. Anxiety and excessive stress can diminish contractions because of elevated adrenaline levels that may cause uterine relaxation (Burke, 2014). Relaxation can facilitate the natural processes.

Intermittent. Labor contractions are intermittent rather than sustained, allowing relaxation of the uterine muscle and resumption of blood flow to and from the placenta.

Contraction Cycle. Each contraction consists of three phases (Fig. 12.1). The **increment** *(period of increasing strength)* occurs as the contraction begins in the fundus and spreads throughout the uterus. The peak, or **acme,** is *the period*

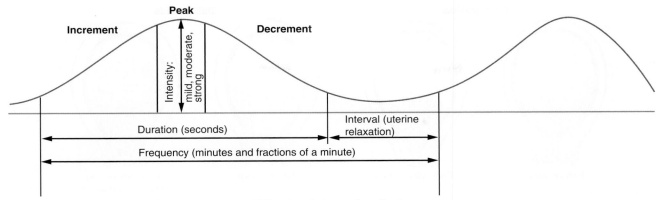

FIG. 12.1 Contraction Cycle.

during which the contraction is most intense. The **decrement** is the *period of decreasing intensity* as the uterus relaxes.

The contraction cycle and pattern of contractions are also described in terms of frequency, duration, and intensity. Frequency may be expressed in minutes and fractions of minutes (e.g., "contractions are 3½ to 4 minutes apart"). The 2008 National Institute of Child Health and Human Development update (Macones, Hankins, Spong, Hauth, & Moore, 2008) recommends that frequency be assessed as the number of contractions in 10 minutes, averaged over 30 minutes ("3 contractions in 10 min."). Duration is usually expressed in seconds (e.g., "contractions last 55 to 65 seconds"). The terms *mild, moderate,* and *strong* describe contraction intensity as palpated by the nurse. Different descriptions of intensity apply when an internal pressure catheter is used to record contractions (see Chapter 14).

The **interval** is *the period between the end of one contraction and the beginning of the next.* The uterus should palpate soft during this time. Most fetal exchange of oxygen, nutrients, and waste products occurs in the placenta at this time.

Uterine Muscle. Uterine activity during labor is characterized by opposing features. The upper two thirds of the uterus contracts actively to push the fetus down. The lower third of the uterus remains less active, promoting downward passage of the fetus. The cervix is passive. The net effect of labor contractions is enhanced because the downward push from the upper uterus is accompanied by reduced resistance to fetal descent in the lower uterus (Cunningham et al., 2014).

Myometrial (pertaining to the uterine muscle) cells in the upper uterus remain shorter at the end of each contraction rather than returning to their original length; myometrial cells in the lower uterus become longer with each contraction. These two characteristics enable the upper uterus to maintain tension between contractions to preserve the cervical changes and downward fetal progress made with each contraction (Norwitz, Mahendroo, & Lye, 2014).

The opposing characteristics of myometrial contraction in the upper and lower uterine segments cause changes in the thickness of the uterine wall during labor. The upper uterus becomes thicker, and the lower uterus becomes thinner and

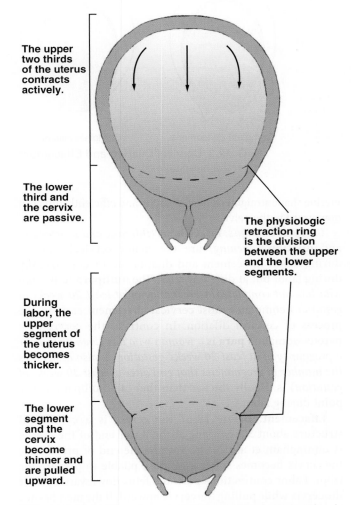

FIG. 12.2 Opposing characteristics of uterine contraction in the upper and lower segments of the uterus.

is pulled upward during labor. The physiologic retraction ring marks the division between the upper and lower segments of the uterus (Fig. 12.2).

The upper and lower uterine segments work opposite of each other, causing the uterine cavity to change shape, becoming more elongated and narrow as labor progresses. This change in

Primigravida

Multigravida

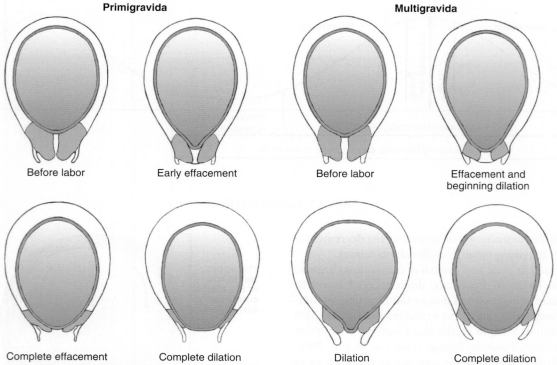

Before labor

Early effacement

Before labor

Effacement and beginning dilation

Complete effacement

Complete dilation

Dilation

Complete dilation

FIG. 12.3 Cervical Dilation and Effacement. During labor the multipara's cervix remains thicker than the nullipara's cervix.

uterine shape straightens the fetal body and efficiently directs it downward in the pelvis.

Cervical Changes. **Effacement** *(thinning and shortening)* and **dilation** *(opening)* are the major cervical changes during labor. Effacement and dilation occur concurrently during labor but at different rates. The **nullipara** *(a woman who has not completed a pregnancy of at least 20 weeks of gestation)* completes most cervical effacement early in the process of cervical dilation. In contrast, the cervix of a parous woman (a **para** *is a woman who has given birth after a pregnancy of at least 20 weeks' gestation; it also designates the number of pregnancies that end after at least 20 weeks of gestation*) is usually thicker than that of a nullipara at any point during labor.

Effacement. Before labor the cervix is a cylindrical structure about 3.5 cm long at the lower end of the uterus (Cunningham et al., 2014). Toward the end of pregnancy, the cervix becomes softer and more pliable to prepare for labor. Labor contractions push the fetus downward against the cervix while pulling the cervix upward. If the membranes are intact, hydrostatic (fluid) pressure of the amniotic sac adds to the force of the presenting part (the part of the fetal body that enters the pelvis first) on the cervix. The cervix becomes shorter and thinner as it is drawn over the fetus and amniotic sac (Fig. 12.3). The cervix merges with the thinning lower uterine segment rather than remaining a distinct structure. Effacement is estimated as a percentage of the original cervical length. A fully thinned cervix is 100% effaced.

Dilation. As the cervix is pulled upward and the fetus is pushed downward, the cervix dilates. Dilation is expressed in centimeters. Full dilation is approximately 10 cm, sufficient to allow passage of the average-size, full-term fetus. At 10 cm, the cervix cannot be felt by an examiner. The action during effacement and dilation can be likened to pushing a ball out through the cuff of a sock.

Cardiovascular System

During each uterine contraction, the muscle fibers of the uterus constrict around the maternal spiral arteries that supply the placenta. This temporarily shunts 300 to 500 mL of blood back into maternal systemic circulation, thereby causing a relative increase in the woman's blood volume (Monga & Mastrobattista, 2014). This temporary change increases her blood pressure slightly and slows her pulse rate. Therefore the woman's vital signs are best assessed during the interval between contractions. Supine hypotension may occur during labor if the woman lies on her back, as a result of aortocaval compression (Monga & Mastrobattista, 2014). The woman should be encouraged to rest in lateral positions to promote blood return to her heart and thus enhance blood flow to the placenta and promote fetal oxygenation.

Respiratory System

The depth and rate of respirations increase during labor, especially if the woman is anxious or in pain. A woman who breathes rapidly and deeply may experience symptoms of hyperventilation. Respiratory alkalosis occurs as she exhales too much carbon dioxide (Monga & Mastrobattista, 2014). She may feel tingling of her hands and feet, numbness, and dizziness. The nurse should help her slow her breathing through relaxation techniques and breathe into a paper bag or her cupped hands to restore normal blood levels of carbon dioxide and relieve these symptoms.

Gastrointestinal System

Gastric motility is reduced during labor, which can result in nausea and vomiting. Controversy exists on whether laboring women should be allowed to eat or drink during labor. Concerns surround the risk for vomiting and aspiration of undigested foods in the event general anesthesia is required. In a Cochrane review, a lack of evidence was found to restrict low-risk laboring women from food and oral fluids during labor (Singata, Tranmer, & Gyte, 2013). The maternal need for calories to perform the work of labor is underappreciated. Increased glucose utilization and oxygen consumption occur during labor, resulting in the need for additional nutrition (American College of Nurse-Midwives [ACNM], 2016). The American Society of Anesthesiologists' (ASA, 2016) *Practice Guidelines for Obstetrical Anesthesia* position statement on aspiration prevention states that oral intake of clear liquids is appropriate in low-risk laboring women; however, solid foods should be avoided. Ice chips, juices, and Popsicles in moderate amounts are common options available to women during labor.

Urinary System

The most common change in the urinary system during labor is a reduced sensation of a full bladder. Because of intense contractions and the effects of regional anesthesia, the woman may be unaware that her bladder is full, yet it may contribute to discomfort. A full bladder can inhibit fetal descent because it occupies space in the pelvis. Bladder status should be evaluated throughout labor for distention.

Hematopoietic System

Most authorities recognize 500 mL as the maximum normal blood loss during vaginal birth. Women usually tolerate this loss well because the blood volume increases during pregnancy by 30% to 60% (Blackburn, 2013; Cunningham et al., 2014). A woman who is anemic at the beginning of labor has less reserve for normal blood loss and a poor tolerance for excess bleeding. A hemoglobin (Hgb) level of 11 grams per deciliter (g/dL) and a hematocrit (Hct) of 33% or higher before birth give most women an adequate margin of safety for blood loss associated with normal birth (Blanchard & Daniels, 2014). The leukocyte count may be 20,000 to 30,000/mm^3 during active labor, with no other evidence of infection (Antony, Pacusin, Aagaard, & Dildy, 2017).

Levels of several clotting factors, especially fibrinogen, are elevated during pregnancy and continue to be higher during labor and after delivery. This increase provides protection from hemorrhage but also increases the mother's risk for a venous thrombosis during pregnancy and after birth.

Fetal Response
Placental Circulation

The exchange of oxygen, nutrients, and waste products between the mother and fetus occurs in the intervillous spaces of the placenta without mixing of maternal and fetal blood. During strong labor contractions, the maternal blood supply to the placenta decreases as the spiral arteries supplying the intervillous spaces are compressed by the uterine muscle. Therefore most placental exchange occurs during the interval between contractions. The placental circulation usually has enough reserve compared with fetal basal needs to tolerate the periodic interruption of blood flow.

Fetal protective mechanisms include the following (Ross & Ervin, 2017):
- Fetal Hgb (Hgb F), which more readily takes on oxygen and releases carbon dioxide when compared to maternal Hgb
- High Hgb and Hct levels that can carry more oxygen than adult Hgb
- A high cardiac output

The fetus may not tolerate labor contractions well in conditions associated with reduced placental function, such as maternal diabetes and hypertension, and conditions associated with reduced fetal oxygen-carrying capacity, such as fetal anemia.

Cardiovascular System

The fetal cardiovascular system reacts quickly to events during labor. Alterations in the rate and rhythm of the fetal heart may result from normal labor effects or suggest fetal intolerance to the stress of labor. The fetal heart rate (FHR) is rapid and ranges from 110 to 160 beats per minute (bpm) at term (Macones et al., 2008). The preterm fetus often has a rate in the higher end of this range.

Pulmonary System

The fetal lungs produce fluid to allow normal development of the airways. The fetus also has breathing motions in utero, breathing in amniotic fluid. Lung fluid must be cleared to allow normal air breathing after birth. As term nears, production of fetal lung fluid decreases to approximately 65% of its maximum production and its absorption into the interstitium of the lungs increases. Labor speeds the absorption of lung fluid. Approximately 35% of the maximum amount remains in the airways at birth (Jobe & Kamath-Rayne, 2014). Some fluid is expelled from the upper airways as the fetal head and thorax are compressed during passage through the birth canal. Most remaining lung fluid is absorbed into the interstitial spaces of the newborn's lungs and then into the circulatory system. A small amount is cleared by the lymphatic circulation (Blackburn, 2013).

Catecholamines (primarily epinephrine and norepinephrine) produced by the fetal adrenal glands in response to the stress of labor appear to contribute to the infant's adaptation to extrauterine life. They stimulate cardiac contraction and breathing, quicken the clearance of remaining lung fluid, and aid in temperature regulation. Infants born by cesarean birth not preceded by labor are more likely to have transient breathing difficulty.

COMPONENTS OF THE BIRTH PROCESS

Four major factors interact during normal childbirth. These factors are often called the *four Ps*: powers, passage, passenger, and psyche.

Powers
Uterine Contractions
During the first stage of labor (onset to full cervical dilation), uterine contractions are the primary force that moves the fetus through the maternal pelvis.

Maternal Pushing Efforts
During the second stage of labor (full cervical dilation to birth of the baby), uterine contractions continue to propel the fetus through the pelvis. In addition, the woman feels an urge to push and bears down as the fetus distends her vagina and puts pressure on her rectum. Her voluntary pushing efforts add to the force of uterine contractions in second-stage labor.

Passage
The birth passage consists of the maternal pelvis and soft tissues. The bony pelvis is usually more important to the outcome of labor than the soft tissue because the bones and joints do not readily yield to the forces of labor. However, softening of the cartilage linking the pelvic bones occurs near term because of increased levels of the hormone relaxin.

The linea terminalis (pelvic brim) divides the bony pelvis into the false pelvis (top) and true pelvis (bottom) (see Chapter 3). The true pelvis is most important in childbirth. The true pelvis has three subdivisions: (1) the inlet, or upper pelvic opening; (2) the midpelvis, or pelvic cavity; and (3) the outlet, or lower pelvic opening. During birth, the true pelvis functions such as a curved cylinder with different dimensions at different levels (Fig. 12.4).

Passenger
The passenger is the fetus, membranes, and placenta. Several fetal anatomic and positional variables influence the course of labor.

Fetal Head
The fetus enters the birth canal in the cephalic **presentation** (*the fetal part that enters the pelvic inlet first*) 96% of the time. The fetal shoulders are also important because of their width, but they usually can be moved to adapt to the diameter of the pelvis.

Bones, Sutures, and Fontanels. The bones of the fetal head involved in the birth process are the two frontal bones on the forehead, two parietal bones at the crown of the head, and one occipital bone at the back of the head (Fig. 12.5). The five major bones are not fused but are connected by **sutures**, which are *narrow areas of flexible tissue that connect fetal skull bones, permitting slight movement during labor*. The **fontanels** are *wider spaces at the intersections of the sutures connecting fetal or infant skull bones*.

The anterior fontanel has a diamond shape formed by the intersection of four sutures: the two coronal, frontal, and sagittal sutures, which connect the two frontal and two parietal bones. The posterior fontanel has a triangular shape formed by the intersection of three sutures: one sagittal and two lambdoid sutures, which connect the two parietal bones and occipital bone. The posterior fontanel is very small and often looks or feels more like a slight indentation in the skull. The sutures and fontanels allow the bones to move slightly, changing the shape of the fetal head so it can adapt to the size and shape of the pelvis by **molding** (*shaping of the fetal head during movement through the birth canal*). The sutures and different shapes of the fontanels provide important landmarks to determine fetal **position** (*relation of a fixed reference point on the fetus to the quadrants of the maternal pelvis*) and head flexion during vaginal examination.

Fetal Head Diameters. Most fetuses enter the pelvis in the cephalic presentation, but several variations are possible. The major transverse diameter of the fetal head is the biparietal diameter, measured between the two parietal bones. The biparietal diameter averages 9.5 cm in a term fetus.

The anteroposterior diameter of the head varies with the degree of flexion. In the most favorable situation, the head becomes fully flexed during labor and the anteroposterior diameter is suboccipitobregmatic, averaging 9.5 cm (see Fig. 12.5, *B*).

Fetal Lie
The orientation of the long axis of the fetus to the long axis of the woman is called the **fetal lie** (Fig. 12.6). In more than 99% of pregnancies, the lie is longitudinal and parallel to the long axis of the woman. In the longitudinal lie, either the head or the buttocks of the fetus enter the pelvis first. A transverse lie exists when the long axis of the fetus is at a right angle to the woman's long axis. This occurs in less than 1% of pregnancies. An oblique lie is at some angle between the longitudinal lie and the transverse lie.

Attitude
The relation of fetal body parts to one another is the **attitude** of the fetus (Fig. 12.7). The normal fetal attitude is one of flexion, with the head flexed toward the chest and the arms and legs flexed over the thorax. The back is curved in a convex C shape. Flexion remains a characteristic feature of the term *newborn*.

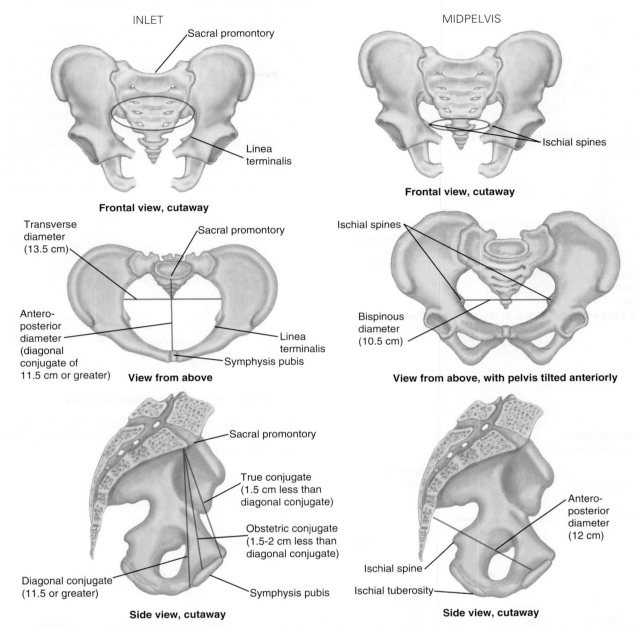

INLET

Sacral promontory

Linea terminalis

Frontal view, cutaway

Transverse diameter (13.5 cm)

Sacral promontory

Antero-posterior diameter (diagonal conjugate of 11.5 cm or greater)

Linea terminalis

Symphysis pubis

View from above

Sacral promontory

True conjugate (1.5 cm less than diagonal conjugate)

Obstetric conjugate (1.5-2 cm less than diagonal conjugate)

Diagonal conjugate (11.5 or greater)

Symphysis pubis

Side view, cutaway

MIDPELVIS

Ischial spines

Frontal view, cutaway

Ischial spines

Bispinous diameter (10.5 cm)

View from above, with pelvis tilted anteriorly

Antero-posterior diameter (12 cm)

Ischial spine

Ischial tuberosity

Side view, cutaway

The boundaries of the inlet are the symphysis pubis anteriorly, the sacral promontory posteriorly, and the linea terminalis on the sides. The inlet is slightly wider in its transverse diameter (13.5 cm) than in its anteroposterior (diagonal conjugate) diameter (11.5 cm or greater).

The diagonal conjugate is slightly larger than both the obstetric and true conjugates. The obstetric conjugate is the narrowest of the three conjugate diameters but cannot be measured directly. The obstetric conjugate is estimated by first measuring the diagonal conjugate and then subtracting 1.5 to 2 cm.

If the inlet is small, the fetal head may not be able to enter it. Because it is almost entirely surrounded by bone, except for cartilage at the sacroiliac joint and symphysis pubis, the inlet cannot enlarge much to accommodate the fetus. The bony measurements are essentially fixed.

The midpelvis, or pelvic cavity, is the narrowest part of the pelvis through which the fetus must pass during birth. Mid-pelvic diameters are measured at the level of the ischial spines. The anteroposterior diameter averages 12 cm.

The transverse diameter (bispinous or interspinous) averages 10.5 cm. Prominent ischial spines that project into the midpelvis can reduce the bispinous diameter.

FIG. 12.4 Pelvic Divisions and Measurements.

Continued

OUTLET

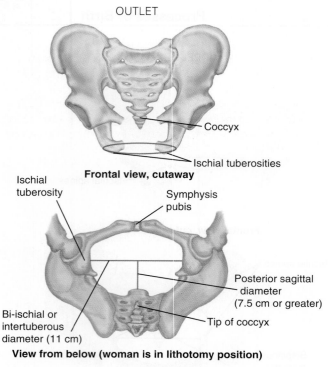

Coccyx

Ischial tuberosities

Frontal view, cutaway

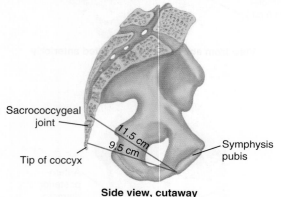

Ischial tuberosity

Symphysis pubis

Posterior sagittal diameter (7.5 cm or greater)

Bi-ischial or intertuberous diameter (11 cm)

Tip of coccyx

View from below (woman is in lithotomy position)

Sacrococcygeal joint

11.5 cm

9.5 cm

Tip of coccyx

Symphysis pubis

Side view, cutaway

Three important diameters of the pelvic outlet are (1) the anteroposterior, (2) the transverse (bi-ischial or intertuberous), and (3) the posterior sagittal. The angle of the pubic arch also is an important pelvic outlet measure.

The anteroposterior diameter ranges from 9.5 to 11.5 cm, varying with the curve between the sacrococcygeal joint and the tip of the coccyx. The anteroposterior diameter can increase if the coccyx is easily movable.

The transverse diameter is the bi-ischial, or intertuberous, diameter. This is the distance between the ischial tuberosities ("sit bones"). It averages 11 cm. The posterior sagittal diameter is normally at least 7.5 cm. It is a measure of the posterior pelvis.

The posterior sagittal diameter measures the distance from the sacrococcygeal joint to the middle of the transverse (bi-ischial) diameter. The angle of the pubic arch is important because it must be wide enough for the fetus to pass under it.

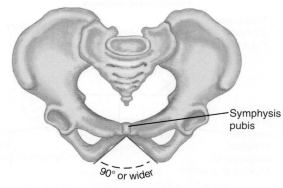

Symphysis pubis

90° or wider

Frontal view, with pelvis tilted anteriorly

The angle of the pubic arch should be at least 90 degrees. A narrow pubic arch displaces the fetus posteriorly toward the coccyx as it tries to pass under the arch.

FIG. 12.4, cont'd

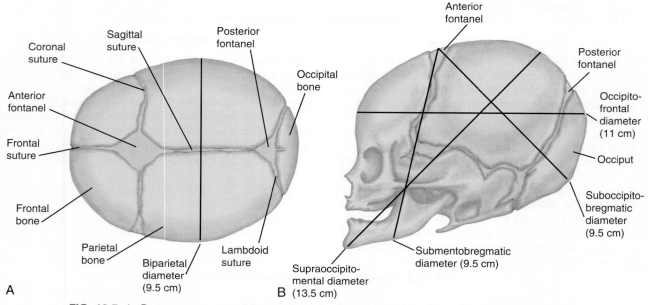

Coronal suture

Sagittal suture

Posterior fontanel

Occipital bone

Anterior fontanel

Frontal suture

Frontal bone

Parietal bone

Biparietal diameter (9.5 cm)

Lambdoid suture

A

Anterior fontanel

Posterior fontanel

Occipitofrontal diameter (11 cm)

Occiput

Suboccipitobregmatic diameter (9.5 cm)

Submentobregmatic diameter (9.5 cm)

Supraoccipitomental diameter (13.5 cm)

B

FIG. 12.5 A, Bones, sutures, and fontanels of the fetal head. Note that the anterior fontanel has a diamond shape, whereas the posterior fontanel is triangular. B, Lateral view of the fetal head demonstrating that anteroposterior diameters vary with the amount of flexion or extension.

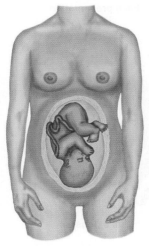
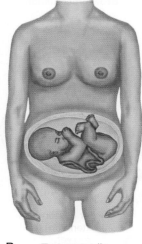

A Longitudinal lie   B Transverse lie

FIG. 12.6 Fetal Lie. A, In a longitudinal lie, the long axis of the fetus is parallel to the long axis of the mother. **B,** In a transverse lie, the long axis of the fetus is at right angles to the long axis of the mother. The woman's abdomen has a wide, short appearance.

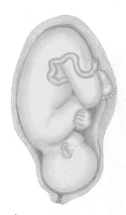
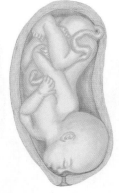

A Flexion   B Extension

FIG. 12.7 Attitude. A, The fetus is in the normal attitude of flexion, with the head, arms, and legs flexed tightly against the trunk. **B,** The fetus is in an abnormal attitude of extension. The head is extended, and the right arm is extended. A face presentation is illustrated.

Presentation

The fetal part that first enters the pelvis is termed the *presenting part*. Presentation falls into three categories: (1) cephalic, (2) breech, and (3) shoulder. The cephalic presentation with the fetal head flexed is the most common. Other presentations are associated with prolonged labor and are more likely to require cesarean birth.

Cephalic Presentation. The cephalic presentation is more favorable than others for the following reasons:
- The fetal head is the largest single fetal part, although the breech (buttocks), with the legs and feet flexed on the abdomen, is collectively larger than the head. After the head is born, the smaller parts follow easily as the extremities unfold.

- During labor, the fetal head can gradually change shape, molding to adapt to the size and shape of the maternal pelvis.
- The fetal head is smooth, round, and hard, making it a more effective part to dilate the cervix, which is also round.

Cephalic presentation has the following four variations (Fig. 12.8):
- Vertex—This is the most common type of cephalic presentation, in which the fetal head is fully flexed. It is called a *vertex* or *occiput presentation* and is the most favorable for normal progress of labor because the smallest suboccipito-bregmatic diameter is presenting.
- Military—The head is in a neutral position, neither flexed nor extended. The longer occipitofrontal diameter is presenting.
- Brow—The fetal head is partly extended. The brow presentation is unstable, usually converting to a vertex presentation if the head flexes or to a face presentation if it extends. The longest supraoccipitomental diameter is presenting.
- Face—The head is extended, and the fetal occiput is near the fetal spine. The submentobregmatic diameter is presenting.

Breech Presentation. A breech presentation occurs when the fetal buttocks or legs enter the pelvis first, which happens in approximately 3% to 4% of births. Breech presentation is more common in preterm births, hydrocephaly (enlargement of the head with fluid), multiple gestations, abnormalities of the maternal uterus and pelvis, and with *placenta previa* (placenta in the lower uterus) (Cunningham et al., 2014).

Breech presentations are associated with the following disadvantages:
- The buttocks are not smooth and firm like the head and are less effective at dilating the cervix.
- The fetal head is the last part to be born. By the time the fetal head is deep in the pelvis, the umbilical cord is outside the mother's body and is subject to compression between the fetal head and the maternal pelvis.
- Because the umbilical cord can be compressed after the fetal chest is born, the head should be delivered quickly to allow the infant to breathe. This does not permit gradual molding of the fetal head as it passes through the pelvis.

The breech presentation has the following three variations, depending on the relationship of the legs to the body (Fig. 12.9):
- Frank breech—This is the most common variation, occurring when the fetal legs are extended across the abdomen toward the shoulders.
- Complete breech—This is a reversal of the usual cephalic presentation. The head, knees, and hips are flexed, but the buttocks are presenting.
- Footling breech—This occurs when one or both feet are presenting.

Shoulder Presentation. The shoulder presentation is a transverse lie and accounts for only 0.3% of births (Cunningham et al., 2014). It occurs more often with preterm birth, high parity, prematurely ruptured membranes, hydramnios, and placenta

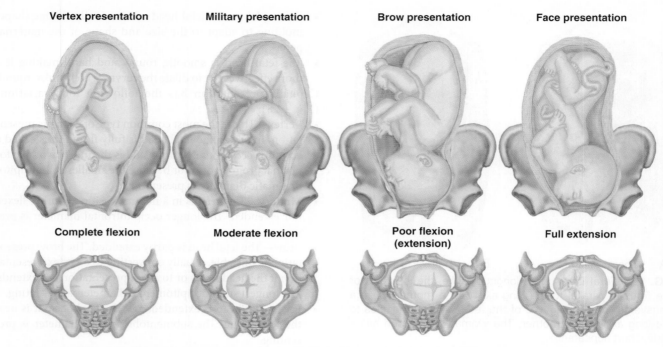

Vertex presentation   **Military presentation**   **Brow presentation**   **Face presentation**

Complete flexion   **Moderate flexion**   **Poor flexion (extension)**   **Full extension**

FIG. 12.8 Four Variations of Cephalic Presentation. The vertex presentation is normal. Note positional changes of the anterior and posterior fontanels in relation to the maternal pelvis.

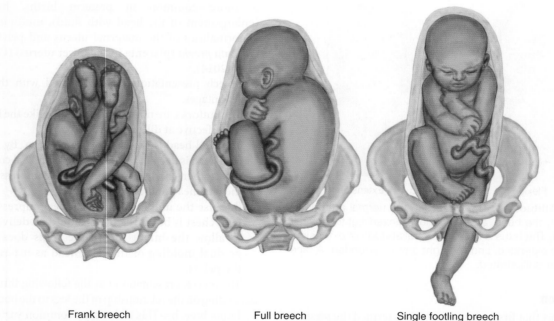

Frank breech   **Full breech**   **Single footling breech**

FIG. 12.9 Three Variations of a Breech Presentation. Frank breech is the most common variation. Footling breeches may be single or double.

previa. A cesarean birth is necessary when the fetus is viable (one of a gestational age that might survive).

KNOWLEDGE CHECK

6. What are the two powers of labor?
7. What are the three divisions of the true pelvis?
8. Why is the vertex presentation best during birth?

Position

Fetal position describes the location of a fixed reference point on the presenting part in relation to the four quadrants of the maternal pelvis (Fig. 12.10). The four quadrants are the right and left anterior and right and left posterior. The fetal position is not fixed but changes during labor as the fetus moves downward and adapts to the pelvic contours.

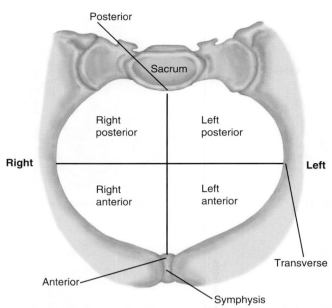

FIG. 12.10 Four quadrants of the maternal pelvis from above, which are used to describe fetal position.

Abbreviations indicate the relationship between the fetal presenting part and maternal pelvis.

Right (R) or Left (L). The first letter of the abbreviation describes whether the fetal reference point is to the right or left of the mother's pelvis. If the fetal reference point is neither to the right nor to the left of the pelvis, this letter is omitted.

Occiput (O), Mentum (M), or Sacrum (S). The second letter of the abbreviation refers to the fixed fetal reference point, which varies with the presentation. The occiput is used in a vertex presentation. The chin, or mentum, is the reference point in a face presentation. The sacrum is used for breech presentations. Letters may also designate the less common brow (F for fronto) and shoulder (Sc for scapula) presentations.

Anterior (A), Posterior (P), or Transverse (T). A, P, and T describe whether the fetal reference point is in the anterior or posterior quadrant of the mother's pelvis. If the fetal reference point is in neither an anterior nor a posterior quadrant, it is described as transverse. If the fetal occiput is in the left anterior quadrant of the mother's pelvis, the position is described as left occiput anterior (LOA). If the occiput is in the mother's anterior pelvis, neither to the right nor to the left, it is described as occiput anterior (OA). If the fetal sacrum is in the mother's right posterior pelvis, the abbreviation is R (right) S (sacrum) P (posterior) (Fig. 12.11).

KNOWLEDGE CHECK

9. For each fetal position listed, describe the fetal landmark. Where is this landmark located in relation to the mother's pelvis: ROP? OA? RSA? LMA?
10. If the fetus is in the face presentation, why is using the occiput to determine position within the pelvis not possible?

Psyche

A woman's psychological response to labor and birth are influenced by anxiety, culture, expectations, life experiences, and support.

Anxiety

Marked anxiety and fear may decrease a woman's ability to cope with pain in labor. Maternal catecholamines secreted in response to anxiety and fear can inhibit uterine contractility and placental blood flow. In contrast, relaxation augments the natural process of labor. Prenatal education or childbirth classes can increase a woman's knowledge, enhancing her ability to work with her body's efforts rather than resist the natural forces. Much of the nurse's care during labor involves reducing anxiety and fear and assisting with coping strategies. Information, a positive sense of control, and mastery over the birth increase the woman's sense of satisfaction with her birth experience (Fair & Morrison, 2012).

Culture and Expectations

A woman's culture affects her values and expectations for and responses to birth and the practices surrounding it. The nurse's familiarity with a group's cultural values and practices provides a framework to care for the woman and her family as individuals. The nurse should assess the personal expectations and values of each woman and her support person related to birth within this general framework. Questions for the intrapartum period might include the following:

- Are they recent immigrants, or have their relatives and friends lived in the area for generations?
- What is the primary language used? Do the woman and her support person speak the same language? Are they comfortable communicating in the nurse's language if that is not their usual language? How does a woman with hearing impairment communicate with people who can hear? If an interpreter is needed, what people would the woman or her family consider unacceptable interpreters (e.g., men or members of certain religious groups)?
- Who is the woman's primary support person for labor? What is that person's role? Will that person actively support the laboring woman (e.g., by coaching her breathing), or will he or she take a less active role? Who will be present at the birth?
- Who is the decision maker, or who should be consulted about important decisions?
- Will another relative (such as a grandmother) assume primary care for the infant?
- Is a professional caregiver (such as a nurse or physician) of the same gender and cultural group essential?
- What are the woman's feelings about touch? Is she comfortable telling the nurse when she does not welcome touch?
- How is pain perceived? What are acceptable pain levels and appropriate pain reduction strategies?
- Are specific symbols, practices, and ceremonies used during the birth period? Who will conduct any ceremonies?

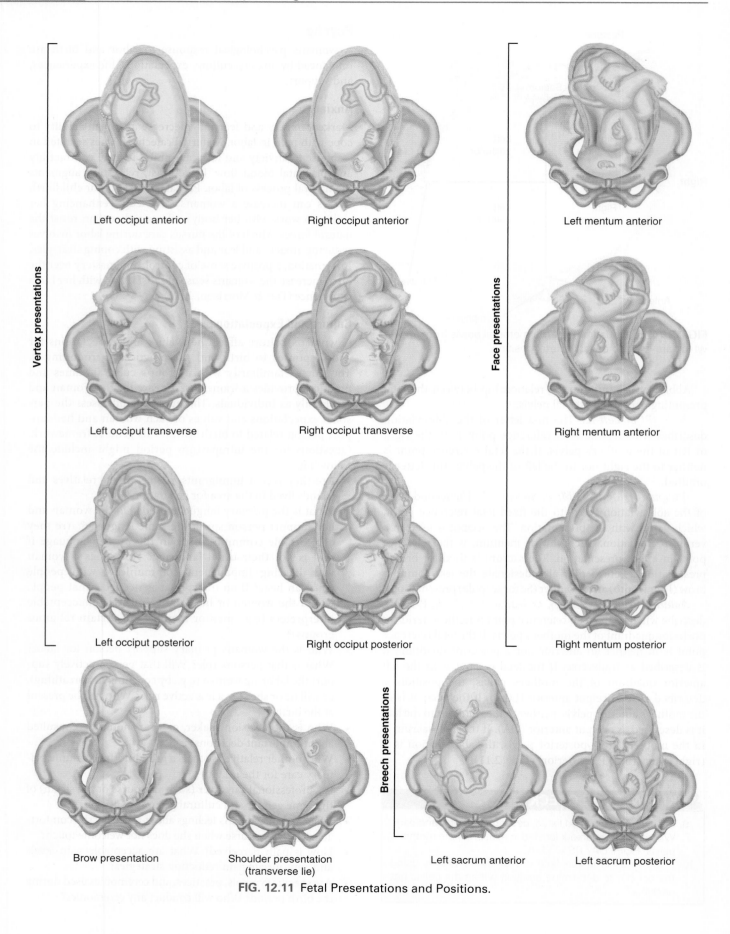

Vertex presentations

Left occiput anterior

Right occiput anterior

Left occiput transverse

Right occiput transverse

Left occiput posterior

Right occiput posterior

Face presentations

Left mentum anterior

Right mentum anterior

Right mentum posterior

Breech presentations

Left sacrum anterior

Left sacrum posterior

Brow presentation

Shoulder presentation
(transverse lie)

FIG. 12.11 Fetal Presentations and Positions.

Birth as an Experience

Childbirth is a physical and an emotional experience. It is an irrevocable event that forever changes a woman and a family. Families describe the births of their children as they describe other pivotal events in life such as marriages, anniversaries, religious events, and even deaths. A woman who has realistic expectations about birth is more likely to have a positive experience. Nursing measures that increase the woman's sense of control and mastery during birth help her perceive the birth as a positive event. The woman's past experiences with childbirth, pain, and personal success and failure will influence her expectations for this birth.

Support

The positive effects of continuous labor support are well documented (Gilliland, 2011; Hodnett, Gates, Hofmeyr, & Sakala, 2013; Kashanian, Javadi, & Haghighi, 2010; Khresheh, 2010). Support includes physical comfort measures, providing information, advocacy, praise and reassurance, presence, and the maintenance of a calm and comfortable environment.

Interrelationships of Components

The four Ps have been described separately but are actually an interrelated whole. For instance, a woman with a small pelvis (passage) and a large fetus (passenger) may be able to have a normal labor and birth if the fetus is ideally positioned and the uterine contractions and maternal bearing-down efforts (powers) are vigorous. The nurse's supportive attitude strengthens positive psychological elements (psyche) and enhances the processes of birth. The nurse can act as an advocate for the laboring woman and her support person to increase their sense of control and mastery of labor, which often reduces anxiety and fear and helps them achieve their desired birth experience.

NORMAL LABOR

Theories of Onset

Despite continuing research, the exact mechanisms that initiate labor remain unknown. Labor normally starts when the fetus is mature enough to adjust easily to extrauterine life but before it grows so large that vaginal birth is impossible. This stage (term gestation) occurs between 37 and 42 weeks after the first day of the woman's last menstrual period (Norwitz et al., 2014). One or more sonograms early in pregnancy may have influenced the "due date," especially for the woman who often has irregular periods.

Natural labor begins when forces favoring continuation of pregnancy are offset by forces favoring its end. Research is ongoing in this area. Factors that appear to have a role in starting labor (Cunningham et al., 2014; Kilpatrick & Garrison, 2017) include the following:

- Changes in the ratio of maternal estrogen to progesterone so that estrogen levels are higher than progesterone levels. Progesterone promotes smooth muscle relaxation of the uterus during most of pregnancy. Relatively higher estrogen levels as progesterone levels fall near the onset of labor enhance uterine sensitivity to substances that stimulate uterine contractions: prostaglandins from the fetal membranes and oxytocin from the maternal posterior pituitary gland. Estrogens increase the number of gap junctions—connections that allow the individual uterine muscle cells to contract as a coordinated unit.

- Prostaglandins produced by the decidua and membranes may have a role in preparing the uterus for oxytocin stimulation at term. Prostaglandins are secreted from the lower area of the fetal membranes (forebag) during labor and may reflect inflammation caused by contact with microorganisms from the woman's vagina.

- Increased secretion of natural oxytocin appears to maintain labor once it has begun. Oxytocin alone does not appear to start labor but may play a part in labor's initiation in conjunction with other substances. Evidence of fetal oxytocin secretion also exists.

- Oxytocin receptors in the uterus increase markedly as labor begins, and the increase continues during labor and peaks at delivery. Oxytocin has little effect on the uterine muscle if the receptors have not developed.

- A fetal role in the initiation of labor appears likely. The fetal membranes release prostaglandin in high concentrations during labor. In addition to fetal oxytocin secretion, large quantities of cortisol are secreted by the fetal adrenal glands, possibly acting as a uterine stimulant.

- Stretching, pressure, and irritation of the uterus and cervix increase as the fetus reaches term size. During early pregnancy the uterus has not reacted to stretching by contracting as smooth muscle normally does. A feedback loop is likely responsible for labor contractions at term: the fetal head stretches the cervix, causing the fundus of the uterus to contract, pushing the fetal head against the cervix, and causing more fundal contractions. Cervical stretching also causes secretion of oxytocin.

Premonitory Signs
Braxton Hicks Contractions

As term gestation approaches, **Braxton Hicks contractions** *(irregular, mild uterine contractions that occur throughout pregnancy and become stronger in the last trimester)* become more noticeable and even painful. Parous women often describe more uterine activity preceding labor than do nulliparous women.

Increased perception of Braxton Hicks contractions often makes sleep difficult at the end of pregnancy. The contractions may become regular at times, only to decrease spontaneously. These contractions are often uncomfortable and sometimes regular, which can cause women to be confused about whether labor has begun.

Lightening

As the fetus descends toward the pelvic inlet ("dropping"), the woman notices that she breathes more easily because upward pressure on her diaphragm is reduced. However, increased pressure on her bladder causes her to urinate more frequently. Pressure of the fetal head in the pelvis also may cause leg cramps and edema. **Lightening** *(descent of the fetus toward the pelvic inlet before labor)* is most noticeable in nulliparas and occurs about 2 to 3 weeks before the natural onset of labor.

Increased Vaginal Mucous Secretions

An increase in clear and nonirritating vaginal secretions occurs as fetal pressure causes congestion of the vaginal mucosa.

Cervical Ripening and Bloody Show

As full term nears, the cervix *softens because of the effects of the hormone relaxin.* These changes (**ripening**) allow the cervix to yield more easily to the forces of labor contractions. As the fetal head descends with lightening, it puts pressure on the cervix, starting the process of effacement and dilation. Effacement and dilation cause expulsion of the mucus plug that sealed the cervix during pregnancy, rupturing small cervical capillaries in the process. **Bloody show** *(mixture of cervical mucus and pink or brown blood from ruptured capillaries in the cervix; often precedes labor and increases with cervical dilation)* may begin several days to a few weeks before the onset of labor, especially in the nulliparous woman, or it may not begin until labor starts.

A recent vaginal examination or sexual intercourse also may result in small amounts of bloody show because it disrupts these small vessels. Bloody show increases during labor as the cervix completes dilation and effacement. Women who have previously had a vaginal birth often have less bloody show than nulliparas.

Energy Spurt

Some women have a sudden increase in energy, which is called "nesting." They should be cautioned to conserve their energy so that they are not exhausted when labor begins.

Weight Loss

A small weight loss of 2.2 to 6.6 kg (1 to 3 lb) may occur because the altered estrogen-to-progesterone ratio causes excretion of some of the extra fluid that accumulates during pregnancy.

True Labor and False Labor

False labor, also called *prodromal labor* or *prelabor,* is common because the exact time of labor's onset is rarely known and usually is gradual. False labor often causes women to go to the birth center, thinking that labor has started, only to be disappointed when it has not. Women may be observed in the labor unit for enough time to have two cervical examinations to evaluate cervical change (American Academy of Pediatrics [AAP] & American College of Obstetricians and Gynecologists [ACOG], 2012). The term *false labor* is discouraging to women because they do not realize that these "false" contractions are preparation for true labor.

Several characteristics distinguish true labor from false labor: contractions, discomfort, and cervical change. The best distinction between true and false labor is that contractions of true labor cause progressive change in the cervix. A more rapid increase in effacement and dilation occurs with true labor contractions.

Some women experience membrane rupture as the first sign of labor onset. If this occurs, the woman should go to the birth center for evaluation. Infection and compression of the fetal umbilical cord are possible complications.

> ### ❓ CRITICAL THINKING EXERCISE 12.1
>
> Alan phones you when you are working in the birth unit of your hospital one night. He says, "My wife's baby is due. Heather has been having some contractions off and on all day, and they're keeping her awake now. Should we come to the hospital?"
>
> **Questions**
> 1. Do you need any other information? If so, what information do you need? (Assume your hospital has a protocol for telephone triage that allows nurses to answer and document similar phone inquiries.)
> 2. How should you explain these symptoms? What advice is appropriate?

PATIENT TEACHING

How to Know Whether Labor Is "Real"

True labor differs from false labor in three categories.

FALSE LABOR	TRUE LABOR
Contractions	
Are inconsistent in frequency, duration, and intensity	Usually have a consistent pattern of increasing frequency, duration, and intensity
Do not change or may decrease with activity (such as walking)	Tend to increase with walking
	Begin in lower back and gradually sweep around to lower abdomen
Discomfort	
Is felt in the abdomen and groin	May persist as back pain in some women
May be more annoying than truly painful	Often resembles menstrual cramps during early labor
Cervix	
Does not significantly change in effacement or dilation	Includes progressive effacement and dilation (most important characteristic)

Labor Mechanisms

The mechanisms (cardinal movements) of labor occur as the fetus is moved through the pelvis during birth. The fetus undergoes several positional changes to adapt to the size and shape of the mother's pelvis at different levels (Fig. 12.12). Although the mechanisms of labor are described separately in Fig. 12.12, some occur concurrently. In a vertex presentation, the mechanisms include the following:

- Descent of the fetal presenting part through the true pelvis
- **Engagement** of the fetal presenting part as its widest diameter reaches the level of the ischial spines of the mother's pelvis (0 station).

DESCENT, ENGAGEMENT, AND FLEXION

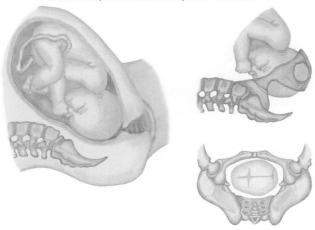

Descent of the fetus is a mechanism of labor that accompanies all the others. Without descent, none of the mechanisms will occur.

Station

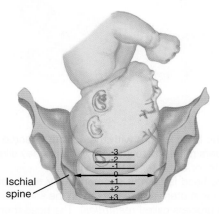

Ischial
spine

Station is a measurement of the descent of the fetal presenting part in relation to the level of the ischial spines of the maternal pelvis. The level of the ischial spines is a zero station. Other stations are described with numbers representing the approximate number of centimeters above (negative numbers) or below (positive numbers) the ischial spines. As the fetus descends through the pelvis, the station changes from higher negative numbers (−3, −2, −1) to zero to higher positive numbers (+ 1, + 2, + 3, etc.). Sometimes the terms *floating* or *ballotable* may describe a fetal presenting part that is so high that it is easily displaced upward during abdominal or vaginal examination, similar to tossing a ball upward.

Engagement

Engagement occurs when the largest diameter of the fetal presenting part (normally the head) has passed the pelvic inlet and entered the pelvic cavity. Engagement is presumed to have occurred when the station of the presenting part is zero or lower. Engagement often takes place before onset of labor in nulliparous women. In many parous women and in some nulliparas, it does not occur until after labor begins.

Flexion

As the fetus descends, the fetal head is flexed farther as it meets resistance from the soft tissues of the pelvis. Head flexion presents the smallest anteroposterior diameter (suboccipitobregmatic) to the pelvis.

Internal Rotation

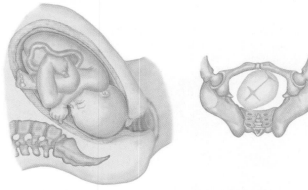

The fetus enters the pelvic inlet with the sagittal suture in a transverse or oblique orientation to the maternal pelvis because that is the widest inlet diameter. Internal rotation allows the longest fetal head diameter (the anteroposterior) to conform to the longest diameter of the maternal pelvis. The longest pelvic outlet diameter is the anteroposterior. As the head descends to the level of the ischial spines, it gradually turns so that the fetal occiput is in the anterior of the pelvis (OA position, directly under the maternal symphysis pubis). When internal rotation is complete, the sagittal suture is oriented in the anteroposterior pelvic diameter (OA). Less commonly, the head may turn posteriorly so that the occiput is directed toward the mother's sacrum (OP).

FIG. 12.12 Mechanisms (Cardinal Movements) of Labor.

Continued

EXTENSION

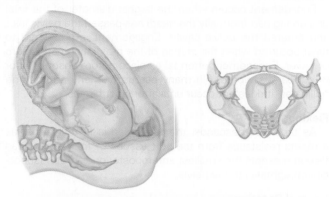

Extension beginning (internal rotation complete)

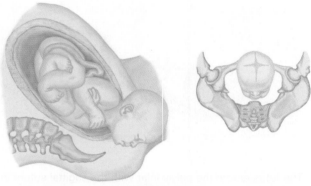

Extension complete

Because the true pelvis is shaped like a curved cylinder, the fetal face is directed posteriorly toward the rectum as it begins its rotation and descent. To negotiate the curve of the pelvis, the fetal head must change from an attitude of flexion to one of extension.

While still in flexion, the fetal head meets resistance from the tissues of the pelvic floor. At the same time, the fetal neck stops under the symphysis, which acts as a pivot. The combination of resistance from the pelvic floor and the pivoting action of the symphysis causes the fetal head to swing anteriorly, or extend, with each maternal pushing effort. The head is born in extension, with the occiput sliding under the symphysis and the face directed toward the rectum. The fetal brow, nose, and chin slide over the perineum as the head is born.

EXTERNAL ROTATION

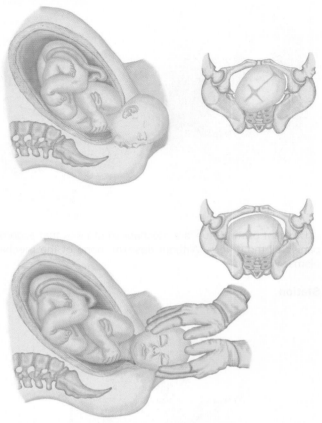

When the head is born with the occiput directed anteriorly, the shoulders must rotate internally so that they align with the anteroposterior diameter of the pelvis.

After the head is born, it spontaneously turns to the same side as it was in utero as it realigns with the shoulders and back (through a process called *restitution*). The head then turns farther to that side in external rotation as the shoulders internally rotate and are positioned with their transverse diameter in the anteroposterior diameter of the pelvic outlet. External rotation of the head accompanies internal rotation of the shoulders.

EXPULSION

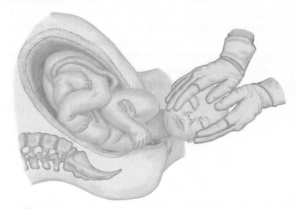

Expulsion occurs first as the anterior, then the posterior, shoulder passes under the symphysis. After the shoulders are born, the rest of body follows.

FIG. 12.12, cont'd

- Flexion of the fetal head, allowing the smallest head diameters to align with the smaller diameters of the midpelvis as the fetus descends
- Internal rotation to allow the largest fetal head diameters to align with the largest maternal pelvic diameters
- Extension of the fetal head as the neck pivots on the inner margin of the symphysis pubis, allowing the head to align with the curves of the pelvic outlet
- External rotation of the fetal head, aligning the head with the shoulders during expulsion
- Expulsion of the fetal shoulders and fetal body

The mechanisms of labor are different in presentations other than the vertex, but the reason is the same: to effectively use the available space in the maternal pelvis.

KNOWLEDGE CHECK

11. What are some signs and symptoms that a woman might experience before labor begins?
12. What are the differences between true and false labor? Which difference is the most significant?
13. Why does the fetus enter the pelvis with the sagittal suture aligned with the transverse diameter of the woman's pelvic inlet?
14. Why does the fetal head turn during labor until the sagittal suture aligns with the anteroposterior diameter of the mother's pelvic outlet?

Stages and Phases of Labor

Labor is divided into four stages. Each stage has unique qualities (Table 12.1). This chapter describes typical physiologic characteristics and maternal behaviors in the average woman. Women vary in their labor patterns and responses to this process. Regional anesthesia may alter some of the maternal behaviors.

First Stage

Cervical effacement and dilation occur in the first stage, or the stage of dilation. It begins with the onset of true labor contractions and ends with complete dilation (10 cm) and effacement (100%) of the cervix. The first stage of labor is the longest for both nulliparous and parous women. Three phases within the first stage are latent, active, and transition. Each phase is characterized by changing maternal behaviors. These behaviors vary with the woman's preparation, use of coping skills, and use of medication.

When the active phase begins, the cervix of the nullipara usually dilates at a slower rate than that of the **multipara** *(a woman who has given birth after two or more pregnancies of at least 20 weeks of gestation; also, informally used to describe a pregnant woman before the birth of her second child)* (Cunningham et al., 2014; Kilpatrick & Garrison, 2017; Thorpe & Laughon, 2014). Historically, labor progress often has been plotted on a labor progress graph called a *Friedman curve* (Fig. 12.13). Current research suggests that normal labor progresses more slowly than previously

believed. Revisions to the labor curve may be made as more data become available.

Latent Phase. Historically, the latent phase has been defined as 0 to 3 cm dilated. However, recent research has suggested that the latent phase be considered to last until 5 to 6 cm dilated (Hanson & VandeVusse, 2014; Spong, Berghella, Wenstrom, Mercer, & Saade, 2012; Zhang et al., 2010). Its length varies among women but may be longer for the nullipara than for the multipara. Latent labor may be quite long, and much of it may pass unnoticed by the pregnant woman as latent labor gradually merges into active labor. Cervical effacement and fetal positional change occur during the latent phase, preparing for the more rapid changes of active labor.

Contractions gradually increase in frequency, duration, and intensity. The interval between contractions shortens until contractions are about 5 minutes apart as the woman progresses to the active phase. Duration increases to 30 to 40 seconds by the end of the latent phase. Initially, the contractions are mild; the contracting uterus can be easily indented with the fingertips, and progress to moderate intensity, during which the uterine muscle is indented with more difficulty (Simpson & O'Brien-Abel, 2014). The contractions gradually build to their peak intensity and remain at the peak briefly before diminishing.

During latent labor, the woman may notice discomfort in her back with each contraction. As labor progresses, back discomfort encircles the lower abdomen with each contraction. Many women describe the discomfort as like menstrual cramps, especially during early labor.

The woman is usually sociable, excited, and cooperative. She is anxious as she realizes that these contractions are not Braxton Hicks contractions but the "real thing"; she is usually relieved that she is close to the birth of her baby.

Active Phase. When the rate of cervical change accelerates, the woman has progressed to active phase (Kilpatrick & Garrison, 2017). The fetus descends in the pelvis, and internal rotation begins. Active and transition phases are linked as one phase enters the next, and references may not distinguish the two.

For more than 50 years, our understanding of the progress of normal labor has been based on the classic research of Dr. Emanuel Friedman in the 1950s (Friedman, 1955). The Friedman labor curve has been used to assess labor progress in the clinical setting. Per Friedman's work, the active phase of first stage labor begins at 4 cm dilation. After this point, a multiparous woman should progress at a rate of 1.5 cm/hr and a nulliparous woman should progress at a rate of 1.2 cm/hr (Kilpatrick & Garrison, 2017).

More recent research (Hanson & VandeVusse, 2014; Laughon, Branch, Beaver, & Zhang, 2012; Spong et al., 2012; Zhang et al., 2010) indicates that for various reasons, modern women progress through labor at a slower rate. Per these findings, the active phase of first-stage labor begins at 5 to 6 cm dilation. The first stage of labor then lasts an average of 6 to 13.3 hours in the nullipara and 5.7 to 7.5 hours in the multipara (Kilpatrick & Garrison, 2017). These findings are supported by the American College of Obstetricians and Gynecologists (ACOG) and the Society for Maternal-Fetal Medicine (SMFM) (ACOG & SMFM, 2014).

TABLE 12.1   Conventional Characteristics of Normal Labor

Characteristics	First Stage	Second Stage	Third Stage	Fourth Stage
Work accomplished	Effacement and dilation of cervix	Expulsion of fetus	Separation of placenta	Physical recovery and bonding with newborn
Forces	Uterine contractions	Uterine contractions and voluntary bearing-down efforts	Uterine contractions	Uterine contraction to control bleeding from placental site
Cervical dilation	*Latent phase*:* 0-3 cm *Active phase*:* 4-7 cm *Transition phase:* 8-10 cm	10 cm (complete dilation)	Not applicable	Not applicable
Uterine contractions	*Latent phase:* Initially mild and infrequent; progress to moderate strength, every 5 min with a regular pattern; duration increases to 30-40 sec by end of latent phase *Active phase:* Increase in frequency, duration, and intensity until every 2-3 min, 40-60 sec, and moderate to strong intensity *Transition phase:* Strong, every 1½-2 min, 60-90 sec	Strong, every 2-3 min, lasting 40-60 sec; may be slightly less intense than during transition phase of first stage; may pause briefly as second stage begins	Firmly contracted	Firmly contracted
Discomfort†	Often begins with a low backache and sensations similar to those of menstrual cramps; back discomfort gradually sweeps to lower abdomen in a girdle-like fashion; discomfort intensifies as labor progresses	Urge to push or bear down with contractions, which becomes stronger as fetus descends; distention of vagina and vulva may cause a stretching or splitting sensation	Little discomfort; sometimes slight cramp is felt as placenta is passed	Discomfort varies; some women have afterpains, more common in multigravidas or those who have had a large baby; as anesthesia wears off, perineal discomfort may become noticeable
Maternal behaviors†	Sociable, excited, and somewhat anxious during early labor; becomes more inwardly focused as labor intensifies; may lose control during transition	Intense concentration on pushing with contractions; often oblivious to surroundings and appears to doze between contractions	Excited and relieved after baby's birth; usually very tired; often cries	Tired, but may find it difficult to rest because of excitement; eager to become acquainted with her newborn

*Conventional cervical dilatation for latent and active phase are shown here. Current research indicates that latent phase may continue until 5-6 cm dilatation.
†Maternal discomfort and behaviors often vary with pain-relief method chosen.

Contractions are about 2 to 5 minutes apart, with a duration of approximately 40 to 60 seconds and an intensity that ranges from moderate to strong (Simpson & O'Brien-Abel, 2014). Active labor contractions resist indenting, reach their peak intensity quickly, and stay at the peak longer than during the latent phase.

As contractions intensify, discomfort also increases if the woman has not had analgesia such as an epidural block. The site of discomfort during the active phase is like that during the latent phase.

The woman's behavior changes. She becomes more anxious and may feel helpless as the contractions intensify. The sociability that characterized early labor is gone and is replaced by a serious, inward focus. She is unlikely to initiate interactions unless she has specific requests. Her behaviors are typical of a person concentrating intently on a demanding task. Women who choose to take pain medication and regional analgesia usually do so during this phase. The nurse helps the woman maintain her concentration, supports her coping techniques, and helps her find alternatives for methods that do not work for her.

Transition Phase. The cervix dilates from 8 to 10 cm in this phase of the first stage, and the fetus descends further into the pelvis. Bloody show often increases with the completion of cervical dilation. Transition is a short but intense phase within the first stage.

Contractions are very strong. They may be as frequent as 1½ to 2 minutes apart, and their duration is 60 to 90 seconds (Simpson & O'Brien-Abel, 2014). Strong contractions combined with fetal descent may cause the woman to have an urge to push and bear down during contractions. Leg tremors, nausea, and vomiting are common.

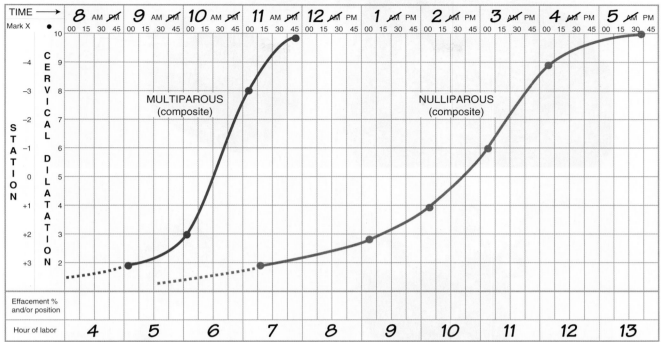

Composite Normal Dilation Curves

FIG. 12.13 A labor curve, sometimes called a *Friedman curve,* has been used to identify whether a woman's cervical dilation progressed at the expected rate. Current research suggests that normal labor progresses more slowly than previously believed. Revisions to the labor curve may be made as more data become available.

The woman who does not choose epidural analgesia often finds the transition phase to be the most difficult part of her labor. She may be irritable and lose control. Her partner may be confused because actions that were helpful just a short time ago now bother her. The nurse can encourage the woman and her support person that the end of labor is near and help them use coping techniques most effectively. If premature bearing down is a problem, the nurse can help the woman blow outward with each breath until the urge passes.

? CRITICAL THINKING EXERCISE 12.2

After examining a woman in labor with her first baby, the nurse-midwife gives you the following information: "Carmelita is 2 to 3 cm, 75%, and 0. The baby is vertex and ROP."

Question

1. What is the correct interpretation of this information? What behaviors would be expected for Carmelita at this time? What behaviors should suggest to you that she has begun making very rapid labor progress?

Second Stage

The second stage (expulsion) begins with complete (10 cm) dilation and full (100%) effacement of the cervix and ends with the birth of the baby. Duration of second stage labor also varies with whether the woman has an epidural. Duration of the second stage for the nullipara with no epidural averages 2.8 hours

whereas the average duration is 3.6 hours with an epidural. Duration of the second stage for the multipara with no epidural ranges from 1.1 to 1.3 hours, and the average duration is 1.6 to 2 hours with an epidural (Zhang et al., 2010).

Contractions may diminish slightly or even pause briefly as the second stage begins. They are still strong and about 2 to 3 minutes apart, with a duration of 40 to 60 seconds.

As the fetus descends, pressure of the presenting part on the rectum and the pelvic floor causes an involuntary pushing response in the mother. She may say that she needs to have a bowel movement or say "the baby's coming" or "I have to push." Her voluntary pushing efforts augment involuntary uterine contractions. As the fetus descends low in the pelvis and the vulva distends with the crowning of the fetal head, she may feel a sensation of stretching or splitting even if no trauma occurs. The maternal urge to push does not always occur the moment the woman is fully dilated. Allowing the woman to "labor down" is beneficial in most cases (see Chapter 15).

The woman often regains a feeling of control during the second stage of labor. Contractions are strong, but she may feel more in control and know that she is doing something to complete the process by pushing with the contractions. The word *labor* aptly describes the second stage. The woman exerts intense physical effort to push her baby out. Between contractions, she may be oblivious to her surroundings and appear to be asleep. She feels tremendous relief and excitement as the second stage ends with the birth of the baby.

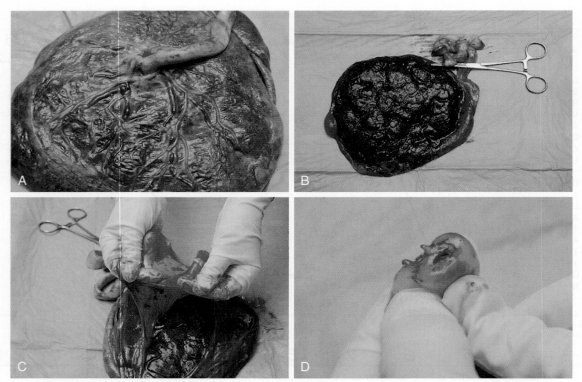

FIG. 12.14 A, Fetal side of the placenta. **B,** Maternal side of the placenta. **C,** Separating membranes. **D,** Umbilical cord vessels: two arteries and one vein.

Third Stage

The third (placental) stage begins with the birth of the baby and ends with the expulsion of the placenta (Fig. 12.14). This stage is the shortest, with an average length of 6 minutes (Kilpatrick & Garrison, 2017). No difference in duration exists between nulliparas and parous women.

When the infant is born, the uterine cavity becomes much smaller. The reduced size decreases the size of the placenta site, causing it to separate from the uterine wall. The following four signs suggest placenta separation:

- The uterus has a spherical shape.
- The uterus rises upward in the abdomen as the placenta descends into the vagina and pushes the fundus upward.
- The cord descends further from the vagina.
- A gush of blood appears as blood trapped behind the placenta is released.

The uterus must contract firmly and remain contracted after the placenta is expelled to compress open vessels at the implantation site. Inadequate uterine contraction after birth may result in hemorrhage.

Pain during the third stage of labor results from uterine contractions and brief stretching of the cervix as the placenta passes through it.

Fourth Stage

The fourth stage of labor is the stage of physical recovery for the mother and infant. It lasts from the delivery of the placenta through the first 1 to 4 hours after birth.

Immediately after birth, the firmly contracted uterus can be palpated through the abdominal wall as a firm, rounded mass approximately 10 to 15 cm (4 to 6 inches) in diameter at or below the level of the umbilicus. Uterine size varies with the size of the infant and parity of the mother and is larger when the infant is large or the mother is a multipara. A full bladder or blood clot in the uterus interferes with uterine contraction, increasing blood loss. A soft (boggy) uterus and increasing uterine size are associated with postpartum hemorrhage because large blood vessels at the placenta site are not compressed (see Chapter 18).

The *vaginal drainage after childbirth* is called **lochia**. The three stages are lochia rubra, lochia serosa, and lochia alba (see Chapter 17). Lochia rubra, consisting mostly of blood, is present in the fourth stage of labor.

Many women are chilled after birth. The cause of this reaction is unknown but may be due to the sudden decrease in effort, loss of the heat produced by the fetus, decrease in intraabdominal pressure, and fetal blood cells entering the maternal circulation. The chill lasts for about 20 minutes and subsides spontaneously. A warm blanket, a hot drink, or soup may help shorten the chill and make the woman more comfortable.

Discomfort during the fourth stage usually results from birth trauma and afterpains. Localized discomfort from birth trauma such as lacerations, an episiotomy, edema, or a hematoma is evident as the effects of local and regional anesthetics diminish. Ice packs on the perineum limit this edema and hematoma formation.

Afterpains are intermittent uterine contractions occurring after birth as the uterus begins to return to the prepregnancy state. The discomfort is like menstrual cramps. Afterpains are more common in multiparas, women who breastfeed, women who have large babies, in cases of uterine overdistention during pregnancy, and in those involving interference with uterine contraction because of a full bladder or blood clot that remains in the uterus.

The mother is simultaneously excited and tired after birth. She may be exhausted but too excited to rest. The fourth stage of labor is an ideal time for bonding of the new family because the interest of both the parents and the newborn is high. It is the best time to initiate breastfeeding if maternal and infant problems are absent. The baby is alert and seeks eye contact with the new parents, giving powerful reinforcement for the parents' attachment to their newborn.

❓ KNOWLEDGE CHECK

15. How do maternal behaviors change during each phase of first-stage labor and the second stage?
16. What are typical characteristics of contractions during each phase of first-stage and second-stage labor?
17. What four signs may indicate that the placenta has separated?
18. What complications may occur if the uterus does not contract firmly and remain contracted after the placenta is expelled?

Duration of Labor

The total duration of labor is significantly different for women who have never given birth and those who have previously given birth vaginally. However, women are individuals. Some nulliparas progress through labor quickly, whereas labor for some parous women resembles that of women who have never given birth.

Because of the high cesarean birth rate and fewer **vaginal births after cesarean** (**VBAC**), a parous woman may have had no vaginal births. In this situation, the woman is likely to have a labor more like that of the nullipara, particularly if she did not labor before her previous cesarean birth.

THE IMPACT OF TECHNOLOGY

The goal of maternity care is to protect the health of the mother, fetus, and newborn and to support and enrich the family's birth experience. Technology helps caregivers identify problems and intervene quickly to promote maternal and fetal well-being. However, extensive use of sophisticated technology may make maternity care seem impersonal. Women may think their feelings are less important than the data from the monitors and infusion pumps attached to them. The nurse should guard against "nursing the machines" or internal feelings of being unnecessary to the woman's birth experience. If the nurse focuses on the woman as the childbearer and the machine as a tool, frustration for all concerned is less likely.

Although normal labor and birth do not require routine use of sophisticated technology, women may quickly agree to suggested interventions and not voice their desire for a low-intervention birth. Other women simply have not thought of a low-technology birth, possibly because many friends and relatives have had a high-technology birth. Communication on the indications and risks and benefits to the use of technology is important in planning each individual's care. The intrapartum nurse can be the bridge between the technology and humanity of the birth experience by keeping the focus on the woman, the fetus, and the support person rather than on the technology.

▌ SUMMARY CONCEPTS

- Labor contractions are intermittent, which allows oxygen, nutrients, and waste products to be exchanged between maternal and fetal circulations during the interval between contractions.
- The upper uterus contracts actively during labor, maintaining tension to pull the more passive lower uterus and cervix over the fetal presenting part. These actions result in cervical effacement and dilation.
- Maternal vital signs are best assessed between contractions because alterations in the woman's blood pressure and pulse rate may occur during a contraction.
- Hyperventilation may occur if the woman breathes deeply and rapidly. Its manifestations include tingling of the hands and feet, numbness, and dizziness.
- The fetal heart rate and rhythm respond rapidly to events occurring during labor.

- Several occurrences during late pregnancy and labor aid the newborn in making adaptations to extrauterine life: reduced production of fetal lung fluid and increased absorption of lung fluid into the interstitium of the fetal lungs; expulsion of fluid from upper airways during the compression forces of labor; and increased catecholamine secretion by the fetal adrenal glands to stimulate cardiac contraction and breathing, speed clearance of remaining lung fluid, and aid in temperature regulation.
- Four interrelated components affecting the process of birth are the powers, passage, passenger, and psyche. Presentation and position further describe the relation of the fetus (passenger) to the maternal pelvis (passage).
- The exact reasons for the beginning of labor are unknown, but several maternal and fetal factors seem to have a role. These include fetal adrenal gland production of cortisol;

increase in the ratio of estrogen to progesterone; increased uterine oxytocin receptors and gap junctions; and stretching of the uterus and cervix.

- As labor approaches, the woman may notice one or more premonitory signs preceding its onset: increase in frequency and intensity of Braxton Hicks contractions, lightening, increased vaginal secretions, bloody show, a spurt of energy, and weight loss.
- The conclusive difference between true labor and false labor is that progressive effacement and dilation of the cervix occur with true labor.

- The four stages and phases of labor are characterized by different physiologic events and maternal behaviors: first stage, cervical dilation and effacement; second stage, expulsion of the fetus; third stage, expulsion of the placenta; and fourth stage, maternal physiologic stabilization and parent–infant bonding.
- Normal labor is characterized by consistent progression of uterine contractions, cervical dilation and effacement, and fetal descent.

REFERENCES & READINGS

American Academy of Pediatrics & American College of Obstetricians and Gynecologists (AAP & ACOG). (2012). *Guidelines for perinatal care* (7th ed.). Elk Grove Village, IL: Author.

American College of Nurse-Midwives. (2016). Clinical bulletin no. 16. Providing oral nutrition to women in labor. *Journal of Midwifery and Womens Health, 61*(4), 528–534.

American College of Obstetricians and Gynecologists & Society for Maternal-Fetal Medicine (ACOG & SMFM). (2014). Safe prevention of the primary cesarean delivery. Obstetric Care Consensus No. 1. *Obstetrics and Gynecology, 123*(3), 693–711.

American Society of Anesthesiologists (ASA). (2016). Practice guidelines for obstetrical anesthesia: an updated report by the American Society of Anesthesiologists Task Force on Obstetrical Anesthesia. *Anesthesiology, 124.*

Antony, K. M., Pacusin, D. A., Aagaard, K., & Dildy, G. A. (2017). Maternal physiology. In S. G. Gabbe, J. R. Niebyl, J. L. Simpson, M. B. Landon, H. L. Galan, R. M. Jauniaux, D. A. Driscoll, et al. (Eds.), *Obstetrics: Normal and problem pregnancies* (7th ed.) (pp. 39–64). Philadelphia, PA: Saunders.

Blackburn, S. T. (2013). *Maternal, fetal, and neonatal physiology: a clinical perspective* (4th ed.). St. Louis, MO: Saunders.

Blanchard, D. G., & Daniels, L. B. (2014). Cardiac diseases. In R. K. Creasy, R. Resnik, J. D. Iams, C. J. Lockwood, & T. R. Moore (Eds.), *Creasy & Resnik's Maternal-fetal medicine: Principles and practice* (7th ed.) (pp. 852–877). Philadelphia, PA: Saunders.

Burke, C. (2014). Labor and birth. In K. R. Simpson, & P. A. Creehan (Eds.), *AWHONN's perinatal nursing* (4th ed.) (p. 494). Philadelphia, PA: Lippincott Williams and Wilkins.

Cunningham, F. G., Leveno, K. J., Bloom, S. L., Spong, C. Y., Dashe, J. S., Hoffman, B. L., & Sheffield, J. S. (2014). *Williams obstetrics* (24th ed.). New York: McGraw-Hill.

Fair, C. D., & Morrison, T. E. (2012). The relationship between prenatal control, expectations, experienced control, and birth satisfaction among primiparous women. *Midwifery, 28*, 39–44.

Friedman, E. A. (1955). Primigravid labor: a graphicostatistical analysis. *Obstetrics and Gynecology, 6*(6), 567–589.

Gilliland, A. L. (2011). After praise and encouragement: emotional support strategies used by birth doulas in the USA and Canada. *Midwifery, 27*(4), 525–531.

Hanson, L., & VandeVusse, L. (2014). Supporting labor progress toward physiologic birth. *Journal of Perinatal & Neonatal Nursing, 28*(2), 101–107.

Hodnett, E. D., Gates, S., Hofmeyr, G. J., & Sakala, C. (2013). Continuous support for women during childbirth. *Cochrane Database of Systematic Reviews, 2013* CD003766.

Jobe, A. H., & Kamath-Rayne, B. D. (2014). Fetal lung development and surfactant. In R. K. Creasy, R. Resnik, J. D. Iams, C. J. Lockwood, & T. R. Moore (Eds.), *Creasy & Resnik's Maternal-fetal medicine: Principles and Practice* (7th ed.) (pp. 175–186). Philadelphia, PA: Saunders.

Kashanian, F., Javadi, J., & Haghighi, M. M. (2010). Effect of continuous support during labor on duration of labor and rate of cesarean delivery. *International Journal of Gynecology and Obstetrics, 109*(3), 198–200.

Khresheh, R. (2010). Support in the first stage of labour from a female relative: the first step in improving the quality of maternity services. *Midwifery, 26*(6), e21–e24.

Kilpatrick, S., & Garrison, E. (2017). Normal labor and delivery. In S. G. Gabbe, J. R. Niebyl, J. L. Simpson, M. B. Landon, H. L. Galan, R. M. Jauniaux, D. A. Driscoll, et al. (Eds.), *Obstetrics: Normal and problem pregnancies* (7th ed.) (pp. 246–270). Philadelphia, PA: Saunders.

Laughon, S. K., Branch, D. W., Beaver, J., & Zhang, J. (2012). Changes in labor patterns over 50 years. *American Journal of Obstetrics and Gynecology, 205*(5), 419.e1–419.e9.

Macones, G. A., Hankins, G. D. V., Spong, C. Y., Hauth, J., & Moore, T. (2008). The 2008 National Institute of Child Health and Human Development workshop report on electronic fetal monitoring: update on definitions, interpretation and research guidelines. *Journal Obstetric, Gynecologic, & Neonatal Nursing, 37*(5), 510–515.

Monga, M., & Mastrobattista, J. M. (2014). Maternal cardiovascular, respiratory, and renal adaptation to pregnancy. In R. K. Creasy, R. Resnik, J. D. Iams, C. J. Lockwood, & T. R. Moore (Eds.), *Creasy & Resnik's Maternal-fetal medicine: Principles and Practice* (7th ed.) (pp. 93–96). Philadelphia, PA: Saunders.

Norwitz, E. R., Mahendroo, M., & Lye, S. J. (2014). Biology of parturition. In R. K. Creasy, R. Resnik, J. D. Iams, C. J. Lockwood, & T. R. Moore (Eds.), *Creasy & Resnik's maternal-fetal medicine: Principles and practice* (7th ed.) (pp. 66–79). Philadelphia, PA: Saunders.

Ross, M. G., & Ervin, M. G. (2017). Fetal development and physiology. In S. G. Gabbe, J. R. Niebyl, J. L. Simpson, M. B. Landon, H. L. Galan, R. M. Jauniaux, D. A. Driscoll, et al. (Eds.), *Obstetrics: Normal and problem pregnancies* (7th ed.) (pp. 26–38). Philadelphia, PA: Saunders.

Simpson, K. R., & O'Brien-Abel, N. (2014). Labor and birth. In K. R. Simpson, & P. A. Creehan (Eds.), *AWHONN's perinatal nursing* (4th ed.) (pp. 343–444). Philadelphia, PA: Lippincott Williams and Wilkins.

Singata, M., Tranmer, J., & Gyte, G. M. L. (2013). Restricting oral fluid and food intake during labour. *Cochrane Database of Systematic Reviews* (1), CD003930.

Spong, C. Y., Berghella, V., Wenstrom, K. D., Mercer, B. M., & Saade, G. R. (2012). Preventing the first cesarean delivery: summary of a joint Eunice Kennedy Shriver National Institute of Child Health and Human Development, Society for Maternal-Fetal Medicine, and American College of Obstetricians and Gynecologists Workshop. *Obstetrics and Gynecology, 120*(5), 1181–1193.

Thorp, J. M., & Laughon, S. K. (2014). Clinical aspects of normal and abnormal labor. In R. K. Creasy, R. Resnik, J. D. Iams, C. J. Lockwood, & T. R. Moore (Eds.), *Creasy & Resnik's Maternal-fetal medicine: Principles and practice* (7th ed.) (pp. 673–706). Philadelphia, PA: Saunders.

Zhang, J., Landy, H. J., Branch, D. W., Burkman, R., Haberman, S., Gregory, K. D., & Reddy, U. (2010). Contemporary patterns of spontaneous labor with normal neonatal outcomes. Consortium on Safe Labor. *Obstetrics and Gynecology, 116,* 1281–1287.

Pain Management During Childbirth

Grace Moodt

Each woman has unique expectations about birth, including expectations about pain and her ability to manage it. The woman who successfully copes with the pain of labor is more likely to view her experience as a positive life event. A woman's experience with labor pain varies with several physical and psychological elements, and each woman responds differently. Nonpharmacologic and pharmacologic methods offer a selection of pain management techniques from which the laboring woman may choose.

UNIQUE NATURE OF PAIN DURING BIRTH

Pain is a universal experience but is difficult to define. It is an unpleasant sensation of distress resulting from stimulation of sensory nerves. Pain involves two components:

- A physiologic component that includes reception by sensory nerves and transmission to the central nervous system (CNS)
- A psychological component that involves recognizing the sensation, interpreting it as painful, and reacting to the interpretation

Pain is subjective and personal. No one can feel another's pain. Evidence of pain is a person's reaction to it. Childbirth pain, however, differs from other types of pain in the following important respects:

- It is part of a normal process—Childbirth pain is part of a normal process, whereas other types of pain relate to injury or illness. Pain may lead a woman to assume different positions in labor, favoring descent of the fetus through her pelvis.
- Preparation time exists—The pregnant woman has several months to prepare for labor, including acquiring skills to help manage pain. Realistic preparation and knowledge about the birth process help her develop skills to cope with labor pain.

- It is self-limiting—Labor pain has a foreseeable end. Although it may be intense, a woman can expect her labor to end in hours, rather than days, weeks, or months. Other kinds of pain may also be brief, but the baby's birth brings a rapid decrease in pain.
- Labor pain is not constant, but rather intermittent—A woman may describe little discomfort with contractions during early labor. Even during late labor, a woman may be relatively comfortable between contractions.
- Labor ends with the birth of a baby—The emotional significance of the child's birth cannot be ignored when trying to understand a woman's response to pain. Care about her fetus often motivates a woman to tolerate more pain during labor than she otherwise might be willing to endure.

ADVERSE EFFECTS OF EXCESSIVE PAIN

Although expected during labor, pain that exceeds a woman's tolerance can have harmful effects on her and the fetus.

Physiologic Effects

Excessive pain can heighten a woman's fear and anxiety, which stimulates sympathetic nervous system activity and results in increased secretion of catecholamines (epinephrine and norepinephrine). Catecholamines stimulate alpha and beta receptors, causing effects on the blood vessels and uterine muscles.

Stimulation of the alpha receptors causes uterine and generalized vasoconstriction and an increase in the uterine muscle tone. These effects reduce uterine blood flow as they raise the maternal blood pressure (Huether, Rodway, & DeFriez, 2014).

Stimulation of the beta receptors relaxes the uterine muscle and causes vasodilation. However, uterine vessels are already dilated in pregnancy, so dilation of other maternal vessels allows the woman's blood to pool in them. The pooling of blood reduces the amount of blood available to perfuse the placenta.

The combined effects of excessive catecholamine secretion are as follows:

- Reduced blood flow to and from the placenta, restricting fetal oxygen supply and waste removal
- Reduced effectiveness of uterine contractions, slowing labor progress

Labor increases a woman's metabolic rate and her demand for oxygen. Pain and anxiety increase her already high metabolic rate. She breathes fast to obtain more oxygen, exhaling too much carbon dioxide in the process. Significant changes, more than those expected during labor, can occur in the woman's partial pressure of oxygen (PaO_2) and partial pressure of carbon dioxide ($PaCO_2$) levels and in her arterial pH. If persistent, these maternal respiratory and metabolic changes alter placental exchange significantly. The fetus may have less oxygen available for uptake and have less ability to unload carbon dioxide to the mother. The net result is that the fetus shifts to anaerobic metabolism, with buildup of hydrogen ions (acidosis). This type of acidosis is metabolic and does not resolve as quickly after birth as respiratory acidosis, which results from shorter periods of hypoxia (Blackburn, 2013).

Psychological Effects

Women have a surprising tolerance for labor pain. However, poorly managed pain lessens the pleasure of this extraordinary life event for both partners. The mother may find it difficult to interact with her infant because she is depleted from a painful labor. Unpleasant memories of the birth may affect her response to sexual activity or another labor. Her support person may feel inadequate during birth. The woman's partner may feel helpless and frustrated when her pain is unrelieved.

> ### ⓘ KNOWLEDGE CHECK
> 1. How does the pain of childbirth differ from other kinds of pain?
> 2. How can excessive pain adversely affect a laboring woman and her fetus?

VARIABLES IN CHILDBIRTH PAIN

A variety of physical and psychosocial factors contribute to a woman's pain response during labor. These factors provide possibilities for nursing interventions for pain relief.

Physical Factors

Childbirth pain is of two types: visceral and somatic. Visceral pain is a slow, deep, poorly localized pain that is often described as dull or aching. Visceral pain dominates during first-stage labor as the uterus contracts and the cervix dilates.

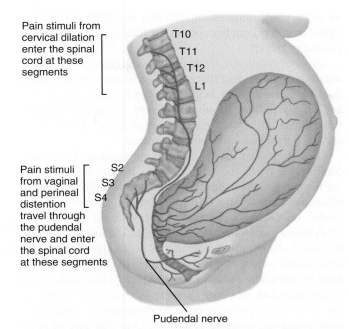

Pain stimuli from cervical dilation enter the spinal cord at these segments

T10
T11
T12
L1

Pain stimuli from vaginal and perineal distention travel through the pudendal nerve and enter the spinal cord at these segments

S2
S3
S4

Pudendal nerve

FIG. 13.1 Pathways of Pain Transmission during Labor.

Somatic pain is a quick, sharp pain that can be precisely localized. Somatic pain is most prominent during late first-stage labor and during second-stage labor as the descending fetus puts direct pressure on maternal tissues.

Sources of Pain

Four sources of labor pain exist in most labors. Other physical factors may modify labor pain, increasing or decreasing it.

Tissue Ischemia. The blood supply to the uterus decreases during contractions, leading to tissue hypoxia and anaerobic metabolism. Ischemic uterine pain has been likened to ischemic heart pain.

Cervical Dilation. Dilation and stretching of the cervix and lower uterus are a major source of pain. Pain stimuli from cervical dilation travel through the hypogastric plexus, entering the spinal cord at the T10, T11, T12, and L1 levels (Fig. 13.1).

Pressure and Pulling on Pelvic Structures. Some pain results from pressure and pulling on pelvic structures such as ligaments, fallopian tubes, ovaries, bladder, and peritoneum. The pain is a visceral pain; a woman may feel it as referred pain in her back and legs.

Distention of the Vagina and Perineum. Marked distention of the vagina and perineum occurs with fetal descent, especially during the second stage. The woman may describe a sensation of burning, tearing, or splitting (somatic pain). Pain from vaginal and perineal distention and pressure and pulling on adjacent structures enters the spinal cord at the S2, S3, and S4 levels (see Fig. 13.1).

Factors Influencing Perception or Tolerance of Pain

Although physiologic processes cause labor pain, a woman's tolerance of pain is affected by other physical influences.

Labor Intensity. The woman who has a short, intense labor may complain of severe pain because each contraction does so much work (effacement, dilation, and fetal descent). A rapid labor may limit her options for adequate pharmacologic pain relief as well.

Cervical Readiness. If prelabor cervical changes (softening, with some dilation and effacement) are incomplete, the cervix does not open as easily as it does when it is soft and dilation and effacement have begun. More contractions are needed to achieve dilation and effacement, resulting in a longer labor and greater fatigue in the laboring woman.

Fetal Position. Labor is likely to be longer and more uncomfortable when the fetus is in an unfavorable position. An occiput posterior position is a common variant seen in otherwise normal labors. In this position, each contraction pushes the fetal occiput against the woman's sacrum. She experiences intense back discomfort (back labor) that persists between contractions. A woman may not be able to deliver the fetus until it rotates to the occiput anterior position. The fetal head must therefore rotate a wider arc before the mechanisms of extension and expulsion occur, so labor is often longer (see Fig. 12.12). Back pain may decrease dramatically when a fetus rotates into the more favorable position. The rate of labor progress usually increases as well. However, back pain may persist in any labor.

Pelvic Anatomy. The size and shape of a woman's pelvis influence the course and length of her labor. Abnormalities may contribute to fetal malpresentation or malposition, resulting in a difficult and longer labor.

Fatigue. Fatigue reduces a woman's ability to tolerate pain and to use coping skills she has learned. She may be unable to focus on techniques that would otherwise help her tolerate labor. An extremely fatigued woman may have an exaggerated response to contractions, or she may be unable to respond to sensations of labor such as the urge to push. Because oral intake is often limited, her energy reserves are also likely to be depleted in a long labor.

Many women find that sleep is difficult during the last weeks of pregnancy. A woman's shortness of breath when lying down, frequent urination, and fetal activity interrupt sleep so she often begins labor with a sleep deficit. If labor begins late in the evening, she may have been awake more than 24 hours by the time she gives birth. Even if a woman begins labor well rested, slow progress may exhaust her.

Caregiver Interventions. Although they may be appropriate for the well-being of a woman and fetus, common interventions often add discomfort to the natural pain of labor.

Intravenous (IV) lines cause pain when inserted and remain noticeable to many women during labor. Fetal monitoring equipment is uncomfortable to some women, but others want to hear the sounds. Both may hamper a woman's mobility, which she might use to assume a more comfortable position. A woman may expect routine electronic fetal monitoring (EFM) and subordinates her own comfort for reassurance of her baby's well-being with technology.

A woman whose labor is induced or augmented often reports more pain and increased difficulty coping with it because contractions reach peak intensity quickly. Labor is more interventional with induction or augmentation

(see Chapter 15). Vaginal examinations, amniotomy, and insertion of internal fetal monitoring devices also increase a woman's discomfort briefly because of vaginal and cervical stretching. Vaginal manipulation often stimulates a contraction because of a reflex known as *Ferguson's reflex.*

Psychosocial Factors

Several psychosocial variables influence a woman's experience of pain.

❓ CRITICAL THINKING EXERCISE 13.1

Truc is a Vietnamese American in labor with her first baby. Her cervix is dilated 6 cm, effacement is 100%, and the fetus is at a +1 station. Truc's contractions occur every 3 minutes, last 50 to 60 seconds, and are of strong intensity. She smiles at the nurse each time the nurse talks to her but does not talk much herself. Truc stiffens her body during contractions and interacts little with her husband or the nurse at those times.

Questions
1. How should the nurse interpret Truc's assessment and behavior?
2. Does the nurse need additional data?
3. What nursing actions are appropriate?

Culture

A woman's sociocultural roots influence how she perceives, interprets, and responds to pain during childbirth. Some cultures encourage loud and vigorous expression of pain, whereas others value self-control. However, women are individuals within their cultural groups. The experience of pain is personal, and caregivers should not make assumptions about how a woman will behave during labor.

Women should be encouraged to express themselves in any way they find comforting, and the diversity of their expressions should be respected. Loud and vigorous expression may be a woman's personal pain coping mechanism, whereas a quiet woman may need medication relief but feels the need to remain stoic. Accepting a woman's individual response to labor and pain promotes a therapeutic relationship. The nurse should avoid praising behaviors (such as stoicism) and belittling others (such as noisy expression).

The unique nature of childbirth pain and women's diverse responses to it make nursing management complex. The nurse can miss important cues if the woman is either stoic or outspoken about her pain. With either extreme, the nurse may not readily identify critical information such as impending birth or symptoms of a complication.

Anxiety and Fear

Mild or moderate anxiety can enhance attention and learning. However, high anxiety and fear magnify sensitivity to pain and impair a woman's ability to tolerate pain. Anxiety and fear consume energy the woman needs to cope with the birth process, including its painful aspects.

Anxiety and fear increase muscle tension, diverting oxygenated blood to the brain and skeletal muscles.

Tension in pelvic muscles counters the expulsive forces of uterine contractions and the laboring woman's pushing. Prolonged tension results in general fatigue, increased **pain perception** or **threshold** (lowest stimulus level perceived as painful), and reduced ability to use skills to cope with pain.

If a previous pregnancy had a poor outcome such as a stillborn infant or one with abnormalities, a woman is probably more anxious during labor and for a time after birth. She is likely to examine and reexamine her infant to assure herself that this baby is normal.

Previous Experiences with Pain

Early in life a child learns that pain means bodily injury. Consequently, fear and withdrawal are natural reactions to pain during labor. Learning about the normal sensations of labor, including pain, helps a woman suppress her natural reactions of fear and withdrawal, allowing her body to do the work of birth.

A woman who has given birth previously has a different perspective. If she has had a vaginal delivery, she is probably aware of normal labor sensations and is less likely to associate them with injury or abnormality. Also, time has a way of blunting the memory of painful experiences. A woman who had a previous long and difficult labor may be anxious about the outcome of the present one. She may be surprised that her second labor moves more quickly than her first. The woman having a second (or higher) vaginal birth may find late first-stage and second-stage labor to be more painful because the fetus descends faster. All women are different and yet similar.

A woman who plans a vaginal birth after cesarean (VBAC) but has never experienced labor may be particularly anxious. The experience of cesarean birth is known to her, even if she does not want to repeat it, whereas labor is unknown. A repeat cesarean birth may seem to be the quicker and less painful option at times, yet she strongly prefers a "normal" vaginal birth, if possible. She may have difficulty yielding to the normal forces of birth.

Previous experiences may positively affect a woman's ability to deal with pain. She may have learned ways to cope with pain during other episodes of pain or during other births and may use these skills adaptively during labor.

Preparation for Childbirth

Preparation for childbirth does not ensure a pain-free labor. A woman should be prepared for pain realistically, including reasonable expectations about analgesia and **anesthesia** (loss of sensation). She may feel that unexpected events during labor may invalidate her childbirth preparation.

Preparation reduces anxiety and fear of the unknown. It allows a woman to rehearse for labor and learn a variety of skills to cope with pain as labor progresses. She and her partner learn about expected behavioral changes during labor, and their knowledge decreases their anxiety when those changes occur.

Support System

An anxious partner is less able to provide the support and reassurance the woman needs during labor. In addition, anxiety in others can be contagious, increasing the woman's anxiety. She may assume that if others are worried, something is wrong.

The birth experiences of a woman's family and friends cannot be ignored. Those individuals can be an important source of support if they express realistic information about labor pain and its control. If they describe labor as intolerable, however, she may have needless distress. Hearing that labor is painless is equally detrimental. No two labors are alike, even in the same woman.

> **❓ KNOWLEDGE CHECK**
>
> 3. How may physical and psychological factors interact in a woman's labor pain experience?
> 4. What four sources of pain are present in most labors?
> 5. How can each of the following physical factors influence the pain a woman experiences during childbirth: Labor intensity? Cervical readiness? Fetal position? Maternal pelvis? Fatigue?
> 6. What psychosocial factors influence a woman's experience with labor pain?

STANDARDS FOR PAIN MANAGEMENT

The Joint Commission (TJC) (2014) has recognized that pain management is an essential part of the care of all people in health care settings and that the patient should be involved in the assessment and management of pain through pharmacologic and nonpharmacologic strategies.

NONPHARMACOLOGIC PAIN MANAGEMENT

The nurse who cares for women in labor and birth can offer many nonpharmacologic and pharmacologic pain management methods. Education about nonpharmacologic pain management is the foundation of prepared childbirth classes, although today's classes contain significant content on pharmacologic pain management, particularly epidural analgesia. Most women use these methods to complement pharmacologic methods, although some use them as their only pain management techniques.

To be most helpful to women and their labor partners, the intrapartum nurse should know methods that are taught in local childbirth classes. Teaching techniques during labor that conflict with what a woman has learned and practiced may confuse her. Other techniques can be reserved for use if a woman finds learned techniques ineffective.

Advantages

Nonpharmacologic methods have several advantages over pharmacologic methods if pain control is adequate. They do not slow labor and have no side effects or risk for allergy (Jones, Whitburn, Davey, & Small, 2015).

The woman who chooses analgesia needs alternative pain management until she receives it, usually after labor is established. Also, some pharmacologic methods may not eliminate labor pain, and a woman needs these techniques to control the pain that remains, even if it is greatly reduced.

Nonpharmacologic methods may be the only realistic option for a woman who enters the hospital in advanced, rapid labor. Drugs might not have enough time to take effect, or there may not be time needed to administer an effective epidural block before birth. The time of peak drug action in terms of newborn respiratory effort should be considered if an **analgesic** (systemic agent to relieve pain) drug is given.

Limitations

Nonpharmacologic methods also have limitations, especially as the sole method of pain control. Women do not always achieve their desired level of pain control using these methods alone. Because of the many variables in labor, even a well-prepared and highly motivated woman may have a difficult labor and need analgesia or anesthesia.

Gate-Control Theory

A discussion of nonpharmacologic pain management techniques would not be complete without discussion of the **gate-control theory** of pain. Per this theory, transmission of nerve impulses is controlled by a neural mechanism in the dorsal horn of the spinal cord that acts like a gate to control impulses transmitted to the brain. Transmission is affected by stimulation of large- or small-diameter sensory nerve fibers and descending impulses from the brain. This mechanism opens or closes the "gate" to pain sensation by allowing or preventing some impulses from reaching the brain, where they are recognized as pain (Huether et al., 2014).

Pain is transmitted through small-diameter sensory nerve fibers. Stimulation of large-diameter fibers in the skin blocks conduction of pain through small-diameter fibers, thereby "closing the gate" and decreasing the amount of pain felt. Examples of this stimulation include tactile stimulation such as massage, thermal stimulation, or hydrotherapy (Blackburn, 2013).

Impulses from the brain have a similar ability to impede transmission through the dorsal horn using visual and auditory stimulation techniques. Examples of visual or auditory stimulation include use of a focal point or breathing techniques.

Memory and cognitive processes affect the perception of stimuli as painful. Education and support during labor are used to increase the woman's relaxation, confidence, and feeling of control. Although these methods may not completely prevent pain, they may decrease the severity of perceived pain (Cunningham et al., 2014).

Preparation for Pain Management

The ideal time to prepare for nonpharmacologic pain control is before labor. During the last few weeks of pregnancy, the woman learns about labor, including its painful aspects, in childbirth classes. She can prepare to confront the pain, learning a variety of skills to use during labor. Her support person learns specific methods to encourage and support her.

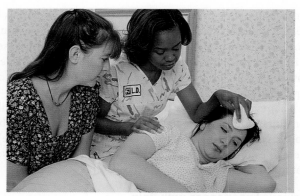

FIG. 13.2 General comfort measures such as the nurse's reassuring presence or a cool cloth applied to the face supplement other methods of nonpharmacologic and pharmacologic pain control.

After admission, the nurse can review and reinforce what the partners learned in class.

The nurse can teach the unprepared woman and her support person nonpharmacologic techniques. The latent phase of labor is the best time for intrapartum teaching because the woman is usually anxious enough to be attentive and interested and yet comfortable enough to understand. The nurse should usually teach one contraction at a time during late labor because the woman's focus is very narrow.

No one method or combination of methods helps every woman. Most methods may become less effective (habituation) after prolonged use, and changing techniques counters this problem. Knowing a variety of methods gives the nurse a selection.

Application of Nonpharmacologic Techniques

Techniques that can be applied during labor include relaxation, cutaneous stimulation, hydrotherapy, mental stimulation, and breathing techniques.

Relaxation

Promoting relaxation is a basis for all other methods, both nonpharmacologic and pharmacologic, because it achieves the following (Cunningham et al., 2014: Huether et al., 2014):
- Promotes uterine blood flow, improving fetal oxygenation
- Promotes efficient uterine contractions
- Reduces tension that increases pain perception and decreases **pain tolerance** (maximum pain one is willing to endure)
- Reduces tension that can inhibit fetal descent

Environmental Comfort. Comfortable surroundings support relaxation. The nurse can reduce irritants such as bright lights and uncomfortable temperature and can change soiled underpads.

Music masks outside noise and provides a background for use of imagery and breathing techniques. This distraction shifts the woman's attention from pain perception. Television has a similar effect for some women.

General Comfort. Promoting the woman's personal comfort helps her focus on using pain management techniques during labor (Fig. 13.2). This includes actions to increase comfort and reduce the effects of irritants.

Reducing Anxiety and Fear. The nurse may reduce a woman's anxiety and increase her self-control by providing accurate information and focusing on the normality of her labor. Hospitals are typically associated with illness or injury, situations that provoke anxiety. Yet in North America, hospitals are the most common site for the normal event of birth.

Simple nursing actions keep the focus on the normality of childbirth regardless of the setting. Empowerment of the woman and her partner by giving them choices, whenever possible, helps them see themselves as competent people who can accomplish the task of giving birth.

Specific Relaxation Techniques. Relaxation techniques work best if they are practiced before labor. During practice sessions at home, couples may practice *progressive relaxation,* in which the woman contracts and then releases specific muscle groups until all muscles are relaxed. *Neuromuscular dissociation* helps the woman learn to relax all muscles except those that are working (e.g., the uterus or the abdominal muscles when pushing). The woman can learn *touch relaxation* in response to her partner's touch, and *relaxation against pain* as the partner deliberately causes mild pain and the woman learns to relax despite the pain.

Even if the woman did not practice these relaxation techniques at home, the nurse can teach her how to consciously relax as labor progresses. The partner can learn to watch for signs of tension, touch that area, and direct the woman to relax.

Cutaneous Stimulation

Cutaneous stimulation has several variations that are often combined with each other or with other techniques.

Self-Massage. The woman may rub her abdomen, legs, or back during labor (effleurage) to counteract discomfort. Some women find abdominal touch irritating, especially near the umbilicus. Women in labor may find firm stroking more helpful than light stroking.

Some women benefit from firm palm or sole stimulation during labor. They may like someone to rub their palms vigorously; independently to rub their hands or feet together; or to bang their palms on or grip a cool surface. They may hold another person's hand tightly during a contraction. The nurse should determine whether these actions indicate excess pain or if they are a woman's way of countering pain and therefore useful.

Massage by Others. Massage increases circulation and reduces muscle tension. The support person or nurse can rub the woman's back, shoulders, legs, or any area where she finds massage helpful. Body powder on the skin reduces friction during massage.

Counterpressure. Sacral pressure may help when the woman has back pain, usually most intense when her fetus is in an occiput posterior position. Sacral pressure may be applied using the palm of the hand, the fist or fists, or a firm object such as two tennis balls in a sock (Fig. 13.3). A variation of sacral pressure is a double hip squeeze, in which the palms are placed on the woman's hips and pressed down and inward toward the symphysis (Cunningham et al., 2014). When pressure is used, the woman should guide the support

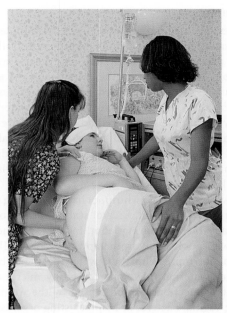

FIG. 13.3 The coach applies sacral pressure to counter back pain, common during labor.

person as to the exact location and amount of pressure. An upright maternal position enhances counterpressure with the fists to the lower back.

Touch. Nonclinical touch by the nurse is a powerful tool if the woman does not object to it. Holding her hand, stroking her hair, or similar actions convey caring, comfort, affirmation, and reassurance at this vulnerable time.

Thermal Stimulation. Many women appreciate warmth applied to the back, abdomen, or perineum during labor. Warmth increases local blood flow, relaxes muscles, and raises the pain threshold. Massage is often more comfortable to a tense woman after her skin is warmed. A warm shower, tub bath, or whirlpool bath is relaxing and provides thermal stimulation. A sock filled with dry rice and microwaved provides gentle warmth and can be used to apply warm pressure to the sacral area (Sullivan & McGuiness, 2015).

Cool, damp washcloths provide comforting coolness if the woman feels hot. She may put them on her head, throat, abdomen, or any place she wants. She also may want to put them in her mouth to relieve dryness. Ice chips cool the mouth and provide hydration.

Acupressure. Acupressure is a directed form of massage in which the support person applies pressure to specific pressure points using hands, rollers, balls, or other equipment. It is related to its invasive counterpart, acupuncture, in which tiny needles are inserted into similar points. Acupuncture and acupressure have data to support effectiveness to relieve nausea and vomiting, including morning sickness of pregnancy. Few controlled studies exist on acupressure's usefulness during birth. For updated objective information on acupressure and other complementary and alternative medicine (CAM) techniques, visit the website for the National Center for Complementary and Alternative Medicine (NCCAM), which is part of the National Institutes of Health (NIH; www.nccam.nih.gov).

Hydrotherapy

Water therapy can supplement any relaxation technique. The buoyancy afforded by immersion supports the body, equalizes pressure on the body, and aids muscle relaxation. In addition, fluid shifts from the extravascular space to the intravascular space, reducing edema as the excess fluid is excreted by the kidneys. Women who used water therapy effectively during the first stage had decreased use of anesthesia, analgesia, decrease in the duration of labor, and improved satisfaction (American Academy of Pediatrics & American College of Obstetricians and Gynecologists [AAP & ACOG], 2014).

A shower, tub bath, or whirlpool bath is relaxing and provides thermal stimulation. Several studies have shown benefits of water therapy during labor, including immersion in a tub or whirlpool (jet hydrotherapy, or Jacuzzi). The major concern about immersion therapy has been newborn and postpartum maternal infections caused by microorganisms in the water. Infections can be caused by the woman's own ascending vaginal bacteria or by preexisting organisms in an improperly cleaned tub. However, several studies failed to find a significant association between newborn or postpartum maternal infections and use of immersion hydrotherapy with proper cleaning (Davies, Davis, Peace, & Wong, 2014; Sullivan & McGuiness, 2015). More research is needed to clarify both the benefits and the concerns about hydrotherapy (Box 13.1). Facility policies should be written to outline specific guidelines based on most recent evidence for use of hydrotherapy.

Mental Stimulation

Mental techniques occupy the woman's mind and compete with pain stimuli. They also aid relaxation by providing a tranquil imaginary atmosphere.

Imagery. If the woman has not practiced a specific imagery technique, the nurse can help her create a relaxing mental scene. Most women find images of warmth, softness, security, and total relaxation most comforting.

Imagery can help the woman dissociate herself from the painful aspects of labor. For example, the nurse can help her visualize the work of labor—the cervix opening with each contraction or the fetus moving down toward the outlet each time she pushes. This technique is like visualizing success or movement toward a goal with each contraction. The nurse can help the woman visualize being in a pleasant and relaxing place.

Focal Point. When using nonpharmacologic techniques, a woman may prefer to close her eyes or may want to concentrate on an external focal point. Childbirth classes may emphasize that keeping the eyes open on a focal point helps her concentrate on something outside her body and thus away from the pain of contractions. She may bring a picture of a relaxing scene or an object to use as a focal point and to aid in the use of imagery. She can use any point in her room as a focal point.

BOX 13.1 Use of Water Therapy during Labor

Use of water therapy has accompanied trends toward a low-intervention approach to intrapartum care. Water therapy can be delivered in the following ways:

- Shower
- Standard tub
- Whirlpool

Benefits

- Associated with a more natural, homelike atmosphere.
- Gives a woman greater control over her labor.
- Upright position facilitates progress of labor.
- Faster labor progress if contractions are frequent when woman enters the tub.
- Buoyancy relieves tired muscles and reduces pressure.
- Facilitates fetal rotation from occiput posterior or transverse positions to the occiput anterior position. The woman also can assume different positions to aid rotation.

Disadvantages

- May reduce frequency of contractions and dilation if used during the latent phase of labor.
- Fetus should be assessed with intermittent auscultation rather than electronic fetal monitoring.

Contraindications and Precautions

No specific contraindications if the woman can safely be out of bed.

- Thick meconium in the amniotic fluid is an indication for continuous electronic fetal monitoring in most birth facilities and would preclude use of water therapy.
- Bleeding.
- Oxytocin induction or augmentation. The use of both oxytocin and water therapy could cause excess uterine activity.
- Maintain water temperature at 36°C to 37°C (96.8°F to 98.6°F) to avoid maternal and fetal hyperthermia that increases demand for oxygen.
- Encourage maternal fluids to prevent dehydration related to greater maternal fluid excretion by the kidneys.

CNS, Central nervous system.

❓ KNOWLEDGE CHECK

7. How does the gate-control theory of pain relate to nonpharmacologic methods of pain control?
8. What are some nursing actions to encourage relaxation during labor?
9. How can the nurse reduce a laboring woman's anxiety or fear?
10. How might each of these cutaneous stimulation techniques be used to aid relaxation during labor: Self-massage? Massage by others? Counterpressure? Warmth or cold?
11. When hydrotherapy is used during labor, why are these cautions required: Adequate maternal hydration? Control of water temperature?

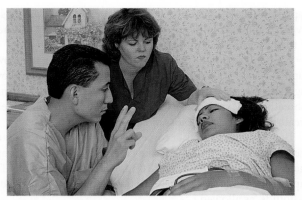

FIG. 13.4 A woman and her partner who are prepared for labor have learned a variety of skills to master pain as labor progresses. The coach uses hand signals to tell the woman how to change her pattern of paced breathing.

Breathing Techniques

Breathing techniques give a woman a different focus during contractions, interfering with pain sensory transmission (Fig. 13.4). They begin with simple patterns and progress to more complex ones as greater distraction is needed. No universal right time exists to change patterns during labor. However, complex patterns are fatiguing if used for a long time.

For best results, the woman and her partner should practice the techniques frequently. If patterns are too complicated or if the woman has not practiced, they may not be helpful during labor. Breathing techniques should be used only when needed, usually when the woman can no longer walk or talk during a contraction. The woman should not change from a simpler technique to the next, more complex technique until necessary so that use of the most complex techniques is limited to the shortest time possible.

First-Stage Breathing. Breathing in the first stage of labor consists of a cleansing breath and progressively more complex techniques of paced breathing, if needed.

Taking a Cleansing Breath. Each contraction begins and ends with a deep inspiration and expiration known as the *cleansing breath*. Like a sigh, a cleansing breath helps the woman release tension. It provides oxygen to help reduce myometrial hypoxia, one cause of pain in labor. The cleansing breath also helps the woman clear her mind to focus on relaxing and signals her labor partner that the contraction is beginning or ending. The woman may inhale through the nose and exhale through the mouth or take her cleansing breath in any way comfortable for her. When electronic monitors are used, a partner may help ease the discomfort of rapid contractions by watching for the rise in the lower part of the strip that signals the beginning of the contraction and telling the woman to take a cleansing breath.

Slow-Paced Breathing. The first breathing is slow-paced breathing, a slow, deep breathing that increases relaxation (Fig. 13.5). The woman should concentrate on relaxing her body rather than on regulating the rate of her breathing. Relaxation naturally triggers slower breathing, like that during sleep. Slow-paced breathing is usually about half of the

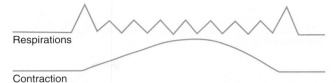

FIG. 13.5 Slow-Paced Breathing. Although a specific rate may or may not be used, slow-paced breathing should be no slower than half the woman's usual respiratory rate to ensure adequate oxygenation. This pace is generally about six to nine breaths per minute.

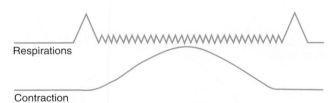

FIG. 13.6 Modified-Paced Breathing. The pattern for modified-paced breathing should be comfortable to the woman and no faster than twice her normal respiratory rate to prevent hyperventilation or interference with relaxation.

woman's normal respiratory rate (in-2-3-4; out-2-3-4). The woman can use nose, mouth, or a combination, depending on which is most comfortable.

Slow-paced breathing should be used as long as possible during labor because it promotes relaxation and oxygenation. Labor nurses often teach the technique to women who enter labor unprepared. It is easy to learn between contractions and, with the support of the nurse, helps even a frightened woman become calm and able to work with her contractions.

As with all techniques, variety prevents habituation. Adding other pain-relief approaches such as effleurage may help prolong the effectiveness of slow-paced breathing. Using another type of breathing for a short time may allow the woman to return to slower breathing again later.

Modified-Paced Breathing. When slow-paced breathing is no longer effective, the woman begins modified-paced breathing (Fig. 13.6). Modified-paced breathing is slightly faster than normal but no more than twice the normal rate (in-2, out-2). This chest breathing at a faster rate matches the natural tendency to use more rapid breathing during stress or physical work such as labor. Although modified-paced breathing is shallower than slow-paced breathing, the faster rate allows oxygen intake to remain about the same. As with slow-paced breathing, the focus is on release of tension rather than on the actual number of breaths taken.

Women sometimes learn to combine slow and modified-paced breathing during a contraction (Fig. 13.7). They begin slowly and use shallow, faster breathing over the peak of the contraction. During labor, women often do this naturally. The most important concern is ensuring that the breathing does not interfere with relaxation but enhances it.

Patterned-Paced Breathing. Patterned-paced breathing (sometimes called *pant-blow breathing*) involves focusing on the pattern of breathing (Fig. 13.8). It is like modified-paced breathing. After a certain number of breaths, however, the

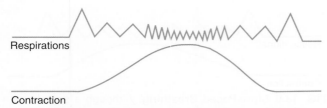

FIG. 13.7 Combining Techniques. Slow and modified-paced breathing can be combined by using the slower breathing at the beginning and end of the contraction and the more rapid breathing over the peak of the contraction.

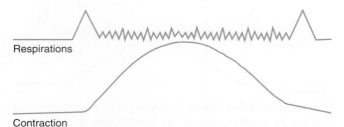

FIG. 13.8 Patterned-Paced Breathing. Patterned-paced breathing adds a slight emphasis or "blow" on the exhalation in a pattern. The diagram shows the emphasis after every third inhalation.

woman exhales with a slight emphasis or blow and then begins the modified-paced breathing again. This addition causes her to focus more on her breathing and reduces habituation. The mouth should remain relaxed, and the woman should not try to make specific sounds that would tighten her vocal cords. Relaxation of her entire body is the goal.

The number of breaths before the blow may remain constant (usually between two and six) or may change in a pattern. Variations include a set pattern such as "3-1, 5-1, 3-1" or a decreasing, "stair-step," pattern such as "6-1, 5-1, 4-1, 3-1." Some couples use a random pattern determined by the coach, who uses hand signals to show the number of breaths the woman should take before each blow. The coach holds up fingers to show the total breaths to be taken or a single finger for each breath. Use of the random pattern, however, may be ineffective without sufficient practice to enable the coach and woman to work together well.

Breathing to Prevent Pushing. If a woman pushes strenuously before the cervix is completely dilated, she risks injury to her cervix and the fetal head. Blowing prevents closure of the glottis and breath-holding, helping to overcome the urge to push strenuously. The woman blows repeatedly using short puffs when the urge to push is strong. The support person may learn to blow along with her to help the woman concentrate. Some women vary the blowing by using one short breath and one blow.

Overcoming Common Problems. Hyperventilation and mouth dryness are common when breathing techniques are used. Hyperventilation results from rapid deep breathing that causes excessive loss of carbon dioxide and therefore respiratory alkalosis. The woman may feel dizzy or lightheaded and may have impaired thinking. Vasoconstriction leads to tingling and numbness in the fingers and lips. If

hyperventilation continues, tetany occurring from decreased levels of calcium in tissues and blood may result in stiffness of the face and lips and carpopedal spasm.

Women are taught to blow into a paper bag or their own cupped hands if they begin to feel dizzy. This kind of blowing increases the carbon dioxide levels by making the woman rebreathe her exhaled air. The woman should slow her rate of breathing to reduce the loss of carbon dioxide.

The woman's mouth becomes dry with prolonged mouth breathing. To avoid dryness, she can place her tongue gently against the roof of her mouth to moisturize entering air. The support person can offer ice, mouthwash, sugarless suckers, or liquids, as allowed.

Second-Stage Breathing. Care in the second stage of labor encourages a physiologic completion of labor, assisting the mother to respond to her urge to push rather than directing her to push as soon as her cervix is completely dilated even if she does not feel the urge. Lengthy pushing in second stage has been shown to result in greater maternal fatigue, more operative births, and nonreassuring fetal heart rate (FHR) patterns and does not significantly shorten the second stage (Association of Women's Health, Obstetric and Neonatal Nurses [AWHONN], 2014).

Research has shown that strenuous directed pushing increases risk for structural and neurogenic injury to a woman's pelvic floor. Closed-glottis pushing causes recurrent increases in intrathoracic pressure with a resulting fall in cardiac output and maternal blood pressure. The woman's lower blood pressure then causes less blood to be delivered to the placenta, resulting in fetal hypoxia that is reflected in nonreassuring fetal heart patterns.

Promoting a physiologic second stage uses nondirected pushing. The woman makes her decision with the nurse about when it is time to start pushing. She may grunt, groan, sigh, or moan as she pushes, and the nurse should validate that these sounds are normal. Pushing three to four times for 6 to 8 seconds is likely to be effective in aiding descent and safe for the baby. Adjust the pushing process depending on fetal status (AWHONN, 2013, 2014). See Chapter 15 for further discussion of second-stage nursing care.

With newer techniques of epidural analgesia, women who choose this method of labor pain control often feel the urge to push, although not as strongly as the urge felt by women who have not had this type of medication. Using their natural urge to push, even if reduced, helps them push with contractions most effectively. Delaying pushing for up to 1 to 2 hours after complete dilation has shown benefits similar to those in women who do not have epidural analgesia.

❓ KNOWLEDGE CHECK

12. Why is it important to avoid advancing to more complex breathing techniques sooner than needed?
13. What is the purpose of a cleansing breath?
14. Is there a valid reason why a woman should push as soon as her cervix is completely dilated? Why, or why not?

PHARMACOLOGIC PAIN MANAGEMENT

Most women choose pharmacologic pain relief at some point in their labor, even if they also use nonpharmacologic methods. Pharmacologic methods for pain management include systemic drugs, **regional** pain management techniques (block of pain in localized area with consciousness), and general anesthesia. Decisions for any method should be made on a risk versus benefit process.

Special Considerations for Medicating a Pregnant Woman

Medicating a woman when she is pregnant is not as simple as before pregnancy, for the following reasons:

- Any drug taken by the woman is likely to affect her fetus.
- Drugs may have effects in pregnancy that they do not have in the nonpregnant person.
- Drugs can affect the course and length of labor.
- Pregnancy complications may limit the choice of pharmacologic pain management methods.
- Women who require other therapeutic drugs, use herbal or botanical preparations, or practice substance abuse may have fewer safe choices for labor pain relief.

Effects on the Fetus

Effects on the fetus of drugs given to the mother may be direct, resulting from passage of the drug or its metabolites across the placenta to the fetus. An example of a direct effect on the fetus is decreased FHR variability after administration of an analgesic to the woman.

Effects on the fetus may be indirect, or secondary to drug effects in the mother. For example, if a drug causes maternal hypotension, blood flow to the placenta is reduced. Fetal hypoxia and acidosis may result.

Maternal Physiologic Alterations

Normal pregnancy changes in four body systems have the greatest implications for pharmacologic pain management methods.

Cardiovascular Changes. Compression of the aorta and inferior vena cava by the uterus can occur when a woman lies in the supine position (aortocaval compression). If the woman must be in the supine position temporarily, the uterus should be displaced to one side with the hands or with a small wedge or towel roll under one hip. Operating room tables are often tilted slightly to one side for a cesarean birth to provide the uterine displacement.

Respiratory Changes. A pregnant woman's full uterus reduces her respiratory capacity. To compensate, she breathes more rapidly and deeply. Thus she is more vulnerable to reduced arterial oxygenation during induction of **general anesthesia** (systemic loss of sensation and consciousness) and is more sensitive to inhalational anesthetic agents. The normal edema of pregnancy is also present in her upper airways and may present difficulty if she must be intubated for general anesthesia.

Gastrointestinal Changes. A pregnant woman's stomach is displaced upward by her large uterus and has a higher internal pressure. Progesterone slows peristalsis and reduces the tone of the sphincter at the junction of the stomach and esophagus. These changes make a pregnant woman vulnerable to regurgitation and aspiration (inhalation) of gastric contents during general anesthesia.

Nervous System Changes. During pregnancy and labor, circulating levels of **endorphins** and **enkephalins**, natural substances with analgesic properties, are high. These substances modify pain perception and reduce requirements for analgesia and anesthesia.

The epidural and **subarachnoid spaces** between the arachnoid mater and pia mater are smaller during pregnancy, enhancing the spread of anesthetic agents used for epidural blocks or subarachnoid blocks (SABs). Cerebrospinal fluid (CSF) pressure is higher during a contraction and when the woman is pushing. Nerve fibers are more sensitive to local anesthetic agents. High intraabdominal pressure causes engorgement of the epidural veins, increasing the risk for intravascular injection of anesthetic agents. The net result of these changes is that a reduced volume of local anesthetic is needed to achieve satisfactory epidural block or SAB (Wong, 2014).

Effects on the Course of Labor

Ideally, analgesics are given when labor is well established to avoid slowing progress. However, caregivers should consider the adverse effects of excessive pain on labor progress, regardless of the cervical dilation. Regional analgesia, primarily the epidural block, can slow progress during the second stage by reducing a woman's spontaneous urge to push.

Effects of Complications

Complications during pregnancy may limit the choices of analgesia or anesthesia. For example, large volumes of IV fluids are infused to prevent hypotension with regional analgesia and anesthesia. If a pregnant woman has heart disease, this fluid load could be detrimental. Yet without it, she is vulnerable to hypotension (Creedon et al., 2013).

Interactions with Other Substances

A woman who ingests drugs (therapeutic, over-the-counter, or illicit), herbal or botanical preparations, or other substances may have fewer options because of interactions between these substances and analgesics or anesthetics. For example, recent alcohol use increases the depressant effects of opioid analgesics, making both the mother and the newborn susceptible to respiratory depression.

❓ KNOWLEDGE CHECK

15. How can drugs taken by the expectant mother affect the fetus?
16. How do changes in the following maternal body systems affect pharmacologic pain management: Cardiovascular system? Respiratory system? Gastrointestinal system? Nervous system?
17. Why is it important to know about a woman's intake of drugs, botanical medicines, legal substances (such as alcohol), and illegal drugs?

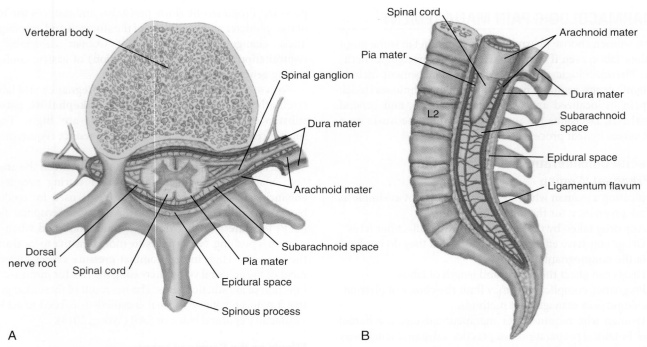

FIG. 13.9 A, Cross-section of spinal cord, meninges, and protective vertebrae. The dura mater and arachnoid mater lie close together. The pia mater is the innermost of the meninges and covers the brain and spinal cord. The subarachnoid space is between the arachnoid mater and pia mater. **B,** Sagittal section of spinal cord, meninges, and vertebrae. The epidural and subarachnoid spaces are illustrated. Note that the spinal cord ends at the L2 vertebra.

Regional Pain Management Techniques

Regional pain control methods may be used for intrapartum analgesia, surgical anesthesia, or both. These methods provide pain relief without loss of consciousness. Depending on the specific technique, it may be used for only labor, for only birth, or for both labor and birth.

Epidural block provides pain control during much of labor and for the birth itself. Intrathecal anesthetic agents and opioids are used for pain control during labor; additional measures are needed during late labor and for the birth. Another regional block, the SAB, is used only at birth. A combined spinal-epidural (CSE) analgesia allows subarachnoid injection of opioids via a spinal needle followed by ongoing pain relief from anesthetics injected through the epidural catheter. Regional anesthetics with a small area of anesthesia are used only for birth and include the local and pudendal blocks (Wong, 2014).

The major advantage of regional pain management methods is that the woman can participate in birth and yet have good pain control. The woman usually feels some pressure and discomfort, although these sensations are greatly reduced. Protective airway reflexes remain. Disadvantages depend on the specific technique. The effects on the fetus depend primarily on how the woman responds rather than on direct drug effects.

Epidural Block

The lumbar epidural block is a popular regional block that provides analgesia and anesthesia for labor and birth without sedation of the woman and fetus. It is used for both vaginal and cesarean births. Epidural blocks are started and maintained by an **anesthesiologist** (physician specialized in administration of anesthesia) or **nurse-anesthetist** (registered nurse with advanced education and certification in anesthetic administration).

The **epidural space** is outside the dura mater, between the dura and the spinal canal. It is loosely filled with fat, connective tissue, and epidural veins that are dilated during pregnancy (Fig. 13.9).

An epidural block is performed by injecting a local anesthetic agent, often combined with an opioid, into the tiny epidural space. It provides substantial relief of pain from contractions and birth canal distention. The level of the epidural block can be extended upward to provide anesthesia for a cesarean birth or tubal ligation after birth. Analgesia, rather than full anesthesia that results in complete loss of movement and sensation, is preferred for labor. Lower concentrations of the anesthetic agent and an epidural opioid provide adequate pain relief without complete **motor block** (loss of voluntary movement) for most women. Higher concentrations of the anesthetic agent used for abdominal surgery result in greater loss of both motor and sensory functions (Wong, 2014).

Technique. The exact time to begin an epidural block is individualized. It is started just before a scheduled cesarean birth. For labor, the best time to start the block is when the woman is in active labor, to avoid slowing progress. Several ways are available to customize the epidural block for different pain management needs. If she is in early labor and needs

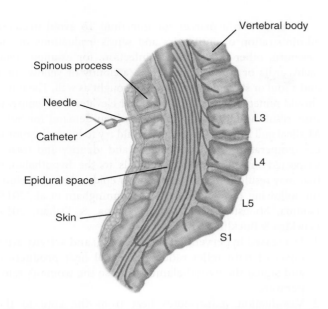

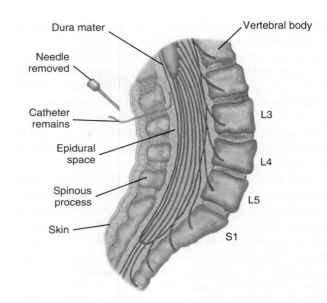

The epidural space is entered with a needle below where the spinal cord ends. A fine catheter is threaded through the needle.

After the catheter is threaded into the epidural space, the needle is removed. Medication can then be injected into the epidural space intermittently or by continuous infusion for pain relief during labor and birth.

FIG. 13.10 Technique for Epidural Block.

pain relief, the woman may be given parenteral opioids until her labor is more active. Or she may be given a preservative-free epidural opioid via the epidural catheter, supplemented with a stronger epidural anesthetic agent when labor becomes more active. In this way, she obtains pain relief and relaxation in early labor with less likelihood that labor progress will be slowed.

The epidural space is entered at about the L3-L4 interspace (below the end of the spinal cord), and a catheter is passed through the needle into the epidural space (Fig. 13.10). The catheter allows continuous infusion or intermittent injection of medication to maintain pain relief during labor and vaginal or cesarean birth. The infusion of epidural medication also may be regulated by a patient-controlled epidural analgesia (PCEA) pump (Hawkins & Bucklin, 2017; Tsen, 2014; Wong, 2014).

Epidural blocks require a larger volume of anesthetic agent because it is outside the meninges. Before the full epidural dose is given, a small test dose of anesthetic is injected by the anesthesia provider to determine whether the epidural catheter has inadvertently punctured a blood vessel or the dura. If a large dose of anesthetic reaches the subarachnoid space instead of the epidural space, the woman experiences rapid, intense motor and **sensory block** (loss of sensation). Numbness of the tongue and lips, lightheadedness, dizziness, and tinnitus may occur with intravascular injection. Epinephrine in the test dose produces tachycardia if injected intravascularly, although the tachycardia can have other causes, such as pain (Hawkins & Bucklin, 2017; Wong, 2014).

Epidural opioids that may be used during labor include fentanyl (Sublimaze), sufentanil (Sufenta), ropivacaine (Naropin),

and morphine (Duramorph, Astramorph) (Wong, 2014). *All drugs injected into the epidural or subarachnoid spaces should be preservative free.*

A single dose of a long-acting epidural analgesic such as morphine is often given after cesarean birth before removal of the epidural catheter to provide long-acting pain relief with a low dose of opiate. The mother may require no added analgesics for almost 24 hours, or oral ones may be sufficient. The mother's respiratory status should be monitored for an extended time after the long-acting epidural analgesic, up to 24 hours based on the duration of action for the specific drug.

Dural Puncture. Because the tough dura and the fragile weblike arachnoid membranes lie close together, dural puncture also punctures the arachnoid. If the dura is unintentionally punctured with the needle used to introduce the epidural catheter, leakage of CSF can occur, which may result in a post–dural puncture ("spinal") headache. Dural puncture and headache also can occur without obvious CSF leakage.

Contraindications and Precautions. Epidural block is not suitable for all laboring women, and some refuse the block. Contraindications include coagulation defects, uncorrected hypovolemia, an infection in the area of insertion or a severe systemic infection, allergy, or a fetal condition that demands immediate birth. Women who have had spinal surgery, such as for scoliosis (spinal curvature), are evaluated individually.

Adverse Effects of Epidural Block. Epidural block can have several adverse effects.

Maternal Hypotension. Sympathetic nerves are blocked along with pain nerves, which may result in vasodilation and hypotension. Maternal hypotension with possible reduction in placental perfusion is most likely to occur within the first 15 minutes of an epidural's initiation or injection of intermittent bolus doses to maintain pain relief. However, a significant percentage of women may have hypotension that occurs within 1 hour of initiation or repeat bolus doses (AWHONN, 2011; Hawkins & Bucklin, 2017; Wong, 2014). In addition, the fetus is more likely to have nonreassuring signs on an EFM strip, for example, a prolonged deceleration, if the mother has hypotension (Dozier et al., 2013). Nonreassuring fetal signs may have other causes, however (see Chapter 14).

Rapid infusion of a nondextrose IV solution, often warmed, such as lactated Ringer's solution or normal saline, before initiation of the block, fills the vascular system to offset vasodilation. Typical preload IV quantities are 500 to 1000 mL infused rapidly (Hawkins & Bucklin, 2017; Wong, 2014). If hypotension occurs and techniques such as rapid nondextrose IV fluid bolus, maternal repositioning, and oxygen administration are ineffective, IV phenylephrine in increments of 50 to 100 mcg or ephedrine in increments of 5 to 10 mg to promote vasoconstriction to raise the blood pressure (Cunningham, et. al, 2014; Hawkins & Bucklin, 2017).

Bladder Distention. A woman's bladder fills quickly because of the large quantity of IV solution, but her sensation to void is reduced. Bladder distention may cause pain that remains after initiation of the block and may interfere with fetal descent in labor.

Prolonged Second Stage. Delayed pushing is often intentional for second-stage labor, and the urge to push may be less intense for the woman who has an epidural block, particularly if she has an intense motor block. The pelvic muscles may be relaxed, which can interfere with the mechanism of internal rotation. These factors increase the chance for vacuum extractor–assisted births or forceps-assisted births.

Catheter Migration. After accurate placement, the epidural catheter may move. A woman may then have symptoms of intravascular injection, an intense block or one that is too high, absence of anesthesia, or a unilateral block. The anesthesia professional should be notified of any question about catheter placement.

Cesarean Births. Early research on whether cesarean births were more likely for women who had epidural blocks did show a risk, but the epidural block was much more intense than current epidurals. More recent research has not shown epidurals to increase the risk for cesarean birth, although the length of the second stage is likely to be longer than for the woman who did not have an epidural (Cunningham et al., 2014; Wong, 2014).

Maternal Fever. For reasons that are not completely clear, fever after epidural analgesia during labor is common. The fever associated with epidural analgesia is usually not caused by infection but may result from the reduced hyperventilation and decreased heat dissipation, for example, reduced sweating, which occur when the woman's pain is relieved. Also, women who are having prolonged labors may be more likely to have epidural block analgesia.

Fever is also a marker for infection. To avoid needless administration of antibiotics and sepsis evaluations in the newborn, other indicators for infection, for example, fetal tachycardia or amniotic fluid with a cloudy or yellow color and a foul or strong odor, should be sought as well. The nurse should remember that maternal fever elevates fetal temperature, resulting in tachycardia and oxygen demand for both. Medical and nursing personnel should try to lower the mother's temperature to a normal level and identify and treat a suspected infection. Possible signals to the hypothalamus that may result in maternal fever after epidural block include the following (AWHONN, 2011; Cunningham et al., 2014; Douma, Stienstra, Middeldorp, Arbous, & Dahan, 2015; Hawkins & Bucklin, 2017):

1. Decreased hyperventilation, sweating, and activity after onset of pain relief reduce maternal heat production and signal the hypothalamus to raise the woman's temperature.
2. Vasodilation redistributes heat from the core to the periphery of the body, where it is lost to the environment. The lower core temperature then signals the hypothalamus to increase heat production.
3. Shivering often occurs with sympathetic blockade accompanied by a dissociation between warm and cold sensations. In effect, the body believes that the temperature is lower than the true temperature and raises the "thermostat" to produce heat by shivering, thus increasing the core temperature.

Adverse Effects of Epidural Opioids. Adverse effects associated with epidural opioids may include nausea and vomiting, pruritus, and delayed maternal respiratory depression.

Nausea and Vomiting. Nausea and vomiting occur during labor. Sometimes it is related to epidural opioid administration. It may be associated with hypotension due to patient position or neuraxial analgesia. Blood pressure should be immediately assessed and the woman repositioned. Adjunctive drugs such as metoclopramide (Reglan), ondansetron (Zofran), or droperidol may be used to reduce nausea and vomiting that can occur with epidural opioids.

Pruritus. Itching of the face and neck is an annoying side effect that may occur with epidural opioids. Although she may not specifically complain of itching, a woman may rub or scratch her face and neck. Diphenhydramine (Benadryl), naloxone (Narcan), nalbuphine (Nubain), or naltrexone (Trexan) may relieve pruritus (Table 13.1) (Wong, 2014).

Shivering. Shivering is common in labor and sometimes is associated with epidural anesthesia. The cause is unknown (Wong, 2014).

Delayed Respiratory Depression. The possibility of late respiratory depression in the woman exists for up to 12 hours after the administration of an epidural opioid, depending on the duration of action of the drug used (Wong, 2014).

Nursing Care. Nurses with proper education who have demonstrated current competence should be able to participate in management of pain relief during labor (ACOG, 2015; American Society of Anesthesiologists [ASA], 2016). The nurse should record baseline maternal vital signs and FHR

TABLE 13.1 Drugs Commonly Used for Intrapartum Pain Management

Drug/Dose	Comments
Opioid Analgesics	
Meperidine (Demerol)	Respiratory depression (primarily in the neonate) is the main side effect.
12.5-50 mg every 1-2 hr IV; may be given by PCA	
Fentanyl (Sublimaze)	Onset is quick (5 min for IV administration), but duration of action is short.
50-100 mcg; may be repeated every hour; may be given by PCA	Less nausea, vomiting, and respiratory depression occurs than with meperidine.
Adjunct to epidural analgesia during labor (dose individualized)	Epidural use may cause pruritus.
Butorphanol (Stadol)	Has some narcotic antagonist effects; should not be given to the opiate-dependent woman (may precipitate withdrawal) or after other narcotics such as meperidine (may reverse their analgesic effects); also a respiratory depressant. 1-3 mg IV may be given to relieve pruritus associated with epidural narcotics.
1-2 mg every 3-4 hr; range 0.5-2 mg IV; may be given by PCA	
Nalbuphine (Nubain)	Same as butorphanol.
10 mg every 3 hr IV; may be given by PCA	2.5-10 mg may be given to relieve pruritus associated with epidural narcotics.
Adjunctive Drugs	
Ondansetron (Zofran)	4-8 mg to relieve pruritus associated with epidural narcotics
4 mg to prevent or treat nausea from opioid administration	
Metoclopramide (Reglan)	Before or during cesarean birth for aspiration prophylaxis
10 mg IV	
Diphenhydramine (Benadryl)	Given to relieve pruritus from epidural narcotics.
10-50 mg every 4-6 hr IV	
Narcotic Antagonists	
Naloxone (Narcan)	Action shorter than that of most narcotics it reverses; observe for recurrent respiratory depression and be prepared to give additional doses.
To reduce respiratory depression induced by opioids: 0.4-2 mg IV (adult)	
To reverse pruritus from epidural opioids: 40 to 80 mcg IV or IV infusion 0.25 to 2 mcg/kg/hr	
Naltrexone (Trexan)	Unlabeled use as a long-acting drug to relieve pruritus from epidural narcotics.
One dose of 3-6 mg PO	May reduce some analgesic effect when given for pruritus.
Vasopressor	
Phenylephrine 50-100 mcg or ephedrine 5-10 mg IV	Corrects hypotension related to epidural or subarachnoid block.

CNS, Central nervous system; *IM,* Intramuscularly; *IV,* intravenously; *PCA,* patient-controlled analgesia; *PO,* orally.

References: Bujedo, B.M. (2016). An update on neuraxial opioid induced pruritus prevention. *J Anesth Crit Care Open Access* 6(2): 00226. DOI: 10.15406/jaccoa.2016.06.00226; Cunningham, F. G., Leveno, K.J., Bloom, S.L., Spong, C.Y., Dashe, J.S., Hoffman, B.L., Casey, B. M., Sheffield, J. S. (2014). *Williams obstetrics* (24th ed.). New York, NY: McGraw-Hill Medical; Hawkins, J. L., & Bucklin, B. A. (2017). Obstetric anesthesia. In S. G. Gabbe, J. R. Niebyl, J. L. Simpson, M.B. Landon, H.L. Galan, R. M. Jauniaux, D.A. Driscoll, et al. (Eds.), *Obstetrics: Normal and problem pregnancies* (7th ed., pp.344–367). Philadelphia, PA: Saunders; Wong, C. A. (2014) Epidural and spinal analgesia/anesthesia for labor and vaginal delivery. In D. Chestnut, C.A. Wong, L.C. Tsen, D.N.K Warwick, Y Beilin, J.M. Mhyre, & V Naveen (Eds.), *Chestnut's obstetric anesthesia: Principles and practice* (5th ed.) Philadelphia, PA: Saunders.

patterns for comparison with prenatal levels and those after the block. IV access is ensured, and the prescribed preload of fluid is given. The nurse supports the woman in the correct position and tells the anesthesia provider when the woman is having a contraction. The woman may feel a brief "electric shock" sensation as the catheter is passed. The nurse should assist her in remaining still while the block is completed. After the medication is injected, the nurse observes for signs of subarachnoid puncture or intravascular injection.

Evidence-based practice guidelines from AWHONN (2011) and the American College of Obstetricians and Gynecologists (ACOG, 2015) suggest assessing the maternal blood pressure and FHR every 5 minutes during the first 15 minutes after initiation of the epidural or any additional bolus doses of epidural medication. Repeat assessment of BP and FHR at 30 minutes and at 1 hour after the procedure. Individual facilities may use these guidelines or develop their own guidelines. As in any labor, maternal and fetal assessments are done more frequently, if needed, in situations such as maternal bleeding or a nonreassuring FHR pattern.

The woman's bladder should be assessed frequently because of the large IV fluid load and her reduced sensation to void. Indwelling catheterization is common, but intermittent catheterization if a woman is unable to void is recommended by the AWHONN (2011). Based on results from varied researchers that support a woman's ability to void or need few, if any, intermittent catheterizations, the goal of labor caregivers should be to support normal urination rather than catheterizing all women with epidural analgesia.

The nurse should observe for signs associated with catheter migration from the epidural space and for adverse effects from epidural opioids, such as nausea and vomiting and pruritus. Reassurance about the harmless and temporary nature of pruritus is often sufficient.

Intrathecal Opioid Analgesics

Intrathecal injection of an opioid analgesic provides another option for pain management without sedation. The drug is injected into the subarachnoid space, where it binds to opiate receptors, allowing much smaller doses than would be adequate if given systemically. The woman can feel her contractions but not the pain they would otherwise cause.

Advantages of intrathecal analgesics include the following:
- Rapid onset of pain relief without sedation
- No motor block, enabling the woman to ambulate during labor
- No sympathetic block, with its hypotensive effects
Disadvantages may include the following:
- Limited duration of action, possibly requiring another procedure for continued pain relief
- Inadequate pain relief for late labor and the birth, requiring added measures to manage pain at these times

Combining intrathecal opioids with epidural block in a combined-spinal epidural (CSE) provides rapid pain control at the time an epidural catheter is placed. Epidural drugs are then given to provide a long-acting block for labor.

Technique. The subarachnoid space is entered with a spinal needle, as in the subarachnoid block (SAB). A preservative-free opioid analgesic is then injected. The drug chosen depends on the expected duration of labor at the time it is given. Drugs that may be used by this route include fentanyl, sufentanil, and morphine.

One technique for performing the CSE is to insert the epidural needle into the epidural space. The much thinner spinal needle is then inserted through the larger epidural needle to reach the subarachnoid space for injection of the intrathecal opioid. The smaller needle is then withdrawn and an epidural catheter placed for injection of epidural medication (Chestnut, 2014).

Adverse Effects of Intrathecal Opioids. As with epidural opioids, nausea, vomiting, and pruritus may occur. Delayed maternal respiratory depression may occur, depending on the drug used.

Nursing Care. Vital signs and FHR are taken at the usual intervals for the woman's stage of labor. Side effects, such as nausea and vomiting or pruritus, are reported and managed similarly to those occurring with the epidural block. Reduced effectiveness suggests that the drug's duration of action is ending or that the woman is in late labor. Other pain management methods may be needed for the remainder of labor and for birth (Creedon et al., 2013).

Care for the woman undergoing a CSE block is the same as that for one receiving a noncombined block.

Subarachnoid (Spinal) Block

An SAB is a simpler procedure than the epidural block and may be performed when a quick cesarean birth is necessary and an epidural catheter is not in place. It is similar to local infiltration and pudendal block. SAB is performed just before birth, providing no pain relief during most of labor.

The physician or nurse-anesthetist injects local anesthetic into the subarachnoid space in a single dose. The woman loses both sensory and motor function below the level of the SAB, with relief of pain from contractions.

Technique. A 25- to 27-gauge spinal needle is placed in the subarachnoid space. Appearance of CSF at the needle hub ensures correct placement, and the local anesthetic is injected (Fig. 13.11).

The level of anesthesia for both epidural blocks and SABs is determined by the volume, concentration, and density of the drug (Fig. 13.12).

Contraindications and Precautions. Contraindications and precautions are similar to those for epidural block: the woman's refusal, coagulation defects, uncorrected hypovolemia, infection in the area of insertion, systemic infection, and allergy.

Adverse Effects. Three adverse effects of an SAB are maternal hypotension, bladder distention, and post–dural puncture headache. Hypotension is more likely with the SAB than with the epidural block and is treated in the same manner, often with a larger volume of preload IV fluid. Bladder distention is managed with ongoing assessments, support of the woman's ability to void and intermittent catheterization if necessary.

Post–Dural Puncture Headache. Post–dural puncture headache may occur after SAB in some women because of CSF leakage at the site of dural puncture. A spinal headache is postural. It is worse when a woman is upright and may disappear when she is lying flat. Headache is less likely if a small-gauge needle is used.

Bed rest with oral or IV hydration helps relieve the post–dural puncture headache. Caffeine is another oral therapy. A blood patch may provide definitive relief. The blood patch involves injection of a small amount of the woman's blood (obtained with sterile technique) into the epidural space. The blood causes a tamponade effect and may form a gelatinous seal over the hole in the dura, stopping spinal fluid leakage (Fig. 13.13) (Hawkins & Bucklin, 2017).

Systemic Drugs for Labor

Systemic drugs have effects on multiple systems because they are distributed throughout the body. These intrapartum drugs include opioid analgesics and adjunctive drugs. Although general anesthesia is also systemic, it is discussed separately because it is used only at birth and causes loss of consciousness.

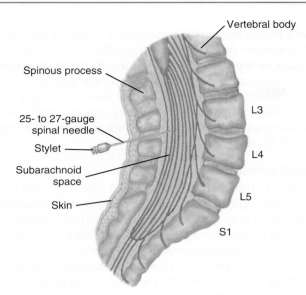

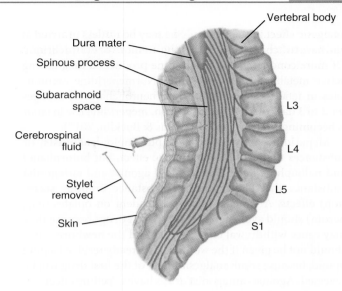

A 25- to 27-gauge spinal needle with a stylet occluding its lumen is passed into the subarachnoid space below where the spinal cord ends.

The stylet is removed, and one or more drops of clear cerebrospinal fluid at needle hub confirm correct needle placement. Medication is then injected, and the needle is removed.

FIG. 13.11 Technique for Subarachnoid Block.

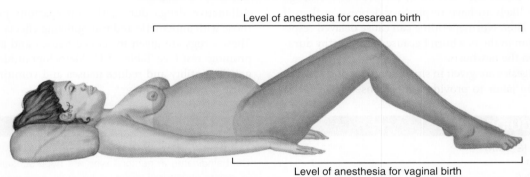

FIG. 13.12 Levels of Anesthesia for Epidural and Subarachnoid Blocks. A level of T10 through S5 is adequate for vaginal birth. A higher level of T4 to T6 is needed for cesarean birth.

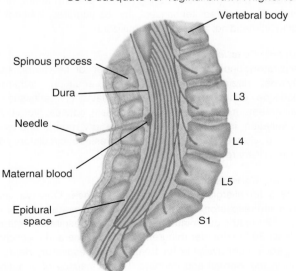

FIG. 13.13 Blood Patch for Relief of Spinal Headache. To seal a dural puncture, a small amount of the woman's blood is injected into the epidural space. Other fluids such as normal saline or dextran may be injected using a similar technique.

Nitrous Oxide

Nitrous oxide ("laughing gas") is used for labor pain management in several Western countries and was used briefly in the United States in the early to mid-1900s. Its use is returning to this country. Nausea, vomiting, and dizziness are some of the possible side effects to consider. For labor pain, the gas is delivered as 50% nitrous oxide and 50% oxygen. Nitrous oxide in labor is self-administered; the woman controls when she takes breaths of the 50:50 combination (El-Wahab, & Fernando, 2014; Stewart & Collins, 2013).

Parenteral Analgesia

Opioid analgesics are the most common parenteral medications given to reduce perception of pain without loss of consciousness. Analgesics that may be used for labor are meperidine (Demerol), fentanyl (Sublimaze), butorphanol (Stadol), and nalbuphine (Nubain) (see Table 13.1) (El-Wahab & Fernando, 2014; Hawkins & Bucklin, 2017).

Although the drug may be prescribed for labor analgesia, meperidine often produces a dysphoric rather than an analgesic effect in the woman. She may be restless or irritable and have twitching, jerking, shaking, tremors, or even delirium. Of more concern is that meperidine produces a long-lasting active metabolite, normeperidine, Normeperidine accumulates in fetal tissue and can cause neurobehavioral changes for 2 to 3 days of life. For this reason, meperidine use in labor is becoming controversial (Hawkins & Bucklin, 2017).

Meperidine and fentanyl are pure opioid **agonists**, or substances that cause a physiologic effect, but butorphanol and nalbuphine have mixed opioid agonist and **antagonist** (substance that blocks another substance or body secretion) effects. A woman who is dependent on opiates (e.g., heroin) should avoid agonist–antagonist drugs because they may cause withdrawal effects in her and the newborn. They should not be given if the woman has already received a pure opioid, because some analgesic effect of the first drug will be reversed. Agonist–antagonist drugs have a "ceiling effect" on the amount of analgesia they provide and are unsuitable for the increasing pain of the entire labor for many women.

The primary side effect of opioids is respiratory depression, which is more likely to affect the newborn. Timing of administration is important to reduce neonatal respiratory depression. An infant who is born at the peak of the drug's action is more likely to have respiratory depression than if born earlier or later. Normeperidine can cause delayed respiratory depression in the newborn because of its lengthy duration of action in the newborn.

Opioid analgesics are given in small, frequent doses by the IV route during labor to provide a rapid onset of analgesia and a predictable duration of action. The woman will benefit from rapid pain control, with less likelihood of neonatal respiratory depression. Starting the injection at the beginning of the contraction, when blood flow to the placenta is normally reduced, limits transfer to the fetus. When placental blood flow resumes, more of the drug is in maternal tissues. The drugs also may be delivered by patient-controlled analgesia (PCA) pump.

Opioid Antagonists

Naloxone (Narcan) reverses opioid-induced respiratory depression. Naloxone does not reverse respiratory depression from other causes such as barbiturates, anesthetics, nonopioid drugs, or pathologic conditions. Naloxone has a shorter duration of action than most of the opioids it reverses, and respiratory depression may recur. In an opiate-dependent woman or newborn, naloxone can induce withdrawal symptoms.

Airway management (i.e., bag-and-mask ventilation) takes precedence over use of naloxone for the newborn, and the drug is not routinely given to the baby for respiratory depression (AAP & ACOG, 2012).

Adjunctive Drugs

Adjunctive drugs during the intrapartum period include those with antiemetic and tranquilizing effects and sedatives. These drugs are given to reduce nausea and anxiety and to promote rest (see Table 13.1). Metoclopramide can increase gastric motility and reduce nausea and vomiting. It also can cause drowsiness.

DRUG GUIDE

Butorphanol (Stadol)

Classification
Opioid analgesic.

Action
Opioid analgesic with some agonist–antagonist effects; exact mechanism of action unknown; produces respiratory depression that does not increase markedly with larger doses.

Indications
Systemic pain relief during labor.

Dosage and Route
Intravenous
1 mg every 3 to 4 hours; range 0.5 to 2 mg; may be given undiluted.

Absorption
Onset of analgesia almost immediate with intravenous administration, peaks after approximately 30 minutes, and lasts about 3 hours; faster onset and shorter duration of action than meperidine or morphine.

Excretion
Excreted in urine; crosses placental barrier; secreted in breast milk.

Contraindications and Precautions
Contraindicated in persons who are hypersensitive; not used in opiate-dependent persons because antagonist activity of the drug may cause withdrawal symptoms in the woman or newborn; cautiously used during birth of preterm infant; drug actions potentiated (enhanced) by barbiturates, phenothiazines, cimetidine, and other tranquilizers.

Adverse Reactions
Respiratory depression or apnea (woman or newborn), anaphylaxis; dizziness, lightheadedness, sedation, lethargy, headache, euphoria, mental clouding, fainting, restlessness, excitement, tremors, delirium, insomnia; nausea, vomiting, constipation, increased biliary pressure, dry mouth, anorexia; flushing, altered heart rate and blood pressure, circulatory collapse; urinary retention; sensitivity to cold.

Nursing Considerations
Assess for allergies and opiate dependence. Observe vital signs and respiratory function in woman (respiratory rate of at least 12 breaths per minute) and newborn (respiratory rate of at least 30 breaths per minute). Have naloxone and resuscitation equipment available for treatment of respiratory depression in the woman and neonate. Report nausea or vomiting to the birth attendant for a possible order for an antiemetic. Antiemetics or other CNS depressants may enhance the respiratory depressant effects of butorphanol.

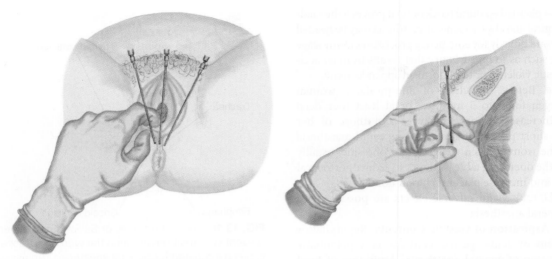

FIG. 13.14 Local infiltration anesthesia numbs the perineum just before birth for an episiotomy or after birth for suturing of a laceration. The birth attendant protects the fetal head by placing a finger inside the vagina while injecting the perineum in a fanlike pattern or as needed.

Sedatives

Sedatives such as barbiturates are not routinely given because they have prolonged depressant effects on the neonate. However, a small dose of a short-acting barbiturate may be given to promote rest if a woman is fatigued from false labor or a prolonged latent phase.

❓ KNOWLEDGE CHECK

18. What is the primary adverse effect of opioid administration? How can this effect be reduced?
19. What is the preferred order of resuscitation for the newborn who has respiratory depression? Does naloxone have any use in an adult?

Vaginal Birth Anesthesia
Local Infiltration Anesthesia

Infiltration of the perineum with a local anesthetic is done by the physician or nurse-midwife before an episiotomy or perineal repair (Fig. 13.14). Local infiltration does not alter pain from uterine contractions or distention of the vagina. The local agent provides anesthesia in the immediate area of the episiotomy or laceration. A short delay occurs between anesthetic injection and onset of numbness, and the drug burns before its anesthetic action begins. Local infiltration rarely has adverse effects on either mother or infant.

Pudendal Block

A pudendal block anesthetizes the lower vagina and part of the perineum. It is often used to provide anesthesia for an episiotomy and vaginal birth, especially one that requires using low forceps. A pudendal block does not block pain from uterine contractions, and the mother feels pressure. The pudendal block is a highly localized type of regional block, like a dental anesthetic that provides numbness for dental procedures.

The physician or nurse-midwife injects the pudendal nerves near each ischial spine with a local anesthetic (Fig. 13.15).

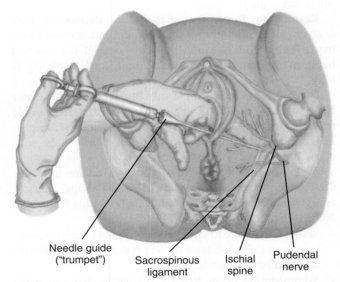

Needle guide ("trumpet")   Sacrospinous ligament   Ischial spine   Pudendal nerve

FIG. 13.15 Pudendal block provides anesthesia for an episiotomy and use of low forceps. A needle guide ("trumpet") protects the maternal and fetal tissues from the long needle needed to reach the pudendal nerve. Only about 1.25 cm (½ inch) of the long needle protrudes from the guide.

The perineum is infiltrated with local anesthetic because the pudendal block does not fully anesthetize this area. As in local infiltration, a brief delay occurs between injection and onset of numbness. Possible maternal complications include a toxic reaction to the anesthetic, rectal puncture, hematoma, and sciatic nerve block. If maternal toxicity is avoided, the fetus usually is not affected.

General Anesthesia

General anesthesia is systemic pain control that involves loss of consciousness. It is rarely used for vaginal births, but it still has a place in cesarean birth. Some women either refuse or are not good candidates for epidural block or SAB for cesarean birth.

Occasionally, a planned epidural block or SAB proves to be inadequate for surgical anesthesia. General anesthesia may be needed unexpectedly and quickly for emergency procedures at any stage of pregnancy, such as to repair injury that results from an accident or domestic violence or to perform an appendectomy.

Technique. Before induction of anesthesia, a woman breathes oxygen for 3 to 5 minutes, or at least four deep breaths, to increase her oxygen stores and those of her fetus for the short period of apnea during rapid anesthesia induction. The woman has a wedge under one side, usually her right (or the operating table is tilted), to reduce aortocaval compression and increase placental blood flow.

Adverse Effects. Major adverse effects are possible with the use of general anesthesia.

Maternal Aspiration of Gastric Contents. Regurgitation with aspiration of acidic gastric contents is a potentially fatal complication of general anesthesia. Aspiration of food particles may result in airway obstruction. Aspiration of acidic secretions results in a chemical injury to the airways—**aspiration pneumonitis**. Infection often occurs after the initial lung injury.

Respiratory Depression. Respiratory depression may occur in either the mother or the infant but is more likely in the baby. This is more likely to occur if the interval between induction of anesthesia and cord clamping is long.

Uterine Relaxation. Some inhalational anesthetics may cause uterine relaxation. This characteristic is desirable for treating some complications, for example, replacing an inverted uterus. However, postpartum hemorrhage may occur if the uterus relaxes after birth.

Methods to Minimize Adverse Effects. Measures to reduce the risk for maternal aspiration or to limit lung injury if aspiration occurs include the following (Hawkins & Bucklin, 2017; Tsen, 2014):
- Restricting intake to clear fluids or maintaining nothing-by-mouth (NPO) status if surgery is expected, such as with a scheduled cesarean birth
- Administering drugs to raise the gastric pH and make secretions less acidic—for example, sodium citrate and citric acid (Bicitra), ranitidine (Zantac), cimetidine (Tagamet), or famotidine (Pepcid)
- Administering drugs to reduce secretions—for example, glycopyrrolate (Robinul)
- Administering drugs to speed gastric emptying, for example, metoclopramide (Reglan)
- Using cricoid pressure (Sellick's maneuver) to block the esophagus by pressing the rigid trachea against it (Fig. 13.16)

Neonatal respiratory depression may be minimized by doing the following:
- Reducing the time from induction of anesthesia to clamping of the umbilical cord
- Keeping use of sedating drugs and anesthetics to a minimum until the cord is clamped

To reduce the time from induction of anesthesia to cord clamping, the woman is prepared and draped and the physicians are ready before anesthesia is induced. The anesthesia is

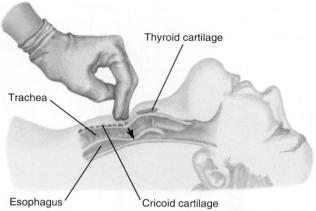

FIG. 13.16 Cricoid pressure, or Sellick's maneuver, is used to prevent vomitus from entering the woman's trachea while she is being intubated for general anesthesia. An assistant applies pressure to the cricoid cartilage to obstruct the esophagus. Once the woman is successfully intubated with a cuffed endotracheal tube, gastric secretions cannot enter the trachea.

kept light until the infant is born and the woman may move slightly on the table, although she usually has no memory of the experience. The anesthesia level is deepened as soon as the cord is clamped.

> **? KNOWLEDGE CHECK**
>
> 20. What are two major advantages of using regional pain management techniques during childbirth?
> 21. What is the major adverse effect of the epidural block or SAB? How can the fetus be affected? How may this effect be reduced?
> 22. What are common side effects of epidural or intrathecal opioid analgesics, and how are these managed?
> 23. What are the major adverse effects of general anesthesia? What measures reduce the risks?

◆ APPLICATION OF THE NURSING PROCESS: PAIN MANAGEMENT

Nursing care related to pain management should be combined with support for normal labor and any complications that arise. Care of the fetus remains important. Two problems that affect many women are pain and care related to epidural analgesia.

PAIN

◆ Assessment

Pain assessment begins at admission and continues throughout labor and postpartum (see Table 15.1). Pain-related assessments include the following:
- Preferences for pain management
- Previous surgeries, type of anesthesia, and any anesthesia-associated problems
- Maternal vital signs
- FHR and EFM patterns

- Allergies, focusing especially on allergy to opioid analgesics, dental anesthetics, and iodine (used in some skin preparation solutions)
- Oral intake—Time and type of last intake
- Evidence of pain—Verbal statement, requests for pain-relief measures, crying, moaning; and nonverbal evidence such as tense, guarded posture or facial expression

Labor Status

In addition to these routine assessments, ask the woman if she needs help with pain management. A stoic woman may give little evidence of pain yet may say she wants pain control, if asked.

When assessing pain, clarify the words a woman uses. When asked if she has "pain," the woman may deny it. Yet changing the word used to "discomfort," "cramping," "aching," "pressure," or other words that may describe labor pain may elicit a different response. Do not assume that everyone uses the same words to describe pain. Pain is an individual experience, and so is the expression of pain.

Asking a woman to rate her pain on a scale of 0 to 10 (or your facility's standard scale) helps clarify her pain's intensity. A zero represents no pain, whereas 10 is the worst possible pain. Ask the woman to rate her pain on this scale before and after pain-relief measures to evaluate their effectiveness. Multilingual and picture scales are available for those who do not speak the dominant language.

A surprising number of women have difficulty using a pain scale because they have little experience with pain. They may underrate current pain, expecting an increase in the amount of pain (and therefore pain number) later in labor, or they may say that they have no idea what the "worst pain imaginable" is and therefore cannot guess how a pain rating of 10 feels. A scale or description by the woman does, however, provide one measure of how pain feels before and after relief measures (Jones et al., 2015).

Body language gives a clue to comfort level. Moaning, crying, thrashing, and an inability to use nonpharmacologic techniques are likely indicators that a woman needs help with pain control, including pharmacologic pain relief. However, more subtle clues such as remaining tense between contractions also suggest difficulty coping with pain.

Evaluate the woman's labor status to help her choose the most appropriate method of pain control. Inform her if she has reached a decision point in labor to use or not use a specific pharmacologic method. No standard time or amount of cervical dilation serves as a guideline for this critical point. This is estimated based on projected time of birth, amount of time needed to establish a specific method, and the pharmacology of the drug or drugs.

Avoid making assumptions about a woman's pain based on her rate of labor progress, cervical dilation, or apparent intensity of contractions. Do not assume that a woman whose cervix is 2 cm dilated has little pain and that a woman whose cervix is dilated 8 cm has intense pain. An obese woman's contractions may be strong, but they may seem mild if they are assessed by palpation or an external monitor because of her thick abdominal fat pad. *Labor progress or contraction intensity cannot be equated with a woman's pain perception or tolerance.*

A woman's need for pain relief should not be based only on her outward expression. A quiet woman may need medication but may be reluctant to ask, whereas an expressive woman may be satisfied with only nonpharmacologic measures. Because women who do not speak the prevailing language may not know what is available, seek an interpreter not related to the laboring woman to communicate most effectively.

Observe for and report pain that is not typical of normal labor. Although labor pain is often intense, it should come and go with each contraction. The uterus should not be tender or boardlike between contractions and should not cause constant intense pain.

◆ Identification of Patient Problems

Analysis of the data collected enables the nurse to identify actual and potential patient problems and develop an individualized plan of care. Pain is expected in normal childbirth, and most laboring women have nursing needs that relate to its management. "Pain from the effects of uterine contractions and fetal descent" may be an appropriate problem.

◆ Planning: Expected Outcomes

Because pain is a subjective experience and expected in labor, two expected outcomes are realistic. The woman will do the following:

1. Describe pain-relief measures, both nonpharmacologic and pharmacologic, as satisfactory during labor.
2. Effectively use breathing and relaxation techniques learned in childbirth class or from the nurse during labor.

◆ Interventions

Nursing care related to intrapartum pain management focuses on reducing factors that hinder the woman's pain control and enhancing those that benefit it. Although epidurals are very common in North American hospitals, do not make the assumption that every woman will want one for birth. Caring contact with a nurse enhances pain management and the overall experience of giving birth.

Promoting Relaxation

Simple attention to details promotes relaxation. Make the environment more comfortable. If noise is a problem, suggest music or television to mask it. A warm blanket, a cool cloth, or a warm pack provides tangible comfort and conveys the nurse's caring attitude. Change linens and underpads as needed to keep the woman reasonably clean and dry.

Offer the woman a warm shower or bath, especially if she is tense and if no contraindications exist (see Box 13.1). In general, walking is good during early labor, and water therapy is better during active labor. The mild nipple stimulation that occurs in a whirlpool or shower may intensify contractions in a woman whose labor has slowed, causing her posterior pituitary gland to secrete oxytocin.

Reduce intrusions as much as possible. For example, wait until a contraction is over before asking questions or performing a procedure. Longer assessments and procedures may span several contractions, but try to stop during each contraction, if possible.

Reducing Outside Sources of Discomfort

Anesthetize the IV site with lidocaine (Xylocaine) before inserting the line if the woman is not allergic and if policy permits. Normal saline infiltration of the site has a similar effect. Remind her to change position regularly to reduce tension and discomfort from constant pressure. Support her with pillows.

Observe the woman's bladder for distention hourly, and encourage her to void every 2 hours or more often if she has received a large quantity of IV fluids. Most intrapartum order sets include an order for catheterization if the woman cannot void and her bladder is full.

Reducing Anxiety and Fear

Accurate information reduces the negative psychological impact of the unknown. Tell the woman about her labor and its progress. You cannot predict when she will give birth, but tell her if labor progress is or is not on course. Sometimes, she needs only the reassurance from an experienced nurse that her intense contractions are, indeed, normal. The woman may be willing to endure more discomfort than she otherwise would if she is making progress.

Be honest if problems do occur. A woman usually knows if a problem exists and is more anxious if she does not know what it is. Explain all measures taken to correct the problem, and inform her of the results.

Helping the Woman Use Nonpharmacologic Techniques

If the nonpharmacologic method is safe for the woman and fetus and if it is effective, do not interfere with its use. Try not to distract the woman from whatever technique she is using.

Massage. Fetal monitor belts hinder abdominal effleurage. Encourage the woman to do effleurage on uncovered areas of her abdomen or to stroke her thighs. Consider using intermittent auscultation or intermittent EFM (see Chapter 14).

Use powder to avoid friction, and seek feedback from the woman about the best location and amount of pressure to use for sacral pressure or other massage. Because this information may change during labor or massage may become uncomfortable rather than helpful, seek the woman's feedback regularly.

Mental Stimulation. Use a low, soothing voice when helping a woman use imagery. Speaking close to her ear is often helpful when trying to create a tranquil imaginary scene or to calm her. Use of a low, soothing voice during an emergency has a calming effect as well. Music can enhance mental stimulation techniques.

Breathing. Women often modify the techniques they learn in class or invent some of their own during labor. Encourage the woman to change techniques when she feels it is necessary but to save the complex ones for later labor. If she has trouble

maintaining her concentration, the nurse or her support person may try to make eye contact (if culturally appropriate) and breathe the pattern with her.

Symptoms of hyperventilation (dizziness, tingling and numbness of the fingers and lips, carpopedal spasm) are likely if a woman breathes fast and deep. If she hyperventilates, she should breathe into her cupped hands, a paper bag, or a washcloth placed over her nose and mouth. Talk to her gently to slow her breathing.

Teach breathing techniques to the unprepared woman and her coach when she is admitted. Review them when she seems to need a different method. If she makes up a breathing technique that works, leave it alone.

When teaching pain management techniques to the unprepared woman who is in advanced labor, follow these guidelines:
- Teach one method at a time.
- Demonstrate the method between contractions.
- Use breathing techniques with the woman while maintaining eye contact.
- Give her control over her labor (e.g., who is present or what technique she will use).
- Speak in a soft, calm tone of voice.

Incorporating Pharmacologic Methods

All pharmacologic methods require collaboration with medical personnel for orders. Tell the woman soon after admission what medication is available if she needs it. This is intended not to undermine her self-confidence but to allow her to make an informed choice about medication, when necessary. Analgesia is most effective if it is given before pain is severe.

Tell the woman that her preferences about pain-relief methods will be honored if possible, but predicting the course of her labor is impossible. Her preferred method of pain management may be inappropriate if labor has unexpected developments. Assure her that no pharmacologic method will be used without her understanding and consent (see Patient Teaching: How Will This Medicine Affect Our Baby?).

PATIENT TEACHING

How Will This Medicine Affect Our Baby?

Women and their partners often ask whether pain medication or anesthesia will harm their baby. The nurse can help parents choose wisely from available options by providing honest information, as follows:
- Pain that you cannot tolerate is not good for you or your baby, and it reduces the joy of this special event.
- Some risk is associated with every type of pain medication or anesthesia, but careful selection and the use of preventive measures minimize this risk. If complications occur, corrective measures can reduce the risk to you and your baby.
- Some pain relievers can cause your baby to be slow to breathe at birth, but carefully controlling the timing and dose of the medication reduces the likelihood that this will occur. We can support your baby's breathing or use another medication to reverse this effect, if needed.

Continued

How Will This Medicine Affect Our Baby?

- Epidural or spinal anesthesia can cause your blood pressure to fall, which can reduce the blood flow to your baby. However, we give you lots of intravenous fluids to reduce this effect. We have other medications to increase your blood pressure if the fluids are not enough.
- General anesthesia can cause your baby to be slow to breathe at birth. To reduce this risk, the anesthesia will not be started until everything is ready for the surgery, and the doctors will clamp the baby's umbilical cord as quickly as possible.

If a woman finds nonpharmacologic methods inadequate, help her try other ones or offer her available medication. When contacting the birth attendant for medication orders, report the fetal and maternal status and vital signs, labor status, and her request for medication. If she has a continuous epidural block, contact the person who inserted it if problems occur. Observe special nursing considerations associated with the method used (Table 13.2).

◆ Evaluation

Labor is not expected to be painless, even with the most effective pharmacologic methods. The first goal or expected outcome is achieved if the woman is satisfied with her ability to manage her pain. Many women have occasional difficulty using breathing or other techniques, even if they have practiced faithfully. The nurse may ask the following questions: How did the woman's pain scale rating change before and after the pain-relief method? Were nonpharmacologic or pharmacologic methods used? Is she satisfied with her level of pain relief?

EPIDURAL ANALGESIA

Many women choose epidural analgesia for pain relief during labor because of its effectiveness without sedation. Epidural block analgesia requires several specific nursing assessments and interventions.

◆ Assessment

The admission assessment focuses on possible allergies to local anesthetics or opioid drugs that might be used in the block. Determine baseline maternal vital signs and the FHR and pattern. Assess for any skin infection of the back where the epidural will be inserted.

◆ Identification of Patient Problems

The primary risks associated with epidural analgesia are maternal hypotension and injury. These result in collaborative problems:

- Potential complication—Maternal hypotension with secondary fetal hypoxia
- Potential complication—Patient injury resulting from reduced sensation and movement secondary to epidural effects

◆ Planning: Expected Outcomes

Appropriate goals or expected outcomes are (1) the woman has achieved the outcome if her blood pressure and the FHR pattern do not change significantly after the epidural, and (2) the woman has achieved the outcome if she does not have a treatment-related injury while her sensation and mobility are reduced.

◆ Interventions

Maternal Hypotension

Maternal hypotension reduces blood supply to the placenta, decreasing fetal oxygen and nutrient supply and waste removal. Birth facilities will have policies that provide specific guidelines for care when women receive epidural block. Infuse the prescribed IV solution, typically 500 to 1000 mL as ordered, before the block's initiation. If the woman has not received the full amount when the block is begun, notify the anesthesia professional.

The epidural may be placed with the woman in the sitting or side-lying position, based on the decision of the anesthesia provider. If she is in a sitting position, hugging a pillow or a small birth ball helps her hold the correct position. Tell the anesthesia clinician when the woman is having a contraction. Warn the woman that she may feel a brief "electric shock" sensation as the catheter is passed. After the epidural is initiated, maintain her position so that aortocaval compression is avoided, for example, by placing a pillow under one hip.

Measure the woman's blood pressure and pulse rate (often an automatic cuff is used) every 2 to 3 minutes or per the facility's protocol for 15 to 20 minutes after the initial injection of medication, comparing the values with her baseline blood pressure and pulse rate. Maintain continuous EFM. A significant blood pressure decrease is a 20% fall from her baseline or a drop to 100 mm Hg or lower systolic. Hypotension of any degree accompanied by FHR decelerations or loss of variability is significant. If hypotension occurs, increase the rate of her IV fluid infusion, keeping her positioned to avoid aortocaval compression. Phenylephrine 50 to 100 mcg (or ephedrine, usually 5 to 10 mg) is ordered if hypotension is significant and a fluid increase does not quickly improve it. When the blood pressure is stable, assess it every 15 minutes. If hypotension occurs, report it to the professional who oversees the anesthetic for definitive treatment. Pulse oximetry identifies a decrease in maternal oxygenation status to below 95%.

Continue observing the FHR. Signs of reduced placental perfusion may be evident before the woman shows signs of hypotension. These include fetal tachycardia (more than 160 beats per minute [bpm]) or bradycardia (less than 110 bpm), prolonged decelerations, and late decelerations (see Chapter 14). Monitor the mother's temperature to identify elevations that also may contribute to fetal tachycardia.

Avoidance of Injury

Epidural block reduces lower extremity sensation and movement to varying degrees. Some women have such a light motor block that their epidural is called a "walking epidural." However, to prevent falls, these women should not walk alone.

TABLE 13.2   Pharmacologic Methods of Intrapartum Pain Management

Method and Uses	Nursing Considerations

Opioid Analgesics
 	
Systemic analgesia during labor and for postoperative pain after cesarean birth.
 	
May be combined with an adjunctive drug to reduce nausea and vomiting that sometimes occur with narcotic use and after surgery.
 	
Often delivered by PCA pump in postoperative period.
	1. Assess the woman for drug use at admission.
	   Women who are opiate-dependent should not receive analgesics having mixed agonist and antagonist actions (butorphanol and nalbuphine).
	2. Observe neonate for respiratory depression, especially if mother had opioid narcotics within 4 hr of birth or at time of drug's peak action, or if mother received multiple opioid doses during labor:
	   • Delay in initiating or sustaining normal depth and rate of respirations
	   • Respiratory rate <30/min
	   • Poor muscle tone: Limp, floppy
	3. Use of adjunctive drugs for nausea, such as metoclopramide, enhances respiratory depressant effects.
	4. Respiratory (bag-and-mask) and cardiac support precede drug administration in neonatal resuscitation. If naloxone is given, observe for recurrent respiratory depression.

Epidural Opioids *Labor:* Mixed with a local anesthetic agent to give better pain relief with less motor block. *Postoperatively:* Gives long-acting analgesia without sedation, allowing mother and infant to interact more easily.	1. Monitor for same nursing implications as with epidural block. 2. Do not give additional opioids or other CNS depressants except as ordered by anesthesia provider. Nonsteroidal antiinflammatory drugs or oral analgesics are often prescribed in routine orders. 3. Maternal respiratory depression may be delayed for up to 24 hr and varies with drug given. Observe respiratory rate and depth, oxygen saturation, and arousability hourly for 24 hr or as ordered. Notify the anesthesia provider of respiratory rate of <12/min, persistent oxygen saturation of <95% on pulse oximetry, reduced respiratory effort, difficulty arousing, or as ordered by provider. Cyanosis is a late sign of respiratory depression. 4. Have naloxone 0.4 mg, an oral airway, and an Ambu bag and mask immediately available, such as on a "crash cart." 5. Observe for pruritus or rubbing of face and neck. Routine postoperative orders to relieve pruritus are usually provided. Notify the anesthesia provider if these are inadequate. 6. Urinary retention may occur after indwelling catheter removal. Observe for adequacy of voiding, as in all postpartum women. 7. Notify the anesthesia provider for relief of nausea or vomiting. 8. Assess sensation and mobility before allowing ambulation.
Intrathecal Opioid Analgesics Provides analgesia for most of first-stage labor without maternal sedation. A very small dose of the drug is needed because it is injected very near spinal cord where sensory fibers enter. Usually not adequate for late labor or birth itself. Often combined with epidural block for CSE technique for labor.	1. Observe for common side effects of nausea, vomiting, and pruritus. Notify the anesthesia provider if these effects occur, and have an antagonist such as naloxone or naltrexone available. 2. Observe for delayed respiratory depression, depending on drug given. Use a pulse oximeter, as indicated. 3. Observe for nonreassuring FHR patterns that may be associated with reduced maternal oxygenation.
Local Infiltration Anesthesia Numbs perineum for episiotomy or repair of laceration at vaginal birth. No relief of labor pain. Not adequate for instrument-assisted birth.	1. Assess for drug allergies, especially to dental anesthetics because they are related to those used in maternity care. 2. Apply ice to perineum after birth to reduce edema and hematoma formation and to increase comfort.
Pudendal Block Numbs lower vagina and perineum for vaginal birth. No relief of labor pain because it is done just before birth. Provides adequate anesthesia for many instrument-assisted births.	1. Use same interventions as for local infiltration. A woman or her partner may be alarmed if the long needle is noticed (about 15 cm [6 inches]). Teach her that it must be long to reach the pudendal nerve through the vagina and that it will be inserted only about 1.25 cm (½ inch) near the location of the nerve. Tell her that a guide ("trumpet") will be used to avoid injuring her vaginal tissue or that of her baby.

TABLE 13.2   Pharmacologic Methods of Intrapartum Pain Management—cont'd

Method and Uses	Nursing Considerations
Epidural Block *Labor:* Insertion of catheter provides pain relief for labor and vaginal birth (T10-S5 levels). *Cesarean birth:* If epidural was used during labor, level of block can be extended upward (T4-T6 level). Also used for cesarean birth that is not preceded by labor.	1. Prehydrate woman with 500-1000 mL warmed nonglucose crystalloid solution such as lactated Ringer's solution or normal saline solution. 2. Displace uterus manually or with a wedge placed under woman's side to enhance placental perfusion. 3. Assess for hypotension at least every 5 min for 15 min after block is begun and with each new dose until vital signs are stable. Report following to anesthesia provider: Systolic BP of <100 mm Hg or a fall of 20% or more from baseline levels, pallor, or diaphoresis. Facility procedures give further guidance. 4. Assess FHR for signs of impaired placental perfusion, and report the following to the anesthesia and obstetric providers: Tachycardia (>160 bpm for 10 min), bradycardia (<110 bpm for 10 min), late decelerations (see Ch 14). 5. If hypotension or signs of impaired placental perfusion occur, increase rate of infusion of nonadditive IV fluid, reposition woman to her side, and administer oxygen by face mask (8-10 L/min). Have phenylephrine or ephedrine available (usually included in epidural tray). 6. Observe for a full bladder, and catheterize if the woman is unable to void. 7. Leg movement and strength vary after an epidural block. Transfer with help to avoid muscle strains to the nurse or the woman. 8. Have the woman ambulate only if adequate sensation and movement are present and with another person's assistance with first ambulation.

Subarachnoid Block
 	
Cesarean birth: Can be established slightly faster than epidural block.
Rarely used for complicated vaginal birth.
Does not provide pain relief for labor because it is done just before birth.
May be combined with an epidural block in a CSE. (See "Intrathecal Opioid Analgesics" for more information.)
	1. See "Epidural Block" for these interventions:
	  • IV prehydration
	  • Uterine displacement
	  • Observation of BP and FHR
	  • Care for hypotension or signs of impaired placental perfusion
	  • Observation and intervention for bladder distention
	  • Transfer and ambulation precautions
	2. Observe for post–spinal puncture headache—a headache that is worse when the woman is upright and that may disappear when she is lying flat. Notify the anesthesia provider if it occurs (a blood patch may be done).
	3. Nursing interventions for post–spinal puncture headache: Encourage bed rest, increase oral fluids if not contraindicated, give oral caffeine, and give analgesics, as ordered.

General Anesthesia Cesarean birth if epidural or spinal block is not possible or if woman refuses regional anesthesia. May be required for emergency procedures.	1. Determine type and time of last food intake on admission. 2. Restrict oral intake to clear liquids or as ordered. Consult with the physician or nurse-midwife if surgical intervention is likely. 3. Report to anesthesia provider: Oral intake before and during labor, vomiting. 4. Displace uterus (see "Epidural Block"). 5. Give ordered drugs such as sodium citrate and citric acid (Bicitra). 6. Maintain cricoid pressure (Sellick's maneuver) during intubation. 7. Woman will remain intubated until protective (gag) reflexes have returned. Have oral airway and suction immediately available. 8. Oxygen by face tent or face mask should be given after extubation. 9. Interventions for postoperative respiratory depression: give positive-pressure oxygen by face mask; observe oxygen saturation with pulse oximetry until woman is awake and alert; have woman take several deep breaths if oxygen saturation falls below 95%. Notify the anesthesia provider.

CNS, Central nervous system; *CSE,* combined spinal-epidural; *FHR,* fetal heart rate; *IV,* intravenous; *PCA,* patient-controlled analgesia.

Most women should remain in bed or sit in a nearby chair after their epidural is begun because of reduced sensation.

Assess the degree of motor block and sensation hourly. If a distinct increase or change is noted, report it to the anesthesia clinician because this may indicate catheter migration or another complication.

A woman who has reduced mobility and sensation should be moved so that she maintains an anatomic position. Avoid prolonged pressure on one area. Remember that changing position often improves labor progress, even if the woman does not need to change positions for comfort. If surgery is needed, pad bony prominences to reduce pressure on those areas.

Before any ambulation, such as for urination after birth, test the woman's ability to raise and move her legs. Have her push her legs against your hands to determine her leg strength. When she ambulates, accompany her and monitor her ability to move and her strength the entire time the epidural is in effect. The woman should sit before standing to evaluate for postural (orthostatic) hypotension, which may occur in any postpartum woman regardless of her pain management methods during labor.

◆ Evaluation

The nurse evaluates the reduction of potential for injury by comparing the woman's baseline blood pressure and FHR to those after the block is begun to identify any significant changes. The goal or expected outcome related to injury is achieved if the woman does not have an injury related to her altered sensation and mobility while the epidural block is exerting its effects.

◆ APPLICATION OF THE NURSING PROCESS: RESPIRATORY COMPROMISE

◆ Assessment

General anesthesia may be needed any time during birth, most often for cesarean birth. Document the type (solids or liquids) and time of the woman's last oral intake. Question her closely if she reports an unusually long interval since her last intake. Anesthesia providers can anticipate and prevent problems better if they know the actual oral intake, although most assume that every woman has food in her stomach and induce general anesthesia accordingly.

◆ Identification of Patient Problems

Analysis of the data collected enables the nurse to identify actual and potential patient problems and develop an individualized plan of care. The woman is at risk for respiratory compromise as a result of aspiration.

◆ Planning: Expected Outcomes

The expected outcome is that the woman will not experience respiratory compromise from aspiration of gastric contents during the perioperative period.

◆ Interventions

Nursing interventions relate to identifying factors that increase a woman's risk for aspiration as well as collaborative and nursing measures to reduce the risk for aspiration or lung injury.

Identifying Risk Factors

Report oral intake both before and after admission to the anesthesia provider. Oral intake during labor may be restricted to medications, clear liquids such as water and ice, clear fruit juices, carbonated drinks, clear tea and coffee, sports drinks, Popsicles, or hard sugar-free candies (ACOG, 2015).

Vomiting is a common occurrence during normal labor, regardless of the mother's oral intake. If vomiting occurs, chart the time, quantity, and character (amount, color, presence of undigested food).

Reducing Risk for Aspiration or Lung Injury

Nurses collaborate with medical personnel to reduce a woman's risk for pulmonary complications.

Perioperative Care

Restrict oral intake, as ordered, if surgery is expected. Give ordered medications such as sodium citrate and citric acid (Bicitra). Depending on when the medications are needed, either the nurse or the anesthesia provider may administer parenteral drugs such as glycopyrrolate (Robinul).

An experienced nurse or a trained anesthesia assistant provides cricoid pressure (Sellick's maneuver) to block the esophagus until the woman is intubated and the cuff of the endotracheal tube is inflated. Successful intubation with the cuffed endotracheal tube blocks passage of any gastric contents into the trachea. However, the value of cricoid pressure has not been thoroughly researched (ASA, 2016; Tsen, 2014).

Postoperative Care

Birth facility protocols guide postoperative care, including preextubation and postextubation care for the woman who has had general anesthesia. The woman is extubated when her protective laryngeal reflexes have returned, often before transfer from the operating table. Suction equipment and an Ambu bag with appropriate-size mask should be immediately available not only in the operating room and postanesthesia care unit but also in standard patient care rooms on the nursing unit. Administer oxygen by mask or face tent for 2 to 5 minutes until the woman is awake and alert because the agents used for general anesthesia are respiratory depressants. Monitor oxygen saturation with a pulse oximeter. If her oxygen saturation falls below 95%, have her take several deep breaths. Deep breathing also helps her eliminate inhalational anesthetics and reduces stasis of pulmonary secretions.

Assess the woman's pulse rate, respiration, and blood pressure every 15 minutes for 1 hour or until stable; then continue per policy. In addition to using pulse oximetry, observe her color for pallor or cyanosis, which, respectively, suggest shock or hypoventilation (ASA, 2016).

◆ Evaluation

Interventions for this patient problem are preventive and short term because it is a temporary high-risk situation. The goal is met if the woman does not aspirate gastric contents during the perioperative period.

SUMMARY CONCEPTS

- Childbirth pain is unique because it is normal and self-limiting, the woman has time to prepare for the pain, and the pain ends with a baby's birth.
- Excess or poorly relieved pain may be harmful to the mother and fetus.
- Pain is a complex physical and psychological experience. It is subjective and personal.
- Four sources of pain are present in most labors, but other physical and psychological factors may increase or decrease the pain felt from these sources. These sources are cervical dilation, uterine ischemia, pressure and pulling on pelvic structures, and distention of the vagina and perineum.
- Relaxation enhances all other pain management techniques.
- Several nonpharmacologic pain management techniques supplement relaxation—cutaneous stimulation, hydrotherapy, mental stimulation, and breathing techniques.
- Physiologic alterations of pregnancy may affect a woman's response to medications.
- Any drug the expectant mother takes, whether therapeutic or abused, including herbal or botanical preparations, also may affect the fetus. Fetal effects may be direct or indirect, and their durations of action may be different from those in an adult.
- The nurse should observe for respiratory depression, primarily in the newborn, if the mother has received opioid analgesics during labor.
- The major advantages of regional pain management methods are that the woman can participate in the birth and that she retains her protective airway reflexes.
- The nurse should monitor and take actions to prevent maternal hypotension that may result from an epidural or subarachnoid block.
- If the woman receives a regional pain management technique that carries the risk for maternal hypotension, the nurse should observe for fetal heart rate changes associated with impaired placental perfusion.
- The primary adverse effects that should be monitored in the woman who receives epidural or intrathecal opioids are nausea and vomiting, pruritus, and delayed respiratory depression.
- Regurgitation with aspiration of acidic gastric contents is the greatest risk for a woman who receives general anesthesia.

REFERENCES & READINGS

American Academy of Pediatrics & American College of Obstetricians and Gynecologists (AAP & ACOG). (2012). *Guidelines for perinatal care* (7th ed.). Elk Grove Village, IL: Author.

American Academy of Pediatrics & American College of Obstetricians and Gynecologists (AAP & ACOG). (2014). Clinical report: Immersion in water during labor and delivery. *Pediatrics, 133*(4), 758–761.

American College of Obstetricians and Gynecologists (ACOG). (2015). *Obstetric analgesia and anesthesia (ACOG Practice Bulletin No. 36, July 2002, reaffirmed 2015).* Washington, DC: Author.

American Society of Anesthesiologists (ASA). (2016). Practice guidelines for obstetric anesthesia: An updated report by the American Society of Anesthesiologists Task Force on Obstetric Anesthesia and the Society for Obstetric Anesthesia and Perinatology. *Anesthesiology, 124*(2), 270–300.

Association of Women's Health, Obstetric and Neonatal Nurses (AWHONN). (2011). *Nursing care and management of the second stage of labor: Evidence-based clinical practice guidelines* (2nd ed.). Washington, DC: Author.

Association of Women's Health, Obstetric and Neonatal Nurses (AWHONN). (2013). *Basic, high-risk and critical-care intrapartum nursing: Clinical competencies and education guide* (5th ed.). Washington, DC: Author.

Association of Women's Health, Obstetric and Neonatal Nurses (AWHONN). (2014). *Second stage of labor: Mother-initiated, spontaneous pushing. In Women's health and perinatal nursing care quality refined draft measures specifications.* Washington, DC: Author.

Blackburn, S. T. (2013). *Maternal, fetal, & neonatal physiology: A clinical perspective* (4th ed.). St. Louis, MO: Saunders.

Chestnut, D. (2014). Alternative regional analgesic techniques for labor and vaginal delivery. In D. Chestnut, C. A. Wong, L. C. Tsen, D. N. K. Warwick, Y. Beilin, J. M. Mhyre, & V. Naveen (Eds.), *(2014) Chestnut's obstetric anesthesia: Principles and practice* (5th ed.). Philadelphia, PA: Saunders.

Creedon, D., Akkerman, D., Atwood, L., Bates, L., Harper, C., Levin, A., & Wingeier, R. (2013). *Management of labor. Institute for Clinical Systems Improvement (ICSI).* Bloomington, MN: Saunders.

Cunningham, F. G., Leveno, K. J., Bloom, S. L., Spong, C. Y., Dashe, J. S., Hoffman, B. L., Casey, B. M., & Sheffield, J. S. (2014). *Williams obstetrics* (24th ed.). New York: McGraw-Hill Medical.

Davies, R., Davis, D., Peace, M., & Wong, N. (2014). The effect of waterbirth on neonatal mortality and morbidity: A systematic review protocol. *Joanna Briggs Institute of Systematic Reviews and Implementation Reports, 12*(7), 1–8.

Douma, M. R., Stienstra, R., Middeldorp, J. M., Arbous, M. S., & Dahan, A. (2015). Differences in maternal temperature during labour with remifentanil patient controlled analgesia or epidural anesthesia: A randomized controlled trial. *International Journal of Obstetric Anesthesia, 24*(4), 313–322. http://dx.doi.org/10.1016/j.ijoa.2015.06.003.

Dozier, A., Howard, C., Brownell, E., Wissler, R., Glantz, J., Ternullo, S., & Lawrence, R. (2013). Labor epidural anesthesia, obstetric factors and breastfeeding cessation. *Maternal & Child Health Journal, 17*(4), 689–698. http://dx.doi.org/10.1007/s10995-012-1045-4.

El-Wahab, N., & Fernando, R. (2014). Systemic analgesia: Parenteral and inhalation agents. In D. Chestnut, C. A. Wong, L. C. Tsen, D. N. K. Warwick, Y. Beilin, J. M. Mhyre, & V. Naveen (Eds.), *Chestnut's obstetric anesthesia: Principles and practice* (5th ed.). Philadelphia, PA: Saunders.

Hawkins, J. L., & Bucklin, B. A. (2017). Obstetric anesthesia. In S. G. Gabbe, J. R. Niebyl, J. L. Simpson, M. B. Landon, H. L. Galan, R. M. Jauniaux, D. A. Driscoll, et al. (Eds.), *Obstetrics: Normal and problem pregnancies* (7th ed.) (pp. 344–367). Philadelphia, PA: Saunders.

Huether, S. E., Rodway, G., & DeFriez, C. (2014). Pain, temperature regulation, sleep and sensory function. In K. L. McCance, S. E. Huether, V. L. Brashers, & N. S. Rose (Eds.), *Pathophysiology: The biologic basis for disease in adults and children* (7th ed.). St. Louis, MO: Mosby.

Joint Commission Online November 12, 2014. (2014). *Revisions to pain management standards effective January, 2015*. Retrieved from www.jointcommission.org/assets/1/23/jconline_November_12_14.pdf.

Jones, L. E., Whitburn, L. Y., Davey, M., & Small, R. (2015). Assessment of pain associated with childbirth: Women's perspectives, preferences and solutions. *Midwifery*, 31(7), 708–712. http://dx.doi.org/10.1016/j.midw.2015.03.012.

Stewart, L. S., & Collins, M. (2013). Nitrous oxide as labor analgesia. *Nursing for Women's Health*, 16(5), 398–409. http://dx.doi.org/10.1111/j.1751-486X.2012.01763.x.

Sullivan, D. H., & McGuiness, C. (2015). Natural labor pain management. *International Journal of Childbirth Education*, 30(2), 20–25.

Tsen, L. C. (2014). Anesthesia for cesarean delivery. In D. Chestnut, C. A. Wong, L. C. Tsen, D. N. K. Warwick, Y. Beilin, J. M. Mhyre, & V. Naveen (Eds.), *Chestnut's obstetric anesthesia: Principles and practice* (5th ed.). Philadelphia, PA: Saunders.

Wong, C. A. (2014). Epidural and spinal analgesia/anesthesia for labor and vaginal delivery. In D. Chestnut, C. A. Wong, L. C. Tsen, D. N. K. Warwick, Y. Beilin, J. M. Mhyre, & V. Naveen (Eds.), *Chestnut's obstetric anesthesia: Principles and practice* (5th ed.). Philadelphia, PA: Saunders.

Intrapartum Fetal Surveillance

Becky Cypher

OBJECTIVES

After studying this chapter, you should be able to:

1. Identify key physiologic principles underlying fetal heart rate (FHR) and uterine activity (UA) assessment in the intrapartum period.
2. Discuss advantages and limitations of each method of intrapartum fetal surveillance: auscultation/palpation and electronic fetal monitoring (EFM).
3. Explain instrumentation types used for auscultation/palpation and EFM.
4. Review principles of FHR and UA interpretation using a standardized approach.
5. Identify specific components of the three FHR categories.
6. Describe clinical interventions performed for normal, indeterminate, and abnormal FHR patterns.
7. Use the nursing process to plan care for a woman undergoing intrapartum fetal assessment.

The primary goal of intrapartum fetal surveillance is to enable clinicians to assess adequacy of fetal oxygenation during labor. Over several decades, the principle method of intrapartum monitoring of fetal well-being and uterine activity (UA) has transitioned primarily from "low-technology," auscultation and palpation, to "high-technology," electronic fetal monitoring (EFM). Approximately 89% of births in the United States are monitored electronically, whereas exclusive use of auscultation and palpation in the intrapartum setting is limited (Chen, Chauhan, Ananth, Vintzileos, & Abuhamad, 2011).

The low-technology method of fetal surveillance requires a clinician to count the fetal heart rate (FHR) with a fetoscope or Doppler in relationship to UA. Counting and palpation occur at specified intervals for a predetermined amount of time depending on the stage of labor and patient risk status. Palpation of the uterus by the clinician provides UA information such as frequency, duration, intensity, and resting tone. Unlike auscultation and palpation, EFM incorporates a complex electronic device that acquires, processes, and displays the FHR and UA with visual and computer interpretation (Ayers-de-Campos & Noguiera-Reis, 2015). This device may provide additional information compared with intermittent auscultation (IA) in identifying fetuses at risk for hypoxic injury that may result in permanent neurologic injury or death (Amer-Wahlin & Kwee, 2016; Miller, 2016).

Each method of fetal surveillance has advantages and limitations. Both approaches can be interchanged depending on pregnancy risk factors, current clinical situation, patient's preference, nurse-to-patient ratio, and institutional policy. When necessary, timely and appropriate corrective measures can be taken to improve fetal oxygenation and avoid unnecessary interventions. Regardless of which method is used for surveillance, information gathered at the bedside during the intrapartum period can assist clinicians with the following:

1. Evaluating fetal oxygenation based on bedside assessments and accurate interpretation of data.
2. Deciding when implementation of physiologically based corrective measures to improve fetal oxygenation is necessary.
3. Providing a continuing mechanism to optimize communication between clinicians and patients.
4. Supporting clinical decision making, which promotes an environment that improves patient safety and health care quality.

FETAL OXYGENATION

The placenta, which contains both maternal and fetal tissue, functions as an extracorporeal fetal support system. In other words, the placenta is responsible for gas, nutrient, and substance exchange for fetal growth, development, and oxygenation. The placenta also plays a vital role in metabolism, endocrine secretion, immunologic safeguards, and protection of the fetus against certain substances in maternal circulation that may be harmful, such as some viruses and medications (Blackburn, 2013; Freeman, Garite, Nageotte, & Miller, 2012; Nageotte, 2015).

An understanding of the dynamics of uteroplacental exchange and maternal-fetal circulation is essential to understanding how fetuses respond to labor stressors such as uterine contractions. As mentioned in Chapter 9, oxygen is carried from the environment to the fetus by a maternal and fetal circulation pathway that includes maternal lungs, heart, vasculature, uterus, placenta, and umbilical cord. Adequate fetal oxygenation requires the following:

1. Sufficient maternal blood flow and volume to the placenta.
2. Normal maternal oxygen saturation.
3. Adequate placental exchange of oxygen and carbon dioxide.
4. An open circulatory path from placenta to fetus through umbilical cord vessels.
5. Normal fetal circulatory and oxygen-carrying functions.

Interruption of the oxygen pathway at one or more points can cause physiologic changes resulting in characteristic FHR changes that may be interpreted on the tracing (Miller, Miller, & Cypher, 2016).

Uteroplacental Circulation

Maternal blood flow to the uterus and placenta originates primarily in the uterine, internal iliac and ovarian arteries. Approximately 85% of uterine blood flow supplies volume for uteroplacental circulation, and the remaining percentage circulates blood to uterine musculature (Freeman et al., 2013). Maternal arterial blood pressure maintains flow of oxygen- and nutrient-rich blood to the uterus, placenta, and finally to the intervillous spaces of the placenta via spiral arteries. In the nonpregnant state, spiral arteries are small vessels supplying blood to the uterine endometrium. In the first few weeks of pregnancy, spiral arteries are remodeled to meet the growing demands of the developing fetus (Freeman et al., 2013; Pijnenborg, Vercruysse, & Hanssens, 2006).

The fetal chorionic villi, which are protrusions of fetal tissue, are located in the intervillous spaces of the placenta where the microscopic branches of the chorionic villi are immersed in maternal blood from the remodeled spiral arteries. The intervillous space allows for exchange of substances, such as oxygen, without mixing of maternal and fetal blood (Fig. 14.1). Simultaneously, maternal blood carrying away carbon dioxide and fetal waste products drains from the intervillous spaces through endometrial veins and returns to maternal circulation for elimination (Blackburn, 2013; Nageotte, 2015; O'Brien-Abel, 2015).

Spiral arterial blood flow can be altered by maternal cardiac output and impact the blood flow to the placenta and fetus. For example, when the uterus contracts, elevated myometrial pressure at the peak of a contraction can exceed intraarterial pressure within the spiral arteries. This causes a temporary cessation of maternal blood flow to the intervillous space. If this interruption is prolonged, acute or chronic episodes of hypoxia can occur. Dramatic changes in maternal blood pressure can affect blood flow in the intervillous space. The fetus responds to these interruptions by redistributing blood flow to the vital organs (heart, brain, and adrenal glands) and decreasing blood flow to the nonvital organs (lungs, kidneys, liver, gastrointestinal tract, and periphery). Persistent redistribution of blood flow may cause a loss of fetal cerebral autoregulation resulting in decreased fetal cardiac output. If this physiologic process continues, a reduction of cerebral blood flow could potentially result in fetal neurologic injury or death (Blackburn, 2013; Nageotte, 2015).

Fetal Placental Circulation

The umbilical cord connects the placenta to the fetus. Within the umbilical cord are three vessels, two arteries, and one vein, which are protected by Wharton's jelly. Oxygenated blood is carried to the fetal heart from the placenta via placental veins that form a single umbilical vein. The fetal heart then circulates oxygenated blood throughout the fetal body. After the blood has circulated, two umbilical arteries return to the placenta then separate into smaller vessels at the umbilical cord insertion site on the placenta. (See Fig. 5.7). An arteriovenous system is created within the chorionic villi allowing for deoxygenated blood from the fetus to be returned (Blackburn, 2013).

> ### ❓ KNOWLEDGE CHECK
>
> 1. What high technology method is primarily used in the United States to assess FHR and UA?
> 2. Describe maternal blood flow to the uterus and placenta.
> 3. Which umbilical cord vessel(s) carry(ies) deoxygenated blood back from the fetus to the placenta?

Fetal Heart Rate Regulation

In the fetal medulla oblongata, a cardioregulatory center acts as the source of FHR regulation via the following:

1. Intrinsic cardiac pacemakers (sinoatrial node, atrioventricular node)
2. Cardiac conduction pathways
3. Sympathetic and parasympathetic branches of the autonomic nervous system
4. Intrinsic factors such as baroreceptors and chemoreceptors
5. Extrinsic factors such as maternal medications or placental abruption
6. Hormonal influences
7. Miscellaneous factors (calcium, potassium)

Changes in fetal oxygen and carbon dioxide (chemoreceptors) or blood pressure (baroreceptors) affect the cardioregulatory center controlling the FHR baseline, variability, accelerations, and decelerations. For example, if the cardioregulatory center detects hypoxia, it signals the heart to alter the cardiac output and redistribute blood flow primarily to the vital organs, such as the brain, heart, and adrenal glands. Thus, the fetal heart rate patterns represent the final product of intrinsic and extrinsic factors (Miller, 2016; O'Brien-Abel, 2015).

Autonomic Nervous System

The autonomic nervous system (ANS) is a neural network that assists with maintaining physiologic stability in such areas as the cardiovascular system when challenged by circumstances that can interrupt normal function. This is also referred to as homeostasis. The ANS is divided into the parasympathetic and sympathetic branches and are the balanced forces regulating the FHR.

The parasympathetic branch is an important mechanism in controlling the heart. Parasympathetic impulses originate in the fetal brainstem and are distributed to the vagus nerve and heart. When the vagus nerve is stimulated, the parasympathetic branch decreases the baseline rate over time. Sympathetic impulses originate in the fetal myocardium and increase the FHR baseline. The sympathetic system also can stimulate the release of catecholamines in response to interruptions in oxygenation and blood pressure changes. This results in an increased FHR and possible peripheral vasoconstriction in the fetus (Blackburn, 2013; Miller & Ruth, 2017).

Fetal heart rate variability is a component of the baseline and reflects changes in variance over time between consecutive heart beats. It is a direct result from the sympathetic and parasympathetic effects on the heart, similar to a push and pull method. This FHR characteristic originates in the brainstem and is conducted to the fetal heart by the vagus nerve. Variability is considered the most critical predictor of adequate fetal oxygenation during labor for the following two reasons (Clark et al., 2013):

1. Adequate oxygenation promotes normal function of the ANS and helps the fetus maintain homeostasis during labor.
2. Variability evaluates the function of the fetal ANS.

Baroreceptors and Chemoreceptors

Located in the carotid arch and aortic sinus, baroreceptors are pressure-sensitive stretch receptors that respond to blood pressure changes. Baroreceptors perceive blood pressure alterations and send a signal to the brainstem. This results

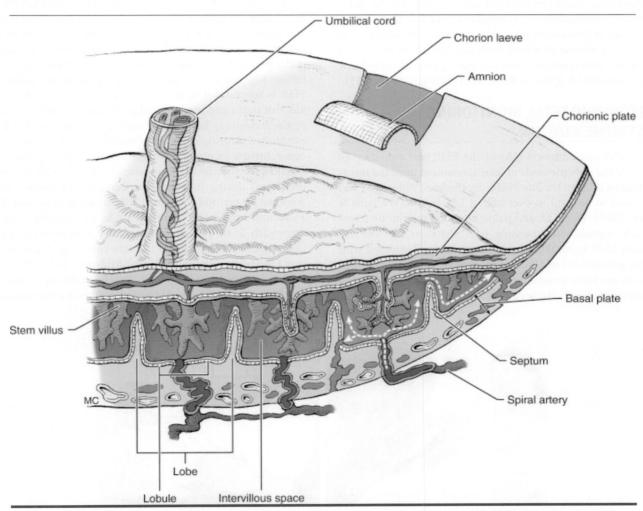

FIG. 14.1 Transverse Section of Placental Structure That Assists with Uteroplacental Circulation. (From Miller, D. A. (2016). Intrapartum fetal evaluation. In S. G. Gabbe, J. R. Niebyl, J. L. Simpson, et al. (Eds), *Obstetrics: Normal and problem pregnancies* (7th ed., pp. 308-343). Philadelphia, PA: Elsevier.)

in either slowing of the FHR to decrease blood pressure or increases the FHR to resolve hypotension in the fetus. Chemoreceptors are located in the medulla oblongata as well as the aortic and carotid bodies. They are less understood but are thought to be sensory nerve endings that are stimulated by alterations in oxygen, carbon dioxide, and fetal blood pH. Chemoreceptors respond to blood pH and oxygen decreases or increases in carbon dioxide by eliciting a sympathetic response. This response increases FHR to improve oxygenation or decrease carbon dioxide (Blackburn, 2013; Miller & Ruth, 2017; O'Brien-Abel, 2015).

Hormonal Influences

Hormones are circulated into the bloodstream by organs such as the adrenal glands, hypothalamus, and pituitary gland. Stressors such as too many contractions trigger the fetus to release hormones that will assist with FHR regulation, maximizing perfusion to the vital organs. The adrenal medulla secretes catecholamines (epinephrine and norepinephrine). Epinephrine and norepinephrine increase myocardial contraction force, accelerate the FHR, and improve arterial blood pressure, comparable to sympathetic branch stimulation. Decreases in fetal blood pressure cause the adrenal cortex to respond by release of aldosterone and retention of sodium and water, which will increase circulating fetal blood volume (Blackburn, 2013; Miller & Ruth, 2017; O'Brien-Abel, 2015).

ELECTRONIC FETAL MONITORING INSTRUMENTATION

Intermittent auscultation (IA) of the FHR and palpation of UA were the only methods of fetal assessment until the introduction of EFM in the late 1960s. By the late 1970s, EFM was estimated to be used in over half of U.S. births (Williams & Hawe, 1979). While IA and palpation continued to be a reasonable approach to assessing fetal status in the low-risk patient, EFM technology gained popularity. Compared with earlier generations of fetal monitoring systems, today's EFM systems are more innovative than previous systems, allowing for more efficient bedside care.

Intermittent Auscultation and Palpation

IA in conjunction with palpation has been found to be an effective method of surveillance if performed in a consistent manner in accordance with professional guidelines. This method of assessing FHR and rhythm is done with a fetoscope, Pinard stethoscope, or hand-held Doppler ultrasound (Fig. 14.2). Unlike Doppler ultrasound, which translates fetal heart motion into a signal, a fetoscope or Pinard stethoscope allows the listener to hear actual fetal heart sounds, which include opening and closing of fetal heart valves. In most facilities, the Doppler is selected to auscultate the FHR intermittently.

There is a lack of evidence of which method of IA and intervals of counting are best for laboring women. One example of determining FHR baseline describes clinicians listening and counting for a set period, usually 15 to 60 seconds. Longer periods of counting may be required depending on the clinical situation. For example, if the FHR is within normal limits but has changed significantly from the previous assessment, a longer listening period or more frequent assessments may clarify whether the rate is a change in baseline or a temporary increase or decrease. Counting is done between contractions and when the fetus is not actively moving. Clinicians should palpate a maternal radial pulse simultaneously to distinguish between maternal heart rate and FHR during auscultation. Rhythm should be noted as regular or irregular. The FHR is auscultated at selected intervals based on the woman's risk status and institutional guidelines. Audible increases or decreases may be detected once a baseline rate has been established. During episodes of audible changes, counting in consecutive 6-second intervals and multiplying the rate by 10 should give the clinician an estimate in the beats per minute (bpm) during increases or decreases (Procedure 14.1). Another IA method includes FHR counting in several 5- to 15-second increments. An increase in the number obtained from each 5- or 15-second count can indicate an acceleration, whereas a decrease in the rate can suggest a deceleration (American College of Nurse-Midwives [ACNM], 2015; Feinstein, Sprague, & Trépanier, 2008). An abrupt decrease in rate from the baseline should be followed with other measures

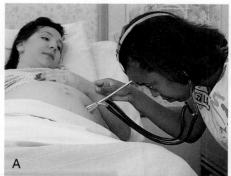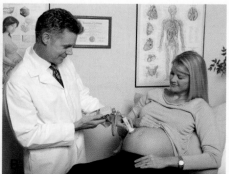

FIG. 14.2 Low-Intervention Methods for Evaluating the FHR during Labor. A, Fetoscope, showing the head attachment that allows for bone conduction to auscultate the opening and closing fetal heart valves to determine fetal heart rate (FHR). **B,** Example of a hand-held Doppler ultrasound being used to detect FHR via sound waves.

NURSING PROCEDURE 14.1 Auscultating the Fetal Heart Rate

Explain the procedure to the woman and support person. Wash your hands with warm water to reduce the transmission of microorganisms and to make your hands more comfortable for the woman when touching her abdomen.

1. Use Leopold's maneuvers to identify the fetal back (see Procedure 15.1).
2. Assess FHR with a fetoscope or Doppler transducer.
3. Fetoscope—Place the bell of the fetoscope over the fetal back with the head plate pressed against your forehead to add bone conduction to the sound coming through the ear-pieces. Move the fetoscope until you locate where the FHR is loudest. Use your forehead to maintain pressure during auscultation.
4. Doppler transducer—Review the manufacturer's instructions for operating the Doppler device. Place water-soluble conducting gel over transducer to allow for clear signal transmission. Place the transducer over the fetal back, and move until audible clear sounds are located.
5. Palpate the woman's radial pulse to verify the maternal heart rate is different from the FHR. If the pulse is synchronized with the sounds from the fetoscope or Doppler transducer, move the instrument to another location. Other sounds that may be represented by the Doppler are the funic souffle (blood flowing through the umbilical cord) or uterine souffle (blood flowing through the uterine vessels). The funic souffle is synchronized with the fetal heart and has the same rate; the uterine souffle is synchronized with the mother's pulse.
6. Auscultating the FHR. Count the baseline FHR for 15 to 60 seconds between contractions. Audible increases or decreases may be detected once a baseline rate has been established. During episodes of audible changes, counting in consecutive 6-second intervals and multiplying the beats by 10 gives clinicians an estimate in beats per minute during increases or decreases. Counting at 6-second intervals and multiplying each result by 10 give a sequence of numbers that can be averaged. This method also provides a better picture of the depth and duration of a decrease in FHR while counting.

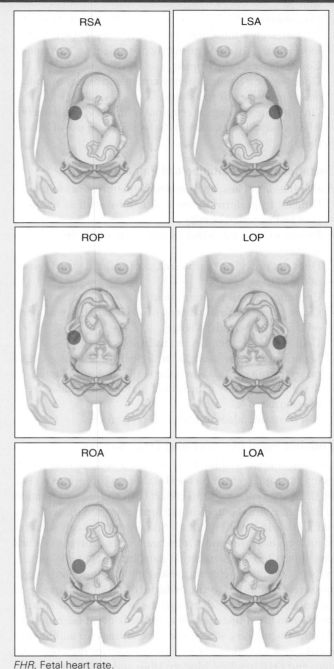

FHR, Fetal heart rate.

to clarify the fetal condition, such as continued assessment or placement of an EFM device.

Palpation is a subjective method of assessing UA. The uterus is a muscle, and as the uterus contracts the muscle gradually becomes firm. After the contraction is over the muscle relaxes and becomes soft. Palpation with the fingertips allows for assessment of UA frequency, duration, intensity, resting tone, and relaxation time. Because palpation is subjective, descriptive terms such as mild, moderate, and strong or firm are used for UA. If a uterine contraction is easily indented it

is described as mild. Some clinicians suggest that a mild contraction feels similar to the tip of the nose. Slight indention of the uterus is described as a moderate contraction, which feels equivalent to the chin. Strong contractions result in a uterus that cannot be indented and palpates similar to the forehead.

Benefits of Auscultation and Palpation

The benefits of auscultation and palpation are as follows:
- Widely available and easy to use with proper training
- Less invasive than EFM

- Outcomes comparable to those with EFM in low-risk women
- Inexpensive
- Promotes an atmosphere for the laboring patient that is more natural than one primarily dependent on technology
- Comfortable for the woman
- Offers women freedom of movement and ability to ambulate to promote normal labor
- One-on-one nursing care promotes "doula effect" benefits
- Allows easy FHR and UA assessment during use of hydrotherapy

Limitations of Auscultation and Palpation

The limitations of auscultation and palpation are as follows:

- Difficult to perform in some situations, such as hydramnios and maternal obesity
- Patient may be intolerant of clinician's touch during contraction
- Does not provide a permanent, documented visual record of the FHR or UA
- Counting of FHR is intermittent
- Cannot assess visual patterns of FHR variability or periodic and nonperiodic changes
- Unable to determine UA intensity objectively
- Significant events such as prolonged decelerations may occur during periods when the FHR is not auscultated
- May not allow early detection of FHR changes reflective of hypoxemia
- Not recommended for high-risk pregnancies

Bedside Fetal Monitor and Transducers

Instrumentation used for EFM include a bedside fetal monitoring unit and transducers with cables to capture data (Fig. 14.3). Fetal monitoring units collect FHR and UA information to provide a visual output in the form of a numerical display and a graphic strip (Fig. 14.4). Some monitors can simultaneously record twin and triplet heart rates. Current systems have inputs to collect maternal data, including temperature, oxygen saturation, electrocardiographic status, and blood pressure. In addition to the bedside, display units may be at the nursing station or other locations to allow remote surveillance when the clinician is not at the bedside. These units display the tracing on a screen and have settings for audible and visual alerts such as upper and lower limits for maternal vital signs and FHR baseline. Modern labor and delivery units may have wireless monitoring systems that transmit data to a base station for interpretation. Wireless systems allow patients the opportunity to ambulate in labor and can be used in water. External FHR is obtained by Doppler (also known as ultrasound), and UA is acquired by a tocodynamometer ("toco"). External monitoring, also called *indirect* or *noninvasive monitoring*, can be used at any time because cervical dilation and ruptured membranes are not necessary for placement. Both devices are held in place with either an elastic belt or adhesive patch that attaches to the transducer. Recording FHR requires ultrasound conduction gel to be applied on the Doppler surface. This gel assists in transmission of high-frequency sound

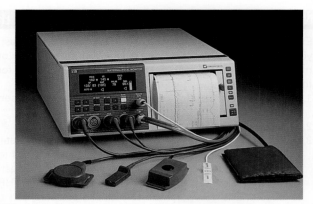

FIG. 14.3 Bedside Unit for Electronic Fetal Monitoring. In addition to fetal heart rate and uterine activity, the unit can evaluate a woman's blood pressure, pulse rate, and oxygen saturation. Twin and triplet gestations can be monitored depending on the device. (Courtesy Corometrics Medical Systems, Wallingford, CT.)

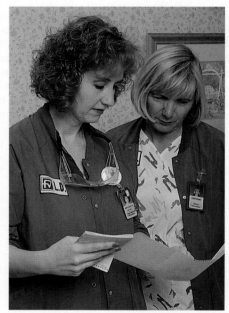

FIG. 14.4 Monitor tracings are often continuous permanent recordings with fetal heart rate (FHR) and uterine activity (UA), either paper or computer based. Regardless of whether the tracing is on paper or a computer screen, both methods allow clinicians to collaborate together to problem solve, make clinical decisions, and set priorities depending on FHR and UA interpretation as well as the stage of labor.

waves to the level of the fetal heart where heart motion is detected. Sound waves then bounce back to be recorded by the bedside unit. After confirming the location of the fetal back with Leopold's maneuver, the ultrasound transducer is placed where the point of maximum intensity of the FHR can be heard (Procedure 14.2). A toco is required to detect UA and is usually placed at the level of the fundus or where contraction intensity is palpable (Fig. 14.5). Tocos do not require ultrasound conduction gel because a pressure-sensitive button identifies changes in uterine shape occurring with contractions or maternal-fetal movement.

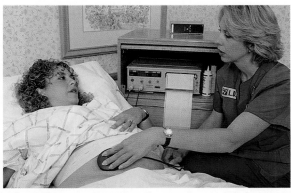

FIG. 14.5 The nurse applies the uterine activity transducer to the top of the woman's fundus. The Doppler transducer is placed where the fetal back is located, which is usually the point of maximum intensity.

NURSING PROCEDURE 14.2 External Fetal Monitor

1. Review institutional policy for EFM and how the device interfaces with computer documentation if necessary. Verify date and time for the equipment are consistent with computer documentation. Become familiar with proper operation of the monitoring equipment by reviewing the manufacturer's guidelines.

2. Perform a function test following manufacturer's instructions. Press the "TEST" button and observe the result. A correct function test ensures the bedside monitor is calibrated properly so accurate data can be interpreted. Each manufacturer sets standards for indicators of proper function.

3. Explain the basic EFM procedure to the woman and support system.

4. Transducer belts should be placed around the maternal abdomen before transducer placement. After Leopold's maneuver, apply ultrasound gel, which improves sound transmission between the Doppler ultrasound transducer and monitoring device. Place the transducer on the woman's abdomen along the fetal back. Move the transducer until a clear signal is heard. Most bedside units have a green light or flashing light to indicate an adequate signal.

5. Place the tocodynamometer in the uterine fundus or the area where contractions are palpated the strongest.

6. Apply transducer belts or adhesive ring to secure transducers in place. Be sure to keep the belts smooth under the patient's back because this will improve maternal comfort and improve transmission contact of external transducers. Adequate contact improves tracing quality and may reduce the number of adjustments needed.

7. Assess FHR and UA in accordance with institutional policies and professional guidelines.

EFM, Electronic fetal monitoring; *FHR,* fetal heart rate; *UA,* uterine activity.

Benefits of Ultrasound and Tocodynamometer Transducers

The benefits of ultrasound and tocodynamometer transducers are as follows:
- Noninvasive
- Easy to apply
- May be used during both the antepartum and intrapartum periods
- Sometimes used with telemetry when available
- Does not require ruptured membranes or cervical dilation
- No known risks to woman or fetus
- Provides continuous recording of the FHR and UA

Limitations of Ultrasound and Tocodynamometer Transducers

The limitations of ultrasound and tocodynamometer transducers are as follows:
- Limit maternal mobility
- Frequent repositioning of transducers often needed to maintain readable accurate tracing
- May double-count a slow FHR of less than 60 bpm, resulting in an apparently normal FHR during a bradycardia or may half-count a FHR greater than 180 bpm, resulting in an apparently normal FHR during tachycardia
- Maternal heart rate may be recorded if ultrasound transducer is placed over maternal arterial vessels, such as the aorta
- Tocotransducer provides information limited to frequency, duration, and relaxation time of uterine contractions but cannot accurately assess strength or intensity of uterine contractions
- Obese women and preterm or multifetal gestations may be difficult to monitor

Internal fetal monitoring requires a fetal spiral electrode (FSE) to record FHR and an intrauterine pressure catheter (IUPC) to document UA. Internal monitoring is referred to as direct or invasive fetal monitoring because this method requires cervical dilatation (usually 2 cm) and ruptured membranes. Electrodes are applied directly to the fetal presenting part (head or buttocks) and never placed on the fetal genitalia, face, or fontanels. Each electrode measures, processes, and records the R-to-R interval in a QRS complex to record the FHR. The opposite end of the electrode is attached to a pad and secured on a woman's thigh or lower abdomen. A cable is attached to the pad and plugged into the fetal monitor (Fig. 14.6). Electrodes should not be placed if there is an unidentifiable presenting part, placenta previa, hemophilia, maternal human immunodeficiency virus (HIV) infection, visible genital herpes lesions, or patient report of prodromal lesions symptoms. In cases of extreme prematurity or in the presence of a maternal infection such as hepatitis, group B hemolytic *Streptococcus* infection, syphilis, or gonorrhea, electrode placement may be acceptable if fetal benefit outweighs risk.

When a tracing warrants better assessment of frequency, duration, intensity, resting tone, and relaxation time, an IUPC may be inserted into the uterus transcervically. This sterile, flexible catheter measures actual intrauterine pressure (Fig. 14.7). Presently there are three IUPC types: fluid-filled, transducer-tipped, and air-coupled sensor tipped. Data are transmitted by an electrical signal that converts uterine pressure data into millimeters of mercury (mm Hg). This pressure is then displayed on the fetal monitor.

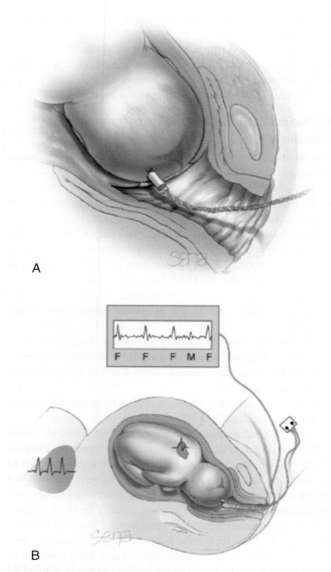

A

B

FIG. 14.6 Fetal Spiral Electrode. A, Diagram representation of a fetal spiral electrode to monitor fetal heart rate. **B,** Graphic representation of a bipolar electrode attached to the fetal scalp for detection of fetal QRS complexes. (From Intrapartum assessment (2014). In F. Cunningham, K. J. Leveno, S. L. Bloom, et al. (Eds), *William's obstetrics* (24th ed., pp. 473-503). New York, NY: McGraw-Hill.)

Benefits of Fetal Spiral Electrodes

The benefits of FSEs are as follows:
- Capable of accurately displaying some fetal cardiac arrhythmias when linked to electrocardiographic recorder
- Accurately displays an FHR between 30 and 240 bpm
- Maternal positional changes do not usually affect quality of FHR tracing

Benefits of Intrauterine Pressure Catheters

The benefits of IUPCs are as follows:
- Only truly accurate measure of all UA (e.g., frequency, duration, intensity, resting tone, and relaxation time)
- Allows for use of amnioinfusion

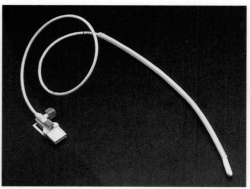

FIG. 14.7 Solid Intrauterine Pressure Catheter with Transducer in its Tip. This model also has a lumen for amnioinfusion and is shown with its introducer over the catheter. (Courtesy Utah Medical Products, Midvale, UT).

Limitations of Fetal Spiral Electrodes

The limitations of FSEs are as follows:
- Requires ruptured membranes
- Cervix must be dilated sufficiently to allow placement
- Improper insertion can cause maternal trauma such as vaginal lacerations
- Presenting part must be accessible and identifiable
- May record maternal heart rate in presence of fetal demise
- May not have adequate electrographic conduction when excessive fetal hair is present
- Possible increased risk for infection

Limitations of Intrauterine Pressure Catheters

The limitations of IUPCs are as follows:
- Requires ruptured membranes
- Cervix must be dilated sufficiently to allow placement
- Improper insertion can cause maternal or placental trauma such as uterine perforation or placental abruption
- Maternal positioning may change uterine hydrostatic pressure, resulting in inaccurate readings
- Different IUPC types may give higher pressure readings than other types
- Possible increased risk for infection

Fetal Monitoring Tracing

Fetal monitors capture FHR and UA data, which prints on a continuous paper tracing similar to an electrocardiogram strip. Some institutions prefer data be recorded on a computer tracing that is viewed at the bedside or a remote location instead of paper. Regardless of the mode, each tracing has an x-axis and y-axis with an upper and lower graph (Fig. 14.8). FHR information is traced on the upper graph, and UA is recorded on the lower graph. The x-axis on the upper and lower graph reveals thin, light, vertical lines that represent 10-second intervals. Every 60 seconds a thick, dark vertical line is printed representing 1-minute intervals. The y-axis also has thin, light horizontal lines with the upper graph recording FHR in intervals of 10 bpm ranging from 30 to 240 bpm. The y-axis on lower graph records uterine pressure in increments of 5 mm Hg ranging from 0 to 100 mm Hg (Miller, 2016).

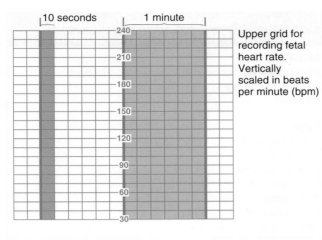

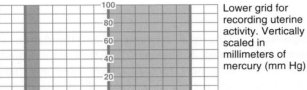

Upper grid for recording fetal heart rate. Vertically scaled in beats per minute (bpm)

Lower grid for recording uterine activity. Vertically scaled in millimeters of mercury (mm Hg)

FIG. 14.8 Recording Electronic Fetal Monitoring Data. Each *dark vertical line* represents 1 minute, and each *lighter vertical line* represents 10 seconds. Paperless computer displays that depict the fetal heart rate and uterine activity patterns have a similar appearance.

KNOWLEDGE CHECK

4. What are the advantages and limitations of each fetal monitoring method?
5. What three descriptive terms are used to characterize UA with palpation?
6. Which grid on the paper tracing or computer monitor is used to record FHR and UA data?
7. Which EFM sensor uses heart motion to measure FHR?
8. What are two factors that may affect tocodynamometry accuracy?

FETAL HEART RATE INTERPRETATION

Fetal monitoring was launched into daily clinical practice without a nationally agreed upon consensus statement regarding FHR patterns and definitions. Clinicians had broad variations in definitions, descriptions, and interpretations of FHR characteristics to communicate findings. For example, a clinician may have described tachysystole (increased uterine activity) as greater than five contractions in 10 minutes whereas another may have described tachysystole as five or more contractions in 10 minutes. The lack of standardization was a key obstacle in effective communication and had the potential to lead to adverse perinatal and neonatal outcomes.

The first consensus statement standardizing definitions was released by the National Institute of Child Health and Development (NICHD) but was slow to be integrated into intrapartum care (NICHD, 1998). In 2006, professional nursing

BOX 14.1 Potential Cause of Fetal Heart Rate Tachycardia

Maternal
Beta-sympathomimetic drugs (terbutaline, epinephrine)
Parasympatholytic drugs
Dehydration
Fever
Hyperthyroidism
Infection (chorioamnionitis, appendicitis)
Cocaine

Fetal
Acute blood loss
Fetal anemia
Heart failure
Hyperthyroidism
Hypoxia/hypoxemia
Increased metabolic rate
Infection and fetal sepsis
Tachyarrhythmias

and physician organizations endorsed the document. In 2008, a panel of experts reaffirmed the 1997 document and added UA definitions and categories of FHR tracings (Macones, Hankins, Spong, Hauth, Moore, 2008). During the intrapartum period, clinicians need to understand and acknowledge three fundamental concepts to using a systematic approach to fetal monitoring: (1) *standardized definitions,* or nomenclature that is used to define FHR and UA characteristics; (2) *interpretation,* or the physiologic significance of the FHR and UA characteristics; and (3) *management,* or the clinical response to FHR and UA characteristics (Miller, 2016).

Baseline Fetal Heart Rate

Baseline FHR is determined by approximating the mean FHR rounded in 5-bpm increments during a 10-minute period. In this 10-minute assessment, periodic and episodic changes (accelerations and decelerations) and periods of marked variability are excluded. During the 10-minute period of observation, there must be at least 2 minutes of identifiable baseline segments that do not need to be contiguous. If a 2-minute period is uninterpretable, the FHR baseline is considered indeterminate. The previous 10-minute period may need to be reviewed to establish a baseline (Macones et al., 2008). Baseline rates are classified as follows:

- Normal FHR baseline—110 to 160 bpm. Preterm fetuses often average a rate at the upper end of normal because the sympathetic branch of the ANS is more dominant. Fetuses at a gestational age that is considered term have a parasympathetic branch that is more dominant. These fetuses may have a baseline rate at the lower end of normal.
- Abnormal baseline FHR
  - *Tachycardia*—Greater than 160 bpm. Physiologically, increases in sympathetic or decreased parasympathetic tone cause tachycardia. Potential causes of FHR tachycardia are presented in Box 14.1.

BOX 14.2   Potential Causes of Fetal Heart Rate Bradycardia

Maternal
Sympatholytic medications (methyldopa)
Beta blockers (labetalol [Normodyne], propranolol)
Sjögren's antibodies
Hypoglycemia
Hypothermia
Viral infection (cytomegalovirus)

Fetal
Cardiac conduction abnormalities
Heart block
Fetal heart failure (hydrops)
Structural cardiac defects
Heterotaxia
Hypothyroidism
Interrupted fetal oxygenation pathway (umbilical cord prolapse)

BOX 14.3   Potential Causes for Absent and Minimal Fetal Heart Rate Variability

Maternal
Medications (narcotics, barbituarates, tranquilizers)
General anesthesia
Infection

Fetal
Fetal sleep cycle
Fetal anemia
Fetal tachycardia
Fetal cardiac arrhythmia
Prematurity
Preexisting neurologic injury
Fetal metabolic acidosis

• *Bradycardia*—Less than 110 bpm. Physiologically, increases in parasympathetic and decreases in sympathetic tone cause bradycardia. The potential causes of FHR bradycardia are presented in Box 14.2.

Baseline Fetal Heart Rate Variability

Baseline FHR variability is determined in a 10-minute window, excluding periodic and episodic changes. Variability is defined as fluctuations in the baseline FHR that are irregular in amplitude and frequency. These fluctuations are visually quantitated as the amplitude of the peak-to-trough in beats per minute. Variability is classified as follows (Fig. 14.9):
• Absent variability—Amplitude range visually undetectable.
• Minimal variability—Amplitude range visually detectable but 5 bpm or less.
• Moderate variability—Amplitude range 6 bpm to 25 bpm.
• Marked variability—Amplitude range 25 bpm or greater.
  Moderate variability reliably predicts the absence of fetal metabolic acidemia at the time it is observed. However, the opposite is not true. Minimal or absent variability does *not* confirm the presence of fetal metabolic acidemia or ongoing hypoxic injury (Macones et al., 2008) because there may be other pathologic and nonpathologic causes, such as fetal sleep (Box 14.3). Marked variability is considered a normal variant or an exaggerated ANS response to the early phase of interrupted fetal oxygenation (Miller, 2016).
  Sinusoidal patterns are excluded from the definition of variability because this pattern is characterized by FHR fluctuations that are regular in amplitude and frequency. This pattern appears as a visually apparent, smooth, sine wave–like undulating pattern in the FHR baseline with a cycle frequency of 3 to 5 per minute that persists for 20 minutes or more (Macones et al., 2008). The pattern may be intermittent or continuous. Accelerations and responses to UA, fetal movement, or stimulation are absent (Mondanlou & Freeman, 1982). True sinusoidal patterns are extremely rare and have been associated with severe fetal anemia as a result of conditions such as Rh alloimmunization, vasa previa, or twin-to-twin transfusion (Mondanlou & Murata, 2004). In the past, the term *pseudosinusoidal* has been used to describe a sinusoidal-appearing pattern after medication administration. This term is not defined in standardized EFM definitions. Common medications associated with this pattern include fentanyl, butorphanol, and meperidine. Sinusoidal patterns that are medication induced are short lived and followed by a FHR with normal characteristics. Clinicians must have the ability to differentiate between a true sinusoidal pattern and one that is related to medication administration. True sinusoidal patterns suggest a compromised fetus, so bedside evaluation is necessary to optimize perinatal outcome.

Periodic and Episodic Fetal Heart Rate Patterns

Periodic FHR patterns are those associated with uterine contractions. Periodic patterns are distinguished on the basis of waveform and are either "abrupt" or "gradual" in onset. Abrupt waveforms are quantified as those that have an onset to nadir (lowest point) of deceleration or peak of acceleration in less than 30 seconds. Gradual waveform takes more than 30 seconds. Episodic (non-periodic) patterns may have an abrupt or gradual onset but are *not* linked with UA.

Accelerations

Accelerations are defined as visually apparent abrupt increases in the FHR and may be periodic or nonperiodic. The peak of the acceleration must be at least 15 bpm above the baseline lasting at least 15 seconds or more from the onset to return (Fig. 14.10). The onset to peak occurs in less than 30 seconds. In gestations that are less than 32 weeks, the peak of the acceleration must be at least 10 bpm above the baseline lasting at least 10 seconds from onset to

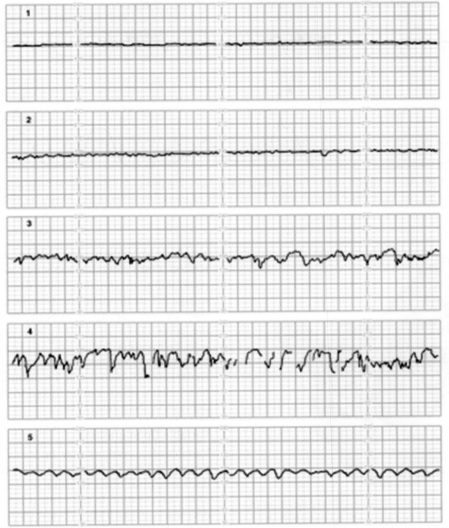

FIG. 14.9 Fetal Heart Rate (FHR) Variability. *1,* Absent variability: Undetectable *2,* Minimal variability: Greater than undetectable but 5 or fewer bpm. *3,* Moderate variability: 6 to 25 bpm. *4,* Marked variability: More than 25 bpm. *5,* Sinusoidal pattern with the classic smooth, sinelike pattern of regular fluctuation. Sinusoidal pattern is excluded from the definition of FHR variability (From Intrapartum assessment. (2014). In F. Cunningham, K. J. Leveno, S. L. Bloom, et al. (Eds), *William's obstetrics* (24th ed., pp 473-503). New York: McGraw-Hill.)

return. Prolonged accelerations have a duration between 2 and 10 minutes. Anything greater than 10 minutes is considered a FHR baseline change. Accelerations often occur with fetal movement but also may be elicited with vibro-acoustic stimulation, uterine contractions, or fetal scalp stimulation during a vaginal examination. Scalp stimulation is used to evaluate fetal response to gentle tactile stimulation through a dilated cervix when an indeterminate FHR tracing is observed (Fig. 14.11). Scalp stimulation should not be attempted during a deceleration. The goal is to elicit an FHR acceleration suggesting normal acid-base balance (Clark, Gimovsky, & Miller, 1984). Accelerations, whether spontaneous or evoked, are predictive of adequate oxygenation and a fetal pH that rules out acidemia (7.19 or greater) at

the time of observation (Parer, 1997; Porter & Clark, 1999; Williams & Galerneau, 2003).

Early Decelerations

Early decelerations are defined as periodic patterns that are visually apparent, are symmetric in shape, and have a gradual decrease and return of FHR baseline that mirrors a uterine contraction. This means the deceleration onset, nadir, and recovery coincides with the beginning, peak, and ending of a contraction (Macones et al., 2008) (Fig. 14.12). The onset of the deceleration to the nadir is equal to or greater than 30 seconds (ACOG, 2009). Early decelerations are thought to represent a vagal response during fetal head compression. This response alters intracranial blood flow

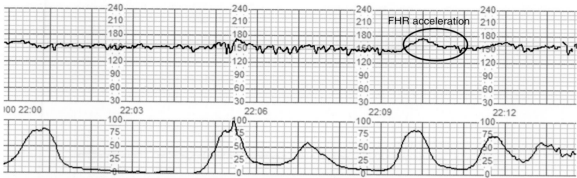

FIG. 14.10 Acceleration of the Fetal Heart Rate. Note the peak of the acceleration is at least 15 bpm above the baseline lasting at least 15 seconds or more from the onset to return. (Courtesy PeriGen, Princeton, NJ.)

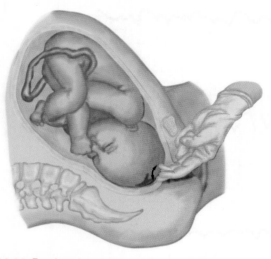

FIG. 14.11 Fetal scalp stimulation helps identify whether the fetus responds to gentle massage. An acceleration in the fetal heart rate peaking 15 beats per minute above the baseline suggests that the fetus is in normal oxygen and acid-base balance.

and leads to cardiac slowing. Early decelerations are benign and not associated with an interruption of fetal oxygenation resulting in fetal hypoxia, acidosis, or low Apgar scores (Nageotte, 2016).

Late Decelerations

Late decelerations are also considered a periodic pattern. They are visually apparent and usually symmetric in shape, with a gradual decrease and return of the FHR baseline. Late decelerations occur when the onset of the deceleration to the nadir is equal to or greater than 30 seconds (ACOG, 2009) and the nadir of the deceleration occurs after the peak of the contraction (Fig. 14.13).

Late decelerations are thought to occur with decreased blood flow through the intervillous space resulting in fetal hypoxia. In most cases, late decelerations appear before the loss of variability (i.e., moderate to minimal) and are a reflex to transient fetal hypoxia caused by an interruption

anywhere along the oxygen pathway, such as maternal hypotension. Once corrective measures, such as maternal lateral positioning, are initiated, these decelerations will typically dissipate. Late decelerations become more concerning when they are recurrent (present with 50% or more of the uterine contractions in a 20-minute period) and associated with tachycardia and a loss of variability. If uncorrected, hypoxic stress will lead to an accumulation of oxygen debt. Deoxygenated blood will be insufficient for myocardial metabolism, which can be linked to acidemia and neonatal depression (Nageotte, 2016).

Variable Decelerations

Variable decelerations may be either periodic or episodic patterns. These decelerations are visually apparent, abrupt decreases from onset to nadir of a deceleration. The onset of the deceleration to the nadir is less than 30 seconds. The decrease is at least 15 bpm below the baseline, with the deceleration lasting at least 15 seconds and no longer than 2 minutes from onset to the return to baseline (Macones et al., 2008; ACOG, 2009) (Fig. 14.14). Deceleration shape, depth, duration, and timing in relationship to contractions may vary. Variable decelerations are the most frequent type of deceleration during first- and second-stage labor.

Variable decelerations are suggestive of an interruption of oxygenation at the level of the umbilical cord where cord vessels may be compressed. Physiologically, the thin-walled umbilical vein is occluded during umbilical cord compression in situations such as umbilical cord prolapse or oligohydramnios. Fetal venous response is decreased, and baroreceptors trigger a rise in FHR that sometimes appears as a "shoulder" before deceleration onset. As the umbilical cord continues to be occluded, the compressed umbilical arteries cause an abrupt increase in fetal peripheral resistance and blood pressure. Baroreceptors detect the abrupt rise in blood pressure and signal the brainstem to increase parasympathetic outflow, which results in an abrupt FHR decrease. Once the umbilical cord is decompressed, umbilical arteries open and an increase in the FHR occurs. Once all the umbilical cord vessels are open, the FHR usually returns to the previous baseline (Miller, 2016; Nageotte, 2015).

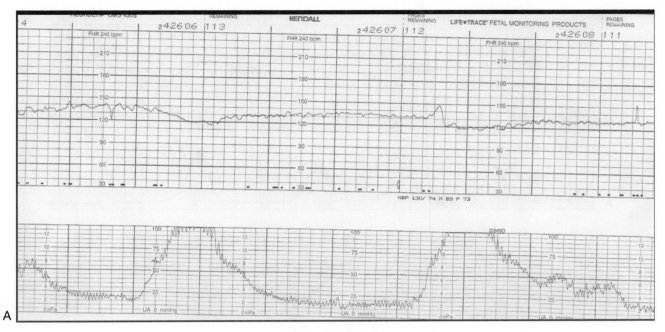

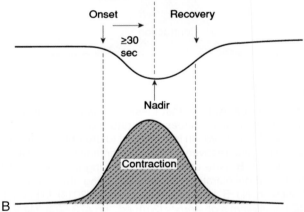

FIG. 14.12 Early Decelerations. A, Note that these decelerations are visually apparent, symmetric in shape, and have a gradual decrease and return of FHR baseline, which "mirrors" a uterine contraction. This deceleration, which is attributed to head compression, has a deceleration onset, nadir, and recovery that coincide with the beginning, peak, and ending of a contraction. **B,** Early deceleration showing gradual onset to nadir in more than 30 seconds, with both onset and recovery coincident with the onset and recovery of the contraction. (A, Courtesy PeriGen, Princeton, NJ. B, Intrapartum assessment, (2014). In F. Cunningham, K. J. Leveno, S. L. Bloom, et al. (Eds), *William's obstetrics* (24th ed., pp 473-503). New York: McGraw-Hill.)

Generally, variable decelerations are not associated with significant hypoxia or acidosis as long as they are intermittent and accompanied by normal baseline rate and variability. If cord compression is recurrent or prolonged, interruption in fetal oxygenation can progress to hypoxemia, hypoxia, metabolic acidosis, and metabolic acidemia if corrective measures are not successful (Miller et al., 2016). Regardless of whether variable decelerations are intermittent or recurrent, they should be evaluated and managed appropriately.

Prolonged Decelerations

Similar to variable decelerations, prolonged decelerations are either periodic or episodic and are generally

isolated on the tracing. These decelerations are defined as a decrease in the FHR that lasts a minimum of 2 minutes and no longer than 10 minutes from onset to return to baseline (Fig. 14.15). After 10 minutes, the deceleration is considered a baseline change. From a physiologic standpoint, prolonged decelerations are difficult to classify. Some experts think the same mechanisms responsible for late or variable decelerations are responsible for FHR changes associated with prolonged deceleration, only they last longer (Miller, 2016). Regardless, a prolonged deceleration reflects interruption of oxygen transfer from the environment to the fetus at one or more points along the oxygen pathway.

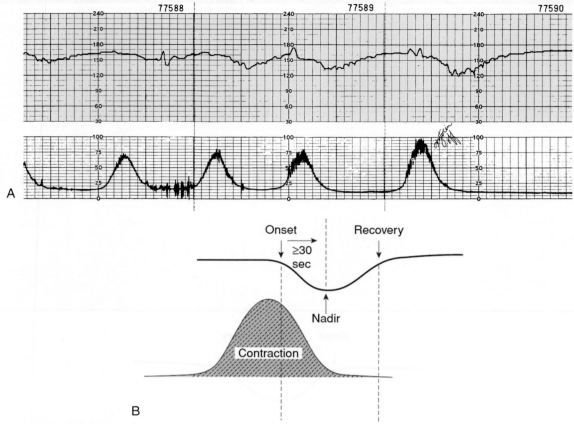

FIG. 14.13 Late Decelerations. **A,** Note that these decelerations are visually apparent, are symmetric in shape, and have a gradual decrease and return of the fetal heart rate baseline that are "late" in timing. This deceleration, which is attributed to uteroplacental insufficiency, has a deceleration with an onset, nadir, and recovery of the deceleration occurring after the beginning, peak, and ending of a contraction. **B,** Late deceleration showing gradual onset to nadir in more than 30 seconds, with nadir and deceleration recovery occurring after the end of the contraction. (A, Courtesy PeriGen, Princeton, NJ. B, Intrapartum assessment (2014). In F. Cunningham, K. J. Leveno, S. L. Bloom, et al. (Eds), *William's obstetrics* (24th ed., pp 473-503). New York: McGraw-Hill.)

CRITICAL THINKING EXERCISE 14.1

Margaret is a 34-year-old (G2P0010) undergoing an oxytocin induction at 39 1/7 weeks for gestational diabetes that has been well controlled with insulin. Presently she has ruptured membranes and is 6 cm dilated, 90% effaced, and at +1 station. An internal fetal spinal electrode and intrauterine pressure catheter were placed earlier in the day. The baseline fetal heart rate is 135 bpm with moderate variability. Uterine contractions are now 2 to 2.5 minutes apart, 70 to 90 seconds in duration, with an intensity of 60 to 80 mm Hg, and uterine resting tone of 10 to 15 mm Hg. Margaret's nurse, Ruth, notes a pattern of uniform decelerations that have an onset, nadir, and recovery that coincides with the beginning, peak, and ending of a contraction. The nadir of the deceleration occurs 35 seconds after its onset.

Questions

1. What pattern does this describe? What is the probable cause?
2. What is the most appropriate corrective measure? Why? Are corrective actions necessary?

Uterine Activity

Standardized definitions are used to describe UA, which is quantified as the number of contractions in a 10-minute window of time, averaged over 30 minutes (Macones et al., 2008; Miller et al., 2016).

- Frequency—Calculated from onset of one contraction to onset of next contraction described in minutes.
- Duration—Calculated from onset of one contraction to end of the contraction described in seconds.
- Intensity—Strength of contraction peak. When palpation or a toco is used, intensity is described as mild, moderate, or strong (firm). Quantitative numbers in the form of millimeters of mercury are used with an IUPC.
- Resting tone—Amount of intrauterine tone when the uterus is at rest described as soft or relaxed when normal and firm or not relaxed when abnormal with palpation or millimeters of mercury with an IUPC. Normal resting tone is approximately 10 mm Hg with an IUPC, and hypertonus is greater than 20 to 25 mm Hg with an IUPC.

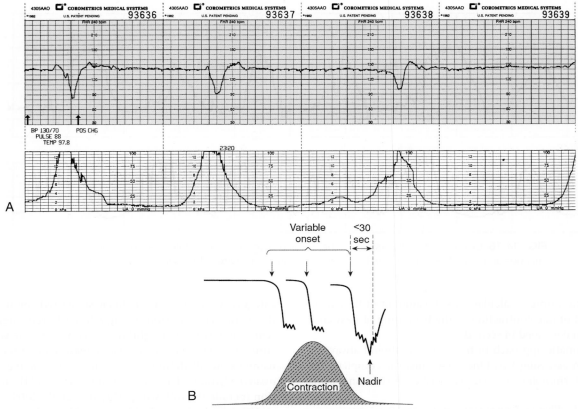

FIG. 14.14 Variable Decelerations. A, Note these decelerations are visually apparent, abrupt decreases from onset to nadir of a deceleration and are attributed to umbilical cord compression. The decrease is at least 15 bpm below the baseline, with the deceleration lasting a minimum of 15 seconds and no longer than 2 minutes from onset to baseline. Deceleration shape, depth, duration, and timing may vary. **B,** Variable deceleration showing abrupt onset to nadir in less than 30 seconds with deceleration measuring 15 bpm or greater 15 seconds or longer; total duration is less than 2 minutes. (A, Courtesy PeriGen, Princeton, NJ. B, Intrapartum assessment (2014). In F. Cunningham, K. J. Leveno, S. L. Bloom, et al. (Eds), *William's Obstetrics* (24th ed., pp 473-503). New York: McGraw-Hill.)

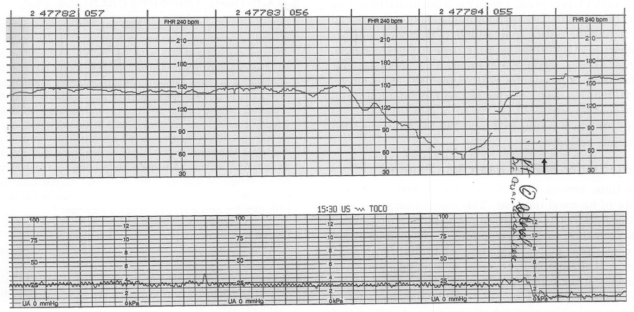

FIG. 14.15 Prolonged Decelerations. Note this deceleration shows a decrease in the fetal heart rate that lasts a minimum of 2 minutes but no longer than 10 minutes from onset to return to baseline. (Courtesy PeriGen, Princeton, NJ.)

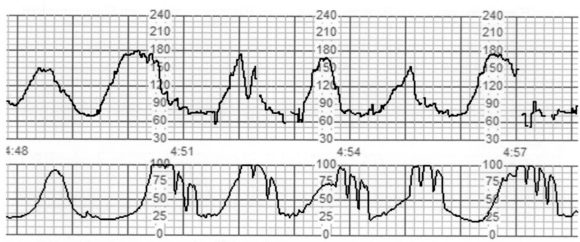

FIG. 14.16 Example of tachysystole in the second stage of labor. Note the presence of periodic changes and lack of relaxation time between contractions. (Courtesy PeriGen, Princeton, NJ)

- Relaxation time—Calculated as the amount of time from the end of one contraction to the beginning of next contraction described in seconds.

A systematic approach to these criteria should always be used when assessing UA. Once assessment is complete, the following terminology is used to describe UA (Macones et al., 2008):

- Normal—Five or fewer contractions in 10 minutes, averaged over a 30-minute period
- Tachysystole—More than five contractions in 10 minutes, averaged over a 30-minute period regardless of whether periodic or episodic changes of the FHR are present (Fig. 14.16). Terminology such as *hyperstimulation* or *hypercontractility* is no longer accepted.

Montevideo units (MVUs) sometimes may be used to describe contraction intensity over a 10-minute period when an IUPC is in place. The MVU is calculated by noting each contraction's intensity in millimeters of mercury and subtracting the resting tone. Numbers are added together to report MVUs during that timeframe (Caldeyro-Barcia, Pose, & Alvarez, 1957). For example, if a woman has four contractions in 10 minutes, with an intensity of 70, 60, 70, and 80 mm Hg, and a uterine resting tone of 10 mm Hg, this would be calculated as (70–10) + (60–10) + (70–10) + (80–10) which results in a total 240 MVUs during that 10-minute period.

Categorization of Fetal Heart Rate Patterns

Over time, certain FHR characteristics have been predictive of neonatal outcome. This continuum starts with FHR characteristics considered normal for an oxygenated fetus. Over time, when interruptions in oxygenation occur, the continuum moves from normal to "indeterminate" patterns that suggest hypoxemia or hypoxia. Finally, if uncorrected, these indeterminate patterns may evolve to abnormal patterns that are predictive of inadequate tissue oxygenation leading to metabolic acidemia. A three-tiered categorization system has been suggested for use during the intrapartum period. Using a three-tiered category system provides a meaningful way to communicate with other clinicians. This system is also a reasonable alternative to using vague, ill-defined terms such as *reassuring* or *nonreassuring* (Miller et al., 2016). Categories of FHR interpretation include the following (Macones et al., 2008):

- Category I—Normal and are strongly predictive of normal fetal acid-base status at the time of observation (Fig. 14.17)
- Category II—Indeterminate and fetal acid-base status is uncertain
- Category III FHR—Abnormal and predictive of abnormal fetal acid status at the time of observation

Patterns associated with each category are presented in Box 14.4.

? CRITICAL THINKING EXERCISE 14.2

Eleanor is a 29-year-old (G3P2002) at 37 1/7 weeks who presented to labor and delivery in active labor. Her cervix on arrival was 8 cm and 75% effaced, and the fetal station was −1. Her amniotic membranes ruptured shortly after arrival. Continuous external electronic fetal monitoring is being used. Eleanor has not had medication for pain relief. The baseline fetal heart rate (FHR) is 140 bpm with moderate variability. Uterine contractions are now 2 to 2.5 minutes apart, are 80 to 100 seconds in duration, and have a palpable intensity of moderate to strong and a uterine resting tone that palpates as soft. After entering Eleanor's labor room, her nurse Natalie notes abrupt decreases from the onset to the nadir of a deceleration. Each decrease is 50 to 60 seconds below the FHR baseline and is lasting 30 to 50 seconds.

Questions

1. What pattern does this describe? What is the probable cause?
2. What is the most appropriate corrective measure? Why? Are corrective actions necessary, and in what order would you perform them?

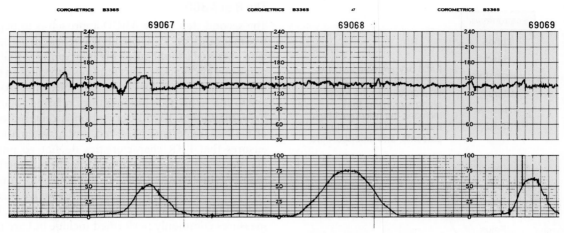

FIG. 14.17 Electronic fetal monitoring tracing showing a category I fetal heart rate (FHR) as evidenced by a baseline FHR of 130 bpm, moderate variability, and an acceleration. There are 3 contractions in 10 min, occurring about every 4 minutes, lasting 60 to 130 seconds. Because this is an external tocodynamometer, intensity and resting tone would need to be palpated.

KNOWLEDGE CHECK

9. What is the significance of FHR accelerations?
10. Describe the differences among early, late, and variable decelerations.
11. Define frequency, duration, intensity, resting tone, and relaxation time.
12. Which category is interpreted as being predictive of abnormal fetal acid-base status?

BOX 14.4   Categories of Fetal Heart Rate Interpretation

Category I—Normal
FHR baseline: 110-160 bpm
Moderate variability
Accelerations present or absent
Variable or late
Decelerations absent
Early decelerations present or absent

Category II—Indeterminate
Tracings not categorized as category I or III

Category III—Abnormal
Absent variability
and
Recurrent late decelerations
or
Recurrent variable decelerations
or
Bradycardia
or
Sinusoidal pattern

STANDARDIZED INTRAPARTUM INTERPRETATION AND MANAGEMENT

In health care and even more so in labor and delivery, a standardized, evidence-based approach to intrapartum FHR interpretation and management necessitates a shared mental model. Shared mental models imply team performance improves if members share an understanding of the task to be performed (Jonker, Van Riemsdijk, & Vermeulen, 2011). For example, if a clinician interprets an FHR tracing as sinusoidal, he or she understands that this pattern is abnormal. The clinician conveys the findings to colleagues, such as a physician who reviews the tracing. After a systematic review of the tracing and clinical situation, a cesarean delivery is called. Because team members used a shared mental model, urgent tasks were performed together with a common goal of optimizing perinatal outcome. In other words, standardized interpretation and management is critical to maternal-fetal well-being as long as effective teamwork and meaningful communication occur. Intrapartum EFM is meant to assess adequacy of oxygen transfer during labor (Fig. 14.18). The following two evidence-based principles in intrapartum FHR interpretation can be inferred when clinicians review a FHR tracing (Miller et al., 2016):

- Principle 1—Variable, late, and/or prolonged decelerations indicate interruption of oxygen transfer from the environment to the fetus at one or more points.
- Principle 2—Moderate variability and/or accelerations reliably exclude ongoing hypoxic injury at the time they are observed.

These evidence-based principles create the groundwork for a standardized approach to FHR management referred to as the *ABCD* approach (Fig. 14.19) (Miller et al., 2016), as follows:

- **A**—Assess oxygen pathway and identify the cause of FHR changes, both maternal or fetal
- **B**—Begin corrective measures

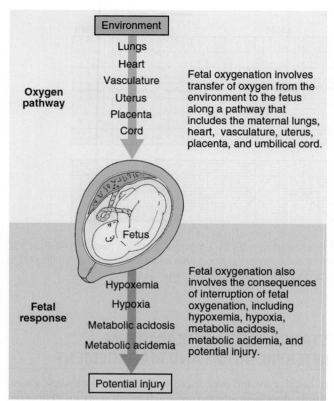

FIG. 14.18 Oxygen Pathway and Fetal Response. (From Miller, D. A. (2016). Intrapartum fetal evaluation. In S. G. Gabbe, J. R. Niebyl, J. L. Simpson, et al. (Eds), *Obstetrics: Normal and problem pregnancies* (7th ed., pp. 308-343). Philadelphia, PA: Elsevier.)

- **C**—Clear obstacles to delivery
- **D**—Determine a delivery plan

This process incorporates the NICHD definitions and principles of interpretation.

The A of ABCD

FHR and UA interpretation requires the availability of reliable and useful data. Clinicians should identify and minimize potential sources of error so data are recorded satisfactorily for interpretation and management. For example, if an external ultrasound transducer is not able to transmit a continuous tracing in a high-risk obese patient, placement of an FSE may be required. Once reliable data are confirmed, a systematic approach to evaluating five FHR characteristics is performed: baseline rate, variability, accelerations, decelerations, and changes or trends over time. Tracing evaluations are completed periodically at reasonable intervals in accordance with institutional policies and procedures. If a category I pattern is identified, the tracing is considered normal because this is reflective of a normally oxygenated fetus. On the other hand, if a category II or III pattern is identified, a prompt, methodical approach to assessing the oxygenation pathway should be completed to identify a potential source of interrupted oxygenation.

The B in ABCD

The second step in the ABCD approach is to begin corrective measures, or "B." Once FHR assessment is complete, the data obtained should guide the interventions that are physiologically appropriate. This requires clinicians to take action to implement procedures that may maximize oxygen delivery to the fetus. This is sometimes referred to as *intrauterine resuscitation*. Each intervention is centered on the type of FHR characteristic observed, and a systematic approach ensures that FHR characteristics do not go unnoticed so decisions are made in a timely manner. Sometimes more than one intervention may be implemented to resolve category II or III pattern, and not all corrective measures will be used in every clinical scenario (Miller, 2016). Corrective measures commonly performed include but are not limited to the following:

- Maternal repositioning
- Intravenous fluid boluses
- Administering oxygen
- Reducing UA
- Correcting maternal hypotension
- Performing amnioinfusion
- Modifying second-stage pushing efforts

Maternal repositioning is a corrective measure. Two situations exist in which a maternal-position change may improve fetal oxygenation and uteroplacental perfusion to return an FHR pattern to one that is considered normal (Garite & Simpson, 2011). First, repositioning to lateral or hands and knees will alter the relationship between the uterine wall, amniotic fluid, fetus, and umbilical cord. In this case, variable or prolonged decelerations related to umbilical cord compression may be reduced. Second, lateral positioning may increase uterine blood flow, which may have been decreased by aortocaval compression during supine positioning. The supine position is associated with an undesirable impact on maternal hemodynamics, including decreased venous return and cardiac output, because the weight of the gravid uterus, amniotic fluid, placenta, and fetus or fetuses compresses the aorta and inferior vena cava. This compression decreases uteroplacental perfusion, which inhibits the delivery of oxygenated blood to the fetus (Garite & Simpson, 2011; Miller, 2016).

Uteroplacental perfusion and fetal oxygenation depend on maternal cardiac output and intravascular volume. An *intravenous (IV) fluid bolus* of 500 to 1000 mL of isotonic fluid such as lactated Ringer's solution can improve cardiac output by increasing circulating volume, venous return, left ventricular end-diastolic pressure, ventricular preload, and stroke volume. Increased volume will affect maternal cardiac output and uteroplacental perfusion, resulting in improved fetal oxygenation. IV boluses of fluids containing glucose should be avoided because of potential maternal and fetal complications. Fluid amounts in high-risk women who are at risk for volume overload and pulmonary edema should be carefully considered (Garite & Simpson, 2011; Miller, 2016). Fetal oxygenation depends on maternal blood oxygenation and flow into the intervillous space.

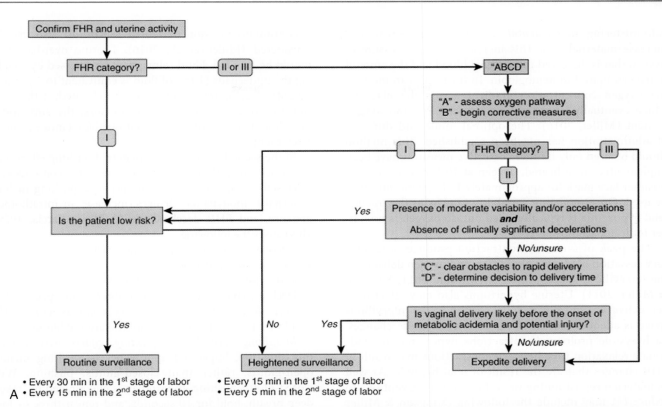

FIG. 14.19 Intrapartum fetal heart rate (FHR) management decision model demonstrating an algorithm for management of electronic fetal monitoring tracings during the intrapartum period. *OR*, Operating room; *SLE*, systemic lupus erythematosus. (From Miller, D. A. (2016). Intrapartum fetal evaluation. In S. G. Gabbe, J. R. Niebyl, J. L. Simpson, et al. (Eds), *Obstetrics: Normal and problem pregnancies* (7th ed., pp. 308-343). Philadelphia, PA: Elsevier.)

Administering *supplemental oxygen* to the woman can increase maternal Po_2. This increases partial pressure of oxygen that is dissolved in maternal blood and the amount of oxygen bound to hemoglobin. In turn, this can increase the oxygen concentration gradient across the placenta, which eventually leads to increased fetal Po_2 and oxygen content (Miller, 2016). The optimal mode and duration of administration has not been established. This method should be used only if other corrective measures have been implemented. If indicated, oxygen at 10 L/min via nonrebreather face mask for approximately 15 to 30 minutes may be used. Once moderate variability returns to the tracing, fetal hypoxemia is typically ruled out, so oxygen is no longer indicated (Simpson, 2015).

The peak of a uterine contraction produces a temporary cessation of uterine blood flow and oxygen delivery to the intervillous space (Garite & Simpson, 2011; Simpson & Miller, 2011). Uterine hypertonus also may affect oxygen delivery. Typically, residual oxygen in the intervillous space is adequate for the fetus to tolerate these changes. Tachysystole, prolonged contractions, hypertonus, or inadequate relaxation time between contractions may result in FHR changes that are the result of fetal hypoxia. As well as maternal repositioning or an IV bolus, interventions to *reduce UA* may include the following (Simpson & Miller 2011):

- Removal of prostaglandin cervical ripening agents
- Decreasing or discontinuing oxytocin
- Assessment to rule out conditions such as chorioamnionitis or placental abruption
- Administration of a tocolytic agent such as a beta-sympathomimetic agent

Correcting maternal hypotension is another measure to be considered to increase uteroplacental perfusion and fetal oxygenation. Hypotension may be caused by supine positioning, inadequate maternal hydration, decreased venous return and reduced cardiac output, and peripheral vasodilation secondary to sympathetic blockade during neuraxial anesthesia such as an epidural (Miller, 2016). Therefore lateral repositioning and IV hydration are usually sufficient to correct hypotension. If these corrective actions do not increase blood pressure, medications such as ephedrine or phenylephrine may be necessary.

Amnioinfusion requires instillation of isotonic fluid, such as lactated Ringer's solution or normal saline, through an IUPC into the uterus to restore amniotic fluid volume to normal or near-normal levels (Miller, 2016). The physiologic principle behind amnioinfusion is that decreased amniotic fluid, or oligohydramnios, can cause interruptions in the oxygen pathways via umbilical cord compression, which can lead to variable or prolonged decelerations. By replacing fluid, umbilical cord compression may be relieved, resulting in optimal blood flow through the umbilical cord vessels with oxygenated blood. Amnioinfusion rates and amounts are directed by institutional policies. One suggested guideline includes an initial bolus of 250 to 500 mL over a 20- to 30-minute timeframe via an infusion pump or gravity flow.

A continuous infusion of 120 to 180 mL/hr also may be considered (Miller et al., 2016). Uterine overdistention should be avoided. Fluid return may be assessed by weighing the underpads (1 mL of fluid is equivalent to 1 gram of weight). Uterine resting tone may be elevated; if there are concerns related to intrauterine pressure, the amnioinfusion should be temporarily discontinued for a more accurate assessment.

In the second stage of labor, maternal pushing efforts can be associated with FHR decelerations. The consequences of closed-glottis pushing or Valsalva-style pushing include maternal hemodynamic changes, increases in intrathoracic pressure, and FHR decelerations (Caldeyro-Barcia, 1979). This causes the following:

- Decrease in venous return to the heart
- Decrease in cardiac output
- Reduction in maternal arterial pressure
- Decline in blood perfusion in the intervillous space, resulting in decreased oxygen supply to the fetus as evidenced by a lower pH and Po_2 of the umbilical arterial blood

Modifying second-stage pushing efforts may correct this situation. Suggested approaches to pushing include open-glottis, rather than closed-glottis, pushing. With closed-glottis pushing, the woman is encouraged to "take a deep breath, hold for 10 seconds, and repeat three or four times with each contraction." Instead, open-glottis pushing encourages women to push when there is an urge to bear down. Rather than holding her breath for a prolonged time, women are asked to push for approximately 6 to 8 seconds, repeating three to five times during each contraction (Association of Women's Health, Obstetric, and Neonatal Nurses [AWHONN], 2008; Caldeyro-Barcia, 1979). Women also should take several breaths between pushes and be reassured rather than chastised if they grunt or make a deep guttural sound while pushing. Alternative pushing efforts also may include shorter individual pushing efforts, pushing with every other or every third contraction, and pushing only with perceived urge (Simpson, 2007; Simpson & James, 2005). In fact, passive descent with the woman who does not have the urge to push may be considered when there are no maternal-fetal conditions that require an expedited delivery. After performing corrective measures, if the pattern returns to category I, continued surveillance is possible as long as surveillance is performed in a reasonable timeframe.

Category II patterns require continued surveillance and further evaluation. In a situation in which moderate variability and/or accelerations without significant decelerations are present, heightened observation is appropriate. In other situations, category II patterns are more challenging, making interpretation difficult. Despite using a shared mental model, the health care team may disagree on interpretation or level of risk. In these cases, a standardized approach to management of category II patterns may be implemented. At the other extreme of the fetal monitoring spectrum are abnormal patterns, or category III. Expedited delivery, whether vaginally or operatively, may be considered for a category III pattern, depending on the entire clinical situation if corrective measures are ineffective.

The C in ABCD

If at any time clinicians are uncertain about the clinical situation, the management model guides clinicians to the next step, "C," clear obstacles for delivery. When moving to this step, there is no obligation to make critical decisions about time or mode of delivery. This part of the management model encourages the entire health care team to focus methodically on potential areas of delay that could prevent a management plan from being performed in a timely manner. Potential obstacles include the hospital, the staff, the woman and her fetus, and the actual labor process.

The D in ABCD

The last step in the ABCD approach, "D," is to determine the decision to delivery time. Clinicians, regardless of their position on the team, should continue to use a shared mental model to ensure all steps of the management approach have been completed. Decisions to expedite delivery via cesarean section or operative vaginal delivery versus waiting for a spontaneous vaginal delivery is based on the best available information. If a decision is made to expedite delivery, the rationale for delivery is documented and the plan is quickly implemented. In these situations, an umbilical cord blood gas sample may be obtained to assess fetal acid-base status and level of oxygenation at the time of delivery. If the decision is made to wait for vaginal delivery, the justification for waiting and the management plan also should be documented. Ultimately the person responsible for the delivery will determine the time and mode of delivery.

Umbilical cord blood gas sampling is a direct method of assessing the level of oxygenation and fetal acid-base after delivery in situations in which a category II or III pattern is observed. A double clamped section of the umbilical cord is obtained at birth. Two heparinized syringes (prevents coagulation) with small-gauge needles are used to draw blood gas samples from the umbilical artery (deoxygenated) and umbilical vein (oxygenated) (Fig. 14.20).

Arterial cord blood best reflects information on blood returning from the fetus to the placenta and best describes fetal status at the time of delivery. A sample from the umbilical vein reflects placental function and the level of oxygenation at the intervillous space going to the fetus (see Fig. 14.20). This sample also confirms the accuracy of the umbilical artery sample. Blood samples are stable for up to 60 minutes and do not need to be kept on ice for analysis. Umbilical cord blood gas samples are analyzed for pH, partial pressure of carbon dioxide (Pco_2), partial pressure of oxygen (Po_2), bicarbonate (HCO_3) levels, and base deficit or excess. This information helps identify the presence or absence of fetal acidosis. If acidosis is present, respiratory (short term) acidosis can be distinguished from metabolic (prolonged), or mixed acidosis (Cypher, 2015).

KNOWLEDGE CHECK

13. Describe the ABCD management approach used in fetal monitoring.
14. List the corrective measures that may be considered to correct a category II or III FHR pattern.
15. How does an IV bolus of fluids benefit fetal oxygenation?
16. What response should be elicited when performing fetal scalp stimulation? What does this tell you about fetal oxygenation?
17. What is the purpose of umbilical cord blood gas sampling? Which umbilical cord vessels reflect oxygenated and deoxygenated blood.
18. What are potential obstacles that may be encountered during the "C" part of the ABCD approach? Describe measures to overcome these obstacles.

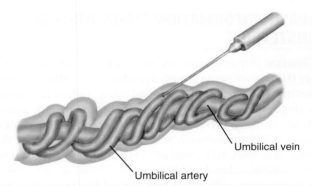

Umbilical vein

Umbilical artery

FIG. 14.20 Umbilical Cord Blood Gas Sampling. Samples are drawn from both the umbilical artery and umbilical vein.

ASSESSMENT FREQUENCY AND DOCUMENTATION

Documentation of clinical care in a medical record is critically important to communicate information that is complete, factual, and an objective report of relevant information and care provided (Miller & Ruth, 2017). Clinical information about the woman and fetus is documented throughout labor. Documentation tools used to chart patient care during the intrapartum period include flowsheets, clinical pathways, checklists, summary notes, or plotted graphs such as vital signs. These tools may be on paper, in an electronic format, or a combination of both methods. Each institution should have a documentation policy that highlights documentation tools to be used, style, format, and frequency interval.

The nursing professional organization, AWHONN, has a position statement that has suggested frequency of assessment and documentation parameters when auscultation, palpation, and EFM are used during the intrapartum period. At a minimum, a systematic approach to assessment and documentation should include the following (AWHONN, 2015; Macones et al., 2008; Miller & Ruth, 2017):

1. An admission evaluation of the woman and fetus at the time of arrival

2. Ongoing systematic maternal-fetal assessments to include FHR and UA data as well as changes or trends over time using standardized definitions that at a minimum must include the following:
   - Baseline FHR
   - Baseline variability
   - Presence or absence of accelerations
   - Presence or absence of decelerations
   - Type of decelerations
   - UA to include frequency, duration, intensity, and resting tone with MVUs if directed by institutional policy
3. Corrective measures used during labor and evaluation of responses
4. Communication with the woman and support system
5. Interactions with providers with response and actions taken

HEALTH INFORMATION TECHNOLOGY IN OBSTETRICS

Clinicians play an integral role in health information technology (HIT), continuing growth in a journey to further improve obstetric patient–centered care and safety. Today's fetal monitoring systems are more comprehensive and include point-of-care charting, FHR and UA pattern interpretation, clinical decision support software, and archiving capabilities. At the most basic level, HIT measures FHR and UA, which is then consolidated and analyzed. Once analyzed, data are interpreted in conjunction with a clinician's clinical knowledge that has been accumulated through hands-on experience and education (Cypher, 2016). This type of computer technology allows clinicians to ask the right questions at the appropriate time, complete structured nursing assessments, accurately determine a correct diagnosis from a multidisciplinary approach, and execute interventions along the decision-making process.

FETAL MONITORING EDUCATION AND COMPETENCY

Fetal assessment during the intrapartum period requires skilled clinicians to be able to interpret FHR and UA patterns as well as make clinical decisions based on these findings. Professional organizations have developed guidelines to promote education and standardization in fetal monitoring. Comprehensive fetal monitoring education should include didactic information, such as FHR physiology, and psychomotor skills, such as FSE placement. Ongoing fetal monitoring education and clinical competency are also important to achieve and maintain sound clinical judgment and thorough decision-making proficiency.

ROLE OF INTRAPARTUM FETAL SURVEILLANCE

Obstetric nurses are typically the primary clinicians who provide patient care in labor and delivery and who are responsible for fetal surveillance. In nursing and in obstetric medicine, standardized definitions, interpretation, and management approaches are continuing to evolve. Both professions, nurses and physicians, agree that monitoring is intended to assess the adequacy of fetal oxygenation during labor. There is also very little argument regarding the difference between normal and abnormal FHR tracings. When there is evidence of an interruption in oxygenation along the oxygenation pathway, fetal surveillance often can alert clinicians to conduct further evaluation and possibly implement corrective measures to improve oxygen delivery. Fetal surveillance also has demonstrated that a tracing often can assist clinicians in determining frequency and severity of interrupted oxygenation so that a management plan can be implemented regarding optimal timing and mode of delivery.

Clear documentation regarding maternal-fetal clinical concerns should be written and shared with the entire health care obstetric and neonatal team. In this era of family-centered care and elevating the standards associated with patient safety and health care quality, clinicians at the bedside and in leadership positions should continue to promote the use of evidence-based guidelines and research in fetal surveillance to ensure quality obstetric care in the intrapartum setting.

◆ APPLICATION OF THE NURSING PROCESS: PATIENT TEACHING WITH LACK OF KNOWLEDGE

Clinicians may identify any number of patient care challenges when fetal surveillance is used during the intrapartum period. A woman may become anxious if EFM is initiated for oxytocin induction when her birth plan stated she preferred IA and palpation for FHR and UA assessment. Pain that was once relieved with ambulation and hydrotherapy may become intolerable if continuous fetal monitoring is necessary. FHR interpretation may be challenging if narcotics are given in the latent phase of labor. Therefore two nursing care responsibilities related to fetal assessment should be considered: assessing the woman's (and support person's) learning needs and expanding nursing care related to fetal oxygenation and potential interruptions along the oxygenation pathway.

◆ Assessment

Identify what the woman and her support person already know about EFM, IA, and palpation (Fig. 14.21). Women who have attended prepared childbirth classes or have given birth before may have a basic understanding of the purpose, benefits, and limitations of fetal surveillance. Identifying what patients already know allows clinicians to build on pre-existing knowledge and correct any inaccurate information.

If the woman is not familiar with either technique of intrapartum fetal assessment, assess her perception and understanding of each method. For example, does the woman believe an EFM will signal the development of a complication? Does the woman expect that she will be able to use a telemetry system during the first stage of labor? Is the woman comfortable with IA for fetal

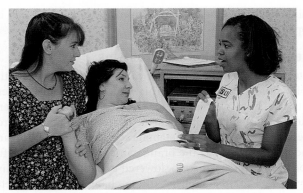

FIG. 14.21 The nurse teaches a woman and her support person about electronic fetal monitoring (EFM) to limit fear and anxiety. The nurse should help the woman understand that EFM is only one method used to evaluate fetal well-being during labor.

assessment or does she worry that something important will be missed?

Lack of knowledge contributes to anxiety. Note the anxiety level of the woman when the monitor is used. For example, is the woman afraid to change positions because the FHR becomes intermittent? Does she frequently question why the monitor is not showing how strong her contractions are? Questions should be answered to the best of the clinician's ability, and then knowledge reassessment will identify information that is still unclear.

◆ Identification of Patient Problems

Because of the prevalence of EFM for labor, one common patient problem is the need for patient education regarding EFM. If IA and palpation are being used, there may also be a need for patient education regarding fetal surveillance.

◆ Planning: Expected Outcomes

An expected outcome criteria for a patient with a need for education is for the woman (and support person) to express an understanding about equipment, procedures, benefits, limitations, and expected data after receiving education about fetal surveillance.

◆ Interventions

Based on the woman's knowledge level, education is provided at the bedside (see Fig. 14.21). This includes but is not limited to the purpose and equipment chosen for monitoring, frequency of assessment, and a brief explanation about what is shown on the tracing. Sometimes clarification about how the equipment functions is necessary. For example, women may not understand that there is no safety risk for being attached to an electrical device, especially when transducers are exposed to amniotic fluid. Women can be reassured that the connections to the device and those to the wall current are isolated from each other.

When EFM is used during the intrapartum period, women may have questions that should be answered. The following are frequently asked questions and suggested answers:

- *Can I move around with all these straps on?*

    "Of course, you can move or reposition yourself in bed because I want you to be comfortable. In fact, I want you to reposition yourself frequently as long as the baby is not having FHR changes that are concerning. Staying in the same position is not only uncomfortable but doesn't promote normal labor. Sometimes the monitor will be unable to record the FHR continuously or record contractions very well. If you notice this, don't panic. Most of the time it's because the transducer on your belly has shifted out of place and lost contact with the heartbeat. Use your call bell to reach me, and I'll come in to readjust the monitor. If we continue to have difficulties recording the FHR or contractions, we may discuss other alternatives."

- *What if I need to go to the bathroom?*

    "If you need to go to the bathroom, we'll unplug the cords from the monitor. We may also be able to roll the monitor to the door of the bathroom."

- *Why is the baby's heart beating so fast? It sounds like a galloping horse!"*

    "A baby's heartbeat is faster than an adult's heartbeat. The normal heart rate for these little ones is about 110 to 160 bpm. If the rate is lower or higher than normal, we'll review the tracing to see what the potential cause is and then make decisions about interventions that may need to be performed."

- *Why do those numbers for the baby's heart rate keep changing so much?*

    "The heart rate of your baby changes because just like at home, your baby takes naps for short periods and then wakes up. When the baby moves, the heart speeds up, just as yours does when you are exercising. When the baby sleeps the rate becomes slow and steady."

- *What do those numbers for contractions mean? They change all the time.*

    "The IUPC we placed earlier is recording the pressure inside your uterus. The numbers change when you are contracting. The numbers will also fluctuate when you are breathing heavily, coughing, laughing, or readjusting your position."

- *My contractions don't look very strong, but they sure feel strong to me!*

    "I know you're discouraged because the contractions on the tracing are not recording as strong as you feel them. Sometimes contractions appear stronger or weaker than they really are because of the position you're in, how big or small your baby may be, the position of the baby, and how much tissue is between the uterus and the transducer. Remember you have an external monitor that has a pressure sensor button. Because it is external and not internal, the monitor will accurately record only your contraction frequency and *duration, but not the actual strength. I'll be palpating your uterus to determine how strong your contractions are. If we need to record the actual uterine pressure, we'll talk to you about placing an IUPC."*

- *Will the FSE hurt my baby?*

"The electrode attaches to the first couple of layers of the baby's skin similar to the thickness of a dime, which is about 1 mm. We already know your baby is head down so were very careful to avoid sensitive areas on the head such as the fontanels (soft spots) or the face."

- *The alarms on the monitor are really annoying. Can you turn down the volume?*

"Thanks for letting me know this information. I know alarms can be distracting to you because I know you want to have a quiet, calming environment for labor. Alarms beep for a variety of reasons. They let me know things like a transducer has slipped out of place and is unable to record the FHR, your blood pressure is too high, or if the FHR becomes too low. Let me lower the volume for you. If it's still too loud, let me know and I can mute the sound in the room. I'll still be able to monitor for problems by visually reviewing the tracing."

◆ Evaluation

Evaluation of knowledge is ongoing because women may think of questions after initial explanations and as clinical conditions change. Achievement of the goal or expected outcome is evident if a woman and her support person indicate an understanding after each explanation. This may be accompanied by a decrease in signs of anxiety.

◆ APPLICATION OF THE NURSING PROCESS: OXYGENATION

◆ Assessment

Assessment of the FHR and UA using standardized definitions and a consistent management approach is critical to intrapartum fetal surveillance. Standardized definitions allow clinicians to answer three questions: what do we call it, what does it mean, and what do we do about it (Miller et al., 2016). In answering the first question, clinicians are able to interpret FHR and UA data to determine whether a tracing is normal, indeterminate, or abnormal. The second question can be answered by simply applying two principles: is there presence or absence of interrupted oxygenation and can hypoxic injury be ruled out based on the existence of moderate variability or accelerations. Assessment of mother and fetus is continuous during the dynamic process of labor. Comparing baseline data with ongoing assessments of FHR patterns and UA will provide an opportunity to observe subtle trends in the data and distinguish between patterns that have similar appearances, for example, early and late decelerations. Once these questions are answered, a standardized management approach

using corrective measures to improve oxygenation can be applied to the clinical situation.

◆ Identification of Patient Problems

Interruption of oxygen transfer can occur at any or all of the points along this pathway. This interruption can interfere with fetal homeostasis, leading to a deterioration in oxygenation. Eventually, if left uncorrected, fetal oxygenation progresses from hypoxia to metabolic acidemia. Multiple organs and systems, such as the brain, can experience hypoperfusion, reduced oxygenation, lowered pH, and reduced delivery of fuel for metabolism. These changes cause the fetal system to cascade through multiple cellular events that lead to cellular and tissue dysfunction, neurologic injury, and potentially death (Miller, 2016). Therefore, an appropriate patient problem is: possible fetal injury because of an interrupted fetal oxygenation pathway.

◆ Planning: Expected Outcome

Clinicians have a responsibility to have a plan if an indeterminate or abnormal FHR pattern is assessed. Based on the pattern observed, clinicians need to articulate a clear and understandable plan. Simply stated, if a pattern is assessed as category I, the plan would include reevaluating the tracing at specific intervals. If a category II or III pattern is observed, the clinician will plan to provide corrective measures that promote adequate fetal oxygenation, report the tracing and outcomes of interventions to the delivering provider, support the woman and support person, and document assessments and care. The expected outcome is that the FHR pattern will maintain evidence of adequate fetal oxygenation, such as a normal baseline rate and variability.

◆ Interventions

Once a thorough assessment of baseline FHR, variability, accelerations, decelerations, UA, and changes or trends over time have been completed, the standardized management model, "ABCD," is implemented. Using this method will provide a safeguard to ensure important steps in the intervention phase are not overlooked and are accomplished in a timely manner.

If the FHR pattern is related to an interruption in the oxygenation pathway and requires corrective measures, the clinician's priority is to identify the cause and take steps to improve fetal oxygenation. Implementing corrective measures in response to FHR and UA data is within the scope of practice of nurses (AWHONN, 2015). Most facilities have protocols to give clinicians a framework for these steps. Corrective measures may include both independent nursing actions and delegated medical actions. Regardless of the situation, the delivering provider should be notified. Women may understandably become anxious when the ABCD approach is implemented. Clinicians should always remain calm at the bedside to avoid increasing a woman's fear and anxiety, which can reduce the woman's ability to grasp what is occurring. Another way to decrease fear and anxiety is to explain the clinical situation and reason for corrective measures in succinct, simple language that the woman will understand.

◆ Evaluation

Ongoing evaluation of the clinical situation is necessary to evaluate the effects of interventions on the maternal-fetal condition. This allows clinicians to determine whether corrective measures were successful. Evaluation will also determine whether the plan was effective and whether an alternative plan should be in place. The outcome is met if the FHR pattern demonstrates adequate fetal oxygenation with a Category I pattern.

■ SUMMARY CONCEPTS

- The goal of intrapartum fetal heart rate surveillance is to assess adequacy of fetal oxygenation so timely and appropriate steps can be taken when necessary to optimize perinatal outcomes.

- The placenta functions as an extracorporeal fetal support system. Critical placental tasks that assist with fetal growth, development, and oxygenation include functioning as a fetal lung for respiratory exchange, kidney for excretion, gastrointestinal tract for nutrition, and skin surface for heat exchange. The placenta also plays a vital role in metabolism, endocrine secretion, immunologic safeguards, and as a protective structure against some medications and viruses that are considered harmful.

- Uteroplacental circulation starts with maternal blood flow into the intervillous space through the spiral arteries. Exchange of oxygen and nutrients take place in the intervillous space as maternal blood bathes the chorionic villi. Simultaneously, maternal blood carrying away carbon dioxide and fetal waste products drain from the intervillous spaces through endometrial veins and returns to maternal circulation.

- Adequate fetal oxygenation depends on the absence of an interruption in the oxygenation pathway because oxygenated maternal blood must flow from the environment to the fetus via the maternal lungs, heart, vasculature, uterus, placenta, and umbilical cord to provide oxygenated blood to the fetus.

- Two approaches to intrapartum fetal heart rate surveillance include intermittent ascultation and palpation or electronic fetal monitoring. Each type has advantages and limitations.

- Intrapartum fetal assessment consists of the assessment and evaluation of fetal status during labor using standardized definitions.

- Two physiologic principles about fetal heart rate changes caused by interrupted oxygenation are important. Fetal oxygenation involves (1) oxygen transfer from the environment to the fetus and (2) the fetal response to any interruption of oxygen transfer.

- A standardized approach to fetal heart rate management is referred to as the ABCD approach. This includes: "A" to assess the oxygen pathway and identify the cause of FHR pattern changes, "B" to begin corrective measures, "C" to clear obstacles to delivery, and "D" to determine a delivery plan.

- A direct method of assessing the level of fetal oxygenation during the intrapartum period is to perform umbilical cord blood gas sampling.

- Suggested frequency of assessment and documentation of FHR and UA during the intrapartum period are directed by nursing professional organizations and institutional policies. At a minimum, documentation should include admission evaluation of the woman and fetus, ongoing systematic maternal-fetal assessments using standardized definitions for FHR and UA, corrective measures used during labor and the maternal-fetal response, communication with the woman and support system, and interactions with providers.

REFERENCES & READINGS

American College of Nurse-Midwives (ACNM). (2015). Intermittent auscultation for intrapartum fetal heart rate surveillance. *Journal of Midwifery & Women's Health, 55*(4), 397–403.

American College of Obstetrics and Gynecology (ACOG). (2009). Intrapartum fetal heart rate monitoring: Interpretation, nomenclature and general management principles. *ACOG Practice Bulletin, No. 106*, 192–202.

Amer-Wahlin, I., & Kwee, A. (2016). Combined cardiotocographic and ST event analysis: A review. *Best Practice & Research: Clinical Obstetrics and Gynaecology, 30*(1), 48–61.

Association of Women's Health, Obstetric and Neonatal Nurses (AWHONN). (2008). *Nursing management of the second stage of labor.* Washington, DC: Author.

Association of Women's Health, & Obstetric and Neonatal Nurses (AWHONN). (2015). Position statement: Fetal heart monitoring. *Journal of Obstetric, Gynecologic, and Neonatal Nursing, 44*(5), 683–686.

Ayers-de-Campos, D., & Nogueira-Reis, Z. (2015). Technical characteristics of current cardiotocographic monitors. *Best Practice & Research: Clinical Obstetrics and Gynaecology, 30*(1), 22–32.

Blackburn, S. T. (2013). *Maternal, fetal & neonatal physiology* (4th ed.). St. Louis, MO: Saunders.

Caldeyro-Barcia, R. (1979). The influence of maternal bearing-down efforts during second stage on fetal well-being. *Birth, 6*(1), 17–21.

Caldeyro-Barcia, R., Pose, S. V., & Alvarez, H. (1957). Uterine contractility in polyhydramnios and the effects of withdrawal of the excess of amniotic fluid. *American Journal of Obstetrics and Gynecology, 73*(6), 1238–1254.

Chen, H. Y., Chauhan, S. P., Ananth, C. V., Vintzileos, A. M., & Abuhamad, A. Z. (2011). Electronic fetal heart rate monitoring and its relationship to neonatal and infant mortality in the United States. *American Journal of Obstetrics and Gynecology, 204*(6) 491–e1–e10.

Clark, S. L., Gimovsky, M. L., & Miller, F. C. (1984). The scalp stimulation test: A clinical alternative to fetal scalp blood sampling. *American Journal of Obstetrics and Gynecology, 148*(3), 274–277.

Clark, S. L., Nageotte, M. P., Garite, T. J., Freeman, R. K., Miller, D. A., Simpson, K. R., Hankins, G. D. (2013). Intrapartum management of category II fetal heart rate tracings: Towards standardization of care. *American Journal of Obstetrics and Gynecology, 209*(2), 89–97.

Cypher, R. L. (2015). Assessment of fetal oxygenation and acid-base status. In A. Lyndon, & L. Usher (Eds.), *AWHONN: Fetal heart monitoring: Principles and practices* (5th ed.) (pp. 191–215). Dubuque, IA: Kendall Hunt.

Cypher, R. L. (2016). Technologies in perinatal nursing: Time to accept & embrace the challenge. Retrieved from www.perigen.com/wpcontent/uploads/2016/07/TechnologyAndPerinatalNursingbyRebeccaCypher.pdf.

Feinstein, N. F., Sprague, A., & Trépanier, M. J. (2008). *Fetal heart auscultation* (2nd ed.). Washington, D.C.: Association of Women's Health, Obstetric and Neonatal Nurses.

Freeman, R. K., Garite, T. J., Nageotte, M. P., & Miller, L. A. (2012). *Fetal heart rate monitoring* (4th ed.). Philadelphia, PA: Lippincott Williams & Wilkins.

Garite, T. J., & Simpson, K. R. (2011). Intrauterine resuscitation during labor. *Clinical Obstetrics and Gynecology, 54*(1), 28–39.

Jonker, C. M., Van Riemsdijk, M. B., & Vermeulen, B. (2011). Shared mental models. In *Coordination, organizations, institutions, and norms in agent systems* (pp. 132–151). Berlin: Springer.

Macones, G. A., Hankins, G. D., Spong, C. Y., Hauth, J., & Moore, T. (2008). The 2008 National Institute of Child Health and Human Development workshop report on electronic fetal monitoring: Update on definitions, interpretation, and research guidelines. *Obstetrics and Gynecology, 112*(3), 661–666.

Miller, D. A. (2016). Intrapartum fetal evaluation. In S. G. Gabbe, J. R. Niebyl, J. L. Simpson, et al. (Eds.), *Obstetrics: Normal and problem pregnancies* (7th ed.) (pp. 308–343). Philadelphia, PA: Elsevier.

Miller, L. A., Miller, D. A., & Cypher, R. L. (2016). *Pocket guide to fetal monitoring: A multidisciplinary approach* (8th ed.). St. Louis, MO: Elsevier.

Miller, L. A., & Ruth, D. J. (2017). In B. B. Kennedy, & S. M. Baird (Eds.), *Intrapartum management modules* (5th ed.) (pp. 140–210). Philadelphia, PA: Lippincott Williams & Wilkins.

Modanlou, H. D., & Freeman, R. K. (1982). Sinusoidal fetal heart rate pattern: Its definition and clinical significance. *American Journal of Obstetrics and Gynecology, 142*(8), 1033–1038.

Modanlou, H. D., & Murata, Y. (2004). Sinusoidal heart rate pattern: Reappraisal of Its definition and clinical significance. *Journal of Obstetrics and Gynaecology Research, 30*(3), 169–180.

Nageotte, M. P. (2015). Fetal heart rate monitoring. *Seminars in Fetal and Neonatal Medicine, 20*(3), 144–148.

National Institute of Child Health and Human Development Research Planning Workshop (NICHD). (1997). Electronic fetal monitoring: Research guidelines for interpretation. *American Journal of Obstetrics and Gynecology, 117*(6), 1385–1390 and *Journal of Obstetric, Gynecologic, and Neonatal Nursing, 26*(6), 635–640.

O'Brien-Abel, N. (2015). Physiological basis for fetal monitoring. In A. G. Lyndon, & L. U. Ali (Eds.), *AWHONN: Fetal heart rate principles and practices* (5th ed.) (pp. 23–47). Dubuque, IA: Kendall Hunt.

Parer, J. T. (1997). *Handbook of fetal heart rate monitoring* (2nd ed.). Philadelphia, PA: WB Saunders.

Pijnenborg, R., Vercruysse, L., & Hanssens, M. (2006). The uterine spiral arteries in human pregnancy: Facts and controversies. *Placenta, 27*(9), 939–958.

Porter, T. F., & Clark, S. L. (1999). Vibroacoustic and scalp stimulation. *Obstetrics and Gynecology Clinics of North America, 26*(4), 657–669.

Simpson, K. R. (2007). Intrauterine resuscitation during labor: Review of current methods and supportive evidence. *Journal of Midwifery & Women's Health, 52*(3), 229–237.

Simpson, K. R. (2015). Maternal oxygen administration as an intrauterine resuscitation measure during labor. *MCN: The American Journal of Maternal/Child Nursing, 40*(2), 136.

Simpson, K. R., & James, D. C. (2005). Efficacy of intrauterine resuscitation techniques in improving fetal oxygen status during labor. *Obstetrics & Gynecology, 105*, 1362–1368.

Simpson, K. R., & Miller, L. (2011). Assessment and optimization of uterine activity during labor. *Clinical Obstetrics and Gynecology, 54*(1), 40–49.

Williams, K. P., & Galerneau, F. (2003). Intrapartum fetal heart rate patterns in the prediction of neonatal acidemia. *American Journal of Obstetrics and Gynecology, 188*(3), 820–823.

Williams, R. L., & Hawes, W. E. (1979). Cesarean section, fetal monitoring, and perinatal mortality in California. *American Journal of Public Health, 69*(9), 864–870.

Nursing Care During Labor and Birth

Kristin L. Scheffer, Kristine DeButy

OBJECTIVES

After studying this chapter, you should be able to:

1. Teach the patient and family when to go to the birth facility.
2. Describe admission and continuing intrapartum nursing assessments.
3. Describe common nursing procedures used when caring for women during the intrapartum period.
4. Prioritize nursing care of the intrapartum patient in emergent situations.
5. Communicate therapeutically with the intrapartum woman and her significant others.
6. Apply the nursing process to care of the woman experiencing false or early labor.
7. Apply the nursing process to care of the woman and her significant others during the intrapartum period.
8. Identify clinical situations in which specific obstetric procedures are appropriate.
9. Explain risks, precautions, contraindications, and nursing considerations for each procedure.
10. Identify methods to provide effective emotional support to the woman undergoing an obstetric procedure.
11. Apply the nursing process to care for the woman having a cesarean birth.

Care of the woman and her family during labor and birth is a rewarding yet demanding specialty within nursing. Birth is more than a physical event. It is a powerful, life-changing event that leaves a lasting impact on the childbearing woman and her family. Every culture recognizes that birth has deep personal and social significance. Roles and relationships are forever altered by this event.

Intrapartum nurse responsibilities include assessing, supporting, documenting, and communicating labor progress to patients, their families, and providers. The nurse must support natural physical processes, promote a meaningful experience for the family, and be alert for complications. Additionally, the nurse cares for two patients, one of whom—the fetus—cannot be observed directly.

Although labor is a normal process, some women require special procedures to help them and their fetuses. This chapter will also address the nursing considerations for some of these procedures.

ADMISSION TO THE BIRTH FACILITY

The Decision to Go to the Birth Facility

During the last trimester of pregnancy, the woman needs to know when she should go to the hospital or birth center. Factors to consider include the following:
- Number and duration of any previous labors
- Distance from the hospital
- Available transportation
- Child care needs
- Risk status

During prenatal care, nurses teach women to distinguish between false (prodromal) and true labor. Nurses teach guidelines for going to the birth center and reinforce those given by the provider (see "Patient Teaching: When to Go to the Hospital or Birth Center"). Not everyone has a typical labor, so a woman should be encouraged to go to the birth center if she is uncertain or has other concerns.

PATIENT TEACHING

When to Go to the Hospital or Birth Center

These are guidelines for providing individualized instruction to women about when to enter the hospital or birth center.
- Contractions—A pattern of increasing regularity, frequency, duration, and intensity.
  - Nullipara—Regular contractions, 5 minutes apart, lasting 1 minute, for 1 hour
  - Multipara—Regular contractions, 10 minutes apart, lasting 1 minute, for 1 hour
- Ruptured membranes—A gush or trickle of fluid from the vagina should be evaluated, regardless of whether contractions are occurring.

Continued

When to Go to the Hospital or Birth Center

- Bleeding—Bright-red bleeding should be evaluated promptly. Normal bloody show is thicker, pink or dark red, and mixed with mucus.
- Decreased fetal movement—A substantial decrease in the baby's normal activity requires evaluation, your physician or nurse-midwife should be notified, or come to the labor unit.
- Other concerns—These guidelines cannot cover all situations and do not replace specific instructions given to you by your physician or nurse midwife. Therefore, go to the hospital for evaluation of any concerns and feelings that something may be wrong.

THERAPEUTIC COMMUNICATIONS

Sandra is a nursing student assigned to the intrapartum unit. A woman walks toward Sandra. The woman is leaning on a man and breathing rapidly. She says to Sandra, "I think I'm in labor, and my water broke on the way to the hospital." The staff nurse greets the woman and asks Sandra to take the woman to a labor room.

Sandra: It sounds like today's the day!

Sandra asks the woman's name (Amy) and that of her provider (Donna, CNM, a nurse-midwife) as they walk slowly to a room.

Sandra: I'm Sandra, a nursing student. What names do you want us to call each of you? *(Questioning for information. Shows respect by not assuming how the couple wants to be addressed.)*

Amy: I'm Amy, and my husband is Jeff.

Sandra: Is this your first baby, Amy, or have you had others? *(Questioning in a way that avoids "yes" or "no" answers.)*

Amy: It's my second, and the first took forever! I've been having contractions off and on since midnight, but they didn't get regular till about 6:00 this morning. They are coming every 3 minutes now and starting to hurt a lot.

Sandra helps Amy put a gown on and prepares the external fetal monitor while they wait for the RN. She does not follow up on Amy's implied concern about having a long labor, however.

Amy: Oh no . . . the monitor. . . .

Sandra: You have a problem about the monitor? *(Clarifying the nonspecific remark that Amy made about the monitor.)*

Amy: I hated having that thing on with my last baby. I had to lie the same way all the time or they couldn't hear the baby. I know it's best for the baby, though.

Sandra: You seem to have mixed feelings about the monitor. *(Reflecting what Amy seems to be feeling.)*

Amy: Yes, I didn't like it, but I do feel better knowing the baby's okay.

Sandra: We can often find ways so it doesn't bother you so much. We don't want you to feel tied down because that will make you more uncomfortable. *(Giving information without promising that Amy will be totally comfortable with the external fetal monitor.)*

Sandra observes that Amy's contractions are every 3 minutes and strong. She seeks an experienced nurse to help evaluate Amy. Sandra uses critical thinking and wisely seeks help from an experienced nurse because Amy seems to be in active labor and this is her second baby. The fact that Amy's first labor "took forever" does not necessarily mean that this labor will be long.

Nursing Responsibilities during Admission

Developing rapport, gaining a sense of birth expectations, and assessment of maternal-fetal status are three key components of the initial interaction during admission.

Establish a Therapeutic Relationship (Developing Rapport)

The nurse should quickly establish a therapeutic relationship with the woman and her significant other. The woman's first impression influences her perception of the quality of her entire birth experience. Even when the unit is busy, the nurse should communicate interest, friendliness, caring, and competence.

Nurses often encounter women who speak a language other than English. Arranging for a culturally acceptable interpreter makes the woman and her family feel welcome, promotes safety through enhanced understanding, and meets regulatory standards (The Joint Commission, 2016). Hospitals offer interpreters via telephone, online device, or in person when available.

Convey Confidence. From the first encounter, the nurse should convey confidence and optimism in the woman's ability to give birth and the ability of her significant other to support her. Women having their first baby may be overwhelmed by the pain associated with labor. The nurse can reassure these women that intense contractions are normal in active labor while helping them manage the pain and watching for complications.

Assign a Primary Nurse. Having one nurse provide all care during labor is ideal but often unrealistic. However, changes in caregivers should be limited. Explanation of caregiver roles is important.

Use Touch for Comfort. Touch can communicate acceptance, offer reassurance, and provide physical and emotional comfort to many laboring women. Women who usually do not welcome touch may appreciate it during labor. Cultural norms and personal history influence a woman's acceptance of touch from an unrelated person. The nurse should not assume the woman desires touch, but instead ask her if she welcomes or benefits from touch. As labor progresses, the woman's desire for touch may change; it may become irritating rather than comforting.

Respect Cultural Values. Cultural beliefs and practices give structure, meaning, and richness to the birth experience. They influence the behavior of both the childbearing family and the professional staff. Most cultural groups have specific practices related to childbearing. The nurse should incorporate a family's cultural practices into care as much as is safe and possible.

Determine Family Expectations about Birth. Regardless of their number of children, women and their partners have expectations about their birth experience. Whereas some women use birth plans describing what they desire, others may not have specific plans but have expectations shaped by contact with relatives, friends, previous birth experiences, and the media. An individualized birth plan brought to the hospital is a great communication tool to help the team meet the woman's birth expectations. If the woman does not have a specific birth plan, the nurse should use open-ended questions to identify the expectations of the woman and her family.

KNOWLEDGE CHECK

1. What communication skills can the nurse use to establish a therapeutic relationship when the woman and her family enter the hospital or birth center?
2. How can the nurse incorporate a couple's cultural practices into intrapartum care?

Assessment of Maternal-Fetal Status

The assessment of the obstetric patient is an ongoing, multidimensional process that begins with admission and continues throughout her hospital stay. The admission process includes performing a physical examination; reviewing the woman's medical, surgical, and obstetric history; performing a psychosocial assessment; and asking about personal preferences for labor and birth. This inquiry includes both the patient's perspective and that of her support system. Assessment does not end with completion of the admission intake process. The obstetric registered nurse (RN) continually assesses maternal-fetal status while supporting the woman and her family throughout the antenatal, birth, and postpartum periods.

The prenatal record serves as a communication tool between the provider and the birth facility. During admission, information obtained from the prenatal record is verified or updated as needed. Women who have not had prenatal care or who have received care from a provider who practices at a different facility need more extensive assessment by the nurse and provider (Table 15.1).

TABLE 15.1 Intrapartum Assessment Guide*

Assessment, Method (Selected Rationales)	Common Findings	Significant Findings and Nursing Action
Interview *Purpose:* To obtain information about the woman's pregnancy, labor, and conditions that may affect her care. The interview is curtailed if delivery is imminent.		
Introduction: Introduce yourself and ask the woman how she wants to be addressed. Ask her if she wants her partner and/or family to remain during the interview and assessment. *(Shows respect for the woman and gives her control over those she wants to remain with her.)*	Many women prefer to be addressed by their first names during labor.	The surname (family name) precedes the given name in some cultures. Clarify which name is used to properly address the woman and to properly identify both mother and newborn. Have the woman verify accuracy of identification bands before placing them on her and baby.
Culture and language: If she is from another culture, ask what her preferred language is and what language(s) she speaks, reads, or verbally understands. *(Identifies the need for an interpreter and enables the most accurate data collection.)*	Common non-English languages of women in the United States are Spanish and some Asian dialects. The most common non-English language varies with location.	Secure an interpreter fluent in the woman's primary language. Ask her if there are people who are not acceptable to her as interpreters (e.g., males or members of a group in conflict with her culture). Family members are not be the best interpreters because they may interpret selectively, adding or subtracting information as they see fit. Online or phone interpreters are available in many facilities. Hearing-impaired women may read lips well, or they may need sign-language interpreters or other assistance.
Communication: Ask the woman to tell you when she has a contraction, and pause during the interview and physical assessment. *(Shows sensitivity to her comfort and allows her to concentrate more fully on the information the nurse requests.)*	Women in active labor have difficulty answering questions or cooperating with a physical examination while they are having a contraction.	If contractions are very frequent, assess the woman's labor status promptly rather than continuing the interview. Ask only the most critical questions.
Nonverbal cues: Observe the woman's behaviors and interactions with her family and the nurse. *(Permits estimation of her level of anxiety. Identifies behaviors indicating that she should have a vaginal examination to determine whether birth is imminent.)*	*Latent phase:* Woman is sociable and mildly anxious. *Active phase:* Woman concentrates intently during contractions; often uses prepared childbirth techniques.	The unprepared or extremely anxious woman may breathe deeply and rapidly, displaying a tense facial and body posture during and between contractions. These behaviors suggest that birth is imminent: 1. Her statement that the baby is coming 2. Grunting sounds (low-pitched, guttural sounds) 3. Bearing down with abdominal muscles 4. Sitting on one buttock Euphoria, combativeness, or sedation suggests recent illicit drug ingestion.

Continued

TABLE 15.1 Intrapartum Assessment Guide*—cont'd

Assessment, Method (Selected Rationales)	Common Findings	Significant Findings and Nursing Action
Reason for admission: "What brings you to the hospital/birth center today?" *(Open-ended question promotes more complete answer.)*	Labor contractions at term, induction of labor, or observation for false labor are common reasons for admission.	Bleeding, preterm labor, pain other than labor contractions. Report these findings to the physician or nurse-midwife promptly.
Prenatal care: "Did you see a doctor or nurse-midwife during your pregnancy?" "Who is your doctor or nurse-midwife?" "How far along were you in your pregnancy when you saw the physician or nurse-midwife?" "Have you ever been admitted here before during this pregnancy?" *(Enables location of prenatal record and prior visit records.)*	Early and regular prenatal care promotes maternal and fetal health.	No prenatal care or care that was irregular or begun in late pregnancy means that complications may not have been identified.
Estimated date of delivery (EDD): "When is your baby due?" *(Determines whether gestation is term.)* "When did your last menstrual period begin?" *(For estimation of EDD if woman did not have prenatal care.)*	*Term gestation:* 37-42 wk. The woman's gestation may have been confirmed or adjusted during pregnancy with an ultrasound or other clinical examination.	Gestations earlier than the beginning of the 37th wk (preterm) or later than the end of the 42nd wk (postterm) are associated with more fetal or neonatal problems. The physician may try to stop labor that occurs earlier than 36 wk if there are no contraindications for mother or fetus.
Gravidity, parity, abortions: "How many times have you been pregnant?" "How many babies have you had? Were they full term or premature?" "How many children are now living?" "Have you had any miscarriages or abortions?" "Were there any problems with your babies after they were born?" *(Helps estimate probable speed of labor and anticipate neonatal problems.)*	Labor may be faster for the woman who has given birth before than for the nullipara. Miscarriage is used to describe a spontaneous abortion because many lay people associate the term *abortion* with only induced abortions.	Parity of 5 or more (grand multiparity) is associated with placenta previa (see Chapter 10) and postpartum hemorrhage (see Chapter 18). Women who have had several spontaneous abortions or who have given birth to infants with abnormalities may face a higher risk for an infant with a birth defect.

Pregnancy History (identifies problems that may affect this birth)

Present pregnancy: "Have you had any problems during this pregnancy, such as high blood pressure, diabetes, infections, or bleeding?"	Complications are not expected.	Women who have diabetes or hypertension may have poor placental blood flow, possibly resulting in fetal compromise. Some complications of past pregnancies, such as gestational diabetes, may recur in another pregnancy.
Past pregnancies: "Were there any problems with your other pregnancy(ies)?" "Were your other babies born vaginally or by cesarean birth?"	Women who had previous cesarean birth(s) may have a trial of labor and vaginal birth (VBAC). A woman who previously had a difficult labor or a cesarean birth may be more anxious than one who had an uncomplicated labor and birth.	Although VBAC is less common, it may be chosen for a variety of reasons. The nurse should be aware of the need for support and for complications that may be more likely in the current pregnancy.
Other: "Is there anything else you think we should know so we can better care for you?"	This open-ended question gives the woman a chance to share information that may not be elicited by other questions.	

TABLE 15.1   Intrapartum Assessment Guide*—cont'd

Assessment, Method (Selected Rationales)	Common Findings	Significant Findings and Nursing Action
Labor status: "When did your contractions become regular?" "What time did you begin to think you might really be in labor?" *(Facilitates a more accurate estimation of the time labor began.)*	Varies among women. Many women go to the birth facility when contractions first begin. Others wait until they are reasonably sure that they are really in labor.	Women who say they have been "in labor" for an unusual length of time (e.g., "for 2 days") have probably had false (prodromal) labor. These women may be very tired from the annoying and apparently nonproductive contractions.
Contractions: "How often are your contractions coming?" "How long do they last?" "Are they getting stronger?" "Tell me if you have a contraction while we are talking." *(Obtains the woman's subjective evaluation of her contractions. Alerts the nurse to palpate contractions that occur during the interview.)*	Varies according to her stage and phase of labor. Labor contractions are usually regular and show a pattern of increasing frequency, duration, and intensity.	Irregular contractions or those that do not increase in frequency, duration, or intensity are more likely to represent false labor. Contractions that are too frequent or too long can reduce placental blood flow. Incomplete uterine relaxation between contractions also can reduce placental blood flow.
Membrane status: "Has your water broken?" "What time did it break?" "What did the fluid look like?" "About how much fluid did you lose—was it a big gush or a trickle?" *(Alerts the nurse of the need to verify whether the membranes have ruptured if it is not obvious. Identifies possible prolonged rupture of membranes, preterm rupture or meconium stained fluid.)*	Most women go to the birth facility for evaluation soon after their membranes rupture. If a woman is not already in labor, contractions usually begin within a few hours after the membranes rupture at term.	If the woman's membranes have ruptured and she is not in labor or if she is not at term, a vaginal examination is often deferred. A speculum examination may be done by the physician or nurse-midwife to identify the woman's admission status. Labor may be induced if she is at term with ruptured membranes.
Allergies: "Are you allergic to any foods, medicines, or other substances?" "Do you have an allergy to latex?" "What kind of reaction do you have?" "Have you ever had a problem with anesthesia when you have had dental work?" *(Determines possible sensitivity to drugs that may be used or history of malignant hyperthermia.)*	Record any known allergies to food, medication, or other substances. As needed, describe how they affected the woman.	Allergy to seafood, iodized salt, or imaging contrast media may indicate iodine allergy. Because iodine is used in many "prep" solutions, alternative ones should be used. Allergy to latex is more common. Allergy to dental anesthetics may indicate possible allergy to the drugs used for local or regional anesthetics. These drugs usually end in the suffix *-caine*. Anesthetics also can cause severe changes in temperature and muscle contraction that can be fatal.
Food intake: "When was the last time you had something to eat or drink?" "What did you have?" *(Provides information needed to most safely administer general anesthesia if required. Identifies possible fluid or energy deficit.)*	Record the time of the woman's last food intake and what she ate. Include both liquids and solids.	If the woman says she has not had any intake for an unusual length of time, question her more closely: "Is there any food you may have forgotten, such as a snack or a drink of water or other liquid?"
Recent illness: "Have you been ill recently?" "What was the problem?" "What did you do for it?" "Have you been around anyone with a contagious illness recently?"	Most pregnant women are healthy. An occasional woman may have had a minor illness such as an upper respiratory tract infection.	Urinary tract infections are associated with preterm labor. The woman who has had contact with someone having a communicable disease may become ill and possibly infect others in the facility.
Medications: "What medications do you take that your doctor or nurse-midwife has prescribed?" "Are there any over-the-counter or herbal drugs that you use?" "I know this may be uncomfortable to discuss, but we need to know about any illegal or abused substances that you use, to more safely care for you and your baby." *(Permits evaluation of the woman's drug intake and encourages her to disclose nonprescribed use.)*	Prenatal vitamins and iron are commonly prescribed. Record all drugs the woman takes, including time and amount of last ingestion. Women often do not consider botanical preparations to be drugs. Women who use illegal substances often conceal or diminish the extent of their use because they fear reprisals.	Drugs may interact with other medications given during labor, especially analgesics and anesthetics. Substance abuse is associated with complications for the mother and infant (see Chapter 11). If the woman discloses that she uses illegal drugs, ask her what kind and the last time she ingested them (often referred to as "taking a hit"). A nonjudgmental approach in private is more likely to result in honest information.

Continued

TABLE 15.1 Intrapartum Assessment Guide*—cont'd

Assessment, Method (Selected Rationales)	Common Findings	Significant Findings and Nursing Action
Tobacco or alcohol: "Do you smoke or use tobacco in any other form? How many cigarettes a day?" "Do you use alcohol? How many drinks do you have each day (or week)?" *(Evaluates use of these legal substances.)*	As in substance abuse, women may underreport the extent of their use of tobacco or alcohol.	Infants of heavy smokers are often smaller and may have reduced placental blood flow during labor. Infants of women who use alcohol may show fetal alcohol effects at birth or later.

Birth Plans (Shows respect for the woman and her family as individuals and promotes achievement of their expectations; enables more culturally appropriate care.)

Coach or primary support person: "Who is the main person you want to be with you during labor?" Ask that person how he or she wants to be addressed, such as "Mr. Ramos" or "Carlos."	This may be the woman's husband, the baby's father, or significant other, but it may be her mother, her sister, or a friend, especially if she is single.	The woman who has little or no support from significant others probably needs more intense nursing support during labor and after the birth.
Other support: "Is there anyone else you would like to be present during labor?"	Women often want another support person present.	
Preparation for childbirth: "Did you attend prepared childbirth classes?" "Did someone go with you?"	Ideally, the woman and a partner have had some preparation in classes or self-study. Women who attended classes during previous pregnancies do not always repeat the classes during subsequent pregnancies.	The unprepared woman may need more support with simple relaxation and breathing techniques during labor. Her partner may need to learn techniques to assist her.
Preferences: "Are there any special plans you have for this birth?" "Is there anything you want to avoid?" "Did you plan to record the birth with pictures or video?"	Some women or couples have strong feelings regarding certain interventions. Common ones are (1) analgesia or anesthesia; (2) intravenous lines; (3) fetal monitoring; (4) use of episiotomy or forceps.	Conflict may arise if the woman has not previously discussed her preferences with her physician or nurse-midwife or if she is unaware of what services are available where she gives birth.
Cultural needs: "Are there any special cultural practices that you plan when you have your baby?" "How can we best help you to fulfill these practices?"	Women from Asian and Hispanic cultures may subscribe to the "hot-and-cold" theory of illness and want specific foods after birth, such as soft-boiled eggs. They may not want their water or other fluids iced.	Try to incorporate all positive or neutral cultural practices. If a practice is harmful, explain why and try to find a way to work around it if the family does not want to give it up.

Fetal Evaluation

Purpose: To determine whether the fetus seems to be healthy and tolerating labor well.		
Fetal heart rate (FHR): Assess by intermittent auscultation, or apply an external fetal monitor if that is the facility's policy (most common in the United States). Document FHR according to the risk status, stage of labor, and facility policy. *Guidelines include:* *Low risk:* Every 1 hr (latent phase), every 30 min (active phase), every 15 min (2nd stage) *High risk:* Every 30 min (latent phase), every 15 min (active phase), every 5 min (2nd stage)	Average rate at term is 110-160 bpm. Rate usually increases when the fetus moves and is reassuring.	These signs may indicate fetal stress and should be reported to the physician or nurse-midwife: 1. Rate outside the normal limits 2. Slowing of the rate that persists after the contraction ends 3. No increase in rate when the fetus moves 4. Irregular rhythm More frequent assessments should be made of the FHR and contractions if any finding is questionable.

TABLE 15.1   Intrapartum Assessment Guide*—cont'd

Assessment, Method (Selected Rationales)	Common Findings	Significant Findings and Nursing Action
Labor Status		
Purpose: To identify whether the woman is in labor and if birth is imminent. If she displays signs of imminent birth, this assessment is done as soon as she is admitted.		
Contractions (yields objective information about labor status): In addition to asking the woman about her contraction pattern, assess the contractions by palpation with the fingertips of one hand. Contractions should be assessed each time the FHR is assessed.	See Interview section earlier in table.	See Interview section earlier in table. Women who have intense contractions or who are making rapid progress should be assessed more frequently.
Vaginal examination *(Determines cervical dilation and effacement; fetal presentation, position, and station; bloody show; and status of the membranes.)*	Varies according to the stage and phase of labor. It may not be possible to determine the fetal position by vaginal examination when membranes are intact and bulging over the presenting part.	A vaginal examination is not performed if the woman reports or has evidence of active bleeding (heavier and redder than bloody show) and may not be done if her gestation is 36 wk or less and she does not seem to be in active labor. Report reasons for omitting a vaginal examination to the physician or nurse-midwife.
Status of membranes: During a vaginal examination, a flow of fluid suggests ruptured membranes. A **pH test** and/or **fern test** may be done, often using a sterile speculum examination. The presence of amniotic fluid will turn pH paper blue. The fern test involves collecting fluid from the vagina during a speculum exam, smearing it on a microscope slide and examining the slide under the microscope. Amniotic fluid will form a fern pattern on the slide when it dries. *(Test is not needed if it is obvious that the membranes have ruptured.)*	Amniotic fluid should be clear, possibly containing flecks of white vernix. Its odor is distinctive but not offensive. The test with a color change of blue-green to dark blue (pH > 6.5) suggests true rupture of the membranes but is not conclusive. The fern test is more diagnostic of true rupture of membranes because it is less likely to be affected by vaginal infections, recent intercourse, or other factors.	A greenish color indicates meconium staining, which may be associated with fetal compromise or postterm gestation and puts the infant at risk for meconium aspiration syndrome (see Chapter 24). Thick green-black meconium may be passed by the fetus in a breech presentation and is not necessarily associated with fetal compromise. Cloudy, yellowish, strong-smelling, or foul-smelling fluid suggests infection. Bloody fluid may indicate partial placental separation (see Chapter 10).
Leopold's maneuvers: Often done before assessing the FHR to locate the best place for assessment. *(Identifies fetal presentation and position. Most accurate when combined with information from vaginal examination.)*	A cephalic presentation with the head well flexed (vertex) is normal. The fetal head is often easily displaced upward ("floating") if the woman is not in labor. When the head is engaged, it cannot be displaced upward with Leopold's maneuvers.	A hard, round, freely movable object in the fundus suggests a fetal head, meaning the fetus is in a breech presentation. Less commonly, the fetus may be crosswise in the uterus—a transverse lie.
Pain: Note discomfort during and between contractions. Note tenderness when palpating contractions. *(Distinguishes between normal labor pain and abnormal pain that may be associated with a complication.)*	There may be verbal or nonverbal evidence of pain with contractions, but the woman should be relatively comfortable between contractions. The skin around the umbilicus is often sensitive.	Constant pain or a tender, rigid uterus suggests a complication, such as placental abruption (separated placenta) or, less commonly, uterine rupture.

Continued

TABLE 15.1 Intrapartum Assessment Guide*—cont'd

Assessment, Method (Selected Rationales)	Common Findings	Significant Findings and Nursing Action
Physical Examination		
Purpose: To evaluate the woman's general health and identify conditions that may affect her intrapartum and postpartum care.		
General appearance: Observe skin color and texture, nutritional state, and appearance of rest or fatigue. Examine the woman's face, fingers, and lower extremities for edema. Ask her if she can take her rings off and put them on.	Women are often fatigued if their sleep has been interrupted by Braxton Hicks contractions, fetal activity, or frequent urination. Mild edema of the lower extremities is common in late pregnancy.	Pallor suggests anemia. Substantial edema of the face and fingers or extreme (pitting) edema of the lower extremities is associated with pre-eclampsia, although it may occur in the absence of this hypertensive disorder (see Chapter 10).
Vital signs: Take the woman's temperature, pulse rate, respirations, and blood pressure. Reassess the temperature every 2-4 hr (every hour after membranes rupture or if temperature is elevated); reassess blood pressure, pulse, and respirations every hour.	*Temperature:* 35.8-37.3°C (96.4-99.1°F) *Pulse rate:* 60-100 bpm *Respirations:* 12-20/min, even and unlabored Blood pressure near baseline levels established during pregnancy. Transient elevations of blood pressure are common when the woman is first admitted, but they return to baseline levels within about 30 min.	Report abnormalities to physician or nurse-midwife. Temperature of 38°C (100.4°F) or higher suggests infection. Pulse rate and respirations also may be elevated. Pulse rate and blood pressure may be elevated if the woman is extremely anxious or in pain. A blood pressure ≥140 mm Hg or ≥90 mm Hg diastolic or higher is considered hypertensive. For women who did not have prenatal care, there is no baseline for comparison.
Heart and lung sounds: Auscultate all areas with a stethoscope.	Heart sounds should be clear with a distinct S_1 and S_2. A physiologic murmur is common because of the increased blood volume and cardiac output. Breath sounds should be clear, with respirations even and unlabored.	The woman who is breathing rapidly and deeply may have symptoms of hyperventilation: tingling and spasm of the fingers, numbness around the lips.
Abdomen: Observe for scars at the same time Leopold's maneuvers and the FHR are assessed. It is usually sufficient to assess the fundal height by observing its relation to the xiphoid process.	Striae (stretch marks) are common. If scars are noted, ask the woman what surgery she had and when. The fundus at term is usually slightly below the xiphoid process but varies with maternal height and fetal size and number.	Report a previous cesarean birth to the physician or nurse-midwife. Transverse uterine scars are least likely to rupture if the woman is in labor. Measure the fundal height (see Chapter 7) if the fetus seems small or if the gestation is questionable.
Deep tendon reflexes (DTRs): Assess patellar reflex (see Chapter 10). Upper extremity DTRs also should be evaluated at admission if epidural block analgesia is planned because they are normally not as strong as the patellar reflex.	A brisk jerk without spasm or sustained muscle contraction is normal. Some women normally have hypoactive reflexes, but at least a slight twitch is expected. Obese women may appear to have diminished reflexes because of the fat tissue over the tendon.	Report absent (uncommon unless the woman is receiving magnesium sulfate) or hyperactive reflexes. Hyperactive reflexes and clonus (repeated tapping when the foot is dorsiflexed) are associated with preeclampsia, hypertension, and often precede a seizure (see Chapter 10).
Midstream urine specimen: Assess protein and glucose levels with a dipstick. Follow instructions on the package for waiting times. Check for ketones if the woman has not eaten for a prolonged period or has been vomiting. Send a separate specimen for urinalysis, if ordered.	Negative or trace of protein and glucose; negative ketones.	Proteinuria is associated with preeclampsia but also may be associated with urinary tract infections or a specimen contaminated with vaginal secretions. Glycosuria is associated with diabetes. Ketonuria is common in poorly controlled diabetes or if the woman does not eat adequate carbohydrates to meet her energy needs.

TABLE 15.1   Intrapartum Assessment Guide*—cont'd

Assessment, Method (Selected Rationales)	Common Findings	Significant Findings and Nursing Action
Laboratory tests: Women who have had prenatal care may not need as many admission tests. Common tests include the following:		
1. Complete blood cell count (or hematocrit done on unit)	1. Hemoglobin at least 11 g/dL (grams per deciliter); hematocrit at least 33%.	1. Values lower than these reduce maternal reserve for normal blood loss at birth.
2. Blood type and Rh factor	2. The woman who is Rh-negative and has had regular prenatal care receives Rh immune globulin at 28 wk of gestation to prevent formation of anti-Rh antibodies.	2. Rh-negative mothers need Rh immune globulin after birth if the infant is Rh-positive.
3. Serum tests for syphilis. Other routine admission tests may include serum HIV, vaginal gonorrhea and chlamydia, or vaginal GBS tests. Drug screens may be ordered for a woman who has not had prenatal care.	3. Negative on all. GBS screening may have been done recently during a prenatal visit late in pregnancy.	3. A positive test indicates the baby could be infected and needs treatment after birth. The mother should be treated if she has not been treated already. Maternal antibiotics are given for positive GBS to reduce newborn infection from organisms within the vagina.

*Women who have had prenatal care have much of this information available on their prenatal record. The nurse need only verify it or update it, as needed.

bpm, Beats per minute; *GBS,* group B *Streptococcus; HIV,* human immunodeficiency virus; *VBAC,* vaginal birth after cesarean.

Focused Assessment. On admission, a focused assessment is performed before the broader database assessment is completed. Assessment priorities are set by the condition of the mother and fetus and whether birth is imminent. (See Box 15.1 for assisting with an emergency birth.) This assessment includes, at a minimum, the patient's chief complaint, assessment of the fetal heart rate, maternal vital signs, and uterine contractions/labor progress (American Academy of Pediatrics AAP & American College of Obstetricians and Gynecologists [AAP & ACOG], 2012; Simpson & O'Brien-Abel, 2014).

Fetal Heart Rate. For assessment of a term fetus using intermittent auscultation, the following fetal heart rate (FHR) guidelines are considered normal, category I (Killion, 2015; Lyndon, O'Brien-Abel, & Simpson, 2014; Miller, Miller, & Cypher, 2017; Freeman et al., 2012):

- A baseline rate of 110 beats per minute (bpm) to 160 bpm
- Regular rhythm
- Absence of decreases from the baseline
- Presence of increases from the baseline

If electronic fetal monitoring (EFM) is used, additional characteristics indicating fetal well-being include the following:

- Presence of accelerations in the FHR baseline may be present
- Absence of pathologic (late, variable, or prolonged) decelerations
- Moderate variability (see Chapter 14).

Maternal Vital Signs. Maternal vital signs provide insight into well-being of both the mother and the fetus. They identify complications such as hypertension or infection.

Hypertension during pregnancy is defined as a sustained blood pressure increase of 140 mm Hg systolic or 90 mm Hg diastolic or higher. Hypertension may be transient, related to pregnancy, or chronic (AAP & ACOG, 2012; Roberts, August, & Bakris, 2013). A temperature of 38°C (100.4°F) or higher suggests infection. Tachypnea, hypotension, and tachycardia also can be associated with varying degrees of maternal complications such as infection, respiratory distress, or blood loss.

Impending Birth. Grunting sounds, bearing down, sitting on one buttock, and saying urgently, "The baby's coming" suggest imminent birth. In this situation, the nurse abbreviates the initial assessment and collects other information after birth. While the nurse cares for the mother, pertinent/critical information can be quickly gathered if birth is imminent:

- Names of mother and support person(s)
- Name of her provider if she had prenatal care
- Number of pregnancies and prior births, including whether the births were vaginal or cesarean
- Status of membranes
- Expected date of delivery
- Problems during this or other pregnancies
- Significant medical and surgical history
- Allergies to medications, foods, or other substances
- Time and type of last oral intake
- Maternal vital signs and FHR
- Pain: Location, intensity, factors that intensify or relieve, duration, whether constant or intermittent, whether the pain is acceptable to the woman

BOX 15.1   Assisting with an Emergency Birth

The inexperienced nurse rarely must deliver a baby in the hospital or birth center but occasionally helps the more experienced nurse do so. Unplanned out-of-hospital births are not common, but they do occur.

Nursing Priorities for an Emergency Birth in Any Setting
Prevent or reduce injury to the mother and infant.
Maintain the infant's airway and temperature after birth.

Preparing for an Emergency Birth
Study the delivery sequence in Figs. 15.7 and 15.8.
Locate the emergency delivery pack ("precip" tray) on the unit.

During the Birth
Remain with the woman to assist her in giving birth. Use the call bell or ask her partner to call for help. Stay calm to reduce the couple's anxiety.
Put on gloves to prevent contact with blood and other secretions. Sterile gloves reduce transmission of environmental organisms to the mother and the infant. However, the nurse will be "catching" the infant in this situation. No invasive procedure is expected, so clean gloves are adequate.

After the Birth
Observe the infant's color and respirations for distress. Wipe excess secretions from the infant's face and mouth with a clean cloth. Suction the mouth and nose with a bulb syringe if necessary.
Dry the infant and place skin-to-skin with the mother. Cover mother and baby with warmed blankets to maintain warmth.
Put the infant to the mother's breast and encourage suckling to promote uterine contraction, which will facilitate placental expulsion and control bleeding, as well as initiate lactation.

The provider is notified promptly if any of the following are identified or suspected (AAP & ACOG, 2012; Simpson & O'Brien-Abel, 2014; Wisner & Gauthier, 2015):

- Imminent birth
- Indeterminate (category II) or abnormal (category III) FHR (see Chapter 14)
- Abnormal vital signs
- Vaginal bleeding
- Preterm labor
- Preterm premature rupture of membranes (PPROM)
- Acute abdominal pain

KNOWLEDGE CHECK

3. What are the three assessment priorities when a woman comes to the intrapartum unit?
4. What FHR characteristics (when auscultated) are normal?
5. What observations suggest that a woman is going to give birth very soon? What should the nurse do in that case?

Database Assessment. If focused assessments of mother and fetus are normal and birth is not imminent, a more complete admission assessment is performed to further assess the mother, fetus, and available maternal support persons.

CRITICAL THINKING EXERCISE 15.1

During a labor admission assessment, a woman quickly denies her use of drugs and herbal preparations other than her prenatal vitamins. She becomes quiet, answering the nurse's questions in a terse manner.

Questions
1. What might explain the woman's change in behavior?
2. Should the nurse alter the assessment interview?

Basic Information. Regulatory agencies and defined standards of care require certain elements to be addressed on admission to the hospital. Intrapartum admission forms guide the nurse to obtain required information. Typical information includes the following:

- Chief complaint—Reason for coming to the hospital or birth center (e.g., contractions, rupture of membranes, decreased fetal movement, headache)
- Prenatal care—When it began, her most recent visit, and the name of her provider
- Estimated date of delivery (**EDD**, also may be abbreviated **EDB** [estimated date of birth])
- Number of pregnancies, births, or spontaneous and elective **abortions**
- Allergies—Medications, food, or other substances such as latex
- Last solid food and oral intake—What time was it consumed
- Medical, surgical, and pregnancy histories
- Recent illness, including treatment
- Medications, including prescription and over-the-counter drugs, tobacco, alcohol, and other substances of abuse
- Complementary or alternative therapy or use of herbal and botanical preparations and their purposes
- The woman's subjective evaluation of her labor
- Birth plans, including planned pain management methods
- Support persons—Who they are and the role of each
- Domestic violence—Risk or history of (ask only when the woman is alone)
- Psychosocial well-being, including history of depression, anxiety, or suicidal risk
- Other important aspects include assessment of nutrition, resources at home, level of education, and learning style

Women often bring several people with them to the birthing room and want them to stay during admission. Caution is prudent when asking sensitive information, such as prior pregnancies, sexually transmitted infections (STIs), and potential abuse, when others are present. The woman's partner and other visitors may be unaware of her history. Delay asking intimate information until the woman is alone for confidentiality, safety, and accuracy.

Physical Examination. A physical examination evaluates the woman's overall health and covers important observations relating to pregnancy, including the presence and location of edema, abdominal scars, and the height of the fundus.

Fetal Assessments. The fetal presentation and position are assessed using a combination of vaginal examination and Leopold's maneuvers (Procedure 15.1). The FHR is assessed

NURSING PROCEDURE 15.1 Leopold's Maneuvers

PURPOSE: Systematic assessment using four distinct maneuvers to determine presentation and position of the fetus and aid in location of fetal heart sounds. Also provides assessment of uterine tone, irritability, tenderness, and presence or absence of contractions.

1. Explain the procedure to the woman and the rationale for each step as it is performed. Tell her what is found at each step. *Gives information, teaches the woman, and reassures her when the assessment findings are normal.*

2. Ask the woman to empty her bladder if she has not done so recently. Have her lie on her back with her knees flexed slightly. Place a small pillow or folded towel under one hip. *Decreases discomfort of a full bladder during palpation and improves ability to feel fetal parts in the suprapubic area. Knee flexion helps the woman relax her abdominal muscles to enhance palpation. Uterine displacement prevents aortocaval compression, which could reduce blood flow to the placenta.*

3. Wash your hands with warm water. Wear gloves if contact with secretions is likely. *Prevents transmission of microorganisms. Warm hands are more comfortable during palpation and prevent tensing of abdominal muscles.*

4. Stand beside the woman, facing her head, with your dominant hand nearest her. *The first three maneuvers are most easily performed in this position.*

5. First maneuver—Palpate the uterine fundus. Use the flat palmar surface of hands, with fingers together using gentle, but firm pressure to perform palpation. The breech (buttocks) is softer and more irregular in shape than the head. Moving the breech also moves the fetal trunk. The head is harder and has a round, uniform shape. The head can be moved without moving the entire fetal trunk. *Distinguishes between a cephalic and breech presentation. If the fetus is in a cephalic presentation, the breech is felt in the fundus. If the presentation is breech, the head is felt in the fundus.*

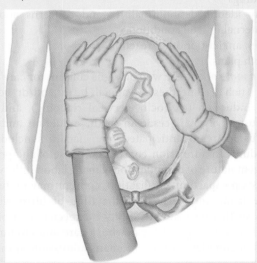

6. Second maneuver—Hold the left hand steady on one side of the uterus while palpating the opposite side of the uterus with the right hand. With the right hand, start palpating at the uterine fundus and progress downward toward the symphysis pubis. Then hold the right hand steady while palpating the opposite side of the uterus with the left hand. The fetal back is a smooth, convex surface. The fetal arms and legs feel nodular, irregular, or protruding, and the fetus often moves them during palpation. *Determines on which side of the uterus is the back and on which side are the fetal arms and legs ("small parts").*

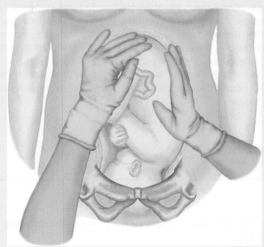

7. Third maneuver (Pallach's maneuver or grip)—Palpate the suprapubic area. Attempt to grasp the presenting part gently between the thumb and middle finger. If the presenting part is not engaged, the grasping movement of the fingers moves it upward in the uterus. If the presenting part is engaged, it remains fixed and difficult to move. If a breech was palpated in the fundus, expect a hard, rounded head in this area. *Confirms the presentation determined in the first maneuver. Determines whether the presenting part is engaged (widest diameter at or below zero station) in the maternal pelvis.*

8. Omit the fourth maneuver if the fetus is in a breech presentation. Is performed only in cephalic presentations to determine whether the fetal head is flexed.

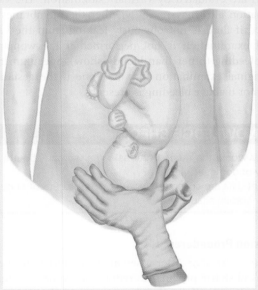

Continued

NURSING PROCEDURE 15.1   Leopold's Maneuvers—cont'd

9. Fourth maneuver—Turn so that you face the woman's feet. *Is most easily performed in this position.*

10. Place your hands on each side of the uterus with fingers pointed toward the pelvic inlet. Slide hands downward on each side of the uterus. On one side, your fingers easily slide to the upper edge of the symphysis. On the other side, your fingers meet an obstruction, the cephalic prominence. *Determines whether the head is flexed (vertex) or extended (face). The vertex presentation is normal. If the head is flexed, the cephalic prominence (the forehead in this case) is felt on the opposite side from the fetal back. If the head is extended, the cephalic prominence (the occiput in this case) is felt on the same side as the fetal back.*

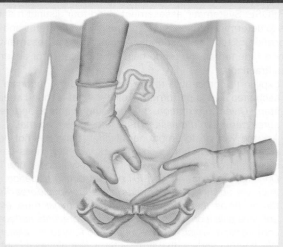

---

by intermittent auscultation or electronic monitoring (see Chapter 14).

Labor Status. The woman's labor status is determined by assessing her contraction pattern, performing vaginal examination, and determining whether her membranes have ruptured. A sudden gush, or steady leakage of fluid from the vagina may indicate ruptured membranes. If there is doubt, vaginal fluid may be tested for pH or examined under a microscope for the presence of ferning (see Table 15.1). The nurse documents the time of rupture, color, amount, and odor of the amniotic fluid. Contractions are assessed by palpation (Procedure 15.2) or via the electronic monitor. Cervical dilation, effacement, station, fetal presentation, and position are evaluated by vaginal examination. The vaginal examination also may reveal whether the membranes have ruptured if fluid is not obviously leaking from the vagina. Vaginal examination is not performed if the woman has active bleeding (other than bloody show). Speculum rather than vaginal examination may be done if the gestation is preterm or if active bleeding is present.

? KNOWLEDGE CHECK

6. Why would the nurse defer asking a woman about a history of domestic violence?
7. What data are collected to determine the current status of the woman's labor?

Admission Procedures

Notify the Provider. After assessment the nurse notifies the woman's obstetric provider to report the woman's status and obtain orders. The following data are provided:

- The woman's name and age
- Gravidity, parity, term and preterm births, abortions (spontaneous and elective), and living children
- EDD and fundal height if it conflicts with the date
- Contraction pattern
- Results of vaginal examination:
  - Cervical dilation and effacement
  - Fetal presentation and position
  - Station of the presenting part
  - Membrane status
- FHR and uterine activity (UA) pattern
- Maternal vital signs
- Relevant history, including medical, surgical, and obstetric findings
- Any identified abnormalities and concerns about the maternal or fetal condition
- Pain, anxiety, or other reactions to labor
- Birth plans

Consent Forms. The woman signs consent for care during labor, such as anesthesia, vaginal birth and/or cesarean birth, induction (oxytocin, cervical ripening), and blood transfusion. Even if cesarean birth, induction and blood transfusion are not anticipated, many facilities include these procedures in admission consents because of the potential emergent nature of complications during labor. If the woman requests postpartum sterilization, consent may be required before labor and verified at the time of birth with the emphasis that permanent sterility is expected after bilateral tubal ligation. Consent for newborn care and circumcision are often completed on the woman's admission to the birth facility.

Laboratory Tests. Common laboratory results needed on admission to the labor and delivery unit include complete blood count, blood type, human immunodeficiency virus (HIV) screen, hepatitis B surface antigen, Venereal Disease Research Laboratory (VDRL) or rapid plasma reagin (RPR) tests for syphilis, rubella titer, and midstream urine specimen to assess protein, glucose, and ketones. Women who receive prenatal care may have laboratory results available on the

NURSING PROCEDURE 15.2 Palpating Contractions

PURPOSE: To determine uterine tone at rest and during contractions; to measure frequency, duration, intensity, relaxation time, and resting tone. Also can provide information about uterine tenderness, fetal size, and fetal movement.

1. Assess at least three contractions in a row at the time the fetal heart rate (FHR) is checked. Guidelines for minimal frequency of assessments for low-risk patients are, therefore, as follows: (Wisner & Ali, 2015)
    a. Latent phase: < 4 cm, at least hourly; 4 to 5 cm, every 30 minutes
    b. Every 30 minutes during active phase and transition
    c. Every 15 minutes during second stage
    Assess more frequently if abnormalities are identified. Assessment of at least three sequential contractions permits better evaluation of the pattern. Palpate contractions periodically when an external fetal monitor is used because it is not accurate for intensity or resting tone because of the thickness of the abdominal fat pad, maternal position, and fetal position.

2. Place fingertips of one hand on the uterine fundus, using light pressure. Keep fingertips relatively still rather than moving them over the uterus. *The fingertips are more sensitive to the first tightening of the uterus. Contractions usually begin in the fundus, although the mother usually feels them in her lower abdomen and back. Constant moving of the hand over the uterus may stimulate contractions and give an inaccurate assessment of their true pattern.*

3. Note the time when each contraction begins and ends.
    a. Determine frequency by noting the average time that elapses from the beginning of one contraction to the beginning of the next one.
    b. Determine duration by noting the average time in seconds from the beginning to the end of each contraction.
    c. Determine relaxation time interval by noting the average time between the end of one contraction and the beginning of the next one.

Contractions are expected to increase in frequency, duration, and intensity as labor progresses. False labor is usually characterized by contractions that are irregular and do not increase in frequency, duration, and intensity.

4. Estimate the average intensity of contractions by noting how easily the uterus can be indented during the peak of the contraction:
    a. With mild contractions, the uterus can be easily indented with the fingertips. The contractions feel similar to the tip of the nose.
    b. With moderate contractions, the uterus is firm and is indented with more difficulty. The contractions feel similar to the chin.
    c. With firm contractions, the uterus feels rigid or board-like and cannot be readily indented. The contractions feel similar to the forehead.
    Contractions during labor are expected to intensify progressively. If they do not, the woman may not be in true labor or she may be experiencing dysfunctional labor. (Report excessive uterine activity, whether spontaneous or stimulated by induction or cervical ripening agent.)
    a. Tachysystole—More than 5 contractions in 10 minutes, averaged over 30 minutes
    b. Tetanic contractions—Series of single contractions with durations longer than 120 seconds
    c. Inadequate relaxation time—Intervals shorter than 60 seconds between contractions in first-stage labor; less than 45 to 50 seconds between contractions in second stage
    d. Hypertonus—Incomplete relaxation of the uterus between contractions as noted by uterine tone that does not return to soft by palpation or a resting tone that exceeds 20 to 25 mm Hg with an intrauterine pressure catheter
    Excessive uterine activity reduces placental blood flow by prolonged compression of the vessels that supply the intervillous spaces.

---

prenatal record. Guidelines for STI testing are recommended by the state health department in collaboration with the Centers for Disease Control and Prevention. The obstetric provider may order additional tests pertinent to the patient's presenting complaint and medical history. When there is no prenatal record available on admission, more extensive testing may be required.

Intravenous Access. If ordered, intravenous (IV) access is started with a large-bore (18-gauge or larger) catheter. A saline lock may be used, or the woman may receive a continuous infusion of fluids. The saline lock allows freedom of movement when walking during early labor but provides quick access if fluids or medications are needed. Continuous fluid infusion reduces dehydration and is necessary if epidural analgesia is used. IV solutions containing electrolytes, such as lactated Ringer's solution, are the most common fluids administered.

Ongoing Assessments. If it is unclear after the initial assessment whether the woman is in true labor, the woman may be observed. After 1 or 2 hours, progressive cervical change (effacement, dilation, or both) strongly suggests true labor.

After the admission assessment, the woman and fetus need ongoing evaluations based on their risk status to promote well-being and minimize the risk for iatrogenic harm and avoid unnecessary interventions. General guidelines for continuing assessments are listed here.

Maternal Assessments
Labor Progress
The frequency of vaginal examinations depends on the woman's parity, status of her membranes, and overall speed of her labor (Fig. 15.1). Vaginal examinations are limited to avoid the introduction of microorganisms from the perineal area into the uterus.

Pressure of the fetal head on the rectum in late labor makes many women feel the need to have a bowel movement. The nurse should look at the perineum for **crowning** (appearance of the fetal scalp or presenting part at the vaginal opening) and perform a sterile vaginal examination if the woman suddenly expresses an urge to push or have a bowel movement during a contraction.

PURPOSES
To determine whether membranes have ruptured.
To determine cervical effacement and dilation.
To determine fetal presentation, position, and station.

METHOD
Vaginal examination is not usually performed by the inexperienced nurse except when training for graduate nursing practice in the intrapartum area.

EQUIPMENT
Sterile gloves, sterile lubricant. If a pH swab or nitrazine paper is being used to test for ruptured membranes, lubricant is not used to avoid altering the test paper.

HAND POSITION

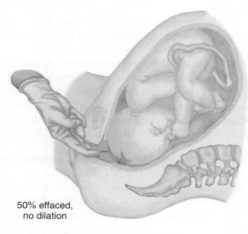

50% effaced,
no dilation

The nurse usually uses the index and middle fingers of the dominant hand for vaginal examination. The thumb and other fingers are kept out of the way to avoid carrying microorganisms into the vagina.

DETERMINING WHETHER MEMBRANES HAVE RUPTURED

Intact membranes feel like a slippery membrane over the fetal presenting part. No leakage of amniotic fluid can be detected.

Bulging membranes feel like a slippery, fluid-filled balloon over the presenting part. It may be difficult to feel the presenting part clearly if the membranes are bulging tensely.

Ruptured membranes show drainage of fluid from the vagina as the nurse manipulates the cervix and presenting part.

DETERMINING CERVICAL EFFACEMENT AND DILATION

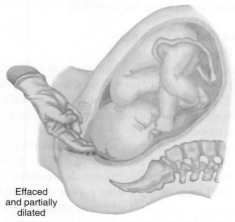

Effaced
and partially
dilated

The nurse determines *effacement* by estimating the thickness of the cervix. The uneffaced cervix is about 2 cm long. If it is 50% effaced, it is about 1 cm long. Effacement is expressed as a percentage (0% to 100%), or it may be described as the length in centimeters.

Dilation is determined by sweeping the fingertips across the cervical opening. The average woman's index finger is about 1.5 cm in diameter.

DETERMINING THE PRESENTING PART

The fetal skull feels smooth, hard, and rounded in a cephalic presentation. The fetal buttocks are softer and more irregular in a breech presentation. If the membranes are ruptured, the fetus in a breech presentation may expel thick, green-black meconium. (Presence of meconium in a breech presentation is *not* necessarily a sign of fetal compromise. The nurse must evaluate other signs of fetal condition.)

DETERMINING THE FETAL POSITION

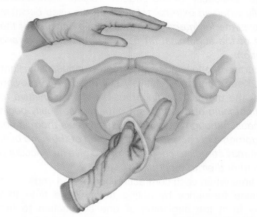

In a cephalic presentation, the nurse feels for the distinctive features of the fetal skull. The posterior fontanel is usually felt in a vertex presentation and is triangular with three suture lines (two lambdoid and one sagittal) leading into it. The anterior fontanel is not felt unless the head is poorly flexed or is in the mechanism of extension in late labor. It feels like a diamond-shaped depression with four suture lines (one frontal, two coronal, and one sagittal) leading into it.

DETERMINING THE STATION

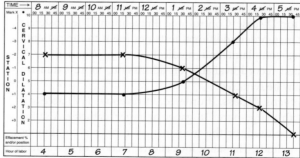

Findings of the vaginal examination may be recorded on a labor flow sheet, narrative, or a graph. The graph may be termed a *Friedman curve*, a *partogram*, or a *labor curve*.

FIG. 15.1 Vaginal Examination during Labor.

Contractions

Normal UA during labor includes less than or equal to 5 contractions in a 10-minute window. Contractions can be assessed by palpation or with the electronic fetal monitor. As defined by National Institute of Child Health and Human Development, excessive UA leads to progressive fetal decompensation secondary to inadequate blood flow to the intervillous space compromising fetal gas exchange and a resultant increased risk for development of fetal acidemia (Bakker, Kurver, Kuik, & VanGeijin, 2007; Macones, Hankins, Spong, Hauth, & Moore, 2008; Miller et al., 2017). The goal is to maintain normal UA by intervening for any cases of excessive UA. (See Chapter 14.)

Intake and Output

Oral and IV intake and each void are recorded. Labor may reduce a woman's urge to void; therefore her suprapubic area should be checked every 2 hours or more frequently to identify bladder distention.

Response to Labor

The woman's behavioral responses change as labor intensifies, especially if she has not had epidural analgesia. Often, this response is determined by cultural expectations. She may withdraw from interactions but need more nursing presence and reassurance. She may experience anxiety for any number of reasons: pain and fear of bodily injury, unknown outcome, loss of control, unresolved psychological issues that influence her readiness to give birth (e.g., sexual abuse, previous birth experiences), or unexpected occurrences during labor. Anxiety has been associated with increased catecholamine release that can cause dysfunctional labor/ineffective UA (Simpson & O'Brien-Abel, 2014).

Women experience a broad range of emotions that can affect their ability to cope with labor. Interventions to assist the woman include both nonpharmacologic and pharmacologic measures. The goal of nursing care is to support the woman's desires and manage her pain, while not interfering with her labor progress or causing adverse outcomes for the woman or fetus. Roberts, Gulliver, Fisher, and Cloyes (2010) developed an algorithm for assessing a woman's ability to cope with labor as an alternative to the traditional pain scale of 0 to 10. Signs of coping include the following:

- States she is coping
- Focused inward
- Has rhythmic motion and breathing patterns
- Able to relax between contractions

Behaviors that suggest the woman may not be coping with labor include the following:

- Specific requests for medication and other pain control measures such as epidural analgesia
- Statements that current measures are ineffective
- Tension of her muscles and arching of her back or panicked activity during contractions
- Crying, tearfulness, tremulous voice
- A tense facial expression, rolling in the bed
- States she is not coping; may use expressions such as "I can't take it anymore"

Labor support plays an integral role in perinatal outcomes. The 2013 Cochrane Database review on Continuous Labor Support during childbirth looked at 22 trials involving over 15,000 women. They found that women who had continuous labor support were more likely to have shorter labors without analgesia that resulted in spontaneous vaginal delivery. They were less likely to have operative vaginal births or infants with low 5-minute Apgar status, or report dissatisfaction with the birth experience. This review also stated that support was most effective when it was delivered by someone other than hospital staff (Hodnett, Gates, Hofmeyr, & Sakala, 2013). Therefore the inclusion of the woman's support system is integral to her labor.

Support Person's Response

Labor can be stressful for the woman's partner/support person. Often, the person may become anxious, fearful, or tired. The person may feel a responsibility to protect and support the woman but may have limited resources for doing so. Watching the woman in pain is difficult, even if the pain is normal. The support person may respond to stress in many ways, including being quiet, suffering silently, or reacting with pacing and anger. At times, the person may respond by leaving the room frequently or for long periods, whereas others resist even short breaks.

Cultural norms may dictate that the father's presence during labor and birth is strictly prohibited. The father may be pulled in two directions, wanting to be included but hesitating because men in his culture are not customarily involved in birth. The nurse should respect the values of each couple and their wishes about paternal involvement.

The support person also may be the woman's parent, another relative, friend, or significant other. The nurse should remember that anyone who assists the woman during labor may have feelings of anxiety and helplessness at times. Reassurance and care for the labor partner strengthen the person's ability to support the woman and enhance the likelihood that both will view the birth experience as positive.

Fetal Assessments

Assessments are performed to identify signs of well-being and those that suggest compromise. The principal fetal assessments include FHR patterns and character of the amniotic fluid. Abnormalities revealed in these assessments may be associated with impaired fetal gas exchange and infection (see Chapter 14).

Fetal Heart Rate

FHR is assessed using either intermittent auscultation or EFM. Frequency of assessment and documentation depends on the risk status of the mother and fetus and the stage of labor. FHR assessments are recommended before and after procedures or interventions that might change the intrauterine environment or the relationship of the fetus to its environment. Some examples include rupture of membranes (spontaneous or artificial), ambulation of the patient, administration of analgesia or anesthesia, administrations of induction agents, or vaginal examinations. This assessment and documentation of fetal status allows the clinician to demonstrate the response of the fetus to procedures/interventions.

❓ CRITICAL THINKING EXERCISE 15.2

Chloe is in labor at term with her second baby. The baby is in a left occiput anterior position, and Chloe's cervix is 5 cm dilated and completely effaced. Her membranes rupture at the end of a strong contraction. You note that the fluid is green and watery.

Question
1. What nursing actions are most important at this time? Why?

Fetal Membranes and Amniotic Fluid

Spontaneous rupture of membranes (SROM) may occur, or the provider may perform an amniotomy. **Amniotomy** (artificial rupture of the membranes or AROM) is usually performed in conjunction with **induction** (artificial initiation) and **augmentation** of labor (artificial stimulation of uterine contractions) and to allow internal EFM.

The time of rupture, FHR, color, odor, and quantity of the amniotic fluid are noted and charted. The fluid should be clear and may include bits of vernix, the creamy white fetal skin lubricant, and have a mild, musty smell. A large amount of vernix in the fluid suggests that the fetus may be preterm. Greenish, meconium-stained fluid may be seen in response to transient fetal hypoxia, postterm gestation, or placental insufficiency. Fluid with a foul or strong odor, cloudy appearance, or yellow color suggests **chorioamnionitis** (inflammation of the amniotic sac, usually caused by bacterial and viral infections).

Quantity of fluid should be described in approximate terms; for example, at term, a "large" amount is more than 1000 mL, a "moderate" amount is approximately 500 to 1000 mL, and "scant" amniotic fluid is a trickle, barely enough to detect. If the fetus is engaged in the pelvis when the membranes rupture, a small amount of fluid in front of the fetal presenting part may be discharged (forewaters or forebag), with the rest lost at birth. **Polyhydramnios** (excessive volume of amniotic fluid) is associated with some fetal abnormalities. **Oligohydramnios** (abnormally small quantity of amniotic fluid) may be associated with placental insufficiency or fetal urinary tract abnormalities.

AROM and SROM are associated with risks that the nurse must observe for, including prolapse of the umbilical cord, infection, and placental abruption.

Prolapse of the Umbilical Cord. The primary risk at the time of rupture is that the umbilical cord will slip down in the gush of fluid. The cord can be compressed between the fetal presenting part and the woman's pelvis, obstructing blood flow to and from the placenta and reducing fetal gas exchange. The FHR is assessed for at least 1 full minute after amniotomy or SROMs. Indeterminate or abnormal patterns or significant changes from previous assessments are reported promptly to the provider. Cord compression is usually accompanied by variable or prolonged decelerations or a bradycardic FHR.

Infection. With interruption of the membrane barrier, vaginal organisms have free access to the intrauterine cavity and may cause chorioamnionitis. The risk is low at first but increases as the interval between membrane rupture and birth increases. Twenty-four percent of patients will develop chorioamnionitis with rupture of 24 hours or longer. Rates of up to 60% incidence are noted in pregnancies that are remote from term (Mercer, 2014). Birth within 24 hours of membrane rupture is desirable, although infection does not occur at any absolute time.

Abruptio Placentae. **Abruptio placentae,** also known as placental abruption (Chapter 10), can occur if the uterus is distended with excessive amniotic fluid when the membranes rupture. As the uterus collapses with discharge of the amniotic fluid, the area of placental attachment shrinks. The placenta then no longer fits its implantation site and partially separates. A large area of placental disruption can significantly reduce fetal oxygenation, nutrition, and waste disposal (Cunningham et al., 2014).

Nursing Considerations: Assisting with an Amniotomy. Obtain a baseline FHR via electronic monitoring or auscultation before amniotomy is performed. The initial fetal assessment provides a baseline to compare with later assessments.

Before amniotomy, two or three underpads should be placed under the woman's buttocks to absorb the fluid; the underpads should be overlapped to extend from her waist to her knees. A folded bath towel under the buttocks absorbs more amniotic fluid. Explain to the woman that amniotomy is no more painful than a vaginal examination because there are no sensory nerves in the amniotic sac.

Other supplies needed are a sterile, disposable plastic hook (such as AmniHook), sterile gloves for the provider, and sterile lubricant. The nurse should partly open the package containing the plastic hook at the handle end and hold back the package until the provider takes the hook. (Fig. 15.2).

The provider performs a vaginal examination to determine cervical dilation, effacement, station, and fetal presenting part. Amniotomy is often deferred if the fetal presenting part is high or the presentation is not cephalic. The risk for a prolapsed cord is higher in these situations. The hook is passed through the cervical opening, snagging the membranes. The opening in the membranes is enlarged with the finger, allowing fluid to drain.

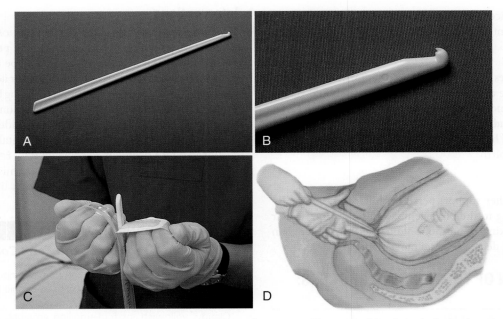

FIG. 15.2 A, Disposable plastic membrane perforator. **B,** Close-up of hook end of plastic membrane perforator. **C,** Correct method to open the package. **D,** Technique for artificial rupture of membranes.

❓ CRITICAL THINKING EXERCISE 15.3

A provider performs an amniotomy on a laboring woman whose cervix is dilated to 5 cm. The amniotic fluid is pale yellow and moderate in amount, and it has a strong odor. The baseline fetal heart rate ranges from 155 to 165 beats per minute (bpm), accelerating when the fetus moves. Maternal vital signs are temperature, 99.7°F (37.6°C); pulse rate, 92 bpm; respirations, 22/min; blood pressure, 116/80 mm Hg. Contractions are moderate to firm in intensity, every 3 to 4 minutes, with a duration of 50 to 60 seconds and with complete uterine relaxation between contractions.

Questions

1. Which of these observations should the nurse regard as normal? Which factors are abnormal?
2. Should the nurse modify routine labor care based on the postamniotomy assessments?

❓ KNOWLEDGE CHECK

8. What observations suggest that the woman may need additional help with pain management during labor?
9. What are three risks associated with amniotomy?
10. Why is the FHR assessed before and after the membranes rupture?
11. What maternal and fetal signs are associated with chorioamnionitis?
12. Describe the significance of each of the following types of amniotic fluid: greenish, cloudy, yellowish, foul-smelling.
13. Why are frequent vaginal examinations undesirable during labor?

◆ APPLICATION OF THE NURSING PROCESS: FALSE OR EARLY LABOR

◆ Assessment

After observation, the nurse may realize that the woman is not in true active labor. If findings are normal and the woman's membranes are intact, she is usually discharged. The woman who is in very early latent labor may be discharged to await active labor, especially if she is a nullipara and lives nearby.

◆ Identification of Patient Problems

A woman may be frustrated because she cannot tell whether labor is real. She may resist returning to the birth center, possibly causing needless delay of care. She often is tired of being pregnant and just wants it to be over. There is often a need for patient teaching regarding the characteristics of true labor.

◆ Planning: Expected Outcomes

An expected outcome for this patient problem is that before discharge the woman and her support person will describe reasons for returning to the birth center for evaluation.

◆ Interventions

Reassurance

A woman sent home after observation may feel foolish and frustrated. She may want to have labor induced simply to "get it over with." Reassure her that even professionals cannot always distinguish true and false labor. Also, tell her that important preparation for labor occurs during late pregnancy, such as softening of the cervix, even if obvious progress such as cervical dilation has not yet occurred. Early latent labor may gradually intensify as it merges into the active phase of first stage. Other women may notice a more abrupt intensity and frequency change as the latent phase becomes active labor.

Teaching

Review guidelines for returning to the birth center and explain that these are only guidelines and she should return if she has any concerns. Returning with false labor is better than entering in advanced labor or developing complications at home. Remind her that her body is often making the final preparations for birth.

◆ Evaluation

The woman and her support person should describe guidelines for returning to the birth center. These include regular contractions, leaking of amniotic fluid, bleeding other than bloody show, and decreased fetal movement.

◆ APPLICATION OF THE NURSING PROCESS: TRUE LABOR

The admission assessment may confirm that the woman is in true labor, or true labor may be evident after observation. Patient problems change during labor because the intrapartum period is an active process. Problems covered in this chapter relate to fetal oxygenation, maternal discomfort, and maternal injury.

Patient problems often have an impact on each other during labor. For example, high anxiety reduces effectiveness of pain-relief measures by interfering with relaxation. Maternal dehydration can alter fetal oxygenation because less blood is available to circulate to the placenta.

FETAL OXYGENATION

◆ Assessment

The critical assessments related to fetal well-being are the following (see Table 15.1):
- FHR evaluation
- Amount and character of amniotic fluid and time of rupture
- Maternal vital signs
- Contractions—Frequency, duration, intensity, relaxation interval, and resting tone

◆ Identification of Patient Problems

Several factors such as maternal hypotension and hypertension, maternal fever, excessively strong and long contractions (tetanic), and compression of the umbilical cord can reduce fetal oxygen, nutrient, and waste exchange. The healthy fetus usually tolerates labor well, and the nurse simply needs to be alert for problems. Therefore the potential for fetal compromise is a patient problem in all labors.

◆ Planning: Expected Outcomes

Planning includes nursing responsibilities to (1) promote normal placental function and (2) observe for and report problems to the provider. The expected outcome is that the fetus does not show signs of compromise such as Category III (abnormal) FHR patterns.

◆ Interventions

Promote Placental Function. Maternal positioning is the primary measure to promote placental perfusion during normal labor. The supine position should be avoided because it causes the woman's uterus to compress her aorta and inferior vena cava (aortocaval compression), reducing blood flow to the placenta. If she must be in the supine position for a procedure such as catheterization, a small pillow or folded blanket under one hip shifts her uterus to maintain placental blood flow.

Observe for Conditions Associated with Fetal Compromise. If conditions associated with fetal compromise are identified, provide interventions directed at the most likely physiologic cause and notify the provider.

CRITICAL TO REMEMBER

Conditions Associated with Fetal Compromise

Fetal heart rate (FHR) outside the normal range of 110 to 160 bpm or loss of FHR variability with electronic FHR monitoring
Meconium-stained (greenish) amniotic fluid
Cloudy, yellowish, or foul-smelling amniotic fluid (suggests infection)
Excessive frequency or duration of contractions (reduces placental blood flow)
Incomplete uterine relaxation and intervals shorter than 45 to 60 seconds between contractions (reduces placental blood flow)
Maternal hypotension (may divert blood flow away from the placenta to ensure adequate perfusion of the maternal brain and heart)
Maternal hypertension (may be associated with vasospasm in spiral arteries, which supply the intervillous spaces of the placenta)
Maternal fever (38°C [100.4°F] or higher)

◆ Evaluation

Throughout labor, compare actual data with the norms for mother and fetus. The outcome criteria has been met if the fetus does not develop signs of compromise.

DISCOMFORT

Women vary in their responses to labor pain and choices of pain management methods. Providing choices for pain management and support for those choices allows an increased sense of control over her birth experience. The woman who successfully masters the pain and other physical demands of labor is more likely to view her experience as positive. Her support person also is likely to feel more satisfaction with the experience. Working with people in pain is difficult, and most nurses feel compelled to relieve pain promptly, yet pain is expected and has a purpose in labor. It cannot be eliminated. The nurse's role is to teach the patient and her support person about various methods of pain management and then support her decisions and evaluate her responses.

◆ Assessment

See Table 15.1 for continuing assessments of the laboring woman. Specific data applicable to discomfort include the birth plan, identification of support persons, and any preparation for childbirth. If the woman has had previous births, assessment of the pain management methods used and their effectiveness is important.

◆ Identification of Patient Problems

Pain and anxiety are related patient problems. Excess anxiety reduces pain tolerance, and pain worsens anxiety. The nurse clusters assessment data to determine the primary problem. For example, several cues such as a previous poor experience during birth and expressions of worry and concern suggest that anxiety is primary. However, if contractions are intense and labor is progressing quickly, the primary problem would be pain. This discussion will focus on the primary problem of pain, which may be due to ineffective use of pain management techniques.

◆ Planning: Expected Outcomes

The elimination of labor's pain is not realistic. Therefore appropriate goals and expected outcomes related to pain include the following:
1. During labor, the woman will state that her chosen method or methods of pain management are satisfactory and will tell the nurse if others are needed.
2. By discharge from the birth facility, the woman's support person will express satisfaction with having provided labor support.
3. By discharge from the birth facility, the woman will describe her birth experience as positive.

◆ Interventions

Labor pain management includes pharmacologic and non-pharmacologic measures such as breathing techniques and medication to promote comfort and specific methods to relieve pain (see Chapter 13).

Provide Comfort Measures. Comfort measures such as environmental control, hygiene, positioning, and assistance with voiding affect the woman's ability to relax, which enhances the effectiveness of all pain management techniques.

Lighting. Soft, indirect lighting is soothing, whereas a bright overhead light is irritating. Bright lights imply a hospital ("sick") atmosphere rather than a normal event such as birth. A bright, overhead light should be used only when needed.

Temperature. Labor is hard work, and the woman in labor is often hot and perspiring. Cool, damp washcloths on the woman's face and neck can promote comfort (Fig. 15.3). Other interventions include placing socks if her feet are cold or using a fan to circulate air in the labor room. Be sure that the fan does not blow on the infant after birth, which might cause hypothermia.

Cleanliness. Bloody show and amniotic fluid leak from the woman's vagina during labor. Change the sheets and gown, as needed, to keep her dry and comfortable and to reduce microorganisms that might ascend into the vagina. A folded towel or bath blanket absorbs larger quantities of amniotic fluid than the pad alone. Patient preferences guide nursing care; therefore interventions to assist the patient may

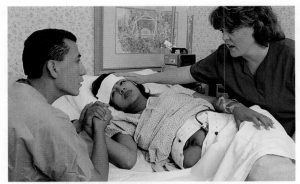

FIG. 15.3 Cool, damp washcloths placed where the woman finds them most comforting help her relax during each contraction.

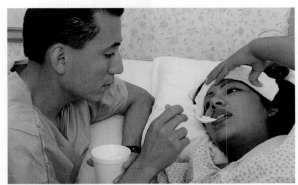

FIG. 15.4 Most laboring women welcome ice chips to ease their dry mouths.

be delayed. For example, during transition many women may not want to be disturbed.

Oral Care. Ice chips (Fig. 15.4), frozen juice bars, and hard candy on a stick reduce the discomfort of a dry mouth. Brushing the teeth and simply rinsing the mouth are helpful to the woman. Lip balm will provide needed moisture to her lips.

Bladder. A full bladder intensifies pain during labor and can delay fetal descent. It may cause pain that remains after an epidural is started. Remind the woman to empty her bladder, and check her suprapubic area at least every 2 hours. Catheterization may be required for some patients.

Positioning. Clinician preferences and the patient's cultural background influence the positioning women choose when laboring. Encourage the woman to assume any position she finds comfortable (other than the supine) and change positions frequently (Fig. 15.5). Movement and frequent position changes in labor decrease pain, improve maternal-fetal circulation, improve the strength and effectiveness of contractions, decrease the length of labor, facilitate fetal descent, and decrease perineal trauma and episiotomies (Association of Women's Health, Obstetric and Neonatal Nurses [AWHONN], 2008; Zwelling, 2010). Zwelling (2010) recommended that nurses follow six physiologic principles related to maternal positioning in labor proposed by Fenwick and Simkin (1987): promote spinal flexion, promote an

POSITIONS FOR FIRST STAGE

Standing

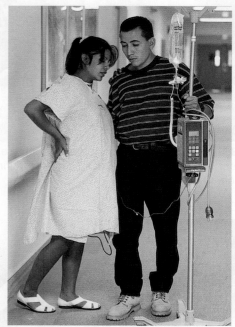

Sitting Upright

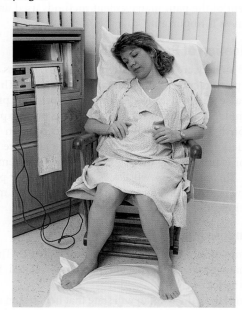

Advantages
Adds gravity to force of contractions to promote fetal descent.
Contractions are less uncomfortable and more efficient.
Variation: Standing, leaning forward with support reduces back pain because fetus falls forward, away from the sacral promontory.

Disadvantages
Tiring over long periods.
Continuous electronic fetal monitoring is not possible without telemetry if woman is walking in the hall.

Nursing Implications
If the woman has IV fluid running, give her a rolling pole. Encourage her to alternate walking with other positions whenever she tires or desires to do so.
Remind the woman and her partner when she should return to the labor area for evaluation of the fetal heart rate and her labor status.

Advantages
Uses gravity to aid fetal descent.
Can be done when sitting on side of bed, in a chair, or on the toilet.
Can be used with continuous fetal monitoring.
Avoids supine hypotension.

Disadvantages
May increase suprapubic discomfort.
Contractions are the most efficient when the woman alternates sitting with other positions.

Nursing Implications
A rocking chair is soothing.
Place a pillow on a chair with a disposable underpad over the pillow to absorb secretions.
Use pillows or a footstool to keep a short woman's legs from dangling.
Encourage the woman to alternate positions periodically. For example, she can alternate walking with sitting or sitting with side-lying.

FIG. 15.5 Common Maternal Positions for Labor. Many maternal labor positions can be adapted for the first stage and second stage of labor.

increase in the uterospinal drive angle, facilitate stronger expulsive forces, promote a good fit, increase pelvic diameter, and facilitate occiput posterior rotation. By encouraging upright positions, frequent position changes, and a C-shaped spine with the mother leaning forward, the nurse can follow these principles.

"Back labor" is common when the back of the fetal head puts pressure on the woman's sacral promontory (occiput posterior position). The discomfort of back labor is difficult to relieve with medication alone. Positions that encourage the fetus to move away from the sacral promontory, such as those in which the mother uses the hands-and-knees position or leans forward over a birthing ball, reduce back pain and

enhance the internal rotation mechanism of labor. Smaller versions of the birthing ball are available for use when the mother is sitting and leaning forward.

Although ambulation and some positions may not be safe for the woman with an epidural, many options are available by using the flexibility of modern birthing beds with leg supports, squatting bars, and multiple positions of the head and foot sections. Utilization of the peanut ball to assist with positioning has been shown to decrease the time of first- and second-stage labor in primiparous women with epidurals and decrease the incidence of cesarean section in these patients (Roth, Dent, Parfitt, Hering, & Bay, 2016; Tussey et al., 2015). Nursing care of the woman with an epidural includes assisting

POSITIONS FOR FIRST STAGE

Sitting, Leaning Forward with Support

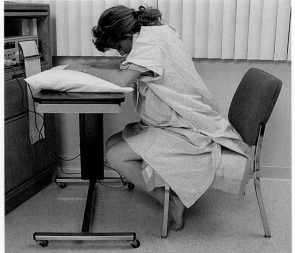

Advantages
Same as for sitting.
Reduces back pain because fetus falls forward, away from sacral promontory.
Partner or nurse can rub back or provide sacral pressure to relieve back pain.

Disadvantages
Same as for sitting.

Nursing Implications
Same as for sitting.

Semisitting

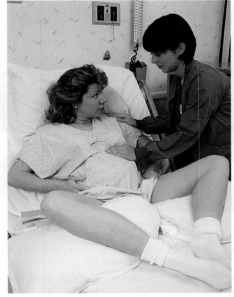

Advantages
Same as for sitting.
Aligns long axis of uterus with pelvic inlet, which applies contraction force in the most efficient direction through pelvis.

Disadvantages
Same as for sitting.
Does not reduce pain as well as the forward-leaning positions.

Nursing Implications
Same as for sitting.
Raise bed to about a 30- to 45-degree angle.
Encourage the woman to use sitting (leaning forward) or side-lying position if she has back pain so the caregiver can rub her back or apply sacral pressure.

FIG. 15.5, cont'd

Continued

the woman with position changes every 30 to 45 minutes (Zwelling, 2010).

Teaching. Teaching the woman in labor is a continuously changing task based on the progress of her labor, preferred pain management methods, and their effectiveness.

First Stage. First-stage labor is divided into two categories: latent and active (see Chapter 12). Many women become discouraged because several hours are needed to reach 4 to 5 cm of cervical dilation. The latent phase of first stage can last from hours to days. From a time standpoint, 5 cm is approximately two thirds of the way through first-stage labor because the rate of dilation increases during the active phase. Patient teaching during the first stage includes keeping the patient informed of the progress of labor, her status, and the status of the fetus. The nurse also should teach the patient about alternative pain management options if her chosen methods do not meet her expectations.

A woman's urge to push can occur on complete dilation and effacement with the fetus at +1 station or lower. However, as she nears the second stage, the fetus may descend enough to give her an urge to push before full cervical dilation. This urge is triggered by the presenting part stretching the pelvic floor muscles and is commonly referred to as the Ferguson reflex. This process releases endogenous oxytocin, stimulating an urge to push (AWHONN, 2008; Simpson & O'Brien-Abel, 2014). The timing of pushing should be individualized to the maternal response.

Pushing against a cervix that does not easily yield to pressure from the presenting part may result in cervical lacerations, or cervical edema, which can block labor progress . If the woman has a strong urge to push, but pushing is likely to injure her cervix or cause cervical edema, teach her to exhale in short breaths.

Second Stage. Discomfort in the second stage of labor is associated with pushing. The woman may need help to trust the sensations from her body and push most effectively. Patient teaching for this stage of labor includes when to start pushing, positions for pushing, and the method for pushing. Nursing research on labor support is increasing and has resulted in inclusion of care based on solid evidence.

Laboring Down. Two hours was once accepted as the upper limit for the duration of the second stage, with little evidence of the benefits of restricting the duration of second

POSITIONS FOR FIRST STAGE

Side-Lying

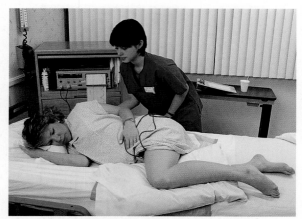

Kneeling, Leaning Forward with Support

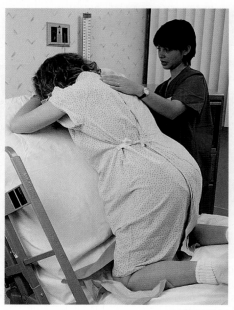

Advantages

It is a restful position.

Prevents supine hypotension and promotes placental blood flow.

Promotes efficient contractions, although they may be less frequent than with other positions.

Can be used with continuous fetal monitoring.

Disadvantages

Does not use gravity to aid fetal descent.

Nursing Implications

Teach the woman and her partner that although the contractions are less frequent, they are more effective.

This position offers a break from more tiring positions.

Use pillows for support and to prevent pressure: at her back, under her superior arm, and between her knees.

Use disposable underpads to protect the pillow between the woman's knees from secretions.

Some women like to put their superior leg on the bed rail. If the woman wants this variation, pad the bed rail with a blanket to prevent pressure.

If she wants to remain recumbent, she should use this position to promote placental blood flow.

Advantages

Reduces back pain because fetus falls forward, away from sacral promontory.

Adds gravity to force of contractions to promote fetal descent.

Can be used with continuous fetal monitoring.

Caregivers can rub her back or apply sacral pressure.

Promotes normal mechanisms of birth.

Disadvantages

Knees may become tired or uncomfortable.

Tiring if used for long periods.

Nursing Implications

Raise the head of the bed and have the woman face the head of the bed while she is on her knees.

Another method is for the partner to sit in a chair, with the woman kneeling in front, facing her partner, and leaning forward on him or her for support.

Use pillow under the knees and in front of the woman's chest, as needed, for comfort.

Encourage her to change positions if she becomes tired.

FIG. 15.5, cont'd

stage or the accuracy of this time limit. A second stage longer than 2 hours is now recognized as safe provided the mother and fetus show no signs of compromise (Spong, Berghella, Wenstrom, Mercer, & Saade, 2012).

Women push most effectively when they feel the reflex urge to do so as the fetus descends. Women with regional analgesia may not have an urge to push. Many women do not immediately feel the urge to push when the cervix is fully dilated, even if no regional analgesia such as an epidural is administered. A brief slowing of contractions often occurs at the beginning of the second stage. Pushing as soon as complete dilation is achieved with no regard to maternal readiness can lead to issues such as maternal exhaustion and pelvic floor injuries (Simpson & O'Brien-Abel, 2014).

The technique of delaying pushing until the reflex urge to push occurs may be called *delayed pushing, laboring down, rest and descend,* and *passive descent.* Active pushing is the most physiologically stressful part of labor for the fetus. Delayed pushing has been shown to result in less maternal fatigue, decreased pushing time, decreased risk for instrument-assisted and cesarean births, and Apgar scores equivalent to those of women who pushed immediately on full cervical dilation (AWHONN, 2008; Miller et al., 2017; Simpson & O'Brien-Abel, 2014).

Simply put, laboring down means allowing uterine contractions to cause most fetal internal rotation and descent after full dilation. The woman rests before actively pushing her baby out. If no fetal descent has occurred after 2 hours, an evaluation by the midwife or physician is necessary.

POSITIONS FOR FIRST STAGE

Hands and Knees

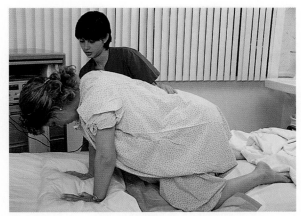

Advantages

Reduces back pain because the fetus falls forward, away
   from the sacral promontory.
Promotes normal mechanisms of birth.
The woman can use pelvic rocking to decrease back pain.
Caregivers can rub the woman's back or apply sacral pres-
   sure easily.

Disadvantages

The woman's hands (especially wrists) and knees can become
   uncomfortable.
Tiring when used for a long time.
Some women are embarrassed to use this position.

Nursing Implications

Encourage the woman to change to less tiring positions occasionally.
Ensure privacy when encouraging the reluctant woman to try
   this position if she has back pain.
A second hospital gown with the opening in front covers her
   back and hips but may be too warm. A variation is for the
   mother to kneel and lean forward against a beanbag or the
   side of the bed. This variation reduces some of the strain
   of wrists and hands.

POSITIONS FOR PUSHING IN SECOND STAGE

Squatting
Standing
This position may be tiring, and access to the woman's
   perineum is difficult. Because the infant could fall to the
   ground if birth occurs rapidly, provide padding under the
   mother's feet. Gravity aids fetal descent.

Hands and Knees
Advantages and disadvantages are similar to those during
   first-stage labor. In addition, caregivers must reorient
   themselves because the landmarks are upside down from
   their usual perspective.

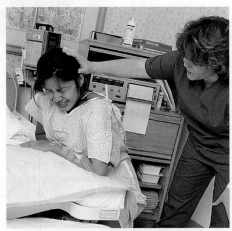

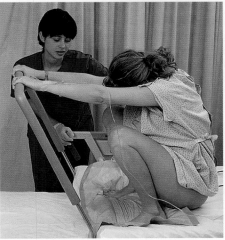

Advantages
Adds gravity to force of contractions to promote fetal descent.
Straightens the pelvic curve slightly for more direct fetal descent.
Increases dimensions of pelvis slightly.
Promotes effective pushing efforts in the second stage.
Caregivers can rub back or provide sacral pressure.
Disadvantages
Knees and hips may become uncomfortable because of pro-
   longed flexion.
Tiring over a long time.
Nursing Implications
Provide support with a squat bar attached to the bed or by
   two people standing on each side of the woman.
If she becomes tired, or between contractions, she can lean
   back into the sitting position.
Variation: Have the woman squat beside the bed as she pushes.

FIG. 15.5, cont'd

Continued

POSITIONS FOR PUSHING IN SECOND STAGE

Semisitting

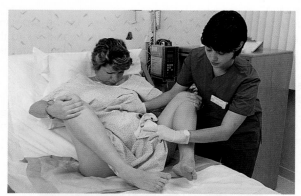

Many women prefer this because they have the security of a back rest; it is also familiar to caregivers and allows easy observation of the perineum. Elevate the woman's back at least 30 to 45 degrees so that gravity aids fetal descent. The woman pulls on her flexed knees (behind or in front of them) as she pushes. She should keep her head flexed and her back in a C curve.

Side-Lying

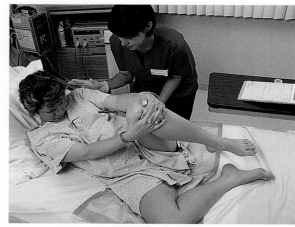

The woman flexes her chin on her chest and curls around her uterus as she pushes. She pulls on her flexed knees or the knee of the superior leg as she pushes.

FIG. 15.5, cont'd

EVIDENCE-BASED PRACTICE

Does delayed pushing versus immediate pushing during a woman's second stage have any physical advantages for her? What about her newborn? Two nursing research articles provide evidence that delaying pushing when a nullipara reaches second stage shortened the duration of pushing compared to the nulliparas in the immediate pushing group. However, the total length of second stage was longer in the delayed pushing group in each study, an expected finding. Primary outcome measures in both studies were the length of pushing during second stage, total length of second stage, and maternal fatigue.

Kelly, Johnson, Lee, et al. (2010) conducted a randomized clinical trial (RCT) for 44 nulliparas: immediate pushing for 28; delayed pushing for 16. Consent was obtained before full dilation and entry into study. All women were receiving epidural anesthesia before reaching complete dilation. Labor was spontaneous or induced electively or was medically indicated. Fetal heart rate (FHR) at the time they entered the study was reassuring, and gestation was ≥38 weeks. Pain scores were ≥3 on a scale of 10 when they entered the study. This study delayed pushing up to 90 minutes at which time pushing with contractions would be encouraged. The study found that length of pushing time in the immediate pushing group (78.7 ± 7.9 min) versus the delayed pushing group (38.9 ± 6.9 min) to be 51% less in the delayed pushing group. The woman pushed sooner if she had a strong urge. The shorter duration of actual pushing time was statistically significant in the delayed pushing group versus the immediate pushing group. Duration of second stage was about 30 min shorter in the immediate pushing group (87.1 ± 8.6 min) versus delayed pushing (117.6 ± 12.1 min) but not statistically significant. Maternal fatigue, measured with the visual analog scale (VAS) was similar in the two groups.

Gillesby, Burns, Dempsey, et al. (2010) had similar results with their group of 77 women, 39 in the immediate pushing group and 38 in the delayed pushing group. Their group was also nulliparas with epidural pain relief as they entered second stage. For the delayed pushing group, this RCT used 120 minutes as the maximum delay for pushing at which time pushing would be encouraged if the woman had no earlier urge. The duration of pushing time in the mothers with immediate pushing (94 ± 57 min) versus mothers with delayed pushing (68 ± 46 min) is also a statistically significant difference. Second stage labor duration averaged 107 ± 56 minutes in the immediate pushing group versus 163 ± 64 minutes in the delayed pushing group. Maternal fatigue scores were also similar with the two groups. Total second stage time was 59 minutes longer for the group who delayed pushing. Fatigue scores with the VAS were similar for the two groups.

These two studies support the benefit of delaying pushing without evidence of fetal compromise. Passive fetal descent and rotation is the likely reason why the second stage, while longer in total length, requires a shorter period of pushing.

Above results were confirmed by two large meta analyses reported in 2014 by M. Kopas. Delayed pushing resulted in longer second stage, but less time spent actively pushing in the group of women who experienced delayed pushing (Kopas, 2014).

References

Gillesby, E., Burns, S., Dempsey, A., Kirby, S., et al. (2010). Comparison of delayed versus immediate pushing during second stage of labor for nulliparous women with epidural anesthesia. *Journal of Obstetric, Gynecologic, and Neonatal Nursing, 39*(6), 635–644.

Kelly, M., Johnson, E., Lee, V., et al. (2010). Delayed versus immediate pushing in second stage of labor. *MCN: The American Journal of Maternal-Child Nursing, 35*(2), 81–88.

Kopas, M. (2014). A review of evidence-based practices for management of the second stage of labor. *Journal of Midwifery and Women's Health, 59*(3), 264–276.

Positions. Although vertical maternal positions enhance fetal descent and shorten labor, often the patient is placed in a recumbent position for provider convenience (Simpson & O'Brien-Abel, 2014). Squatting is an ideal position for pushing because it enlarges the pelvic outlet slightly and adds the force of gravity to the mother's efforts, which is an advantage if she has a small pelvis or the fetus is large. If the mother is too tired to squat, the toilet can be used for support while maintaining an upright, open pelvis position (Simpson & O'Brien-Abel, 2014). Pushing while sitting on a birthing ball, pulling against a squatting bar on the bed, or playing "tug of war" with another person provides a similar gravitational advantage. Women may find that pulling on something from above is efficient. Her upper torso should be in front of her pelvis to allow her coccyx to move backward as the fetus descends deeply into her pelvis (Zwelling, 2010). Epidural analgesia may limit the positions a woman can assume for pushing; however, with modern birthing beds, many modified positions are safe and effective with or without epidural analgesia.

If the mother pushes in the sitting or semisitting position, teach her to curve her body around her uterus in a C shape rather than arching her back. For greatest effectiveness, the woman should pull on her knees, handholds, or a squat bar while pushing. She should maintain a similar C shape to her upper body if she pushes on her side.

Method and Breathing Pattern. Support the woman's spontaneous pushing techniques if they are effective. The woman should push with her abdominal muscles while relaxing her perineum. If she needs coaching, teach her to begin by taking a breath and exhaling and then taking another breath and exhaling while pushing for 6 seconds at a time. Sustained pushing while holding a breath (Valsalva maneuver or "purple pushing") or pushing more than four times per contraction reduces blood flow to the placenta, increases intrathoracic pressure, is fatiguing, and should be discouraged (Simpson & O'Brien-Abel, 2014). Another deep breath that is more like a sigh helps her relax after the contraction.

A woman who is modest or fears losing control may inhibit her best pushing efforts if she is instructed to push as if she were having a bowel movement, particularly if she is in a bed or chair. An anatomically correct image is to teach the woman to push down and out under her symphysis (pubic bone), following the pelvic curve. Seeing a diagram or model of the pelvis helps her visualize the curve.

Encouragement. Women who receive continuous support in labor have improved outcomes compared with women who do not have support (Hodnett et al., 2013). Laboring women need the support of a skilled, empathic, and intuitive nurse at the bedside—coaching them, reassuring them, and, most of all, being there for them. Tell the woman when her labor is progressing. If she can see that her efforts are effective, she has more courage to continue. Help her touch or see the baby's head with a mirror as crowning occurs. Praise the woman

and her support person when they use breathing and other coping techniques effectively. This reinforces their actions, gives them a sense of control, and conveys the respect and support of the nurse. If one technique is not helpful after a reasonable trial (three to five contractions), encourage them to try other techniques.

Although the woman and her support person may have prepared for childbirth, they often welcome suggestions and affirmation from the nurse. They are more likely to use the techniques they learned if the nurse helps them. The nurse's presence, gentle coaching, and encouragement help the woman have confidence in her own body and fitness to give birth.

Offering Pharmacologic Measures. Childbirth is a normal process; however, many women desire pharmacologic pain management. The nurse must be informative but neutral when explaining available pain medication.

Some women may have a firm goal to avoid pain medication during labor. A woman who planned an unmedicated birth may interpret the nurse's information about available medication as pressure for her to take medication. Careful review of the woman's birth plan and specific teaching or review of available options establish a therapeutic relationship with the woman, her coach, and the nurse. This should be done as early in the labor as possible while the woman is still in control and can think critically. The discussion should include the option for the woman to change her mind and how that will be communicated.

Other women may plan to use a specific method such as epidural analgesia. At times, labor does not go as "planned" and the woman may be upset about this unexpected development in her birth experience. Although the event may not be what she wanted, encouraging the woman to express her feelings helps her put it into perspective.

Care for the Birth Partner. The woman's support person is an integral part of her labor care. Her labor partner can provide care and comfort that support the woman's ability to give birth. Some partners are coaches in the true sense of the word, actively assisting the woman through labor. Others want the woman and nurse to lead them and tell them how to help. They are eager to do what they can but expect instructions about methods and timing. Many couples see the partner's role as encouraging, offering moral support, and simply being there for the woman. Caring for the support person includes respect for the couple's wishes about partner involvement in the birth process. The nurse should provide support that the partner cannot and should consider the partner's physical needs for food and rest.

◆ **Evaluation**

Achievement of the three goals or expected outcomes occurs if the following conditions are met:
1. The woman indicates satisfaction with her method of pain management or requests nursing assistance to find other, more satisfactory methods.

2. The woman's support person expresses satisfaction with having provided labor support by the time of discharge.
3. The woman describes her birth experience as positive by the time of discharge.

The first goal regarding pain management is continually reevaluated throughout labor. The ability of the woman's support person is also continually evaluated. The last goal, describing the birth experience as positive, is evaluated after the woman and her significant other have had time to begin putting the birth experience into perspective.

PREVENT INJURY

◆ Assessment

Nursing assessments of the mother and fetus continue as the woman nears birth. During the second stage, observe the woman's perineum to determine when to make final birth preparations.

The exact time for final birth preparations varies according to the woman's parity, overall speed of labor, and fetal station. Preparations are usually completed when fetal head begins to crown in the nullipara. The multipara is prepared sooner, usually when her cervix is fully dilated and the fetal head is well down in the pelvis, typically before crowning has occurred.

◆ Identification of Patient Problems

The woman is vulnerable to injury immediately before and after birth for several reasons: (1) altered physical sensations such as intense pressure and effects of medication, (2) positional changes for birth, and (3) unexpectedly rapid progress.

◆ Planning: Expected Outcomes

The nurse's primary objective is to prevent and minimize potential injuries. The goal or expected outcome for this problem is that the woman does not have a preventable injury such as muscle strains, thrombosis, and lacerations during birth.

◆ Interventions

Positioning the woman in the birthing bed is the first step in the sequence of events that culminates in the birth of the baby (Figs. 15.6 to 15.8). During the period around birth, the nurse reduces factors that contribute to maternal injuries.

Transferring to a Delivery Room. Most vaginal births occur in a combination labor, delivery, and recovery room. Occasionally the woman must be transferred to a separate room for the birth. If so, she should be transferred early to avoid rushed, last-minute preparations that cause anxiety for everyone.

Positioning for Birth. Upright positions promote effective pushing and take advantage of gravity. Squatting is a good position for uncomplicated birth but limits accessibility to

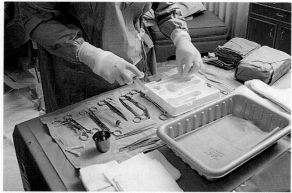

FIG. 15.6 The provider arranges instruments in final preparation for birth. Although the vagina is not sterile, a sterile table is prepared to limit introduction of outside organisms into the birth canal. Included on the sterile table are infant care materials (e.g., cord clamp, cord blood tube), instruments for repair of maternal injury or episiotomy, and anesthesia materials (if needed).

the woman's perineum and may not be an option for women with epidural analgesia. Maternal positions with the upper body leaning forward promotes expulsive efforts, directs the fetus efficiently toward the pelvic outlet, and increases the diameters of the pelvic outlet.

Other upright positions for the birth include standing and kneeling upright positions. The semirecumbent position limits movement of the coccyx as the fetus descends during birth but maintains some advantages of gravity. Sitting on a birthing bed with a cutout for the perineal area maintains many advantages of squatting and may be less tiring. The hands-and-knees position may be helpful for the fetus in the occiput posterior position and to rotate wide fetal shoulders.

Many women and providers are more comfortable using stirrups and foot rests to support the woman's legs and feet and make her perineum more accessible. If she cannot move her legs because of motor block from anesthesia, raise and lower her legs together, and do not separate them too widely. Surfaces that contact the popliteal space behind the knee should be padded because pressure on veins near the surface could lead to thrombus formation. The woman's upper body should be in the semi-Fowler's or sitting position rather than the supine position.

Observe the Perineum. The exact time at which a woman is ready to give birth is an educated guess. Birth is near when the fetal head progresses anteriorly in the mechanism of extension and the occiput moves under the symphysis pubis. Observe the woman's perineum, especially during late second-stage labor.

A classic sign of imminent birth is the mother's urgent cry, "The baby's coming!" Look at her perineum, and if the baby will be born before the provider arrives, remain calm, and support the infant's head and body with gloved hands as it emerges. Ask the support person to push the call button to summon help.

Transfer and Positioning for Birth

Action: When the woman is almost ready to give birth, transfer her to the delivery room or position the birthing bed. The exact time varies with several factors (such as overall speed of labor and rate of fetal descent). *Rationale:* Rushed, last-moment preparations are anxiety-producing for the woman, her partner, and the nurse. Remaining in the birth position for a long time can be tiring.

Action: Continue observing her perineum while making final preparations for birth. *Rationale:* Birth may occur unexpectedly, and the nurse should be prepared to "catch" the infant if the attendant (physician or nurse-midwife) is not in the room.

Action: Continue observing the fetal heart rate (FHR) with continuous monitoring or intermittent auscultation. *Rationale:* Detects changes in fetal condition that may require interventions by the attendant to speed birth.

Action: Elevate the woman's back, shoulders, and head with a wedge (on a delivery table) or by raising the head of the birthing bed. *Rationale:* Allows more effective maternal pushing and uses gravity to aid fetal descent.

Action: Stirrups or foot rests to support the woman's legs and feet may be used on a birthing bed. Pad the surface. *Rationale:* Padding reduces pressure, preventing venous stasis and possible thrombus formation.

Action: When placing the woman's legs in stirrups, elevate them and remove them simultaneously. Do not separate her legs widely. *Rationale:* Reduces strain on muscles and ligaments.

Prepping and Draping

Action: After the woman is in position, cleanse the perineal area with a sterile iodophor and water preparation unless she is allergic. Use warm water to dilute the iodophor scrub. *Rationale:* Removes secretions and feces from perineal area.

Action: After handwashing, apply sterile gloves for the prep procedure. Take a fresh sponge to begin each new area, and do not return to a clean area with a used sponge. Six sponges are needed. The proper order and motions are as follows:

1. Use a zig-zag motion from clitoris to lower abdomen just above the pubic hairline.

2, 3. Use a zig-zag motion on the inner thigh from the labia majora to about halfway between the hip and knee. Repeat for the other inner thigh.

4, 5. Apply a single stroke on one side from clitoris over labia, perineum, and anus. Repeat for the other side.

6. Use a single stroke in the middle from the clitoris over the vulva and perineum.

Rationale: Prevents cross-contamination or recontamination of an area that is already clean.

Action: The attendant may apply sterile drapes if desired. *Rationale:* A vaginal birth is a clean procedure rather than a sterile one because the vagina is not sterile. Sterile drapes are unnecessary, but some attendants may prefer to use them.

Birth of the Head

Action: If an episiotomy is needed, the attendant will perform it when the head is well crowned. *Rationale:* Minimizes blood loss from the episiotomy.

Action: As the vaginal orifice encircles the fetal head, the attendant applies gentle pressure to the woman's perineum with one hand while applying counterpressure to the fetal head with the other hand (Ritgen's maneuver). The attendant may ask the mother to blow so that she avoids pushing, or to push gently. *Rationale:* Controls the exit of the fetal head so that it is born gradually rather than popping out; this minimizes trauma to the maternal tissues.

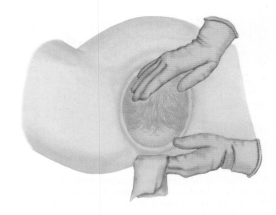

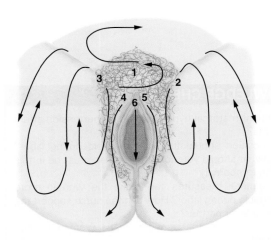

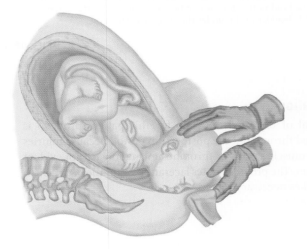

FIG. 15.7 Sequence for Delivery.

Continued

Action: The attendant wipes secretions from the infant's face and suctions the nose and mouth with a bulb syringe. If needed *Rationale:* Removes blood and secretions, preventing the infant from aspirating them with the first breaths.

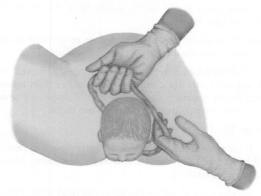

Action: The attendant feels for a cord around the fetal neck (nuchal cord). If it is loose, it is slipped over the head. If tight, it is clamped and cut between two clamps before the rest of the baby is born. *Rationale:* Allows the rest of the birth to occur and prevents stretching or tearing the cord.

Birth of the Shoulders

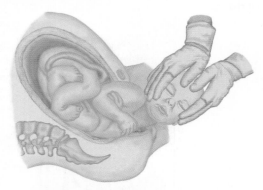

Action: After external rotation, the attendant applies gentle traction on the fetal head in the direction of the mother's perineum. *Rationale:* External rotation allows the shoulders to rotate internally and aligns their transverse diameter with the antero-posterior diameter of the mother's pelvic outlet. Traction on the head in the direction of her perineum allows the anterior fetal shoulder to slip under the symphysis pubis.

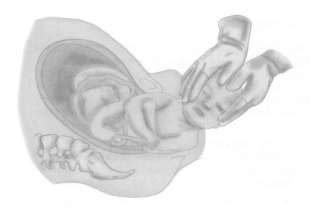

Action: The attendant then lifts the head toward the mother's symphysis pubis. *Rationale:* Permits the posterior fetal shoulder to be eased over the perineum, minimizing trauma to the maternal tissues.

Clearing the Infant's Airway and Cutting the Cord

Action: The rest of the infant's body is born quickly after the sholders are born. The attendant maintains the infant in a slightly head down position while wiping excess secretions away. If needed, a bulb syringe may be used to gently suction the mouth and nose. The infant is often placed on the mother's abdomen. *Rationale:* Gravity aids spontaneous drainage of secretions and prevents aspiration of oral mucus and seretion.

Action: The attendant clamps the cord. Either the father or the attendant cuts the cord above the clamp. *Rationale:* Allows parents to interact more freely with their infant. Prevents flow of blood between placenta and infant, which might result in anemia (if infant is higher than placenta) or polycythemia (if infant is below the placenta).

Delivery of the Placenta

Action: After the placenta separates, it can usually be delivered if the mother bears down. The attendant may pull gently on the cord. *Rationale:* Excess traction on the cord may cause it to break, making the placenta harder to deliver.

Action: The attendant inspects both sides of the placenta. *Rationale:* Ensures that no fragments remain inside the uterus that might cause hemorrhage and infection.

After the infant and placenta are born, the attendant inspects the birth canal for injuries. If needed, any injuries and the episiotomy (if one was done) are repaired.

FIG. 15.7, cont'd

◆ Evaluation

The goal or expected outcome for this patient problem is evaluated throughout the postpartum period because injuries such as muscle strains or thrombus formation are not evident until later. The provider notes lacerations after the baby's birth and makes necessary repairs.

KNOWLEDGE CHECK

14. How might maternal hypotension or hypertension affect the fetus?
15. What position should the woman avoid during labor? Why? What should you do if the woman must be in this position temporarily?
16. What general measures can make the woman more comfortable during labor? How can the nurse support the woman's labor partner?
17. Why is watching the perineum as a woman pushes important?

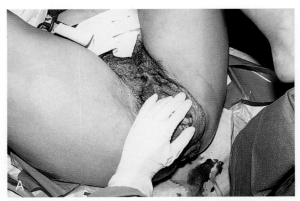

A, Crowning. The fetal head distends the labial and perineal tissues. The anus is stretched wide, and it is not unusual to see the woman's anterior rectal wall at this time. Any feces expelled are wiped posteriorly to avoid contaminating the vulva. The attendant (physician or nurse-midwife) is not holding the fetal head back but rather controlling its exit by using gentle pressure on the fetal occiput.

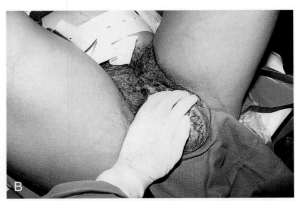

B, Ritgen Maneuver. Pressure is applied to the fetal chin through the perineum at the same time pressure is applied to the occiput of the fetal head. This action aids the mechanism of extension as the fetal head comes under the symphysis.

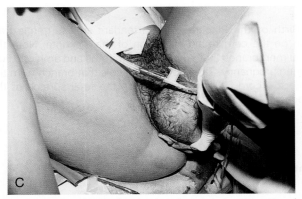

C, Birth of the Head. As the head emerges, the attendant prepares to wipe the mouth and nose to avoid aspiration of secretions when the infant takes the first breath.

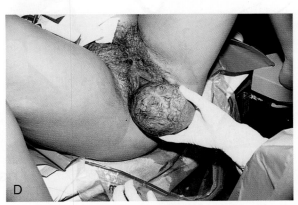

D, Restitution and External Rotation. After the head emerges, it realigns with the shoulders (restitution). External rotation occurs as the fetal shoulders internally rotate, aligning their transverse diameter with the anteroposterior diameter of the pelvic outlet.

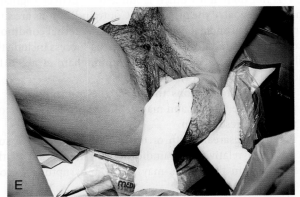

E, Birth of the Anterior Shoulder. The attendant gently pushes the fetal head toward the woman's perineum to allow the anterior shoulder to slip under her symphysis. The bluish skin color of the fetus is normal at this point; it becomes pink as the infant begins air breathing.

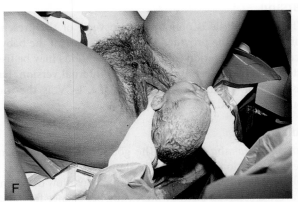

F, Birth of the Posterior Shoulder. The attendant now pushes the fetal head upward toward the woman's symphysis to allow the posterior shoulder to slip over her perineum.

FIG. 15.8 Vaginal Birth.

Continued

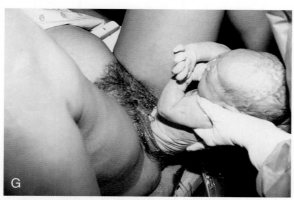

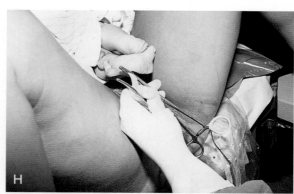

G, Completion of the Birth. The attendant supports the fetus during expulsion. Note that the fetus has excellent muscle tone, as evidenced by facial grimacing and flexion of the arms and hands.

H, Cord Clamping. While the infant is in skin-to-skin contact on the mother's abdomen, the attendant doubly clamps the umbilical cord. The cord is then cut between the two clamps. Samples of cord blood are collected after it is cut. If the parents have chosen to bank cord blood, the health care team follows the instructions in the cord blood banking collection kit.

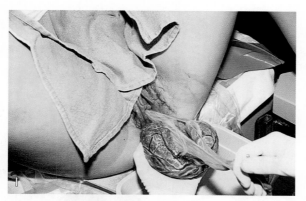

I, Birth of the Placenta. The attendant applies gentle traction on the cord to aid expulsion of the placenta. Note the fetal membranes that surrounded the fetus and amniotic fluid during pregnancy. The chorionic vessels that branch from the umbilical cord are readily visible on the fetal surface of the placenta.

FIG. 15.8, cont'd

ALTERATIONS IN NORMAL LABOR

Although labor is a normal process, some women may require interventions such as versions, labor induction, or labor augmentation.

Version

When the fetal lie is oblique or transverse or the presentation is breech, the provider may attempt to turn the baby to a cephalic presentation. Either of two methods may be used: **external cephalic version (ECV)** and internal version. Each has different indications and technique. ECV is the more common method.

Indications

External Cephalic Version. The goal of ECV is to change the fetal position from a breech, shoulder (transverse lie), or oblique presentation. Successful version may allow the woman to avoid a cesarean birth by increasing her chance for vaginal birth. Version of a fetus with a transverse lie has a higher success rate than breech presentations (Cunningham et al., 2014). Research has shown that, in many cases, spontaneous version occurs by 36 to 37 weeks of gestation (ACOG, 2016; Cunningham et al., 2014).

Internal Version. Malpresentation in twin gestations is usually managed by cesarean birth, but internal version is sometimes used for the vaginal birth of the second twin.

Contraindications

ECV is not done if a woman is unlikely to deliver vaginally, which is the goal of the procedure. Contraindications are similar for internal and external procedures. Maternal conditions that may contraindicate ECV or reduce its success include the following (AAP & ACOG, 2012; Cunningham et al., 2014; Thorp & Laughon, 2014):

- Uterine malformations that limit the room available to perform the version and may be the reason for the abnormal fetal presentation.
- Previous cesarean birth or other significant uterine surgery is a relative contraindication. Manipulation of the fetus within the uterus may strain and rupture the old incision.
- Placenta abnormalities (abruption or previa). Manipulation of the fetus within the uterus may cause hemorrhage, endangering both mother and fetus.
- Third-trimester bleeding.
- Disproportion between fetal size and maternal pelvic size.

Fetal conditions that may contraindicate the use of version include the following:

- Multifetal gestation, which reduces the room available in which to turn the fetus or fetuses. Version may be attempted after the first twin is born vaginally in a cephalic presentation.
- Oligohydramnios, ruptured membranes, and a cord around the fetal body or neck (**nuchal cord**). These conditions limit the room to turn the fetus and may lead to cord compression and fetal hypoxia.
- Intrauterine growth restriction.
- Uteroplacental insufficiency. Uterine contractions occurring during the version and labor may worsen the insufficiency and cause fetal compromise.
- Engagement of the fetal head into the pelvis.

Risks

Complications occur in 1% to 2% of attempted versions (Thorp & Laughon, 2014). Changes to FHR pattern are common, but the pattern usually returns to normal after the version. Serious risks involving the fetus include umbilical cord entanglement, compressing its vessels and resulting in hypoxia, and placental abruption if fetal manipulation disrupts the placental site, leading to fetal compromise and even death (Cunningham et al., 2014; Thorp & Laughon, 2014). Fetal and maternal blood could become mixed within placental vessels, possibly resulting in maternal sensitization to the fetal blood type. Cesarean birth may be needed for fetal compromise at the time of the version or later if the fetus returns to an abnormal presentation.

Technique

External Cephalic Version. ECV is performed at a location and time to allow emergency cesarean delivery if necessary (ACOG, 2016; Cunningham et al., 2014). A nonstress test or biophysical profile is done before the procedure to evaluate fetal health and placental function. If fetal well-being is not present, the version is not performed. An ultrasound examination confirms fetal gestational age and presentation and identifies adequacy of amniotic fluid and placental location (Cunningham et al., 2014).

ECV usually is attempted at 37 weeks or longer of gestation but before the woman is in labor, for the following reasons:

- The fetus may spontaneously turn to a cephalic presentation before 37 weeks.
- The fetus is more likely to return to an abnormal presentation if version is attempted before 37 weeks of gestation.
- If fetal compromise and onset of labor occur, a fetus born after 37 weeks of gestation is not likely to have major problems associated with preterm birth, such as respiratory distress syndrome.

The woman often is given a tocolytic to relax the uterus while the version is performed. Epidural or spinal block may be given to reduce the mother's discomfort as the physician manipulates the fetus. Ultrasonography guides fetal manipulations during ECV and monitors the FHR. The physician gently pushes the breech out of the pelvis in a forward or

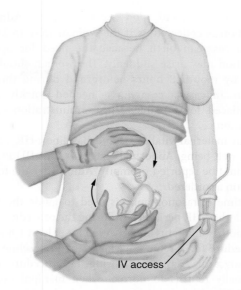

FIG. 15.9 External Cephalic Version. Intravenous access is established, if needed. If terbutaline is used as a tocolytic or uterine relaxant medication, it is given by subcutaneous injection.

backward roll (ACOG, 2016; Thorp & Laughon, 2014) (Fig. 15.9).

Rh immunoglobulin (RhoGAM) is given to the Rh-negative woman after external version to prevent Rh sensitization.

Labor induction may be done immediately after successful ECV, or the woman may await spontaneous labor or a later induction. EFM is performed for a minimum of 1 hour after the version for evaluation of fetal condition (Thorp & Laughon, 2014).

Internal Version. Internal version is an uncommon procedure, most often for the second twin after the first delivers in the cephalic presentation. The physician reaches into the uterus with one hand and, with the other hand on the maternal abdomen, moves the fetus into a longitudinal lie (cephalic or breech) to allow vaginal birth (Cunningham et al., 2014).

Nursing Considerations

When caring for the woman having external version, the nurse provides information, assesses the woman and fetus, and helps reduce her anxiety.

Provide Information. The provider explains the indications and risks for ECV to the woman before she signs an informed consent. Purposes and side effects of any planned tocolytic drug are reviewed. If epidural or other analgesia is planned, its purposes and side effects are explained by the person who will administer the treatment, and the woman signs additional consents. The nurse verifies the woman's understanding of the purposes, risks, and limitations of the procedure and related treatments. Because cesarean birth may be required suddenly, permits to allow the surgery and initial care of her newborn are signed.

Promote Maternal and Fetal Health. Admission information is collected as if the woman were in labor or having a cesarean birth because the need for operative intervention may arise suddenly. The woman should have nothing by mouth 8 hours before and during this short procedure in case a cesarean is needed quickly. An IV line is placed for possible drug administration or fluid resuscitation.

Obtain maternal vital signs and baseline FHR values to establish well-being. Abnormal (category II or III) FHR patterns should be reported promptly. Administer the tocolytic medication as ordered.

Real-time ultrasonography is used to guide the version and check the FHR periodically during the procedure.

The mother and fetus are observed for at least 1 hour after the procedure for a return of vital signs to baseline values. Fetal bradycardia may occur during the procedure, but the FHR usually returns to normal when manipulation ends (Thorp & Laughon, 2014). Reassuring fetal signs are a heart rate within the same range as on admission, resolution of any bradycardia, and the presence of moderate variability and FHR accelerations.

Maternal vital signs are taken every 15 to 30 minutes until they return to baseline. The woman's pulse rate should be no higher than 120 bpm. Discomfort should diminish quickly after the version, regardless of whether fetal position changes are successful. Persistent and continuous pain suggests a complication such as placental abruption.

If epidural or spinal analgesia was used and is now discontinued, observe for return of sensation before ambulation. Accompany the woman while ambulating until she is steady on her feet.

Regular contractions suggest onset of labor. SROM sometimes occurs, with leakage of fluid from the mother's vagina. Rh immunoglobulin is given if indicated. The IV line is discontinued after the maternal and fetal conditions return to normal unless labor will be induced the same day.

Because the woman having ECV is near term, the nurse should review the signs of true labor and membrane rupture with her and explain guidelines for returning to the hospital if she will be discharged.

Reduce Anxiety. The woman may be anxious before version because its success is not certain and complications may require emergency cesarean delivery. Afterward, she still may be anxious because the fetus can return to its previous position and vaginal birth is not certain. The nurse should keep the woman informed about what is occurring during the version to reduce her fear of the unknown.

The nurse can point out reassuring fetal monitor patterns such as a normal rate and rate accelerations to help reduce anxiety about the baby. If a problem such as bradycardia develops, the nurse should explain what has happened, what steps are being done to relieve it, and the result of these interventions.

KNOWLEDGE CHECK

18. Why is observing the FHR important before, during, and after ECV?
19. Why should the UA be monitored after ECV?

Induction and Augmentation of Labor

Induction and augmentation of labor use artificial methods to stimulate uterine contractions. Techniques and nursing care are similar for both induction and augmentation.

Induction of labor is an increasingly common procedure in intrapartum units. Induction rates more than doubled from 1990 to 2010, reaching an all-time high of 23.8% (Osterman & Martin, 2014). Data from the National Vital Statistics System shows that after nearly 20 years of steady increases, the rate is declining, as seen in the 2015 induction rate of 23.9% (Osterman & Martin, 2014, National Center for Health Statistics - NCHS, 2017).

Inductions have been associated with a higher cesarean birth rate. This increased risk for cesarean section can be mitigated if the cervix is dilated (at least 2 cm) and somewhat effaced before labor (Thorp & Laughon, 2014). Induction is more likely to be successful at term because prelabor cervical changes favor dilation. In 2014, the cesarean rate was 32.2% for women of all racial origins, which was 2% lower than the rate in 2013 (Hamilton, Martin, Osterman, Curtin, & Mathews, 2015). This decline is partly attributed to the focus on reducing nonmedically indicated (elective) cesarean sections and induction of labor before 39 weeks.

Indications

Induction of labor may be medically necessary for an obstetric, fetal, or other medical indication or it may be elective (i.e., performed at the convenience of the patient and/or provider). Labor induction is not done if the fetus must be delivered more quickly than the process permits, in which case a cesarean birth is performed. Induction is indicated in the following conditions (ACOG, 2015a; Thorpe & Laughon, 2014):

- The intrauterine environment is hostile to fetal well-being (e.g., intrauterine fetal growth restriction, isoimmunization [maternal-fetal blood incompatibility], oligohydramnios)
- SROM at or near term without onset of labor, also called **premature rupture of the membranes** (PROM). If pregnancy is preterm, less than 37 weeks, the term **preterm premature rupture of the membranes** (PPROM) is used (see Chapter 16)
- Postterm pregnancy
- Chorioamnionitis (infection and inflammation of the amniotic sac)
- Hypertension associated with pregnancy or chronic hypertension, both of which are associated with reduced placental blood flow
- Placental abruption (large abruptions require immediate delivery)

- Maternal medical conditions that worsen with continuation of the pregnancy (e.g., diabetes, hypertension, renal disease, pulmonary disease, heart disease, antiphospholipid syndrome)
- Fetal demise

Induction solely for convenience is not recommended. Factors such as having a history of rapid labor and living a long distance from the hospital may be valid reasons to induce labor because of the real possibility that the baby would be born in uncontrolled circumstances. (ACOG, 2015a; Simpson & O'Brien-Abel, 2014). Elective inductions have two major risks: twofold increase in cesarean section compared with spontaneous labor and increased risk for neonatal respiratory complications (Thorp & Laughon, 2014). Therefore confirmation of fetal gestational age is paramount before elective induction. Recent recommendations suggest waiting until 40 to 41 weeks before considering elective induction (AWHONN, 2012; Spong et al., 2012; Thorp & Laughon, 2014). This gestational age is associated with decreased risk for cesarean delivery and neonatal respiratory morbidity.

Prenatal testing sometimes identifies a fetal anomaly that will require specialized neonatal care at a distant facility. The mother may be transported to that facility for labor induction or cesarean birth.

Augmentation of labor with oxytocin is considered when labor has begun spontaneously but progress has slowed or stopped, even if contractions seem to be adequate. Nonpharmacologic augmentation may be possible with nipple stimulation (Cunningham et al., 2014; Thorp & Laughon, 2014).

Contraindications

Any contraindication to labor and vaginal birth is a contraindication to induction or augmentation of labor. Possible contraindications and cautions associated with induction may include the following (ACOG, 2015a; Benirschke, 2014; Simpson & O'Brien-Abel, 2014; Thorpe & Laughon, 2014):

- **Placenta previa**, placental implantation in the lower uterine segment, which could result in hemorrhage during labor
- **Vasa previa**, a velamentous insertion of the umbilical cord (umbilical cord vessels branch over the amniotic membrane rather than inserting into the placenta, therefore lacking protection of Wharton jelly); these vessels cross the cervical os; fetal hemorrhage is a possibility if the membranes rupture
- Umbilical cord prolapse, because immediate cesarean is indicated to stop cord compression
- Abnormal fetal presentation for which vaginal birth is often more hazardous (i.e., transverse fetal lie)
- Active genital herpes
- Previous uterine surgery, such as a previous classical cesarean incision or myomectomy (removal of uterine fibroids) that entered the endometrial cavity

Other maternal or fetal conditions are not contraindications to induction but require individual evaluation, such as the following (ACOG, 2015b; Thorpe & Laughon, 2014):

- One or more previous low transverse cesarean deliveries
- Breech presentation
- Conditions in which the uterus is overdistended, such as a multifetal pregnancy and polyhydramnios, because the risk for uterine rupture is higher
- Severe maternal conditions such as heart disease and severe hypertension
- Fetal presenting part above the pelvic inlet, which may be associated with cephalopelvic disproportion or a preterm fetus
- Inability to adequately monitor the fetal status during labor or presence of indeterminate or abnormal FHR

Risks

Induction and augmentation of labor, like spontaneous labor, are associated with the following risks (ACOG, 2015a; Cunningham et al., 2014; Simpson & O'Brien-Abel, 2014):

- Excessive UA (increased frequency, duration, or insufficient relaxation time or resting tone) can reduce placental perfusion and fetal oxygenation. Uterine tachysystole may or may not be accompanied by an indeterminate or abnormal FHR pattern.
- Uterine rupture may occur, which is more likely with overdistention of the uterus with excess amniotic fluid or a multifetal pregnancy or in cases of excessive UA.
- Maternal water intoxication can occur, which is more likely if a hypotonic IV solution is used to dilute the oxytocin and with rates greater than 20 milliunits/min.
- Chorioamnionitis and cesarean birth.
- Postpartum hemorrhage.

Elective labor induction at term is associated with increased risk for cesarean birth and newborn respiratory problems. Studies have demonstrated that nulliparous women who have their labor induced are two to three times more likely to have a surgical birth. A Bishop score (Table 15.2) of 7 or less is associated with an increased risk for cesarean birth compared with spontaneously laboring patients (Cunningham et al., 2014). The risk for cesarean after failed induction was similar whether women had medical or elective inductions. Risk for chorioamnionitis increases as the duration of ruptured membranes increases (Cunningham et al., 2014).

Technique

Pharmacologic and mechanical methods may be used for labor induction and augmentation. Cervical assessment estimates whether the cervix is favorable for induction. The Bishop scoring system (see Table 15.2) is used to estimate cervical readiness for labor with five factors: cervical dilation, effacement, consistency, position, and fetal station. Vaginal birth is more likely to result if a Bishop score is higher than 8 (ACOG, 2015a).

TABLE 15.2   Bishop Scoring System to Evaluate the Cervix*

	SCORE			
Factor	0	1	2	3
Dilation	0 cm	1-2 cm	3-4 cm	5-6 cm
Effacement	0-30%	40%-50%	60%-70%	≥80%
Fetal station	−3	−2	−1 or 0	+1 or +2
Cervical consistency	Firm	Medium	Soft	
Cervical position	Posterior	Middle	Anterior	

Modified from Bishop, E. H. (1964). Pelvic scoring for elective induction. *Obstetrics & Gynecology, 24*(2), 266–268.
*This system is used to estimate how easily a woman's labor can be induced. Higher scores are associated with a greater likelihood of successful induction because her cervix has undergone prelabor changes, often called *ripening*. A woman who has given birth before usually has a successful induction when her Bishop score is 5 or higher. Delivery in a woman who is having her first baby is most successfully induced if her score is 7 or higher.

Cervical Ripening. Cervical ripening is a process used to ripen (soften) the cervix and make it more likely to dilate with the forces of labor. Typically, this procedure is performed before the scheduled induction. Cervical ripening is recommended for Bishop score of 4 or less (Cunningham et al., 2014).

Pharmacologic Methods. Prostaglandin is a drug that may be used to cause cervical ripening. Prostaglandin E_2 (PGE_2) preparations may be given as an intravaginal gel, an intracervical gel, or a timed-release vaginal insert (Table 15.3). PGE_2 preparations are administered in a setting where fetal monitoring and emergency care, including immediate cesarean birth, are readily available.

Misoprostol (Cytotec) is a prostaglandin E_1 (PGE_1) analog usually given for gastric ulcers. Misoprostol can be used for both cervical ripening and induction of labor. Misoprostol for cervical ripening is currently an off-label use, and its manufacturer does not plan to seek U.S. Food and Drug Administration (FDA) approval for these purposes. In addition to its effectiveness, misoprostol is attractive for its lower cost and stability at room temperature (ACOG, 2015a; Cunningham et al., 2014; FDA, 2015). However, it should not be given to a woman who has had a previous cesarean birth or major uterine surgery (ACOG, 2015b; Simpson & O'Brien-Abel, 2014).

Misoprostol is available in 100- and 200-mcg tablets. The usual dose is 25 or 50 mcg vaginally, one quarter or one half of an unscored 100-mcg tablet (ACOG, 2015a). A pharmacist should prepare the tablet to ensure dose accuracy when using an unscored tablet. The 25-mcg preparation of misoprostol is placed high in the vagina. An oral dose of misoprostol 100 mcg has also been reported to be effective (ACOG, 2015a; Cunningham et al., 2014).

Because the major adverse effect of prostaglandins is tachysystole, the drug is administered in a setting in which fetal monitoring and emergency care, including cesarean birth, are immediately available. After vaginal insertion of prostaglandins, the patient should remain recumbent for at least 30 minutes. The FHR and UA should be monitored continuously for a period of 30 minutes to 2 hours (ACOG, 2015a).

Mechanical Methods. Mechanical methods for cervical ripening are efficacious and have decreased risk for excessive UA. These methods include placement of a transcervical balloon catheter, membrane stripping, or placement of hydroscopic inserts (i.e., *Laminaria*—sterile cone-shaped preparations of dried seaweed).

Transcervical catheters are placed through the internal cervical os, and downward tension is created by either taping the catheter to the thigh or attaching the catheter to a dependent IV bag (Cunningham et al., 2014; Simpson & O'Brien-Abel, 2014).

Membrane stripping is the digital separation of the amniotic membrane from the wall of the cervix and the lower uterine segment. Spontaneous labor may occur within 48 hours and reduces the need for other induction methods (ACOG, 2015a; Simpson & O'Brien-Abel, 2014).

Hydroscopic inserts (Laminaria) are placed into the cervical canal, where they absorb water and swell, gradually dilating the cervix. Placement requires a speculum and can be cumbersome and uncomfortable (Cunningham et al., 2014).

Oxytocin Administration. Oxytocin is the most common drug given for induction and augmentation of labor (see Drug Guide). Oxytocin is a powerful drug, and predicting a woman's response to it is impossible. Several precautions reduce the chance of adverse reactions in the mother and fetus.

- Oxytocin is diluted in an isotonic solution and given as a secondary (piggyback) infusion so it can be stopped quickly if complications develop.
- The oxytocin line is inserted into the primary (nonadditive or maintenance) IV line as close as possible to the venipuncture site (the proximal port) to limit the amount of drug infused if discontinued.
- Oxytocin is started slowly, increased gradually, and regulated with an infusion pump. The primary line is also regulated with an infusion pump.
- UA, FHR, and fetal heart patterns are monitored before induction for a baseline, when oxytocin is started, and throughout labor.

Oxytocin receptor sites become desensitized from prolonged exposure. Continual rate increases can result in abnormal UA (tachysystole), coupling or tripling of contractions, or

TABLE 15.3 Prostaglandin Preparations for Cervical Ripening at Term

Prostaglandin Gel (Dinoprostone [Prepidil])	Vaginal Insert (Dinoprostone [Cervidil])	Misoprostol (Cytotec)
Dosage*		
0.5 mg applied in the cervix; may be repeated 6-12 hr later. Maximum recommended dose is 1.5 mg applied in the cervix in a 24-hr period. 2.5 mg applied in the vagina.	10 mg in a time-release vaginal insert left in place for up to 12 hr. Remove with onset of active labor, membrane rupture, or uterine tachysystole.	One quarter to one-half of 100-mcg tablet vaginally (~25-50 mcg; see following precautions). Also used for labor induction by repeating 25-mcg dose every 3-6 hr. A 50-mcg dose has been associated with excessive uterine activity.
Actions for Hypertonic Contractions, with or without Nonreassuring Fetal Heart Rate Pattern		
Place woman in side-lying position. Provide oxygen by nonrebreather face mask at 10 L/min. Administer tocolytic drug such as terbutaline. Typically begins 1 hr after gel application. Higher incidence with vaginal application.	Same as for dinoprostone gel. Remove insert. Hypertonic uterine activity may occur up to 9.5 hr after insert placement. Greater incidence than with lower dose intracervical dinoprostone gel.	Same as for dinoprostone gel. Higher dose or more frequent administration is more likely to cause excessive contractions, which may or may not be accompanied by a nonreassuring fetal heart rate pattern.
When Oxytocin Induction May Begin		
Safe interval has not been established. Delaying oxytocin administration for 6-12 hr after total intracervical dose of 1.5-mg or 2.5-mg vaginal dose recommended.	30-60 min after removal of insert.	At least 4 hr after last dose.
Precautions and Comments		
Limit dinoprostone gel to maximum of 1.5 mg in the cervix in 24 hr. Woman should remain recumbent with lateral uterine displacement for 15-30 min after application. Has increased effect if combined with other oxytocics such as oxytocin (Pitocin). Increases hypertensive effect of the herb ephedra. Use caution in women with asthma, hypertension, glaucoma, severe renal or hepatic dysfunction, or ischemic heart disease.	Remove after 12 hr or when active labor begins. Adverse effects can be reduced within 15 min of removal. Most expensive of prostaglandin options.	Misoprostol is currently FDA-approved only for treatment of peptic ulcers but is widely used for cervical ripening and induction of labor. Manufacturer does not intend to seek approval, but the ACOG supports its use for these purposes. 100-mcg tablet is not scored. The hospital pharmacy should prepare the 25- or 50-mcg dose for greater accuracy. Cost is ~1%-2% that of other prostaglandin preparations. Contraindicated in woman with a previous cesarean or other uterine surgery.

From American Academy of Pediatrics & American College of Obstetricians and Gynecologists (AAP & ACOG). (2012). *Guidelines for perinatal care* (7th ed.). Elk Grove Village, IL: Authors; American College of Obstetricians and Gynecologists (ACOG). (2015a). *Induction of labor.* Practice Bulletin 107. Washington, DC: Author; Sheibani, L., & Wing, D. A. (2017). Abnormal labor and induction of labor. In S. G. Gabbe, J. R. Niebyl, & J. L. Simpson, M.B. Landon, H.L. Galan, R. M. Jauniaux, D.A. Driscoll, et al. (Eds.), *Obstetrics: Normal and problem pregnancies* (7th ed., pp. 271–288). Philadelphia, PA: Saunders.
ACOG, American College of Obstetricians and Gynecologists; *FDA,* U.S. Food and Drug Administration.
*Doses may be higher in cases of fetal death.

🔷 DRUG GUIDE

Oxytocin (Pitocin)
Classification
Oxytocic.

Action
Synthetic compound identical to the natural hormone released from the posterior pituitary. Stimulates uterine smooth muscle, resulting in increased strength, duration, and frequency of uterine contractions. Uterine sensitivity to oxytocin increases gradually during gestation. Oxytocin has vasoactive and antidiuretic properties.

Indications
Induction or augmentation of labor at or near term. Maintenance of firm uterine contractions after birth to control postpartum bleeding. Management of inevitable or incomplete abortion.

Continued

Dosage and Route

Induction or Augmentation of Labor

1. Intravenous (IV) infusion via a secondary (piggyback) line. Oxytocin infusion is controlled with a pump. Various dilutions of oxytocin and balanced electrolyte solution may be used. Mixtures having 60 milliunits/mL are convenient because the milliliters per hour setting on the infusion pump is the same number as the milliunits per minute infused, reducing the chance for errors. Common mixtures that provide 60 milliunits/mL of oxytocin include (1) 15 units of oxytocin (1.5 mL) plus 250 mL of solution; (2) 30 units (3 mL) of oxytocin plus 500 mL of solution; and (3) 60 units (6 mL) of oxytocin plus 1000 mL of solution. Lower concentrations such as 10 to 20 units of oxytocin plus 1000 mL of solution also may be used. Oxytocin solutions may be standardized and premixed in the pharmacy to reduce risk for error.

2. Guidelines for oxytocin administration from ACOG (2015a) provide examples of low-dose and high-dose oxytocin labor induction protocols. Depending on the protocol followed, the following recommendations are provided: (1) starting doses of 0.5 to 2 milliunits/min for the low dose protocol and 6 milliunits/min for the high dose protocol, and (2) increasing the dose in 1 to 2 milliunits/min increments every 15 to 40 minutes for low dose; high-dose protocols may increase the dose in increments of up to 6 milliunits/min. The actual oxytocin dose is based on uterine response and absence of adverse effects. Higher starting doses, higher dose increases, and shorter intervals between dose increases are most likely to result in uterine tachysystole. A lower starting dose and lower rate increase increments are usually required to augment labor.

3. Once active labor is achieved and an adequate contraction pattern exists, oxytocin may be reduced by similar increments.

Control of Postpartum Bleeding

IV infusion: Dilute 10 to 40 units in 1000 mL of IV solution. The rate of infusion must control uterine atony. Begin at a rate of 20 to 40 milliunits/min, increasing or decreasing the rate according to uterine response and the rate of postpartum bleeding. Any identifiable cause of the hemorrhage should also be corrected.

Intramuscular Injection

Inject 10 units after delivery of the placenta often used if no IV access.

Inevitable or Incomplete Abortion

Dilute 10 units in 500 mL of IV solution and infuse at a rate of 10 to 20 milliunits/min. Other dilutions are acceptable.

Absorption

IV, within 1 minute; intramuscular (IM), 3 to 5 minutes.

Excretion

Renal (urine).

Contraindications and Precautions

Include, but are not limited to, placenta previa, vasa previa, indeterminate or abnormal fetal heart rate (FHR) patterns, abnormal fetal presentation, prolapsed umbilical cord, previous classic or other fundal uterine incision, active genital herpes infection, pelvic structural deformities, invasive cervical carcinoma.

Adverse Reactions

Most result from hypersensitivity to drug or excessive dosage. Adverse reactions include excessive uterine activity (UA) (tachysystole, hypertonus, inadequate relaxation time, etc.), impaired uterine blood flow, uterine rupture, and placental abruption. Uterine hypertonicity may result in fetal bradycardia, fetal tachycardia, reduced FHR variability, and late or prolonged decelerations. Fetal arrhythmias (including premature ventricular contractions) may also occur. Fetal asphyxia may occur with diminished uterine blood flow. Fetal or maternal trauma, or both, may occur from rapid birth. Prolonged administration may cause maternal fluid retention, leading to water intoxication. Hypotension (seen with rapid IV injection), tachycardia, cardiac arrhythmias, and subarachnoid hemorrhage are rare adverse reactions.

Drug interactions include vasopressors and the herb ephedra, causing hypertension.

Nursing Considerations

Intrapartum

Assess the FHR for at least 20 minutes before induction to identify fetal well-being. Perform Leopold's maneuvers, a vaginal examination, or both to verify a cephalic fetal presentation. If indeterminate or abnormal FHR patterns are identified or if fetal presentation is other than cephalic, notify the physician and do not begin induction until an ultrasound is done to ascertain fetal presentation and fetal well-being.

Observe UA for establishment of effective labor pattern: contraction frequency every 2 to 3 minutes, duration of 40 to 90 seconds. Observe for excessive UA: contractions less than 2 minutes apart, rest interval shorter than 60 seconds in first-stage labor and 45 to 50 seconds in second-stage labor, duration longer than 120 seconds, or an elevated resting tone firm by palpation or greater than 20 to 25 mm Hg (if measured with an intrauterine pressure catheter).

Observe FHR for patterns such as tachycardia, bradycardia, decreased variability, and pathologic (late, variable, or prolonged) decelerations. If uterine tachysystole or FHR patterns as indicated previously occur, intervene to reduce UA and increase fetal oxygenation: stop the oxytocin infusion, increase the rate of nonadditive solution, position the woman in a side-lying position, and administer oxygen by nonrebreather face mask at 10 L/min. Notify the provider of adverse reactions, nursing interventions, and patient response. Record the maternal blood pressure, pulse rate, and respirations every 30 to 60 minutes or with each dose increase. Record intake and output.

Postpartum

Observe the uterus for firmness, height, and deviation. Massage until firm if uterus is soft ("boggy"). Observe lochia for color, quantity, and presence of clots. Notify the provider if the uterus fails to remain contracted or if lochia is bright red or contains large clots. Assess for cramping. Assess vital signs every 15 minutes or according to protocol for the recovery period. Monitor intake and output and breath sounds to identify fluid retention or bladder distention.

Inevitable or Incomplete Abortion

Observe for cramping, vaginal bleeding, clots, and passage of products of conception. Observe maternal vital signs and intake and output as noted under postpartum nursing implications.

Oxytocin: Drug information. (2016). UpToDate. Retrieved from www.uptodate.com/contents/oxytocin-drug-information?source=-search_result&search=oxytocin

low-intensity contractions (Simpson & O'Brien-Abel, 2014). The rate of oxytocin infusion may be gradually reduced once the active phase of labor is reached (4 to 6 cm of cervical dilation) to decrease the receptor site saturation (Simpson & O'Brien-Abel, 2014). It may be stopped, or the rate reduced after the patient's membranes rupture. When labor is augmented with oxytocin, a lower total dose usually is needed to achieve adequate contractions compared to the dose needed for labor induction.

Nursing Considerations. When providing care during cervical ripening and labor induction or augmentation, the nurse observes the woman and fetus for complications and takes corrective actions if abnormalities are noted. The nurse has a great responsibility when administering uterine stimulants to a pregnant woman. The nurse decides when to start, change, and stop an oxytocin infusion using the facility's protocols and medical orders. Facility policies related to oxytocin must clearly support correct nursing and medical actions.

! SAFETY CHECK

Signs of Excessive Uterine Activity

- Contraction duration longer than 120 seconds
- Less than 60 seconds relaxation time between contractions in first-stage labor and 45 to 50 seconds in second-stage labor
- Uterine resting tone firm by palpation or higher than 20 to 25 mm Hg (with intrauterine pressure catheter)
- Montevideo units (MVUs; unit of measure for uterine contraction intensity) exceeding 300 to 400 (Killion, 2015)
- More than 5 contractions in a 10-minute window, averaged over 30 minutes

Nursing Actions for Excessive Uterine Activity
(ACOG, 2015c; Simpson & O'Brien-Able, 2014)
With Normal Fetal Heart Rate Patterns
- Position the woman on her side.
- Administer an IV fluid bolus of at least 500 mL.
- If the tachysystole does not resolve in 10 to 15 minutes, the oxytocin infusion rate should be decreased by half.
- If tachysystole persists after another 10 to 15 minutes, the oxytocin infusion should be stopped until the uterine activity is normal.

With Abnormal Fetal Heart Rate Patterns
- Stop the oxytocin infusion and administer bolus of at least 500 mL of the primary nonadditive infusion.
- Keep the woman in a side-lying position to prevent aortocaval compression and increase placental blood flow.
- Consider oxygen administration at 10 L/min via nonrebreather face mask until FHR pattern improves.
- Notify the provider; anticipate order for terbutaline (Brethine 0.25 mg subcutaneously) if no improvement occurs with other interventions.

In both cases, oxytocin may be restarted when the tachysystole resolves and the FHR pattern returns to normal. The oxytocin should be restarted at no more than half the previous rate if it has been turned off for less than 20 to 30 minutes. If more than 30 to 40 minutes has elapsed, it should be restarted at the initial dose.

? CRITICAL THINKING EXERCISE 15.4

A woman is having term labor induced with oxytocin. Her cervix is 4 cm dilated and fully effaced, and the fetal head is at station 0. The nurse notes that the fetal heart rate (external monitor) is near its baseline of 120 to 130 beats per minute (bpm), with a variability of 10 bpm (moderate variability). Contractions are firm to palpation and occur every 2 minutes (every 120 seconds), and the duration is usually 100 seconds. With palpation the nurse notes that the woman's uterus does not fully relax before another contraction begins.

Questions
1. What is the correct interpretation of these assessments?
2. What are appropriate nursing actions in this situation, and why are they done?

Observe the Fetal Response. Oxytocin stimulates uterine contractions, and they may become too frequent (tachysystole). Tachysystole may reduce placental blood flow (uteroplacental insufficiency), which decreases exchange of fetal oxygen and waste products. Before induction and augmentation of labor, the nurse assesses the FHR and contraction pattern to ensure fetal well-being is present. ACOG and AWHONN set forth standards for FHR assessment based on risk-stratification of the patient (Simpson, 2013). Individual facilities set documentation guidelines incorporating those recommendations.

The nurse remains alert for FHR patterns that suggest reduced placental exchange secondary to excessive UA. Examples are fetal bradycardia, tachycardia, pathologic decelerations, and decreased FHR variability. The nurse should assess the woman and fetus carefully to identify the most likely cause of the problem and institute corrective actions. See Chapter 14 for more detailed information on fetal monitoring.

If indeterminate or abnormal patterns occur with tachysystole, the nurse takes the following steps to reduce UA and increase fetal oxygenation (ACOG, 2015c; Simpson & O'Brien-Abel, 2014):
- Stop the oxytocin infusion and administer a bolus of at least 500 mL of the primary nonadditive infusion.
- Keep the woman in a side-lying position to prevent aortocaval compression and increase placental blood flow.
- Consider oxygen administration at 10 L/min via nonrebreather facemask until FHR pattern improves.
- Notify the provider; anticipate order for terbutaline (Brethine), a smooth muscle relaxant, 0.25 mg subcutaneously, if no improvement with other interventions.
- Oxytocin may be restarted when the tachysystole resolves and the FHR pattern returns to normal. The oxytocin should be restarted at no more than half the previous rate if it has been turned off for less than 20 to 30 minutes. If more than 30 to 40 minutes have elapsed, it should be restarted at the initial dose.

Observe the Mother's Response. The uterus must be assessed for excessive UA that may reduce fetal oxygenation and contribute to uterine rupture. Contractions are assessed for frequency, duration and intensity, uterine resting tone, and relaxation time of at least 60 seconds between contractions in first-stage labor and 45 to 50 seconds in second-stage labor (Miller et al., 2017). UA observations are charted at the same intervals as the FHR. Corrective actions for excessive UA with normal FHR patterns include positioning the woman on her side and administering an IV fluid bolus of at least 500 mL. If the tachysystole does not resolve in 10 to 15 min, the oxytocin infusion rate should be decreased by half. If tachysystole persists after another 10 to 15 minutes, the oxytocin infusion should be stopped until the UA is normal. Provided that the FHR pattern has remained normal, the oxytocin infusion may be restarted as described previously in the discussion of the fetal response (ACOG, 2015c; Simpson & O'Brien-Able, 2014).

If the oxytocin must be discontinued, the medical decision about resuming is individualized. The oxytocin infusion may be restarted at the same or a lower dose if the contractions are no longer too frequent and the FHR is reassuring. If the oxytocin has been discontinued for 40 minutes or longer, the drug that was in the woman's system has been metabolized. Therefore it should be restarted at the beginning dose ordered and advanced more slowly to prevent a recurrence of uterine tachysystole and indeterminate or abnormal FHR patterns.

The woman's blood pressure and pulse rate are taken every 30 minutes or with each oxytocin dose increase to identify changes from her baseline. Her temperature is assessed every 2 hours, unless ruptured, and then it is assessed hourly to identify infection (Simpson & O'Brien-Abel, 2014).

The woman may need to use pharmacologic and non-pharmacologic pain management techniques sooner than in a spontaneous labor. Although the goal of induced and augmented labor is to mimic natural labor, stimulated contractions often increase in intensity more quickly. Cervical ripening may increase the discomfort felt by the woman.

Recording intake and output identifies fluid retention, which may precede water intoxication. Signs and symptoms of water intoxication include headache, blurred vision, behavioral changes, increased blood pressure and respirations, decreased pulse rate, auscultatory crackles and wheezing, and coughing.

After birth the mother is observed for postpartum hemorrhage caused by uterine relaxation. Postpartum uterine atony is more likely if she had prolonged use of oxytocin. The uterine muscle becomes fatigued and does not contract effectively to compress vessels at the placental site, and the oxytocin receptor sites may be saturated and less responsive. Atony is manifested by a soft uterine fundus and excess amounts of lochia, usually with large clots. Hypovolemic shock may occur with hemorrhage.

? KNOWLEDGE CHECK

20. What precautions are taken to enhance the safety of oxytocin administration for the woman and fetus?
21. How may oxytocin administration differ if labor is being augmented rather than induced?
22. What signs may indicate a nonreassuring fetal response to oxytocin stimulation?
23. What are the signs of excessive uterine activity?
24. How can induction of labor with oxytocin contribute to postpartum hemorrhage?

NURSING CARE: PREPARATION AND BIRTH

Responsibilities during Birth

The nurse's responsibilities during birth may include the following:

- Preparation of a delivery table with sterile gowns, gloves, drapes, solutions, and instruments (see Fig. 15.6)
- Perineal cleansing preparation
- Ongoing assessments of woman and fetus
- Supporting the woman and partner with final pushing efforts
- Initial care and assessment of the newborn
- Administration of medications (usually oxytocin) to contract the uterus and control blood loss.

A nurse or resuscitation team from the nursery is usually present if the newborn is at risk for problems such as respiratory depression and if problems occurred during labor. A person certified to provide neonatal resuscitation should be present at all births (AAP & ACOG, 2012).

Personal protective equipment, including eye shields, should be worn as protection from fluid splashing and blood spurting. The newborn is covered with blood, amniotic fluid, vernix, and other body substances. The first bath usually occurs several hours after birth, so persons involved in infant care should wear gloves and other needed protective equipment to avoid contact with potentially infectious secretions.

Operative Vaginal Birth

Operative vaginal birth, also called *forceps* or *vacuum extraction,* may be used by the provider to apply traction to or assist descent of or rotation of the fetal head during birth, aiding the woman's expulsive efforts. As the rate of cesarean birth has increased, vaginal births assisted by either forceps or vacuum extractor have declined. Among vaginal births in 2013, 3.3% were delivered with instrumentation, with 0.59% of the women delivered with forceps and 2.72% with vacuum extraction. Use of either method is down from 9.01% in 1990 (Martin et al., 2015; Simpson & O'Brien-Abel, 2014).

A vacuum extractor uses suction to grasp the fetal head while traction is applied (Fig. 15.10). Its use is similar to that of forceps and carries the following contraindications to use:

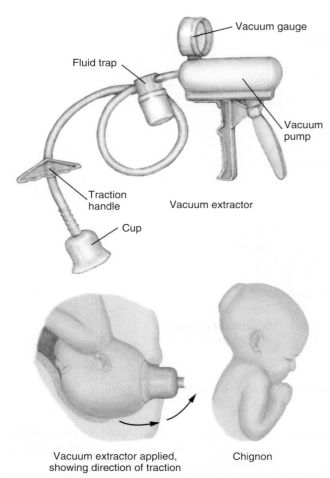

Vacuum gauge

Fluid trap

Vacuum pump

Traction handle   Vacuum extractor

Cup

Vacuum extractor applied,   Chignon
showing direction of traction

FIG. 15.10 Birth Assisted with a Vacuum Extractor. The chignon is scalp edema that often forms under the suction cup when the vacuum extractor is used.

breech, face, or brow presentation; cephalopelvic dispro-portion; unengaged fetal head; incompletely dilated cervix; suspected bone demineralization condition (i.e., osteogen-esis imperfecta); bleeding disorder (i.e., hemophilia, von Willebrand's disease); or premature infant. The fetus of 34 weeks or less of gestation is more likely to injure the head, scalp, and intracranial vessels from vacuum suction (ACOG, 2015d; Thorp & Laughon, 2014). No more than three "pop-offs" of the vacuum extractor should be allowed, and they should not be followed by attempts to deliver with forceps (ACOG, 2015d; Simpson & O'Brien-Abel, 2014; Thorp & Laughon, 2014).

Forceps are curved, metal instruments with two curved blades that can be locked in the center. Many styles are avail-able for different needs. The blades may be closed or open and are shaped to grasp the fetal head (Fig. 15.11). Foam pads are available to cushion the fetal head from the blades. Piper forceps are a special type used to assist birth of the head, as it is born last in a vaginal breech birth. Forceps and a vacuum extractor also may be used during cesarean birth if assistance is needed in delivering the head.

Indications

Forceps or vacuum extraction is considered if the second stage should be shortened for the well-being of the woman, fetus, or both and if vaginal birth can be accomplished quickly without undue trauma. Maternal indications may include exhaustion, inability to push effectively, infection, and cardiac or pulmo-nary disease (Cunningham et al., 2014). Fetal indications may include failure of the fetal presenting part to fully rotate and descend in the pelvis, partial separation of the placenta, or abnormal FHR patterns near the time of birth.

Contraindications

Cesarean birth is preferable if the maternal and fetal condi-tions mandate a more rapid birth than can be accomplished with forceps or vacuum extraction or if the procedure would be too traumatic. Examples of these conditions are severe fetal compromise, acute maternal conditions such as conges-tive heart failure and pulmonary edema, a high fetal station, and disproportion between the size of the fetus and maternal pelvis.

Risks

The main risk in forceps and vacuum extraction is trauma to maternal and fetal tissues. Because of the relative safety of cesarean birth, the attempt at an instrumental birth usually is abandoned if the fetal head does not descend easily.

Maternal risks include laceration and hematoma of the vagina, pelvic floor disorders, anal sphincter disruption, and infection (Simpson & O'Brien-Abel, 2014). The infant may have ecchymoses, facial and scalp lacerations and abrasions, facial nerve injury, cephalohematoma, subgaleal hemorrhage, and intracranial hemorrhage. A vacuum extractor may create scalp edema called a *chignon* at the application area (see Fig. 15.10).

Technique

Preparation for vacuum extraction or forceps is similar to that for any vaginal birth. The presentation, position, and station of the fetal presenting part are verified. Membranes must be ruptured and the cervix completely dilated for forceps or vac-uum extraction birth. The woman needs adequate anesthesia, usually a regional block such as an epidural.

Forceps and vacuum extractor–assisted births are classi-fied according to the extent of descent of the fetal head into the pelvis during the procedure and necessary degree of rota-tion for the fetal head to be born. Describing descent in cen-timeters below the ischial spines is preferred (AAP & ACOG, 2012; ACOG, 2015d; Simpson & O'Brien-Abel, 2014; Thorp & Laughon, 2014).

- Outlet operative vaginal delivery—The fetal head is at or on the perineum, with the scalp visible at the vaginal opening without separating the labia. The position is either right or left occiput anterior (ROA, LOA) or right or left occiput posterior (ROP, LOP).
- Low operative vaginal delivery—The leading edge of the fetal skull is at station +2 cm or lower and not on the pelvic floor. Low operative vaginal birth is subdivided according

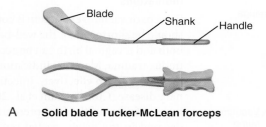

A   **Solid blade Tucker-McLean forceps**

Application of forceps with an open (fenestrated) blade

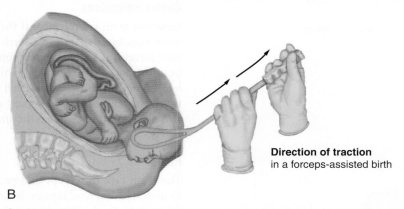

Direction of traction
in a forceps-assisted birth

B

FIG. 15.11 Obstetric Forceps and Their Application. A, Solid-blade Tucker-McLean forceps.
B, Direction of traction in a forceps-assisted birth.

to the amount of rotation of the fetal head needed. Births requiring 45 degrees or less of fetal head rotation are simpler.

• Midpelvis operative vaginal delivery—The leading edge of the fetal skull is between 0 (at the level of the ischial spines or engaged) and +2 cm station.

The physician determines the presentation, position, and station of the fetal head and amount of cervical dilation. When the blades are correctly applied, the long axis of the blades lies over the fetal cheeks and parietal bones. After checking for proper application, the physician locks the two blades in the center and pulls gently as the woman pushes, following the curve of the pelvis. An **episiotomy** (surgical incision of the perineum) may be performed as the fetal head distends the perineum. The physician may keep the forceps on until the head is born or may remove the blades just before expulsion. The rest of the fetus is born in the usual way.

For vacuum extraction, a hand pump is used to create suction to hold the vacuum cup on the fetal head in the midline of the occiput. The physician applies traction intermittently, as in a forceps-assisted birth. A vacuum release allows easy removal of the cup. Hospital policies usually limit to three the number of times the vacuum cup can be applied.

Nursing Considerations

When a forceps or vacuum extraction birth is anticipated, a catheter is often added to the instrument table for the birth to empty the bladder before the procedure. The physician specifies the type of vacuum cup or forceps. If the nurse must

apply the suction to the cup, suction should not go outside the green zone on the suction indicator. FHR should be assessed and any rate lower than 100 bpm reported.

After birth the mother and infant are observed for trauma. The mother may have vaginal wall lacerations or hematoma (see Chapter 18). Cold applications for the first 12 hours reduce pain by numbing the area and limit bruising and edema of the tissues. Heat applications after 12 hours aid resolution of the edema and bruising.

The infant often has reddening and mild bruising of the skin where the forceps were applied. These areas do not need treatment. Cold treatment is not done for an infant because of hypothermia. Skin breaks that allow entry of microorganisms should be noted and kept clean. Facial asymmetry, which is most obvious when the infant cries, suggests facial nerve injury. Temporary caput or scalp edema (**chignon**) is common at the location of the vacuum extractor cup.

After a forceps birth a parent may ask why the baby's cheeks are reddened or bruised. A good response is to explain that the pressure of the forceps on the baby's delicate skin may cause minor bruising that usually resolves without treatment. Point out improvement in the area during the postpartum stay. Parents may need an explanation for the scalp edema, or chignon, after a vaginal birth assisted with a vacuum extractor.

Episiotomy

Episiotomy, or incision of the perineum just before birth, was once routine for vaginal births, but the incidence has remarkably decreased over the past 30 years (Cunningham et al.,

Median or Midline

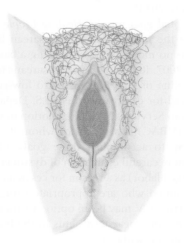

Mediolateral

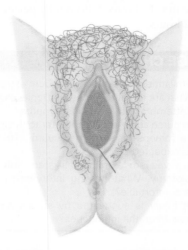

Advantages	*Disadvantages*
Minimal blood loss	An added laceration may
Neat healing with little	extend the median
scarring	episiotomy into the
Less postpartum pain	anal sphincter
than the mediolateral	Limited enlargement of the
episiotomy	vaginal opening because
	perineal length is limited
	by the anal sphincter

Advantages	*Disadvantages*
More enlargement of	More blood loss
the vaginal opening	Increased postpartum
Little risk that the	pain
episiotomy will	More scarring and
extend into the anus	irregularity in the
	healed scar
	Prolonged dyspareunia
	(painful intercourse)

FIG. 15.12 Types of Episiotomies.

2014). The presumed maternal benefits of reducing pain, perineal tearing, and later pelvic relaxation with incontinence have not proved true (Cunningham et al., 2014). However, the birth attendant must decide if one is needed, and indications are not always clear.

Indications

Examples of situations in which the birth attendant may perform an episiotomy are as follows (Cunningham et al., 2014):
- Rapid resolution of fetal shoulder dystocia, in which the shoulder of a fetus becomes lodged under the mother's symphysis during birth
- Vacuum extractor–assisted or forceps-assisted births
- Birth with the fetus in an occiput posterior (face-up) position
- Breech delivery
- Macrosomic fetus

Risks

Infection is the main risk in episiotomy. Perineal pain occurs with both episiotomy and spontaneous tears. However, perineal pain may last longer with episiotomy, mainly because of its tendency to extend into deeper lacerations. Prolonged perineal pain impairs resumption of sexual intercourse and makes it uncomfortable for the woman.

Data since the 1980s have confirmed that midline episiotomies, more frequently done than mediolateral episiotomies, increase a woman's risk for the more extensive third-degree (into the anal sphincter) or fourth-degree (through the rectal sphincter) tear. Fecal incontinence was increased fourfold to

sixfold compared with women who delivered with an intact perineum (Cunningham et al., 2014). Spontaneous lacerations are more likely to occur if a woman had an episiotomy with a previous pregnancy. However, despite data confirming maternal benefits of avoiding episiotomies, approximately 12% of vaginal deliveries have routine episiotomies performed (ACOG, 2013; Cunningham et al., 2014).

Technique

An episiotomy is done when the fetal presenting part has crowned to a diameter of approximately 3 to 4 cm. The two types of episiotomies, median (midline) and mediolateral, have different advantages and disadvantages (Fig. 15.12).

Nursing Considerations

An episiotomy sometimes can be avoided or limited in length with nursing measures. An upright position while pushing promotes gradual stretching of the woman's perineum. Delaying pushing until the urge is felt also gradually distends the soft tissue of the pelvic floor. Pushing with an open-glottis technique rather than prolonged breath-holding when pushing also promotes gradual perineal stretching.

Daily perineal massage and stretching by the woman from 36 weeks until birth has been shown to reduce the risk for perineal trauma during birth (Cunningham et al., 2014). Women older than 30 years having their first baby and adhering to the daily 10-minute perineal massage showed greatest benefit.

Nursing interventions during the recovery and postpartum periods are similar for episiotomy and perineal laceration. The perineum should be observed for hematoma and edema. As with use of forceps, perineal cold applications are done for at least the first 12 hours, followed by perineal heat applications after 12 hours.

Cesarean Birth

In 1965, the cesarean birth rate in the United States was approximately 5% of all births, rising to almost 21% in 1996, when the percentage dropped slightly. From 1996 to 2009 the number of cesareans steadily increased among all maternal age groups, with a peak in 2009 at 32.9%. Data for 2015 show that cesarean deliveries have continued the steady downward trend started in 2010, with the current rate being 31.8% of all births (Hamilton et al., 2015 NCHS, 2017).

Many factors contribute to the rise in the national cesarean birth rate, including the following (Hamilton et al., 2015; Simpson & O'Brien-Abel, 2014; Thorp & Laughon, 2014):

- Women having their first baby are more likely to deliver by cesarean than women who have had one or more previous births vaginally.
- Women having labor induction with their first baby have a greater risk for a cesarean.
- The 26% primary (first) cesarean rate adds to the overall rate because more women will have repeat cesareans rather than attempting vaginal birth for subsequent children.
- Women are having children later, and cesareans are more common in the older pregnant woman.
- Increasing maternal body mass index.
- Cesarean birth may be chosen if the baby remains in a breech presentation.
- A high threat of litigation if birth outcomes are not good causes physicians to opt for surgery quickly if the maternal or fetal condition or both seem to be at risk.
- Cesarean on maternal request rather than medical need.

Evidence linking labor induction to increased risk for cesarean birth continues to accumulate. Studies have demonstrated that women who have their labor induced are two to three times more likely to have a surgical birth. Women having a Bishop score of less than 6 at the time of induction, indicating a cervix that is not favorable, had a greater risk for cesarean than women who had a score of 8 or more. The likelihood of a cesarean increases as the duration of induced labor increases. The risk for cesarean after failed induction was similar whether women had medical or elective inductions (Simpson & O'Brien-Abel, 2014; Thorp & Laughon, 2014).

A national goal for the *Healthy People 2020* initiative is to reduce the rate of first-time cesarean births in low-risk women to no more than 23.9% using a baseline of 27.4% of births in 2007. Reducing repeat cesareans to 81.7% from the 2007 baseline of 90.8% of births to low-risk women is the second goal for cesarean births (U.S. Department of Health and Human Services, 2010). Promotion of vaginal birth after cesarean (VBAC) in women for whom it is appropriate is a major way to accomplish these goals. Other possibilities include more careful evaluation of **dystocia** of labor (difficult or prolonged labor) as a reason for cesarean and careful selection of women who are appropriate candidates for vaginal breech birth. ECV may be an option to attempt to change the presentation of a near-term fetus in the breech presentation to a cephalic presentation.

Vaginal Birth after Cesarean

With the high cesarean rate and the desire to lower the incidence, the decision about whether to have a trial of labor after a cesarean (TOLAC), hopefully resulting in a VBAC, has never been more difficult than now. At one time, the dictum "once a cesarean, always a cesarean" was accepted without question (ACOG, 2015b; Cunningham et al., 2014). For many years after this dictum, having no research backup, the only women who had VBACs were those who entered the hospital in such advanced labor that there was no time for a repeat cesarean. Current literature states VBAC is associated with decreased maternal morbidity and decreased risk for complications in future pregnancies. Yet a failed TOLAC is associated with more complications than a repeat cesarean section (American Academy of Family Physicians [AAFP], 2015; ACOG, 2015b).

As low transverse uterine incisions became the norm for almost all women having cesarean births, the safety of a trial of labor became established. VBAC gradually became an accepted way to lower the rise in cesarean births. Research continues on the safety of VBAC.

The AAP and ACOG (2012) have affirmed their support for VBAC (Box 15.2) but have urged caution when considering a TOLAC because VBAC is associated with a small but significant risk for uterine rupture. The risks and benefits of VBAC must be considered by the woman and her physician. For example, the risk for uterine rupture increases as the number of prior uterine incisions increases, and a woman who has had two cesarean deliveries might be reluctant to attempt VBAC for her third birth because of this added risk (Cunningham et al., 2014; Thorp & Laughon, 2014). She and her infant are more likely to have infections that further complicate their recovery and add to costs. The hospital also incurs greater costs for personnel and supplies.

When making the decision about whether to attempt VBAC, women need to know that surgical birth has risks just as all surgeries have risks. Besides risks common to any surgery, multiple cesarean births have risks such as greater risk for placental abnormalities such as placenta previa (low-lying placenta) or placenta accreta (abnormal adherence of the placenta to the uterine wall, often along the previous incision area) (AAFP, 2015; ACOG, 2015b; Cunningham et al., 2014). Therefore the woman and her physician must consider the risks and benefits of both.

Women may be anxious about attempting vaginal birth in a later pregnancy. A woman may know that she is a good candidate for VBAC but find it impossible to disregard even small risks. Scheduling a repeat cesarean may seem safer and simpler. The prospect of laboring and perhaps still needing a cesarean birth is worrisome as well.

The physician discusses VBAC during prenatal care if it is a reasonable option. The nurse reinforces these explanations and identifies misunderstandings. If the woman chooses VBAC, the nurse should reinforce the appropriateness of attempting VBAC and advantages of a vaginal birth, such as fewer overall complications individually. VBAC should be presented in a positive way if it is a real option, yet the possibility of cesarean delivery should be acknowledged because the surgery can be needed unexpectedly in any birth (see Box 15.2).

Cesarean Section Indications

Cesarean birth is performed when awaiting vaginal birth would compromise the mother, the fetus, or both. Possible indications for cesarean birth include, but are not limited to, the following (Cunningham et al., 2014; Simpson & O'Brien-Abel, 2014):

- Dystocia
- Cephalopelvic disproportion
- Hypertension, if prompt delivery is necessary
- Maternal diseases such as diabetes, heart disease, or cervical cancer, if labor is not advisable
- Active genital herpes
- Some previous uterine surgical procedures such as a classic cesarean incision or removal of fibroid tumors
- Persistent indeterminate or abnormal FHR patterns
- Prolapsed umbilical cord
- Fetal malpresentations such as breech or transverse lie
- Hemorrhagic conditions such as placental abruption or placenta previa
- Maternal request

Contraindications

Few absolute contraindications exist, but cesarean birth in some conditions is not desirable because the risks to the woman are too great compared with the potential benefits to the woman and fetus. These conditions include a fetus that is too immature to survive, a current fetal demise, or maternal coagulation defects that could cause harm to the mother in surgery.

Risks

Cesarean birth is one of the safest major surgical procedures. However, it poses greater risk for the mother compared with vaginal birth. Maternal risks include the following (Thorp & Laughon, 2014):

- Infection
- Hemorrhage
- Urinary tract trauma or infection

BOX 15.2   Vaginal Birth after Cesarean

1. Approximately 60% to 80% of women with one low transverse uterine incision from a previous cesarean birth have successful vaginal births.
2. Women who had their previous cesarean for a nonrecurring reason, such as breech presentation, are more likely to have a successful vaginal birth after cesarean birth (VBAC) than women who had their previous cesarean because of dystocia ("failure to progress").
3. Women who have had a vaginal birth, before or since the prior cesarean birth, are more likely to have successful VBAC.
4. There is a higher probability of success in the woman who has spontaneous labor.

Possible Candidates and Requirements for Vaginal Birth after Cesarean

1. A woman who has one previous low transverse uterine incision.
2. A woman with two prior cesarean deliveries may have a low risk of uterine rupture with VBAC.
3. Absence of other uterine scars (e.g., removal of fibroid tumors) or a previous uterine rupture.
4. A pelvis that is clinically adequate for the estimated fetal size.
5. Immediate availability of a physician during active labor if an emergency cesarean is needed.
6. Availability of anesthesia and personnel to perform an emergency cesarean.

Management of Women Who Plan Vaginal Birth after Cesarean

1. External cephalic version is not contraindicated for the woman with a previous cesarean.
2. Epidural analgesia and anesthesia may be used.
3. Induction and augmentation of labor with oxytocin may be done. Misoprostol (Cytotec) should not be used.
4. Most authorities recommend continuous electronic fetal monitoring.

Data from American College of Obstetricians and Gynecologists (2015b). *Vaginal delivery after previous cesarean birth.* Practice Bulletin 115. Washington, DC: Author; American Academy of Pediatrics & American College of Obstetricians and Gynecologists (AAP & ACOG). (2012). *Guidelines for perinatal care* (7th ed.). Elk Grove Village, IL: Authors; Picklesimer, A. M., & Dorman, K. (2013). Maternal obesity: Effects on pregnancy. In N. H. Troiano, C. J. Harvey, & B. F. Chez (Eds.), *AWHONN high-risk & critical care obstetrics* (3rd ed., pp. 357–367). Philadelphia, PA: Lippincott Williams & Wilkins.

- Thrombophlebitis, thromboembolism
- Paralytic ileus
- Atelectasis
- Endomyometritis
- Anesthesia complications

Cesarean delivery poses added risks to the infant, which may include the following (Thorp & Laughon, 2014):

- Inadvertent preterm birth
- Transient tachypnea of the newborn caused by delayed absorption of lung fluid
- Persistent pulmonary hypertension of the newborn

- Injury such as laceration, bruising, fractures, or other trauma

Lung immaturity is the greatest risk if the fetus is delivered preterm. Therefore tests for fetal lung maturity are done if elective cesarean birth is planned. Other criteria for assuring fetal lung maturity at the time of cesarean birth include the following (AAP & ACOG, 2012):

- Documentation of fetal heart tones for 30 weeks by Doppler
- Passage of 36 weeks since positive results from a pregnancy test performed by a laboratory
- Ultrasound measurement at less than 20 weeks that supports a gestation of 39 weeks or more

Technique

Preparation. Routine laboratory studies vary with the mother's condition and type of anesthesia but may include a complete blood count and blood typing and screening. The physician may order one or more units of blood to be typed and screened or crossmatched to have available for transfusion if the woman's hemoglobin and hematocrit values are low or she has a high risk for hemorrhage, such as grand multiparity (five or more births).

Epidural or combined spinal-epidural block is common for cesarean birth. General anesthesia may be required for either known or unexpected reasons. For emergency cesarean with no epidural in place, a general anesthetic may be chosen because it can be established the most quickly. A drug such as famotidine (Pepcid) or sodium citrate with citric acid (Bicitra) may be given to reduce gastric acidity before surgery.

Additional preoperative care includes a "time out," in which all members of the team validate the woman's identity, surgical site, and consents. Staff members identify themselves and their roles during this process (Cunningham et al., 2014; Simpson & O'Brien-Abel, 2014).

Fetal surveillance continues until just before the sterile abdominal skin preparation (intermittent auscultation or external monitor) or just after the preparation (internal monitor) (AAP & ACOG, 2012). A wedge placed under one hip prevents aortocaval compression and promotes placental blood flow (Cunningham et al., 2014; Simpson & O'Brien-Abel, 2014; Thorp & Laughon, 2014).

A single IV dose of a prophylactic antibiotic such as ampicillin or a cephalosporin is given to the mother during surgery (Simpson & O'Brien-Abel, 2014). There is insufficient evidence to support optimal timing of antibiotic administration; many providers administer around the time the cord is clamped (Thorp & Laughon, 2014). Additional antibiotic doses for 24 hours are common to prevent postoperative infections in patients with an increased infection risk (i.e., prolonged rupture of membranes or a lengthy labor).

If a Pfannenstiel (transverse or "bikini") skin incision is planned, the woman's lower abdominal hair is clipped from about 3 inches above the pubic hairline to the mons pubis, about where her legs come together. The fronts of the upper thighs are also clipped. For a vertical skin incision, the upper border of the abdominal hair clipping is near the umbilicus.

Cordless electric clippers with disposable heads reduce skin nicks that provide an entry point for microorganisms.

An indwelling catheter inserted after the regional block is established but before the surgery allows comfortable insertion and keeps the bladder away from the operative area to reduce the risk for injury (Cunningham et al., 2014). The catheter also may be placed before the block. The catheter allows accurate observation of urine output during and after surgery, which helps evaluate circulatory status. The catheter also allows delay of ambulation to the restroom for urination until the woman can safely ambulate.

A grounding pad for the electrocautery is applied to an area with no bony prominences, usually the thigh. After application of the pad, the woman's legs are secured to the operating table with a wide, padded strap.

Risk for thromboembolism almost doubles for the patient undergoing cesarean delivery. Therefore sequential pneumatic compression devices are applied before surgery initiation (Cunningham et al., 2014; Simpson & O'Brien-Abel, 2014; Witcher & Hamner, 2013).

A sterile abdominal skin preparation is done just before sterile draping and allowed to dry before sterile drapes are applied. Surgical skin preparations vary in methods of application (friction vs. paint). Application begins at the center of the operative site outward and from the pubic area downward on each upper thigh. It may be necessary to secure excess abdominal fat (the pannus, or "apron") away from the skin incision area. Methods include using tape or a commercially prepared retraction device for this process.

If a general anesthetic is required, preoperative preparations are completed before anesthesia is begun to reduce newborn exposure to anesthesia. The team scrubs, dons gowns and gloves, and drapes the woman before general anesthesia is induced.

Incisions. Two incisions are made, one in the abdominal wall (skin incision) and the other in the uterine wall. Either of two skin incisions are used: a midline vertical incision between the umbilicus and the symphysis or a low transverse (Pfannenstiel) incision just above the symphysis (Cunningham et al., 2014) (Fig. 15.13).

Three types of uterine incisions are possible, each with different indications and limitations: (1) low transverse, (2) low vertical, and (3) classic, a vertical incision into the upper uterus (Cunningham et al., 2014) (Fig. 15.14). The low transverse uterine incision is preferred because of its low risk for rupture in subsequent pregnancies. The uterine incision does not always match the skin incision. For example, a woman may have a vertical skin incision and a low transverse uterine incision, particularly if she is obese or has a preexisting vertical scar.

The low transverse uterine incision may not be suitable if the fetus is very large. The length of this incision is limited because the uterine artery and vein enter the uterus at its lower right and left sides. The low transverse incision may not be large enough to deliver a large fetus without tearing these large vessels. Sometimes, a vertical uterine incision must be added to a transverse one (making an inverted T or a J) to deliver a very

Vertical

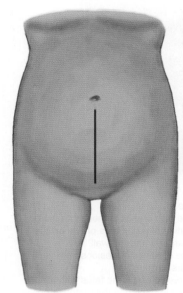

Advantages
Quicker to perform
Better visualization of the
  uterus
Can quickly extend upward
  for greater visualization if
  needed
Often more appropriate for
  obese women

Disadvantages
Easily visible when healed
Greater chance of dehis-
  cence and hernia formation

Pfannenstiel

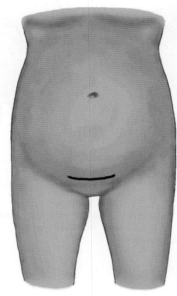

Advantages
Less visibility when healed
  and the pubic hair grows
  back
Less chance of dehiscence
  or formation of a hernia

Disadvantages
Less visualization of the
  uterus
Cannot be done as quickly,
  which may be important in
  an emergency cesarean
  birth
Cannot easily be extended to
  give greater operative exposure
Reentry at a subsequent cesarean birth may require
  more time

FIG. 15.13 Skin (Abdominal Wall) Incisions for Cesarean Birth.

large baby. If an additional vertical incision is needed bilaterally, a U incision is formed (Cunningham et al., 2014).

A classic uterine incision occasionally must be used when the other two incisions are not possible, such as when a placenta previa is located in the lower anterior uterus. The vertical uterine incision, especially the classic one, is more likely to rupture during later pregnancies.

Sequence of Events in a Cesarean Birth. The sequence of events in a cesarean birth is similar to that in a vaginal birth. When the woman is anesthetized and draped, the physician makes the skin incision. If general anesthesia is required, the level is very light until the fetus is delivered and is deepened after the umbilical cord is clamped.

The bladder is separated from the uterine wall and held downward with a wide bladder retractor. The uterus is incised, usually in a low transverse incision. If the membranes are intact, they are ruptured with a sharp instrument and amniotic fluid is suctioned from the operative field. As in vaginal births, the color, odor, and quantity of the amniotic fluid are noted and the time of rupture is recorded.

The physician lifts the fetal presenting part through the uterine incision. An assistant may push on the uterine fundus to help deliver the fetus through the abdominal incision. A vacuum extractor or forceps may be needed to facilitate birth of the fetal head.

The infant's face is wiped, and the mouth and nose may be suctioned to remove secretions that would impair breathing. The cord is clamped and cut. Evidence suggests that a 60-second delay in cord clamping increases total body iron stores, expands blood volume, decreases anemia, and decreases rate of intraventricular hemorrhage in the preterm infant (Cunningham et al., 2014). The physician collects cord blood for analysis.

After the infant's birth, the physician removes the placenta. IV oxytocin is given to contract the uterus. The physician then closes the uterine and abdominal incisions, approximating each layer separately. Physicians may flush the operative area with saline before abdominal closure.

Nursing care for the infant is similar to that after vaginal birth. Resuscitation equipment should be readied for use before delivery. Professional personnel who care for the infant born by cesarean vary with the baby's anticipated condition and facility policy. A pediatrician, neonatal nurse practitioner, or neonatal team usually attends the at-risk infant at the time of cesarean birth (Cunningham et al., 2014). Newborn care personnel must be prepared for unexpected resuscitation measures as in any birth.

Nursing Considerations

Nursing care for a woman who has a cesarean birth varies according to the situation. She may be planning a cesarean birth, or a surgical birth may be unexpected. Even in these two situations, women differ. For example, is the planned cesarean her first or has she had a cesarean birth before? Was her previous cesarean planned? An unplanned cesarean birth may occur after hours of unsuccessful labor or may be needed quickly in an emergency.

Nursing care for women having cesarean childbirth is similar to that for vaginal birth, but the approach in each situation is different (Box 15.3). For example, although preoperative teaching is important, it must be abbreviated or even omitted in a true emergency.

Emotional Support. Emotional support may begin before and extend after the birth. A mother who has had a previous cesarean birth may harbor unresolved feelings of grief, guilt, or inadequacy because she perceives that she somehow

Low Transverse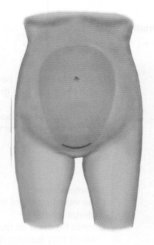

Low Vertical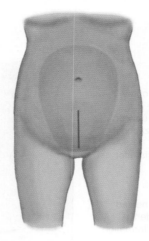

Classic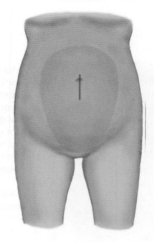

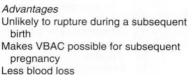

Advantages
Unlikely to rupture during a subsequent birth
Makes VBAC possible for subsequent pregnancy
Less blood loss
Easier to repair
Less adhesion formation

Disadvantage
Limited ability to extend laterally to enlarge the incision

Advantage
Can be extended upward to make a larger incision if needed

Disadvantages
Slightly more likely to rupture during a subsequent birth
A tear may extend the incision downward into the cervix

Advantage
May be the only choice in these situations:
  Implantation of a placenta previa on the lower anterior uterine wall
  Presence of dense adhesions from previous surgery
  Transverse lie of a large fetus with the shoulder impacted in the mother's pelvis

Disadvantages
Most likely of the uterine incisions to rupture during a subsequent birth
Eliminates VBAC as an option for birth of a subsequent infant

FIG. 15.14 Uterine Incisions for Cesarean Birth. The abdominal and uterine incisions do not always match. *VBAC,* Vaginal birth after cesarean.

BOX 15.3 Nursing Care for a Woman Having Cesarean Birth

Before the Cesarean Birth
1. Assess the time of last oral intake and what was eaten.
2. Assess for allergies. Include drug, food, and substance (e.g., latex) allergies.
3. Determine medications taken and last dose. Include herbal preparations.
4. Have the woman sign informed consents for surgery, anesthesia, and usually blood transfusion.
5. Obtain the ordered laboratory work.
6. Do preoperative teaching: what the woman can expect in the operating and recovery rooms, infant care, and who will be present, recovery routine (monitoring, assessments, coughing and deep breathing).
7. Start the ordered intravenous infusion, and begin a fluid bolus for the regional anesthetic at the appropriate time (see the discussion on epidural block in Chapter 13).
8. Clip body hair from the skin area needed for planned incision.
9. Administer the ordered medication to control gastric secretions if not done by the anesthesiologist.
10. Insert an indwelling urinary catheter (or insert in operating room [OR] after regional block).
11. Assist the woman to the operating table, positioning her with a wedge under her hip to displace the uterus if the table is flat.
12. Apply the grounding pad for electrocautery and sequential compression devices (SCDs)
13. Perform sterile preparation of abdomen.
14. Call the infant care team if it is routine in the facility or if newborn complications are anticipated.

During the Recovery Period
1. Begin anesthesia-related interventions: Pulse oximeter, oxygen administration, cardiac monitor.
   a. Assess for return of sensation and movement if regional anesthesia was used.
   b. Assess level of consciousness if general anesthesia was used.
2. Do routine assessments every 15 minutes for the first hour, every 30 minutes during the second hour, and hourly thereafter until the woman is transferred to the postpartum unit. Assess:
   a. Vital signs, oxygen saturation
   b. Electrocardiogram pattern
   c. Uterine fundus for firmness, height, and deviation (massage if poorly contracted)
   d. Lochia for color, quantity, and presence of large clots
   e. Urine output for color, quantity, and patency of the catheter and tubing
   f. Abdominal dressing for drainage
   g. Return of lower body movement if regional block
3. Assess need for analgesia, and administer as ordered.
4. Change position hourly if no contraindication exists. Have the woman breathe deeply and cough at each routine assessment time. Provide a small pillow to support her incision when coughing or turning if sensation is present.
5. Continue SCD function, if used during surgery

failed in her expected birth experience. She may feel anxious about choosing repeat cesarean when given the choice of a VBAC. Therapeutic communication techniques help identify stressors and misunderstandings to promote a positive childbirth experience.

Anxiety is an expected and normal reaction to surgery and is useful within limits. The staff's behavior can either reduce or increase the woman's anxiety. A calm and confident manner helps her feel she is being cared for by competent professionals. A quiet, low voice is calming. The nurse and the woman's significant others are important sources of emotional support. The nurse should remain with the woman and let her express her fears. Therapeutic communication helps clarify her concerns, so explanations to reduce her fear of the unknown can be most effective.

The support person should be encouraged to remain with her during surgery if she has regional anesthesia. In some hospitals, the support person may come into the operating room after the woman is intubated for general anesthesia to foster attachment with the infant and help the mother integrate her birth experience afterward.

Nurses also support a woman's partner and significant others during the cesarean birth. The partner may be as anxious as the woman but afraid to express it because the woman needs so much support. The partner may be physically exhausted after hours of labor coaching. The staff should not expect more support from partners than can be reasonably provided.

Although cesarean births are routine in the intrapartum unit, they are not routine to women who undergo them and to their families. Avoid belittling their fears by telling women and their families not to worry and that everything will be all right, especially if an emergency occurs.

After birth, in the postanesthesia care unit (PACU), the nurse begins to answer questions about the surgery and fill in any gaps in the mother and her family's understanding. This helps them understand the experience and promotes a positive perception of the birth.

Teaching. Knowledge may reduce fear of the unknown and increase a woman's sense of control over her infant's birth. The nurse cannot assume that a woman who had a previous cesarean birth already knows what will happen and why. If her previous surgery was done after a long labor or in an emergency, a woman may recall only parts and not understand those parts she does remember. Teaching should be given in simple language and include her support person.

The nurse explains preoperative procedures such as hair clipping in the incisional area, indwelling catheter, IV lines, and dressings and their purposes. The catheter and IV lines usually remain in place no longer than 24 hours after birth. Sequential compression devices (SCDs) may be used throughout surgery and until ambulating well to reduce the risk for deep vein thrombosis.

Women who have regional anesthesia such as an epidural or a subarachnoid block often fear they will feel pain during surgery. They do feel pressure and pulling, but these sensations do not mean that the anesthesia is wearing off. The nurse reassures the woman that her pain management is regularly assessed by the anesthesia provider.

If a woman is having general anesthesia, the nurse explains why operative preparations are completed before she is anesthetized. The patient should be reassured that her surgery will not begin until she is asleep and she will not wake up during the procedure.

The nurse describes the operating room (OR) and who will be present to make it less intimidating to her. Staff in the OR should introduce themselves, if possible. The patient's labor nurse often is the circulating nurse during surgery and reassures her with a familiar face and voice. The OR is very cool in most cases, and the surgery table is narrow.

The support person should be told when to expect to come into the OR. If it is not already in place, an epidural block often is established after the woman goes to the OR. The partner may not be brought in until the regional block and other preparations such as the indwelling catheter are complete. These preparations may take 30 to 45 minutes if no rush exists. Support persons should be told that they will not be forgotten and that apparent delays do not indicate problems. Surgery preparation time that moves quickly and efficiently for staff often moves very slowly for family and the main support person.

The PACU and any equipment that will be used, for example, a pulse oximeter, electrocardiogram monitor, and automatic blood pressure cuff, are explained to the woman. The nurse reviews routine assessments and interventions such as fundus and lochia checks, coughing, and deep breathing. The woman is taught simple exercises to promote normal circulation. The nurse reassures her that every effort will be made to promote her comfort with medication, positioning, and other interventions.

Promoting Safety. The woman's food intake is assessed for type and time on admission because general anesthesia occasionally is necessary. Oral intake and emesis during labor are recorded and reported to the anesthesia clinician. Oral intake other than ordered medications and possibly ice chips is discontinued if a cesarean birth becomes likely. Drugs to control gastric and respiratory secretions are administered, as ordered.

The woman is transferred and positioned carefully to prevent injury, especially if she has received regional anesthesia that reduces motor control and sensation. Bariatric operating tables are used for women with increased body mass index. Bony prominences are cushioned. A safety strap placed across her thighs secures her on the narrow operating table. A wedge under one hip or a tilted operating table avoids aortocaval compression and reduced placental blood flow. During positioning the drain tube of the indwelling catheter should be routed under her leg to promote drainage and keep the tubing away from the operative area. The catheter bag is placed near the head of the table so that the anesthesia provider can monitor urine output, an important measure of fluid balance.

The nurse verifies proper function of equipment such as suction devices, monitors, and electrocautery. Leads for the cardiac monitor, temperature, and pulse oximeter are placed to observe vital functions. A grounding pad permits safe use of electrocautery.

After the surgery, the incision area is cleansed with sterile water and a sterile dressing is applied. Blood and amniotic fluid are cleaned from the woman's abdomen, buttocks, and back before she is transferred to a bed. Lateral transfer devices are available to assist with transition off the operating table. Smooth transfers reduce pain and hypotension.

NURSING CARE AFTER BIRTH

Intrapartum nursing care extends through the fourth stage of labor and includes care of the infant, the mother, and the family unit.

Care of the Infant

Nursing care of the newborn includes supporting cardiopulmonary and thermoregulatory function and identifying the infant. In addition, assess the infant for approximate gestational age and examine for obvious anomalies and birth injuries. A full neonatal assessment may be delayed for about 1 hour to allow time for uninterrupted skin-to-skin contact with the mother after delivery. Much of the initial assessment can be done while new parents are bonding with their infant.

Maintain Cardiopulmonary Function

Assess the infant's Apgar score (Table 15.4) at 1 and 5 minutes and every 5 minutes thereafter until the Apgar score is greater than 7 (Fraser, 2014). This scoring system after birth allows for rapid evaluation of early cardiopulmonary adaptation. If the Apgar score is 8 or higher, no intervention is needed other than supporting thermoregulation and promoting normal respiratory efforts by positioning and wiping secretions from the mouth and nose. If the infant is obviously in distress (no or low heart rate and respirations, limp muscle tone, lack of response to stimulation, blue or pale color), interventions to correct the problem are instituted immediately rather than waiting for the 1-minute Apgar score (AAP & American Heart Association [AHA], 2016).

A baby with a vigorous cry and minimal secretions is usually sufficiently warmed by skin-to-skin contact with the parents, but a prewarmed warmer should be available. Avoid an extended time with the infant in a head-dependent position because upward pressure from the intestines limits diaphragmatic movement. An infant in a warmer should be placed in the flat position or turned to one side with the head flat or slightly elevated. Wipe secretions from the infant's face and mouth. Suction the infant's mouth and nose with a bulb syringe, if needed. Suctioning with a catheter may be necessary for more copious secretions.

Support Thermoregulation

Hypothermia raises the infant's metabolic rate and oxygen consumption, worsening any respiratory problems. When necessary to evaluate a transitioning infant separate from the mother,

TABLE 15.4   Apgar Score*

Assessment	POINTS		
	0	**1**	**2**
Heart rate	Absent	Below 100 beats per minute (bpm)	100 bpm or higher
Respiratory effort	No spontaneous respirations	Slow respirations or weak cry	Spontaneous respirations with strong, lusty cry
Muscle tone	Limp	Minimal flexion of extremities; sluggish movement	Flexed body posture; spontaneous and vigorous movement
Reflex response	No response to suction or gentle slap on soles	Minimal response (grimace) to suction or gentle slap on soles	Responds promptly to suction or gentle slap to sole with cry or active movement
Color	Pallor or cyanosis	Bluish hands and feet only (acrocyanosis)	Pink (light skinned) or absence of cyanosis (dark skinned); pink mucous membranes

0	1	2	3	4	5	6	7	8	9	10
Infant needs resuscitation.†			Gently stimulate by rubbing infant's back while administering oxygen. Determine whether mother received narcotics, which may have depressed infant's respirations.				Provide no action other than support of infant's spontaneous efforts and continued observation.			

*The Apgar score is a method for rapid evaluation of the infant's cardiorespiratory adaptation after birth. The nurse scores the infant at 1 minute and 5 minutes in each of five areas. The assessments are arranged from most important (heart rate) to least important (color). The infant is assigned a score of 0 to 2 in each of the five areas, and the scores are totaled. Resuscitation should not be delayed until the 1-minute score is obtained. However, general guidelines for the infant's care are based on three ranges of 1-minute scores: 0 to 2, 3 to 6, 7 to 10.

†*Note:* Neonatal resuscitation measures, if needed, do not await 1-minute Apgar scoring but are instituted at once.

place the infant on a prewarmed warmer, and quickly dry with warm towels to reduce evaporative heat loss. The head should be dried well because substantial heat loss can occur from the head, which is about one fourth of the neonate's body surface area. The stimulus of drying the skin promotes vigorous crying and lung expansion in most healthy infants.

Skin-to-skin contact with a parent also maintains the infant's temperature and promotes bonding between the infant and parent. Delaying the first bath for several hours allows the temperature to stabilize. Avoid positioning yourself between the infant and the radiant heat source in the warmer. The infant should be wrapped in dry, warm blankets when not in the warmer or making skin-to-skin contact. Remove wet linens, replacing them with warm and dry ones. A stockinette cap further reduces heat loss if it is placed on the baby's *dry* head. A cap is not worn while the infant is in the radiant warmer because the cap slows transfer of heat to the baby.

Identify the Infant

Bands with matching imprinted numbers and identifying information are the primary means to ensure that the right baby goes to the right mother after any separation. Check that the imprinted band number and mother's name are identical on each set of bands, and have the parent(s) verify this information at the time of banding. Apply identification band(s) on the infant, preferably on the ankle to prevent facial scratching. Infant bands are applied more snugly than those worn by an adult, with about one adult finger width of slack in the bands. Trim the excess band ends and apply the longer band to the mother's wrist. The mother's primary support person usually wears a fourth band. The infant will not be released to any adult who is not wearing a band with a matching name and number. A set of bands is needed for each baby in a multiple

birth. Some facilities take an early photo of the infant, when the infant is often alert, which serves two purposes: as a keepsake for the parents and identification in the event of abduction. Other facilities use footprints for the same purposes.

Care of the Mother

Nursing care of the mother during the fourth stage of labor focuses on observing for hemorrhage and relieving discomfort (Table 15.5).

Observe for Hemorrhage

Important assessments related to hemorrhage are the woman's vital signs, uterine fundal location and tone, bladder, lochia, and perineal and labial areas.

Vital Signs

Assess the woman's temperature when fourth-stage care begins. Blood pressure, pulse, and respirations should be assessed every 15 minutes during the first hour or as indicated (James, 2014). A rising pulse rate is an early sign of excessive blood loss because the heart pumps faster to compensate for reduced blood volume. The blood pressure falls as the blood volume diminishes, but this is a late sign of hypovolemia. A rising pulse rate also may reflect medications administered.

Fundus

The most common reason for excessive postpartum bleeding is that the uterus does not firmly contract and compress open vessels at the placental site. Assess the firmness, height, and positioning of the uterine fundus while supporting the lower uterine segment during uterine massage to prevent inversion or prolapse (James, 2014). Uterine assessment is typically performed with each vital sign assessment. The fundus should

TABLE 15.5	Maternal Problems during the Fourth Stage of Labor	
Sign	**Potential Problem**	**Immediate Nursing Action**
Rising maternal pulse rate and/or falling blood pressure; possibly accompanied by low or no urine output	An early sign of hypovolemia caused by excessive blood loss (visible or concealed)	Identify probable cause of blood loss, usually a poorly contracted uterus. Take steps to correct it (see later). Indwelling catheter may be inserted to observe urine output.
Soft (boggy) uterus	A poorly contracted uterus does not adequately compress large open vessels at placental site, resulting in hemorrhage	With one hand securing uterus just above symphysis and other hand on fundus, massage uterus until firm. Push downward on *firm* uterus to expel any clots. Empty woman's bladder (by voiding or catheterization) if that is contributing to uterine atony.
High uterine fundus, often displaced to one side	Suggests a full bladder, which can interfere with uterine contraction and result in hemorrhage	Massage uterus if it is not firm. Help woman urinate in bathroom or on bedpan. If she cannot void, catheterize her (usually a routine postpartum order).
Lochia exceeding one saturated perineal pad per hour during fourth stage	Suggests hemorrhage; however, perineal pads vary in their absorbency, and this must be considered	Identify cause of hemorrhage, usually uterine atony, which is manifested by a soft uterus. Correct cause. If lacerations are suspected cause (excess bleeding with a firm fundus), notify provider. Keep woman on NPO status until birth attendant evaluates her.
Intense perineal or vaginal pain, poorly relieved with analgesics	Hematoma, usually of vaginal wall or perineum; signs of hypovolemia may occur with substantial blood loss into tissues	If hematoma is visible, apply cold packs to area to slow bleeding into tissues. Notify provider and anticipate possible surgical drainage. Keep woman on NPO status.

NPO, Nothing by mouth.

be firm, in the midline, and below the umbilicus (about the size of a large grapefruit). If the fundus is firm, no massage is needed, but if it is soft (boggy), it should be massaged until it is firm. Nipple stimulation from the infant's suckling releases oxytocin from the mother's posterior pituitary gland to maintain firm uterine contraction. IV or intramuscular (IM) oxytocin has the same effect.

Bladder

A full bladder interferes with contraction of the uterus and may lead to hemorrhage. A full bladder is suspected if the fundus is above the umbilicus or displaced to one side, usually the right. The first two to three voidings are often measured until it is evident that the mother voids without difficulty and empties her bladder completely. Each voiding is usually at least 300 to 400 mL if she is emptying her bladder. If no contraindication, such as altered sensation is present, the mother can walk to the bathroom (with assistance the first few times). She should sit on the side of the bed to make sure she is not lightheaded, move her legs back and forth, and raise her knees to be sure she has adequate strength and movement before ambulation.

Lochia

Assess for lochia with each vital sign and fundal assessment. The amount of lochia seems large to the inexperienced nurse and new mother. Perineal pads vary in their absorbency, but saturation of one standard pad (one that does not contain a cold pack) within the first hour is a guideline for the maximal normal lochia flow. Turn the mother to check for lochia pooling under her buttocks and back. Small clots may be present, but the presence of large clots is not normal, and the provider should be notified.

Perineal and Labial Areas

Observe perineal and labial areas for bruising and hematoma formation. Small hematomas usually are easily limited by ice packs that are also applied for comfort. Large and rapidly expanding hematomas may cause significant enlargement of the tissues involved, a bluish color, and pain. Observe the episiotomy using the acronym REEDA (redness, edema, ecchymosis, discharge, approximation of edges of episiotomy) for assessment guidelines (James, 2014).

Promote Comfort

Uterine contractions (afterpains) and perineal trauma are common causes of pain after birth. A postpartum chill often adds to discomfort. Pain usually is mild and readily relieved by simple measures. Notify the birth attendant if pain is intense or does not respond to common relief measures.

Ice Packs. Apply an ice pack to the perineum promptly after vaginal birth to reduce edema and limit hematoma formation. Some perineal pads include chemical cold packs. These pads absorb less lochia than ordinary pads, so this should be considered when estimating pad saturation. Evidence shows that ice applied for the first 24 to 48 hours in 10- to 20-minute intervals, rather than continuously, is most beneficial (James, 2014).

Analgesics. Afterpains and perineal pain respond well to mild oral analgesics. Regular urination reduces the severity of afterpains because the uterus contracts most effectively when the bladder is empty. The nurse should encourage the woman to take analgesics as needed for both perineal and afterpain discomfort.

Warmth. A warm blanket shortens the chill common after birth. A portable radiant warmer provides warmth to both the mother and infant. The mother may enjoy warm drinks initially.

Postoperative Care

Postoperative care for the mother who has had a cesarean birth is like that for one who has had a vaginal birth, with additional assessments and interventions related to the incision and anesthesia. Her temperature is assessed on admission to the PACU and according to protocol thereafter. If her condition is stable, other assessments are done every 15 minutes during the first hour and progress to every 30 minutes to 1 hour until she is transferred to her postpartum room. In addition to temperature, routine postoperative assessments include the following:

- Vital signs, respiratory character, and oxygen saturation
- Return of motion and sensation if a regional block was given
- Level of consciousness, particularly if general anesthesia and sedating drugs were given
- Abdominal dressing
- Uterine firmness and position (midline or deviated to one side)
- Lochia (color, quantity, presence, and size of any clots)
- Urine output (quantity, color, other characteristics)
- IV infusion (fluid, rate, condition of IV site)
- Pain relief needs
- Function of the SCD

The nurse observes for return of motion and sensation if the woman had epidural or subarachnoid block anesthesia. The level of consciousness and respiratory status (skin and mucous membrane color, rate and quality of respirations, pulse oximeter readings) are important observations if she had general anesthesia. Respiratory observations also are important if the woman received epidural opioid narcotics, which can cause delayed respiratory depression. Naloxone (Narcan) should be available to reverse opioid-induced respiratory depression.

The pulse rate, respirations, blood pressure, and oxygen saturation level provide important clues to the woman's circulatory and respiratory status. If oxygen saturation falls below 92%, it usually can be raised with several deep breaths. A persistent respiratory rate of less than 12 breaths per minute suggests respiratory depression. Deep breathing and coughing move secretions out of the lungs. A small pillow to support her incision reduces pain when she coughs. Position changes every 2 hours improve ventilation, reduce pooling of lung secretions, and decrease discomfort from constant pressure.

As with vaginal birth, the fundus is assessed for height, firmness, and position. This examination is painful after regional anesthesia wears off, but the postcesarean mother also can have uterine atony. To relax her abdominal muscles and thus reduce pain from fundus checks, she should flex her knees and take slow, deep breaths. The nurse can gently "walk" the fingers toward the fundus to determine uterine firmness. The woman who has a Pfannenstiel skin incision usually has less pain with fundus checks than the woman with a vertical skin incision. A firm fundus does not need massage. The dressing is checked for drainage with each fundus check.

The nurse assesses the lochia and urine output with other assessments. Lochia may pool under the mother's buttocks and lower back. Urine may be bloody temporarily if the cesarean delivery was done after a long labor or an attempted forceps delivery. The urine drain tubing should be observed for gradual clearing of the blood. Urine should drain freely to prevent bladder distention, which worsens pain and increases the risk for postpartum hemorrhage. The nurse must remember that falling urine output is an early sign of hypovolemia.

The woman's needs for pain relief should be regularly assessed. The woman who received an epidural opioid may not need other analgesia during the early postpartum period. If she needs added pain relief while the epidural opioid is still in effect, the dose ordered often is lower than if she had not had that form of analgesia. Oral analgesics usually replace parenteral ones the day after surgery. A nonsteroidal antiinflammatory drug, such as ibuprofen, provides long-acting analgesia to supplement the epidural opioid. If she did not receive an epidural opioid, analgesia usually is given by patient-controlled analgesia pump.

KNOWLEDGE CHECK

29. Why is the low transverse uterine incision preferred for cesarean birth?
30. What should a woman who expects a cesarean birth be taught about the operating room? The recovery room or the PACU?
31. How should the nurse modify recovery room care of the mother who had a cesarean birth from that of the mother who had a vaginal delivery?

Promote Early Family Attachment

The first hour after birth is ideal for parent–infant attachment because the healthy neonate is alert and responsive. Provide privacy while unobtrusively observing the parents and infant. The infant can remain in the parent's arms while the nurse takes vital signs, administers IM medications as ordered, and suctions small amounts of secretions. Many newborn admission assessments can be performed while the parent holds the baby.

Assist the mother to nurse during the recovery period if she plans to breastfeed. The infant is usually attentive and nurses briefly. Early nipple stimulation helps initiate milk production and contract the uterus.

When the parents are ready, siblings, other family members, and friends should be allowed to visit. Help siblings see and touch their new brother or sister by putting a stool at the bedside or letting them sit on the bed.

Toddlers are often upset by the separation from their mother and may not be interested in the new baby. With supervision, children of preschool age or older may sit in a chair and hold the baby. School-age children are often fascinated by the new baby and surroundings and ask many questions. Adolescents react in various ways. They may be excited and eager to be a substitute parent, or they may be embarrassed about their parents' obvious sexuality "at their age." Observe for signs of early parent–infant attachment. Parent behaviors are tentative at first, progressing from fingertip touch to palm touch to enfolding of the infant. Parents usually make eye contact with the infant and talk to the baby in higher-pitched, affectionate tones.

Cultural variations should be considered when assessing early attachment. The nurse should be knowledgeable about the typical practices of the populations commonly served. In some cultures, great attention to the newborn is considered unlucky ("evil eye").

SUMMARY CONCEPTS

- Some women do not have symptoms typical of true labor. They should enter the birth center for evaluation if they are uncertain and have concerns other than those listed in the guidelines.
- The childbearing family's first impression on admission to the intrapartum unit is important to promote a therapeutic relationship with caregivers and a positive birth experience.
- Initial intrapartum assessments quickly evaluate maternal and fetal health and labor status.
- The fetus is the more vulnerable of the maternal–fetal pair because of complete dependence on the mother's physiologic systems.
- The normal fetal heart rate at term averages 110 to 160 beats per minute. Other reassuring signs include regular rhythm, presence of accelerations, absence of decelerations, and presence of moderate variability.
- A maternal supine position can reduce placental blood flow because the uterus compresses the aorta and inferior vena cava (aortocaval compression).
- General comfort measures promote the woman's ability to relax and cope with labor.
- Regular changes in position during labor promote maternal comfort and help the fetus adapt to the pelvis.
- Prolapse and compression of the umbilical cord are the primary risks of amniotomy. As the fluid gushes out, the cord can become compressed between the fetal presenting part and the woman's pelvis.
- Infection is more likely to occur when membranes have been ruptured for a long time (e.g., 24 hours or longer).
- The nurse must be alert for signs of impending birth: The woman may state, "The baby's coming," make grunting sounds, and bear down.

- Induction of labor may be done if continuing the pregnancy is more hazardous to the maternal and fetal health than the induction. It is not done if a maternal or fetal contraindication to labor and vaginal birth exists.
- Oxytocin-stimulated uterine contractions may be excessive, decreasing placental perfusion.
- External cephalic version is done to promote vaginal birth by changing the fetal presentation from a breech or transverse lie to a cephalic presentation. Internal version sometimes is used to change presentation of a second twin after the birth of the first twin.
- Trauma to maternal and fetal tissue is the primary risk associated with use of forceps and vacuum extraction. Possible trauma to the mother includes vaginal wall laceration and hematoma. Trauma to the infant may include ecchymoses, lacerations, abrasions, facial nerve injury, and intracranial hemorrhage.
- The median episiotomy is less painful but more likely to extend into the rectum than the mediolateral episiotomy.

- The preferred uterine incision for cesarean birth is the low transverse incision because it is least likely to rupture in a subsequent pregnancy. The skin incision does not always match the uterine incision and is unrelated to the risk for later uterine rupture.
- Some women have feelings of guilt and inadequacy if they have a cesarean birth or if they choose not to try VBAC when given that choice. Therapeutic communication and sensitive, family-centered care are essential to help them achieve a positive perception of their birth experience.
- The priority nursing care of the newborn immediately after birth is to promote normal respirations, maintain normal body temperature, and promote attachment.
- The priority nursing care of the mother after birth is to assess for hemorrhage and promote firm uterine contraction, promote comfort, and promote parent–infant attachment.

REFERENCES & READINGS

Academy of American Family Physician (AAFP). (2015). *Planning for Labor and Vaginal Birth After Cesarean Delivery: Guidelines from the AAFP.* Retrieved from www.aafp.org/afp.

American Academy of Pediatrics & American College of Obstetricians and Gynecologists (AAP & ACOG). (2012). *Guidelines for perinatal care* (7th ed.). Elk Grove Village, IL & Washington, DC: Author.

American Academy of Pediatrics & American Heart Association (AAP & AHA). (2016). *Neonatal resuscitation textbook* (7th ed.). Elk Grove Village, IL: Authors.

American College of Obstetricians and Gynecologists (ACOG). (2013). *Prevention and Management of Obstetric Lacerations at Vaginal Delivery.* ACOG Practice Bulletin 165. Washington, DC: Author.

American College of Obstetricians and Gynecologists (ACOG). (2015a). *Induction of Labor.* ACOG Practice Bulletin 107. Published 2009, reaffirmed 2015. Washington, DC: Author.

American College of Obstetricians and Gynecologists (ACOG). (2015b). *Vaginal Birth After Previous Cesarean Delivery.* ACOG Practice Bulletin 115. Published 2010, reaffirmed 2015. Washington, DC: Author.

American College of Obstetricians and Gynecologists (ACOG). (2015c). *Management of intrapartum fetal heart rate tracing.* ACOG Practice Bulletin 116. Published 2010, reaffirmed 2015. Washington, DC: Author.

American College of Obstetricians and Gynecologists (ACOG). (2015d). *Operative Vaginal Delivery.* ACOG Practice Bulletin 154. Washington, DC: Author.

American College of Obstetricians and Gynecologists (ACOG). (2016). *External Cephalic Version.* ACOG Practice Bulletin 161. Washington, DC: Author.

Association of Women's Health, Obstetric and Neonatal Nurses (AWHONN). (2008). *Nursing care and management of the second stage of labor: Evidence-based clinical practice guidelines* (2nd ed.). Washington, DC: Author.

Association of Women's Health, Obstetric and Neonatal Nurses (AWHONN). (2012). *Go the Full 40.* Retrieved from www.health4mom.org/wp-content/uploads/2015/03/Go-The-Full-40-Implementation-Toolkit_2015-1.pdf.

Bakker, P. C., Kurver, P. H., Kuik, D. J., & Van Geijin, H. P. (2007). Elevated uterine activity increases the risk of fetal acidosis at birth. *American Journal of Obstetrics and Gynecology, 196*(4), 313.e1–313.e6.

Benirschke, K. (2014). Multiple gestation: The biology of twinning. In R. K. Creasy, R. Resnik, J. D. Iams, C. Lockwood, T. Moore, & M. Green (Eds.), *Creasy & Resnik's Maternal-fetal medicine: Principles and practice* (7th ed.) (pp. 53–65). Philadelphia, PA: Saunders.

Bishop, E. H. (1964). Pelvic scoring for elective induction. *Obstetrics & Gynecology, 24*(2), 266–268.

Cunningham, F. G., Leveno, K. J., Bloom, S. L., Spong, C. Y., Dashe, J. S., Hoffman, B. L., & Sheffield, J. S. (2014). *Williams obstetrics* (24th ed.). New York: McGraw-Hill Medical.

Fenwick, L., & Simkin, P. (1987). Maternal positioning to prevent or alleviate dystocia in labor. *Clinical Obstetrics and Gynecology, 30*(1), 83–89.

Fraser, D. (2014). Newborn adaptation to extrauterine life. In K. R. Simpson, & P. A. Creehan (Eds.), *AWHONN's perinatal nursing* (4th ed.) (pp. 581–596). Philadelphia, PA: Lippincott Williams & Wilkins.

Freeman, R. K., Garite, T. J., Nageotte, M. P., & Miller, L. A. (2012). *Fetal Heart Rate Monitoring* (4th ed.) (pp. 85–111). Philadelphia, Lippincott Williams & Wilkins.

Hamilton, B. E., Martin, J. A., Osterman, M. J. K., Curtin, S. C., & Mathews, T. J. (2015). Births: Final data for 2014. *National Vital Statistics Report, 64*(12). Retrieved from www.cdc.gov/nchs/nvss/births.htm.

Hodnett, E. D., Gates, S., Hofmeyr, G. J., & Sakala, C. (2013). Continuous support for women during childbirth. *Cochrane Database of Systematic Reviews, 2013*(7), CD003766.

James, D. C. (2014). Postpartum care. In K. R. Simpson, & P. A. Creehan (Eds.), *AWHONN's perinatal nursing* (4th ed.) (pp. 530–580). Philadelphia, PA: Lippincott Williams & Wilkins.

Joint Commission. (2016). Retrieved from www.jointcommission.org/standards_information/jcfaqdetails.aspx?StandardsFaqId=995

Killion, M. M. (2015). Techniques for fetal heart and uterine activity assessment. In A. Lyndon, & L. U. Ali (Eds.), *Fetal Heart Monitoring Principles and Practices* (5th ed.) (pp. 85–124). Washington D.C: Kendall Hunt Publishing.

Lyndon, A., O'Brien-Abel, N., & Simpson, K. R. (2014). Fetal assessment during labor. In K. R. Simpson, & P. A. Creehan (Eds.), *AWHONN's perinatal nursing* (4th ed.) (pp. 445–492). Philadelphia, PA: Lippincott Williams & Wilkins.

Macones, G. A., Hankins, G. D., Spong, C. Y., Hauth, J., & Moore, T. (2008). The 2008 National Institute of Child Health and Human Development workshop report on electronic fetal monitoring: Update on definitions, interpretation, and research guidelines. *Journal of Obstetric, Gynecologic, and Neonatal Nursing, 37*(5), 510–515.

Martin, J., Hamilton, B., Osterman, M., Curtin, S., & Mathews, T. (2015). Births: Final data for 2013. *National Center for Health Statistics, 64*(1) Hyattsville, MD: National Center for Health Statistics.

Mercer, B. M. (2014). Premature rupture of the membranes. In R. K. Creasy, R. Resnik, J. D. Iams, C. Lockwood, T. Moore, & M. Green (Eds.), *Creasy & Resnik's Maternal-fetal medicine: Principles and practice* (7th ed.) (pp. 663–672). Philadelphia, PA: Saunders.

Miller, L. A., Miller, D. A., & Cypher, R. L. (2017). *Mosby's Pocket Guide to Fetal Monitoring: A multidisciplinary approach* (8th ed.) (pp. 75–102). St. Louis, MO: Mosby.

National Center for Health Statistics. (2017). *Data File Documentations, Natality, 2015.* Hyattsville, MD: Author.

Osterman, M. J. K., & Martin, J. A. (2014). Recent declines in induction of labor by gestational age. *National Center for Health Statistics Data Brief.* No. 155. Retrieved from www.cdc.gov/nchs/data/databriefs/db155.pdf.

Oxytocin: Drug Information. (2016). *UpToDate.* Retrieved from www.uptodate.com/contents/oxytocin-drug-information?-source=search_result&search=oxytocin.

Roberts, J. M., August, P. A., & Bakris, G. (2013). *Task Force on Hypertension in Pregnancy.* Washington D.C.: American College of Obstetricians and Gynecologists.

Roberts, L., Gulliver, B., Fisher, J., & Cloyes, K. G. (2010). The coping with labor algorithm: An alternative pain assessment tool for the laboring woman. *Journal of Midwifery & Women's Health, 55*(2), 107–116.

Roth, C., Dent, S. A., Parfitt, S. E., Hering, S. L., & Bay, R. C. (2016). Randomized control trial of use of the peanut ball during labor. *The American Journal of Maternal Child Nursing, 41*(3), 140–146.

Sheibani, L., & Wing, D. A. (2017). Abnormal labor and induction of labor. In S. G. Gabbe, J. R. Niebyl, J. L. Simpson, M. B. Landon, H. L. Galan, R. M. Jauniaux, D. A. Driscoll, et al. (Eds.), *Obstetrics: Normal and problem pregnancies* (7th ed.) (pp. 271–288). St. Louis, MO: Elsevier.

Simpson, K. R. (2013). *Cervical ripening and induction and augmentation of labor* (4th ed.). Washington D.C.: Association of Women's Health, Obstetric and Neonatal Nurses.

Simpson, K. R., & O'Brien-Abel, N. (2014). Labor and birth. In K. R. Simpson, & P. A. Creehan (Eds.), *AWHONN's perinatal nursing* (4th ed.) (pp. 343–444). Philadelphia, PA: Lippincott Williams & Wilkins.

Spong, C. Y., Berghella, V., Wenstrom, K. D., Mercer, B. M., & Saade, G. R. (2012). Preventing the first cesarean delivery: Summary of a joint Eunice Kennedy Shriver National Institute of Child Health and Human Development, Society for Maternal-Fetal Medicine, and American College of Obstetricians and Gynecologists Workshop. *Obstetrics and Gynecology, 120*(5), 1181–1193.

Thorp, J. M., & Laughon, S. K. (2014). Clinical aspects of normal and abnormal labor. In R. K. Creasy, R. Resnik, J. D. Iams, C. Lockwood, T. Moore, & M. Green (Eds.), *Creasy & Resnik's Maternal-fetal medicine: Principles and practice* (7th ed.) (pp. 673–706). Philadelphia, PA: Saunders.

Tussey, C. M., Botsios, E., Gerkin, R. D., Kelly, L. A., Gamez, J., & Mensik, J. (2015). Reducing length of labor and cesarean surgery rate using a peanut ball for women laboring with an epidural. *Journal of Perinatal Education, 1*(24), 16–24.

U.S. Department of Health and Human Services. (2010). *Healthy People 2020. Reduce cesarean births among low-risk (full term, singleton, vertex presentation) women.* Retrieved from www.healthypeople.gov/2020/topics-objectives/topic/maternal-infant-and-child-health/objectives.

U.S. Food and Drug Administration. (2015). *Misoprostol (marketed as Cytotec) information (2015).* Retrieved from www.fda.gov/Drugs/DrugSafety/PostmarketDrugSafetyInformationforPatientsandProviders/ucm111315.htm.

Wisner, K., & Ali, L. (2015). Documentation of fetal heart monitoring information. In A. Lyndon, & L. U. Ali (Eds.), *Fetal Heart Monitoring Principles and Practices* (5th ed.) (pp. 249–283). Washington D.C.: Kendall Hunt Publishing.

Wisner, K., & Gauthier, D. (2015). Maternal-fetal assessment. In A. Lyndon, & L. U. Ali (Eds.), *Fetal Heart Monitoring Principles and Practices* (5th ed.) (pp. 51–84). Washington D.C.: Kendall Hunt Publishing.

Witcher, P. M., & Hamner, L. (2013). Venous thromboembolism in pregnancy. In N. H. Troiano, C. J. Harvey, & B. F. Chez (Eds.), *AWHONN High-risk & critical care obstetrics* (3rd ed.) (pp. 285–299). Philadelphia, PA: Lippincott Williams & Wilkins.

Zwelling, E. (2010). Overcoming the challenges: Maternal movement and positioning to facilitate labor progress. *MCN: American Journal of Maternal-Child Nursing, 35*(2), 72–80.

Intrapartum Complications

Cheryl Roth

After studying this chapter, you should be able to:

1. Explain abnormalities that may result in dysfunctional labor.
2. Describe maternal and fetal risks associated with premature rupture of the membranes.
3. Analyze factors that increase a woman's risk for preterm labor.
4. Explain maternal and fetal problems that may occur if pregnancy persists beyond 42 weeks.
5. Describe the intrapartum emergencies discussed in this chapter.
6. Explain management of each intrapartum complication.
7. Apply the nursing process to care of women with intrapartum complications and their families.

For most women, birth is a normal process that is free of major complications. However, complications sometimes make childbearing hazardous for the woman or her baby. The nurse's challenge is to identify complications promptly and provide effective care for such mothers while nurturing the entire family at this significant time of life.

The complications addressed in this chapter are often interrelated. For example, a dysfunctional labor is likely to be prolonged, and the woman is more vulnerable to infection, psychological distress, and fetal compromise. Also, women who have complications are more likely to need interventions such as lengthy hospitalization before vaginal or cesarean birth. The nurse should provide nursing care that relates to all problems experienced by the woman.

DYSFUNCTIONAL LABOR

Normal labor is characterized by progression of cervical effacement, dilation, and fetal descent. Dysfunctional labor is one that does not result in normal progress. A dysfunctional labor may result from problems with the powers of labor, the passenger, the passage, the psyche, or a combination of these. Often this type of labor is prolonged but may be unusually short and intense.

An operative birth (assisted with a vacuum extractor or forceps, or cesarean birth) may be needed if dysfunctional labor does not resolve or compromise occurs with the fetus or mother. Signs of possible compromise include persistent abnormal fetal heart rate (FHR) patterns (see Chapter 14), fetal acidosis, and meconium passage. Maternal infection or exhaustion can also occur with a long labor. Nursing measures

that enhance labor progress, maternal comfort, and promote fetal well-being are discussed in this chapter.

Problems of the Powers

The powers of labor may not be adequate to expel the fetus because of ineffective contractions or maternal pushing efforts.

Ineffective Contractions

Effective uterine activity is characterized by coordinated contractions that are strong and numerous enough to propel the fetus past the resistance of the woman's bony pelvis and soft tissues. It is not possible to say how frequent, long, or strong labor contractions must be. One woman's labor may progress with contractions that would be inadequate for another woman. Possible causes of ineffective contractions include the following:

- Maternal fatigue
- Maternal inactivity
- Fluid and electrolyte imbalance
- Hypoglycemia
- Excessive analgesia or anesthesia
- Maternal catecholamines secreted in response to stress or pain
- Disproportion between the maternal pelvis and fetal presenting part
- Uterine overdistention such as with multiple gestation or **hydramnios** (excess volume of amniotic fluid)
- Poor application of the presenting part to the cervix

Two patterns of ineffective uterine contractions are labor dystocia and tachysystole. The characteristics and management of each are different, but either results in poor labor progress if it persists.

Labor Dystocia. **Labor dystocia** means a difficult labor and may be used to describe any form of dysfunctional labor. However, it is most often used to describe labor that does not progress as expected. When labor dystocia, or "failure to progress," occurs, contractions are coordinated but too weak to be effective. They are infrequent, brief and when palpated, they can be indented easily with fingertip pressure at the peak.

Labor dystocia, or secondary arrest, occurs during the active phase of labor, when progress normally quickens. The active phase usually begins by 6 cm of cervical dilation. Uterine overdistention is associated with labor dystocia because the stretched uterine muscle contracts poorly.

The woman may be fairly comfortable due to weaker contractions. However, she often is frustrated because labor slows at a time when she expects to be making faster progress. Labor dystocia is tiring as a result of the duration of labor. Fetal hypoxia is not usually seen with dystocia.

Management depends on the cause. Many women respond to simple measures. Administration of adequate intravenous (IV) or oral fluids corrects maternal fluid and electrolyte imbalances or hypoglycemia. Maternal position changes, particularly different upright positions, favor fetal descent and promote effective contractions. The woman who actively changes positions typically has better labor progress and is more comfortable than the woman who remains in one position. Standing or sitting in a shower provides the comfort of warm water and an upright position. Pain management techniques such as epidural block may have outcomes that reduce the effectiveness of contractions, requiring interventions specific to that factor. Effective pain management may, however, improve the progress of labor.

The nurse should use therapeutic communication to help the woman identify anxieties or beliefs about labor and its progress. Identifying her anxieties is important because the stress response could slow her labor. For example, the nurse might ask, "What do you think is making your labor slow?" or "How do you feel your labor is going?"

Measures such as amniotomy and oxytocin infusion may be needed to promote labor progress. The birth attendant evaluates the woman's labor to confirm she is having labor dystocia rather than a prolonged latent phase of labor or false labor. The maternal pelvis, fetal presentation, and position are evaluated to identify abnormalities. Reducing undesired maternal effects of a prolonged latent phase such as exhaustion or infection is a goal of the birth attendant. However, the birth attendant should consider the possibility a woman is in false labor rather than in a prolonged latent phase when choosing interventions to correct the labor progress.

Amniotomy or augmentation, usually with oxytocin, may be used to stimulate an established, yet slow labor pattern. The risks of amniotomy include umbilical cord prolapse, infection, and placental abruption (premature separation of placenta). Reduced placental perfusion caused by excessive uterine contractions is the most common risk for labor augmentation using oxytocin (Simpson, 2013; Sheibani, & Wing, 2017) (see Chapter 15).

Tachysystole. Tachysystole can be either spontaneous or induced and is defined as excessive uterine activity. Tachysystole is more than 5 contractions in 10 minutes, averaged over 30 minutes (Macones, Hankins, Spong, Hauth & Moore, 2008). In addition to tachysystole, contractions lasting 2 minutes or longer, contractions with less than 1 minute resting time between, or failure of the uterus to return to resting tone between contractions via palpation or intrauterine pressure above 25 mm Hg measured by an intrauterine pressure catheter (IUPC) may also be of concern. Contractions may be uncoordinated and erratic in their frequency, duration, and intensity (Simpson, 2013).

Although each contraction varies in its intensity, the **uterine resting tone** (uterine muscle tone when not having contraction) between contractions may be higher than normal, reducing uterine blood flow. The reduction of blood flow to the uterus decreases fetal oxygen supply and causes the woman to have almost constant cramping pain. With a high uterine resting tone and complaints of continuous pain, the nurse should be alert to a possibility of placental abruption as the symptoms can be the same.

The mother becomes very tired because of nearly constant discomfort. She may lose confidence in her ability to give birth and cope with labor. She often thinks, "If it hurts this much so early, I must be a real baby about pain." Frustration and anxiety further reduce her pain tolerance and interfere with the normal processes of labor. Cervical dilation should not be equated with the amount of pain a woman "should" experience.

Management of uterine tachysystole depends on the cause. If oxytocin is being administered, the dose should be decreased or stopped. Oxytocin can intensify the already high uterine resting tone. Secondly, relief of pain is an important intervention to promote a normal labor pattern. In the latent phase of labor, warm showers and baths promote relaxation and rest, often allowing a normal labor pattern to ensue. Systemic analgesics or, occasionally, low-dose epidural analgesia may be required to achieve this purpose.

Tocolytic drugs (drugs that inhibit uterine contractions) may be ordered to reduce uterine resting tone and improve placental blood flow. The decision to order uterine stimulant or relaxant drugs is very individualized, based on each woman's labor pattern.

Ineffective Maternal Pushing

A reflexive urge to push with contractions usually occurs as the fetal presenting part reaches the pelvic floor during second-stage labor. However, ineffective pushing may result from the following:

- Use of nonphysiologic pushing techniques and positions
- Fear of injury because of pain and tearing sensations felt by the mother when she pushes
- Decreased or absent urge to push
- Maternal exhaustion
- Analgesia or anesthesia that suppresses the woman's urge to push
- Psychological unreadiness to "let go" of her baby

Management focuses on correcting causes contributing to ineffective pushing. There is no limit for the duration of the second stage of labor as long as the woman and fetus are stable with normal vital signs and FHR patterns. Each woman is evaluated individually by her birth attendant to determine whether labor should be ended with an operative delivery or can continue safely.

Nursing care to promote effective pushing helps the mother make each effort more productive. Most women, including those with epidural analgesia, can detect the urge to push. The practice of laboring down, or delayed pushing—encouraging the woman to wait until she feels the reflexive urge to push—has shown a lower incidence of adverse effects than pushing immediately on full cervical dilation. (See Chapter 15 for more information about the nursing practice of laboring down.)

Upright positions such as squatting add gravity to the woman's pushing efforts. Semisitting, side-lying, and pushing while sitting on the toilet are other options. If she prefers to lie in bed on her side, she should pull her upper leg toward her chest with each push. Leaning forward while in the sitting or squatting position maintains the best alignment of the fetal head with the pelvis.

The woman who fears injury because of the sensations she feels when pushing may respond to accurate information about the process of fetal descent. If she understands that sensations of tearing often accompany fetal descent but her tissues can expand to accommodate the baby, she may be more willing to push with contractions.

Epidural analgesia for labor uses a mixture of a local anesthetic agent and an epidural opioid analgesic to provide pain control without the major loss of sensation that is likely if local anesthetic is used alone. However, if a woman cannot feel the urge to push at all or cannot feel it strongly after the fetus has descended, she can be coached to push with each contraction.

The woman who is exhausted may push more effectively if she is encouraged to rest and push only when she feels the urge, or she may push with every other contraction. Oral and IV fluids can provide energy for the strenuous work of second-stage labor. Reassuring her about fetal well-being and the fact that she has no absolute deadline to meet helps her work with her body's efforts most effectively. This reassurance also helps the woman who may be emotionally readying herself to "let go" of her fetus in exchange for a newborn as she labors.

Problems with the Passenger

Fetal problems associated with dysfunctional labor are related to the following:

- Fetal size
- Fetal presentation or position
- Multifetal pregnancy
- Fetal anomalies

These variations may cause mechanical problems and contribute to ineffective labor.

Fetal Size

Macrosomia. The **macrosomic** infant weighs more than 8 lb 13 oz (4000 g) at birth, although some authorities define it as a weight of 9 lb, 15 oz (4500 g) or greater. The head or shoulders may not be able to adapt to the pelvis if they are too large (**cephalopelvic disproportion**). In addition, distention of the uterus by the large fetus reduces the strength of contractions both during and after birth.

Size, however, is relative. The woman with a small or abnormally shaped pelvis may not be able to deliver an average-size or small infant. The woman with a large pelvis may easily give birth to an infant heavier than 8 lb 13 oz (4000 grams). Fetal position as the baby descends through the pelvis is another important factor in terms of fetal size and maternal pelvic size.

Use of different maternal positions that open the pelvis may promote vaginal delivery. Positions that promote the C curve of the spine, in which the patient leans the shoulders forward and causes the spine to curve forward, direct the fetal pressure toward the back of the pelvis rather than the front, narrower part of the pelvis. Use of labor balls, large inflated physiotherapy balls, or a firm foundation to sit on will cause the pelvic diameter to increase. Use of side-lying positions with the peanut ball (a peanut shaped labor ball) between the knees can allow the sacrum and coccyx to fall farther back, increasing the pelvic diameter.

Shoulder Dystocia. Delayed or difficult birth of the shoulders may occur as they become impacted above the maternal symphysis pubis. Shoulder dystocia is more likely to occur when the fetus is large or the mother has diabetes, but many cases occur in pregnancies with no identifiable risk factors. Labor may be long, but shoulder dystocia also may occur after a normal labor (American College of Obstetricians and Gynecologists (ACOG), 2017a; Lanni, Gherman, & Gonik, 2017).

Shoulder dystocia is an urgent situation because the umbilical cord can be compressed between the fetal body and the maternal pelvis. One of the initial signs of shoulder dystocia is known as the "turtle sign." After the head is born, it retracts against the perineum, much like a turtle's head drawing into its shell. When the turtle sign is identified, the delivery team should make preparations for surgical delivery, which should be anticipated while taking immediate steps to deliver the baby vaginally. Although the infant's head is out of the vaginal canal, the chest is inside, preventing respirations. Any of several methods may be used to quickly release the impacted fetal shoulders (Fig. 16.1). McRobert's maneuver is a nursing action that should be taken immediately, pulling the mother's knees up as far toward the shoulders as possible. Fundal pressure should be avoided so that the shoulders are not pushed even harder against the symphysis. Suprapubic pressure may assist in moving the impacted shoulder past the symphysis. The provider will take other measures to affect delivery. After delivery of the infant, the clavicles should be checked for crepitus, deformity, and bruising, each of which suggests fracture (see Chapter 20). Documentation of all care is essential, including a clear description of the maneuver used to assist with delivery. One person is usually designated the "timekeeper" for accuracy of records (Lanni, Gherman, & Gonik, 2017; Simpson, 2014).

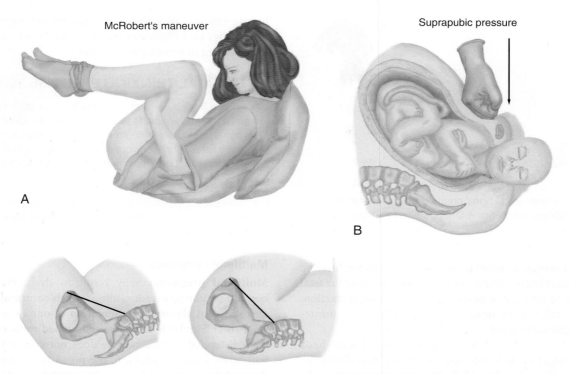

McRobert's maneuver

Suprapubic pressure

A

B

FIG. 16.1 Methods That May Be Used to Relieve Shoulder Dystocia. **A**, McRobert's maneuver. The woman flexes her thighs sharply against her abdomen, which straightens the pelvic curve somewhat. **B**, Suprapubic pressure by an assistant pushes the fetal anterior shoulder downward to displace it from above the mother's symphysis pubis. Fundal pressure should not be used because it will push the anterior shoulder even more firmly against the mother's symphysis.

Abnormal Fetal Presentation or Position

An unfavorable fetal presentation or position may interfere with cervical dilation or fetal descent.

Rotation Abnormalities. Persistence of the fetus in the occiput posterior (OP) or occiput transverse (OT) position can contribute to dysfunctional labor. These positions prevent the mechanisms of labor (cardinal movements) from occurring normally. Most fetuses that begin in the occiput posterior position rotate spontaneously to the occiput anterior (OA) position, promoting normal extension and expulsion of the head. The fetus may not rotate or may partly rotate and remain in the OT position. Although many women cannot readily deliver a fetus in the OP position, the woman with a pelvis larger than the fetal size may be able to do so.

Labor usually is longer and more uncomfortable when the fetus remains in the OP or OT position. Intense back or leg pain that may be poorly relieved with analgesia makes coping with labor difficult for the woman. "Back labor" aptly describes the sensations a woman feels when her fetus is in the OP position. Some women who had a fetus in the OP position during labor continue to feel more pain in the back or coccyx during the postpartum period.

Maternal position changes promote fetal head rotation to the OA position and descent (see other examples in Chapter 15). Examples include the following:

- Hands and knees—Rocking the pelvis back and forth while on hands and knees promotes rotation. The woman's knees should be slightly behind her hips in this position. A peanut ball may aid in helping a patient feel supported. A dense epidural may interfere with the use of this position.
- Side-lying (on the opposite side of the fetal occiput)— Especially when in the far side-lying position with the posterior shoulder pulled behind the patient and the upper knee touching the bed. A peanut ball may be used in the side-lying position to open the pelvis.
- Squatting (for second-stage labor)—Sitting on a slightly underinflated birth ball gives a similar effect.
- Sitting, kneeling, or standing while leaning forward.

Upright maternal positions promote descent, which usually is accompanied by fetal head rotation. The hands-and-knees and side-lying positions promote rotation because the mother's abdomen is dependent in relation to her spine. In the hands-and-knees position, the convex surface of the fetal back tends to rotate toward the convex anterior uterus, similar to nesting of two spoons (Fig. 16.2). The side-lying position has a similar effect, although not quite as pronounced. These positions decrease the mother's discomfort by reducing the pressure of the fetal head on her sacrum.

All variations of the squatting position aid rotation and fetal descent by straightening the pelvic curve and enlarging the pelvic outlet. They add gravity to the force of maternal pushing.

If spontaneous rotation does not occur, the physician may assist with the rotation and descent of the head by manual rotation or using forceps. The vacuum extractor cannot always be applied to the fetal head when it remains in the OP

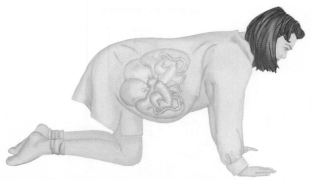

FIG. 16.2 A hands-and-knees position helps this fetus rotate from a left occiput posterior (LOP) position to an occiput anterior position.

position. However, some styles of vacuum extractors may be used to correct minor degrees of malrotation because the fetal head tends to rotate as it descends with downward traction. Cesarean birth may be needed if these methods are unsuccessful or cannot be used.

Deflexion Abnormalities. The poorly flexed fetal head presents a larger diameter to the pelvis than if flexed with the chin on the chest (see Fig. 12.8). In vertex presentation, the head diameter is smallest. In military and brow presentations, the head diameter is larger. In face presentation, the head diameter is similar to that of vertex presentation but the maternal pelvis can be traversed only if the fetal chin (mentum) is anterior.

Breech Presentation. Cervical dilation and effacement often are slower when the fetus is in breech presentation because the buttocks or feet do not form a smooth, round dilating wedge like the head. The greatest fetal risk is that the head—the largest fetal part—is the last to be born. By the time the lower body is born, the umbilical cord is well into the pelvis and may be compressed. The shoulders, arms, and head should be delivered quickly so that the infant can breathe.

A breech presentation is common well before term, but only 3% to 4% of term fetuses remain in this presentation. Reasons for breech presentation may include the following:

- Low birth weight as a result of preterm gestation, multifetal pregnancy, or intrauterine growth restriction
- Fetal anomalies contributing to breech presentation, such as hydrocephalus
- Complications secondary to placenta previa or previous cesarean birth

External cephalic version (ECV) may be attempted to manually move the fetus in breech presentation or transverse lie to cephalic presentation (see Chapter 15). If the fetus remains in the abnormal presentation, cesarean section usually is performed to avoid complications. Birth for the nulliparous woman with a fetus that remains in breech presentation is almost always by cesarean section. The fetus remaining in a transverse lie is delivered by cesarean section as well.

Some women are admitted in advanced labor with the fetus in breech presentation, so birth attendants and intrapartum nurses should be prepared to care for the woman having either a planned or an unexpected vaginal breech birth. (Fig. 16.3 illustrates the mechanisms of vaginal birth for an infant in breech presentation.)

❓ CRITICAL THINKING EXERCISE 16.1

A woman having her first baby has been in labor for several hours. Her nurse-midwife performs a vaginal examination and says that the cervix is 6 cm dilated and completely effaced, with the fetus in right occiput posterior position. The mother is having persistent back pain that worsens during contractions.

Questions
1. How should the nurse interpret this information?
2. Should the nurse take any specific action based on this examination?

Multifetal Pregnancy

Multifetal pregnancy may result in dysfunctional labor because of uterine overdistention, which contributes to labor dystocia, and abnormal presentation of one or both fetuses (Fig. 16.4). Similar to a large overstretched rubber bands, the over distended uterine muscle does not contract evenly or with great force. In addition, the potential for fetal hypoxia during labor is greater because the mother must supply oxygen and nutrients to more than one fetus. She is at greater risk for postpartum hemorrhage resulting from uterine atony because of uterine overdistention.

Some patients with twin A in the vertex position may have a vaginal delivery. Because of risk for cord prolapse, placental shearing, and potential bleeding problems, many women with multifetal pregnancies opt for cesarean birth. If three or more fetuses are involved, the birth is almost always cesarean. The physician considers fetal viability, fetal presentations, maternal pelvic size, and presence of other complications such as preeclampsia or chronic hypertension when determining the best plan of care for the patient and her fetuses.

Each twin's FHR is monitored during labor. When in bed, the woman should remain in the lateral position to promote adequate placental blood flow. After vaginal birth of the first twin, assessment of the second twin's FHR continues until birth (Newman & Unal, 2017).

The delivery staff should be prepared for the care and possible resuscitation of multiple infants. Radiant warmers, resuscitation equipment, medications, and identification materials should be prepared for each infant. One or more neonatal nurses, a neonatal nurse practitioner, and a pediatrician or a neonatologist should be available to care for each infant. One nurse should be dedicated to caring for the mother.

❓ KNOWLEDGE CHECK

1. How does labor dystocia differ from tachysystole?
2. How can maternal position changes favor rotation of the fetus from the OT or OP position to the OA position?
3. Why is cesarean birth usually the delivery method of choice for infants in breech presentation?
4. How does preparation for the birth of multiple infants (vaginal or cesarean) differ from preparation for a single infant's birth?

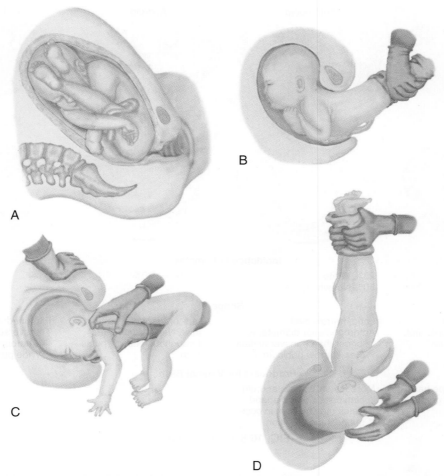

FIG. 16.3 Sequence for Vaginal Birth in a Frank Breech Presentation. A, Descent and internal rotation of the fetal body. **B,** Internal rotation complete; extension of the fetal back and neck as the trunk slips under the symphysis pubis. The birth attendant uses a towel for traction when grasping the fetal legs. **C,** After the birth of the shoulders, the attendant maintains flexion of the fetal head by using the fingers of the left hand to apply pressure to the lower face. The fetal body straddles the attendant's left arm. An assistant provides suprapubic pressure to help keep the fetal head well-flexed. **D,** After the fetal head is brought under the symphysis pubis, an assistant grasps the fetal legs with a towel for traction while the attendant delivers the face and head over the mother's perineum.

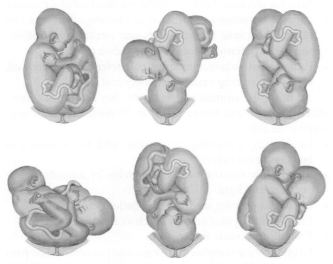

FIG. 16.4 Twins can present in any combination of presentations and positions.

Fetal Anomalies

Fetal anomalies such as hydrocephalus or a large fetal tumor may prevent normal descent of the fetus. Abnormal presentations such as breech or transverse lie also are associated with fetal anomalies. These abnormalities often are discovered by ultrasound examination before labor. Cesarean birth is scheduled if vaginal birth is not possible or is inadvisable.

Problems with the Passage

Dysfunctional labor may occur because of variations in the maternal bony pelvis or soft tissue problems that inhibit fetal descent.

Pelvis

A small (contracted) or abnormally shaped pelvis may retard labor and obstruct fetal passage. The woman may experience

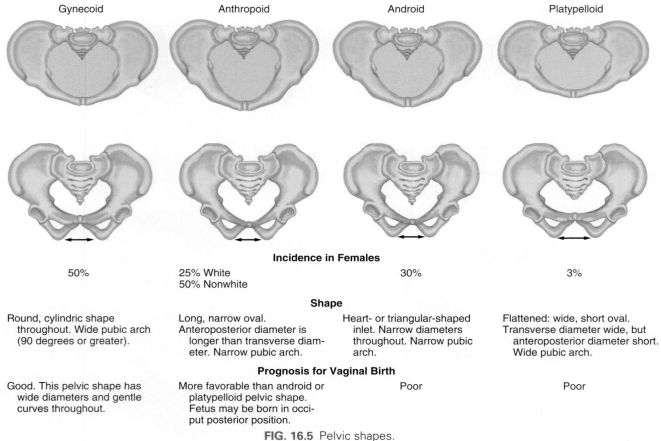

Gynecoid	Anthropoid	Android	Platypelloid

Incidence in Females

50%	25% White 50% Nonwhite	30%	3%

Shape

Round, cylindric shape throughout. Wide pubic arch (90 degrees or greater).	Long, narrow oval. Anteroposterior diameter is longer than transverse diameter. Narrow pubic arch.	Heart- or triangular-shaped inlet. Narrow diameters throughout. Narrow pubic arch.	Flattened: wide, short oval. Transverse diameter wide, but anteroposterior diameter short. Wide pubic arch.

Prognosis for Vaginal Birth

Good. This pelvic shape has wide diameters and gentle curves throughout.	More favorable than android or platypelloid pelvic shape. Fetus may be born in occiput posterior position.	Poor	Poor

FIG. 16.5 Pelvic shapes.

poor contractions, slow dilation, slow fetal descent, and a long labor.

Four basic pelvic shapes exist, each with different implications for labor and birth (Fig. 16.5). Most women do not have a pure pelvic shape but instead have mixed characteristics from two or more types.

Maternal Soft Tissue Obstructions

During labor, a full bladder is a common soft tissue obstruction. Bladder distention reduces available space in the pelvis and intensifies maternal discomfort. The woman should be assessed for bladder distention regularly and encouraged to void every 1 to 2 hours. Catheterization may be needed if she cannot urinate or if epidural analgesia depresses her urge to void. There are mixed opinions in the literature as to whether intermittent catheterization or Foley placement is more appropriate.

Problems of the Psyche

Labor is a stressful event for most women. A perceived threat caused by pain, fear, nonsupport, or personal situation can result in impaired coping ability and interfere with normal labor progress. Responses to excessive or prolonged stress interfere with labor in the following several ways:

- Increased glucose consumption reduces the energy supply available to the contracting uterus.
- Secretion of catecholamines (epinephrine and norepinephrine) by the adrenal glands stimulates uterine beta receptors, which inhibit uterine contractions (an action similar to that of tocolytic drugs such as terbutaline).
- Adrenal secretion of catecholamines diverts blood supply from the uterus and placenta to the woman's skeletal muscles.
- Labor contractions and maternal pushing efforts are less effective because these powers are working against the resistance of tense abdominal and pelvic muscles.
- Pain perception is increased and pain tolerance is decreased, further increasing maternal anxiety and stress.

Assisting the woman to relax helps her body work more effectively with the forces of labor. Nursing measures may involve the following:

- Establishing a trusting relationship with the woman and her significant other
- Making the environment comfortable by adjusting temperature and light
- Identifying coping measures the patient finds useful
- Promoting physical comfort such as cleanliness
- Providing accurate information
- Implementing nonpharmacologic and pharmacologic pain management

Abnormal Labor Duration

An unusually long or abnormally short, or precipitous, labor may result in maternal, fetal, or neonatal problems.

Prolonged Labor

Reasons for prolonged labor are multifaceted. If a previous birth was by cesarean section before significant cervical dilation occurred, the criteria for labor progress of a nullipara may be most appropriate. Effects of epidural analgesia on labor characteristics and the rate of progress and descent should also be considered by the birth attendant when deciding if interventions are needed to increase progress (Kilpatrick & Garrison, 2017; Sheibani & Wing, 2017).

Traditional thought based on the Friedman curves developed in the 1970s indicated that after the woman reached the active phase of labor, cervical dilation should proceed at a minimum rate of 1.2 cm/hr in the nullipara and 1.5 cm/hr in the parous woman. The fetal presenting part was expected to descend at a minimal rate of 1 cm/hr in the nullipara and 2 cm/hr in the parous woman.

New data have come to light with the results of a study by Zhang, Landy, Branch. et al. (2010), with the Consortium for Safe Labor, a 2010 trial funded by the National Institute of Child Health and Human Development (NICHD). This multicenter retrospective study abstracted detailed labor and delivery information from electronic medical records in 19 hospitals across the United States. A total of 62,415 patients were selected who had a singleton term gestation, spontaneous onset of labor, vertex presentation, vaginal delivery, and a normal perinatal outcome. They found that normal labor may take over 6 hours to progress from 4 to 5 cm and over 3 hours to progress from 5 to 6 cm of dilation. Nulliparas and multiparas appeared to progress at a similar pace before 6 cm. However, after 6-cm, multiparas accelerated much faster than nulliparas. The 95th percentile of the 2nd stage of labor in nulliparas with epidural analgesia was 3.6 hours and without epidural analgesia was 2.8 hours. They concluded that allowing labor to continue for a longer period before 6 cm of cervical dilation may reduce the rate of intrapartum and subsequent repeat cesarean births in the United States. Although these data are becoming increasingly more accepted in the obstetrics community, no practice changes have been made with standards for fetal monitoring assessment and documentation because there is no evidence that a change is indicated.

Possible maternal and fetal problems in prolonged labor include the following:

- Maternal infection, intrapartum or postpartum
- Neonatal infection, which may be severe or fatal
- Maternal exhaustion

- Higher levels of anxiety and fear during a subsequent labor

Maternal and neonatal infections are more likely if the membranes have been ruptured for a prolonged time, because organisms ascend from the vagina.

Nursing measures for the woman who has prolonged labor include promotion of comfort, conservation of energy, emotional support, position changes that favor normal progress, and assessments for infection. Nursing care for the fetus includes observation for signs of intrauterine infection and compromised fetal oxygenation.

Precipitous Labor

Precipitous labor is one in which birth occurs within 3 hours of its onset. Intense contractions often begin abruptly rather than gradually increasing in frequency, duration, and intensity, as is typical of most labors.

Precipitous labor is not the same as a precipitous birth. A **precipitous birth** occurs after a labor of any length, in or out of the hospital or birth center, when a trained attendant is not present to assist. However, a woman in precipitous labor also may have a precipitous birth. If the physician or nurse-midwife will not arrive in time for the baby's birth, the nurse should wear gloves and simply support the infant's body as it emerges. If the maternal pelvis is adequate and the soft tissues yield easily to fetal descent, little maternal injury is likely. However, if the soft tissues are firm and resist stretching, trauma (vaginal wall lacerations, cervical lacerations, sulcus or vulvar tears, and hematoma) of the vagina or vulva may occur.

Several conditions that can be associated with precipitous labor include placental abruption, fetal meconium, infection, maternal cocaine use, postpartum hemorrhage, and low Apgar scores for the infant (Cunningham et al., 2014). Trauma from rapid labor may result in genital tract lacerations in the mother and neonatal birth injuries (Francois & Foley, 2017; Rozance & Rosenberg, 2017). The fetus may become hypoxic because intense contractions with a short relaxation period reduce the time available for gas exchange in the placenta. Abnormal electronic fetal monitoring (EFM) patterns may include bradycardia and late decelerations. The fetus may suffer direct trauma such as intracranial hemorrhage or nerve damage during a precipitous birth from the sudden release of pressure on the fetal head.

Priority nursing care of the woman in precipitous labor includes promotion of fetal oxygenation and maternal comfort. The side-lying position enhances placental blood flow and reduces the effects of aortocaval compression. An added benefit of the side-lying position is to slow the rapid fetal descent and minimize perineal tears. Additional measures to enhance fetal oxygenation include administering oxygen to the mother and maintaining adequate blood volume with nonadditive IV fluids. If oxytocin is being used, it should be stopped. A tocolytic drug may be ordered.

Promoting comfort is difficult in a precipitous labor because intense contractions give the woman little time to prepare and use coping skills such as breathing techniques. Pharmacologic measures such as analgesics or epidural block may not be useful if rapid labor progress does not allow time for them to become effective. Possible newborn respiratory depression should be considered if opioid analgesia is given near birth. The nurse assists the woman to focus on techniques to cope with pain, one contraction at a time. The nurse should remain with her to provide support and assist with an emergency birth if it occurs.

? KNOWLEDGE CHECK

7. Using traditional thought based on Friedman's curve, what is the dilation and fetal descent rate expected for a nulliparous woman during the active phase of labor? For the parous woman? How has new data effected this belief?
8. What is the priority nursing care for a woman in prolonged labor?
9. What are the maternal and fetal risks when labor is unusually short?

◆ APPLICATION OF THE NURSING PROCESS: DURING DYSFUNCTIONAL LABOR

Several patient problems may be appropriate when caring for a woman having dysfunctional labor. The potential complication of fetal compromise should be part of all intrapartum management (see Chapter 14). Pain management is especially important to women in labor because they may find their coping skills are inadequate or difficult to use because of fatigue, possibly to the point of exhaustion. Anxiety or fear often is higher with abnormal labor, which limits the woman's ability to cope with labor. Anxiety or fear may reduce the effectiveness of pain medications or regional block analgesia.

In addition to these problems, nursing care is directed toward two other patient problems: "Possible Intrauterine Infection" and "Maternal Exhaustion."

POSSIBLE INTRAUTERINE INFECTION

Infection can occur with both normal and dysfunctional labors. The labor nurse should be familiar with the criteria for **Triple I** (intrauterine inflammation or infection, or both) (Huggins, et.al., 2016) and the protocols or order sets that are in place in their institution. Triple I is also known as *chorioamnionitis, intra-amniotic infection (IAI) or intra-uterine infection (IUI)*. Triple I is proposed as the preferred term as it is more general and descriptive (Huggins, et.al., 2016).

The following parameters meet the criteria for a diagnosis of Triple I for the mother (Higgins et al., 2016):
- Maternal fever – defined as an oral temperature of 39.0°C or greater (102.2°F) on one reading or 38.0°C (100.4° F) or greater but less than 39.0°C (102.2° F) on 2 readings, 30 minutes apart

  with one or more of the following:
- Fetal tachycardia—Baseline greater than 160 bpm × at least 10 minutes
- Maternal white blood cell (WBC) count greater than 15,000 in the absence of corticosteroids
- Purulent fluid emanating from the cervical os

- Cloudy, yellowish, thick discharge confirmed visually on sterile speculum examination (SSE) to be coming from the cervical canal
- Biochemical or microbiologic amniotic fluid results consistent with microbial invasion of the amniotic cavity (confirmed testing), includes the following:
  - Positive Gram stain for bacteria
  - Low amniotic fluid glucose

NOTE: If *only* maternal temperature is elevated, with no other markers, it is not Triple I.

Fever plus one indicator = Suspected Triple I

Fever plus confirmed testing = Confirmed Triple I

◆ Assessment

Assess maternal temperature every 2 to 4 hours in normal labor and every 2 hours after the membranes have ruptured. Assess the temperature hourly if elevated or other signs of infection are present.

Assess maternal pulse, respirations, and blood pressure hourly if elevated temperature.

Assess amniotic fluid for normal clear color and mild odor. Small flecks of white vernix are normal in amniotic fluid. Yellow or cloudy fluid or fluid with a foul or strong odor suggests infection. The strong odor may be noted before birth or afterward on the infant's skin.

◆ Identification of Patient Problems

For the woman without signs of infection but with risk factors, the patient problem identified is potential for infection because of the presence of favorable conditions for development. The nurse may specify the patient-specific conditions that may cause infection when choosing this patient problem.

◆ Planning: Expected Outcomes

Expected outcomes relate to detecting the onset of infection:
- Maternal temperature will remain below 38°C (100.4°F).
- The FHR will remain near the baseline with an average baseline rate no higher than 160 bpm.
- The amniotic fluid will remain clear and without a foul or strong odor.

◆ Interventions
Reducing the Risk for Infection

Nurses should wash their hands before and after each contact with all patients to reduce transmission of organisms. Limit vaginal examinations to reduce transmission of vaginal organisms into the uterine cavity and maintain aseptic technique during essential vaginal examinations. The intrapartum nurse learns to estimate a woman's progress with few vaginal examinations. For example, increased bloody show and heightened anxiety may occur when the cervix is approximately 6 cm dilated. The patient may have nausea or vomit at 7 cm. The woman may become irritable and lose control at about 8 cm dilation if she has chosen not to have epidural analgesia.

Keep underpads as dry as possible to reduce the moist, warm environment that favors bacterial growth. Periodically clean excess secretions from the vaginal area in a front-to-back direction to limit fecal contamination and promote the mother's comfort. Use personal protective equipment to avoid contact with body secretions.

> **! SAFETY CHECK**
>
> Signs associated with Triple I include the following:
> - Maternal fever – defined as an oral temperature of 39.0°C or greater (102.2°F) on one reading or 38.0°C (100.4° F) or greater but less than 39.0°C (102.2° F) on 2 readings, 30 minutes apart *with one or more of the following:*
> - Fetal tachycardia—Baseline greater than 160 × at least 10 minutes.
> - Maternal white blood cell count greater than 15,000 in the absence of corticosteroids
> - Purulent fluid emanating from the cervical os
>   - Cloudy, yellowish, thick discharge confirmed visually on SSE to be coming from the cervical canal
> - Biochemical or microbiologic amniotic fluid results consistent with microbial invasion of the amniotic cavity (confirmed testing), includes the following:
>   - Positive Gram stain for bacteria
>   - Low amniotic fluid glucose

Identifying Infection

Assess the woman and fetus for signs of infection. Increase the frequency of assessments if labor is prolonged, if other risk factors are present, or if any signs of infection are found. If signs of infection are noted, report them to the birth attendant for further evaluation and treatment. Note the time at which the membranes ruptured to identify prolonged rupture, which adds to the risk for infection.

After birth, the attendant may collect specimens from the uterine cavity or placenta for culture to identify infectious organisms and determine antibiotic sensitivity. Aerobic and anaerobic culture specimens may be collected in containers specifically made for these two types of organisms. Follow directions on the container for proper handling and prevention of contamination with extraneous organisms, which would result in inaccurate results. Transport specimens to the laboratory promptly because living organisms are required for culture and sensitivity study. Antibiotic therapy is started without delay after collecting specimens.

Inform the newborn nursery staff if signs of infection are noted or increased maternal risk factors exist. Specimens of infant secretions also may be obtained for testing before administration of antibiotics. The infant may receive prophylactic antibiotics to prevent neonatal sepsis. If results of maternal or infant cultures indicate that no infection is present, the antibiotic is discontinued. Culture and sensitivity testing may reveal an infection and indicate that a different antibiotic would be more effective, in which case the antibiotic is changed.

◆ Evaluation

The goals and expected outcomes are achieved if the following occur:
- The woman's temperature remains below 38°C (100.4°F).

- The amniotic fluid has no abnormal characteristics that are typical of infection (cloudiness, yellow color, foul or strong odor).
- The FHR remains within the expected range, not showing tachycardia, whether sudden or gradual in onset.

Even if the woman has no signs of infection, she remains at higher risk for postpartum infection and should be observed for signs and symptoms of infection.

MATERNAL EXHAUSTION

◆ Assessment

Many women begin labor with a sleep deficit because of fetal movement, frequent urination, and shortness of breath associated with advanced pregnancy. As labor drags on, the mother's reserves are further depleted. Some women do not choose to or cannot have epidurals. Even with epidural analgesia, a long labor drains the mother's energy. Therefore the labor nurse should be prepared to deal with exhaustion.

Assess the mother for the following signs of exhaustion:
- Verbal expression of tiredness, fatigue, or exhaustion
- Verbal expression of frustration with a prolonged, unproductive labor ("I can't go on any longer. Why doesn't the doctor just take the baby?")
- Ineffectiveness of or inability to use coping techniques (e.g., patterned breathing) that she previously used effectively
- Changes in her pulse rate, respiration, and blood pressure (increased or decreased)

◆ Identification of Patient Problems

The intense energy demands of a dysfunctional labor may exceed a woman's physical and psychological ability to meet them. For this reason, exhaustion due to depletion of maternal energy reserves is an appropriate patient problem.

◆ Planning: Expected Outcomes

Contractions must continue for labor to progress. Two realistic goals or expected outcomes are that the woman will do the following:
- Rest between contractions with her muscles relaxed
- Use coping skills such as breathing and relaxation techniques effectively

◆ Interventions
Conserving Maternal Energy

Reduce the factors that interfere with the woman's ability to relax. Lower the light level, and turn off overhead lights. Reduce noise by closing the door or using soft music, water sounds, or other comforting sounds. Maintain a comfortable maternal temperature with blankets or a fan. If not contraindicated, a warm shower or bath is soothing.

Position the woman to encourage comfort, promote fetal descent, and enhance fetal oxygenation. Support her with pillows or birth balls to reduce muscle strain and added fatigue. Help her change positions regularly (about every 30 minutes) to reduce muscle tension from constant pressure.

A soothing back rub reduces muscle tension and thus decreases fatigue. Firm sacral pressure and use of some maternal positions discussed in the section on fetal occiput posterior positions may reduce back pain. Using the birthing ball can relax and support her in some positions. Warmth to her back can reduce back pain. (See Chapters 13 and 15 for added comfort measures.)

Maintain IV fluids at the rate ordered to provide fluid, electrolytes, and possibly glucose. Assess intake and output to identify dehydration, which may accompany prolonged labor. Dehydration also may cause maternal fever. If not contraindicated, provide juice, lollipops, frozen juice bars, or other clear liquids, as ordered by the physician or nurse-midwife, to moisten the woman's mouth and replenish her energy.

Promoting Coping Skills

When position changes or medical therapies are used to enhance labor, explain their purpose and expected benefits. Encourage the woman to visualize her baby passing downward smoothly through her pelvis as a result of her efforts. Provide mental images that allow her to "see" herself giving birth.

Generous praise and encouragement of the woman's use of skills such as breathing and visualization techniques motivate her to continue them even when she is discouraged. As with any laboring woman, tell her when she is making progress. Tell her that FHRs and patterns are reassuring if this is true. Knowing that her efforts are having the desired results and her fetus is doing well gives the woman courage to continue.

◆ Evaluation

Goals are met if the woman does the following:

- Rests and relaxes between contractions. If she is unable to relax, and feels she needs help, discuss alternative coping methods, including analgesia options with her.
- Continues to demonstrate adequate use of learned skills to cope with labor.

PREMATURE RUPTURE OF THE MEMBRANES

Rupture of the amniotic membranes before onset of true labor is called *premature rupture of the membranes* (PROM), regardless of gestational age. A precise term, *preterm premature rupture of the membranes* (PPROM, sometimes abbreviated as pPROM), refers to the rupture of membranes earlier than 37 weeks, with or without contractions. PPROM is associated with preterm labor and birth. The greatest risks to the newborn occur with birth before completion of 32 to 34 weeks of gestation (ACOG, 2016d; Mercer, 2017).

Etiology

Several conditions are associated with PROM and PPROM, but the exact cause often remains unclear. Conditions associated with preterm ruptured membranes include the following:

- Triple I may be associated with group B *Streptococcus* (GBS), *Neisseria gonorrhoeae, Listeria monocytogenes,* or species from the genera *Mycoplasma, Bacteroides,* and *Ureaplasma* in the amniotic fluid

- Infections, possibly asymptomatic, of the vagina or cervix, such as *N. gonorrhoeae, Chlamydia trachomatis, Trichomonas vaginalis,* GBS, or *Gardnerella vaginalis* (bacterial vaginosis)
- Amniotic sac with a weak structure
- Previous preterm birth, especially if preceded by PPROM
- Fetal abnormalities or malpresentation
- Incompetent cervix or a short cervical length (30 mm or less)
- Overdistention of the uterus, such as multiple gestation or polyhydramnios
- Maternal hormonal changes
- Maternal stress or low socioeconomic status
- Maternal nutritional deficiencies and diabetes

Complications

Both mother and newborn are at risk for infection during the intrapartum and postpartum periods. Infection can be both a cause and a result of PROM. Organisms that cause Triple I weaken the amniotic membrane, leading to the rupture. The mother is at higher risk for postpartum infection, and the newborn is vulnerable to neonatal sepsis.

Triple I, characterized by maternal fever and uterine tenderness, is most likely to precede preterm birth in the infant born before 34 weeks of gestation. Preterm infants with the lowest maturity, such as 23 weeks of gestation, have higher risk for the infection than preterm infants who are even a few weeks more mature. The exact time at which infection occurs cannot be predicted for either term or preterm infants. Frequent performance of digital examination of the cervix increases the risk for all gestations. If Triple I does not precede PROM, it is more likely to occur if a long time elapses between membrane rupture and birth because vaginal organisms can readily enter the uterus. The risk for Triple I is known to increase when the membranes are ruptured for 24 hours or longer.

Membranes that rupture before term may form a seal, stopping the fluid leak and allowing the amniotic fluid to become reestablished. However, membranes may continue to leak, resulting in low levels of amniotic fluid (**oligohydramnios**), prolonging the loss of the amniotic fluid cushion for the fetus. Umbilical cord compression, reduced lung volume, and deformities resulting from compression may occur. The earlier in gestation the rupture occurs, the greater the risks associated with prolonged oligohydramnios.

If preterm birth occurs, the infant is more likely to have respiratory distress syndrome (RDS) and complications related to prematurity. The hazards of prematurity are greatest before 34 weeks of gestation, especially if the woman did not receive steroids to accelerate fetal lung maturation before birth.

Therapeutic Management

Management of PROM depends on the gestation and whether evidence of infection or other fetal or maternal compromise exists. If the fetus is less than 36 weeks, therapeutic management is more complex and may involve short-term tocolytic medications to delay delivery until steroids can be administered to enhance fetal lung maturity and antibiotics can be started to reduce transmission of bacteria, including GBS. Risks for infection or preterm birth complications are weighed against risks of labor induction or cesarean birth. For a woman at or near term (37 weeks or more of gestation), PROM may herald the imminent onset of true labor.

Determining True Membrane Rupture

The first step is to verify ruptured membranes. Urinary incontinence, increased vaginal discharge, or loss of the mucus plug can be mistaken for ruptured membranes. A digital vaginal examination is avoided, particularly if the gestation is preterm and no evidence of labor exists. Instead, a sterile speculum exam is performed to look for a pool of fluid near the cervix and estimate cervical dilation and effacement. A pH test or fern test may be done on the fluid to verify that the liquid is amniotic fluid. Tests are available that check for the presence of placental alpha microglobulin-1 (PAMG-1), found only in amniotic fluid. Tests to assess fetal lung maturity and identify infection are often performed. A transvaginal ultrasound examination may be performed to measure cervical length. A short (25 mm or less) cervix is more likely to continue effacement and dilation even if the gestation is far from term. Serial abdominal ultrasounds will follow fluid levels and fetal growth status.

Gestation Near Term. If labor does not begin spontaneously, the woman's pregnancy is at or near term, her cervix is favorable, and fetal lungs are mature, labor is usually induced (see Chapter 15). If the cervix is not favorable and no infection is evident, induction may be delayed 24 hours or longer to allow cervical softening and administration of antibiotics. Steroids to accelerate fetal lung maturity are not indicated if the fetus is 37 or more weeks of gestation (ACOG, 2017b). If induction is unsuccessful or if infection or other complications develop, a cesarean birth is most common. The nurse should remember, however, that cesarean birth also increases the risk for maternal infection after birth.

Preterm Gestation. If the gestation is preterm, the physician weighs the risks for maternal-fetal infection against the newborn's risk for complications of prematurity. Many variables should be considered by the physician and woman to determine the best course of management. Medical management changes as fetal maturation and conditions of the mother and fetus change with the continuation of pregnancy.

The cervix usually is not favorable for induction far from term. Factors such as gestational age, amount of amniotic fluid remaining, fetal lung maturity, and any signs of fetal compromise are considered. A **cerclage** (suture encircling the cervix) may have been placed earlier in the pregnancy to prevent premature cervical dilation. If infection is not already present, the physician should consider whether leaving the cerclage in place is likely to increase the risk for infection.

If no evidence of infection exists and the fetal lungs are immature, the woman usually is observed for infection or onset of labor in the hospital (**expectant management**). Daily

nonstress tests are performed to watch for FHR nonreactivity, which may occur with intraamniotic infection. Biophysical profiles, in which sonographic evaluation is added to the nonstress test, may be done one or more times per week. Fetal lung maturity testing may be done as term approaches to identify the best time for delivery unless other complications require delivery before fetal lung maturity. Antibiotics are given during labor.

Maternal Antibiotics

A seven-day course of parental and oral maternal antibiotics are usually prescribed for preterm premature membrane rupture because of the increased likelihood that an infection caused or further complicated the rupture for both mother and fetus or newborn. Antibiotics may stop the infection that caused or will occur with the rupture, thereby delaying the onset of labor and allowing the fetus to mature. Drugs to stop infection if early membrane rupture occurs usually include ampicillin, amoxicillin, and erythromycin (ACOG, 2016d; Mercer, 2017). Drugs effective against GBS are common. Guidelines for specific drugs to correct infection associated with early membrane rupture may vary with culture and sensitivity test results, other maternal laboratory results, or changes in the drugs most currently recommended for this purpose.

Nursing Considerations

The woman may remain hospitalized until birth, or she may return home after a few days of hospital observation. If she is hospitalized, the nurse observes for signs of infection. Preparation for home management includes teaching the woman the following:

- Avoid sexual intercourse, orgasm, or insertion of anything into the vagina, which increases the risk for infection caused by ascending organisms and can stimulate contractions.
- Avoid breast stimulation if the gestation is preterm because it may cause release of oxytocin from the posterior pituitary and thus stimulate contractions.
- Take your temperature at least four times a day, reporting any temperature of more than 37.8°C (100°F).
- Maintain any activity restrictions.
- Note and report uterine contractions or a foul odor to vaginal drainage.

❓ KNOWLEDGE CHECK

10. How does PROM differ from PPROM?
11. What is the relationship of infection to PROM?
12. What is the usual therapeutic management of PROM if the woman is at or near term? What if the gestation is preterm?
13. What are the nursing considerations for a woman with PPROM?

PRETERM LABOR

In 2015, the preterm birth rate in the United States was 9.6% (March of Dimes, 2016), down from a high of 12.8% in 2006

(National Center for Health Statistics, 2016). **Preterm labor** begins after the 20th week but before the start of the 37th week of pregnancy. The physical risks to the mother are no greater than labor at term unless complications such as infection, hemorrhage, or the need for a cesarean delivery also exist. Preterm labor, however, may result in the birth of an infant who is ill equipped for extrauterine life, particularly if earlier than 32 weeks of gestation. Adverse effects of prematurity may include cerebral palsy, developmental delay, and vision and hearing impairment. Families may suffer heavy emotional and economic burdens.

There is a significant disparity in the preterm birth rate between races in the United States. Non-Hispanic Black mothers had the highest rate of preterm births followed by Native American, Hispanic and White mothers. Asian mothers had the lowest rate (March of Dimes, 2016).

Many possible risk factors exist that might trigger preterm labor (Box 16.1). A woman who has previously delivered a preterm infant is more likely to have preterm labor. Having a multifetal pregnancy or use of assisted reproductive technology carries higher risks for both mothers and their infants, such as cesarean birth, prematurity, and infant disability or death. Smoking of cigarettes when combined with smoking of marijuana has an 85% increased risk for delivering preterm (Conner, et al., 2016).

Infants born at "early term," 37 $^{0/7}$ weeks of gestation to 38 $^{6/7}$ weeks of gestation, have an increased risk for poor outcomes in both the immediate and longer term period (Craighead, 2012; Simhan, Iams, & Romero, 2017). The Association of Women's Health, Obstetric and Neonatal Nurses (AWHONN) has launched an online campaign to promote the benefits of term pregnancy to women (www.gothefull40.com).

Associated Factors

Just as all causes of onset of labor at term are not known, the causes of preterm labor are not fully known. Over half of the women who have preterm labor and birth do not have known risk factors. Other women who have many risk factors deliver at term.

Preterm labor is thought to be initiated by multiple factors, including infection or inflammation, uteroplacental ischemia or hemorrhage (abruption or previa), uterine overdistention as with multiple gestations, stress, and other immunologically mediated processes. Some of the possible causes of preterm labor are the following (Simhan, Iams, & Romero, 2017):

- Maternal medical conditions, including infections of the urinary tract, reproductive organs, or systemic organs; dental disorders (periodontal disease); preexisting or gestational diabetes; connective tissue disorders; chronic hypertension; and drug abuse
- Conceptions enhanced by assisted reproductive technology, including conceptions resulting in a single fetal gestation rather than a multifetal gestation
- Present and past obstetric conditions such as short cervical length (25 mm or less), multifetal gestation, preterm membrane rupture, preeclampsia, and bleeding disorders that involve the woman, fetus, or placental implantation area

> ### BOX 16.1   Maternal Risk Factors for Preterm Labor
>
> **Medical History**
> Low weight for height
> Obesity
> Uterine or cervical anomalies, uterine fibroids
> History of cone biopsy
> Diethylstilbestrol (DES) exposure as a fetus
> Chronic illness (e.g., cardiac, renal, diabetes, clotting disorders, anemia, hypertension)
> Periodontal disease
>
> **Obstetric History**
> Previous preterm labor
> Previous preterm birth
> Previous first-trimester spontaneous abortion (more than 2)
> Previous second-trimester spontaneous abortion
> History of previous pregnancy losses (2 or more)
> Incompetent cervix
> Cervical length 25 mm (2.5 cm [1 inch]) or less at midtrimester of pregnancy
> Number of embryos implanted (assisted reproductive techniques)
>
> **Present Pregnancy**
> Uterine distention (e.g., multifetal pregnancy, hydramnios)
> Abdominal surgery during pregnancy
> Uterine irritability
> Uterine bleeding
> Dehydration
> Infection
> Anemia
> Incompetent cervix
> Preeclampsia
> Preterm premature rupture of membranes
> Fetal or placental abnormalities
>
> **Lifestyle and Demographics**
> Little or no prenatal care
> Poor nutrition
> Age younger than 18 years or older than 40 years
> Low educational level
> Low socioeconomic status
> Smoking more than 10 cigarettes daily
> Nonwhite
> Employment with long hours and/or long time standing
> Chronic physical or psychological stress
> Domestic violence
> Substance abuse

- Fetal conditions such as growth restriction, inadequate amniotic fluid volume, chromosome abnormalities, and other birth defects
- Social and environmental factors such as inadequate or absent prenatal or dental care, maternal domestic violence episodes, maternal smoking, and housing deficiency such as homelessness
- Demographic factors such as race and ages of the parents, financial stability, and the number and birth intervals of the woman's other children

Signs and Symptoms

Signs and symptoms of early preterm labor are more subtle than those of labor at term and often occur in normal pregnancies as well. Prenatal visits and routine ultrasounds may reveal evidence of cervical changes that have been occurring over several weeks during the second and third trimesters. The woman may be only vaguely aware that something seems different, or she may not detect that anything is amiss. Only when preterm labor reaches the active phase is it likely to have characteristics typical of term labor. Symptoms vary among women, but common ones are as follows:

- Uterine contractions that may or may not be painful (the woman may not feel contractions at all)
- A sensation that the baby is frequently "balling up"
- Cramps similar to menstrual cramps
- Constant low backache; irregular or intermittent low back pain
- Sensation of pelvic pressure or a feeling that the baby is pushing down
- Pain, discomfort, or pressure in the vagina or thighs
- Change or increase in vaginal discharge (increased, watery, "spotting," bleeding)
- Abdominal cramps with or without diarrhea
- A sense of "just feeling bad" or "coming down with something"

Preventing Preterm Birth
Community Education

Preterm birth can impose substantial physical, emotional, and financial burdens on the child, family, and society. Ideally, nursing strategies to prevent preterm birth begin before conception, with community education. Topics may include the following:

- Role of early and regular prenatal care, including dental care, in preventing preterm birth
- Duration of normal pregnancy
- Consequences of preterm birth
- Conditions that increase risk for preterm birth
- Signs and symptoms of preterm labor
- Consequences of preterm birth for mother, baby, and family members

Women who are aware of the consequences of preterm birth may be more likely to take action to prevent it. If they recognize that they have risk factors, they may seek prenatal care earlier in pregnancy. Recognizing that onset of labor in early gestation has subtle signs and symptoms compared with labor near term makes the woman aware that she should seek care promptly rather than waiting for more definite signs of labor.

During Pregnancy

During pregnancy, measures to prevent preterm birth include the following:

- Reducing barriers and improving access to early prenatal care for all women
- Assessing for risk factors to permit changes, if possible
- Promoting adequate nutrition

- Promoting cessation of the use of tobacco and recreational drugs
- Teaching women and their partners about the subtle signs and symptoms of preterm labor and ways in which they differ from normal pregnancy changes
- Empowering women and their partners to take an active approach in seeking care if they have signs and symptoms of preterm labor

Improving Access to Care. Improving access to prenatal care should be customized for the community. What works in one area may be inappropriate for another. Difficult access is a serious problem for women who rely on public clinics for their care. Long waits, fragmented care, language barriers, and insensitivity of caregivers discourage women from obtaining care. Expanding the number of caregivers by using advanced practice nurses such as certified nurse-midwives and nurse practitioners can reduce waits for care significantly. Nurses can help coordinate various aspects of care to limit the number of different appointments a woman needs to obtain complete care.

Identifying Risk Factors. Identification of risk factors may allow reduction or elimination of these factors. Women should be rescreened regularly to identify new risks that emerge as pregnancy progresses. Women with high-risk factors benefit from care such as more frequent prenatal care appointments, reinforcement of the symptoms of preterm labor, telephone contacts, and added assessments of fetal growth and health.

Some risk factors can be reduced or eliminated if the woman changes her lifestyle. Many pregnant women stop smoking or using nontherapeutic drugs, changes that may be difficult for them, to benefit their babies. A woman may need to rest more or stop working, which may be difficult or impossible for many. Nurses and social workers can help the woman reduce her risks as much as possible by helping her identify sources of support.

Infections of the urinary and reproductive tracts are associated with PPROM and preterm labor. Screening at the appropriate times for pathogenic organisms in the urine, vagina, and cervix identifies women who may benefit from antibiotic therapy.

Promoting Adequate Nutrition. An adequate maternal diet contributes positively to the length of gestation and the infant's birth weight. The mother's height should be measured at the first prenatal visit, and her weight should be taken at each visit to evaluate adequacy of weight gain. Every pregnant woman should be offered culturally sensitive dietary counseling. The Special Supplemental Nutrition Program for Women, Infants, and Children (WIC) is available to supplement the diet of some women from low-income groups. Anemia can be corrected with appropriate supplements. Women carrying more than one fetus need additional food intake.

Educating Women and Their Partners about Preterm Labor. All pregnant women and their partners should be taught about symptoms of preterm labor, because half of preterm births occur in women with no identified risk factors. Interpreters who are culturally acceptable to the woman and printed materials in her primary language should be used.

Diagrams should supplement the words of any language for women of limited reading skills. Respecting cultural norms of the woman and her family is an essential part of prenatal care that encourages her to maintain care to identify possible problems early.

Information about the vague signs and symptoms of early preterm labor should be reinforced regularly as part of prenatal care. Women who often have uterine irritability may be given guidelines to observe at home before they should go to the hospital. Preterm labor often has vague sensations to the woman, so any home care guidelines are individualized according to the woman's risk for a preterm birth, the gestation and prenatal status, and the likelihood that specific interventions are beneficial to mother and baby. In addition, women are taught to enter the hospital for evaluation if they are not sure about the seriousness of their sensations. Examples of home care guidelines include the following:

- Drink an adequate amount of water to improve hydration or reduce bladder irritation that may accompany a urinary tract infection (UTI).
- Empty the bladder frequently because a full bladder may be associated with uterine irritability and contractions.
- Rest in the side-lying position to promote uterine blood flow. Limiting physical activity may increase diuresis. Prolonged limitation of physical activity is not usually beneficial or safe for prevention of premature labor, although it may be required for serious maternal disorders such as cardiac disease.
- Palpate contractions for 1 hour or as instructed. However, notify the birth attendant or go directly to the labor unit for assessment if contractions increase in frequency, duration, or sensitivity.

The nurse should verify the woman's understanding by seeking feedback such as having her restate the signs and symptoms of preterm labor and the appropriate responses to them.

Empowering Women and Their Partners. Delaying birth depends critically on early identification of preterm labor. Women should be encouraged to seek treatment promptly if they suspect preterm labor. The woman must communicate her concerns clearly when she arrives at the clinic or hospital. She should tell the triage person that she should be checked for labor, regardless of the subtlety of the symptoms. Caregivers should not make the woman feel foolish if she reports signs and symptoms that could be preterm labor but turn out to be a false alarm. Otherwise she may not seek care for recurrent episodes when she truly is in labor, and the opportunity to delay preterm birth may be lost.

The nurse might suggest that a woman who is seeking care for possible preterm labor say, "I'm not due for 8 more weeks, but I think I may be in labor. I need to be seen right away, or I might have a premature baby."

Therapeutic Management

Management focuses on identifying those at risk for preterm birth, identifying preterm labor early and delaying birth if possible. If preterm birth is likely, the emphasis is accelerating fetal lung maturity and providing neonatal neuroprotection.

Predicting Preterm Birth

Onset of changes that lead to preterm labor and birth may be subtle. The woman may not perceive any changes in her pregnancy. Research has focused on predicting which women will deliver early. Better identification of these women would allow more intensive treatment, ideally before preterm labor or rupture of membranes occurs. Also, many signs and symptoms of preterm labor occur in women who deliver at term, possibly exposing them to unneeded treatment. The key is to identify which women are really at risk for preterm birth and treat those women intensively while continuing regular prenatal care for women who are not truly at risk. A good screening test would provide quick results and would be inexpensive, usable for all pregnant women, noninvasive, and highly specific for predicting preterm birth. No screening test meeting these criteria is currently available. For this reason, many evaluations may be used in an attempt to determine the best medical management for a woman.

Cervical Length. A short cervix (25 mm or less) measured by transvaginal ultrasound at 22 to 24 weeks gestation is associated with an increase in preterm birth. Although the pathologic process is not clearly understood, current evidence suggests that it is not a weakness in cervical resistance to uterine contractions (Simhan et al., 2017). An updated metaanalysis and systematic review following and including the OPPTIMUM study (Norman et al., 2016), showed evidence that vaginal progesterone reduces the risk for both preterm birth and neonatal morbidity and mortality, when studying women with a singleton gestation and a midtrimester cervical length of 25 mm or less, without negative effects on neurodevelopmental outcome (Romero et al., 2016). The study recommends that universal transvaginal cervical length screening be done at 18 to 24 weeks of gestation in women with a singleton gestation and vaginal progesterone offered to those with a cervical length 25 mm or less (Romero et al., 2016). However, ACOG (2016a) cautions that the predictive value of a short cervix as the only indicator of preterm labor is limited and recommends against its exclusive use to direct management of women with symptoms of preterm labor.

Preterm Premature Rupture of Membranes in a Previous Birth. Some women may have a predisposition to weak amniotic membrane structure that predates the actual leaking of fluid. This predisposition seems to repeat in subsequent pregnancies (Mercer, 2017).

Fetal Fibronectin. Fetal fibronectin (fFN) is a protein present in the layers of the amniotic membrane. It is normally found in cervical and vaginal secretions until 16 to 20 weeks of gestation and again at or near term. If it appears too early, it suggests that labor may begin early, similar to the way elevated cardiac enzymes rise in the person experiencing a myocardial infarction. Maternal or fetal infections may be present if the fFN is positive during midpregnancy. Cervical examination, recent sexual intercourse, and vaginal bleeding can result in a false-positive test when preterm labor is not truly present. To reduce false-positive results, the test specimen should be collected at least 24 hours after significant vaginal manipulation from examination. Some research indicates that the fFN test has a high degree of negative predictive value, with a negative result indicating there is a less than 1% chance of delivery in the next 2 weeks. The positive predictive value, indicating the patient will deliver in the next 2 weeks, is much lower, at 12% to 17% (Hologic, 2009). However, because these findings have not been supported by randomized clinical trials, and due to the low positive predictive value of the test, ACOG (2016a) does not support the exclusive use of fFN to direct the medical management of a woman with preterm contractions.

Infections. Infections often increase the risk for preterm membrane rupture or birth, even if the woman does not initially have clinical signs or symptoms with the preterm labor. A UTI is common with preterm labor, so catheterized or midstream urine is often obtained for urinalysis and for culture and sensitivity testing. Tests for other infections associated with increased risk for preterm birth include those that often are found if membranes rupture prematurely.

A woman with an infection that is not related to pregnancy may seek care. Relevant testing may relate to acute gastrointestinal or respiratory tract infections that affect pregnant women as well as other people of both genders. More serious maternal infections may require cultures of maternal blood or respiratory tract or other secretions to determine the ideal treatment. Maternal pneumonia, although rare during pregnancy, increases the risk for fetal or maternal death as well as increasing the risk that a woman will give birth to a living preterm infant. Other poor health conditions during pregnancy (such as crowded living conditions) or a chronic medical condition (such as asthma) may increase a woman's risk for pneumonia as well.

Identifying Preterm Labor

The reason to predict risk for preterm birth or to identify preterm labor early is to delay birth, thereby promoting further fetal maturation.

Frequent Prenatal Visits. Women at risk for preterm labor should have more frequent prenatal visits. In addition to normal prenatal care, they are evaluated for evidence of preterm labor and their ability to follow preventive therapy. They should be assessed for development of new risk factors with each visit. Gentle cervical examinations, possibly with sterile speculum, are done if indicated by other signs or symptoms. A transvaginal ultrasound examination may identify the shortened, thinned cervix that often precedes onset of labor in the asymptomatic woman. Infections of any kind should be identified and treated promptly before rupture of membranes or onset of labor occurs.

Stopping Preterm Labor

Once the diagnosis of preterm labor is made, management focuses on stopping uterine activity. Preterm delivery may be inevitable, but steroid therapy promotes earlier fetal lung maturation. Particularly for very early gestations, such as 25 weeks, treatment may add enough time for the steroids to be effective. Even one more day of fetal maturation may make a great difference in the outcome for the very premature infant.

Initial Measures. The physician initially determines whether any maternal or fetal problems exist that contraindicate continuing the pregnancy. Some examples are maternal complications such as hypertension or hypotension, hypovolemia, hypoxemia, cardiac disease, and pyelonephritis. Fetal problems needing prompt delivery may be demonstrated by persistent abnormal FHR patterns.

Initial measures to stop preterm labor include identifying and treating infections, identifying other causes of preterm labor that may be treatable, and reducing activity.

Identifying and Treating Infections. Infection, both systemic and local, has a strong association with preterm birth and premature rupture of the membranes. However, it may be unclear whether various microorganisms found at diagnosis of preterm labor are significant if the membranes remain intact. Blood studies identify signs of infection and also conditions such as anemia that are associated with preterm labor or affect its management. Common studies include a complete blood cell count with differential white blood cell analysis and cultures for GBS, *Chlamydia*, gonorrhea, or other suspected infections. **Amniocentesis** (transabdominal puncture of amniotic sac) may be done to obtain amniotic fluid for culture if Triple I is suspected, because this infection would contraindicate stopping preterm labor. Fetal lung maturity testing will likely be done on an amniotic fluid specimen as well. (Simhan, Iams, & Romero, 2017) Urinalysis with culture and sensitivity testing may be performed to determine whether treatment for a UTI is indicated.

Culture results require a minimum of 24 to 48 hours to complete, therefore antibiotics that are effective against probable organisms are started as soon as the specimen is obtained. The medication can be changed if culture results indicate that a different antibiotic would be more effective.

Prompt treatment of acute infections such as pyelonephritis improves maternal and fetal outcomes. Broad-spectrum antibiotics (e.g., ampicillin, penicillin) and an aminoglycoside (e.g., gentamicin), which are effective against many organisms, may be ordered. Medications such as clindamycin or metronidazole may be prescribed for a woman who requires a cesarean birth and is at risk for infection from anaerobic organisms (Higgins et al., 2016).

Identifying Other Causes for Preterm Contractions. The woman with polyhydramnios, identified by ultrasonography, may have preterm contractions because her uterus is stretched more than normal. Therapeutic amniocentesis to remove some amniotic fluid can reduce uterine irritability. Multifetal gestations also can be identified by ultrasonography if not previously diagnosed. These mothers may benefit from improved nutrition, stress reduction, assistance with household care, and other interventions.

Limiting Activity. Activity limits, usually by relaxing in the side-lying or semisitting position, increase placental blood flow and reduce fetal pressure on the cervix. However, lengthy and substantial activity restriction (e.g., complete bed rest) has not been shown to significantly prolong pregnancy (ACOG, 2016a). As in other individuals, activity restriction is associated with serious maternal side effects, some of which develop within as little as 24 hours. Adverse effects of substantial activity restriction during pregnancy may include the following:

- Muscle weakness, including aching, muscle atrophy, and bone loss
- Diuresis as the body tries to reduce the normally higher fluid level of pregnancy
- Poor nutrition as a result of appetite loss, lower food intake, and increased indigestion; weight loss or inadequate weight gain
- Orthostatic hypotension caused by the change in blood pressure regulation by baroreceptors
- Psychological effects such as increased stress about separation from her family, anxiety about the pregnancy's outcome, depression, boredom from a decreased activity level and reduced contact with other people, and concerns about finances if her income is essential to her family
- Sleep changes as depression increases or usual activities that direct her sleep-wake cycles are not present

Because of the adverse effects and lack of benefits for most women, bedrest is no longer routine. If necessary, individualized activity reductions may be prescribed. Changes may be relatively simple, such as a change in work hours or duties or finding ways to help the woman meet the needs for her other children, for example, transportation to school or other activities. Several rest periods during the day may be prescribed. Positions for rest may include the semisitting position with the feet and legs elevated. If lying down for rest, a mother's frequent change of the side-lying position reduces discomfort from the pressure of remaining on one side for a prolonged time. Frequent position changes are also beneficial to women who require hospitalization for their preterm labor.

Women hospitalized for care of preterm labor may have a greater activity restriction. Ambulating to the bathroom may be limited because of maternal sedative effects from medications. If preterm labor stops, the woman may usually walk to the restroom for showers, voiding, and bowel movements. If she remains hospitalized for longer term care, she may have activity orders that include sitting in a chair periodically or taking occasional short trips to another area in a wheelchair that her family or friends push.

Whether the woman is expected to be hospitalized briefly or for a longer time, the following services may improve her adherence to care measures:

- Physical therapy to help maintain muscle strength and coordination and to reduce muscle aching, fatigue, and bone loss
- Recreational therapy to identify appropriate activities to relieve boredom
- Occupational therapy to help the woman cope physically with lifestyle changes, particularly if discharge home is anticipated
- Complementary therapy to reduce stressors and enhance physical care measures
- Social work to identify how needs such as financial and child care can be met

- Consultation with a psychologist to help the woman and family cope with the added stressors

Hydrating the Woman. Hydration to stop preterm contractions has not been shown to be beneficial for all women. High-volume IV infusions may cause maternal respiratory distress if tocolytic medications are also administered, especially if given in combination with steroids.

However, dehydration may contribute to uterine irritability for some women. This is often the case in those who have had an infection such as an acute gastrointestinal infection, in which loss of fluid through diarrhea may exceed the nauseated woman's ability to drink water or other fluids. Infections with maternal fever (temperature of 38°C [100.4°F] or greater) increase the patient's metabolic rate and may result in dehydration. IV fluids are ordered according to their expected benefit. Oral fluids are usually encouraged because hydration may reduce uterine irritability and the risk for UTIs.

Tocolytics. Tocolytic medications have not demonstrated a decrease in the rate of preterm birth. However, they may successfully delay the birth of a preterm infant. Delay of preterm birth with tocolysis may provide time for the following (ACOG, 2016a; Simhan et. al, 2017):

- to give maternal corticosteroids to reduce respiratory distress in the newborn
- to give antibiotics to prevent neonatal infection with GBS
- to transfer the mother to a facility with a neonatal intensive care unit (NICU) that is appropriate for the gestation of her fetus at the time of birth
- to give magnesium sulfate for neuroprotection of a fetus less than 32 weeks gestation

Tocolysis is considered appropriate for women, 24 to 34 weeks gestation with regular uterine contractions and cervical change.

Because tocolytic drugs have significant side effects, the decision about whether to treat for preterm labor is individualized, based on risk factors, cervical dilation, and other signs and symptoms. EFM helps identify uterine contractions or irritability and establish fetal status. An fFN test may be done to determine whether the woman is likely to be in preterm labor. Ultrasound imaging provides information that may be useful to determine fetal age, adequacy of placental supply, and status of the cervix. Tests for infection are done if indicated.

Current tocolytic drugs are used primarily for conditions other than preterm labor and therefore have effects on body systems other than the reproductive system. Risks and possible benefits of the drug chosen should be considered and communicated clearly to the woman. The lowest possible dose that inhibits contractions is used. Four types of drugs are used for tocolysis: (1) magnesium sulfate, (2) calcium antagonists, (3) prostaglandin synthesis inhibitors, and (4) beta-adrenergics. (Table 16.1 summarizes doses and routes of administration for each of these drugs.)

Magnesium sulfate. Magnesium sulfate is used in management of pregnancy-associated hypertension to prevent seizures. Because of its added effect of smooth muscle relaxation, including quieting uterine activity, it may be used

TABLE 16.1 Drugs Used in Preterm Labor

Drug and Purpose	Common Dose Regimens*	Side or Adverse Effects
Magnesium sulfate (use as tocolytic) Therapeutic range: 4.5–8.0 mEq/L. ~10 mEq/L = Depression of DTRs ~12 mEq/L = Respiratory depression ~18 mEq/L = Cardiac depression	IV: Loading dose: 4–6 g over 30 min Maintenance dose for tocolysis: 1–4 g/hr When contraction frequency is no higher than 1 per 10 min (≤6 per hr), maintain infusion rate for 12–48 hr, then discontinue drug.	Side and adverse effects are dose-related, occurring at higher maternal serum levels. Depression of DTRs, which should be present, although less active Respiratory or cardiac depression if serum levels are high; greatest risk is in woman with poor urinary elimination of drug Less serious side effects: Lethargy, weakness, visual blurring, headache, sensation of heat, nausea, vomiting, constipation Fetal-neonatal effects: Reduced FHR variability in the first 24 hr, labor dystocia
Nifedipine (Procardia), nicardipine (Cardene) (calcium channel blockers for tocolysis)	Oral loading dose: 10–20 mg Continued oral therapy (if needed): 10–20 mg every 3–6 hr for a maximum of 72 hours	Maternal flushing, dizziness, headache, nausea Transient maternal tachycardia Mild hypotension Modest increases in blood glucose levels
Prostaglandin synthesis inhibitors (NSAIDS) Includes indomethacin (Indocin), sulindac (Clinoril), and ibuprofen	Limit use to preterm labor before 32 wk of gestation. Use indomethacin for no longer than 48–72 consecutive hr. Indocin: Loading dose: 50 mg (oral) Maintenance dose: 25 mg orally every 6 hr for 48 hr Ibuprofen: 600 mg (oral) every 6 hr (used ≤32 wk gestation) Ultrasound examinations and fetal echocardiography help determine whether maternal indomethacin has adverse effects on fetus.	Epigastric pain, nausea, gastrointestinal bleeding Asthma in aspirin-sensitive woman Increased BP in hypertensive woman Fetus: Adverse fetal effects may include constriction of ductus arteriosus, particularly if mother receives indomethacin for more than 48–72 hr and gestation is later than 32 wk; impairs fetal renal function, which may reduce volume of amniotic fluid and result in cord compression.
Terbutaline (beta-adrenergic for tocolysis); should not be used beyond 48–72 hr for preterm labor	Subcutaneous (most common parenteral route): Intermittent injections, 0.25 mg, initially every 20–30 min × 3, followed by rescue doses only.	Terbutaline is not approved by the FDA for inhibiting uterine activity and now carries a *boxed warning and contraindications* ("black box") against use as a tocolytic rather than its intended use as a bronchodilator. Dose may be held if maternal pulse rate exceeds 120 bpm or systolic BP falls below 80–90 mm Hg or FHR <180. Adverse reactions: 1. Cardiovascular: Maternal and fetal tachycardia, palpitations, cardiac dysrhythmias, chest pain, wide pulse pressure 2. Respiratory: Dyspnea, chest discomfort 3. Central nervous system: Tremors, restlessness, weakness, dizziness, headache 4. Metabolic: Hypokalemia, hyperglycemia 5. Gastrointestinal: Nausea, vomiting, reduced bowel motility 6. Skin: Flushing, diaphoresis
Corticosteroids (betamethasone and dexamethasone)	See Drug Guide: Betamethasone, Dexamethasone (p. 445)	
17-P alpha-hydroxyprogesterone caproate (Makena)	IM: 250 mg (1 mL) every 7 days Begin treatment between 16 wk, 0 days and 20 wk, 6 days Continue until 37 wk or delivery	Drug is a progestin indicated to reduce the risk for preterm birth in a woman who had a previous preterm birth; not intended for women with multiple gestation or other risk factors for preterm birth.

Data from American Academy of Pediatrics & American College of Obstetricians and Gynecologists (AAP & ACOG). (2012). *Guidelines for perinatal care* (7th ed.). Elk Grove Village, IL, and Washington, DC: Author; Blackburn, S. T. (2013). *Maternal, fetal, & neonatal physiology: a clinical perspective* (4th ed.). St. Louis, MO: Saunders; *Creasy & Resnik's Maternal-fetal medicine: Principles and practice* (7th ed.). Philadelphia: Saunders; Simhan, H. N., Iams, J. D., & Romero, R. (2017). Preterm birth. In S. G. Gabbe, J. R. Niebyl, J. L. Simpson, M.B. Landon, H.L. Galan, R. M. Jauniaux, D.A. Driscoll, et al. (Eds.), *Obstetrics: normal and problem pregnancies* (6th ed., pp. 627–658). Philadelphia: Saunders; and U.S. Food and Drug Administration (FDA). (2011). FDA drug safety communication: new warnings against use of terbutaline to treat preterm labor. Retrieved from www.fda.gov.
*Doses and frequency of administration are examples; actual protocols may vary.
BP, Blood pressure; *bpm,* beats per minute; *DTRs,* deep tendon reflexes; *FDA,* U.S. Food and Drug Administration; *FHR,* fetal heart rate; *IM,* intramuscularly; *IV,* intravenously; *NSAIDs,* nonsteroidal antiinflammatory drugs.

to inhibit preterm labor. Magnesium sulfate therapy has a well-established record of safety during pregnancy. When given to suppress preterm labor, magnesium sulfate has side effects (such as lethargy and sedation) similar to those seen in its use to prevent seizures related to hypertension. The ACOG Practice Bulletin 171: Management of Preterm Labor supports use of magnesium sulfate as a short-term tocolytic to provide for steroid therapy and for neonatal neuroprotection; long-term therapy is not supported (ACOG, 2016a).

Common hospital criteria for magnesium sulfate therapy include the following:

- Urine output of at least 30 milliliters per hour (mL/hr)
- Presence of deep tendon reflexes
- At least 12 breaths per minute

In addition, the nurse should assess heart and lung sounds with vital signs because fluid overload and electrolyte imbalances can lead to pulmonary edema or cardiac dysrhythmias. Oxygen saturations are often included with vital signs and other assessments. Bowel sounds are checked when therapy begins and every 4 to 8 hours because the smooth muscle in the intestinal tract may be relaxed just as the uterus is relaxed. Serum magnesium level measurements guide maintenance of therapeutic levels (4.5 to 8.0 milligrams per deciliter [mg/dL]). EFM identifies fetal drug effects such as reduced variability.

Calcium gluconate (10%) should be available to reverse magnesium toxicity and prevent respiratory arrest, which can occur if serum levels rise above 12 mg/dL. Excess serum levels of magnesium are less likely when the drug is given for preterm labor, compared to when it is given for pre-eclampsia, because the renal function of the woman in preterm labor is usually normal. However, the nurse should remain alert for this complication of magnesium sulfate therapy.

Calcium Antagonists. Nifedipine (Adalat, Procardia) is a calcium channel blocker usually given for hypertension. Calcium is essential for muscle contraction in smooth muscles such as the uterus, so blocking calcium reduces the muscular contraction. Flushing of the skin, headache, and a transient increase in the maternal and FHR are common side effects. Headache generally resolves in 48 hours. Because nifedipine is a vasodilator, the woman may have postural hypotension.

The nurse should observe for side effects of nifedipine and report a maternal pulse rate greater than 120 bpm. The woman should be given information about possible dizziness or faintness with nifedipine's hypotensive effects. She should sit or stand slowly and call for assistance, if needed. Serial blood pressures should be assessed for evaluation of dosage changes.

Prostaglandin Synthesis Inhibitors. Because prostaglandins stimulate uterine contractions, drugs can be used to inhibit their synthesis. Indomethacin (Indocin) and ibuprofen are the prostaglandin synthesis inhibitors most often used for tocolysis.

Maternal side effects are minimal because of the brief duration of therapy. Gastrointestinal side effects are usually limited to nausea, vomiting, and heartburn. The nurse should observe the woman for gastrointestinal side effects. Because indomethacin and ibuprofen can prolong bleeding time, the nurse observes for abnormal bleeding such as prolonged bleeding after injections and bruising with no apparent cause. The antiinflammatory effect of these medications can mask infection.

Fetal adverse effects are more serious and may include constriction of the ductus arteriosus, pulmonary hypertension, and oligohydramnios. The ductus arteriosus should remain open before birth and will functionally close 12 to 48 hours after birth. Fetal adverse effects of prostaglandin synthesis inhibitors are unlikely if treatment is no longer than 48 to 72 hours and the gestation is less than 32 weeks. Amniotic fluid levels should be monitored and the drug stopped if volume is trending downward. The amniotic fluid volume usually returns to its previous level when treatment is discontinued. Regular ultrasound examinations and fetal echocardiography help determine whether the medication is having adverse effects on the fetus. Decreased fetal movements and absent FHR accelerations with fetal movement may occur if the fetal condition deteriorates. After birth, assessment of the infant may be performed for other complications such as pulmonary hypertension or intracranial hemorrhage, depending on the duration of treatment and the infant's gestation.

Beta-adrenergic Drugs. Ritodrine (Yutopar) was once the only beta-adrenergic medication approved by the U.S. Food and Drug Administration (FDA) for tocolysis, however it has been discontinued in the United States because of significant side effects, cost, and minimal increase in the length of pregnancy. Terbutaline (Brethine), a bronchodilator, is the most frequently used beta-adrenergic for treatment of preterm labor. It is used to delay preterm birth to allow administration of corticosteroids and antibiotics (approximately 48 hours).

The main side effects for beta-adrenergic drugs, including terbutaline, involve the cardiorespiratory system. Maternal and fetal tachycardia are common (see Table 16.1). Propranolol (Inderal), an agent that blocks beta-adrenergic drugs, should be available to reverse severe adverse effects.

Because of reported cardiovascular events, terbutaline now carries a *boxed warning and contraindications* ("black box") against prolonged parenteral use for more than 48 to 72 hours, for use of oral terbutaline for treatment of preterm labor, or to prevent recurrence of preterm labor. (See www.fda.gov for the FDA drug safety report.)

The nurse should assess a woman's apical heart rate and lung sounds before administering each intermittent dose of terbutaline. A maternal heart rate over 120 bpm or respiratory findings such as "wet" lung sounds or tachypnea, possibly accompanied by shortness of breath, suggest drug toxicity and may be a reason to discontinue terbutaline. Abnormal maternal and fetal assessments should be promptly reported to the physician.

Accelerating Fetal Lung Maturity

ACOG (2017b) recommends administration of a single course of corticosteroids to pregnant women, 24 to 34 weeks gestation who are at risk of preterm birth within

7 days. It may be administered as early as 23 weeks gestation, based on the family's decisions regarding resuscitation of an extremely preterm newborn. Administration of a single course may also be considered for a woman at risk of preterm birth within 7 days who is between 34 and 37 weeks gestation. Steroid therapy may reduce the incidence and severity of RDS and intraventricular hemorrhage in the preterm infant (ACOG, 2017b). Betamethasone (Celestone) or dexamethasone (Decadron) may be used for this purpose (ACOG, 2017b).

🔖 DRUG GUIDE

Betamethasone and Dexamethasone

Classification

Corticosteroids.

Indications

Acceleration of fetal lung maturity to reduce the incidence and severity of respiratory distress syndrome. Studies suggest that antenatal steroids can reduce the incidence of intraventricular hemorrhage and neonatal death in the preterm infant. Greatest benefits accrue if at least 24 hours elapses between the initial dose and birth of the preterm infant, but the drug is indicated if birth is not imminent.

Dosage and Route

Betamethasone: 12 mg intramuscularly (IM) for two doses, 24 hours apart.
Dexamethasone: 6 mg IM every 12 hours for four doses.

Absorption

Rapid and complete after IM administration.

Excretion

Metabolized in the liver. Excreted in urine.

Contraindications

Active infection such as Triple I is a relative contraindication. The American College of Obstetricians and Gynecologists (ACOG) recommends use of corticosteroids for the woman who has preterm rupture of the membranes (24 to 34 weeks of gestation) (ACOG, 2017b).

Precautions

Possible infection. Pregnancies complicated by diabetes.

Adverse Reactions

Few, owing to the short-term use of the drug. Pulmonary edema is possible secondary to sodium and fluid retention.

Nursing Considerations

Explain to the woman the potential benefits of corticosteroid administration to the preterm neonate. Explain that the drug cannot prevent or lessen the severity of all complications of prematurity. If the woman has diabetes, explain that more frequent blood glucose determinations are common because these levels are often elevated for up to 7 to 10 days after taking either of the corticosteroids. A temporary rise in platelet and WBC levels may last 72 hours. WBC levels greater than 20,000/mm³ may indicate infection. Assess lung sounds. Report chest pain or heaviness or dyspnea.

Corticosteroids are indicated if the gestation period is between 24 and 34 weeks because of the high incidence of problems such as RDS that affect an infant born at this gestation. Delay of preterm birth for at least 24 hours after initiation of corticosteroid therapy provides the greatest benefit in reducing the incidence and severity of RDS associated with prematurity. Thus one indication for tocolytic therapy is to delay preterm birth to allow the fetus to receive the benefits of the corticosteroid. Evidence shows that an infant born sooner than 24 hours after administration of corticosteroid may have some fetal lung maturation benefits. Therefore concerns regarding the probability of delaying the birth should not prevent administration of corticosteroids.

Vital signs should be assessed to identify fever and elevated pulse rate that may indicate infection. Lung sounds should be assessed with vital signs because corticosteroids can cause sodium retention with accompanying fluid retention and pulmonary edema. The nurse should observe for symptoms of pulmonary edema. The woman is taught to report any chest pain or heaviness or any difficulty breathing because these symptoms could indicate pulmonary edema.

Neuroprotection

Neonatal complications of preterm birth include neurological problems such as cerebral palsy (CP). Current evidence supports the administration of Magnesium Sulfate to the mother before birth to decrease this risk. The ACOG and the Society for Maternal Fetal Medicine (SMFM) recommend its use for women at less than 32 weeks gestation and with anticipated preterm birth (ACOG 2016e). Protocols for the administration of magnesium sulfate for fetal neuroprotection are similar to protocols for its use in pre-eclampsia or as a tocolytic agent (Cunningham, et. al, 2014; Sinham, Iams & Romero, 2017).

Periviable Birth

The ACOG and SMFM Obstetric Care Consensus No. 4 addresses "Periviable Birth," which is defined as birth at 20 $^{0/7}$ weeks to 25 $^{6/7}$ weeks gestation. Prenatal and postnatal counseling regarding the anticipated neonatal outcome based on the specific circumstances of each patient should be provided. If the family desires resuscitative efforts of a periviaible neonate, management strategies may include "short-term tocolytic therapy to allow time for administration of antenatal steroids, antibiotics to prolong latency after preterm premature rupture of membranes or for intrapartum group B streptococci (GBS) prophylaxis, and delivery, including cesarean delivery, for concern regarding fetal well-being or fetal malpresentation" (p. 1, ACOG, 2016c). If birth of a periviable neonate is anticipated, administration of Magnesium Sulfate for fetal neuroprotection is supported. It is recommended that periviable births occur in hospitals with expertise and support services for high-risk maternal and neonatal care (ACOG, 2016c).

◆ APPLICATION OF THE NURSING PROCESS: PRETERM LABOR

Nursing care for the woman experiencing preterm labor often includes interventions related to tocolytic, corticosteroid, or antibiotic drug therapy. If labor cannot be halted, care is similar to that for other laboring women, with additional care to prepare for a preterm infant's needs at birth. Support for anticipatory grieving may be needed if the infant is very immature and not expected to live.

Care for the family when an extremely preterm infant (~20 through 24 weeks of gestation) is expected to be born can be heavily laden with ethical and legal issues. For example, what is the true accuracy of the gestational age? Has a corticosteroid to accelerate fetal lung maturity been administered? Has magnesium sulfate been administered for neuroprotection? If labor cannot be halted, is fetal monitoring beneficial? Abnormal fetal monitoring patterns in the very immature fetus can distress parents and caregivers alike. However, knowledge of the fetal response to labor helps the neonatologist make better decisions about how to treat the infant. In addition, ultrasound estimates of gestational age at this time have shown considerable variations. A fetus presumed to be 23 weeks of gestation before birth may be assessed to be 25 weeks or older after birth and suited to more intense treatment than planned, especially if the woman had no prenatal care before entering the hospital.

Much of the general nursing care for a woman having preterm labor also applies to women experiencing other types of high-risk pregnancies. Women may need multiple hospitalizations that occur in the middle of the night, disrupting sleep and family routines. Other women may have attended a routine prenatal visit and be shocked to discover that they may be in preterm labor. These women often have some activity modifications and may have to stop working if the best outcome for their pregnancy is to be achieved. Therefore this section focuses on the family's psychosocial concerns, management of home care, and the woman's boredom.

PSYCHOSOCIAL CONCERNS

◆ Assessment

The entire family is affected by stressors associated with a high-risk pregnancy. Assess how the woman and her family usually cope with crisis situations and how they are coping with this one. Identify their greatest concerns to prioritize care. For example, the nurse might say, "This development in your pregnancy must have been a shock." The following are other questions the nurse might ask: "How are you handling things?" "In what ways do you usually handle crisis situations in your family?" "What concerns you the most right now?" Rather than asking questions in a rapid-fire manner, the nurse should give the woman time to answer assessment questions because stress has narrowed her focus.

The woman or her family may have physical, emotional, and cognitive impairments because of the unexpected problems. Physical signs of emotional distress such as tremulousness, palpitations, and restlessness also are side effects of beta-adrenergic drugs and corticosteroids. The woman may express fear, helplessness, or disbelief. She may be irritable and tearful. Her ability to concentrate may be impaired at a time when she needs to absorb new information.

Her partner often feels at loose ends. He struggles to keep the household running if she should decrease her activity level. Young children recognize their parents' anxiety and may misbehave or regress. They may feel abandoned if they must be temporarily placed with relatives or friends.

The woman may need to stop working, straining family finances. If she does not have sick time or other benefits, the family sustains an abrupt drop in income at a time when medical expenses are mounting. A woman may be transferred to a distant hospital having a better capacity to care for her and her preterm baby. A distant transfer to a higher-level maternity care facility makes it more difficult for the woman to receive support from friends, family, or support groups.

Overlaid on the sudden change in lifestyle is the family's concern for their baby's well-being. A woman may feel pulled in many directions by the needs of all her children—those already born and the fetus she is trying to mature. She may be concerned about the effects of drug therapy on the fetus and her own body.

◆ Identification of Patient Problems

Unexpected development of complications during pregnancy can prevent a woman and her family from using their normal coping mechanisms. Therefore the patient problem selected for the woman and family is apprehension due to uncertain outcome of the pregnancy, disruption of relationships with family and friends, and financial concerns.

◆ Planning: Expected Outcomes

The outcome of any pregnancy is never certain, especially when the pregnancy is a high-risk one. Goals and expected outcomes should focus on the family's ability to cope with the crisis of preterm labor. The appropriate goal is: The woman and family will identify one or more constructive methods to cope with this temporary disruption in their lives.

◆ Interventions
Providing Information

Knowledge decreases anxiety and fear related to the unknown. Include appropriate family members so they are more likely to be supportive. Appropriate family members may include the woman's partner, mother or mother-in-law, adult siblings, and others, but this may vary according to culture. Determine the extent of the woman's knowledge about preterm birth and the specific therapy recommended. Determine what information the parents need about problems that a preterm infant may face. Use this opportunity to correct misinformation and reinforce accurate information.

Initially, the woman for whom activity modification is prescribed may be highly motivated. Because contractions often diminish, even if for only a short time, she may become restless. She may think there is now no need for any restriction. Explain what is currently known about the benefits of activity modification for her pregnancy complication and assure her that recommendations to restrict her activity often lessen as her pregnancy progresses. Initiate consultations from caregivers such as physical, occupational, and recreational therapists; social workers; and other professionals whose services might benefit the woman.

The Sidelines National Support Network (www.sidelines.org) is an online network of local groups across the country for women experiencing high-risk pregnancy, including the risk for preterm birth. The site has information for women "sidelined" by pregnancy complications, including articles, information about reimbursement from insurance, and contact via e-mail with others who have been "sidelined."

Promoting Expression of Concerns

Encourage the woman and her family to express their concerns. Begin by exploring common concerns of women with problem pregnancies. For example, "Most women are worried when they must adjust their work schedules. How has this affected your family?" An open-ended question gives the woman and her family a chance to express their feelings so they can take the next step—identifying constructive methods to cope with the situation. Collaboration with a social worker may identify financial or other community resources available. Ask her if she would like a visit from a chaplain.

Teaching What May Occur During a Preterm Birth

Because preterm birth often occurs despite all interventions, a pregnant woman and her partner should be prepared for this possibility. If the hospital has a NICU, a nurse often visits the parents to explain what might occur if their baby is born early. One or both parents may tour the unit to see the equipment and care given to preterm infants.

In hospitals with NICUs, one or more neonatal nurses, a neonatal nurse practitioner, a neonatologist, or a combination of these are present at birth to care for the infant. The woman who has planned to give birth in a hospital without a NICU may be transferred to a facility with this type of unit before the birth to allow immediate care and stabilization of her newborn. The infant also may be transferred after birth if there is no time to transfer the woman before birth or the infant has more problems than were anticipated. Hospitalization of the mother, infant, or both at a distant location adds to the stress on the family and can impair the attachment process.

◆ Evaluation

The expected outcome for this patient problem is achieved if the woman and her family can identify one or more constructive methods to deal with their anxiety.

MANAGEMENT OF HOME CARE

◆ Assessment

Care of women with high-risk pregnancies, including a risk for preterm birth, often occurs in their homes if the gestation is sufficiently advanced and the signs and symptoms of preterm labor and birth have diminished significantly. Many daily household activities are managed by the woman, even if only by her directions to others. However, when labor complication becomes greater, family roles are again disrupted because of the changed relationships among family members. Multiple professionals are likely to be involved in home care, including home care nurses and assistants, social workers, therapists (physical, occupational), and others.

Clarify the level of activity prescribed by the physician, and identify the role of each member of the household. A good way to do this is to have the woman describe a usual day before any limitations were recommended. Determine the number and ages of children in the home.

Evaluate the home itself, either by visual inspection or by questioning the family. Does the home or apartment have more than one level? Determine whether a telephone is available for emergency contact. If the woman works, can she do her work online?

Evaluate the family's resources and their willingness to use them. Ask whether family members and friends in the area are available to help. Explore local support groups such as churches or mother-to-mother networks, that the family might contact for assistance. Determine financial reimbursement that may be available through insurance coverage.

◆ Identification of Patient Problems

Activity limitations for the woman may require adjustment in roles and responsibilities of all members of the family resulting in possible changes in the home environment because of altered roles and responsibilities.

◆ Planning: Expected Outcomes

Two goals and expected outcomes are appropriate for this patient problem. The short-term goal may change over time if the woman remains pregnant.

- Short-term goal—The family will identify methods for management of daily household routines.
- Long-term goal—The woman will be able to maintain the prescribed levels of activity and drug therapy.

◆ Interventions

The pregnancy threatened by preterm labor or other complications that require activity modification is a self-limiting situation, making temporary adjustments somewhat easier.

Needed changes in home routines may be brief but sometimes extend over several weeks. Even if the restriction consists only of added rest periods during the day, the woman still is unable to fulfill all her usual roles. For the woman who is prescribed more restricted activity, the disruptions are greater.

Caring for Children

The woman who has children has different concerns from the woman who does not. Toddlers and preschoolers rarely understand why their mother does not play with them as usual. If they already are in daycare, this can continue if the family can afford it. They may temporarily live with a relative or friend. Toddlers may feel that their parents have abandoned them if they are sent away, although this may be the only realistic solution if no one except the mother is available to supervise them.

School-age children can understand the situation better and often are quite helpful. They may assist with care of other children, but they should not be put into the role of an adult. They may resent responsibility that is excessive for their age. School-age children often enjoy learning new facts about their mother's pregnancy and tests the baby may need.

Adolescents may welcome their parents' trust but also resent the intrusion on independent activities with their peers. Teenagers who drive can be very helpful in taking younger siblings to school and other activities. They may be enlisted for grocery shopping and meal preparation. If resentment flares, a reminder that the situation is temporary and they are valuable contributors to the health of the new baby may defuse the situation.

Maintaining the Household

The first step to household maintenance during this time may be for the woman to lower her standards of housekeeping. Things may not be as clean or organized as she would like. The partner may take over some household tasks, but these may compete with responsibilities outside the home. Talk to the woman about ignoring chores that are not performed exactly as she wants and tell her to remember that it is temporary.

Advise the woman to have a list of tasks ready when friends and family ask, "Can I do anything to help?" If they offer to bring a meal or do laundry, encourage her to accept this help. Remind her that people who offer to help mean it and that she may be able to return the favor to someone else. Homemaker services may be an option to help the family deal with the woman's temporary disability.

Transportation of school-aged children may be a concern. If no family or friends are available, the school nurse or the Parent-Teacher Association (PTA) may help find someone willing to take the children to school each day.

◆ Evaluation

Identification of short-term goals and expected outcomes helps the nurse and patient, often including the family, identify resolution of immediate needs. Longer term outcomes may be evaluated over a series of days or weeks as the prescribed therapy for the complicated pregnancy changes.

- The short-term goal is met if the family can identify realistic ways to manage minimal household care.
- The long-term goal is met if the woman can maintain the prescribed therapy until birth.

BOREDOM

◆ Assessment

If activity is restricted, determine what skills the woman has for coping with boredom. Although bed rest to prolong gestation is often brief because of the questionable benefits and known problems, some reduction in activity may be prescribed. The nurse should consider helping the woman choose appropriate activities, whether she is at home or hospitalized.

Ask about a usual day to identify activities that are still appropriate within the restrictions prescribed. Ask about hobbies, present and past. What type of leisure activities does the woman enjoy? Which activities are available or possible? Does she have more than one resting place to still give her a change of scenery and surrounding activity?

Assess her personality. Is she calm and composed, taking whatever comes with serenity? Or does she need to be busy most of the time? No matter how motivated, the woman who finds inactivity tiresome will find even limited activity restriction difficult to maintain.

◆ Identification of Patient Problems

The patient problem is boredom due to lack of knowledge about appropriate activities.

◆ Planning: Expected Outcomes

A possible expected outcome is that the woman will do the following:
- Pursue (with help of others) appropriate activities to relieve boredom while maintaining recommended activity limits.

◆ Interventions
Identifying Appropriate Activities

Determine the woman's understanding about needed activity restrictions to identify misunderstandings and reinforce correct information. Help her identify which usual activities are reasonable and which ones should not be done and why. If she understands the rationale, she may be more willing to maintain restrictions.

Some women continue work activities such as paperwork or phone calls that can be accomplished with minimal physical exertion. Work among colleagues and clients sometimes may be accomplished online. Workplace deadlines can increase stress, even at home. However, the feeling of usefulness gained by such activities may be beneficial because it reduces some financial concerns.

Computer connections can be used for work activities in some jobs and may also provide support from other women with similar problems or entertainment such as games played with other users. Internet sites, if carefully chosen, may provide health information about what she might expect with diagnostic tests and treatment for preterm labor, care of her baby in the special care nursery setting, providing breast milk for her preterm newborn, and comfort measures that have been effective for others in her situation.

Help the woman identify appropriate activities to stay busy and productive. These may include household activities that can be done at rest, volunteer activities such as phone calls, and leisure activities such as puzzles, games, and hand needlework. Instructions for hobbies such as knitting are often available online. Help the woman identify someone who can obtain the necessary supplies for her. This might be a good time to reactivate an old (quiet) hobby or read books that she has previously delayed until "later."

The woman can participate in many activities with her children while she rests. She can read to them and play board or card games. Encourage her to help the children with their homework and stimulate their development with thought-provoking discussions. Working with children on video games may help them learn during their playtime.

Changing the Physical Surroundings

Encourage the woman to identify at least two areas in which she can maintain her prescribed rest periods. A change of location helps the woman be more willing to reduce her activities and still feel part of the family activities. Each area should include pillows, blankets, and a clipboard with writing materials. A laptop computer can be taken from place to place. Small rolling carts made of plastic help keep small things organized and together. The carts may be used after the baby is born for any kind of household need. Ideally, the telephone is within reach and is cordless or she has a cell phone. Either programming or writing important phone numbers such as those of family, friends, and physicians and emergency numbers helps assure the family that phone contacts are easily available for emergency as well as social needs.

◆ Evaluation

The goal is met over time if the woman actually pursues only appropriate activities.

POSTTERM PREGNANCY

The normal length of a pregnancy is 41⁶⁄₇ weeks, with term being regarded as delivery between weeks 39⁰⁄₇ to 40⁶⁄₇ weeks (ACOG, 2014; Cunningham et al., 2014). The late-term pregnancy is defined as the period between 41⁰⁄₇ weeks and 41⁶⁄₇ weeks (ACOG, 2014; Cunningham et al., 2014). A postterm pregnancy is one that lasts longer than 42⁰⁄₇ weeks (ACOG, 2014; Cunningham et al, 2014). Most women in the United States who receive prenatal care and have reliable dates are induced before 42 weeks gestation. Average gestational age at term birth is now 39 weeks rather than 40 weeks. Some apparent cases of prolonged pregnancy are actually miscalculations of the estimated date of delivery (EDD) because the woman has irregular menstrual periods or forgot the date of her last normal period. Late or no prenatal care limits the accuracy of clinical methods such as ultrasound for determining EDD and avoiding potential problems associated with prolonged gestation. Although patients should be encouraged to allow their babies to develop as much as possible, there are risks that can occur to the baby should a pregnancy go past 42 weeks.

Complications

The greatest physical risk in prolonged pregnancy is to the fetus or newborn. Insufficiency of the placental function secondary to aging and infarction reduces transfer of oxygen and nutrients to the fetus and removal of waste. Because the fetus with placental insufficiency has less reserve to tolerate uterine contractions, signs of fetal compromise such as late decelerations and decreased variability may develop during labor. In addition, reduced amniotic fluid volume (oligohydramnios) that often accompanies placental insufficiency can result in umbilical cord compression. The infant may have late growth restriction and appear to have lost weight, with a normal-size head and thin body. **Meconium aspiration syndrome** caused by the aspiration of meconium in the amniotic fluid before or during birth may result in respiratory distress in the newborn.

Many postterm fetuses do not suffer from placental insufficiency and may continue growing. If the fetus becomes large, the woman and fetus then may have complications related to dysfunctional labor, inadequate postpartum uterine contraction to control bleeding, and lacerations or infections (ACOG, 2014). Although the absolute risk for stillbirth and neonatal mortality in postterm pregnancy is low, late-term and postterm pregnancies have an increase in fetal mortality after 41 weeks of gestation compared with 40 weeks of gestation (ACOG, 2014)

Psychologically, the woman often feels as though her pregnancy will never end. The added fatigue imposed by a pregnancy that extends significantly beyond her due date diminishes her resources for tolerating the added stress and anxiety about labor and birth.

Therapeutic Management

If the woman has no prenatal care or receives care late in pregnancy, therapeutic management begins by determining her gestation as accurately as possible. Several markers used to determine gestation, such as ultrasound examination, fundal height measurements, dates of quickening, and first identification of fetal heart tones, may be less accurate or lost if a woman begins prenatal care very late. Also, the woman may have forgotten the date of her last menstrual period or may have irregular menstrual cycles.

Another factor in management decisions is whether the fetus is thriving in the uterus. If antepartum tests such as a biophysical profile indicate that the fetus is doing well and placental function is not diminished, the birth attendant can take a more conservative approach and allow labor to begin naturally. According to the Cochrane review, data are insufficient to define the optimal type or frequency of antepartum testing (ACOG, 2014).

Women are at risk for oligohydramnios with late-term and postterm pregnancies. Oligohydramnios is defined as an amniotic fluid index of 5 cm or less or a single deep pocket of amniotic fluid of 2 cm or less on ultrasound. With decreased amniotic fluid, the risk for stillbirth is increased. Additionally, there is an increased rate of meconium-stained fluid and FHR abnormalities such as decelerations and bradycardia associated with oligohydramnios (ACOG, 2014)

If the gestation appears to be truly postterm, induction is usually indicated as a result of an increased risk for perinatal morbidity and mortality (ACOG, 2014). Many physicians or midwives may choose to perform membrane sweeping to begin the process of labor. Membrane sweeping or "stripping of membranes" involves the provider digitally separating the membranes from the lower uterine segment when the cervix is dilated. According to the Cochrane review, stripping of membranes was associated with significant reductions in the number of pregnancies that progressed beyond 41 weeks of gestation (ACOG, 2014; Boulvain, Stan, & Irion, 2005)

Nursing Considerations

Nursing care for the woman with a prolonged pregnancy is tied to the medical management. The nurse's role may include the following:

- Teaching the woman about antepartum testing to include fetal movement counting
- Supporting the woman's psychological and physical fatigue
- Providing nursing care related to specific procedures such as induction of labor

---

❓ KNOWLEDGE CHECK

18. What are three risks to the fetus or neonate when pregnancy lasts longer than 42 weeks?

INTRAPARTUM EMERGENCIES

Placental Abnormalities

Women with placental abnormalities may experience hemorrhage during the antepartum or intrapartum period. Placental abnormalities include placenta accreta, placenta increta, or placenta percreta. It is unknown as to why the placenta embeds into the uterine tissue as deep as it does, but the theory is a defective decidua basalis. The strongest risk for abnormal placentation is prior uterine surgery, usually one or more cesarean births. Additional risk factors include smoking, advanced maternal age, and a short interconceptual period (Sosa, 2014). Abnormal placentation may cause immediate intrapartum hemorrhage, or hemorrhage may occur immediately after birth because the placenta does not separate cleanly, often leaving small fragments that prevent full uterine contraction. Placenta accreta occurs when the placenta is implanted into the uterine wall (ACOG, 2016b). All or part of the placenta may be involved. Placenta increta occurs when the chorionic villi invade the myometrium (ACOG, 2016b). Placenta percreta is described as complete perforation through the

uterine musculature and onto the adjacent organs such as the bladder (ACOG, 2016b).

A hysterectomy may be required if a large portion of the placenta is abnormally adherent (Foley, Strong, & Garite, 2014; Jauniaux, Bhide & Wright, 2017). An ultrasound evaluation to determine placental location and rule out an implantation abnormality is useful for a pregnant woman with a history of a previous cesarean birth. If placental adherence is suspected, magnetic resonance imaging is recommended to further determine the extent of placental abnormality. Multidisciplinary planning for delivery is crucial and involves the obstetrician, perinatologist, interventional radiologist, urologist, and neonatologist. The additional gynecologic oncologists or a general surgeon may need to be available at delivery. The average blood loss at delivery can be significant, ranging from 3000 to 5000 mL. It is important to have blood products and clotting factors on hold in the blood bank for use in the operating room. An additional IV line should be started for emergency use. Women who are diagnosed with placental abnormalities are at an increased risk for maternal mortality, reported as high as 7% (ACOG, 2016b).

Prolapsed Umbilical Cord

A **prolapsed umbilical cord (prolapsed cord)** slips downward after the membranes rupture, subjecting it to compression between the fetus and pelvis (Fig. 16.6). It may slip down immediately with the fluid gush or long after the membranes rupture. Interruption in blood flow through the cord interferes with fetal oxygenation and is potentially fatal for the fetus.

Causes

Prolapse of the umbilical cord is more likely when the fit is poor between the fetal presenting part and the maternal pelvis. When the fit is good, the fetus fills the pelvis, leaving little room for the cord to slip down. Although prolapse of the cord is possible during any labor, it is more likely if the following conditions are present:

- A fetus that remains at a high station
- A very small or preterm fetus
- Breech presentations (the footling breech is more likely to be complicated by a prolapsed cord because the feet and legs are small and do not fill the pelvis well)
- Transverse lie
- Hydramnios (often associated with abnormal presentations; also, the unusually large amount of fluid exerts more pressure to push the cord out)

Signs of Prolapse

Prolapse may be complete, with the cord visible at the vaginal opening, or it may not be visible but may be palpated on vaginal examination as it pulsates synchronously with the fetal heart. An **occult prolapse** of the cord is one in which the cord slips alongside the fetal head or shoulders. The prolapse cannot be palpated or seen but is suspected because of changes in the FHR, such as sustained bradycardia, variable decelerations or prolonged decelerations.

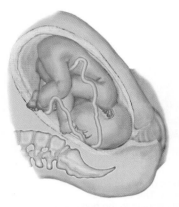

Occult (hidden) prolapse

The cord is compressed between the fetal presenting part and pelvis but cannot be seen or felt during vaginal examination.

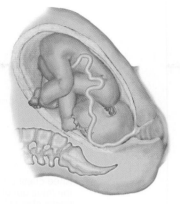

Cord prolapsed in front of the fetal head

The cord cannot be seen but can probably be felt as a pulsating mass during vaginal examination.

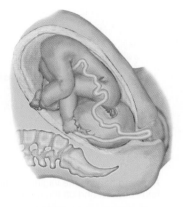

Complete cord prolapse

The cord can be seen protruding from the vagina.

FIG. 16.6 Variations of prolapsed umbilical cord.

> **! SAFETY CHECK**
>
> Factors that increase a woman's risk for a prolapsed umbilical cord include the following:
> - Ruptured membranes *and*
>   - The fetal presenting part at a high station
>   - A fetus that poorly fits the pelvic inlet because of small size or abnormal presentation
>   - Excessive volume of amniotic fluid (hydramnios)

Therapeutic Management

Medical and nursing management often overlap, as they do in many emergency situations. Either the nurse or the birth attendant may be the first to discover umbilical cord prolapse. Birth is almost always cesarean unless vaginal delivery can be accomplished more quickly and less traumatically. If fetal death has occurred, usually before patient arrival, management will focus on the best care for the mother based on other complications.

When cord prolapse occurs, the priority is to relieve pressure on the cord to improve umbilical blood flow until delivery. Interventions should not delay the prompt delivery of a living fetus. Have someone push the call light to summon help. Others should call the physician and prepare for birth while the nurse caring for the woman relieves pressure on the cord vaginally, if the physician or nurse-midwife is not doing so. Neonatal nurses and a pediatrician or neonatologist should be notified, and the staff should prepare for neonatal resuscitation.

Prompt actions reduce cord compression and increase fetal oxygenation:
- Position the woman's hips higher than her head to shift the fetal presenting part toward her diaphragm. Any of these methods (Fig. 16.7) may be used:
  - Knee-chest position
  - Trendelenburg position
  - Hips elevated with pillows, with side-lying position maintained
- Maintain vaginal elevation of the presenting part using a gloved hand while the woman is transferred to the operating room (OR) until the physician orders cessation of vaginal elevation, usually just before cesarean birth. Minimize cord compression from the hand that is elevating the presenting part as much as possible during the woman's transport to the OR.
- Avoid or minimize manual palpation or handling of the cord as much as possible to minimize cord vessel vasospasm.
- Ultrasound examination may be used to confirm presence of fetal heart activity before cesarean delivery.

While preparing for surgery, give the woman oxygen at 8 to 10 liters per minute (L/min) by face mask to increase maternal blood oxygen saturation, making more available for the fetus.

Other actions may be used to enhance fetal oxygenation, but prompt delivery is the priority. A tocolytic drug such as terbutaline inhibits contractions, increasing placental blood flow and reducing intermittent pressure of the fetus against the pelvis and cord.

Prognosis for the woman is good because the only additional risks are those associated with cesarean birth. Prognosis for the infant depends on how long and how severely blood flow through the cord has been impaired. With prompt recognition and corrective actions, the infant usually does well.

Nursing Considerations

In addition to taking prompt corrective actions, the nurse should consider the woman's anxiety. The nurse should remain calm while working quickly during this time and acknowledge the woman's anxiety. Explanations should be simple because anxiety interferes with the woman's ability to comprehend them. Her partner and family should be included as much as possible.

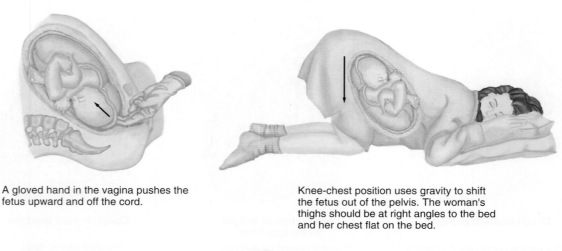

A gloved hand in the vagina pushes the fetus upward and off the cord.

Knee-chest position uses gravity to shift the fetus out of the pelvis. The woman's thighs should be at right angles to the bed and her chest flat on the bed.

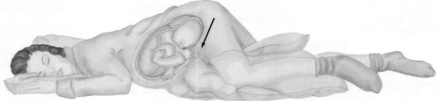

The woman's hips are elevated with two pillows; this is often combined with the Trendelenburg (head down) position.

FIG. 16.7 Measures that may be used to relieve pressure on a prolapsed umbilical cord until delivery can take place.

Uterine Rupture

Sometimes a tear in the wall of the uterus occurs because the uterus cannot withstand the pressure against it (Fig. 16.8). Uterine rupture may occur at home rather than in the hospital. Uterine rupture may precede labor's onset. Three variations of uterine rupture exist:

- *Complete rupture* is a direct communication between the uterine and peritoneal cavities.
- *Incomplete rupture* is a rupture into the peritoneum lining of the uterus or into the broad ligament but not the peritoneal cavity.
- *Dehiscence* is a partial separation of an old uterine scar. Little or no bleeding may occur. No signs or symptoms may exist, and the rupture ("window") may be found incidentally during a subsequent cesarean birth or other abdominal surgery.

Causes

Uterine rupture is rare and is usually associated with previous uterine surgery such as cesarean birth or surgery to remove fibroids. However, there have been incidences of uterine rupture on an unscarred uterus. The risk for rupture in a woman who has had a prior cesarean birth depends on the type of uterine incision. The risk for rupture is greater in women with a classic uterine incision (vertical into the upper uterine segment) than in women with a low transverse incision. For this reason, vaginal birth after cesarean (VBAC) is not recommended for women who have had a previous birth through a classic cesarean incision (see Fig. 15.14 [types of uterine

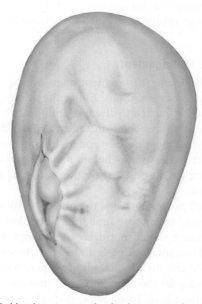

FIG. 16.8 Uterine rupture in the lower uterine segment.

incisions]). The decision about choosing a VBAC is made by the woman and her physician after discussion of the benefits as well as potential problems associated with vaginal birth that follows a previous cesarean (Foley et al., 2014; Landon & Grobman, 2017).

Rupture of the unscarred uterus is more likely for women of high parity with a thin uterine wall, women sustaining blunt abdominal trauma, and women having intense contractions, especially if fetopelvic disproportion is present. Excessively strong contractions may cause the intrauterine pressure to exceed the tensile strength of the uterine wall. If the fetus cannot be expelled downward through the pelvis, contractions may push it through the lower uterine segment. Intense contractions are more likely to occur when uterine stimulants such as oxytocin and misoprostol are administered for induction or augmentation of labor, but they also may occur spontaneously.

Signs and Symptoms

Dehiscence does not have symptoms initially and may not interfere with labor or vaginal birth if the area is small. However, labor progress may stop because the open area prevents efficient expulsion of the fetus. Intrauterine pressures may have little change during contractions. A larger area of dehiscence may cause abdominal pain that persists despite analgesia.

Manifestations of uterine rupture vary with the degree of rupture and may mimic other complications. Possible signs and symptoms of uterine rupture are as follows:

- Abdominal pain and tenderness—The pain may not be severe; it may occur suddenly at the peak of a contraction. The woman may describe a feeling that something "gave way" or "ripped." This may be blunted if the patient has epidural analgesia.
- Chest or shoulder pain, pain between the scapulae, or pain on inspiration—Pain occurs because of the irritation of blood below the woman's diaphragm.
- Hypovolemic shock caused by hemorrhage—Tachycardia, tachypnea, falling blood pressure, pallor, cool and clammy skin, and anxiety. Signs of shock may not occur until after birth. The fall in blood pressure is often a late sign of hemorrhage.
- Signs associated with impaired fetal oxygenation, such as late decelerations, reduced variability, tachycardia, and bradycardia.
- Absent fetal heart sounds with a large disruption of the placenta; absent fetal heart activity by ultrasound examination.
- Cessation of uterine contractions.
- Palpation of the fetus outside the uterus (usually occurs only with a large, complete rupture).

If the rupture is incomplete, blood loss is slower and signs of shock, chest pain, or intrascapular pain may be delayed. Complete rupture results in massive blood loss. Signs of shock and pain develop quickly. External bleeding may not be impressive, however, because most blood is lost into the peritoneal cavity. The fetus often dies in complete rupture because the placental blood supply is disrupted.

Therapeutic Management

Initial management is to stabilize the woman and the fetus for a cesarean birth. If the rupture is small and the woman wants other children, it may be repaired. A woman with a large uterine rupture may require hysterectomy. Blood and blood products are replaced as needed.

Nursing Considerations

The nurse should be aware of women who are at increased risk for uterine rupture and should stay alert for the signs and symptoms. Administer uterine stimulant drugs cautiously to reduce the likelihood of excessive contractions. The nurse should keep in mind that tachysystole also can occur spontaneously. Notify the birth attendant if tachysystole occurs. A tocolytic drug may be needed to reduce excessive contractions.

Uterine rupture may not be detected before birth. If postpartum bleeding is excessive and the fundus is firm, injury to the birth canal, including uterine rupture, is possible. Bleeding may be concealed if the ruptured area bleeds into the broad ligament. In this case, signs of hypovolemic shock are likely to develop quickly.

> **? KNOWLEDGE CHECK**
>
> 19. What is the immediate management of prolapse of the umbilical cord?
> 20. How can contractions stimulated with drugs such as oxytocin or misoprostol increase the risk for uterine rupture?

Uterine Inversion

An inversion occurs when the uterus completely or partly turns inside out, usually during the third stage of labor. Such an event is uncommon but potentially fatal.

Causes

Often, no single cause is identified. Predisposing factors are as follows:

- Excessive traction on the umbilical cord before the placenta detaches from the uterine wall spontaneously
- Fundal pressure during birth
- Fundal pressure on an incompletely contracted uterus after birth
- Increased intraabdominal pressure
- An abnormally adherent placenta
- Congenital weakness of the uterine wall
- Fundal placenta implantation

Signs and Symptoms

The birth attendant notes that either the uterus is absent from the abdomen or a depression in the fundal area is present. The interior of the uterus may be seen through the cervix or protruding into the vagina, appearing as a red, beefy mass. Massive hemorrhage, shock, and pain quickly become evident. The woman has severe pelvic pain.

Management

Quick action by nursing and medical personnel is essential to reduce maternal morbidity and mortality. The physician tries to replace the uterus through the vagina into a normal position. Anesthesia may be required to produce enough relaxation to allow the uterus to be replaced. If replacement is not possible, a laparotomy may be necessary. Several units of blood are usually ordered immediately (Creasy et al., 2014; Francois & Foley, 2017).

Nursing Considerations

Nursing care during the emergency supplements that provided by other staff members. Postpartum nursing care is directed toward observing and maintaining maternal blood volume and correcting shock. The woman may be transferred to the intensive care unit after birth.

Assess the uterine fundus (if a hysterectomy was not required) for firmness, height, and deviation from the midline. Assess vital signs every 15 minutes or more frequently until stable and then according to recovery room routine. Observe for tachycardia and falling blood pressure, which are associated with shock. Remember that the fall in blood pressure is often a late sign of hemorrhagic shock. A cardiac monitor identifies dysrhythmias, which may occur with shock; a pulse oximeter indicates the woman's pulse rate and oxygen saturation. Invasive hemodynamic monitoring with central venous pressure and arterial lines is common to directly evaluate functions such as heart rate, venous and arterial pressures, blood gases, circulation to the lungs, venous functions, and other tests that may be needed.

An indwelling catheter usually is inserted to observe fluid balance and keep the bladder empty so the uterus can contract well. Assess the catheter for patency, and record intake and output. Urine output should be at least 30 mL/hr. A fall in urine output may indicate hypovolemia or an obstructed catheter.

The woman is allowed nothing by mouth until her condition is stable. She usually can receive fluids and progress to solid foods quickly because **uterine inversion** does not usually recur in the current postpartum period. It may recur in a future pregnancy if conditions favor its development.

Anaphylactoid Syndrome

Anaphylactoid syndrome of pregnancy, often called **amniotic fluid embolism** syndrome (AFE), occurs when amniotic fluid is drawn into the maternal circulation and carried to the woman's lungs. Fetal particulate matter (skin cells, vernix, hair, meconium) in the fluid obstructs pulmonary vessels. Failure of the right ventricle occurs early and can lead to hypoxemia. Left ventricular failure follows. Abrupt respiratory distress, depressed cardiac function, and circulatory collapse may occur rapidly. Disseminated intravascular coagulation (DIC) (see Chapter 10) is likely because thromboplastin-rich amniotic fluid interferes with normal blood clotting. This infrequent disorder is often fatal, and survivors may have neurologic deficits (Foley et al., 2014; Cunningham et. al., 2014).

Entry of amniotic fluid containing fetal cells and other matter such as vernix is more likely if labor is very strong. High intrauterine pressure forces amniotic fluid into open uterine or cervical veins. The meconium that often accompanies a stressed fetus in such a labor adds to the particulate matter forced into the woman's circulation.

Rapid therapeutic management of a pregnancy-related anaphylactoid syndrome is primarily medical and includes the following (Cunningham et al., 2014; Foley et al., 2014):
- Cardiopulmonary resuscitation and support
- Oxygen with mechanical ventilation
- Correction of hypotension
- Blood component therapy (e.g., fibrinogen, packed red blood cells, platelets, fresh-frozen plasma) to correct coagulation defects
- Investigation is being done on a new protocol for AFE treatment, called the A-OK Protocol, which involves administering atropine 0.8 mg, ondansetron 4 mg, and ketorolac 30 mg at minute 5 of the event.

If the pregnant mother is in cardiac arrest, following the Advanced Cardiovascular Life Support (ACLS) obstetric protocol for cesarean birth by 4 to 5 minutes after the maternal code begins is likely to improve survival odds for the baby.

TRAUMA

Most trauma during pregnancy occurs because of motor vehicle accidents, assault, or suicide. Battering, or interpersonal violence, is a significant cause of maternal-fetal trauma during pregnancy. Trauma may be blunt, such as that sustained in an automobile accident, or penetrating, such as gunshot and knife wounds. Burns and electrical injuries also may occur. Trauma is the leading cause of nonobstetric maternal death (Brown, 2017; Cunningham et al., 2014).

Although injury may not be fatal, infant neurologic deficits may be found after birth. Direct fetal trauma such as skull fracture or intracranial hemorrhage may occur from maternal pelvic fracture, penetrating wounds, or blunt trauma. Indirect causes of fetal injury or death include placental abruption and disruption of the placental blood flow secondary to maternal hypovolemia or uterine rupture. The most common cause of fetal death resulting from trauma is death of the mother.

The anatomic and physiologic changes of pregnancy make trauma care unique. During early pregnancy, the uterus is surrounded by the pelvis and is well protected from direct damage. As the uterus grows, it protrudes and becomes a large target for trauma. At the same time, it acts as a shield for other maternal organs such as the kidneys, often protecting them from direct trauma.

Normal alterations of pregnancy can affect maternal and fetal outcomes after traumatic injury and can affect the interpretation of diagnostic studies that may be done. Pregnant women have a greater blood volume than nonpregnant women, which gives them a cushion against blood loss. However, the fetus may suffer if the woman hemorrhages because maternal blood is diverted from the placenta to increase her blood volume. Fetal hypoxia, acidosis, and death may then occur.

Maternal fibrinogen levels are higher during pregnancy (300 to 600 mg/dL). A decrease to lower levels is associated with placental abruption and may indicate that disseminated intravascular coagulation is developing.

Management

Care of the pregnant trauma victim first focuses on injuries that threaten her life. Management of the fetus depends on whether the fetus is living and on the gestational age. Cesarean birth is opted for if the fetus is mature enough to survive and if the maternal or fetal condition is likely to be improved by prompt delivery. The fetus that is dead or too immature to survive is not usually delivered unless delivery will improve the mother's outcome. A Kleihauer-Betke (K-B) test may be ordered at intervals to identify placental disruptions that allow fetal blood to leak into the circulation.

Nursing Considerations

Motor vehicle accidents are the leading cause of blunt trauma during pregnancy. Nonuse or incorrect use of automobile restraints such as seat belts or air bags may result in greater trauma or fatality in mother and fetus. Visit the website for the National Highway Traffic Safety Administration for information on correct use of seat belts and air bags during pregnancy (www.nhtsa.dot.gov).

Nursing care of the pregnant trauma victim focuses first on maternal and then on fetal stabilization. A wedge is placed under one side of the mother to tip her uterus away from her major blood vessels. Placing her in a lateral tilt position to displace the uterus may prevent supine hypotension and improve placental blood flow. Vital signs are taken as needed, based on the woman's condition. Vital signs and urine output (at least 30 mL/hr) provide information about the adequacy of her blood volume. Bloody urine suggests bladder or renal damage. Other nursing care is directed toward specific injuries and implementation of medical care.

Signs suggesting placental abruption (vaginal bleeding with uterine pain and tenderness) should be reported because this complication may occur with abdominal trauma. Vaginal bleeding may not be apparent if the edges of the placenta remain attached but the center portion is detached. The uterine height may increase as the uterus fills with blood. Tachycardia usually precedes a fall in blood pressure if hypovolemia is the cause. Fetal tachycardia or cessation of the FHR is likely to occur in more extensive uterine trauma or maternal hemorrhage. Fetal hemorrhage may occur with trauma to the placenta or the umbilical cord.

Once the woman's condition is stable, nursing care for the fetus is intensified. External monitoring is appropriate if the fetus has reached a viable gestational age. Preterm labor may occur but may not be recognized if the woman is unconscious or if pain from injuries overshadows discomfort from contractions. Recurrent restlessness or moaning may accompany contractions. The nurse should palpate the woman's uterus for contractions periodically because they may not be evident on the fetal monitoring strip, especially if the fetus is small.

? KNOWLEDGE CHECK

21. What are the primary complications of a uterine inversion? How are they managed?
22. What are important nursing considerations for each kind of intrapartum emergency: Prolapsed umbilical cord? Uterine rupture? Uterine inversion? Amniotic fluid embolism?
23. What kinds of fetal injury may occur with maternal trauma during pregnancy?

◆ APPLICATION OF THE NURSING PROCESS: INTRAPARTUM EMERGENCIES

Nursing care of the woman with an intrapartum emergency overlaps with care in other situations discussed elsewhere. Much of the nursing care is collaborative and supports medical management. Parents may suffer loss if the fetus dies or the mother loses her ability to bear future children, as may occur with uterine rupture. One problem expected in any emergency situation is the emotional distress of the woman and her family.

◆ Assessment

When an emergency occurs, the woman and her family have little time to absorb what has happened, simply because of its suddenness. In umbilical cord prolapse, for example, labor often has been uneventful up to that point. Suddenly, nurses place the woman in a strange position, administer oxygen, and pull her toward the operating room. The staff is clearly excited as well.

Under such circumstances, the woman and her family have a very narrow focus. They are obviously apprehensive and feel out of control. The woman or her partner may be immobilized by fear.

◆ Identification of Patient Problem

The patient problem is "Apprehension because of the sudden development of complications." This problem is expected to differ from the anxiety associated with preterm labor because the onset is acute. The apprehension also may lessen more quickly because the emergency is sometimes resolved quickly. Grief may occur because of ill effects of the emergency on mother and baby.

◆ Planning: Expected Outcomes

The focus of a goal is very narrow in an emergency situation. Two appropriate outcomes, during and after the emergency, are that the woman and her family will do the following:
- Indicate an understanding of emergency procedures.
- Express their feelings about the complication.

◆ Interventions

Although little time for discussion exists, explain honestly and simply what is occurring. To reduce fear and anxiety of the unknown, tell the woman what is happening and why. Include her partner and family, if appropriate. Provide continued reassurance and support to the woman because her partner often must be excluded from the emergency or operating room when an emergency occurs.

The infant born in an emergency situation may need resuscitation or other supportive measures. Nurses and a neonatal nurse practitioner or pediatrician from the NICU, usually are present at the birth to attend the infant. A neonatologist also may be present. Explain to the family who the other professionals are and their roles. If possible, explain what is being done to care for the baby.

After the emergency, give the woman and her family a chance to ask questions. The ability to absorb new knowledge during periods of severe anxiety is very limited. Adequate explanations afterward help them understand and assimilate the experience.

Although the nurse is usually anxious in an emergency situation, keeping a calm attitude is important. The woman and her family quickly pick up on the staff's anxiety, and consequently their anxiety escalates. Remain with the woman to reduce fears of abandonment. If possible, hold her hand. Speak in a low, calm voice. Debriefing after the occurrence is key to help the nurse assimilate the event.

◆ Evaluation

Evaluation of the goals is probably impossible until the emergency is over and the woman's physical condition stabilizes. Expected outcomes for this patient problem are achieved if the woman and her family do the following:

- Indicate they understand the problem and the rationale for emergency procedures.
- Express, possibly over several days, their feelings about what has occurred.

SUMMARY CONCEPTS

- Dysfunctional labor may occur because of abnormalities in the powers, the passenger, the passage, or the psyche. Combinations of abnormalities are common.
- Nursing care in labor focuses on prevention or prompt identification and action to correct additional complications such as fetal hypoxia, infection, injury to the mother or fetus, and postpartum hemorrhage.
- Premature rupture of the membranes is associated with infection as both a cause and a complication.
- Early indications of preterm labor are often vague. Prompt identification of preterm labor enables the most effective therapy to delay preterm birth.
- Nursing care for the woman at risk for a preterm birth before 37 weeks of gestation focuses on helping her delay birth long enough to provide time for fetal lung maturation with corticosteroids, administration of antibiotics to decrease the risk of neonatal GBS infection, allow transfer to a facility that has neonatal intensive care, or reach a gestation at which the infant's problems with immaturity are less.
- The main risk in prolonged pregnancy is reduced placental function. This may compromise the fetus during labor and result in meconium aspiration in the neonate. Dysfunctional labor may occur if a fetus continues growing during the prolonged pregnancy.
- The key intervention for umbilical cord prolapse is to relieve pressure on the umbilical cord and to expedite delivery.
- Be aware of women at risk for uterine rupture, and observe for signs and symptoms such as signs of shock, abdominal pain, a sense of tearing, chest pain, shoulder pain, pain between the scapulae, abnormal fetal heart rate patterns,

cessation of contractions, and palpation of the fetus outside the uterus. However, lesser degrees of uterine rupture or dehiscence may have minimal symptoms.
- Uterine inversion can be accompanied by massive blood loss and shock. Recovery care promotes uterine contraction and maintenance of adequate circulating volume.
- Anaphylactoid syndrome of pregnancy (amniotic fluid embolism syndrome) is more likely to occur when labor is intense and the membranes have ruptured. The true causes of anaphylactoid syndrome of pregnancy are not known because it is uncommon.
- The uterus is protected by the maternal pelvis during early pregnancy. As the uterus enlarges and ascends out of the pelvis, it is more vulnerable to trauma from direct impact. The fetus may be injured by disruption of the placenta, direct trauma, or either fetal or maternal hemorrhage.
- Medical and nursing care of the pregnant trauma victim focuses on stabilization of the mother first. Management of the fetus depends on gestational age and whether the fetus is alive. Placental abruption and uterine rupture are obstetric complications that may occur with direct abdominal trauma.
- Motor vehicle accidents are a major cause of blunt force trauma that may cause premature separation of the placenta, hemorrhage, fractures, and internal injuries. Penetrating injuries caused by knife or gunshot wounds are particularly dangerous for the fetus.
- Treatment of trauma in the pregnant woman is similar to that in a nonpregnant woman. Cardiopulmonary resuscitation and controlling bleeding are the priorities. Careful evaluation of the uterus and fetus also is essential after even minor trauma.

REFERENCES & READINGS

American Academy of Pediatrics (AAP) and American College of Obstetricians and Gynecologists (ACOG). (2012a). *Guidelines for Perinatal Care* (7th ed.). Elk Grove, IL: Authors.

American College of Obstetricians and Gynecologists (ACOG). (2014). *Management of late-term and postterm pregnancies.* Practice Bulletin No. 146. Washington, DC: Author.

American College of Obstetricians and Gynecologists (ACOG). (2016a). *Management of preterm labor.* Practice Bulletin No. 171. Washington, DC: Author.

American College of Obstetricians and Gynecologists (ACOG). (2016b). *Placenta accreta.* Practice Bulletin No. 529. Washington, DC: Author.

American College of Obstetricians and Gynecologists (ACOG). (2016c). *ACOG obstetric care consensus no. 4. Periviable birth.* Washington, DC: Author.

American College of Obstetricians and Gynecologists (ACOG). (2016d). *Premature rupture of membranes.* Practice Bulletin No. 172. Washington, DC: Author.

American College of Obstetricians and Gynecologists (ACOG). (2016e). Committee opinion no. 652: Magnesium sulfate use in obstetrics. *Obstet Gynecol, 127,* e52–e53.

American College of Obstetricians and Gynecologists (ACOG). (2017a). *Shoulder dystocia.* Practice Bulletin No. 178. Washington, DC: Author.

American College of Obstetricians and Gynecologists (ACOG). (2017b). *Antenatal corticosteroid therapy for fetal maturation.* Committee Opinion No. 713. Washington, DC: Author.

Boulvain, M., Stan, C. M., & Irion, O. (2005). Membrane sweeping for induction of labour. *Cochrane Database of Systematic Reviews,* (1), CD000451.

Brown, H. L. (2017). Trauma & related surgery in pregnancy. In S. G. Gabbe, J. R. Niebyl, J. L. Simpson, M. B. Landon, H. L. Galan, R. M. Jauniaux, D. A. Driscoll, et al. (Eds.), *Obstetrics: Normal and problem pregnancies* (7th ed.) (pp. 565–577). Philadelphia: Saunders.

Conner, S., Bedell, V., Lipsey, K., Macones, G. A., Cahill, A. G., & Tuuli, M. G. (2016). Maternal marijuana use and adverse neonatal outcomes: a systematic review and meta-analysis. *Obstetrics & Gynecology,* 128(4), 713–723.

Craighead, D. V. (2012). Early term birth: Understanding the health risks to infants. *Nursing for Women's Health,* 16(2), 136–144.

Craighead, D. V., & Elswick, R. K. (2014). The influence of early-term birth on NICU admission, length of stay, and breastfeeding initiation and duration. *JOGNN: Journal of Obstetric, Gynecologic & Neonatal Nursing,* 43(4), 409–421.

Creasy, R. K., Resnick, R., Iams, J. D., Lockwood, C. J., Moore, T., & Greene, M. (2014). *Creasy and Resnik's maternal-fetal medicine: Principles and practice* (7th ed.). Philadelphia: Saunders.

Cunningham, F. G., Leveno, K. J., Bloom, S. L., Spong, C. Y., Dashe, J. S., Hoffman, B. L., Casey, B. M., & Sheffield, J. S. (2014). *Williams obstetrics* (24th ed.). New York: McGraw-Hill.

Foley, M., Strong, T., Jr., & Garite, T. (2014). *Obstetric intensive care manual* (4th ed.). New York: McGraw-Hill Medical Education.

Francois, K. E., & Foley, M. R. (2017). Antepartum and postpartum hemorrhage. In S. G. Gabbe, J. R. Niebyl, J. L. Simpson, M. B. Landon, H. L. Galan, R. M. Jauniaux, D. A. Driscoll, et al. (Eds.), *Obstetrics: Normal and problem pregnancies* (7th ed.) (pp. 395–424). Philadelphia: Saunders.

Higgins, R. D., Saade, G., Polin, R. A., Grobman, W. A., Buhimschi, I. A., Watterberg, K., Raju, T. K. (2016). Evaluation and management of women and newborns with a maternal diagnosis of chorioamnionitis: summary of a workshop. *Obstetrics & Gynecology,* 127(3), 426–436.

Holigic. (2009). *Enzyme immunoassay and rapid fFN™ for the TLiIQ® System.* Retrieved from www.ffntest.com/pdfs/rapid_ffn_product_insert_lettersize.pdf.

Jauniaux, E. R. H., Bhide, A., & Wright, J. D. (2017). Placenta accreta. In S. G. Gabbe, J. R. Niebyl, J. L. Simpson, M. B. Landon, H. L. Galan, R. M. Jauniaux, D. A. Driscoll, et al. (Eds.), *Obstetrics: Normal and problem pregnancies* (7th ed.) (pp. 456–466). Philadelphia: Saunders.

Kilpatrick, S., & Garrison, E. (2017). Normal labor and delivery. In S. G. Gabbe, J. R. Niebyl, J. L. Simpson, M. B. Landon, H. L. Galan, R. M. Jauniaux, D. A. Driscoll, et al. (Eds.), *Obstetrics: Normal and problem pregnancies* (7th ed.) (pp. 246–269). Philadelphia: Saunders.

Landon, M. B., & Grobman, W. A. (2017). Vaginal birth after cesarean delivery. In S. G. Gabbe, J. R. Niebyl, J. L. Simpson, M. B. Landon, H. L. Galan, R. M. Jauniaux, D. A. Driscoll, et al. (Eds.), *Obstetrics: Normal and problem pregnancies* (7th ed.) (pp. 444–455). Philadelphia: Saunders.

Lanni, S. M., Gherman, R., & Gonik, B. (2017). Malpresentations. In S. G. Gabbe, J. R. Niebyl, J. L. Simpson, M. B. Landon, H. L. Galan, R. M. Jauniaux, D. A. Driscoll, et al. (Eds.), *Obstetrics: Normal and problem pregnancies* (7th ed.) (pp. 368–394). Philadelphia: Saunders.

Macones, G. A., Hankins, G. D., Spong, C. Y., Hauth, J., & Moore, T. (2008). The 2008 National Institute of Child Health and Human Development workshop report on electronic fetal monitoring: Update on definitions, interpretation, and research guidelines. *Journal of Obstetric, Gynecologic, & Neonatal Nursing,* 37(5), 510–515 and *Obstetrics and Gynecology,* 112, 661–666.

March of Dimes. (2016). *2015 Premature birth report card.* March of Dimes. Retrieved from www.marchofdimes.org.

Mercer, B. M. (2017). Premature rupture of the membranes. In S. G. Gabbe, J. R. Niebyl, J. L. Simpson, M. B. Landon, H. L. Galan, R. M. Jauniaux, D. A. Driscoll, et al. (Eds.), *Obstetrics: Normal and problem pregnancies* (7th ed.) (pp. 647–660). Philadelphia: Saunders.

National Center for Health Statistics. (2016). *Final natality data.* Retrieved from www.marchofdimes.org/peristats.

Newman, R., & Unal, E. R. (2017). Multiple gestations. In S. G. Gabbe, J. R. Niebyl, J. L. Simpson, M. B. Landon, H. L. Galan, R. M. Jauniaux, D. A. Driscoll, et al. (Eds.), *Obstetrics: Normal and problem pregnancies* (7th ed.) (pp. 706–736). Philadelphia: Saunders.

Norman, J. E., Marlow, N., Messow, C., Shennan, A., Bennett, P. R., Thornton, S., Norrie, J. (2016). Vaginal progesterone prophylaxis for preterm birth (the OPPTIMUM study): A multicentre, randomised, double-blind trial. *Lancet,* 387 North American Edition. (10033), 2106–2116.

Romero, R., Nicolaides, K. H., Conde-Agudelo, A., O'Brien, J. M., Cetingoz, E., Da Fonseca, E., Hassan, S. S. (2016). Vaginal progesterone decreases preterm birth ≤ 34 weeks of gestation in women with a singleton pregnancy and a short cervix: An updated meta-analysis including data from the OPPTIMUM study. *Ultrasound in Obstetrics & Gynecology,* 48(3), 308–317.

Rozance, P. J., & Rosenberg, A. A. (2017). The neonate. In S. G. Gabbe, J. R. Niebyl, J. L. Simpson, M. B. Landon, H. L. Galan, R. M. Jauniaux, D. A. Driscoll, et al. (Eds.), *Obstetrics: Normal and problem pregnancies* (7th ed.) (pp. 468–498). Philadelphia: Elsevier Saunders.

Sheibani, L., & Wing, D. A. (2017). Abnormal labor and induction of labor. In S. G. Gabbe, J. R. Niebyl, J. L. Simpson, M. B. Landon, H. L. Galan, R. M. Jauniaux, D. A. Driscoll, et al. (Eds.), *Obstetrics: Normal and problem pregnancies* (7th ed.) (pp. 271–288). Philadelphia: Elsevier Saunders.

Simhan, H. N., Iams, J. D., & Romero, R. (2017). Preterm labor and birth. In S. G. Gabbe, J. R. Niebyl, J. L. Simpson, M. B. Landon, H. L. Galan, R. M. Jauniaux, D. A. Driscoll, et al. (Eds.), *Obstetrics: Normal and problem pregnancies* (7th ed.) (pp. 615–646). Philadelphia: Saunders.

Simpson, K. R. (2013). *Cervical ripening and labor induction and augmentation* (4th ed.). Washington, DC: AWHONN.

Simpson, K. R., & Abel, N. O. (2014). Labor and birth. In K. R. Simpson, & P. A. Creehan (Eds.), *AWHONN's perinatal nursing* (4th ed.) (pp. 343–444). Philadelphia: Lippincott.

Sosa, M. E. B. (2014). Bleeding in pregnancy. In K. R. Simpson, & P. A. Creehan (Eds.), *AWHONN's perinatal nursing* (4th ed.) (pp. 143–165). Philadelphia: Lippincott.

U.S. Food and Drug Administration (FDA). (2011). *FDA drug safety communication: New warnings against use of terbutaline to treat preterm labor.* Retrieved from www.fda.gov.

Zhang, J., Landy, H. J., Branch, D. W., Burkman, R., Haberman, S., Gregory, K. D., Reddy, U. (2010). Contemporary patterns of spontaneous labor with normal neonatal outcomes. Consortium on Safe Labor. *Obstetrics and Gynecology,* 116, 1281–1287.

17

Postpartum Adaptations and Nursing Care

Emily Drake, Mary Suzanne White

OBJECTIVES

After studying this chapter, you should be able to:

1. Explain the physiologic changes that occur during the postpartum period.
2. Explain maternal psychosocial adaptation to childbirth, including the process of bonding and attachment and the stages of maternal role attainment.
3. Discuss the cause, manifestations, and interventions for postpartum blues.
4. Describe the processes of family adaptation to the birth of a baby and factors that may affect that process.
5. Discuss cultural influences on family adaptation.
6. Apply the nursing process to the care of the postpartum family.

7. Discuss expected outcomes and interventions for common postpartum patient problems.
8. Explain the role of the nurse in health education of the postpartum family and identify important areas of teaching.
9. Compare postpartum nursing assessments and care for women who have undergone cesarean birth and vaginal birth.
10. Describe criteria for postpartum discharge and available follow up health care services.

The first 6 weeks after the birth of an infant are known as the *postpartum period,* or **puerperium**. During this time, mothers experience physiologic and psychosocial changes. The family also experiences psychosocial changes as they adapt to the new family member.

PHYSIOLOGIC CHANGES

Many of the physiologic changes are retrogressive: Changes that occurred in body systems during pregnancy are reversed as the body returns to the nonpregnant state. Progressive changes such as the initiation of lactation also occur.

Reproductive System
Involution of the Uterus

Involution refers to the changes the reproductive organs, particularly the uterus, undergo after childbirth to return to their nonpregnant size and condition. Uterine involution involves three processes: (1) contraction of muscle fibers, (2) **catabolism** (the process of converting cells into simpler compounds), and (3) regeneration of the uterine epithelium. Involution begins immediately after delivery of the placenta, when uterine muscle fibers contract firmly around maternal

blood vessels at the area where the placenta was attached. This contraction controls bleeding from the area left denuded when the placenta separated. The uterus decreases in size as muscle fibers, which have been stretched for many months, contract and gradually regain their former contour and size.

Regeneration of the uterine epithelial lining begins soon after childbirth. The outer portion of the endometrial layer is expelled with the placenta. Within 2 to 3 days, the remaining **decidua** (the endometrium during pregnancy) separates into two layers. The first layer is superficial and is shed in the lochia. The basal layer containing the residual endometrial glands and blood vessels remains to provide the source of new endometrium. Regeneration of the endometrium, except at the site of placental attachment, occurs by 2 to 3 weeks after birth (Blackburn, 2013).

Healing at the placental site occurs more slowly and requires approximately 6 weeks (Blackburn, 2013). The site, which is approximately 9 cm (3.5 in) in diameter immediately postpartum, heals by a process of *exfoliation* (scaling off of dead tissue) (Isley & Katz, 2017). New endometrium is generated at the site from glands and tissue that remain in the lower layer of the decidua after separation of the placenta (Cunningham et al., 2014). This process leaves the endometrial layer smooth and spongy, as it was before pregnancy, and the uterine lining is free of scar tissue unless the birth was cesarean. Scarring of the uterine lining may interfere with implantation of future pregnancies.

Descent of the Uterine Fundus. The location of the uterine fundus helps determine whether involution is progressing normally. Immediately after delivery, the uterus is about the size of a large grapefruit or softball and weighs approximately 1000 grams (g) (2.2 pounds [lb]). The fundus can be palpated midway between the symphysis pubis and umbilicus and in the midline of the abdomen. Within 12 hours the fundus rises to approximately the level of the umbilicus (Blackburn, 2013).

The fundus descends by approximately 1 cm, or one fingerbreadth, per day. By the 14th day, it has descended into the pelvic cavity and cannot be palpated abdominally (Fig. 17.1) (Blackburn, 2013). When the process of involution does not occur properly, **subinvolution** occurs. Subinvolution can cause postpartum hemorrhage (see Chapter 18).

Descent of the fundus is documented in relation to the umbilicus. For example, *U-1* or ↓1 indicates that the fundus is palpable about 1 cm (a fingerbreadth) below the umbilicus. Within 1 week, the weight of the uterus decreases to approximately 500 g (1 lb); at 4 weeks, the uterus weighs 100 g (2 to 3 oz) or less (Cunningham, et al., 2014).

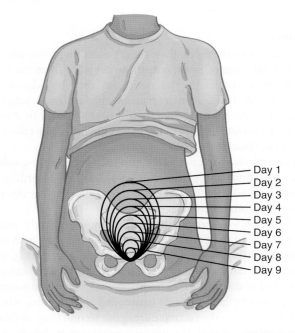

Day 1
Day 2
Day 3
Day 4
Day 5
Day 6
Day 7
Day 8
Day 9

FIG. 17.1 Involution of the Uterus. Height of the uterine fundus decreases by approximately 1 cm per day. The fundus is no longer palpable by 14 days.

Afterpains

Etiology. Intermittent uterine contractions, known as **afterpains**, are a source of discomfort for many women. The discomfort is more acute for multiparas because repeated stretching of muscle fibers leads to loss of muscle tone that causes repeated contraction and relaxation of the uterus.

The uterus of a primipara tends to remain contracted, but she may experience severe afterpains if her uterus has been overdistended or if retained blood clots are present. Afterpains are particularly severe during breastfeeding. Oxytocin, released from the posterior pituitary to stimulate the **milk-ejection reflex** (release of milk from the ducts of the breasts), causes strong contractions of uterine muscles.

Nursing Considerations. Analgesics are frequently used to lessen the discomfort of afterpains. Many breastfeeding mothers are reluctant to take medication for fear it will pass into the breast milk and harm the infant. However, health care experts generally agree that most common analgesics may be used for short-term pain relief without harm to the infant. The benefits of pain relief such as comfort and relaxation facilitate the milk-ejection reflex and usually outweigh the small effect of the medication on the infant. The woman should check with her health care provider before taking any medication. The nurse can reassure the mother that afterpains are self-limiting and decrease in frequency and intensity by the third day (Cunningham et al., 2014).

Lochia. Changes in the color and amount of lochia (the vaginal drainage after childbirth) also provide information about whether involution is progressing normally. Table 17.1 summarizes the characteristics of normal and abnormal lochia.

Changes in Color. On days 1 to 3 after childbirth, lochia consists almost entirely of blood, with small particles of decidua and mucus. It is called **lochia rubra** because of its dark red or red-brown color. The amount of blood decreases when leukocytes begin to invade the area, as they do in any healing surface. The color of lochia then changes from red to pink or brown-tinged (**lochia serosa**). It lasts from days 3 to 10. Lochia serosa is composed of serous exudate, erythrocytes, leukocytes, and cervical mucus. By about the 10th day, the erythrocyte component decreases. The discharge becomes white, cream, or light yellow in color (**lochia alba**). Lochia alba contains leukocytes, decidual cells, epithelial cells, fat, cervical mucus, and bacteria. It may end by day 14 or persist until the end of the 3rd to the 6th week (Blackburn, 2013; Whitmer, 2016).

Amount. Because estimating the amount of lochia on a peripad (perineal pad) is difficult, nurses frequently document lochia in terms that are difficult to quantify,

TABLE 17.1 **Characteristics of Lochia**		
Time and Type	**Normal Discharge**	**Abnormal Discharge**
Days 1-3: Lochia rubra	Bloody; small clots; fleshy, earthy odor; dark red or red-brown	Large clots; saturated perineal pads; foul odor
Days 3-10: Lochia serosa	Decreased amount; serosanguineous; pink or brown-tinged	Excessive amount; foul smell; continued or recurrent reddish color
Days 10-14 (or up to 3rd-6th week): Lochia alba	White, cream, or light yellow color; decreasing amounts	Persistent lochia serosa; return to lochia rubra; foul odor; discharge continuing

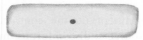

Scant: <2.5 cm (1-inch) stain

Light: 2.5 to 10 cm (1 to 4-inch) stain

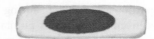

Moderate: 10 to 15 cm (4 to 6-inch) stain

Heavy: Saturated in 1 hour

FIG. 17.2 Guidelines for Assessing the Amount of Lochia on the Perineal Pad.

such as *scant, moderate,* and *heavy.* Agreement on the meanings of terms in an agency is important to make charting accurate. One method for recording the amount of lochia in 1 hour uses the following labels (Whitmer, 2016):

- Scant—Less than a 2.5-cm (1-inch) stain on the peripad
- Light—Less than 10-cm (4-inch) stain
- Moderate—Less than 15-cm (6-inch) stain
- Heavy—Saturated peripad in 1 hour
- Excessive—Saturated peripad in 15 minutes

Determining the time a peripad has been in place is important when assessing lochia. What appears to be a light amount of lochia may be a moderate flow if the peripad has been in use for less than an hour (Fig. 17.2).

The time between delivery and assessment of lochia also is important. Lochia flow will be greater immediately after delivery but will gradually decrease. It is less after cesarean birth because some of the endometrial lining is removed during surgery. The lochia of the woman who had a cesarean birth will go through the same phases as that of the woman who had a vaginal birth, but the amount will be reduced.

Lochia flow is often heavier when the new mother first gets out of bed after birth or after sleeping because gravity allows blood that pooled in the vagina during the hours of rest to flow freely when she stands.

Some women have a sudden, short episode of bleeding 7 to 14 days after birth. This bleeding occurs when the eschar over the placental site sloughs. Increased bleeding lasting longer than 1 to 2 hours should be evaluated by the health care provider (Isley & Katz, 2017).

Cervix

Immediately after childbirth the cervix is dilated, edematous, and bruised. Small tears or lacerations may be present. Rapid healing takes place, and by the end of the first week the external cervical os is 1 cm in diameter (Whitmer, 2016). There

may be some edema for as long as 3 to 4 months (Blackburn, 2013). The internal os closes as before pregnancy, but the shape of the external os is permanently changed. It remains slightly open and appears slitlike rather than round, as in the nulliparous woman.

Vagina

The vagina and vaginal introitus are greatly stretched during birth to allow passage of the fetus. Soon after childbirth, the vaginal walls appear edematous and multiple small lacerations may be present. Very few vaginal rugae are present.

Although rugae begin to reappear by 3 to 4 weeks, 6 to 10 weeks are needed for the vaginal epithelium to be restored. The vagina regains tone and decreases in size, although it does not completely return to the prepregnancy state (Blackburn, 2013).

During the postpartum period, vaginal mucosa becomes atrophic and vaginal walls do not regain their thickness until estrogen production by the ovaries is reestablished. Because ovarian function, and therefore estrogen production, is not well established during lactation, breastfeeding mothers are likely to experience vaginal dryness and may experience **dyspareunia** (discomfort during intercourse).

Perineum

The muscles of the pelvic floor stretch and thin greatly during the second stage of labor, a result of pressure from the fetal head. After childbirth, the perineum may be edematous and bruised. If the woman had an **episiotomy**, a surgical incision of the perineal area, it will begin to heal in 2 to 3 weeks. Complete healing of the episiotomy site may take 4 to 6 months (Blackburn, 2013).

Lacerations of the perineum also may occur during delivery. Lacerations and episiotomies are classified according to tissue involved (Box 17.1). See Chapter 15 for further discussion of episiotomies and lacerations.

Discomfort. Although the episiotomy is relatively small, the muscles of the perineum are involved in many activities (walking, sitting, stooping, squatting, bending, urinating, and defecating). An incision or laceration in this area can cause a great deal of discomfort. In addition, many pregnant women are affected by hemorrhoids (distended rectal veins), which are pushed out of the rectum during the second stage of labor. Hemorrhoids, as well as perineal trauma, can make physical activity or bowel elimination difficult during the postpartum period. Relief of perineal discomfort is a nursing priority. It includes teaching self-care measures such as applying ice, taking sitz baths, performing perineal care, using topical anesthetics and cooling astringent pads, and taking ordered analgesics.

Resumption of Ovulation and Menstruation

Although the first few menstrual cycles for both lactating and nonlactating women are often anovulatory, ovulation may occur before the first menses (Cunningham et al., 2014). For some women, ovulation may resume before their postpartum

BOX 17.1 Lacerations of the Birth Canal

Perineum

Perineal lacerations are classified in degrees to describe the amount of tissue involved. Some physicians or nurse-midwives also use degrees to describe the extent of midline episiotomies.

First-degree—Involves the superficial vaginal mucosa or perineal skin.

Second-degree—Involves the vaginal mucosa, perineal skin, fascia, and muscles of the perineum.

Third-degree—Same as second-degree lacerations but extends into or through the external anal sphincter.

Fourth-degree—Extends through the anal sphincter and into the rectal mucosa.

Periurethral Area

A laceration in the area of the urethra may cause a woman to have difficulty urinating after birth.

An indwelling catheter may be necessary for a day or two.

Vaginal Wall

A laceration involves the mucosa of the vaginal wall.

Cervix

Tears in the cervix may be a source of significant bleeding after birth.

? KNOWLEDGE CHECK

1. Which three processes are involved in involution of the uterus?
2. How is the fundus expected to descend after childbirth?
3. Which mothers are most likely to experience afterpains? How are they treated?
4. What are the differences among lochia rubra, lochia serosa, and lochia alba in appearance and expected duration?
5. When should a woman who is formula feeding her infant expect her menses to resume? When should a woman who is breastfeeding expect her menses to resume?
6. How does breastfeeding affect the resumption of ovulation and menstruation?

---

follow-up appointment. Therefore contraceptive measures are important considerations when sexual relations are resumed for both lactating and nonlactating women. Nonnursing mothers will usually resume menstruation in 6 to 10 weeks (Whitmer, 2016).

Breastfeeding delays the return of both ovulation and menstruation. Menses usually resumes between 10 weeks and 6 months for these mothers (Whitmer, 2016). Generally, women who breastfeed more frequently and use fewer supplements are likely to ovulate and menstruate later than women who breastfeed less often, use more supplements, and wean earlier (Kennedy, 2010). For the woman who is breastfeeding frequently and without supplements, contraception should be used by the time the infant is 6 months old or earlier because ovulation and menses are increasingly likely by that time (Isley & Katz, 2017).

Lactation

During pregnancy, estrogen and progesterone prepare the breasts for lactation. Although prolactin also rises during pregnancy, lactation is inhibited at this time by the high level of estrogen and progesterone. After expulsion of the placenta, estrogen and progesterone levels decline rapidly and prolactin initiates milk production within 2 to 3 days after childbirth. Once milk production is established, it continues because of frequent suckling by the infant and removal of milk from the breast. That is, the more the infant nurses, the more milk the mother produces.

Oxytocin is necessary for milk ejection or "let-down." This hormone causes milk to be expressed from the alveoli into the lactiferous ducts during suckling (see Chapter 22).

Cardiovascular System

Hypervolemia, which produces an average 30% to 45% increase in blood volume at term, allows the woman to tolerate a substantial blood loss during childbirth without ill effect. Up to 500 milliliters (mL) of blood is lost in vaginal deliveries, and up to 1000 mL is lost in cesarean births (Blackburn, 2013).

Cardiac Output

Despite the blood loss, a transient increase in maternal cardiac output occurs after childbirth. This increase is caused by (1) an increased flow of blood back to the heart when blood from the uteroplacental unit returns to the central circulation, (2) decreased pressure from the pregnant uterus on the vessels which increases blood return to the heart, and (3) the mobilization of excess extracellular fluid into the vascular compartment.

The rise in cardiac output returns to prelabor values within an hour after delivery. Gradually, cardiac output returns to prepregnancy levels in most women by 6 to 12 weeks after childbirth (Blackburn, 2013).

Plasma Volume

The body rids itself of the excess plasma volume needed during pregnancy by diuresis and diaphoresis.

- Diuresis (increased excretion of urine) is facilitated by a decline in the adrenal hormone aldosterone and a decrease in oxytocin. A urinary output of up to 3000 mL/day may occur, especially on days 2 through 5 postpartum (Blackburn, 2013).
- Diaphoresis (profuse perspiration) also rids the body of excess fluid. It can be uncomfortable and unsettling for the mother who is not prepared for it. Explanations of the cause and provision of comfort measures such as showers and dry clothing are generally sufficient.

Hematologic System

Several components of the blood change during the postpartum period. Marked leukocytosis may occur, with the white blood cell (WBC) count increasing to as high as 30,000/mm³ during labor and the immediate postpartum period (Cunningham et al., 2014). Although the increased WBC count is not usually caused by infection, an increase of over 30% within 6 hours may indicate infection (Whitmer, 2016). The WBC count falls to normal values by 6 days after birth (Blackburn, 2013).

Maternal hemoglobin (Hgb) and hematocrit (Hct) values are difficult to interpret during the first few days after birth because of the remobilization and rapid excretion of excess body fluid. The Hct is low when plasma increases and dilutes the concentration of blood cells and other substances carried by the plasma. As excess fluid is excreted, the dilution is gradually reduced. The Hct should return to normal limits within 4 to 6 weeks unless excessive blood loss has occurred (Blackburn, 2013).

Coagulation

During pregnancy, plasma fibrinogen and other factors necessary for coagulation increase. As a result the mother's body has a greater ability to form clots and thus prevent excessive bleeding. Fibrinolytic activity is decreased during pregnancy. Elevations in clotting factors continue for several days or longer, causing a continued risk for thrombus formation. It takes 4 to 6 weeks before the hemostasis returns to normal nonpregnant levels (Blackburn, 2013). Although the incidence of thrombophlebitis has declined greatly as a result of early postpartum ambulation, new mothers are still at increased risk for thrombus formation (see Chapter 18). If needed, thromboprophylaxis can be pharmacologic with the use of anticoagulation agents or mechanical agents such as intermittent pneumatic compression devices or graduated compression stockings (Bain et al., 2014).

Gastrointestinal System

Soon after childbirth, digestion begins to be active. The new mother is usually hungry because of the energy expended in labor. She is thirsty because of decreased oral intake during labor and fluid loss from exertion, mouth breathing, and early diaphoresis.

Constipation is a common problem during the postpartum period for a variety of reasons. Bowel tone and motility, which were diminished during pregnancy as a result of progesterone, remain sluggish for several days. In addition, relaxation of the abdominal muscles increases constipation and distention with gas. Decreased food and fluid intake during labor often results in small, hard stools. Perineal trauma, episiotomy, and hemorrhoids cause discomfort and interfere with effective bowel elimination. Many women anticipate pain when they attempt to defecate and are unwilling to exert pressure on the perineum. Women who are taking iron have an added cause of constipation.

Temporary constipation is not harmful, although it can cause a feeling of abdominal fullness and flatulence. Stool softeners and laxatives frequently are prescribed to prevent or treat constipation. The first stool usually occurs within 2 to 3 days postpartum. Normal patterns of bowel elimination generally resume by 8 to 14 days after birth (Blackburn, 2013).

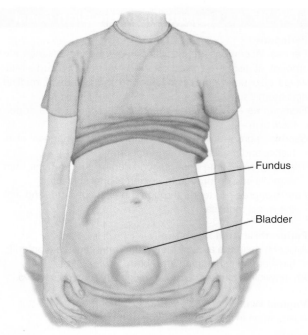

FIG. 17.3 A full bladder displaces and prevents contraction of the uterus.

Urinary System

The kidneys return to normal function by 4 weeks after delivery (Whitmer, 2016). The dilation of the renal pelvis and the ureters that occurs during pregnancy ends within 2 to 8 weeks (Cunningham et al., 2014). Both protein and acetone may be present in the urine for the first few postpartum days secondary to the catabolic processes involved in uterine involution and dehydration that often occurs during the exertion of labor.

Changes during pregnancy cause the bladder of postpartum women to have increased capacity and decreased muscle tone. During childbirth, the urethra, bladder, and tissue around the urinary meatus may become edematous and traumatized. The result is often diminished sensitivity to fluid pressure, and many new mothers have little or no sensation of needing to void even when the bladder is distended.

The bladder fills rapidly because of the diuresis that follows childbirth. It is not unusual for a postpartum woman to void 500 to 1000 mL at a time (Blackburn, 2013). The woman is at risk for overdistention of the bladder, incomplete emptying of the bladder, and retention of residual urine. Urinary retention is more common after the first vaginal delivery, regional anesthesia, and catheterization before delivery. Retention occurs in 1.7% to 17.9% of postpartum women (Blackburn, 2013).

Urinary retention and overdistention of the bladder may cause urinary tract infection (UTI) and increased postpartum bleeding. UTI occurs when urinary stasis allows time for bacteria to multiply. Risk for bleeding increases because uterine ligaments, which were stretched during pregnancy, allow the uterus to be displaced upward and laterally by the full bladder (Fig. 17.3). The displacement results in decreased contraction of the uterine muscles (uterine **atony**), a primary cause of excessive bleeding.

Stress incontinence may occur during pregnancy or after giving birth. Approximately one-third of women have urinary incontinence at 8 weeks postpartum, but only approximately 15% of postpartum women still have a problem at 12 weeks (Isley & Katz, 2017). For some women, the problem resolves with pelvic floor exercises and time for healing. Others may have continued problems.

Musculoskeletal System
Muscles and Joints

In the first 1 to 2 days after childbirth, many women experience muscle fatigue and aches, particularly of the shoulders, neck, and arms, because of exertion during labor. Warmth and gentle massage increase circulation to the area and provide comfort and relaxation.

During the first few days, levels of the hormone relaxin gradually subside, and ligaments and cartilage of the pelvis begin to return to their prepregnancy positions. These changes can cause hip and joint pain that interferes with ambulation and exercise. The mother should be told that the discomfort is temporary and does not indicate a medical problem. Good body mechanics and correct posture are important during this time to help prevent low back pain and injury to the joints.

Abdominal Wall

During pregnancy, the abdominal walls stretch to accommodate the growing fetus and muscle tone is diminished. Many women, expecting the abdomen to return to the prepregnancy condition immediately after childbirth, are dismayed to find the abdominal muscles weak, soft, and flabby.

In addition, the longitudinal muscles of the abdomen may separate (**diastasis recti**) during pregnancy (Fig. 17.4). The separation may be minimal or extensive but is usually 2 to 4 cm (1 to 2.5 inches) (Whitmer, 2016). The new mother may benefit from gentle exercises to strengthen the abdominal wall, which usually returns to normal position by 6 weeks after birth (Whitmer, 2016; Fig. 17.5).

Integumentary System

Many skin changes that occur during pregnancy are caused by an increase in hormones. When estrogen, progesterone, and melanocyte-stimulating hormones decline after childbirth, the skin gradually reverts to the nonpregnant state. This change is particularly noticeable when melasma, the "mask of pregnancy," and linea nigra fade and disappear for many women. In addition, spider nevi and palmar erythema, which may develop during pregnancy as a result of increased estrogen level, gradually disappear.

Striae gravidarum (stretch marks), which develop during pregnancy when connective tissues in the abdomen and breasts are stretched, gradually fade to silvery lines but do not

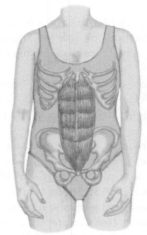
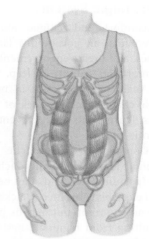

Normal location of rectus muscles of the abdomen

Diastasis recti: separation of the rectus muscles

FIG. 17.4 Diastasis recti occurs when the longitudinal muscles of the abdomen separate during pregnancy.

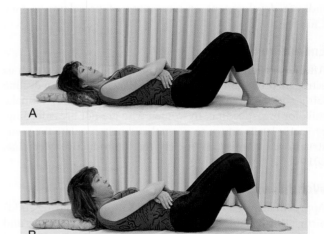

FIG. 17.5 Abdominal Exercises for Diastasis Recti. **A,** The woman inhales and supports the abdominal wall firmly with her hands. **B,** Exhaling, the woman raises her head as she pulls the abdominal muscles together.

disappear. Loss of hair may especially concern the woman. This is a normal response to the hormonal changes that caused decreased hair loss during pregnancy. Hair loss begins at 4 to 20 weeks after delivery and is regrown in 4 to 6 months for two-thirds of women and by 15 months for the remainder of women (Blackburn, 2013).

> ### KNOWLEDGE CHECK
>
> 7. Should the nurse be concerned if a woman who delivered a baby yesterday has a WBC count of 16,000/mm³? Why, or why not?
> 8. Why is the mother at risk for urinary retention? Which two complications may result?
> 9. Why does hyperpigmentation decrease after childbirth?

Neurologic System

Discomfort and fatigue after childbirth are common. Afterpains, an episiotomy, laceration, or incision, muscle aches, and breast engorgement may increase a woman's discomfort and inability to sleep.

Analgesia or anesthesia may cause temporary neurologic changes such as lack of feeling in the legs and dizziness. During this time, prevention of injury from falling is a priority.

Complaints of headache require careful assessment. Frontal and bilateral headaches are common in the first postpartum week and may be a result of changes in fluid and electrolyte balance (Blackburn, 2013). Severe headaches are not common but may be postdural puncture headaches resulting from regional anesthesia (see Chapter 13). They may be most severe when the woman is in an upright position and are relieved by assuming the supine position. They should be reported to the appropriate health care provider, usually an anesthesiologist. Headache, along with blurred vision, photophobia, proteinuria, and abdominal pain, may indicate development or worsening of preeclampsia (see Chapter 10).

Endocrine System

After expulsion of the placenta, placental hormones such as estrogen, progesterone, and human placental lactogen decline fairly rapidly. High prolactin levels trigger the body to make milk for breastfeeding. In women who are not breastfeeding, prolactin levels return to normal and help regulate the menstrual cycle (American Society for Reproductive Medicine, 2014).

Weight Loss

Approximately 4.5 to 5.8 kg (10 to 13 lb) is lost during childbirth. This includes the weight of the fetus, placenta, and amniotic fluid and blood lost during the birth. An additional 2.3 to 3.6 kilograms (kg) (5 to 8 lb) are lost as a result of diuresis and 0.9 kg to 1.4 kg (2 to 3 lb) from involution and lochia by the end of the first week (Blackburn, 2013).

Weight loss continues with the greatest loss during the first 3 months. If the mother's weight gain during pregnancy has not been excessive, she will probably lose all but about 1 kg (2.2 lb) within a year if she follows a well-balanced diet. Younger women with lower prepregnant weight lose more weight and lose it sooner than other women (Blackburn, 2013).

Many mothers are frustrated because they want an immediate return to prepregnancy weight. Nurses can provide information about diet and exercise that will produce an acceptable weight loss without depleting the mother's energy or impairing her health (see Chapter 8).

> **? KNOWLEDGE CHECK**
>
> 10. How much weight will the woman lose during childbirth? How much can she expect to lose by the end of the first week after childbirth?

NURSING CARE OF THE POSTPARTUM FAMILY

Postpartum Assessments

Providing essential, cost-effective postpartum care to new families is a challenge for maternity nurses. Most women stay in the birth facility for 48 hours after an uncomplicated vaginal birth and 96 hours after a cesarean birth. Some women choose to go home at an earlier time. Although the length of stay is short, the family's need for care and information is extensive.

Initial Assessments

Postpartum assessments begin during the fourth stage of labor (the first 1 to 2 hours after childbirth). The mother is examined to determine whether she is physically stable. Initial assessments include the following:

- Vital signs
- Skin color
- Location and firmness of the fundus
- Amount and color of lochia
- Perineum (edema, episiotomy, lacerations, hematoma)
- Presence, degree, and location of pain
- Intravenous (IV) infusions—Type of fluid, rate of administration, type and amount of added medications, patency of the IV line, and redness, pain, or edema of the site
- Urinary output—Time and amount of last void or catheterization, presence of a catheter, color and character of urine
- Status of abdominal incision and dressing, if present
- Level of feeling and ability to move if regional anesthesia was administered

Chart Review

When the initial assessments confirm the mother's physical condition is stable, nurses should review the chart to obtain pertinent information and determine whether there are factors that increase the risk for complications during the postpartum period. Relevant information includes the following:

- Gravida, para
- Time and type of delivery (use of vacuum extractor, forceps, cesarean)
- Presence and degree of episiotomy or lacerations
- Anesthesia or medications administered
- Significant medical and surgical history, such as diabetes, hypertension, heart disease
- Medications given during labor or delivery or routinely taken and the reasons for their use
- Food and drug allergies
- Chosen method of infant feeding
- Condition of the baby

Laboratory data also are examined. Of particular interest are the prenatal Hgb and Hct values, blood type and Rh factor, hepatitis B surface antigen, rubella immune status, syphilis screen, and group B *Streptococcus* status.

Risk Factors for Hemorrhage and Infection. Nurses should be aware of conditions that increase the risk for hemorrhage and infection, the two most common complications of puerperium. These risk factors should be identified in hand-off report and in chart review.

CRITICAL TO REMEMBER

Postpartum Risk Factors

Hemorrhage
- Grand multiparity (five or more)
- Overdistention of the uterus (large baby, twins, hydramnios)
- Precipitous labor (less than 3 hours)
- Prolonged labor
- Retained placenta
- Placenta previa or accreta or placental abruption
- Drugs (tocolytics, magnesium sulfate, general anesthesia, prolonged use of oxytocin)
- Operative procedures (cesarean birth, vacuum extraction, forceps)

Infection
- Operative procedures (cesarean birth, vacuum extraction, forceps)
- Multiple cervical examinations
- Prolonged labor
- Prolonged rupture of membranes
- Manual extraction of placenta or retained fragments
- Diabetes
- Catheterization
- Bacterial colonization of lower genital tract

Need for Rho(D) Immune Globulin. Prenatal and neonatal records are checked to determine whether Rho(D) immune globulin should be administered. It may be necessary if the mother is Rh-negative, the newborn is Rh-positive, and the mother is not already sensitized. Rho(D) immune globulin should be administered within 72 hours after childbirth to prevent the development of maternal antibodies that would affect subsequent pregnancies.

Immunizations

Rubella Vaccine. A prenatal rubella antibody screen is performed on each pregnant woman to determine whether she is immune to rubella. If she is not immune, rubella vaccine is recommended after childbirth to prevent her from acquiring rubella during subsequent pregnancies, when it can cause serious fetal anomalies.

There is a theoretic risk for fetal defects if the rubella vaccine is administered during pregnancy because the vaccine is a live virus. Therefore women are advised not to become pregnant for at least 28 days after receiving the vaccine (Centers for Disease Control and Prevention [CDC], 2016; Hamborsky, Kroger, & Wolfe, 2015). The nurse should document in the chart that the risk has been explained and the parents have verbalized their understanding.

DRUG GUIDE

Rubella Vaccine
Classification
Attenuated live virus vaccine.

Action
Produces a modified rubella (German measles) infection that is not communicable, causing the formation of antibodies against rubella virus.

Indications for Childbearing Women
Administered at least 28 days before pregnancy or after childbirth or abortion to women whose antibody screen shows they are not immune to rubella. This vaccine prevents rubella infection and possible severe congenital defects in the fetus during a subsequent pregnancy.

Dosage and Route
0.5 mL subcutaneously.

Absorption
Well absorbed.

Contraindications and Precautions
The vaccine is contraindicated in women who are immuno-suppressed, pregnant, or sensitive to vaccine component or have a moderate or severe illness. The attenuated virus may appear in breast milk, and some infants may develop a rash, but this is not a contraindication to vaccination of lactating women. It can be given near the time of Rho(D) immune globulin administration. Women receiving the vaccine should be tested for immune status at 6 to 8 weeks to verify immunity.

Adverse Reactions
Transient stinging at site, fever, lymphadenopathy, arthralgia, and transient arthritis are most common.

Nursing Implications
Vials should be refrigerated. Reconstitute only with diluent supplied with the vial. Use immediately after reconstitution and discard if not used within 8 hours. Protect from light. Check with health care provider before giving near time of administration of Rho(D) immune globulin. Birth of infants with congenital rubella syndrome has not been documented when the vaccine has been given inadvertently during pregnancy, but women are advised to avoid pregnancy for at least 4 weeks after vaccination.

From Centers for Disease Control and Prevention [CDC]. (2015). *Epidemiology and prevention of vaccine-preventable diseases* (13th ed.). In J. Hamborsky, A. Kroger, & S. Wolfe (Eds.). Washington, DC: Public Health Foundation.

Pertussis Vaccine. Recent outbreaks of pertussis have had serious effects in infants and young children. Although most adults were vaccinated as children, the effectiveness fades with time. Full protection of vaccinated infants does not occur until the entire series is completed. The CDC (2015) recommends that all adults in contact with infants and young children get a booster dose of pertussis vaccine. It is usually administered along with diphtheria and tetanus vaccines

(Tdap). (See the CDC website at www.cdc.gov/vaccines for current information.)

Varicella Vaccine. Varicella (chicken pox) in pregnant women can cause infection and serious complications in the fetus and newborn. Therefore the American Association of Pediatricians (AAP) and American College of Obstetricians and Gynecologists (AAP & ACOG, 2012) recommend that women who are not immune to varicella should receive the first dose of varicella vaccine after delivery and before discharge from the birth facility. They should be advised not to become pregnant for 1 month after receiving the vaccine.

Focused Assessments after Vaginal Birth

Nurses perform postpartum assessments according to facility protocol. For example, a protocol might require assessment as follows:

- Every 15 minutes for the first hour
- Every 30 minutes for the second hour
- Every 4 hours for the first 24 hours
- Every 8 to 12 hours thereafter

Assessments are made more frequently if findings are abnormal or the mother has additional risk factors. Although assessments vary depending on the particular problems presented, a focused assessment for a vaginal delivery generally includes the vital signs, fundal height and tone, lochia, perineum, bladder elimination, breasts, and lower extremities. The assessment for women who had a cesarean birth is more extensive.

Vital Signs

Blood Pressure. Blood pressure (BP) varies with position and the arm used. To obtain accurate results BP should be measured on the same arm with the mother in the same position each time. Postpartum BP should be compared with that of the predelivery period so that deviations from what is normal for the mother can be quickly identified. An increase from the baseline may be caused by pain or anxiety. If the BP is 140/90 mm Hg or higher, preeclampsia may be present. A decrease may indicate dehydration or hypovolemia resulting from excessive bleeding.

Orthostatic Hypotension. After birth a rapid decrease in intraabdominal pressure results in dilation of blood vessels supplying the viscera. The resulting engorgement of abdominal blood vessels contributes to a rapid fall in BP of 15 to 20 mm Hg systolic when the woman moves from the recumbent position to the sitting position. This change causes mothers to feel dizzy or lightheaded or to faint when they stand.

Hypotension also may indicate hypovolemia. Careful assessments for hemorrhage (location and firmness of the fundus, amount of lochia, pulse rate for tachycardia) should be made if the postpartum BP is significantly less than the prenatal baseline.

Pulse. Bradycardia, defined as a pulse rate of 40 to 50 beats per minute (bpm), may occur. The lower pulse rate may reflect the large amount of blood that returns to the central circulation after delivery of the placenta. The increase in central circulation results in increased stroke volume and allows a slower heart rate to provide adequate maternal circulation.

Tachycardia may indicate pain, excitement, anxiety, fatigue, dehydration, hypovolemia, anemia, or infection. If tachycardia is noted, additional assessments should include degree of pain, BP, location and firmness of the uterus, amount of lochia, estimated blood loss at delivery, and Hgb and Hct values. The objective of the additional assessments is to rule out excessive bleeding and to intervene at once if hemorrhage is suspected.

Respirations. A normal respiratory rate of 12 to 20 breaths per minute should be maintained. Assessing breath sounds is especially important for mothers who have a cesarean birth, are smokers, or have frequent or recent upper respiratory tract infections or asthma or are receiving magnesium sulfate.

Temperature. A temperature of up to 38°C (100.4°F) is common during the first 24 hours after childbirth and may be caused by dehydration or normal postpartum leukocytosis. If the elevated temperature persists for longer than 24 hours, it exceeds 38°C (100.4°F), or the woman shows other signs of infection, the nurse should report it to the physician or nurse-midwife.

Pain. Pain should be assessed along with other vital signs to determine the type, location, and severity on a pain scale. Some new mothers are too excited by the birth of their child to complain of discomfort. Others do not want to "bother the nurse" or may be from cultures in which complaining is not acceptable. Nurses should remain alert to signs of pain or discomfort. Nonspecific signs of discomfort include an inability to relax or sleep, a change in vital signs, restlessness, irritability, and facial grimaces. The nurse should encourage women to take prescribed medications as needed and should also assess the effectiveness of pain-relief measures.

Fundus. The fundus should be assessed for consistency and location (Procedure 17.1). It should be firmly contracted and at or near the level of the umbilicus. If the uterus is above the expected level or shifted from the middle of the abdomen or midline position (usually to the right), the bladder may be distended. The location of the fundus should be rechecked after the woman has emptied her bladder.

If the fundus is difficult to locate or is soft or "boggy," the nurse stimulates the uterine muscle to contract by gently massaging the uterus. The nondominant hand should support and anchor the lower uterine segment during palpation and massage. Uterine massage is not necessary if the uterus is firmly contracted.

The uterus can continue to contract only if it is free of intrauterine clots. To expel clots, the nurse should support the lower uterine segment and massage the fundus until firm, as illustrated in Procedure 17.1. This support helps prevent inversion of the uterus (turning inside out) when the nurse applies firm pressure downward toward the vagina to express clots that have collected in the uterus. Nurses should observe the perineum for the number and size of clots expelled. If lochia is excessive or large clots are expelled, they should be weighed to estimate amount of blood loss (see Chapter 18). Table 17.2 describes normal and abnormal findings of the

NURSING PROCEDURE 17.1   Assessing the Uterine Fundus

PURPOSE: To determine the location and firmness of the uterus.

1. Explain the procedure and rationale before beginning the procedure. *Explanations reduce anxiety and elicit cooperation.*
2. Ask the mother to empty her bladder if she has not voided recently. *A distended bladder lifts and displaces the uterus.*
3. Place the mother in the supine position with her knees flexed. *This relaxes the abdominal muscles and permits accurate location of the fundus.*
4. Put on clean gloves and lower the perineal pad to observe lochia as the fundus is palpated. *Gloves are recommended whenever contact with body fluids may occur.*
5. Place your nondominant hand above the woman's symphysis pubis. *This supports and anchors the lower uterine segment.*

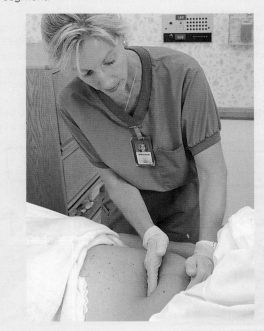

6. Use the flat part of your fingers (not the fingertips) for palpation. Palpation may be painful, particularly for the mother who had a cesarean birth. *The larger surface of the fingers provides more comfort.*
7. Begin palpation at the umbilicus and palpate gently until the fundus is located. It should be firm, in the midline, and approximately at the level of the umbilicus. Locating the fundus is more difficult if the woman is obese or if the abdomen is distended. *Palpation helps determine the firmness and location of the fundus.*
8. If the fundus is difficult to locate or is "boggy," (soft) keep the nondominant hand above the woman's symphysis pubis and massage the fundus with the dominant hand until the fundus is firm. *The nondominant hand anchors the lower segment of the uterus and prevents inversion while the uterus is massaged. The uterus contracts in response to tactile stimulation, and this helps control excessive bleeding.*
9. After massaging a boggy fundus until it is firm, press firmly to expel clots. Do not attempt to expel clots before the fundus is firm. Keep one hand pressed just above the symphysis (over the lower uterine segment) throughout. *Removing clots allows the uterus to contract properly. Attempting to expel clots in a boggy uterus might result in uterine inversion. A firm fundus and pressure over the lower uterine segment help prevent uterine inversion.*
10. If the fundus is above or below the umbilicus, use your fingers to determine the number of fingerbreadths between the fundus and the umbilicus. *Using the fingers to measure allows an approximation of the number of centimeters.*
11. Document the consistency and location of the fundus. Record consistency as "fundus firm," "firm with massage," or "boggy." Record fundal height in fingerbreadths or centimeters above or below the umbilicus. For example, "fundus firm, midline, ↓1" (one fingerbreadth or 1 cm below the umbilicus); "fundus firm with light massage, U +2 (two fingerbreadths or 2 cm above the umbilicus), displaced to right." *This promotes accurate communication and identifies deviations from expected so that potential problems can be identified early.*

TABLE 17.2   Assessments of the Uterine Fundus and Nursing Actions

Normal Findings	Abnormal Findings	Nursing Actions
Fundus is firmly contracted.	Fundus is soft, "boggy," uncontracted, or difficult to locate.	Support lower uterine segment. Massage until firm.
Fundus remains contracted when massage is discontinued.	Fundus becomes soft and uncontracted when massage is stopped.	Continue to support lower uterine segment. Massage fundus until firm; then apply pressure to express clots. Notify health care provider, and begin oxytocin or other drug administration, as prescribed, to maintain a firm fundus.
Fundus is located at or below the level of umbilicus and midline.	Fundus is above umbilicus and/or displaced from midline.	Assess bladder elimination. Assist mother in urinating, or catheterize, if necessary, to empty bladder. Recheck the position and consistency of fundus after bladder is empty.

uterine fundus and includes follow-up nursing actions for abnormal findings.

Drugs are sometimes needed to maintain contraction of the uterus and thus prevent postpartum hemorrhage. The most commonly used drug is oxytocin (Pitocin). Other drugs for excessive postpartum bleeding are discussed in Chapter 18.

Lochia. Important assessments include the amount, color, and odor of lochia. Nurses observe the lochia on peripads and while checking the perineum. They also assess vaginal discharge while palpating or massaging the fundus to determine the amount of lochia and the number and size of any clots expressed during these procedures. Important guidelines include the following:

- A constant trickle, dribble, or oozing of lochia indicates excessive bleeding and requires immediate attention.
- Excessive lochia in the presence of a contracted uterus suggests lacerations of the birth canal. The health care provider should be notified so that lacerations can be located and repaired.

The odor of lochia is usually described as fleshy, earthy, or musty. A foul odor suggests endometrial infection, and assessments should be made for additional signs of infection. These signs include maternal fever, tachycardia, uterine tenderness, and pain.

Absence of lochia, like the presence of a foul odor, may indicate infection. If the birth was cesarean, lochia may be scant because the uterine cavity was wiped by sponges, removing some of the endometrial lining. Lochia should not be entirely absent, however.

Perineum. The acronym REEDA is used as a reminder that the site of an episiotomy or a perineal laceration should be assessed for five signs: redness (R), edema (E), ecchymosis (E), discharge (D), and approximation (A). Redness of the wound may indicate the usual inflammatory response to injury. If accompanied by excessive pain or tenderness, however, it may indicate the beginning of localized infection. Ecchymosis or edema indicates soft tissue damage that can delay healing. No discharge should come from the wound. Rapid healing requires that the edges of the wound be closely approximated (Procedure 17.2 describes the perineal examination.)

Bladder Elimination. Because the mother may not experience the urge to void even if the bladder is full, nurses should rely on physical assessment to determine whether the bladder is distended. Bladder distention often produces an obvious or palpable bulge that feels like a soft, movable mass above the symphysis pubis. Other signs include an upward and lateral displacement of the uterine fundus and increased lochia. Frequent voids of less than 150 mL suggest urinary retention. Signs of an empty bladder include a firm fundus in the midline and a nonpalpable bladder.

Two to three voids should be measured after birth or the removal of a catheter to determine whether normal bladder function has returned. When the mother can void at least 300 to 400 mL, the bladder is usually empty. Regardless of the amount voided, if the fundus was displaced when assessed, it should be assessed again after the woman voids to confirm

NURSING PROCEDURE 17.2   Assessing the Perineum

PURPOSE: To assess perineal trauma and the state of healing.

1. Provide privacy and explain the purpose of the procedure. *This elicits cooperation and reduces anxiety.*
2. Put on clean gloves. *Implements standard precautions to provide protection from possible contact with body fluids.*
3. Ask the mother to assume the Sims (side-lying) position and flex her upper leg. Lower the perineal pads, and lift her superior buttock. If necessary, use a flashlight to inspect the perineal area. *Position provides an unobstructed view of the perineum and allows assessment of lochia that may be under the mother; light allows better visualization.*
4. Note the extent and location of edema or bruising. *Extensive bruising or asymmetric edema may indicate formation of a hematoma.*
5. Examine the episiotomy or laceration for redness, ecchymosis, edema, discharge, and approximation (REEDA). *Redness, edema, or discharge may indicate infection of the wound; extensive bruising may delay healing; wound edges should be in direct contact for uncomplicated healing to occur.*
6. Note the number and size of hemorrhoids. *Swollen, painful hemorrhoids interfere with activity and bowel elimination.*

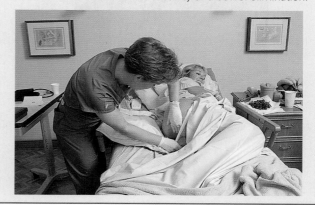

that the bladder is empty. Subjective symptoms of urgency, frequency, or dysuria suggest UTI and should be reported to the health care provider.

Breasts. For the first day or two after delivery, the breasts should be soft and nontender. After that, breast changes depend largely on whether the mother is breastfeeding. The breasts should be examined even if she chooses formula feeding because engorgement may occur despite preventive measures. The size, symmetry, and shape of the breasts should be observed. The skin should be inspected for dimpling or thickening, which, although rare, can indicate a breast tumor.

The areola and nipple should be carefully examined for potential problems such as flat or retracted nipples, which may make breastfeeding more difficult. Signs of nipple trauma (redness, blisters, or fissures) may be noted during the first days of breastfeeding, especially if the mother needs assistance in positioning the infant correctly (see Chapter 22).

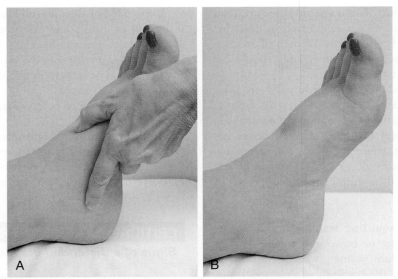

FIG. 17.6 Pedal Edema. A, Apply pressure to foot. B, "Pit" appears when fluid moves into adjacent tissue and away from point of pressure.

The breasts should be palpated for firmness and tenderness, which indicate increased vascular and lymphatic circulation that may precede milk production. The breasts may feel "lumpy" as various lobes begin to produce milk.

The breast assessment is an excellent opportunity to provide information or reassurance about breast care and breastfeeding techniques. It is also an opportunity to teach the mother how to assess her own breasts so she can continue after discharge.

Lower Extremities. The legs are examined for varicosities and signs or symptoms of thrombophlebitis. Indications of thrombophlebitis include localized areas of redness, heat, edema, and tenderness. Pedal pulses may be obstructed by a thrombus and should be palpated with each assessment (see Chapter 18).

Edema and Deep Tendon Reflexes. Pedal or pretibial edema may be present for the first few days, until excess interstitial fluid is remobilized and excreted. (Fig. 17.6 shows how to assess for pitting edema.) Diuresis is highest between the 2nd and 5th days after birth. Fluid and electrolyte balance should return to nonpregnant status by 21 days (Blackburn, 2013).

Deep tendon reflexes should be 1+ to 2+. Report brisker-than-average and hyperactive reflexes (3+ to 4+), which suggest preeclampsia (see Procedure 10.1 for a description of assessing deep tendon reflexes).

❓ KNOWLEDGE CHECK

11. What causes orthostatic hypotension? What are the typical signs and symptoms of orthostatic hypotension?
12. What additional assessments are necessary when tachycardia is noted? Why?
13. When is uterine massage necessary? How is the uterus supported during massage?
14. What does excessive bleeding suggest when the uterus is firmly contracted?

Interventions in the Immediate Postpartum Period

Care of the mother during the immediate postpartum period focuses on physiologic safety of the mother (discussed previously), comfort measures, bladder elimination, and health education.

Providing Comfort Measures

Both cold and warmth are used to alleviate perineal pain after childbirth.

Ice Packs. Ice causes vasoconstriction and is most effective if applied soon after the birth to prevent edema and numb the area. Chemical ice packs and plastic bags or nonlatex gloves filled with ice may be used after a vaginal birth. The ice pack is wrapped in a washcloth or paper before it is applied to the perineum. It should be left in place until the ice melts. It is removed for 10 minutes before a fresh pack is applied. Some peripads have cold packs incorporated in them. Condensation from ice may dilute lochia and make it appear heavier than it actually is.

Although some women may prefer to use cool gel pads or ice, there is limited evidence of the overall effectiveness of these to relieve pain (East, Begg, Henshall, Marchant, & Wallace, 2012) and women may need to combine the use of topical applications with analgesia. Care should be taken for women who are still numb from an epidural as they cannot feel how cold the area becomes.

Sitz Baths. In some facilities, sitz baths may be offered two to four times a day to women with episiotomies, painful hemorrhoids, or perineal lacerations or edema. Sitz baths provide continuous circulation of water, cleansing and comforting the traumatized perineum. Cool water reduces pain caused by edema and may be most effective within the first 24 hours. Ice can be added to cool the water to a comfortable level as the woman sits in it. Warm water increases circulation, promotes healing, and may be most effective after 24 hours. Nurses should be sure that the emergency call light is within easy reach in case the mother feels faint during the sitz bath. Women often take the disposable sitz bath container home. They should be instructed to clean it well between uses.

Analgesics. Mothers should be encouraged to take prescribed medications for afterpains and perineal discomfort. Many analgesics are combinations that include acetaminophen. The nurse should be careful that the woman receives no more than 4 grams of acetaminophen in a 24-hour period. Nonsteroidal antiinflammatory drugs such as ibuprofen are often prescribed because of their antiinflammatory effects.

Perineal Care

Perineal care consists of squirting warm water over the perineum after each voiding or bowel movement. This is important for all postpartum women whether the birth was vaginal or by cesarean. The bottle should not touch the perineum. Perineal care cleanses, provides comfort, and prevents infection of an area that often has an episiotomy or lacerations. The perineum is gently patted dry rather than wiped dry.

Topical Medications. Local anesthetic decreases surface discomfort. It is available as a spray or foam. The mother is instructed to hold the nozzle of the spray 6 to 12 inches from her body and direct it toward the perineum. The spray should be used after perineal care and before clean pads are applied. Foam is placed directly on the clean perineal pad. Astringent compresses should be placed directly over the hemorrhoids to relieve pain. Hydrocortisone ointments may also be applied over hemorrhoids to increase comfort.

Sitting Measures. The mother should be advised to squeeze her buttocks together before sitting and to lower her weight slowly onto her buttocks. This measure prevents stretching of the perineal tissue and avoids sharp impact to the traumatized area. Sitting slightly to the side is also helpful to prevent the full weight from resting on the episiotomy site.

Promoting Bladder Elimination

Many new mothers have difficulty voiding because of edema and trauma of the perineum and diminished sensitivity to fluid pressure in the bladder. As soon as they are able to ambulate safely, mothers should be assisted to the bathroom. Providing privacy and allowing adequate time for the first voiding are important. Common measures to promote relaxation of the perineal muscles and stimulate the sensation of needing to void include the following:

- Medicating the woman for pain to help her relax
- Running water in the sink or shower, placing the mother's hands in warm water, and pouring water over the vulva
- Providing hot tea or fluids of choice
- Asking the mother to blow bubbles through a straw
- Helping the woman into the shower or sitz bath and encouraging her to void there

A nonpalpable bladder and firm fundus at or below the umbilicus and in the midline confirm that the bladder is empty and rule out urinary retention with overflow.

A distended bladder lifts and displaces the uterus, making it difficult for it to remain contracted. The resulting uterine atony permits excessive bleeding. In addition, stasis of urine in the bladder predisposes the woman to UTI. Therefore the mother should be catheterized in the following situations:

- She is unable to void.
- The amount voided is less than 150 mL, and the bladder can be palpated.
- The fundus is elevated or displaced from the midline.

Repeated catheterizations increase the chance of UTI. An indwelling catheter may be ordered for 24 hours if edema is excessive or catheterization is necessary more than once or twice.

CRITICAL TO REMEMBER

Signs of a Distended Bladder

Location of the fundus above the baseline level (determined when the bladder is empty)
Fundus displaced to the side from midline
Excessive lochia
Bladder discomfort
Bulge of bladder above symphysis
Frequent voidings of less than 150 mL of urine, which may indicate urinary retention with overflow

---

❓ CRITICAL THINKING EXERCISE 17.1

Lani has made good progress since she delivered her first baby yesterday morning by cesarean. Her patient-controlled analgesia was discontinued 4 hours ago. Her Foley catheter was removed 3 hours ago, and she was medicated with two Vicodin (hydrocodone 5 mg/acetaminophen 500 mg) tablets for pain 1 hour ago. Now she is wincing and moaning with pain and asking for more pain medication. She says she ambulated to the bathroom with her husband's help a short time after her catheter was removed and urinated but did not measure it. Her fundus is slightly above the umbilicus and slightly to the right. A thick pressure dressing covers the lower abdomen making it difficult to palpate the bladder. Lani says she does not have to urinate.

Questions
1. What other assessments should the nurse make?
2. What should the nurse do?
3. What are possible causes of Lani's pain?

Providing Fluids and Food

Adequate fluids help restore the balance altered by fluid loss during labor and the birth process. Women should be encouraged to drink approximately 2500 mL of fluids each day. Offering ice water or cold drinks may be culturally inappropriate for some women, others may prefer hot or room-temperature water instead. If a woman is unable to tolerate oral fluids, IV administration may be necessary. Women usually are able to have ice chips soon after cesarean birth, and, although protocols vary, most are able to progress to a regular diet in a short time.

New mothers generally have a hearty appetite, and nurses should encourage healthy food choices with respect for ethnic background. Meals and snacks should be available at all times.

Preventing Thrombophlebitis

The woman should be assisted to ambulate early after childbirth to prevent the development of thrombi. Frequent trips to the bathroom will help accomplish this.

Nursing Care after Cesarean Birth

In 2015, 32% of births in the United States were by cesarean delivery (Martin, Hamilton, Osterman, Driscoll, & Mathews, 2017). These mothers must recover from childbirth as well as from major surgery and need special care. The usual length of stay after a cesarean birth is 72 to 96 hours after surgery.

Pain Relief

Assessment of pain and the effectiveness of pain relief is important to the nursing care of women after cesarean birth. These women differ from typical postoperative patients in four important ways. First, they often are eager to be alert so they can interact with their newborn infants. Second, they are concerned the analgesics they receive may pass into their breast milk and harm their infants. Third, compared with other postoperative patients, after cesarean births, the women want to have more input and control of their care. Fourth, they are often healthier than patients who had surgery to correct a problem.

Pain relief is provided in various ways. Patient-controlled analgesia (PCA) is administered by continuous IV infusion of a low-concentration narcotic solution using a pump specifically designed for that purpose. If analgesia is insufficient, the woman can self-administer intermittent small doses of narcotic from the infusion pump. The machine limits the amount of narcotic available within a specified time interval to prevent an overdose. This allows the woman to have pain relief immediately when she needs it without waiting for a nurse to administer it. Side effects include respiratory depression, itching (pruritus), nausea and vomiting, and urinary retention. Patient-controlled epidural analgesia (PCEA) is also used in the same way.

A single dose of opioid (such as preservative-free morphine or fentanyl) injected into the epidural or subarachnoid space immediately after surgery provides 18 to 24 hours of postcesarean analgesia (see Chapter 13). Itching and nausea are the major side effects. Other side effects are the same as for PCA use. Oral analgesics usually are effective if women need additional pain-relief measures. Occasionally, intramuscular analgesics are needed for one or two doses.

Assessment

In addition to the usual postpartum evaluation, after cesarean birth the mother should be assessed as any other postoperative patient.

Respirations. When mothers receive epidural narcotics for postoperative pain relief, respirations should be assessed

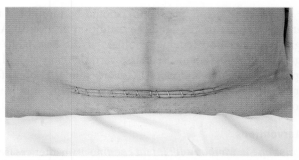

FIG. 17.7 This cesarean incision is closed with staples. Note the absence of all signs of infection, such as redness, edema, bruising (ecchymosis), discharge, and loss of approximation.

frequently because narcotics depress the respiratory center. A pulse oximeter or apnea monitor is used for 18 to 24 hours to detect decreased oxygen saturation from a decreased respiratory rate or depth. Oxygen saturation or respiratory rate is documented hourly or according to facility policy. If a woman receiving epidural narcotics has a respiratory rate of 12 to 14 breaths per minute or less or the pulse oximeter shows a persistent oxygen saturation less than 95%, the nurse should do the following:

- Notify the anesthesia provider..
- Elevate the head of the bed to facilitate lung expansion, and instruct the woman to breathe deeply.
- Administer oxygen, and apply a pulse oximeter (if not already in place).
- Follow facility protocol to administer narcotic antagonists, such as naloxone hydrochloride (Narcan).
- Observe for recurrence of respiratory depression because the duration of naloxone is only approximately 30 minutes.
- Recognize that naloxone may reduce the level of pain relief.

In addition to observing the respiratory rate and depth, the nurse should auscultate the women's breath sounds because depressed respirations and a longer period of immobility allow secretions to pool in the bronchioles.

Abdomen. Nurses assess gastrointestinal function by auscultating for bowel sounds until normal peristalsis is noted in all abdominal quadrants. Although paralytic ileus (lack of movement in the intestines) is rare after cesarean birth, nurses should be aware of the signs. They include abdominal distention, absent or decreased bowel sounds, and failure to pass flatus or stool.

If a surgical dressing is present, it should be assessed for intactness and drainage. When the dressing is removed, nurses observe the incision, which should be approximated, and use the acronym REEDA to assess for signs of infection such as redness and edema (Fig. 17.7). A topical skin adhesive may be used instead of staples. Assessment of the wound is the same.

It is just as important to assess the fundus after cesarean birth as it is with vaginal birth. However, palpation should be gentle because of increased discomfort caused by the abdominal incision.

Intake and Output. The IV line should be monitored for patency, the rate of flow, and the condition of the site. Any signs of infiltration (edema, coolness at the site, pain) or signs of infection (edema, redness, warmth, pain) should be reported. Ice chips and clear fluids are allowed soon after birth. The amount, color, and clarity of urine should be monitored.

Interventions

Assisting the Mother with Infant Feeding. Pain after cesarean may interfere with the mother's ability to breastfeed and care for her infant. Ensuring adequate pain relief is important so the mother can focus on her infant.

It is important to help the mother find a comfortable position for holding and feeding her infant. Some mothers prefer sitting with a pillow on the lap to protect the incisional area. A side-lying position or football hold may be more comfortable because the infant is not putting pressure against the incision (see Chapter 22). A support person or the nurse should be available to help the mother with infant care until she is able to take over herself.

The First 24 Hours. Nursing care for the mother who gave birth by cesarean is similar to that for other postoperative patients.

Providing Pain Relief and Comfort Measures. The nurse should determine the need for pain relief on a regular basis. If a woman has a PCA, the nurse should check how often she is using it. The effectiveness of analgesics should be evaluated. Pain relief enhances the woman's ability to increase her activity, helps prevent thrombophlebitis, and promotes attachment with the baby and healing. For women with epidural or spinal opioids, the nurse should continue to assess the respiratory status. Placing a pillow behind her back and one between her knees prevents strain and discomfort when the woman is lying on her side. Excellent physical care (oral hygiene, perineal care, a sponge bath, clean linen) comforts and refreshes her.

Overcoming Effects of Immobility. The new mother who delivered by cesarean is usually on bed rest for the first 8 to 12 hours. To prevent pooling of secretions in the airways, she should be assisted to turn, cough, and expand the lungs by breathing deeply at least every 2 hours while she is awake. Splinting the abdomen with a small pillow reduces incisional discomfort when she coughs. Incentive spirometers help expand the lungs to prevent hypostatic pneumonia that can result from immobility and shallow, slow respirations.

The woman should be encouraged to flex her knees and to move her legs and feet frequently while she is in bed to improve peripheral circulation and to prevent thrombi. Compression stockings and pneumatic compression devices may be used to prevent the pooling of blood in the lower extremities.

Activity will be gradually increased. The woman needs assistance to sit and dangle her feet for the first few times before she gets out of bed. She should be helped to get out of bed and walk a short distance within 24 hours to decrease risk for thrombi. She will need support ambulating when the IV line and catheter are still in place.

After 24 Hours

Resuming Normal Activities. After 24 hours following a cesarean birth, several normal functions return, and women are able to participate more actively in their own care, as follows:

- Both the indwelling catheter and the IV line are usually discontinued.
- The dressing, if present, is removed in 24 hours. Staples (if present) are removed before discharge. Steri-Strips (small strips of adhesive) may be placed over the incision when staples are removed. A small nonstick dressing may be placed over the incision to protect it from friction from clothing or adipose tissue, or the incision may be left open to air.
- The woman is helped to ambulate by the first postpartum day and is comfortable sitting in a chair for brief periods.
- Clear liquids are changed to a soft or regular diet when bowel sounds are audible or the woman is passing flatus. In some agencies, solids are provided earlier.

Nurses should encourage the woman to increase her activity and ambulation each postpartum day. By the second day, she usually is allowed to shower.

Preventing Abdominal Distention. Abdominal distention is a major source of discomfort. Measures to prevent or minimize it include the following:

- Early, frequent ambulation
- Tightening and relaxing the abdominal muscles
- Avoidance of carbonated beverages and the use of straws, which increase the accumulation of intestinal gas
- Pelvic lifts—Lying supine with her knees bent, the woman lifts her pelvis from the bed and repeats the exercise up to 10 times, several times each day
- Simethicone, as ordered, to help disperse upper gastrointestinal flatulence
- Rectal suppositories, as ordered, to help stimulate peristalsis and passage of flatus

Teaching for Discharge. After cesarean births, mothers receive the same overall teaching as those who had vaginal births. Information about care of the incision and signs to report to the health care provider are added. In addition, women should have support at home because they are recovering from major surgery as well as childbirth.

❓ KNOWLEDGE CHECK

15. What additional assessments are necessary for the mother after a cesarean birth?
16. How can hypostatic pneumonia be prevented?
17. Which nursing measures are used to prevent or minimize abdominal distention?

◆ APPLICATION OF THE NURSING PROCESS: KNOWLEDGE OF SELF-CARE

◆ Assessment

Regardless of the method of birth, nurses are responsible for providing health education before the family is discharged from the birth facility. Much should be taught during this short time, which is not ideal for teaching mothers who are not fully recovered from the birth process.

Before beginning teaching, determine the learning needs and major concerns of the family. Multiparas remember some aspects of self-care but often benefit from a review. Primiparas may be anxious about self-care measures and all aspects of infant care. They may need more thorough teaching and more time for practice. Identify the effects of the most common barriers to learning: age and developmental level, cultural factors, and difficulty understanding the language.

◆ Identification of Patient Problems

In general, women adapt well to the physiologic changes after childbirth, and most nursing care is wellness oriented. A common patient problem is a lack of knowledge of personal care, signs of complications, and preventive measures.

◆ Planning: Expected Outcomes

Expected outcomes for this problem are that the woman will do the following:
- Verbalize or demonstrate understanding of self-care instructions by discharge.
- Verbalize understanding of practices that promote maternal health by discharge.
- Describe plans for follow-up care and signs and symptoms that should be reported to the health care provider by discharge.

◆ Interventions
Preparing for Teaching

Before beginning teaching sessions, be sure the woman is comfortable. Give pain medication, if needed. Schedule the teaching in such a way that it does not interfere with meals, infant care needs, or visiting. Make a teaching plan with the woman to include topics most important to her. Identifying the woman's educational needs ensures her interest in the topics selected and makes best use of the short time available. Topics of less interest may require just a brief review. The review may elicit questions from the mother and interest in more in-depth information.

Teaching about the Process of Involution

Provide the woman with basic information about involution, including how to assess lochia and locate and palpate the fundus. This information allows her to recognize abnormal signs such as prolonged lochia, reappearance of bright-red lochia after lochia rubra has ended, and uterine tenderness, which should be reported to the health care provider. If the mother is a young adolescent, another family member also may need the information.

Teaching Self-Care

Handwashing. Emphasize the importance of thoroughly washing her hands before the woman touches her breasts, after diaper changes, after bladder and bowel elimination, before and after handling peripads, and always before handling the infant. Observing nurses model this behavior reinforces this teaching for parents.

Breast Care for Lactating Mothers. Instruct the breastfeeding mother to avoid using soap on her nipples because it will remove the natural lubrication secreted by the Montgomery's glands. Keeping the nipples dry between feedings helps prevent tissue damage, and wearing a good bra provides necessary support as breast size increases.

Measures to Suppress Lactation. If the mother chooses not to breastfeed, initiate measures to minimize lactation and increase the mother's comfort. Techniques such as binding the breasts, applying an infrared lamp, fluid and diet restrictions, external application of jasmine flower and ice packs have all been used to suppress lactation without convincing evidence. Current recommendations include instructing the woman to wear a firm bra 24 hours a day and express only a small amount of milk if absolutely necessary for pain relief. The woman may use cold compresses or gel packs inside the bra for comfort. Cold cabbage leaves also promote comfort. They should be washed and dried. The large, lumpy veins should be cut out or rolled flat with a rolling pin. The cabbage leaves should then be refrigerated. The woman should place the chilled leaves in her bra and change them out every 2 hours or as they become limp. Analgesic medications may be recommended by the provider (Australian Breastfeeding Association, 2015).

Care of the Cesarean Incision. If the birth was by cesarean, the woman may have concerns about care of the incision. Staples, if used, are usually removed before the woman is discharged. The obese woman may go home with staples and have them removed by the health care provider after discharge. If adhesive strips have been applied over the incision, teach the woman that she can shower with them in place and that they will gradually detach.

If a topical skin adhesive was applied in surgery instead of staples or adhesive strips, there is no dressing, and the woman is generally allowed to shower. For each method, explain that the incision is closed and is unlikely to come apart. There should be little or no drainage from the incision. Instruct her to call her provider if the incision separates or drainage increases or has a foul odor.

Perineal Care. Teach the woman how to clean her perineum. The most common method is to fill a squeeze bottle with warm water and spray the perineal area from the front toward the back. Remind the new mother not to separate the labia during this procedure to avoid allowing water to enter the vagina. The tip of the bottle should not touch the perineum.

Toilet paper or moist antiseptic towelettes are used in a patting motion to dry the perineum. Teach the mother to dry from front to back to prevent fecal contamination of the vaginal introitus from the anal area. She should perform perineal cleansing and change peripads after each voiding or defecation.

Some women do not use peripads for menstrual protection and should be taught how to use them correctly. Mesh panties and adhering pads are used in most facilities. Careful handling to avoid contamination of the pads is important to prevent perineal infection.
- Thorough handwashing is a must before and after changing pads.
- Unused pads should be stored inside their packages.
- Pads should be applied without touching the side that comes into contact with the perineum.

- The pads should be applied and removed in a front-to-back direction to prevent contamination of the vagina and the perineum.
- Used pads should be wrapped and disposed of in a covered container.

Kegel Exercises. All women should become familiar with Kegel exercises. These movements strengthen the muscles that surround the vagina and urinary meatus. The exercise helps prevent the loss of muscle tone that can occur after childbirth and may decrease urinary incontinence.

Promoting Rest and Sleep

Many women experience fatigue after childbirth that continues for weeks or months. Women are often tired when they begin the postpartum period because they slept poorly during the third trimester and are further exhausted by the exertion of labor. Feelings of excitement and euphoria after childbirth interfere with rest. Numerous visitors and phone calls, hospital routines, noise, frequent interruptions, and an unfamiliar environment also interfere with rest. Afterpains, discomfort from an episiotomy or incision, muscle aches, and breast **engorgement** (swelling from increased blood flow, edema, and presence of milk) further contribute to a woman's discomfort and inability to sleep.

Most mothers are discharged from the facility within 24 to 48 hours after vaginal birth or 72 to 96 hours after cesarean birth, and they go home with a tremendous deficit in sleep and energy. Yet new parents may be unprepared for the conflict between their need for sleep and the infant's need for care and attention.

A telephone call to screen mothers for prolonged postpartum fatigue may be helpful in the days after discharge. Anemia, infection, and thyroid dysfunction also may cause postpartum fatigue. Women at risk for these conditions or suffering postpartum fatigue after the first 2 weeks should be evaluated and treated, if necessary.

Rest at the Birth Facility. Hospital routines continue around the clock, making undisturbed rest difficult to obtain during the birth facility stay. Make every effort to avoid interruptions and allow mothers adequate time for unbroken rest periods and relaxed time with their infants.

Cluster assessments and care and try to correlate them with times when the mother will be awake, such as just before or after meals, infant feeding times, and visiting hours

Make plans with the mother for napping. Suggest she restrict phone calls and visitors during planned nap times. Encourage the mother to use a side-lying position for breastfeeding to allow her to rest during feedings. A quiet, softly lit environment also promotes sleep.

Rest at Home. Help the mother understand the impact her physical discomfort and the demands of the newborn and other family members will have on her energy during the first few weeks. If she understands that fatigue is normal and will continue for some time, she can plan ways to obtain extra help and conserve her energy. Suggest energy-saving measures such as the following:

- Maintain a relaxed, flexible routine that focuses on care of the mother and infant.
- Nap or rest when the infant sleeps

- Plan simple meals and flexible meal times.
- Limit visitors.
- Accept assistance with food shopping, meal preparation, laundry, and housework.
- Ask family or friends to care for the infant to provide nap times for the mother.
- Put off housework that is not absolutely necessary.
- Postpone major household projects.
- Involve friends and family to provide care for other children.
- Avoid heavy meals or vigorous exercise near bedtime.

Advise the mother to restrict intake of caffeine or to use caffeine-free versions for the first few weeks. Suggest relaxation exercises (lying quietly, alternately tightening and relaxing the muscles of the neck, shoulders, arms, legs, and feet), when a nap is not possible.

Emphasize to the mother the importance of asking for help when she begins to feel exhausted or overwhelmed. Encourage her to share these feelings with her partner, other family members, friends, and other new mothers.

Infant Sleep and Feeding Schedules. Many families require information about infant sleep cycles, frequency of feeding, and probable crying episodes during the first weeks. Although newborns sleep much of the time, they may awaken every 2 to 3 hours for feeding. If possible, having the father or another helper assist with nighttime care of the infant allows the mother longer sleep periods. For the breastfeeding mother, this would mean that the helper gets up, changes the baby's diaper, and brings the baby to the mother to nurse and returns the baby to the crib or bassinet after nursing.

Providing Nutrition Counseling

Food Supply. Low-income families might benefit from referral to government-sponsored programs such as Temporary Assistance for Needy Families (TANF) or the Special Supplemental Nutrition Program for Women, Infants, and Children (WIC). Determining the facilities available for cooking and storing food also may be necessary. The new family may need referral to a social worker to identify the best solutions for their unique problems.

Diet. Although many women are unsatisfied with slow weight loss, they should avoid severe restriction of caloric intake. A balanced, low-fat diet with adequate protein, complex carbohydrates, fruits, and vegetables provides the energy and nutrients needed.

Promoting Regular Bowel Elimination

Explain the role of progressive exercise, adequate fluid, and dietary fiber in preventing constipation. Walking is an excellent exercise, and the distance can be increased as strength and endurance increase. Drinking at least eight glasses of water daily helps maintain normal bowel elimination. Unpeeled fruits and vegetables are high in fiber, and prunes are natural laxatives. Additional fiber is found in whole-grain cereals, bread, and pasta.

A regular schedule of bowel elimination is important in overcoming constipation. For example, bowel elimination after breakfast allows the mother to take advantage of the gastrocolic reflex (stimulation of peristalsis induced in the colon when food is consumed on an empty stomach). Measures that reduce perineal and hemorrhoid pain include witch hazel astringent compresses and hydrocortisone ointments, which also facilitate bowel elimination.

Promoting Good Body Mechanics

Exercise. Exercise has beneficial physical and psychological effects during the postpartum period. Teach exercises in the early postpartum period to strengthen the abdominal muscles and firm the waist (Fig. 17.8). These mild exercises can be started soon after childbirth with five repetitions, twice a day. The number of exercises is increased gradually as the mother gains strength.

Exercise routines may be resumed gradually after pregnancy as soon as medically safe, depending on the mode of delivery, vaginal or cesarean, and the presence or absence of medical or surgical complications. Some women are capable of resuming physical activities within days of delivery. In the absence of medical or surgical complications, rapid resumption of these activities has not been found to result in adverse effects. Pelvic floor exercises could be initiated in the immediate postpartum period (ACOG, 2015). Walking is a common exercise, and women can take the infant with them on walks. Women who exercise with a friend are more likely to fit it into their schedules.

Counseling about Sexual Activity

The couple may have concerns about resuming sexual intercourse and contraceptive choices. Some couples will ask questions; for others, the nurses should be sensitive to unasked questions and provide anticipatory guidance. Many new parents are reluctant to ask about when to resume sexual activity and potential changes in sexuality resulting from pregnancy and childbirth. Fatigue, pain, fear of pregnancy, concerns about the baby, and a feeling of unattractiveness may interfere with a woman's sexual desire. Some women who breastfeed have nipple tenderness and should be advised that this should subside after the first week and that ongoing nipple pain is not normal (Buck, Amir, Cullinane, & Donath, 2014).

Couples usually can begin intercourse as early as 2 weeks after giving birth, if desire and comfort allow (Cunningham et al., 2014). Low estrogen levels during the early postpartum period and during lactation cause vaginal dryness. Application of a water-soluble vaginal lubricant may increase comfort during intercourse. Women with third- or fourth-degree lacerations or episiotomies may need more time for healing to be complete.

Cultural or religious convictions may restrict the choice of contraceptive method for some couples. The availability of health care or limited finances may dictate the choice for others. Discuss previous experience with contraceptives and the satisfaction with those methods.

Instructing about Follow-Up Appointments

Remind the new mother to make an appointment with her provider for a postpartum examination at the time suggested. This is often 4 to 6 weeks after vaginal birth and 2 weeks after cesarean birth.

Emphasize the importance of the postpartum examination. It allows early assessment of postpartum healing and identification and treatment of problems that may develop. It also provides an opportunity for contraceptive counseling and planning for future pregnancies. Women who have had complications during the pregnancy or postpartum period may need to see their health care provider sooner or have more extensive follow-up than those without complications.

Teaching about Signs and Symptoms That Should Be Reported

Teach new mothers and at least one family member which physical signs and symptoms should be reported to the health care provider immediately. These include the following:

- Fever
- Localized area of redness, swelling, or pain in either breast
- Persistent abdominal tenderness
- Feelings of pelvic fullness or pelvic pressure
- Persistent perineal pain
- Frequency, urgency, or burning on urination
- Abnormal change in character of lochia (increased amount, resumption of bright red color, passage of clots, foul odor)
- Localized tenderness, redness, edema, or warmth of the legs
- Redness, separation or edema of, or foul drainage from an abdominal incision

Ensuring That All Elements Have Been Taught

Organize information so that it can be presented and absorbed in the time available. Many facilities have a television channel for patient teaching. If this format is used, the nurse should follow up, clarifying any misunderstandings and answering any questions. In some cases, women are given information pertaining to postpartum self-care during the prenatal period. During the hospital stay, the nurse reviews and rechecks the mothers' understanding of previous teaching.

Although there are many topics to discuss in parent teaching, avoid covering too much information at a time. Interspersing small segments of teaching into normal care throughout the day will keep the woman from being overwhelmed and help her remember information better. Written instructions, including a phone number for questions, should also be provided at discharge for the family's reference.

Documenting Teaching

Documentation is an important aspect of teaching, just as it is for other aspects of nursing care. Documentation that discharge teaching was performed and that the patient has indicated comprehension of teaching is required by accrediting agencies. To prevent omissions, many hospitals use teaching checklists to record topics that should be taught (Box 17.2) (see Chapter 21 for teaching about infant care).

ABDOMINAL BREATHING

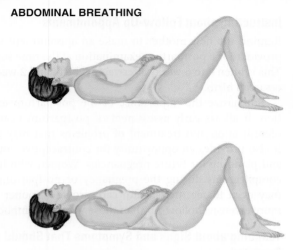

This is one of the simplest exercises and can be started on the first postpartum day. The woman assumes a supine position with knees bent. She inhales through the nose, keeps the rib cage as stationary as possible, and allows the abdomen to expand. She then contracts the abdominal muscles as she exhales slowly through the mouth.

MODIFIED SIT-UPS

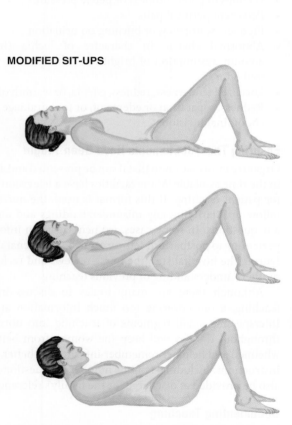

Head lifts may progress to modified sit-ups with the approval of the health care provider; the mother should follow the advice of the health care provider about the number of repetitions.

The exercise begins with the mother supine with arms outstretched and the knees bent. She raises her head and shoulders as her hands reach for her knees. She raises the shoulders only as far as the back will bend; her waist remains on the floor.

HEAD LIFT

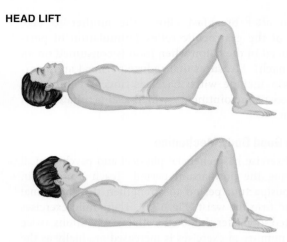

This exercise can be started within a few days after childbirth. The mother is supine with knees bent and arms outstretched at her side. She inhales deeply to begin, then exhales while lifting the head slowly; she holds the position for a few seconds and relaxes.

KNEE AND LEG ROLLS

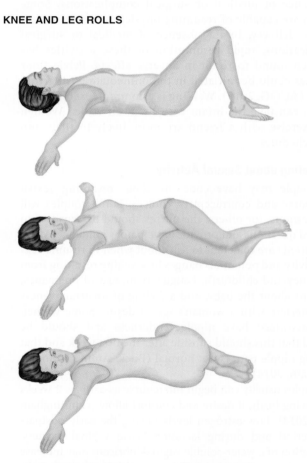

This is an excellent exercise to begin firming the waist. The mother lies flat on her back with knees bent and feet flat on the floor or bed; she keeps the shoulders and feet stationary and rolls the knees to touch first one side of the bed, then the other. She maintains a smooth motion as the exercise is repeated five times. Later, as flexibility increases, the exercise can be varied by the rolling of one knee only. The mother rolls her left knee to touch the right side of the bed, returns to center, and rolls the right knee to touch the left side of the bed.

FIG. 17.8 Postpartum Exercises. Exercises should be approved by the woman's physician, nurse-midwife, or nurse practitioner before she begins them.

CHEST EXERCISES

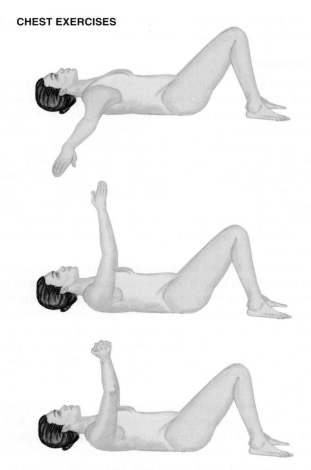

This is an excellent exercise to strengthen the chest muscles. The mother lies flat with arms extended straight out to the side; she brings the hands together above the chest while keeping the arms straight; she holds for a few seconds and returns to the starting position. She repeats the exercise five times initially and follows the advice of the health care provider for increasing the number of repetitions.

Isometric exercises also increase strength and tone; the mother bends her elbows, clasps her hands together above her chest, and presses her hands together for a few seconds. This is repeated at least five times.

FIG. 17.8, cont'd

◆ Evaluation

The mother's demonstration of correct breast and perineal hygiene provides evidence of her ability to perform self-care measures. Her ability to discuss practices that promote health in the areas of diet, exercise, rest, and sleep confirms her understanding of these measures. Her plan for future appointments with the health care provider for examinations or follow-up of complications increases the likelihood that she will experience an uncomplicated recovery.

❓ KNOWLEDGE CHECK

18. How is lactation suppressed when the mother elects not to breastfeed?
19. What is the major challenge nurses have in preparing new mothers for discharge?

BOX 17.2   Postpartum Discharge Teaching Topics

Uterine massage
Lochia norms
Involution
Episiotomy care
Care of abdominal incisions
Breast care for lactating and nonlactating women
Bowel function
Urinary function
Nutrition
Rest
Exercise
Sexual activity
Contraception
Postpartum danger signs
Follow-up care
Medications
Emotional responses and postpartum depression
Infant care and feeding
Family adjustment
Available resources

POSTPARTUM DISCHARGE AND COMMUNITY-BASED CARE

Criteria for Discharge

Most women leave the hospital when they are just beginning to recover from giving birth and starting to learn how to care for themselves and their infants. Criteria for discharge of mothers have been developed by the AAP and ACOG (2012) and include the following:

- The mother has no complications, and assessments (including vital signs, pain level, lochia, fundus, urinary output, incisions, ambulation, ability to eat and drink, and emotional status) are normal.
- Pertinent laboratory data, including blood type and Hgb or Hct have been reviewed, and Rho(D) immune globulin has been administered, if necessary.
- The mother has received instructions on self-care, deviations from normal, and proper response to danger signs and symptoms.
- The mother demonstrates knowledge, ability, and confidence to care for herself and her baby.
- The mother has received instructions on postpartum activity, exercises, and relief measures for common postpartum discomforts.
- Arrangements have been made for postpartum follow-up care.
- Family members or other support persons are available to the mother for the first few days after discharge.

Community-Based Care

Many assessments and interventions of postpartum women occur in the clinic or outpatient setting. Mothers leave the birth facility when they are not fully recovered from the childbirth experience. New parents should be made aware of local community care services. Information lines, websites, telephone calls from birth facility staff, nurse-managed post-partum outpatient clinics, and, in some areas, home visits provide information and guidance for postpartum families. Breastfeeding and parenting classes, "baby and me" walks or exercise sessions, and postpartum support groups also may be available.

 KNOWLEDGE CHECK

20. What are the criteria for discharge of the mother?

PSYCHOSOCIAL ADAPTATIONS

Perhaps no other event requires such rapid change in family structure and function as the birth of a baby. The addition of a new baby requires that all family members adjust their roles. The mother progresses through restorative phases to replenish the energy lost during labor and childbirth and to gain confidence in her role as mother. Both the mother and the father continue the process of attachment with the newborn that began during pregnancy. Siblings must adapt to a new standing in the family structure. Numerous factors such as previous experience, available support system, and culture influence the family's adaptation.

The role of maternity nurses includes not only the care of the mother-infant dyad but also the well-being of the entire family. Nurses are concerned with the family's adjustment to childbearing during the hospital stay and during the early weeks at home. The first 12 weeks, as the family makes the transition to parenthood and adapts to changes in the family structure, are often called the **fourth trimester**.

The Process of Becoming Acquainted

Nursing literature has described how parents and newborns become acquainted and progress to develop feelings of love, concern, and deep devotion that last throughout life. The terms *bonding* and *attachment* are commonly used to describe the initial steps. Although the terms are sometimes used interchangeably, their meanings differ.

Bonding

Bonding refers to the rapid initial attraction felt by parents for their infant. It is unidirectional, from parent to child, and is enhanced when parents and infants are permitted to touch and interact during the first 30 to 60 minutes after birth. During this time the infant is in a quiet, alert state and seems to gaze directly at the parents (Fig. 17.9).

Infants should be placed skin-to-skin on the mother's chest or abdomen for bonding time immediately after delivery, if possible. Nurses frequently delay procedures, such as measurements and medication administration that would interfere with this time, so parents can focus on their newborn baby.

Early and sustained contact between the parents and infant can enhance bonding and attachment. However, if early contact between parent and infant is limited because of an obstetric emergency or neonatal illness, bonding and attachment can still occur at a later time.

Attachment

Attachment is the process by which an enduring bond between a parent and child is developed through pleasurable, satisfying interaction. The process begins in pregnancy and extends for many months after childbirth. The infant receives warmth, food, and security from the parent. The parent accepts responsibility for the infant's care and places the child's needs above his or her own for years to come. In return, the parent receives enjoyment and establishes his or her identity as a father or mother. Both infant and parent benefit from the formation of irreplaceable links that continue long after the child ceases to be dependent.

Attachment follows a progressive or developmental course that changes over time. It is rarely instantaneous. Attachment behaviors of inexperienced or first-time mothers do not differ significantly from those of experienced mothers (Mercer & Ferketich, 1994). Attachment occurs through mutually satisfying experiences. Therefore if the newly delivered mother is in pain or physically exhausted, she needs pain relief and assistance so she is able to enjoy the early experiences with the baby.

Attachment is reciprocal—it occurs in both directions between parent and infant. It is facilitated by positive feedback, either real or perceived, from the infant. For example, an infant's grasp reflex around a parent's finger means "I love you" to the parent. Alert infants have a repertoire of responses called **reciprocal attachment behaviors**. These behaviors are the infant's part in the process of early attachment that progresses to lifelong, mutual devotion.

CRITICAL TO REMEMBER
Reciprocal Attachment Behaviors

Newborn infants have the ability to do the following:
Make eye contact and engage in prolonged, intense, mutual gazing.
Move their eyes and attempt to "track" the parent's face.
Grasp and hold the parent's finger.
Move synchronously in response to rhythms and patterns of the parent's voice (called **entrainment**).
Root, latch onto the breast, and suckle.
Be comforted by the parent's voice or touch.

Maternal Touch

Maternal behavior, particularly maternal touch, changes rapidly as the mother progresses through a discovery phase with her infant. Initially the mother may not reach for the infant, but if the infant is placed in her arms, she holds the baby in an **en face** position with the infant's face in the same vertical plane as her own so they can have eye contact. When the infant is awake, the two engage in prolonged, mutual gazing (see Fig. 17.9).

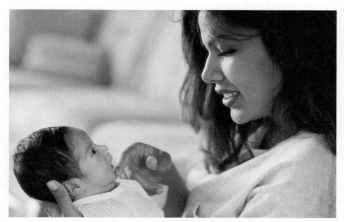

FIG. 17.9 The infant is quiet and alert during the initial sensitive period. The newborn gazes at the mother and responds to her voice and touch. The mother fingertips her infant by touching only with the fingertips.

The mother needs time to get acquainted with the tiny stranger. She may gently explore the infant's face, fingers, and toes with her fingertips only.

After using fingertips to explore the new infant, the mother begins to stroke the baby's chest and legs with her palm. Next, she uses her entire hand and arms to enfold the infant and to bring her baby close to her body. She holds the newborn closer, strokes the baby's hair, presses her cheek against the infant's cheek, and finally feels comfortable enough to engage in a full range of consoling behaviors.

The mother next begins to identify specific features of the newborn: "Look how bright his eyes are." Then she begins to relate features to family members: "He has his father's chin and nose" (Fig. 17.10). This identification process has been called **claiming** or binding-in (Rubin, 1977).

Verbal Behaviors

Verbal behaviors are also important indicators of maternal attachment. Most mothers speak to the infant in a high-pitched voice. Although many mothers have been calling the baby by name since seeing it on an ultrasound scan during pregnancy, others wait until after the birth to progress from calling the baby "it" to "he" or "she," and then to using the given name. "I can't believe it's here" rapidly becomes "Michele is such a good baby." Verbal behaviors may provide clues to a mother's early psychological relationship with her infant. Nurses observe the interactions of mothers and their infants and, if necessary, teach and model interactions that foster early attachment between them. Refer to social worker or home visit if needed to further assess bonding behaviors.

KNOWLEDGE CHECK

21. How do bonding and attachment differ?
22. How does maternal touch change over time?
23. How does verbal interaction change over time?

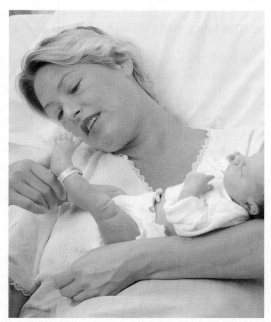

FIG. 17.10 During the binding-in or claiming process the mother identifies her baby's specific features and relates them to other family members. This mother states, "His long toes are exactly like mine."

The Process of Maternal Adaptation
Puerperal Phases

Rubin (1961) identified restorative phases that mothers go through to replenish the energy lost during labor and attain comfort in their new role. The puerperal phases are called *taking-in, taking-hold,* and *letting-go* and provide one method to observe progressive change in maternal behavior. Although they should not be used as strict guidelines for maternal assessment, the phases can help the nurse anticipate maternal needs and intervene to meet those needs.

Taking-In Phase. During the **taking-in** phase, the mother is focused primarily on her own need for fluid, food, and sleep. Inexperienced nurses may be puzzled by the mother's passive, dependent behavior as she takes in or receives attention and physical care. She also takes in every detail of the neonate but seems content to allow others to make decisions.

A major task for the mother during this time is to integrate her birth experience into reality. To do this, she discusses her labor and delivery many times on the telephone or for visitors. She attempts to piece together all the details from those who were involved in the birth. This process helps the mother realize that the pregnancy is over and the newborn is now a separate individual.

Although Rubin believed that the taking-in phase lasted for approximately 2 days, it probably lasts a day or less today. The phase may be prolonged when a cesarean birth, especially in an emergency, has been necessary. These women may have difficulty assimilating the unfamiliar and intrusive procedures that occurred in rapid succession and may have negative perceptions of the birth experience. Women who have had cesarean births need continued attention and sensitive care that takes into account their physical and psychological needs.

Taking-Hold Phase. The mother becomes more independent during the **taking-hold** phase. She exhibits concern about managing her own body functions and assumes responsibility for her own care. When she feels more comfortable and in control of her body, she shifts her attention to the behaviors of the infant. She compares her infant with other infants to validate wellness and wholeness. She welcomes information about the wide variety of behaviors exhibited by newborns.

During the taking-hold phase, the mother may verbalize anxiety about her competence as a mother. She may compare her caretaking skills unfavorably with those of the nurse.

Nurses should be careful not to assume the mothering role in caring for the infant. Instead they should encourage the mother to perform as much of the caretaking as possible. Fathers also should be encouraged to participate in caretaking as they take on a new role. Nurses should praise each attempt, even if the parents' early care is awkward.

The taking-hold phase, which extends over several days, has been called the *teachable, reachable, referable moment.* Nurses who provide home or clinic care can take advantage of this ideal time to review previously taught material and provide additional instructions and demonstrations.

Letting-Go Phase. The **letting-go** phase is a time of relinquishment for the mother and often for the father. If this is their first child, the couple must give up their previous role as a childless couple and acknowledge the loss of their more carefree lifestyle. Many mothers must also give up idealized expectations of the birth experience. For example, they may have planned to have a vaginal birth with minimal or no anesthesia but instead required a cesarean birth.

In addition, some mothers and fathers are disappointed in the size, gender, or characteristics of the infant who does not "match up" with the fantasy baby of pregnancy. They must relinquish the infant of their fantasies and accept the real infant.

These losses often provoke feelings of grief that are so subtle they may be unexamined or unacknowledged. Both parents may benefit, however, if given the opportunity to discuss unexpected feelings and realize that these feelings are common. If the mother is very young or the pregnancy was unplanned, the feelings of loss and grief may be acute.

During this phase, the mother refocuses on her relationship with her partner. She also may return to work at this time. This requires relinquishing part of the care of the infant to a caretaker.

❓ CRITICAL THINKING EXERCISE 17.2

Callie, a 35-year-old primipara, had an infant daughter, Eloina, by cesarean birth after failure to progress in labor. She is very tired, although she is relatively comfortable. Her husband, Xavier, was present during the labor and birth and is excited about being a father. He expresses concern because he and Callie have no experience with children, and his job requires almost constant travel.

On the day of delivery, Callie readily accepts attention and assistance with hygiene. She passively follows the nurse's requests to turn, cough, and breathe deeply. She discusses the details of her labor with friends on the telephone. She examines Eloina closely and touches the face and hands gently with her fingertips. She remarks that she plans to breastfeed and is surprised that the infant sleeps so much.

Questions
1. What are Callie's priority needs at this time?
2. What phase of recovery is she manifesting? Why does she "fingertip" the infant?

The first postoperative day, Callie's catheter is removed and intravenous fluids are discontinued. Callie ambulates with minimal assistance and is pleased to be able to urinate without difficulty. She asks about bowel function and requests the prescribed stool softener. She spends a great deal of time getting the baby to breastfeed. She is very frustrated that Eloina does not breastfeed well and asks for assistance from the lactation consultant.

Questions
3. What are Callie's priority needs now?
4. How have her behaviors changed?

Before discharge, Callie is breastfeeding well. The infant latches on and nurses for 10 to 15 minutes on each breast, and Callie's nipples are free of tenderness or signs of trauma. She has no relatives in the area, and her husband is home for the weekend only. She states that she will just have to get along by herself.

Questions
5. What anticipatory guidance should Callie receive before she goes home?
6. What further nursing interventions would be most helpful to her?

Maternal Role Attainment and Role Conflict

Role attainment is a process by which the mother achieves confidence in her ability to care for her infant and becomes comfortable with her identity as a mother. The process begins during pregnancy and continues for several months after childbirth.

The transition to the maternal or paternal role includes the following four stages (Mercer, 1995b):

1. The anticipatory stage begins during the pregnancy when the pregnant woman chooses a physician or nurse-midwife and a location for the infant's birth. She may attend childbirth classes to be prepared and feel she has some control over the birth experience. She seeks out role models to help her learn the mother role.

2. The formal stage begins with the birth of the infant and continues for approximately 4 to 6 weeks (Mercer, 1995a). During this stage, behaviors are largely guided by others, such as health professionals, close friends, and parents. A major task during this stage is for parents to become acquainted with their infants so that the parents can mesh their caregiving with infant cues.

3. The informal stage, which may overlap the formal stage, begins when mothers have learned appropriate responses to their infants' cues and signals. The mothers begin to respond according to the unique needs of their infants and develop the maternal role that fits them rather than following textbooks or health professionals' directives.

4. The personal stage is attained when the mother feels a sense of harmony in the role, enjoys the infant, sees the infant as a central person in her life, and has internalized the parental role. The mother accepts the role of parent and feels comfortable in this role. The range of time for achieving the maternal role is highly variable, with some mothers reaching that point in the first month and others taking much longer.

Maternal role attainment implies an end point when the woman adjusts to motherhood. However, the process could better be called *becoming a mother* because it continues throughout motherhood. The mothering role grows and evolves as the mother responds to the challenges of her child's growth and development (Mercer, 2004). Most mothers do not feel competent and self-confident in the mothering role until about 4 months after childbirth (Mercer & Walker, 2006).

Role conflict occurs when a person's perception of role responsibilities differs significantly from reality. For example, if the mother perceives her responsibility as providing most of the care and comfort for the infant, but reality dictates that she must place the infant with a caregiver and return to full-time employment, role conflict may occur. In the United States, 64% of women with children under 6 years of age and 58% of mothers with infants younger than 1 year were employed in 2015 (U.S. Department of Labor, 2016). The amount of maternity leave, now often called parental or family leave, may vary. In the United States the Family and Medical Leave Act (FMLA) entitles most workers to up to 12 weeks of unpaid leave for birth or adoption. Most other countries offer paid maternity leave for 14 weeks up to a year or more to care for the new child. Many mothers feel guilty and experience intense "separation grief" when they first leave the infant with a caregiver. Some report feeling jealous of the caregiver, whom they fear will supplant them in the infant's affection.

The nurse can help by acknowledging these feelings and reassuring the mother that her emotions are normal. Anticipatory guidance from the nurse is important. The mother needs to plan for time to reestablish feelings of closeness when she comes home from work. She needs to develop a schedule that allows maximum time with the infant when she is at home. She may have to negotiate with another family member to take over some of the household tasks until she feels more comfortable with the situation (see Nursing Care Plan).

◎ NURSING CARE PLAN

Adaptation of the Working Mother

Assessment

Claire, a 30-year-old single mother, gave birth to a baby boy, Drew, by cesarean delivery 6 days ago. She has made a good recovery, and breastfeeding is going well. During her visit to a nurse-managed postpartum clinic, Claire discusses her need to return to work as a sales executive in 6 weeks. She states that she hates the thought of leaving baby with someone else while she works. "I've always planned to stay home for at least 6 months when I had a baby, but it's impossible. How can I be a mother and work full time?"

Identification of Patient Problems

Emotional distress as a result of inability to perform the role of mother as she wishes because of the need to return to full-time employment.

Critical Thinking

Emotional distress or grief may be related to loss. What has Claire lost, or what must she give up?

Answer

Claire must give up her idealized picture of motherhood. She also must give up mothering tasks and time with the infant to a caregiver. She will have to modify her self-concept based on the perception of these losses.

Expected Outcomes

Claire will do the following:
1. Describe her concerns and feelings about leaving Drew with a caregiver.
2. Verbalize plans to achieve maximal satisfaction in her role as mother by the time she returns to work.

Continued

NURSING CARE PLAN—cont'd

Adaptation of the Working Mother

Interventions and Rationales

1. Allow Claire to describe her perception of her role as a mother and express concerns about how employment will interfere with her ability to fulfill this role. *Venting can help Claire cope with the role conflict, stress, and grief that can result when a mother who envisions her role as the primary caregiver must leave her infant with another caregiver and return to her job.*

2. Suggest Claire openly express her feelings of anxiety, guilt, and jealousy to significant others and to her baby's care provider. *Candid expression of feelings helps resolve them and allows for a discussion of measures that will help overcome the intense feelings that cause conflict.*

3. Acknowledge that Claire's feelings are difficult and reassure her that they are common. *Knowledge that the feelings are not trivial and are experienced by others reinforces their validity and importance.*

4. Suggest that Claire delay her return to employment, if possible, until Drew is at least 12 to 16 weeks old. Part-time work also may be a possibility for a time. *By 12 to 16 weeks most infants are able to sleep through the night, reducing the sleep deprivation that often adds to the stress of working and infant care.*

5. Recommend that Claire investigate several daycare providers before choosing one. She should check references, make unannounced visits, see required licenses and certification, discuss the number and ages of children cared for and the daily schedule, ask about the provider's philosophy of infant care and training in emergency measures, and know what emergency plans are in place. *A great deal of stress is eliminated if parents feel confident that a competent and nurturing daycare provider has been found. Mothers are more content with their return to work if they are satisfied with their child care arrangements.*

6. Suggest that she leave the infant with the chosen daycare provider for 2 to 3 days before resuming full-time employment. *Allowing both mother and infant to "practice separating" while their schedules are still somewhat flexible helps ease the transition and makes it less traumatic.*

7. Recommend that Claire pump her breasts and feed Drew by bottle at least once per day in the week or two before returning to work. *Becoming proficient at pumping the breasts and introducing the infant to bottle feeding prepares both the mother and the infant for all-day separation.*

8. Help Claire develop a schedule that allows her maximum time with Drew. *Feelings of frustration and stress can be alleviated if the mother has a plan that allows her long periods of uninterrupted time with the infant.*
   a. Make a list of errands and supplies needed to avoid frequent stops that delay getting home from work.
   b. Double the recipe when cooking and freeze half for future use.
   c. Pick up nutritious takeout meals to avoid cooking every evening.
   d. Purchase nutritious prepackaged frozen meals to have available when needed.
   e. Schedule appointments on the same day when possible.
   f. Include Drew in daily walks, exercise, and social visits.

9. Recommend that Claire allow 30 to 45 minutes to hold Drew when she first gets home. Delay all other activities until this need is met for both mother and infant. *Time is needed to make the transition between work and home. It helps to reestablish feelings of closeness, comfort, and attachment.*

10. Advise Claire to try to get more rest in the early weeks after returning to work. *The return to work may increase fatigue. Extra rest will help Claire avoid undue fatigue or illness.*

Evaluation

Claire freely expressed her feelings of guilt, anxiety, and concern about leaving Drew. She made a plan to investigate daycare in her area and discussed plans to reorganize her work and social schedule so that she can spend as much time as possible with her son.

Major Maternal Concerns

As the mother gains confidence in her ability to care for the infant and her physical discomfort decreases, emotional concerns related to the self become more important. Body image and the experience of postpartum blues are particularly important.

Body Image. Women are very concerned about regaining their normal figures. Some mothers have unrealistic expectations about weight loss and the time it takes for the body to regain its nonpregnant shape. Nurses should emphasize that weight loss should be gradual. Rigid restriction of calories can lead to depleted energy and decreased immunity.

In addition, nurses should teach the importance of safe activities such as walking and graduated exercises to regain muscle tone. Some birth facilities offer classes for postpartum mothers that include exercise and nutrition, as well as the opportunity to share concerns with other postpartum women.

Smoking. Many women give up smoking during pregnancy to protect the health of the fetus. However, the majority of women resume smoking at some point during the

THERAPEUTIC COMMUNICATIONS

Body Image

Mary Kay gave birth to her first baby 48 hours ago. Aubrey, her nurse, is reviewing self-care measures before Mary Kay's discharge from the birth facility.

Mary Kay: Look at me! I still look pregnant, and my husband calls me Tubby.

Aubrey: You were looking forward to your abdomen being flat after the baby was born. *(This clarifies the woman's concern by reflecting content.)*

Mary Kay: Well, I never had a big belly before. I thought it would all go away after I had the baby. I can't believe I look this fat.

Aubrey: Remember, it took 9 months for those muscles to stretch. You can't expect them to snap back in a few days. *This blocks communication by ignoring the feeling expressed. A more helpful response would be to acknowledge Mary Kay's distress and to delay giving information until feelings have been expressed. For example: "How disappointing for you! If you like, we can discuss some exercises that will help."*

first 6 months postpartum (Jones, Lewis, Parrott, Wormall & Coleman, 2016). Factors that increase the likelihood of relapse include weight concerns, failure to breastfeed, depression, living with a smoker, stress, and planning to quit only during the pregnancy.

Nurses should discuss smoking with postpartum women to offer resources for those who stopped smoking prenatally and are at risk for relapse in the postpartum period. Explanations of the hazards to the infant from smoking also may be helpful because some mothers may think the harmful effects occur only during pregnancy.

Exposure to secondhand smoke increases the risk for sudden infant death syndrome (SIDS) and has been associated with cognitive impairments, behavior problems, ear infections, asthma, and other respiratory problems in children. Cigarettes themselves present a poisoning risk for small children; the amount of nicotine in just one cigarette butt is enough to poison a child. In addition, children of smokers are more likely to grow up to become smokers themselves.

There are many reasons to quit smoking after the baby is born. Nurses can provide support for smoking cessation, reducing smoking, and avoiding environmental tobacco smoke and nicotine exposure around the baby. Provide encouragement and information. Refer patients to quit lines, support groups, and their primary health care provider for further assistance.

Postpartum Blues. **Postpartum blues,** *baby blues,* or *maternity blues* is a frequent concern for new mothers. This mild, transient condition affects 60% to 80% of women who have given birth (Whitmer, 2016). The condition begins in the first week, peaks around day 5, and ends within 2 weeks. If it lasts beyond 2 weeks, it may be a more serious condition (McCall-Hosenfeld, Phiri, Schaefer, Zhu, & Kjerulff, 2016).

Postpartum blues is characterized by irritability, fatigue, tearfulness, mood swings, and anxiety. The symptoms are usually unrelated to events, and the condition does not seriously affect the mother's ability to care for the infant. Nurses should prepare women and their family members for the occurrence of postpartum blues symptoms, let them know it is normal, and offer emotional support and encouragement. Explain the difference between the transient postpartum blues and more serious postpartum depression and anxiety that may require treatment.

Although the direct cause is unknown, postpartum blues may be a result of the emotional letdown that occurs after birth, postpartum discomforts, sleep deprivation, anxiety about her ability to care for the infant, and body image concern. Hormonal fluctuations have not been proved to be a cause, but associations with thyroid dysfunction, serotonin, and progesterone levels have been suggested.

Although postpartum blues is self-limiting, mothers benefit greatly when empathy and support are freely given by the family and the health care team. Because the condition is so common in postpartum women, caregivers or family members may not be as empathetic as they would be for a condition deemed more serious. Yet the mother needs adequate attention to move through this period. She should be encouraged to rest, take time for herself, and discuss her feelings. In addition, reassurance should be given that such feelings are normal and generally last less than 2 weeks.

Postpartum blues should be distinguished from postpartum depression and postpartum psychosis, which are disabling conditions and require therapeutic management for full recovery. Screening for risk factors (e.g., previous history of depression or mental illness or limited social support) along with initial screening and education about early warning signs and symptoms is important during the birth facility stay (see Chapter 11). Many hospitals conduct a baseline Edinburgh Postnatal Depression Screen (EPDS) before discharge. Nurses should teach the woman and the family to call the health care provider if depression becomes severe or lasts longer than 2 week, or if she is unable to cope with daily life. Early detection and early intervention improve treatment success. Nurse home visits, parenting support groups, talk therapy, or medication can be options for treating postpartum depression.

❓ KNOWLEDGE CHECK

24. How do maternal behaviors in the taking-in phase differ from those in the taking-hold phase?
25. What does the mother (and the father) relinquish in the letting-go phase?
26. How do the parents progress through the stages of role attainment?
27. How is postpartum blues different from postpartum depression? How can nurses intervene for this common emotional response?

The Process of Family Adaptation

The birth of an infant requires the reorganization of roles and relationships within the family. The previously childless couple now must integrate a new member into the family unit. Fathers or partners must learn new skills and often adjust to new roles. Siblings must adapt to a new standing in the family structure. Expectations and involvement of grandparents vary widely. Each family member is affected.

Fathers

The father's developing bond with the newborn is facilitated by engrossment. **Engrossment** is an intense fascination and face-to-face observation between the parent and newborn. It is characterized by the father's intense interest in how the infant looks and responds and a desire to touch and hold the baby. Many parents comment on the baby's distinctive features and view the baby as perfect. They experience strong attraction to the infant and elation after the birth. The father's attachment behaviors increase when the infant is awake, makes eye contact, and responds to the father's voice (Fig. 17.11).

Many fathers eagerly look forward to co-parenting with their mate. However, they may lack confidence in providing infant care and are sensitive to being left out of instructions

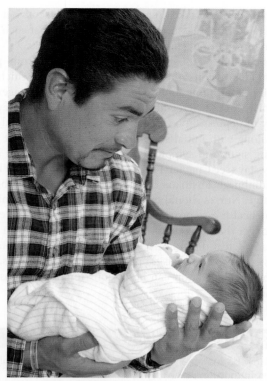

FIG. 17.11 Fathers' behaviors during initial contact with their infants often correspond to maternal behaviors. The intense fascination that fathers exhibit is called *engrossment*. Note eye-to-eye contact between the father and the infant.

and demonstrations of infant care. They may feel that others expect them only to provide support to the mother. Nurses can assist fathers by involving them in child care activities soon after birth to help them feel more confident and competent.

Although first-time fathers may attend prenatal classes about parenting, they often do not know what to expect from infants and need more information about normal growth and development during infancy. A review of information about child care presented in the prenatal period is helpful after the baby is born, when the information seems more relevant and the father is ready to learn.

The additional work involved in care of a newborn may be a source of concern for both mothers and their partners. Parents should be encouraged to negotiate the division of household chores during pregnancy or shortly after delivery.

Siblings

Siblings' response to the birth of a new brother or sister depends on their age and developmental level. Toddlers usually are not completely aware of the impending birth. When the baby arrives, they may view the infant as competition and fear they will be replaced in the parents' affection. They may have feelings of jealousy and resentment when they must share time and attention with a baby. Some toddlers exhibit

hostile behaviors toward the mother, particularly when she holds or feeds the newborn. Sleep problems, an increase in attention-seeking efforts, and regression to more infantile behaviors such as renewed bed-wetting and thumbsucking are common. These behaviors show the jealousy and frustration young children feel as they observe the mother's attention being given to another.

The parents can be taught to accept without judgment the strong feelings expressed by the toddler and to continue to reinforce the child's feelings of being loved. Plans for changes in routine, such as beginning toilet training, should be postponed until family adjustments have been made. Expecting 2-year-olds to welcome a "stranger" is not realistic until they feel secure in the affection of their parents.

Preschool siblings may engage in more looking than touching. Most spend at least some time in proximity to the infant and talk to the mother about the infant (Fig. 17.12). Older children may adapt more easily. All siblings need extra attention from the parents and reassurance that they are loved and important. Sibling classes, available in many agencies, may help ease the transition. Siblings are often allowed to visit the mother on the postpartum unit, where they can interact with the new baby.

At home a relaxed approach without time constraints may facilitate interactions between young children and infants. Special care should be taken by the parents, visitors, and nurses to pay as much attention to the sibling as to the new baby. Parents can emphasize the advantages of being an older sibling and allow siblings to participate in age-appropriate aspects of infant care.

Grandparents

The involvement of grandparents with grandchildren depends on many factors. One of the most important is proximity. Grandparents who live near the child frequently develop a strong attachment. This evolves into unconditional love and a special relationship that brings joy to the grandparents and an added sense of security to the grandchildren (Fig. 17.13).

When grandparents live many miles from grandchildren and have sporadic contact, forming a close attachment is more difficult. Grandparents must try to devise ways to foster a relationship with grandchildren they seldom see.

Expectations of the role of grandparents are also a factor in their adaptation to the birth of a grandchild. Many grandparents strive to be fully involved in the care and upbringing of the child, but others desire less involvement. The degree of grandparent involvement may cause some conflict with parents, or it may be a comfortable arrangement for both families.

Grandparents are often a major part of the support system that new parents need. Grandmothers, in particular, provide assistance with household tasks and infant care, which helps the mother recover from childbirth and make the transition to parenthood. Grandfathers who were very busy providing for their own children may enjoy the opportunity to nurture their grandchildren.

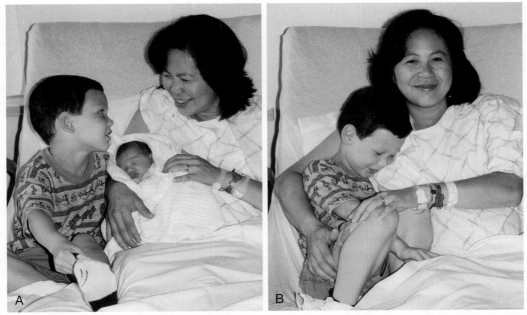

FIG. 17.12 A, Although they may hesitate to touch the infant, children often want to be close. B, This boy's relief and joy are obvious as he reclaims a favorite spot.

CRITICAL TO REMEMBER

Factors That Affect Adaptation

Lingering discomfort or pain
Chronic fatigue
Knowledge of infant needs
Available support system
Expectations of the newborn
Previous experience with infants
Maternal temperament
Infant characteristics
Other factors: Cesarean birth, preterm or ill infant, or birth of more than one infant (e.g., twins or triplets)
Other life events occurring during this time

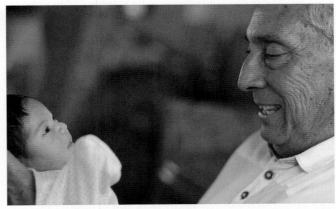

FIG. 17.13 Grandparents may develop strong bonds with grandchildren.

Factors That Affect Family Adaptation

Numerous factors influence the family's adjustment. Some, such as discomfort and fatigue, can be anticipated because they are so common. Additional factors include knowledge of infant needs, expectations of the infant, previous experience, age of the parents, and temperaments of the mother and infant. Other events such as cesarean birth, birth of a preterm or ill infant, and birth of more than one infant also affect the ease and speed with which the family adjusts.

Discomfort and Fatigue

Normally, discomforts associated with childbirth resolve within the first days after birth but may make it difficult to focus on the newborn's needs. Fatigue often remains a problem during the first few weeks and months, when the infant's schedule is erratic and the chance for uninterrupted sleep is minimal. When the infant begins to sleep through the night (usually by 3 to 4 months), the parents can reestablish familiar patterns, and fatigue often becomes less of a factor.

Knowledge of Infant Needs

Parents experience powerful feelings of protectiveness when they discover they can console their infant and the infant responds to their care. First-time parents, who are often unsure about how to care for a newborn, become very anxious if they are unable to console a crying infant. In addition, many are concerned about feeding and specific procedures such as care of the umbilical cord or circumcision. Breastfeeding benefits both the mother and the infant but may add to the stress initially experienced by parents who lack sufficient knowledge and support.

Some parents have concerns about spoiling the infant. They may think that responding each time the infant cries causes the baby to cry to get attention. It may be necessary to teach parents that infants cry to indicate hunger, cold, wetness, and a need for cuddling or gentle stimulation and that responding to crying does not spoil the child. Suggesting a variety of methods to cope with crying may be helpful. Prompt, gentle response to crying helps the infant develop trust in the world as a safe, secure place. Trust is a basic developmental task of infancy and depends on the child learning that caregivers respond consistently and gently in meeting his or her needs.

Previous Experience

Previous experience with newborns also may affect family adjustment. Multiparas are more comfortable with infants and exhibit attachment behaviors earlier than primiparas, who may spend many more hours in the early discovery phase of attachment. Because they know what to expect, multiparas are more relaxed in caring for the new baby but have to establish new routines that fit the expanded family. The mother may find it more difficult to have time alone with her partner. She may need more help from family and friends than the primipara because of the lack of sleep and the time and energy involved in meeting the needs of all family members. Women with other children may need encouragement to take time for themselves and time alone with their partner. Support groups for multiparas may be helpful.

Mothers who have had a long interval between pregnancies may have forgotten much of the teaching received with the last birth and may need more instruction. Those who previously gave birth to infants with anomalies or infants who did not survive may need more time to feel comfortable with this infant.

Expectations about the Newborn

Unrealistic expectations of the infant may influence adjustment. Parents who have little experience with newborns may be surprised and disappointed at the newborn's appearance. They may be unprepared for normal newborn characteristics such as cranial molding, blotchy skin, and newborn rash.

Nurses should teach normal newborn characteristics and early growth and development. They should assist parents in working through misconceptions about newborn behavior. For example, the capacity of an infant's stomach is small, and the infant should be fed frequently. Also, infants are neurologically unable to sleep through the night during the early weeks. Increasing the time the mother spends with the infant during the postpartum stay provides extra opportunities for her to gain comfort with the physical characteristics as well as to learn infant care while a nurse is available to help her.

Some mothers may be very disappointed in the gender of their infants or sense that their partners are disappointed. These feelings should be acknowledged and resolved before attachment can take place. For example, a mother of four sons might be so disappointed that the fifth child is a boy that she cries and refuses to pick out a boy's name at first. Later, when she holds the baby and begins to observe differences between this infant and her other sons, she can begin her discovery period with this unique child.

Maternal Age

Adjustment to parenthood is a challenge for the teenager who has not achieved a strong sense of her own identity. In general, the adolescent may talk less, respond less, and appear more passive or less affectionate with her infant than older parents. She needs special assistance to develop necessary parenting skills that promote optimal development of the infant (see Chapter 11).

Maternal Temperament

Maternal personality traits greatly influence attachment. Mothers who are calm, secure in their ability to learn, and free from unnecessary anxiety adjust more easily to the demands of motherhood. Conversely, mothers who are excitable, insecure, and anxious have more difficulty.

Temperament of the Infant

The infant's temperament also affects maternal adjustment. Infants who are calm, easily consoled, and enjoy cuddling increase parental confidence and feelings of competence. In contrast, irritable infants who are difficult to console and do not respond to cuddling increase parental frustration and interfere with attachment.

Availability of a Strong Support System

A strong, consistent support system is a major factor in the adjustment of the new mother and the family. Friends and relatives who are parents can provide role modeling that is particularly important to first-time parents. They also can provide encouragement, praise, and reassurance that they are good parents. That others see the baby as special and demonstrate love and affection is very important to the new parents. Support may be needed for an extended period after childbirth. In addition, the mother needs practical assistance with household tasks such as meal preparation, laundry, and shopping.

Postpartum support groups are often available and can help the mother with early concerns of this period. They provide an opportunity for women to share their experiences with women who are having similar experiences. Some groups are focused on breastfeeding or exercise, but others simply provide an opportunity for interacting with other new mothers. Fathers may be included at all meetings or occasionally. There are also support groups just for new fathers.

Other Factors

Cesarean Birth. A cesarean birth, especially one that was unexpected, can make parental adjustment more difficult. Cesarean childbirth includes a longer recovery time and additional discomfort for the mother, increased stress for the family, and possible financial strain. The mother's needs for recovery and attachment with her newborn should be considered in planning nursing care.

Preterm or Ill Infant. Birth of a preterm or ill infant results in additional concerns about the condition of the infant. Prolonged separation of parents and child may be necessary. Although attachment can occur in these situations, the separation may delay the process and create stress on the normally functioning family.

Birth of Multiple Infants. The birth of twins or triplets often follows a high-risk pregnancy in which the mother was confined to limited activity. There may have been one or more hospitalizations for preterm labor or other complications. The infants may be preterm and have health problems. Financial strain may occur because the mother had to stop work earlier than expected and expenses associated with the birth and future health care are higher. In addition, birth of more than one infant makes family relationships more complex, especially if there are other children.

Problems of attachment may occur when there is more than one newborn. Rooming-in helps the parents gain confidence in caretaking and facilitates the attachment process. If infants are in a neonatal intensive care unit, early, frequent contacts should be arranged.

Parents attach to the infants separately as they get to know each infant's unique characteristics. They need help to relate to each infant as an individual rather than part of a unit by pointing out the individual responses and characteristics of each infant. Arranging time for the parents to interact with each child alone, especially in the early, getting-acquainted period, is important.

Mothers may be overwhelmed at the prospect of breast-feeding more than one infant. They need reassurance that they will produce an ample supply of milk for each infant because supply increases with demand.

KNOWLEDGE CHECK

28. What does a father mean when he says he feels "out of place"?
29. What feelings may siblings experience when a new baby is born into the family?

Cultural Influences on Adaptation

A major goal of nursing practice in the postpartum period is to provide culture-specific nursing care that fits the health beliefs, values, and practices of each woman. This can be difficult because of the wide ethnic diversity in countries such as the United States and Canada. A major challenge for nurses is to be aware of cultural beliefs and acknowledge their importance in family adaptation. The postpartum period often is thought to be a time of vulnerability for the woman and infant (Mattson, 2015). Many cultural factors relevant to this time can be grouped into communication, health beliefs, and dietary practices.

Communication

Verbal communication may be difficult because of the numerous dialects and languages spoken. An interpreter should be fluent in the language, of the same religion, and of the same country of origin, if possible.

Care of the non–English speaking patient will be challenging for the English-speaking nurse and health care team. Patients who are not able to speak or understand the primary language spoken at the hospital require extra vigilance and support. Extra time and patience may be needed to provide the best possible care. Making an effort by speaking a few words in their language, demonstrating a caring attitude, and using nonverbal communication is a first step. Using an interpreter will improve adherence to discharge instructions, satisfaction with care, and outcomes.

Hospitals are required to provide professionally trained health care interpreter services and translated printed materials for limited English-proficient patients. Culturally and linguistically appropriate services may include telephone or video interpreters, trained volunteer interpreters, or computer-assisted translation. Using the patient's family and friends, children under 18, other patients or visitors, or untrained volunteers is not best practice. Try to meet briefly with the interpreter in advance to make a plan. Speak slowly and in short segments; speak directly to the patient, not to the interpreter; and ask the patient or family member to repeat back what he or she understands.

When the nurse and family speak different primary languages, verifying the family's understanding is important. Nodding or saying "Yes" may be a sign of courtesy rather than understanding or agreement. To be certain the message has been received, the nurse should ask family members to repeat in their own words what they have been told.

A woman may not indicate that she disagrees with what the nurse tells her to do because she does not want to show disrespect. She may simply not follow the nurse's instructions. She might also follow cultural requirements that differ from nursing expectations. Even if she does not really believe the requirements are necessary, she may follow them to avoid offending close relatives.

Respect for privacy and modesty of all people is important, but modesty is especially important in Hispanic, Middle-Eastern, and Asian cultures. Laws of modesty require that Muslim women cover their hair, body, arms, and legs except when at home with family or in all-female company (Giger, 2013).

Health Beliefs

Cultural beliefs and practices provide a sense of security for new mothers. Provision of care for the mother and baby by female relatives is a common thread among cultures.

For many Southeast Asians the postpartum period is important to ensure health in later years. New mothers are expected to rest for 1 to 3 months while the grandmother or other female relatives assume the mother's usual responsibilities of cooking or housework and care for the mother, her baby, and other children. Care for the Korean mother and baby is traditionally performed by the mother-in-law (Callister, 2014).

Women's activities are often restricted for a period after birth to allow rest and recuperation. The time involved varies. Laotian women stay home for 1 month near a fire or heater to help "dry up the womb" (Callister, 2014). Native American women and their infants stay indoors and rest for 20 days or until the umbilical cord falls off (Callister, 2014).

"Doing the month" is very important for Chinese women. Mothers and their babies are cared for by a grandmother. They do not go outside and must keep warm to avoid "wind chill." They wear long sleeves and long pants and restrict bathing and washing their hair (Liu, Petrini, & Maloni, 2015).

Many Southeast Asian and Hispanic women believe the mother should be kept warm to avoid upsetting the balance of hot and cold (Callister, 2014). Use of ice for perineal edema or breast engorgement may not be acceptable to these women.

Many Mexican women follow the customs of *la cuarentena*. This 40-day period is a time when the woman is considered at risk because the entire body is open and subject to entrance of air, which would cause illness and various body aches. The woman may bind her abdomen and wear more clothes than usual to avoid becoming cold, even when the weather is hot. Sexual intercourse is avoided to prevent serious illness to the mother, father, and infant (Waugh, 2011).

When women are unwilling to take baths or showers in the postpartum period, nurses may be concerned about hygiene. Perineal cleansing is generally acceptable. If a sitz bath is indicated and this is explained to the mother, she may agree if she is kept warm throughout the process. Although an opportunity to wash or shower should be offered, it is up to the woman to decide her preference. Tact and sensitivity are necessary to determine what care is appropriate for each woman and to find a compromise, if necessary. In some cultures, baths are an important part of postpartum recovery. Navajo women take a ritual bath on the fourth postpartum day (Mattson, 2015).

Specific religious practices should be accepted and supported. For instance, Muslim mothers are exempted from their obligation to pray while they are bleeding. However, the father and other family members kneel, place their heads on the floor, and pray five times per day. If possible, a clean, quiet room should be provided so that this obligation can be fulfilled without having to leave the birthing center.

Dietary Practices

Some cultural dietary practices to consider center on the hot-cold theory of health and diet. This theory refers to the intrinsic properties of certain foods instead of the temperature or spiciness of foods. For example, some Asians believe that after childbirth the woman should eat only "hot" foods such as chicken, meat, and fish. Others eat warm, salty foods and avoid fruits and green vegetables after childbirth (Mattson, 2015).

Although ice water is commonly given to hospital patients, it is not acceptable to many Asians. For example, Southeast Asian women may refuse cold or ice water and prefer hot water or other warm beverages to keep warm.

Food brought from home is a welcome sign of caring in many cultures. This is especially true if traditional foods are eaten after a woman gives birth. Nurses should encourage this practice and discuss any dietary restrictions with the family.

Home and Community-Based Care

Because many mothers and infants are discharged from the birth facility soon after childbirth, some assessments and interventions described in this chapter occur in the home or clinic setting. Mothers may leave the birth facility when they still have discomfort and are just beginning to recover from the childbirth experience. Consequently, most psychosocial concerns such as family adaptation and postpartum blues surface later, when support from health care professionals is not as readily available.

Methods currently used to provide care for mothers and infants after discharge include telephone calls, nurse-managed postpartum clinics, home visits, and "baby lines" staffed by nurses who provide information and guidance for callers. Comprehensive psychosocial support including telephone calls, home and clinic visits, and breastfeeding and parenting education may decrease the incidence of hospital readmission of normal newborns. Some programs use postpartum doulas or paraprofessionals to help extend the work of nurses in providing support to postpartum women. All methods have advantages and disadvantages.

The overlap between nursing care in the birth facility and home makes communication among nurses extremely important. Nurses in the birth facility, who perform the initial assessments, should make information available to nurses who provide follow-up care.

◆ APPLICATION OF THE NURSING PROCESS: MATERNAL ADAPTATION

◆ Assessment

Several factors such as the mother's progress through the puerperal phases, her mood, her interaction with the infant, and unanticipated events affect maternal adaptation to the birth (Table 17.3).

◆ Identification of Patient Problems

Adjustment to parenting may be altered when one or more caregivers experience difficulty creating or continuing a nurturing environment. Multiple factors such as fatigue, discomfort, and lack of knowledge of infant care may interfere with parent and family adaptation.

◆ Planning: Expected Outcomes

Expected outcomes are that the mother will do the following:
- Verbalize feelings of comfort and support as she progresses through the phases of recovery
- Demonstrate progressive attachment behaviors (enfolding the infant, calling the infant by name, and responding gently when the infant cries) by discharge
- Participate in care of the newborn (diapering, feeding, and care of the umbilical cord and circumcision) by discharge

◆ Interventions

Assisting the Mother through Recovery Phases

"Mother" the Mother. The early, taking-in phase is a time to "mother" the mother to help her transition to more complex tasks of maternal adjustment. During the first few hours after childbirth, she has a great need for physical care and comfort. Provide ample fluids and favorite foods. Keep linens dry, tuck warm blankets around her until chilling has stopped, and use warm water for perineal care.

TABLE 17.3   Assessing Maternal Adaptation

Assessments	Nursing Considerations
Progression through Puerperal Phases	
Taking-in (passive, dependent)	Consider mother's need to rest, her need to tell the details of her labor and child-
Taking-hold (autonomous, seeks information)	birth, and her readiness to learn infant care and assume control of her own care.
Letting-go (relinquishes fantasy baby, begins to see self as mother)	Avoid taking over the mothering role in care of the infant. Praise and encourage mother's efforts. Ideal time to teach.
Maternal Mood	
Mood and energy level, eye contact, posture, and comfort	Tense body posture, crying, or anxiety (may indicate fatigue, discomfort, or beginning of postpartum blues).
Factors That Affect Maternal Adaptation	
Age of mother	May need additional support if under 18 years of age.
Previous experience	Primiparas progress through puerperal phases more slowly and may need more assistance than multiparas. Previous birth of an infant with anomalies or death of an infant may delay adaptation.
Maternal and infant temperaments	Mothers who are calm, secure, and free from anxiety need less assistance. More teaching is necessary for parents of infants who are difficult to console.
Other factors	Cesarean birth causes increased discomfort and longer recovery. Attachment challenges may occur with birth of a preterm or ill infant or more than one infant.
Interaction with Infant	
Maternal touch	Progresses from fingertipping to enfolding and other comforting behaviors.
Verbal interaction	Mother may call infant "it" initially but progresses quickly to using given name and identifying specific characteristics.
Response to infant cues or signals	Prompt, gentle, consistent response indicates progressive adaptation to parenting role.
Preparation for Parenting	
Classes in breastfeeding, parenting, and infant care	Many mothers feel more prepared after completing classes and participate in care sooner.

Monitor and Protect. The new mother depends on nurses to monitor and protect her. Remind her of the need to void, and assist her to ambulate. Assess her level of comfort frequently and offer analgesia before discomfort is severe and analgesia is less effective. Instruct her not to delay requesting analgesia because it is more effective and the postpartum course is smoother if her pain stays well controlled. Encourage her to sleep.

Listen to the Birth Experience. Be prepared to listen to details of the birth experience and offer sincere praise for her efforts during labor. Use open-ended questions to determine the woman's perception of the birth. The opportunity to discuss her feelings about the experience helps her integrate it and clarify concerns. Many mothers spend so much time on the telephone that completing nursing care is difficult. The mother's need to relate her experiences to family and friends is important, and nurses may be reluctant to interrupt. When assessments and care are necessary for the mother's physical safety, a compromise can be effective. Offering a choice is often helpful: "Excuse me for a moment. I need to check you soon. I can do it now or come back in 10 minutes."

Foster Independence

As the mother becomes more independent, allow her to schedule her care as much as possible. Collaborate with her to plan when such care as ambulation or a shower will be performed. Encourage her to assume responsibility for her self-care, and emphasize that the nurse's role at this point is to assist and teach.

Promote Bonding and Attachment

Early, unlimited contact between parents and infants is of primary importance to facilitate the attachment process. In most hospitals and birth centers, infants remain in the room with the parents unless complications intervene. This arrangement may be called *rooming-in, mother-baby care, couplet care,* or *dyad care.* One nurse is responsible for both the mother and the baby and provides teaching and help with bonding as part of ongoing nursing care (Fig. 17.14). The mother participates as she is able. The nurse assists as the mother learns to care for her baby and gradually takes over all care. This provides continuity of care and helps prepare the parents for discharge.

Prolonged contact between mothers and infants leads to more touching and caring for infants as mothers learn their infants' characteristics and needs. Nursing measures to promote bonding and attachment include the following:

- Assist the parents in unwrapping the baby to inspect the toes, fingers, and body. Inspection fosters identification and allows the parents to become acquainted with the "real" baby, which must replace the fantasy baby that many parents imagined during the pregnancy.

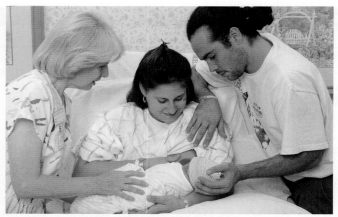

FIG. 17.14 By teaching about the newborn and family, the nurse helps parents develop confidence in their ability to provide care for the infant.

- Position the infant in an en face position and discuss the infant's ability to see the parent's face. Face-to-face and eye-to-eye contact is a first step in establishing mutual interaction between the infant and parent.
- Point out the reciprocal bonding activities of the infant: "Look how she holds your finger." "He hasn't taken his eyes off you."
- Encourage the parents to take as much time as they wish with the infant. This allows them to progress at their own speed through the discovery or getting-acquainted phase.
- Encourage and assist the mother in putting the infant to the breast. Provide positive reinforcement. Answer her questions about feeding.
- Model behaviors by holding the infant close, making eye contact with the infant, and speaking in high-pitched, soothing tones.
- Point out the characteristics of the infant in a positive way: "She has such pretty little hands and beautiful eyes."
- Provide comfort and ample time for rest because the mother must replenish her energy and be relatively free of discomfort before she can progress to initiating care of the infant. A mother who seems uninterested may just need a period of rest or pain intervention to be comfortable enough to focus on the infant.

Involve Parents in Infant Care

Providing care for the infant fosters feelings of responsibility and nurturing and is an important component of attachment. In addition, it allows parents to develop confidence in their ability to care for their infant before they go home. Begin with demonstrations, as necessary, and provide assistance while the parents gradually assume all infant care as their confidence in their abilities grows.

Although teaching begins during pregnancy, review information and repeat demonstrations. Demonstrate the simpler tasks such as care of the cord before progressing to more complicated procedures such as bathing.

Agreement among the entire staff about how to teach basic care is important. Mothers seek confirmation of information, and they become confused and lose faith in the credibility of the staff if information varies. Allow time for practice and repeated encouragement. Parents become easily discouraged if they feel unsuccessful with early attempts to care for their infants.

Suggestions for care should be tactfully phrased to avoid the implication that the parents are inept. "You burped that baby like a professional. There are a couple of little hints I can share about diapering."

◆ Evaluation

The expected outcomes are met when the mother independently performs self-care and verbalizes feelings of comfort and support during her progression through the phases of recovery. She should show progressive attachment behaviors, including enfolding the infant, calling the infant by name, and responding gently when the infant cries. Her participation in infant care should include diapering, feeding, and care of the umbilical cord and circumcision.

◆ APPLICATION OF THE NURSING PROCESS: FAMILY ADAPTATION

◆ Assessment
Partners

The partners' emotional status and interaction with the infant are particularly important because they usually serve as the mother's primary support person. Are the partners involved with the mother and infant? How do they interact with the infant? How much information do they have about infant characteristics and care? What are their expectations about their partner's recovery? Unrealistic expectations of the infant (will sleep through the night, smile, be easily consoled) may lead to problems. In addition, if partners expect the mother to recover her energy and libido rapidly, they may become resentful if her recovery takes longer than anticipated.

TABLE 17.4   Assessing Family Adaptation

Assessment	Nursing Considerations
Characteristics of Infant That May Affect Family Adaptation	
Gender and size of infant	Disappointment about gender or concern about small size may interfere with bonding.
Unexpected characteristics (cephalhematoma, jaundice, cranial molding, newborn rash)	Explain unexpected appearance or behavior in language parents can comprehend. Reassure normalcy and temporary nature, if accurate.
Congenital anomaly or illness	Explain the condition to parents; assist them during visits and in learning care.
Infant behavior (irritable, easily consoled, cuddles)	Infants who are easy to manage increase bonding and attachment.
Paternal Adaptation	
Response to the mother and the infant	The father often provides the most important support for the mother. His involvement with the infant indicates acceptance of parenting role.
Knowledge of infant care	The father's knowledge determines the teaching he will need.
Response to infant cues or signals (crying, fussing)	Many fathers feel awkward handling infant but want to become proficient in infant care.
Ages and Developmental Levels of Siblings	
Reaction of siblings	Young children often fear the newborn will replace them in the affection of the parents. Parents may need anticipatory guidance about sibling rivalry.
Support System	
Interest and availability of family or friends to assist during early weeks	Families may need assistance in identifying available support.
Plans for first few days at home	Suggest that parents plan for support and rest. Provide resources such as telephone "baby lines," postpartum clinics, or support groups.
Follow-up plans	Appointments for the mother and infant are generally scheduled at 2 to 6 weeks with clinic or health care provider.
Cultural Factors	
Cultural beliefs and practices that may affect nursing care	Culture-specific care can be planned for hygiene, dietary preferences, usual care and feeding of infants, and role of the partner and family in child care.
Expectations of health care team	Expectations may vary in different cultures.

Siblings

Note the ages of siblings and their reactions to the newborn. Are they interested and helpful? Are they hostile and aggressive? How do the parents respond to sibling behaviors?

Support System

Family members often provide a powerful support system, and their involvement is important to the adaptation of the family. Are grandparents available and involved? Do sisters and brothers live nearby? Are they available to help the new parents? If the family is unavailable, who provides support? What arrangements have been made for assistance?

Nonverbal Behavior

Nonverbal behavior is equally important. Are the parents' words congruent with their actions?

Validate impressions and conclusions during a psychosocial assessment. One of the best ways to do this is to ask questions such as, "How much experience have you had with newborns?" "How are newborns fed in Vietnam until the mother's milk comes in?" "What are your plans when you go home?" "How long can your mother stay?"

Intersperse questions over time during normal caregiving. The mother should not be made to feel she is being interrogated because the nurse asks so many questions at once. Table 17.4 summarizes family assessment.

◆ Identification of Patient Problems

Family assessment identifies family strengths and areas in which nursing interventions could promote family adaptation or prevent disruptions in family functioning. Sometimes a family that usually functions effectively is unable to cope because of a specific event, such as the birth of a baby. Lack of knowledge of an infant's needs and behaviors, stress during the early weeks at home, and sibling rivalry can interfere with the usual family functioning.

◆ Planning: Expected Outcomes

Goals and expected outcomes may overlap with care after discharge because they often cannot be evaluated before the family leaves the birth facility. By (specific date) the family will do the following:

- Verbalize understanding of the infant's needs and behaviors
- Identify methods for reducing stress during the early weeks at home

- Describe measures to reduce sibling rivalry
- Identify external resources and the family's support system

◆ Interventions

Teaching the Family about the Newborn

Many families access the Internet for information about infant care. Mobile phones also can be used for obtaining information. A free service from the National Healthy Mothers, Healthy Babies Coalition provides texts with information about pregnancy and infants through 1 year. The service can be accessed by going to the website at www.text4baby.org or texting BABY to 511411 on a mobile phone.

Infant Needs. Some new parents have unrealistic expectations of the newborn. Provide them with information about the infant's capabilities as well as the infant's emotional and physical needs.

Infant Signals. Discuss the importance of responding promptly and gently to cues such as crying and fussing that indicate the infant needs attention. Reassure parents that responding to cues does not "spoil" their baby but helps the infant learn to trust that the world is a safe, secure place.

Help parents recognize signals that indicate when their infant has had enough interaction and wants to avoid further stimulation. These avoidance cues, such as looking away, splaying the fingers, arching the back, and fussiness, indicate that the infant needs a quiet time.

Helping the Family Adapt

Providing Anticipatory Guidance about Stress Reduction. Help the family plan for the demands of the first weeks at home by providing anticipatory guidance. This is a time when the need for rest is great but the opportunity for uninterrupted sleep is minimal. As a result, fatigue is a common problem for both parents. The nurse should do the following:

- Emphasize that the priority during the first 4 to 6 weeks should be caring for the mother and the baby.
- Recommend that mothers establish a relaxed home atmosphere and flexible meal schedule because attempts to maintain a rigid schedule or meticulous environment increase tension within the family.
- Recommend that the mother sleep when the infant sleeps and conserve her energy for care of the baby.
- Encourage parents to let friends and relatives know sleep and nap times and request that they telephone and visit at other times.
- Advise parents to place a "Do Not Disturb" sign on the door and to silence the ring on their phones during rest times.
- Suggest the parents limit coffee, tea, colas, and chocolate because they contain caffeine and will interfere with rest.
- Teach breathing exercises and progressive relaxation to reduce stress and energize, especially when a nap is not possible.
- Encourage both parents to delay tiring projects until the infant is older. Remind them that although schedules are chaotic for a while, the infant's behavior is generally more predictable by 12 to 16 weeks of age.
- Encourage open expression of feelings between parents as a first step in coping with stress.

- Remind parents of the need for healthy nutrition and recreation. Fatigue and tension easily can overwhelm the anticipated joys of parenting if no respite is available from constant care.
- Suggest that new parents enlist grandparents, other relatives, and friends to help with cooking, cleaning, shopping, and care of other children.

Helping the Partner Co-Parent. Help the partner become involved with his infant by including him in teaching. Provide opportunities for him to participate in diapering, comforting activities, and feeding or helping the mother breastfeed. Offer frequent encouragement and praise. If classes or chat rooms for men who are new parents are available, refer the father to them.

Providing Ways to Reduce Sibling Rivalry. Suggest that parents plan time alone with older children. Frequent praise and expressions of love and affection help reassure older children of their places in the family. Suggest that visitors and relatives do not focus exclusively on the infant but include older children in their gift giving and attention.

Emphasize the importance of responding calmly and with understanding when a sibling regresses to more infantile behaviors or expresses hostility toward the infant. Acknowledging the child's feelings and offering prompt reassurance of continued love are the most valuable actions.

Some children, particularly those older than 3 years of age, enjoy being a big brother or sister and respond well when they are included in infant care. This participation may not be possible with younger children, and setting aside separate time with them to participate in a favorite activity may be more worthwhile for the parents.

Identifying Resources. In many homes, women assume the major responsibilities of day-to-day homemaking. With the birth of an infant, this task becomes more difficult. A division of labor should be negotiated to prevent undue stress and fatigue. This division of labor is particularly important when other children in the home also need time, attention, and comfort.

Although the mother's primary support often is the father of the baby, extended family members, particularly grandmothers and sisters, also provide valuable support. Community resources such as daycare centers, parenting classes, and breastfeeding support groups are available in many areas. In addition, close friends and neighbors often share solutions to specific problems. Remind the mother that resources are available when she begins to feel isolated and exhausted.

◆ Evaluation

A prompt, gentle response to infant crying and fussing and verbalizations of acceptance of normal newborn behaviors indicate parental understanding of the infant's need. Devising a plan for obtaining rest and lessening anxiety in siblings is a first step in reducing stress and sibling rivalry. Identifying resources in the family, neighborhood, and community may help the family function to meet its needs during the early weeks at home.

SUMMARY CONCEPTS

- After childbirth the uterus returns to its nonpregnant size and condition by involution.
- The site of placental attachment heals by a process of exfoliation, which leaves the endometrium smooth and without scars.
- Involution can be evaluated by measuring the descent of the fundus (~1 cm/day). By about the 14th day after childbirth the fundus should no longer be palpable abdominally.
- Afterpains, or intermittent uterine contractions, cause discomfort for many women, particularly multiparas who breastfeed.
- Vaginal discharge (lochia) progresses from lochia rubra (dark red or red-brown) to lochia serosa (pink or brown-tinged) to lochia alba (white, cream, or light yellow) in a predictable timeframe. Lochia should be assessed for amount, type, and odor. Foul odor suggests endometrial infection.
- Orthostatic hypotension occurs when the mother moves from the supine to standing position quickly.
- Tachycardia may be caused by pain, excitement, anxiety, fatigue, dehydration, hypovolemia, anemia, or dehydration. Additional assessments (e.g., lochia, fundus) are required to determine whether excessive bleeding is the cause.
- The postpartum woman should be afebrile, but her temperature may be higher during the first 24 hours after delivery because of dehydration and leukocytosis.
- Hemorrhoids and perineal trauma can cause a great deal of discomfort and interfere with activity and bladder and bowel elimination.
- Cardiac output increases when blood from the uterus and placenta returns to the central circulation, uterine pressure on the vessels decreases, and extracellular fluid moves into the vascular compartment. Excess fluid is excreted by diuresis and diaphoresis.
- Increased clotting factors predispose the postpartum woman to thrombus formation. Early, frequent ambulation helps prevent thrombophlebitis.
- Constipation may occur from decreased food and fluid intake during labor, reduced activity, decreased muscle and bowel tone, and fear of pain during defecation.
- Increased bladder capacity and decreased sensitivity to fluid pressure may result in urinary retention. Stasis of urine allows time for bacteria to grow and can lead to urinary tract infection. A distended bladder displaces the uterus and can interfere with uterine contraction and cause excessive bleeding.

- Exercises to strengthen the abdominal muscles, good posture, and body mechanics may reduce musculoskeletal discomfort.
- Breastfeeding may delay the return of ovulation and menstruation, but ovulation may occur before the first menses. All mothers need information about family planning.
- After cesarean birth, the woman requires postoperative and postpartum assessments and care. She may have problems with immobility and discomfort.
- Bonding and attachment are gradual processes that begin before childbirth and progress to feelings of love and deep devotion lasting throughout life.
- Nurses foster bonding and attachment by providing early, unlimited contact between the parents and infant and modeling attachment behaviors.
- Maternal touch changes over time as many mothers progress from exploratory "fingertipping" to enfolding and finally demonstrating a full range of comforting behaviors.
- Verbal behaviors are important indicators of maternal attachment. Nurses often model how to speak to the infant and point out the infant's response to the verbal stimulation.
- Maternal adjustment to parenthood is a gradual process involving restorative phases of taking-in, taking-hold, and letting-go. Nurses play a valuable role in the process by first "mothering the mother" and then fostering independence as the mother becomes ready.
- Parents usually progress through four stages of role attainment—anticipatory, formal, informal, and personal—before they attain a sense of comfort and can structure their parenting behaviors to mesh with the infant's unique needs.
- Postpartum blues is a temporary, self-limiting period of tearfulness and mood instability. It should not last longer than 2 weeks.
- The birth of a baby requires reorganization of family structure and renegotiation of family responsibilities. Nurses can assist the partner in co-parenting the infant and help the new parents identify family resources.
- Siblings may be jealous and fearful that they will be replaced by the newborn in the affection of the parents. Nurses can lessen the negative feelings by providing information about ways to reduce sibling rivalry.
- Attention to cultural concerns of postpartum women is important in helping them meet cultural, physical, and psychosocial needs.

REFERENCES & READINGS

American Academy of Pediatrics & American College of Obstetricians and Gynecologists (AAP & ACOG). (2012). *Guidelines for perinatal care* (7th ed.). Elk Grove Village, IL: Author.

American College of Obstetricians and Gynecologists (ACOG). (2015). *Committee Opinion. Physical activity and exercise during pregnancy and the postpartum period.* Retrieved from www.acog.org.

American Society for Reproductive Medicine. (2014). *Hyperprolactinemia (high prolactin levels) fact sheet.* Retrieved from www.asrm.org.

Australian Breastfeeding Association. (2015). *Lactation suppression.* Retrieved from www.breastfeeding.asn.au/bfinfo/lactation-suppression.

Bain, E., Wilson, A., Tooher, R., Gates, S., Davis, L.J., & Middleton, P. (2014). Cochrane Database Systematic Reviews: Prophylaxis for venous thromboembolic disease in pregnancy and the early postnatal period. (5), CD001689. Retrieved from www.cochranelibrary.com.

Blackburn, S. T. (2013). *Maternal, fetal, and neonatal physiology: a clinical perspective* (4th ed.). St. Louis, MO: Saunders.

Buck, M. L., Amir, L. H., Cullinane, M., & Donath, S. (2014). Nipple pain, damage, and vasospasm in the first 8 weeks postpartum. *Breastfeeding Medicine*, 9(2), 56–62.

Callister, L. C. (2014). Integrating cultural beliefs and practices when caring for childbearing women and families. In K. R. Simpson, & P. A. Creehan (Eds.), *AWHONN perinatal nursing* (4th ed.) (pp. 41–70). Philadelphia: Wolters Kluwer Lippincott Williams & Wilkins.

Centers for Disease Control and Prevention. (2015). *Pertussis*. Retrieved from www.cdc.gov.

Centers for Disease Control and Prevention (CDC). (2016). *Pregnancy and rubella*. Retrieved from www.cdc.gov.

Cunningham, F. G., Leveno, K. J., Bloom, S. L., Spong, C. Y., Dashe, J. S., Hoffman, B. L., Sheffield, J. S. (2014). *William's obstetrics* (24th ed.). New York: McGraw-Hill Education, 668–683.

Doering, J. J. (2013). The physical and social environment of sleep in socioeconomically disadvantaged postpartum women. *Journal of Obstetric, Gynecologic, and Neonatal Nursing*, 42(1), E33–E43.

East, C. E., Begg, L., Henshall, N. E., Marchant, P. R., & Wallace, K. (2012). Local cooling for relieving pain from perineal trauma sustained during childbirth. *Cochrane Database of Systematic Reviews* (5), CD006304. Retrieved from www.cochranelibrary.com.

Giger, J. N. (2013). *Transcultural nursing: assessment and intervention* (6th ed.). St. Louis, MO: Mosby.

Hamborsky, J., Kroger, A., & Wolfe, C. (2015). Centers for Disease Control and Prevention. *Epidemiology and prevention of vaccine-preventable diseases* (13th ed.). Washington DC: Public Health Foundation.

Hamilton, B. E., Hoyert, D. L., Martin, J. A., et al. (2013). Annual summary of vital statistics: 2010–2011. *Pediatrics*, 131(3), 548–558.

Isley, M. M., & Katz, V. L. (2017). Postpartum care and long-term health considerations. In S. G. Gabbe, J. R. Niebyl, J. L. Simpson, M. B. Landon, H. L. Galan, R. M. Jauniaux, D. A. Driscoll, et al. (Eds.), *Obstetrics: normal and problem pregnancies* (7th ed.) (pp. 499–516). Philadelphia: Saunders.

Jones, M., Lewis, S., Parrott, S., Wormall, S., & Coleman, T. (2016). Restarting smoking in the postpartum period after receiving smoking cessation intervention: a systematic review. *Addiction*, 111(6), 981–990.

Kennedy, K. I. (2010). Fertility, sexuality, & contraception during lactation. In J. Riordan, & K. Wambach (Eds.), *Breast-feeding and human lactation* (4th ed.) (pp. 705–736). Boston, MA: Jones & Bartlett.

Kennedy, K. I., & Trussell, J. (2011). Postpartum contraception and lactation. In R. A. Hatcher, J. Trussell, A. L. Nelson, et al. (Eds.), *Contraceptive technology* (20th ed.) (pp. 483–511). New York: Ardent Media.

Liu, Y. Q., Petrini, M., & Maloni, J. A. (2015). 'Doing the month': Postpartum practices in Chinese women. *Nursing & Health Sciences*, 17(1), 5–14.

Martin, J. A., Hamilton, B. E., Osterman, M. J. K., Driscoll, A. K., & Mathews, T. J. (2017). Births: Final data for 2015. *National vital statistics report: Vol 66, no 1*. Hyattsville, MD: National Center for Health Statistics. 2017.

Mattson, S. (2015). Ethnocultural considerations in the childbearing period. In S. Mattson, & J. E. Smith (Eds.), *AWHONN core curriculum for maternal-newborn nursing* (5th ed.) (pp. 61–79). St. Louis, MO: Mosby.

McCall-Hosenfeld, J., Phiri, K., Schaefer, E., Zhu, J., & Kjerulff, K. (2016). Trajectories of depressive symptoms throughout the peri- and postpartum period: Results from the first baby study. *Journal of Women's Health*.

Mercer, R. T. (1995a). *Becoming a mother: Research on maternal identity from Rubin to the present*. New York: Springer.

Mercer, R. T. (1995b). Predictors of maternal role attainment. *Nursing Research*, 34(4), 198–204.

Mercer, R. T. (2004). Becoming a mother versus maternal role attainment. *Journal of Nursing Scholarship*, 36(3), 226–232.

Mercer, R. T., & Ferketich, S. L. (1994). Maternal-infant attachment of experienced and inexperienced mothers during infancy. *Nursing Research*, 43(6), 344–351.

Mercer, R. T., & Walker, L. O. (2006). A review of interventions to foster becoming a mother. *Journal of Obstetric, Gynecologic, and Neonatal Nursing*, 35(5), 568–582.

Oladapo, O. T., & Fawole, B. (2012). Treatments for suppression of lactation. *Cochrane Database of Systematic Reviews* (9), CD005937. Retrieved from www.cochranelibrary.com.

Rubin, R. (1961). Puerperal change. *Nursing Outlook*, 9(12), 743–755.

Rubin, R. (1977). Binding-in in the postpartum period. *MCN: American Journal of Maternal/Child Nursing*, 6(1), 65–75.

U.S. Department of Labor, Bureau of Labor Statistics. (2016). *Employment characteristics of families—2015*. Retrieved from www.bls.gov.

Waugh, L. J. (2011). Beliefs associated with Mexican immigrant families' practice of La Cuarentena during postpartum recovery. *Journal of Obstetric, Gynecologic, and Neonatal Nursing*, 40(6), 732–741.

Whitmer, T. (2016). Physical and psychological changes. In S. Mattson, & J. E. Smith (Eds.), *AWHONN core curriculum for maternal-newborn nursing* (5th ed.) (pp. 301–314). St. Louis, MO: Mosby.

Postpartum Maternal Complications

Karen S. Holub

Pregnancy and childbirth are natural events from which most women recover without complication. However, nurses should be aware of problems that may occur and their effect on the family. The most common physiologic complications during the postpartum period are hemorrhage, thromboembolic disorders, and infection. Peripartum mood and anxiety disorders, the major psychological disorders during childbearing, are discussed in Chapter 11.

POSTPARTUM HEMORRHAGE

Postpartum hemorrhage is a major cause of maternal death and morbidity in the United States and the world (Abdul-Kadir et al., 2014; Main et al., 2015). Traditionally, postpartum hemorrhage was defined as blood loss greater than 500 mL for a vaginal birth and greater than 1000 mL for a cesarean birth (Cunningham et al., 2014; Main et al., 2015). However, the nomenclature consensus conference of the American College of Obstetricians and Gynecologists (ACOG) revised the definition of early postpartum hemorrhage as, "Cumulative blood loss of >= 1000 mL or blood loss accompanied by sign/symptoms of hypovolemia within 24 hours following the birth process (includes intrapartum loss)" (ACOG, 2014a, p. 1). Blood loss is frequently underestimated. Estimates are often only about half the actual loss (Cunningham et al., 2014), and therefore blood loss should be quantified by weighing or measuring and records of cumulative loss maintained (Association of Women's Health, Obstetric and Neonatal Nurses [AWHONN], 2015b; Main et al., 2015). Hemorrhage in the first 24 hours after childbirth is called *early postpartum hemorrhage*. Hemorrhage after 24 hours or up to 6 to 12 weeks after birth is called *late postpartum hemorrhage*.

Early Postpartum Hemorrhage

Early postpartum hemorrhage usually occurs during the first hour after birth and is most often caused by uterine atony (ACOG, 2015b; Cunningham et al., 2014). **Atony** refers to lack of muscle tone that results in failure of the uterine muscle fibers to contract firmly around blood vessels when the placenta separates. Trauma to the birth canal during labor and birth, **hematomas** (localized collections of blood in a space or tissue), retention of placental fragments, and abnormalities of coagulation are other causes. Hemorrhage from disseminated intravascular coagulation and placenta previa are discussed in Chapter 10. Other causes of hemorrhage include **placenta accreta** (abnormal adherence of the placenta to the uterine wall) and inversion of the uterus, which are described in Chapter 16.

Uterine Atony

With uterine atony, the relaxed muscles allow rapid bleeding from the endometrial arteries at the placental site. Bleeding continues until the uterine muscle fibers contract to stop the flow of blood. Fig. 18.1 illustrates the effect of uterine contraction on the size of the placental site and the amount of bleeding that occurs.

Predisposing Factors. Knowledge of factors that increase the risk for uterine atony helps the nurse anticipate and therefore reduce excessive bleeding. Overdistention of the uterus from any cause such as multiple gestation, a large infant, or **hydramnios** (excessive volume of amniotic fluid) makes it more difficult for the uterus to contract with enough firmness to prevent excessive bleeding. Multiparity results in muscle fibers that have been stretched repeatedly, and these

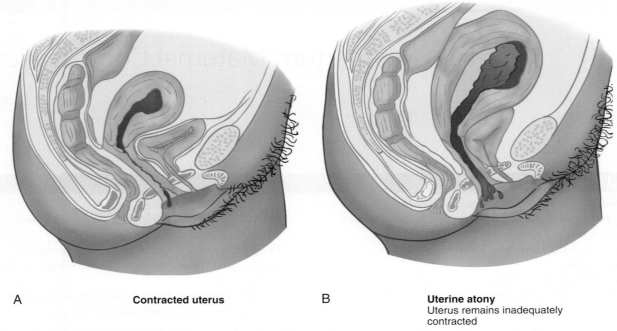

A   **Contracted uterus**   B   **Uterine atony**
                                               Uterine remains inadequately
                                               contracted

FIG. 18.1 A, When the uterus remains contracted, the placental site is smaller, so bleeding is minimal. **B,** If uterine muscles fail to contract around the endometrial arteries at the placental site, hemorrhage occurs.

flaccid muscle fibers may not remain contracted after birth. Obesity also increases the risk for postpartum hemorrhage (Cunningham et al., 2014). Intrapartum factors include contractions that were minimally effective, resulting in prolonged labor; contractions that were excessively vigorous, resulting in precipitous labor; and labor that was induced or augmented with oxytocin. Retention of a large segment of the placenta does not allow the uterus to contract firmly and therefore can result in uterine atony. Box 18.1 summarizes predisposing factors for postpartum hemorrhage.

Clinical Manifestations. Major signs of uterine atony include the following:

- A uterine fundus that is difficult to locate
- A soft or "boggy" feel when the fundus is located
- A uterus that becomes firm as it is massaged but loses its tone when massage is stopped
- A fundus that is located above the expected level
- Excessive lochia, especially if it is bright red
- Excessive clots expelled, either with or without uterine massage

For the first 24 hours after childbirth the uterus should feel like a firmly contracted ball roughly the size of a large grapefruit. It should be easily located at about the level of the umbilicus. Lochia should be dark red and scant to moderate in amount. Saturation of one peripad in 15 minutes represents an excessive blood loss (Whitmer, 2016). The nurse should realize that although bleeding may be profuse and dramatic, a constant steady trickle, dribble, or slow seeping is just as dangerous.

Therapeutic Management. Early administration of oxytocin is recommended for all births as a prophylaxis

---

> **BOX 18.1   Common Predisposing Factors for Postpartum Hemorrhage**
>
> Overdistention of the uterus (multiple gestation, large infant, hydramnios)
> Multiparity (five or more)
> Precipitate labor or birth
> Prolonged labor
> Use of forceps or vacuum extractor
> Cesarean birth
> Manual removal of the placenta
> Uterine inversion
> Placenta previa, placenta accreta, or low implantation
> Drugs: Oxytocin, prostaglandins, tocolytics, or magnesium sulfate
> General anesthesia
> Chorioamnionitis
> Clotting disorders
> Previous postpartum hemorrhage or uterine surgery
> Disseminated intravascular coagulation
> Uterine leiomyomas (fibroids)

against postpartum hemorrhage (Abdul-Kadir et al., 2014; AWHONN, 2015b; Main et al., 2015). Intravenous (IV) infusion of dilute oxytocin (not IV push) should be given during the third stage of labor. Oxytocin also may be administered intramuscularly (AWHONN, 2015b) (see Drug Guide: Oxytocin in Chapter 15). Nurses are with the mother during the hours after childbirth and are responsible for assessments and initial management of uterine atony. If the uterus is not firmly contracted, despite preventive measures, the first intervention is to massage the fundus until it is firm and to express clots

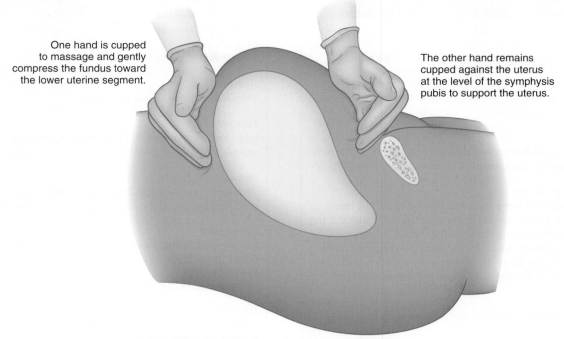

One hand is cupped to massage and gently compress the fundus toward the lower uterine segment.

The other hand remains cupped against the uterus at the level of the symphysis pubis to support the uterus.

FIG. 18.2 Technique for Fundal Massage.

that may have accumulated in the uterus. One hand is placed just above the symphysis pubis to support the lower uterine segment while the other hand gently but firmly massages the fundus in a circular motion (Fig. 18.2).

Clots that may have accumulated in the uterine cavity interfere with the ability of the uterus to contract effectively. They are expressed by applying firm but gentle pressure on the fundus in the direction of the vagina. It is critical that the uterus is contracted firmly before attempting to express clots. *Pushing on a uterus that is not contracted could invert the uterus and cause massive hemorrhage and rapid shock.*

If the uterus does not remain contracted as a result of uterine massage or if the fundus is displaced, the bladder may be distended. A full bladder lifts the uterus, moving it up and to the side, preventing effective contraction of the uterine muscles. Assist the mother to urinate or catheterize her to correct uterine atony caused by bladder distention. Note urine output.

If atony persists despite prophylactic oxytocin and uterine massage, further pharmacologic measures may be necessary. Initially, additional oxytocin may be ordered. Methylergonovine (Methergine) is a common second drug of choice when oxytocin is not effective. Methergine elevates blood pressure and should not be given to a woman who is hypertensive. The usual route of administration is intramuscularly (see Drug Guide: Methylergonovine). Misoprostol (Cytotec), a synthetic prostaglandin E1 (PGE$_1$) given orally or sublingually also may be used to control bleeding (California Maternal Quality Care Collaborative [CMQCC], 2015; Cunningham et al., 2014). Analogs of prostaglandin F2-alpha (PGF$_2\alpha$; carboprost tromethamine [Hemabate; Prostin/15M]) are also effective when given intramuscularly

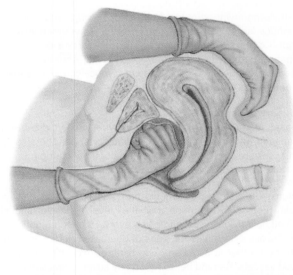

FIG. 18.3 **Bimanual Compression.** One hand is inserted in the vagina, and the other compresses the uterus through the abdominal wall.

or into the uterine muscle (CMQCC, 2015). (See Drug Guide: Carboprost Tromethamine.)

If uterine massage and pharmacologic measures are ineffective in stopping uterine bleeding, the health care provider may use bimanual compression of the uterus. In this procedure, one hand is inserted into the vagina and the other compresses the uterus through the abdominal wall (Fig. 18.3). A balloon may be inserted into the uterus to apply pressure against the uterine surface to stop bleeding (Cekmez, Ozkaya, Ocal, & Kucukozkan, 2015; Martin et al., 2015). Uterine

DRUG GUIDE

Methylergonovine (Methergine)
Classification
Ergot alkaloid, uterine stimulant.

Action
Stimulates sustained contraction of the uterus and causes arterial vasoconstriction.

Indications
Used for the prevention and treatment of postpartum or post-abortion hemorrhage caused by uterine atony or subinvolution.

Dosage and Route
Usual dosage is 0.2 mg intramuscularly every 2 to 4 hours for a maximum of five doses. Change to the oral route 0.2 mg every 6 to 8 hours for a maximum of 7 days. Intravenous use not recommended; use in life-threatening emergency only and give over at least 60 seconds with close monitoring of blood pressure (BP) and pulse; may cause severe hypertension.

Absorption
Well absorbed after oral or intramuscular route.

Excretion
Metabolized by the liver; excreted in the feces and urine.

Contraindications and Precautions
Methylergonovine should not be used during pregnancy or to induce labor. Do not use if the mother is hypersensitive to ergot. Contraindicated for women with hypertension, severe hepatic or renal disease, thrombophlebitis, coronary artery disease, peripheral vascular disease, hypocalcemia, or sepsis or before the fourth stage of labor.

Adverse Reactions
Nausea, vomiting, uterine cramping, hypertension, dizziness, headache, dyspnea, chest pain, palpitations, peripheral ischemia, seizure, and uterine and gastrointestinal cramping.

Nursing Considerations
Before administering the medication, assess the BP. Follow facility protocol to determine at what BP level medication should be withheld. Monitor BP and pulse every 15 minutes until stable. Assess extremities for signs of decreased perfusion. Caution the mother to avoid smoking because nicotine constricts blood vessels. Remind her to report any adverse reactions.

DRUG GUIDE

Carboprost Tromethamine (Hemabate, Prostin/15M)
Classification
Prostaglandin, oxytocic.

Action
Stimulates contraction of the uterus.

Indications
Used for the treatment of postpartum hemorrhage caused by uterine atony. Also used for pregnancy termination.

Dosage and Route
Postpartum hemorrhage: 250 mcg intramuscularly. May repeat at 15- to 90-minute intervals. Maximum total dose 2 mg.

Absorption
Metabolized by the liver and by enzymes in the lungs.

Excretion
Primarily excreted in urine.

Contraindications and Precautions
Contraindicated for women with hypersensitivity to carboprost or other prostaglandins or who have acute pelvic inflammatory disease or cardiac, pulmonary, renal, or hepatic disease. Use caution if the woman has a history of asthma, hypotension or hypertension, anemia, jaundice, diabetes, epilepsy, or previous uterine surgery.

Adverse Reactions and Side Effects
Excessive dose may cause tetanic contraction and laceration or uterine rupture. May cause uterine hypertonus if used with oxytocin. Nausea, vomiting, diarrhea (frequent), fever, chills, facial flushing, headache, hypertension or hypotension, tachycardia, pulmonary edema.

Nursing Considerations
Should be refrigerated. Give via deep intramuscular injection. Rotate sites if repeated. Monitor vital signs. Administer antiemetics and antidiarrheals as ordered.

---

packing also may be used. It may be necessary to return the woman to the birthing area for exploration of the uterine cavity and removal of placental fragments that interfere with uterine contraction.

A laparotomy may be necessary to identify the source of the bleeding. Uterine compression sutures may be placed to stop severe bleeding. Ligation of the uterine or hypogastric artery or embolization (occlusion) of pelvic arteries may be required if other measures are not effective. Hysterectomy is a last resort to save the life of a woman with uncontrollable postpartum hemorrhage.

Hemorrhage requires prompt replacement of intravascular fluid volume. Lactated Ringer's solution, whole blood, packed red blood cells, normal saline, or other plasma extenders are used. Enough fluid should be given to maintain a urine flow of at least 30 milliliters per hour (mL/hr) (Cunningham et al., 2014). Typically, the nurse is responsible for obtaining properly typed and cross-matched blood and inserting large-bore IV lines capable of carrying whole blood.

Trauma

Trauma to the birth canal is the second most common cause of early postpartum hemorrhage. Trauma includes vaginal, cervical, or perineal lacerations and hematomas.

Predisposing Factors. Many of the same factors that increase the risk for uterine atony increase the risk for soft tissue trauma during childbirth. For example, trauma to the birth canal is more likely to occur if the infant is large or if labor and birth occur rapidly. Induction and augmentation of labor and use of assistive devices, such as a vacuum extractor or forceps, increase the risk for tissue trauma.

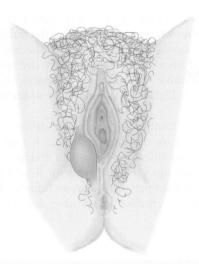

FIG. 18.4 A vulvar hematoma is caused by rapid bleeding into soft tissue, and it causes severe pain and feelings of pressure.

Lacerations. The perineum, vagina, cervix, and area around the urethral meatus are the most common sites for lacerations. Small cervical lacerations occur frequently and generally do not require repairs. Lacerations of the vagina, perineum, and periurethral area usually occur during the second stage of labor, when the fetal head descends rapidly or when assistive devices such as a vacuum extractor or forceps are used to in birth.

Lacerations of the birth canal should be suspected if excessive uterine bleeding continues when the fundus is contracted firmly and is at the expected location. Bleeding from lacerations of the genital tract often is bright red, in contrast to the darker red color of lochia. Bleeding may be heavy or may appear to be minor with a steady trickle of blood.

Hematomas. Hematomas occur when bleeding into loose connective tissue occurs while overlying tissue remains intact. Hematomas develop as a result of blood vessel injury in spontaneous deliveries and deliveries in which vacuum extractors or forceps are used. Hematomas may be found in vulvar, vaginal, and retroperitoneal areas.

The rapid bleeding into soft tissue may cause a visible vulvar hematoma, a discolored bulging mass that is sensitive to touch (Fig. 18.4). Hematomas in the vagina or retroperitoneal areas cannot be seen. Hematomas produce deep, severe, unrelieved pain and feelings of pressure that are not relieved by usual pain-relief measures. Formation of a hematoma should be suspected if the mother demonstrates systemic signs of concealed blood loss, such as tachycardia or decreasing blood pressure, when the fundus is firm and lochia is within normal limits.

Therapeutic Management. When postpartum hemorrhage is caused by trauma of the birth canal, surgical repair is often necessary. Visualizing lacerations of the vagina or cervix is difficult, and it is necessary to return the mother to the birthing area, where surgical lights are available. She is placed in a lithotomy position and carefully draped. Surgical asepsis is required while the laceration is being visualized and repaired.

Small hematomas usually reabsorb naturally. Large hematomas may require incision, evacuation of the clots, and location and ligation of the bleeding vessel.

Late Postpartum Hemorrhage

Late postpartum hemorrhage, also called *secondary postpartum hemorrhage,* is defined as hemorrhage occurring between 24 hours and 12 weeks after birth (ACOG, 2015b). The most common causes of late postpartum hemorrhage are **subinvolution** (delayed return of the uterus to its nonpregnant size and consistency), retained placental fragments, and infection (Cunningham et al., 2014; Doussou, Debost-Legrand, Dechelotte, Lemery, & Venditelli, 2015). Normally the uterus descends at the rate of approximately 1 cm (one fingerbreadth) per day. By 14 days, it is no longer palpable above the symphysis pubis. The endometrial lining has sloughed off as part of the lochia, and the site of placental attachment is well healed by 6 weeks after childbirth. When placental fragments are retained, clots form around the retained fragments, and excessive bleeding can occur when the clots slough away several days after birth.

Clinical Manifestations

Signs of subinvolution include prolonged discharge of lochia, irregular or excessive uterine bleeding, and sometimes profuse hemorrhage. Pelvic pain or feelings of pelvic heaviness, backache, fatigue, and persistent malaise are reported by many women. On bimanual examination the uterus feels larger and softer than normal for that time of the puerperium.

Predisposing Factors

Attempts to deliver the placenta before it separates from the uterine wall, manual removal of the placenta, placenta accreta, previous cesarean birth, and uterine leiomyomas are primary predisposing factors for retention of placental fragments. Debost-Legrand, Riviere, Dossou, and Vendittelli (2015) found that early postpartum hemorrhage and advanced maternal age (35 years or older) were also risk factors.

Therapeutic Management

Late postpartum hemorrhage caused by retained placental fragments is generally preventable. When the placenta is delivered, the health care provider carefully inspects it to determine whether it is intact. If a portion of the placenta is missing, the provider manually explores the uterus, locates the missing fragments, and removes them.

Initial treatment for late postpartum hemorrhage is directed toward control of the excessive bleeding. Oxytocin, methylergonovine, and prostaglandins are the most commonly used pharmacologic measures. Placental fragments may be dislodged and swept out of the uterus by the bleeding, and if the bleeding subsides when oxytocin is administered, no other treatment is necessary. Sonography may identify placental fragments that remain in the uterus. If bleeding continues or recurs, **dilation and curettage** (stretching of the cervical os to permit suctioning or scraping of the walls of the uterus) may be necessary to remove fragments. Broad-spectrum antibiotics may be given if postpartum infection is suspected because of uterine tenderness, foul-smelling lochia, or fever.

Nursing Considerations

In most cases, subinvolution is not obvious until the mother has returned home after childbirth. Nurses should teach the mother and her family how to recognize its occurrence. Demonstrate how to locate and palpate the fundus and how to estimate fundal height in relation to the umbilicus. The uterus should become smaller each day (by approximately one fingerbreadth). Explain the progressive changes from lochia rubra to lochia serosa and then to lochia alba (see Chapter 17).

Instruct the mother to report any deviation from the expected pattern or duration of lochia. A foul odor often indicates uterine infection for which treatment is necessary. Additional signs include pelvic or fundal pain, backache, and feelings of pelvic pressure or fullness. The mother should be able to verbalize the warning signs before leaving the facility.

EVIDENCE-BASED PRACTICE

Obstetric hemorrhage is one of the most common serious complications related to childbirth and one of the most preventable. Many hospitals are adopting massive transfusion protocols (MTP) in order to treat patients with severe hemorrhage. A recent randomized control trial of MTP in patients with severe trauma compared transfusion of plasma, platelets, and packed red blood cells (PRBCs) in a ratio of 1:1:1 versus 1:1:2, respectively (Holcomb et al., 2015). This study showed no significant difference in mortality in 24 hours and 30 days for each of the two ratios. The study did prove the 1:1:1 ratio group achieved hemostasis and fewer deaths due to exsanguination by 24 hours. Butelow et al. (2007) reported the use of high volumes of crystalloid or colloid fluid infused with PRBCs can lead to dilutional coagulopathy. This study discusses the importance of plasma, platelets and PRBCs to replace blood volume in patients with severe postpartum hemorrhage. Replacing severe blood loss with whole blood products restores not only the blood volume but also essential clotting factors. Massive transfusion protocols use a specific ratio of blood products to prevent the mother from developing life-threatening coagulopathy and DIC (disseminated intravascular coagulation).

Massive transfusion guidelines encourage practitioners to guide their resuscitation efforts during a severe postpartum hemorrhage based on their clinical observation of the patient during the acute phase (Burtelow et al., 2007). Laboratory studies may be unavailable in the immediate period of a severe postpartum hemorrhage. Stat labs for coagulation (PT, APTT, fibrinogen, and D-dimer) should be sent as soon as possible and results should guide the maintenance phase of the resuscitation.

These studies conclude that a specific ratio of blood products as well as timely administration can help improve outcomes for patients with severe postpartum hemorrhage.

Questions

1. What assessment questions about the patient's history would alert the nurse that a patient would be at higher risk for postpartum hemorrhage?
2. What type of orders from the provider would the nurse anticipate if a patient is at high risk for hemorrhage?
3. What type of abnormalities in lab values would the nurse anticipate in a patient with severe hemorrhage and possible DIC?

References

Burtelow, M., Riley, E., Druzin, M., Fontaine, M., Viele, M., & Goodnough, L. T. (2007). How we treat: Management of life-threatening primary postpartum hemorrhage with a standardized massive transfusion protocol. *Transfusion, 47*(9), 1564–1572.

Holcomb, J. B., Tilley, B. C., Baraniuk, S., Fox, E. E., Wade, C. E., Podbielski, J. M., van Belle, G. (2015). Transfusion of plasma, platelets, and red blood cells in a 1:1:1 vs a 1:1:2 ratio and mortality in patients with severe trauma: The PROPPR randomized clinical trial. *Journal of American Medical Association, 313*(5), 471–482.

? KNOWLEDGE CHECK

1. Why does the nurse examine the mother's prenatal record and her labor and delivery record?
2. Why is a mother who has given birth to twins at increased risk for postpartum hemorrhage?
3. Can the nurse be positive that bleeding is controlled when the fundus is firm and the lochia is moderate? Why or why not?
4. How is uterine atony treated?
5. How are hematomas treated?
6. What are the major signs of subinvolution?
7. What is the nurse's primary responsibility in the management of subinvolution?

Hypovolemic Shock

During and after giving birth, the woman can tolerate blood loss that approaches the volume of blood added during pregnancy (~1500 to 2000 mL). A woman who was anemic before birth has less reserve than a mother with normal blood values. The amount of blood lost can be estimated by comparing the hematocrit (Hct) before labor to that after birth. If the Hct is lower after birth, the woman lost the amount of blood added during pregnancy plus an additional 500 mL for each 3% drop in the Hct value (Cunningham et al., 2014).

When blood loss is excessive, **hypovolemic shock** (acute peripheral circulatory failure resulting from loss of circulating blood volume) can ensue. **Hypovolemia** (abnormally decreased volume of circulating fluid in the body) endangers vital organs by depriving them of oxygen. The brain, heart, and kidneys are especially vulnerable to hypoxia and may suffer damage in a brief period.

Pathophysiology

Recognition of hypovolemic shock may be delayed because the body activates compensatory mechanisms that mask the severity of the problem. Baroreceptors are stimulated to constrict peripheral blood vessels. This shunts blood to the central circulation and away from less essential organs, such as the skin and extremities. The skin becomes pale and cold, but cardiac output and perfusion of vital organs are maintained.

The adrenal glands release catecholamines, which compensate for decreased blood volume by promoting vasoconstriction in nonessential organs, increasing the heart rate and raising the blood pressure. As a result, blood pressure remains normal initially, although a decrease in **pulse pressure** (difference between systolic and diastolic blood pressures) may be noted. The tachycardia that develops is an early sign of compensation for excessive blood loss.

As shock worsens, the compensatory mechanisms fail and physiologic insults spiral. Inadequate organ perfusion and decreased cellular oxygen for metabolism result in a buildup of lactic acid and the development of metabolic acidosis. Acidosis results in vasodilation, which further increases bleeding. Eventually, circulating volume becomes insufficient to perfuse cardiac and brain tissue. Cellular death occurs as a result of anoxia, and the mother dies.

Clinical Manifestation

Early signs of blood loss such as mild tachycardia or hypotension may not appear until 25% to 30% of the woman's blood volume has been lost (Robbins, Martin, & Wilson, 2014). Tachycardia is one of the earliest signs of hypovolemic shock; even gradual increases in the pulse rate should be noted. A decrease in blood pressure and narrowing of pulse pressure occur when the circulating volume of blood is sufficiently decreased. The respiratory rate increases as the woman becomes more anxious and attempts to take in more oxygen to overcome the need created when hemoglobin (Hgb) is inadequate to transport oxygen adequately.

Skin changes also provide early clues. Vasoconstriction in the skin causes it to become pale and cool to the touch. As hemorrhage worsens, the skin changes become more obvious as pallor increases and the skin becomes cold and clammy.

As shock progresses, changes occur in the central nervous system. The mother becomes anxious, then confused, and finally lethargic as blood loss increases. Urine output decreases and eventually stops.

Therapeutic Management

The goals of therapy are to control bleeding and prevent hypovolemic shock from becoming irreversible. A second IV line should be inserted with a large-bore (14- to 18-gauge) catheter capable of carrying whole blood. Central IV catheters may be placed. Sufficient fluid volume is infused to produce a urinary output of at least 30 mL/hr. Vasopressors may be needed for low blood pressure. The health care team makes every effort to locate the source of bleeding and to stop the loss of blood.

Nursing Considerations

Immediate Care. Multidisciplinary work groups of the National Partnership for Maternal Safety under the guidance of the Council on Patient Safety in Women's Health Care outlined critical clinical practices called *safety bundles* that should be implemented in every maternity unit to address obstetric hemorrhage. These practices fall into four categories: *Readiness* (immediate access to supplies and medications, identification of a response team and the method for immediate communication, protocols for emergency blood transfusions, staff education with regular drills), *Recognition and Prevention* (risk assessment at multiple times during the antepartum, intrapartum, and postpartum periods, quantification of blood loss, early postpartum administration of oxytocin), *Response* (an emergency management plan for obstetric hemorrhage, support programs for patient, families, and staff), and *Reporting and System Learning* (culture of safety, including huddles and debriefs, multidisciplinary quality reviews of hemorrhages with ongoing monitoring of outcomes and practice changes) (Council on Patient Safety in Women' Health, 2015; Main et al., 2015). These practices should be used to facilitate implementation of evidence-based practices to decrease severe maternal morbidity and mortality.

When postpartum hemorrhage is identified, the response team should be notified. One person should be assigned to evaluate and record vital signs. Blood pressure and pulse should be assessed every 3 to 5 minutes. The location and consistency of the fundus, amount of lochia, skin temperature and color, and capillary return are assessed. Oxygen may be administered by tight face mask at 8 to 10 L/min to increase the saturation of fewer red blood cells. Oxygen saturation levels are carefully monitored. Nurses often follow protocols that allow them to draw blood for Hgb, Hct, clotting studies, and type and crossmatch. Nurses administer fluids, blood products, whole blood, and medications as directed and report their effectiveness. A urinary catheter is inserted to measure hourly urinary output. The catheter is also necessary if a surgical procedure to control the hemorrhage is required. In addition, nurses should make every effort to provide information and emotional support to the woman and her family.

> **! SAFETY CHECK**
>
> Signs of postpartum hemorrhage include the following:
> A uterus that does not contract or does not remain contracted
> Large gush or slow, steady trickle, ooze, or dribble of blood from the vagina
> Saturation of one peripad per 15 minutes
> Severe, unrelieved perineal or rectal pain
> Tachycardia

◆ APPLICATION OF THE NURSING PROCESS: THE WOMAN WITH EXCESSIVE BLEEDING

◆ Assessment

The initial postpartum assessment includes a chart review to determine whether risk factors for hemorrhage are present. This alerts the nurse to a woman at increased risk for hemorrhage.

TABLE 18.1 Nursing Assessments for Postpartum Hemorrhage

Assessments	Abnormal Signs and Symptoms	Nursing Implications
Chart review	Presence of predisposing factors	Perform more frequent evaluations.
Fundus	Soft, boggy, displaced	Massage, express clots, and assist to void or catheterize; notify primary health care provider if measures are ineffective.
Lochia	Bleeding (steady trickle, dribble, oozing, seeping, or profuse flow); heavy: saturation of 1 pad/hr; excessive: 1 pad/15 min	Assess for trauma; save and weigh pads, linen savers, and bed linens so estimation of blood loss will be more accurate. Notify health care provider.
Vital signs	Tachycardia, decreasing pulse pressure, falling blood pressure, decreasing oxygen saturation level	Report signs of excessive blood loss.
Urine output	Decreased urine output (should be at least 30 mL/hr)	Report decrease in output.
Comfort level	Severe pelvic or rectal pain	Assess for signs of hematoma, usually perineal or vaginal; examine vulva for masses or discoloration; report findings.
Skin	Cool, damp, pale	Look for signs of hypovolemia; vigilant assessment and management by entire health care team is necessary.

Uterine Atony

Priority assessments for uterine atony include the fundus, bladder, lochia, vital signs, skin temperature, and color. Assess the consistency and the location of the uterine fundus. The fundus should be firmly contracted at or near the level of the umbilicus and midline. If the fundus feels soft (boggy), the uterus is not firmly contracted and bleeding from the placental site may be rapid and continuous. If the fundus is above the level of the umbilicus and displaced, a full bladder may be the cause of excessive bleeding. Assist the mother to urinate or obtain an order and catheterize her. Note urine output and then reassess the uterus (see Procedure 17-1, for assessing the fundus).

Obese women have an increased risk for uterine atony with subsequent postpartum hemorrhage (Wetta et al., 2013); however, assessment of the fundus is difficult in this population. Monitor these women frequently for other signs of uterine atony and attempt to assess the uterine fundus while watching for increased lochia flow or clots to be expelled.

Remember to check under the woman's legs, buttocks, and back for lochia drainage by asking the woman to turn on her side. Although bleeding may be profuse and dramatic, a continuing small but steady trickle also may lead to significant blood loss that becomes increasingly life threatening.

It is difficult to estimate the volume of lochia by visual examination of peripads. More accurate information is obtained by weighing peripads, linen savers, and, if necessary, bed linens before and after use and subtracting the difference. One gram (weight) equals approximately 1 mL (volume).

Measure vital signs at least every 15 minutes or more often if necessary. Apply a pulse oximeter to determine oxygen saturation levels. Because the body initially compensates for excessive bleeding by constricting the peripheral blood vessels and shunting blood to vital organs, the vital signs may remain normal at first, even though the woman is becoming hypovolemic The skin should be warm and dry, mucous membranes of the lips and mouth should be pink, and capillary return should occur within 3 seconds when the nails are blanched. These signs confirm adequate circulating volume to perfuse the peripheral tissue.

! SAFETY CHECK

The following are used to determine the amount of blood loss:
Weigh all blood-soaked items (e.g., peripads, linens).
Weigh similar clean items.
Subtract the weight of the dry items from that of the wet items.
1 g weight = 1 mL of blood.

Trauma

If the fundus is firm but bleeding is excessive, the cause may be lacerations of the cervix or birth canal. Inspect the perineum to determine whether a laceration is visible. Lacerations of the cervix or vagina are not visible, but bleeding in the presence of a firmly contracted uterus suggests a laceration. This warrants examination of the vaginal walls and the cervix by the health care provider.

Assess comfort level. If the mother complains of deep, severe pelvic or rectal pain or if vital signs or skin changes suggest hemorrhage but excessive bleeding is not obvious, the cause may be concealed bleeding and the formation of a hematoma. Examine the vulva for bulging masses or discoloration. However, a hematoma developing in the vagina or in the retroperitoneal area will not be obvious when the vulva is examined. Table 18.1 summarizes assessments, abnormal signs and symptoms, and nursing implications for postpartum hemorrhage.

◆ Identification of Patient Problems

Inadequate fluid volume and reduced tissue perfusion are examples of problems faced by a woman with postpartum hemorrhage. These problems require a team approach to prevent further complications such as hypovolemic shock.

◆ Planning: Expected Outcomes

Hemorrhage requires an interprofessional approach; therefore the nursing plan of care will reflect both dependent and independent nursing care. Planning should reflect the nurse's responsibility to do the following:

- Monitor for signs of postpartum hemorrhage
- Perform actions that minimize postpartum hemorrhage and prevent hypovolemic shock
- Notify the provider if signs of excessive blood loss are observed or if the woman does not respond as desired

◆ Interventions

Preventing Hemorrhage

The key to successful management of early postpartum hemorrhage is early recognition and response. All postpartum women are at risk for hemorrhage. However, be aware of factors that increase this risk further and be particularly vigilant in monitoring these women so that excessive bleeding can be anticipated and minimized.

When predisposing factors are present, initiate frequent assessments. Many hospitals and birth centers have a protocol that calls for assessments every 15 minutes during the first hour after birth, every 30 minutes for the next 2 hours, and hourly for the next 4 hours. This plan may not be adequate for the woman at known risk for postpartum hemorrhage. A delay in assessment could result in excessive blood loss.

Collaborating with the Health Care Provider

When excessive bleeding is suspected and the fundus is boggy, begin uterine massage. Check the woman's bladder for distention and have her empty it if necessary. If she is not able to void and the bladder is distended, obtain an order and catheterize the woman. Weigh blood-soaked pads, linen savers, and linens to accurately determine the amount of blood lost. If massage is not effective in controlling bleeding promptly, notify the provider. Save any tissue or clots passed.

Follow facility protocols to initiate specific laboratory studies, such as Hgb and Hct levels and type and crossmatch of blood, so that blood is available should transfusions become necessary. Coagulation studies that may be ordered include fibrinogen, prothrombin time, partial thromboplastin time, fibrin split products, fibrin degradation products, platelets, D-dimer, and blood chemistry. Many protocols also allow the nurse to increase the flow rate of an existing IV line or insert a large-bore catheter to start IV fluids while the health care provider is being informed of the mother's condition. These actions do not substitute for notifying the provider, but they do allow nurses to make initial interventions quickly.

Keep the woman on bed rest to increase venous return and maintain cardiac output. The full Trendelenburg's position may interfere with cardiac and pulmonary function and is not advised. A modified Trendelenburg's position may be used with the legs elevated 10 to 30 degrees to increase blood return from the legs, the trunk horizontal, and the head slightly elevated. Continue assessments, call for assistance, and save all blood-soaked materials so an accurate estimation of blood loss can be made. Assistance is necessary; one nurse should continue to massage the uterus and perform and record assessments while another notifies the health care provider of the mother's condition and gathers medications and supplies needed.

Administer medications, fluids, and treatments as ordered by the health care provider or as stated in the facility's protocol. Evaluate the effects and relay the information to the provider. Because of oxytocin's antidiuretic effect, listen to breath sounds to identify signs of pulmonary edema from fluid overload if large amounts of oxytocin are given. Document blood pressure if methylergonovine is given. If measures fail to control bleeding, notify the health care provider so additional procedures can be initiated. These may include preparation for operative intervention.

Providing Support for the Family

The unusual activity of the hospital staff may make the mother and her family anxious. Be alert to their nonverbal cues, and acknowledge their feelings when they appear frightened. Keeping the family informed is one of the most effective ways of reducing anxiety.

Acknowledge the anxiety and provide simple appropriate explanations of the activity. "I know all this activity must be frightening. She is bleeding a little more than we would like and we are doing several things at once."

Posthemorrhage Care

After the hemorrhage is controlled, continue to assess the woman frequently for a resumption of bleeding. The woman may be anemic and fatigued. Allow rest periods and organize work to help her conserve energy. Because the woman may experience orthostatic hypotension, assist her in getting out of bed after dangling her legs and assess for dizziness and low blood pressure. Encourage intake of fluids and foods high in iron. She may need assistance feeding her newborn.

Home Care

Nurses who work in home care or nurse-managed postpartum clinics should be aware that women who have had postpartum hemorrhage are subject to a variety of complications. In general, they are exhausted; it may take weeks for them to feel well again. Anemia often results, and a course of iron therapy may be prescribed to restore Hgb levels. Activity may be restricted until strength returns. Some women need extra assistance with housework and care of the new infant. Fatigue may interfere with attachment. Because extensive blood loss increases the risk for postpartum infection, the woman should be taught to observe for specific signs and symptoms.

◆ Evaluation

The nurse collects and evaluates data with established norms and judges whether the data are within normal limits. If problems arise, the nurse acts to minimize hemorrhage and notifies the health care provider.

❓ KNOWLEDGE CHECK

8. Why is it sometimes difficult to recognize that the woman is becoming hypovolemic?

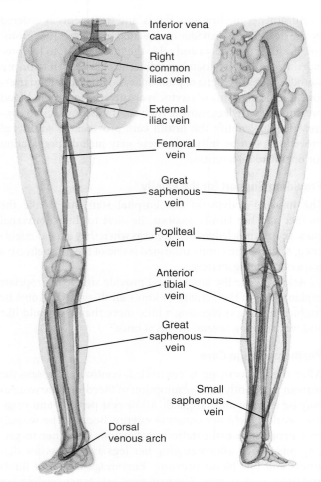

FIG. 18.5 The venous system of the leg is affected when deep venous thrombosis occurs.

Labels: Inferior vena cava; Right common iliac vein; External iliac vein; Femoral vein; Great saphenous vein; Popliteal vein; Anterior tibial vein; Great saphenous vein; Small saphenous vein; Dorsal venous arch

? CRITICAL THINKING EXERCISE 18.1

Dawn, a 26-year-old gravida 5, para 4, is admitted to the hospital. She has a rapid labor and delivers a baby boy weighing 4000 g (8 lb, 13 oz). Two hours later, she is transferred to the postpartum unit. At the initial postpartum assessment, Dawn's fundus is firm, at the level of the umbilicus. Lochia is heavy, with occasional small clots expressed. Vital signs are unchanged from prenatal norms.

Questions

1. Do any "red flags" suggest a potential problem or complication? What actions should the nurse take?
2. At the next assessment, the nurse observes that the fundus is soft and lochia is excessive. What are the priority interventions? Why?
3. Within an hour the fundus becomes "boggy" again and is located 3 cm above the umbilicus and displaced to the right. What is the priority nursing action? Why?
4. Dawn voids 500 mL. The fundus is difficult to locate, however, and lochia is excessive. What is the next nursing action? Why?

THROMBOEMBOLIC DISORDERS

A **thrombus** is a collection of blood factors, primarily platelets and fibrin, on a vessel wall. **Thrombophlebitis** occurs when the vessel wall develops an inflammatory response to the thrombus. This further occludes the vessel. An **embolus** is a mass that may be composed of a thrombus or amniotic fluid released into the bloodstream that may cause obstruction of capillary beds in another part of the body, frequently the lungs. A **pulmonary embolus** is a potentially fatal complication that occurs when the pulmonary artery is obstructed by a blood clot that was swept into circulation from a vein or by amniotic fluid. The three most common thromboembolisms encountered during pregnancy and the postpartum period are superficial venous thrombophlebitis (SVT), deep vein thrombosis (DVT), and occasionally pulmonary embolism (PE). SVT generally involves the saphenous venous system and is confined to the lower leg. DVT can involve veins from the foot to the iliofemoral region. It is a major concern because it predisposes to PE. Fig. 18.5 illustrates the venous system of the leg.

Incidence and Etiology

Approximately 1 per 1000 pregnancies are complicated by thromboembolic events (Cunningham et al., 2014). Thrombi can form whenever the flow of blood is impeded. Once started, the thrombus can enlarge with successive layering of platelets, fibrin, and blood cells as the blood flows past the clot. Thrombus formation is often associated with thrombophlebitis.

The three major causes of thrombosis are venous stasis, hypercoagulable blood, and injury to the endothelial surface (the innermost layer) of the blood vessel (Pettker & Lockwood, 2017). Two of these conditions—venous stasis and hypercoagulable blood—are present in all pregnancies; the third, blood vessel injury, is likely to occur during birth.

Venous Stasis

During pregnancy, compression of the large vessels of the legs and pelvis by the enlarging uterus causes venous stasis. Stasis is most pronounced when the pregnant woman stands for prolonged periods. It results in dilated vessels that increase the potential for continued postpartum pooling of blood. Relative inactivity and activity restriction because of complications during pregnancy lead to venous pooling and stasis of blood in the lower extremities. Prolonged time in stirrups for birth and repair of the episiotomy also may promote venous stasis and increase the risk for thrombus formation.

Hypercoagulation

Pregnancy is characterized by changes in the coagulation and fibrinolytic systems that persist into the postpartum period. During pregnancy the levels of many coagulation factors are elevated. In addition, the fibrinolytic system, which causes clots to disintegrate (lyse), is suppressed. The result is that factors that promote clot formation are increased and factors that prevent clot formation are decreased to prevent maternal

BOX 18.2 Factors That Increase the Risk for Thrombosis

Inactivity
Prolonged bed rest
Obesity
Cesarean birth
Sepsis
Smoking
History of previous thrombosis
Varicose veins
Diabetes mellitus
Trauma
Prolonged labor
Prolonged time in stirrups in second stage of labor
Maternal age older than 35 years
Increased parity
Dehydration
First-degree relative with thrombosis
Use of forceps
Antiphospholipid antibody syndrome
Inherited thrombophilias
Air travel

hemorrhage, resulting in a higher risk for thrombus formation during pregnancy and the postpartum period.

Blood Vessel Injury

Endothelial damage may occur during pregnancy, especially at birth. Lower extremity trauma, operative birth, and prolonged labor can cause vascular damage (Rhode, 2016). Cesarean birth significantly increases the risk for thromboembolic disease (Leung & Lockwood, 2014). Women with varicose veins, obesity, a history of thrombophlebitis, and a history of smoking are at additional risk for thromboembolic disease (Box 18.2). Age older than 35 years doubles the risk (Leung & Lockwood, 2014).

Superficial Venous Thrombosis
Clinical Manifestations

Superficial thrombophlebitis is most often associated with varicose veins and limited to the calf area. It also can occur in the arms as a result of IV therapy. Signs and symptoms include swelling of the involved extremity and redness, tenderness, and warmth. It may be possible to palpate an enlarged, hardened, cordlike vein. The woman may experience pain when she walks, but some women have no signs at all.

Therapeutic Management

Treatment includes analgesics, rest, and elastic support. Elevation of the lower extremity improves venous return. Warm packs may be applied to the affected area. Anticoagulants are not usually needed, but antiinflammatory medications may be used. After a period of bed rest with the leg elevated, the woman may ambulate gradually if symptoms have disappeared. She should avoid standing for long periods and should continue to wear support hose to help prevent venous stasis and a subsequent episode of superficial

thrombosis. Little chance of pulmonary embolism exists if the thrombosis remains in the superficial veins of the lower leg.

Deep Vein Thrombosis

Signs and symptoms of deep vein thrombosis (DVT) or PE are absent in most women affected (Leung & Lockwood, 2014). Those that occur are caused by an inflammatory process and obstruction of venous return. The woman may report pain in the leg, groin, lower back, or right lower quadrant (Rhode, 2016). Swelling of the leg, erythema, heat, and tenderness over the affected area are the most common signs. Homan's sign is nonspecific and may be caused by other conditions such as a strained muscle (Cunningham et al., 2014, Pettker & Lockwood, 2017). Reflex arterial spasms may cause the leg to become pale and cool to the touch with decreased peripheral pulses. Additional symptoms may include pain on ambulation, chills, general malaise, and stiffness of the affected leg.

Diagnosis

Venous ultrasonography with vein compression and Doppler flow analysis of the deep veins of the upper legs is most commonly used to detect alterations in blood flow that are diagnostic of DVT. Noncontrast magnetic resonance imaging (MRI) is considered very sensitive and accurate in diagnosing pelvic and leg thrombosis (Leung & Lockwood, 2014). D-Dimer tests may be performed, but the results are normally higher during pregnancy and postpartum and the test may not be as accurate as at other times (Cunningham et al., 2014; Leung & Lockwood, 2014).

Therapeutic Management

Preventing Thrombus Formation. Women who have had a previous DVT or PE are at risk for another. These women and others at high risk may receive prophylactic heparin, which does not cross the placenta. Either standard unfractionated heparin (UH) or a low-molecular-weight heparin (LMWH) such as enoxaparin (Lovenox) or tinzaparin (Innohep) may be used. LMWH is longer acting and can be given less frequently and with fewer laboratory tests. It has fewer side effects and is less likely to cause bleeding. However, LMWH is more expensive than UH and must be given subcutaneously. UH is given intravenously or subcutaneously.

Women receiving LMWH during pregnancy are changed to UH at approximately 36 weeks of gestation. The change is necessary because UH has a shorter half-life and epidural anesthesia, which may be needed in labor, is contraindicated within 24 hours of the last dose of LMWH. Heparin is discontinued during labor and birth and resumed approximately 6 to 12 hours after uncomplicated birth and 12 hours after the epidural catheter is removed (ACOG, 2014b).

If stirrups must be used during the birth, they should be padded to prevent prolonged pressure against the popliteal angle during the second stage of labor. If possible, the time in stirrups should be no more than 1 hour.

All new mothers are encouraged to ambulate frequently and as early as possible. Ambulation prevents stasis of blood in the legs and decreases the likelihood of thrombus formation. If the woman is unable to ambulate, range-of-motion and gentle leg exercises, such as flexing and straightening the knee and raising one leg at a time, should begin within 8 hours after childbirth. The mother should not use pillows under her knees or the knee gatch on the bed. These devices may cause sharp flexion at the knees and pressure against the popliteal space, leading to pooling of blood in the lower extremities.

Graduated compression stockings or sequential compression devices are used for mothers with varicose veins, a history of thrombosis, or a cesarean birth. Sequential compression devices should be applied preoperatively for a woman undergoing a cesarean birth who is not on anticoagulant therapy and should be continued until she begins to ambulate postpartum (ACOG, 2014b). Compression stockings should be applied before the mother gets out of bed to prevent venous congestion, which begins as soon as she stands. It is important that she understands the correct way to put on the stockings. Improperly applied stockings can roll or bunch and slow venous return from the legs.

Initial Treatment. Anticoagulant therapy is started to prevent extension of the thrombus. Clotting studies should be monitored to ensure a safe but therapeutic levels. The woman is placed on bed rest, with the affected leg elevated to decrease interstitial swelling and to promote venous return from the leg. Analgesics may be prescribed to control pain, and antibiotics will be used as necessary to prevent or control infection. Moist heat provides relief of pain and increases circulation.

Gradual ambulation is allowed when symptoms have disappeared. Sitting with the legs dependent should be avoided.

Subsequent Treatment. The long-term management of DVT depends on whether the woman is pregnant or in the postpartum period. The pregnant woman with a DVT receives anticoagulation therapy until labor begins. It is resumed 6 to 12 hours after birth and continued for 6 weeks to 6 months after birth (ACOG, 2014b). Warfarin (Coumadin) is contraindicated during pregnancy because of teratogenic effects and the risk for fetal hemorrhage. Therefore pregnant women are given UH or LMWH, which do not cross the placenta.

During the postpartum period, warfarin is started before heparin is stopped to provide continuous anticoagulation. Heparin is discontinued when the international normalized ratio (INR) has been at therapeutic levels for 2 days. Warfarin is safe for use during lactation. The INR is used to monitor coagulation time when warfarin is used.

Before discharge from the birth facility, the mother should be taught about lifestyle changes that can improve peripheral circulation. This includes avoiding clothing that is constricting around the legs and prolonged sitting. If sitting for long periods is necessary, walking for a short time hourly or moving her feet and legs frequently will help prevent circulatory stasis.

? KNOWLEDGE CHECK

9. Why is the risk for thrombus formation increased in pregnancy and in the postpartum period?
10. What are the signs and symptoms of SVT?
11. How does the long-term treatment for DVT in the pregnant woman differ from that in the woman who is in the postpartum period?
12. Why is bed rest prescribed for the woman with DVT?

PATIENT TEACHING

How To Prevent Thrombosis (Blood Clots)

The following methods to improve peripheral circulation will help prevent the occurrence of thrombophlebitis:

Improve your circulation with a regular schedule of activity, preferably walking.

Avoid prolonged standing or sitting in one position.

When sitting, elevate your legs and avoid crossing them. This will increase the return of venous blood from the legs.

Maintain a daily fluid intake of 12 or more 8-oz glasses to prevent dehydration and consequent sluggish circulation.

Stop smoking. Smoking is a risk factor for thrombosis and can cause respiratory problems in you and your newborn.

◆ APPLICATION OF THE NURSING PROCESS: THE MOTHER WITH DEEP VENOUS THROMBOSIS

◆ Assessment

Assessment focuses on determining the status of the venous thrombosis. Inspect both legs at the same time so that the affected leg can be compared with the unaffected leg. DVT is most often unilateral, usually affecting the woman's left side (Leung & Lockwood, 2014). Warmth or redness indicates inflammation; coolness or cyanosis indicates venous obstruction. Palpate the pedal pulses, comparing the strength of the right and left. Measure the affected and unaffected legs, comparing the circumferences to obtain an estimation of the edema that may be present in the affected leg. Record the measurements for ongoing assessment. It may be helpful to mark the woman's legs at the location of the measurement for consistency in assessments. Assess for pain. Pain is caused by tissue hypoxia, and increasing pain indicates progressive obstruction.

Evaluate the laboratory reports of clotting studies. Thrombocytopenia is a concern when heparin is administered for a prolonged time.

◆ Identification of Patient Problems

The treatment of DVT includes the administration of anticoagulants for a prolonged time. For many women, a lack of knowledge of anticoagulant precautions places them at an increased risk.

◆ Planning: Expected Outcomes

Expected outcomes for this problem are that the woman will do the following:

- Remain free of bleeding from anticoagulant therapy
- Verbalize precautions necessary when taking anticoagulants
- Verbalize her plan for changes necessary as a result of anticoagulant therapy

◆ Interventions

Monitoring for Signs of Bleeding

At least twice a day, inspect the mother for the appearance of bruising or petechiae. Instruct her to report any signs of bleeding: bruises, bloody nose, blood in urine or stools, bleeding gums, or increased vaginal bleeding. Be alert for signs of hemorrhage, such as tachycardia, falling blood pressure, or other signs that may indicate internal bleeding.

Observe for excessive or bright red lochia. If the uterus is boggy, the cause is uterine atony. Massage the uterus and express clots. If the fundus is firm, bleeding may be from trauma or anticoagulant therapy. In either case the provider should be notified.

Unless frank hemorrhage is present, the usual treatment for excessive anticoagulation is temporary discontinuation of the anticoagulant. Protamine sulfate, which is the antidote for UH and is partially effective against LMWH, should be available. The antidote for warfarin is vitamin K.

Explaining Continued Therapy

Teach the woman how to prevent excessive anticoagulation. Carefully explain the treatment regimen, including the schedule of medication. Help her develop a method for remembering to take the medication as directed. Caution her not to "double up" if a dose is missed. If necessary, teach her and another family member how to inject heparin or enoxaparin. Explain the need for repeated laboratory testing to regulate the anticoagulant dose. Emphasize the importance of careful attention to dosage changes to keep the medication at the appropriate blood levels.

Oral anticoagulants are associated with many clinically significant drug interactions; emphasize the importance of keeping the health care provider informed about any medications she takes. Caution the woman that common over-the-counter medications, such as aspirin and other nonsteroidal antiinflammatory drugs, increase the risk for hemorrhage. Explain that many herbs and dietary supplements may affect the potency of anticoagulants, and the woman should check with her health care provider before using them.

Instruct the woman taking warfarin that eating large amounts of vitamin K–containing foods may interfere with anticoagulation. These foods include broccoli, cabbage, lettuce, spinach, and lentils. Caution her against drinking alcohol, which inhibits the metabolism of oral anticoagulants. The woman should use effective contraception as long as she is taking warfarin because the drug can cause fetal defects.

Suggest that the mother use a soft toothbrush and floss her teeth gently to prevent bleeding from the gums. An electric toothbrush may be too vigorous and may cause bleeding. She should postpone dental appointments until the therapy is completed. Using a depilatory or waxing product or shaving with an electric razor to remove unwanted hair is safer than using a blade razor during anticoagulant therapy. Remind the mother not to go barefoot and to avoid activities that could cause injury. Emphasize the importance of reporting unusual bleeding.

Helping the Family Adapt to Home Care

Assess the family structure and function to determine how prepared the family is to cope with the mother's illness. Determine the ages of any children and availability of family members or friends to help while the mother is confined to bed or on limited activity. Help the family develop a plan of care that includes the temporary assistance needed.

Note interactions between the mother and the newborn and between the father and the newborn. Although the health of the mother is of primary importance, care should be taken that the attachment process between her and the infant progresses normally.

◆ Evaluation

The expected outcomes are met when:

- The mother demonstrates no signs of unusual bleeding or other side effects of the medication.
- The woman discusses precautions she has taken to prevent hemorrhage.
- Necessary changes have been made in the home.

Pulmonary Embolism

Pathophysiology

Pulmonary embolism (PE) is a serious complication of DVT that can lead to maternal mortality. PE occurs when fragments of a blood clot dislodge and are carried to the lungs. An embolus can also consist of amniotic fluid and its debris, a condition called *anaphylactoid syndrome* (Chapter 16). The embolus lodges in a vessel and partially or completely obstructs the flow of blood into the lungs. If pulmonary circulation is severely compromised, death may occur within a few minutes. If the embolus is small, adequate pulmonary circulation may be maintained until treatment can be initiated.

Clinical Manifestations

Clinical signs and symptoms depend on how much the flow of blood is obstructed. Dyspnea, chest pain, tachycardia, tachypnea, and hemoptysis are the most common signs (Rhode, 2016). Syncope is uncommon and may indicate massive emboli (Leung & Lockwood, 2014). Pulmonary crackles, cough, abdominal pain, and low-grade fever also may occur. Pulse oximetry shows decreased oxygen saturation. Arterial blood gas determinations show decreased partial pressure of oxygen, and chest radiography reveals areas of atelectasis and pleural effusion.

Other diagnostic tests may include computed tomographic pulmonary angiography (CPTA) or ventilation-perfusion (V/Q) scan. A venous ultrasound is also performed to identify a DVT (Leung & Lockwood, 2014).

Therapeutic Management

Treatment of PE is aimed at dissolving the clot and maintaining pulmonary circulation. Oxygen is used to decrease hypoxia, and narcotic analgesics are given to reduce pain and apprehension. Bed rest with the head of the bed elevated is used to help reduce dyspnea. The level of care, including support of ventilation, depends on the woman's pulmonary status. Pulse oximetry and arterial blood gases are evaluated. Heparin therapy is initiated and continued throughout pregnancy if the embolism occurs before birth. Therapy may be continued with warfarin for months after birth to prevent further emboli.

Nursing Considerations

Monitoring for Signs. When caring for a woman with DVT, nurses should be aware of the danger of PE and focus the assessment for early signs and symptoms. This includes frequent assessment of respiratory rate and thorough and frequent auscultation of breath sounds. Abnormalities such as diminished or unequal breath sounds or coughing should be reported immediately to the health care provider. Additional signs that require immediate attention include air hunger, dyspnea, tachycardia, pallor, and cyanosis.

Facilitating Oxygenation. Oxygen should be administered at 8 to 10 L/min by tight face mask. The nurse should remain with the mother to allay fear and apprehension. The head of the bed should be raised to facilitate breathing. Narcotic analgesics, such as morphine, may be used to relieve pain. Sedatives may be given to help control anxiety.

Seeking Assistance. The woman's condition is precarious until the clot is lysed or until it adheres to the pulmonary artery wall and is reabsorbed. The primary nurse should call for assistance to initiate interventions. These include continuous assessment of vital signs and administration of IV heparin and emergency drugs that may be needed. The woman requires critical care nursing skills and is usually transferred to an intensive care unit.

? KNOWLEDGE CHECK

13. What additional nursing assessments are necessary when the mother is receiving anticoagulants?
14. In addition to assessment, physical care, and teaching, what should the nurse consider for the mother with a DVT being treated at home?

PUERPERAL INFECTION

Puerperal infection is a term used to describe bacterial infections after childbirth. Until the advent of antibiotics, puerperal infection often resulted in death. It remains a cause of maternal death, especially in developing nations. The most common postpartum infections are **endometritis** (an infection of the inner lining of the uterus), wound infections, urinary tract infections (UTIs), **mastitis** (infection of the breast), and septic pelvic thrombophlebitis. **Endomyometritis** is an infection of the muscle and inner lining of the uterus. If the surrounding tissues are also involved, **endoparametritis**

is present. **Metritis** is the infection of the decidua, myometrium, and parametrial tissues of the uterus.

Definition

The definition of **puerperal infection** is a temperature of 38°C (100.4°F) or higher after the first 24 hours and occurring on at least 2 of the first 10 days after childbirth (Adair, 1935). Although a slight elevation of temperature may occur during the first 24 hours because of dehydration or the exertion of labor, any mother with fever should be assessed for other signs of infection.

Effect of Normal Anatomy and Physiology on Infection

Every part of the reproductive tract is connected to every other part, and organisms can move from the vagina, through the cervix, into the uterus, and through the fallopian tubes to infect the ovaries and peritoneal cavity. The entire reproductive tract is particularly well supplied with blood vessels during pregnancy and after childbirth. Bacteria that invade or are picked up by the blood vessels or lymphatics can carry the infection to the rest of the body, which can result in life-threatening septicemia.

The normal physiologic changes of childbirth increase the risk for infection. During labor and birth the acidity of the vagina is reduced by the amniotic fluid, blood, and lochia, which are alkaline. An alkaline environment encourages growth of bacteria.

Necrosis of the endometrial lining and the presence of lochia provide a favorable environment for the growth of anaerobic bacteria. Many small lacerations, some microscopic in size, occur in the endometrium, cervix, and vagina during birth and allow bacteria to enter the tissue. Although the uterine interior is not sterile until 3 to 4 weeks after childbirth, infection does not develop in most women, partly because granulocytes in the lochia and endometrium help prevent infection. Scrupulous aseptic technique during labor and birth and careful handwashing during the postpartum period are also major preventive factors.

Other Risk Factors

Other factors may predispose a woman to infection (Table 18.2). Cesarean birth is a major predisposing factor (Mackeen, Packard, Ota, & Speer, 2015) because of the tissue trauma that occurs in surgery, the incision that provides an entrance for bacteria, the possibility of contamination during surgery, and foreign bodies such as sutures that can promote infection. In addition, women who must have a surgical birth because of a problem that develops during labor may have other risk factors, such as prolonged labor, that raise the chances of infection. Colonization of the vagina with organisms such as group B *Streptococcus*, *Chlamydia trachomatis*, *Mycoplasma hominis*, and *Gardnerella vaginalis* also predisposes the woman to the development of infection after childbirth.

Any trauma to maternal tissues increases the hazard of infection. Trauma during vaginal birth may occur with rapid birth, birth of a large infant, use of a vacuum extractor or

TABLE 18.2   Risk Factors for Puerperal Infection

Risk Factor	Reason
History of previous infections (urinary tract infection, mastitis, thrombophlebitis)	May be more vulnerable to infectious process.
Colonization of lower genital tract by pathogenic organisms	Infections usually caused by several microbes that have ascended to the uterus from the lower genital tract.
Cesarean birth	Provides increased portals of entry for bacteria.
Trauma	Provides entrance for bacteria and makes tissues more susceptible.
Prolonged rupture of membranes	Removes barrier of amniotic membranes and allows access by organisms to interior of uterus.
Prolonged labor	Increases number of vaginal examinations; allows time for bacteria to multiply.
Catheterization	Could introduce organisms into bladder.
Excessive number of vaginal examinations	Increases chance that organisms from the vagina or outside source are carried into the uterus.
Retained placental fragments	Provide growth medium for bacteria and may interfere with flow of lochia.
Hemorrhage	Results in loss of infection-fighting components of blood.
Poor general health (excessive fatigue, anemia, frequent minor illnesses)	Increases vulnerability to infections and complications of labor.
Poor nutrition (decreased protein, vitamin C)	Less able to repair tissue and defend against infection.
Poor hygiene	Increases exposure to pathogens.
Medical conditions such as diabetes mellitus	Decreases ability to defend against infections of any kind; diabetes increases glucose level in urine.
Low socioeconomic status	More likely to have poor nutrition and inadequate prenatal care.

forceps, manual delivery of the placenta, or lacerations and episiotomies. Catheterization during labor increases the chance of introduction of organisms into the bladder and adds to the trauma to the urinary tract that occurs during normal childbirth.

When prolonged rupture of membranes occurs during labor, organisms from the vagina are more likely to ascend into the uterine cavity. A long labor or many vaginal examinations during labor increases the danger of infection. Each vaginal examination increases the possibility of contamination from organisms in the vagina that are carried through the open cervix. Use of a fetal scalp electrode or intrauterine pressure catheter has the same effect. If part of the placenta remains inside the uterus after birth, the tissue becomes necrotic and provides a good place for bacteria to grow.

Additional factors include postpartum hemorrhage, which causes loss of infection-fighting components of the blood, such as leukocytes, and leaves the mother in a weakened condition. Prenatal conditions (poor nutrition, anemia) interfere with the mother's ability to resist infection. Lack of knowledge of hygiene or lack of access to facilities that permit adequate hygiene increases the risk for postpartum infection.

KNOWLEDGE CHECK

15. Why is the woman who had an assisted birth or cesarean birth at increased risk for postpartum infection?
16. Why do the normal physiologic changes of childbearing make a mother especially susceptible to infection of the reproductive system?
17. Why is infection more likely to develop in a mother who had prolonged labor?

Specific Infections

Endometritis

Incidence and Etiology. Endometritis occurs in 1% to 3% of women after vaginal birth and 5% to 15% of women after scheduled cesarean birth. If extended labor and rupture of membranes precede cesarean birth, infection occurs in 30% to 35% of women who have no prophylactic antibiotics and 10% or less of those who receive prophylactic antibiotics (Cunningham et al., 2014; Duff, 2014).

Endometritis is usually caused by organisms that are normal inhabitants of the vagina and cervix. Most infections are polymicrobial with both aerobic and anaerobic organisms involved. Organisms most often found include aerobic and anaerobic streptococci, *Escherichia coli, Klebsiella pneumoniae, Proteus, Bacteroides,* and *Gardnerella.* (Cunningham et al., 2014). *C. trachomatis* is associated with late-onset infections 2 or more weeks after birth (Rhode, 2016).

Clinical Manifestations. The mother with severe endometritis looks sick. She presents a different picture from the typical happy new mother. The major signs and symptoms are temperature of 38°C (100.4°F) or higher, chills, malaise, anorexia, abdominal pain and cramping, uterine tenderness, and purulent, foul-smelling lochia. Additional signs include tachycardia and subinvolution. In most cases, the signs and symptoms occur within 36 hours after birth (Duff, 2014).

Laboratory data may confirm the diagnosis. The results of a complete blood count may show an elevation in the number of leukocytes (15,000/mm^3 to 30,000/mm^3). Leukocyte levels are normally elevated to as high as 30,000/mm^3 during early postpartum (Blackburn, 2013); however, leukocytosis that is not decreasing should prompt further evaluation. A blood culture and catheterized urine specimen may be obtained. Cultures of the vagina or endometrium are not usually helpful.

Therapeutic Management. Administration of IV antibiotics is the initial treatment for endometritis. The goal is to confine the infectious process to the uterus and prevent spread of the infection throughout the body. Broad-spectrum antibiotics, such as the cephalosporins, clindamycin plus gentamicin, or ampicillin plus aminoglycosides, are often used. Metronidazole with penicillin also may be given. Antibiotics are continued until the woman has been afebrile and asymptomatic for 24 hours (Duff, 2014).

To decrease the incidence of endometritis and wound infections, a single prophylactic IV dose of an antibiotic should be given before skin incision for any woman who is having a cesarean birth (Duff, 2014). Other medications include antipyretics for fever and oxytocics such as methylergonovine to increase drainage of lochia and promote involution.

Complications. If the infection spreads outside the uterine cavity, it may affect the fallopian tubes (salpingitis) or the ovaries (oophoritis), which could result in sterility. Peritonitis (inflammation of the membrane lining the walls of the abdominal and pelvic cavities) may occur and lead to formation of a pelvic abscess. In addition, the risk for pelvic thrombophlebitis is increased when pathogenic bacteria enter the bloodstream during episodes of endometritis. Fig. 18.6 illustrates complications of metritis.

Signs and symptoms that the infection is spreading may be similar to those of endometritis but more severe. Fever and

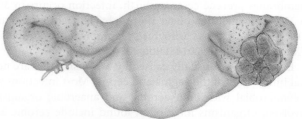

Salpingitis: Infection in fallopian tubes causes them to become enlarged, hyperemic, and tender.

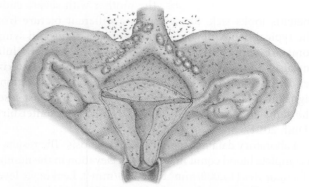

Peritonitis: Infection spreads through the lymphatics to the peritoneum; a pelvic abscess may form.

FIG. 18.6 Areas of Spread of Uterine Infection.

abdominal pain will be particularly pronounced. Peritonitis may result in paralytic ileus and abdominal distention with absent bowel sounds.

Nursing Considerations. The woman with endometritis should be placed in a Fowler's position to promote drainage of lochia. She should be medicated as needed for abdominal pain or cramping, which may be severe. Monitor the woman's response to treatment, and note signs of improvement or of continued infection (nausea and vomiting, abdominal distention, absent bowel sounds, and severe abdominal pain). Assess vital signs every 2 hours while fever is present and every 4 hours afterward. Comfort measures include warm blankets, cool compresses, cold or warm drinks, or use of a heating pad. Foods high in vitamin C and protein to aid healing are encouraged along with oral fluids to maintain hydration.

Teaching should include signs and symptoms of worsening condition, side effects of therapy, and the importance of adhering to the treatment plan and follow-up care. If the woman is so sick that she must be separated from her infant or her infant is discharged before the mother, there is a risk for alteration in attachment. If the mother is breastfeeding, she will need help to pump her breasts to establish and maintain lactation.

Wound Infection

Wound infections are common types of puerperal infection because any break in the skin or mucous membrane provides a portal of entry for organisms. The most common sites are cesarean surgical incisions, episiotomies, and lacerations. Infection of the incision occurs along with endometritis in 3% to 5% of women after cesarean (Duff, 2014). Risk factors include obesity, diabetes, hemorrhage, anemia, chorioamnionitis, corticosteroid therapy, and multiple vaginal examinations.

Clinical Manifestations. Signs of wound infection are edema, warmth, redness, tenderness, and pain. The edges of the wound may pull apart, and seropurulent drainage may be present. If the wound remains untreated, generalized signs of infection, such as fever and malaise, also may develop. As with other puerperal infections, cultures may reveal mixed aerobic and anaerobic bacteria. Necrotizing fasciitis is a rare infection that may occur at any incision site. The necrosis may spread and the condition may be fatal.

Therapeutic Management. An incision and drainage of the affected area may be necessary. The wound exudate is cultured, and broad-spectrum antibiotics are ordered until a report of the organism is returned. Analgesics are often necessary, and warm compresses or sitz baths may be used to provide comfort and promote healing by increasing circulation to the area. Surgical debridement is performed for necrotizing fasciitis.

Nursing Considerations. Despite their small size, wound infections are painful and annoying to the mother. Perineal infections cause discomfort during many activities, such as walking, sitting, or defecating, and are particularly troublesome because they are not expected by the new mother.

Wound infections may require readmission to the hospital or home health care visits. The woman requires reassurance and supportive care. Comfort measures include sitz baths, warm compresses, and frequent perineal care. She should be taught to wipe from front to back and to change perineal pads frequently. Good handwashing techniques are emphasized. Adequate fluid intake and a healthy diet are important. Activity may be modified depending on the site, severity, and treatment of the wound infection.

The infant is not routinely isolated from the mother with a wound infection, but she should be advised how to protect her infant from contact with contaminated articles such as dressings. Anticipatory guidance should include teaching side effects of medications, signs of worsening condition, self-care measures, and the importance of handwashing.

> ### ? KNOWLEDGE CHECK
> 18. What are the signs and symptoms of endometritis? How is it usually treated?
> 19. What are the most common sites for wound infections?
> 20. How does the nurse assess for wound infection?

Urinary Tract Infections

Etiology. During childbirth, the bladder and urethra are traumatized by pressure from the descending fetus. Insertion of a catheter, with its risk for infection, also may occur during labor. After childbirth the bladder and urethra are hypotonic, with urinary stasis and retention common problems. Residual urine and reflux of urine may occur during voiding.

Women who had bacteria in the urine during pregnancy, often without symptoms, are at increased risk for cystitis and pyelonephritis, which may result in preterm labor. Asymptomatic bacteriuria may be discovered during urine screens in 2% to 11% of pregnant women (Duff, 2014). UTIs are most often caused by coliform bacteria, such as *E. coli.* Other organisms include *K. pneumoniae* and *Proteus* species (Duff & Birsner, 2017).

Clinical Manifestations. Symptoms typically begin on the first or second postpartum day. They include dysuria, urgency, frequency, and suprapubic pain. Hematuria also may occur. A low-grade fever is sometimes the only sign. On the third or fourth day, some women may develop an upper UTI, such as pyelonephritis, with chills, spiking fever, costovertebral angle tenderness, flank pain, and nausea and vomiting. This infection of the renal pelvis may result in permanent damage to the kidney if not promptly treated.

Therapeutic Management. Most UTIs can be treated with antibiotics on an outpatient basis. Asymptomatic bacteriuria during pregnancy increases the risk for pyelonephritis 20 to 30 times. Treatment reduces the incidence of pyelonephritis significantly (Duff, 2014). Pyelonephritis during pregnancy may require hydration and IV administration of broad-spectrum antibiotics. In addition, the woman should be observed for signs of preterm labor. If the postpartum woman is only mildly ill, she can be treated with oral antibiotics at home. Urinary analgesics such as phenazopyridine (Pyridium) also may be ordered. Antibiotics that are safe for use during lactation are given if the mother is breastfeeding.

Nursing Considerations. The woman with a UTI should be instructed to take the medication for the entire time it is prescribed and not stop when symptoms abate. In addition, she should drink at least 2500 to 3000 mL of fluid each day to help dilute the bacterial count and flush the infection from the bladder. Acidification of the urine inhibits multiplication of bacteria, and drinks that acidify urine, such as apricot, plum, prune, and cranberry juices, are frequently recommended. Grapefruit and carbonated drinks should be avoided because they increase urine alkalinity. Teaching also should include measures to prevent UTI, such as using proper perineal care, increasing fluid intake, and urinating frequently.

Mastitis

Incidence and Etiology. Mastitis, an infection of the breast, occurs most often 2 to 4 weeks after childbirth, although it may develop at any time during breastfeeding. Approximately 5% to 10% of lactating women are affected (Duff, 2014). It usually affects only one breast. Mastitis is often caused by *Staphylococcus aureus,* methicillin-resistant *Staphylococcus aureus* (MRSA), *E. coli,* and streptococci (Lawrence & Lawrence, 2016). The bacteria are most often carried on the skin of the mother or in the mouth or the nose of newborn. The organism may enter through an injured area of the nipple, such as a crack or blister, although no obvious signs of injury may be apparent. Soreness and pain of a nipple may result in insufficient emptying of the breast during breastfeeding.

Engorgement and stasis of milk may precede mastitis. This may occur when a feeding is skipped, when the infant begins to sleep through the night, or when breastfeeding is suddenly stopped. Constriction of the breasts by a bra that is too tight may interfere with emptying of all the ducts and may lead to infection. The mother who is fatigued or stressed or who has other health problems that might lower her immune system is also at increased risk for mastitis.

Clinical Manifestations. Initial symptoms may be flulike with fatigue and aching muscles. Symptoms progress to include a temperature of 39°C (102.2°F) or higher, chills, malaise, and headache. Mastitis is characterized by a localized lump or wedge-shaped area of pain, redness, heat, inflammation, and enlarged axillary lymph nodes. A hard, tender area may be palpated (Fig. 18.7). Untreated mastitis may progress to breast abscess.

Therapeutic Management. Antibiotic therapy and continued emptying of the breast by breastfeeding or breast pump constitute the first line of treatment. With early antibiotic treatment, mastitis usually resolves within 24 to 48 hours. Antibiotics should be continued for 7 to 10 days (Duff, 2014). Women who develop a breast abscess are treated with surgical drainage and antibiotics.

Supportive measures include application of moist heat or ice packs, breast support, bed rest, fluids, and analgesics.

Early mastitis   Acute mastitis

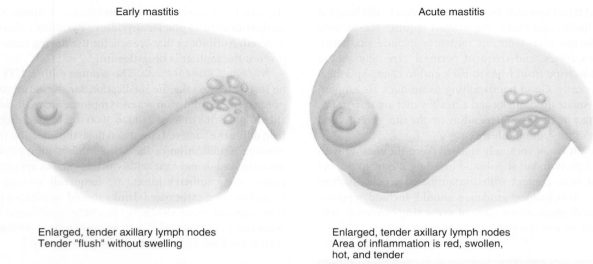

Enlarged, tender axillary lymph nodes   Enlarged, tender axillary lymph nodes
Tender "flush" without swelling   Area of inflammation is red, swollen,
                                                 hot, and tender

FIG. 18.7 Mastitis typically occurs after 2 to 3 weeks after birth in the breast of a woman who breastfeeds.

The mother should continue to breastfeed from both breasts. Regular and thorough emptying of the breast is important in preventing abscess formation. If an abscess forms and is surgically drained, breastfeeding can be continued as long as the incision is not near the areola and the mother is comfortable. If an abscess ruptures into the milk ducts, breastfeeding on that side should be discontinued temporarily and a breast pump used to empty the breast (Lawrence & Lawrence, 2016).

Nursing Considerations. Because mastitis rarely occurs before discharge from the birth facility, the nurse should provide adequate information for prevention. Measures to prevent mastitis include positioning the infant correctly and avoiding nipple trauma and milk stasis. The mother should breastfeed every 2 to 3 hours and avoid formula supplements. Nursing pads should not have a plastic layer and should be changed as soon as they are wet. She should also avoid continuous pressure on the breasts from tight bras or infant carriers.

Once mastitis occurs, nursing measures are aimed at increasing comfort and helping the mother maintain lactation. Moist heat promotes comfort and increases circulation. A disposable diaper, wet with warm water and placed over the breast, is an easy way to apply heat. The thickness helps maintain the temperature, and the plastic cover prevents dripping. A shower or hot packs should be used before feeding or pumping the breasts. The woman should complete the entire course of antibiotics to prevent recurrence or a breast abscess.

The breast should be completely emptied at each feeding to prevent stasis of milk. If the mother is too sore to breastfeed on the affected side, she should be shown how to express the milk or use a pump to empty the breasts.

Breastfeeding or pumping every 1.5 to 2 hours makes the mother more comfortable and prevents stasis. Starting the feeding on the unaffected side causes the milk-ejection reflex to occur in both breasts, making milk available in the painful breast as soon as the infant begins to nurse on that side. Massage over the affected area before and during the feeding helps ensure complete emptying. The mother should stay in bed during the acute phase of her illness. Her fluid intake should be 2500 to 3000 mL per day. Analgesics may be required to relieve discomfort.

The mother with mastitis is likely to be very discouraged. Some mothers decide to stop breastfeeding because of the discomfort involved. Weaning during an episode of mastitis may increase engorgement and stasis, leading to abscess formation or recurrent infection. The mother may need much encouragement, and she will need help in arranging care for other children or with other responsibilities so she can rest.

Septic Pelvic Thrombophlebitis

Incidence and Etiology. Septic pelvic thrombophlebitis is the least common of the puerperal infections, occurring in 1 in 2000 pregnancies (Duff, 2014). It usually is not seen until 2 to 4 days after childbirth. It occurs when infection spreads along the pelvic venous system and thrombophlebitis develops.

Clinical Manifestations. The primary symptom is pain in the groin, abdomen, or flank. Fever, tachycardia, gastrointestinal distress, and decreased bowel sounds may be present. The only sign may be fever that does not respond to antibiotic therapy.

Laboratory data may be used to exclude other diagnoses and usually include complete blood count with differential, blood chemistries, coagulation studies, and cultures. Pelvic ultrasound, computed tomography, or MRI may be performed to confirm the diagnosis.

Therapeutic Management. Readmission to the hospital is usually necessary. Primary treatment includes anticoagulation therapy with IV heparin and IV antibiotics. Warfarin may be given when heparin is discontinued. Supportive care is similar to that for DVT and includes monitoring for safe levels of anticoagulation therapy and for signs and symptoms of PE.

◆ APPLICATION OF THE NURSING PROCESS: INFECTION

◆ Assessment

Although all women are observed for indications of infection as part of routine nursing assessments, the nurse should practice increased vigilance for mothers who are at increased risk for infection.

Pay particular attention to signs that may be expected in infection, such as fever, tachycardia, pain, or unusual amount, color, or odor of lochia. Generalized symptoms of malaise and muscle aching may be significant. Examine all wounds each shift for signs of localized infection, such as redness, edema, tenderness, discharge, or pulling apart of incisions or sutured lacerations. Ask the mother if she has difficulty emptying her bladder or discomfort related to urination.

Assess the mother's knowledge of hygiene practices that prevent infections, such as proper handwashing, perineal care, and handling of perineal pads. Evaluate her knowledge of breastfeeding and any problems that might result in breast engorgement and stasis of milk in the ducts. Examine the nipples for signs of injury that might provide a portal of entry for organisms.

◆ Identification of Patient Problems

Because all women have a potential for infection to occur after childbirth, most facilities have developed protocols and procedures that protect postpartum women from infection. When predisposing factors increase the likelihood of infection, however, routine assessments and care should be modified and preventive measures intensified. Therefore a postpartum woman may have an increased potential for infection because of her specific risk factors.

◆ Planning: Expected Outcomes

The expected outcomes for this patient problem are that the mother will do the following:

- Remain free of signs of infection during the postpartum period
- Describe methods to prevent infection
- List signs of infection that should be reported immediately

---

! SAFETY CHECK

Signs and symptoms of postpartum infection include the following:

Fever, chills
Pain or redness of wounds
Purulent wound drainage or wound edges not approximated
Tachycardia
Uterine subinvolution
Abnormal duration of lochia, foul odor
Elevated white blood cell count
Frequency or urgency of urination, dysuria, or hematuria
Suprapubic pain
Localized area of warmth, redness, or tenderness in the breasts
Body aches, general malaise

◆ Interventions
Preventing Infection

Promoting Hygiene. Nursing responsibilities for the woman at risk for puerperal infection focus on prevention of initial infection. Preventive measures include using aseptic technique for all invasive procedures and paying attention to meticulous handwashing. Handwashing is important for the nursing staff and the mother. She should wash her hands before and after changing pads or touching the perineum. Instruct her on care of the perineum and episiotomy site (see Chapter 17). Make sure that she can demonstrate cleansing methods before she is discharged.

Preventing Urinary Stasis. An adequate intake of fluids (at least 2500 to 3000 mL/day) is important for preventing stasis of urine. Encourage the woman to empty her bladder at least every 2 to 3 hours during the day. Measure the first two voids after childbirth or removal of a urinary catheter, and assess the bladder and fundus to be certain the bladder is empty. Instruct her to report any signs of UTI immediately so that early treatment can be initiated.

Use appropriate measures to promote bladder emptying if she has difficulty. Drinking hot fluids, such as tea, helps some mothers void. Running water or having the mother blow bubbles in a glass of water uses the sound of water to stimulate the urge to urinate. Pouring warm water over the perineum or having the mother void in a sitz bath or shower may help relax the urinary sphincter. Administration of analgesics may help her relax enough to urinate.

Teaching Breastfeeding Techniques. Mothers often need assistance in establishing an effective pattern of breastfeeding that results in complete emptying of the breasts at each feeding and that reduces the risk for nipple trauma (see Chapter 22).

Providing Information

Advise mothers to obtain adequate rest and sufficient food of high nutritive value to replenish their energy and prevent infection. Identify foods high in protein and vitamin C, necessary for repair of damaged tissue. Red meat, poultry, fish, cheese, eggs, whole-grain breads, cereals, and pasta are some of the best sources of protein. This is particularly important if the mother is breastfeeding.

Obtaining adequate rest is a problem for many mothers. Nursing interventions focus on helping them plan a schedule that allows them to rest while the infant sleeps and to identify family members or friends who are available to provide support and assistance.

Teaching Signs and Symptoms That Should Be Reported

Before discharge, teach the woman signs and symptoms of infection that should be reported to her health care provider. These include fever, chills, dysuria, and redness and tenderness of a wound. Malodorous lochia, discharge from a wound, and prolonged lochial discharge also should be reported.

⊙ NURSING CARE PLAN

Postpartum Infection

Assessment

Lisa, a thin, pale, 16-year-old primipara, is admitted to the postpartum unit after a cesarean birth because of fetal distress. She was in labor for 16 hours and her membranes were ruptured for 14 hours before the birth. She was catheterized twice during labor, with insertion of an indwelling catheter shortly before her surgery. She plans to breastfeed her infant.

Critical Thinking

What data indicate that Lisa is at increased risk for infection? What additional data should be obtained?

Answer

Factors that increase the risk for endometritis include a cesarean birth and rupture of membranes 14 hours before the surgery was performed. Catheterization increases the risk for urinary tract infection. Additional necessary data to better evaluate the risks for infection include estimated blood loss and prenatal conditions such as anemia or other infections.

Identification of Patient Problems

Potential for infection as a result of presence of favorable conditions for infections

Planning: Expected Outcomes

Before discharge Lisa will do the following:
1. Demonstrate no signs of infection
2. Discuss methods she will use to prevent infections
3. List signs of infection she will report to her health care provider

Interventions and Rationales

1. Assess vital signs every 4 hours. *Temperature above 38°C (100.4°F) or tachycardia suggests an infectious process and should be reported.*
2. Observe the surgical incision for redness, tenderness, edema, drainage, and approximation and note the odor of lochia every 4 hours. Determine the character of urine and whether Lisa experiences frequency, urgency, or pain with urination after the catheter is removed. *Redness, pain, or edema of the incision suggests wound infection. Drainage could be bleeding or a sign of infection. Separation also can indicate infection. Foul odor of lochia suggests endometrial infection. Frequency, urgency, or painful urination may indicate urinary tract infection.*
3. Instruct Lisa in the following hygienic practices to prevent infection:
   a. Careful handwashing before and after perineal care. *Handwashing is the most important defense against infection and its spread.*

   b. Perineal cleansing after elimination. *Perineal cleansing helps prevent growth of bacteria.*
   c. Changing peripads frequently. *Frequent pad changes remove accumulated lochia, an excellent culture medium for bacteria.*
   d. Wiping the perineum from front to back. *Wiping from front to back prevents fecal contamination of the vagina.*
4. Initiate the following measures to reduce the risk for urinary tract infection.
   a. Provide fluids of Lisa's choice when she is able to take them, and emphasize the importance of drinking 2500 to 3000 mL/day. *Adequate hydration helps prevent stasis of urine, which increases the risk for urinary tract infection.*
   b. Monitor bladder distention to prevent overfilling. Teach Lisa the importance of emptying her bladder every 2 to 3 hours during the first days after childbirth. *Frequent emptying of the bladder helps prevent stasis of urine.*
   c. Use methods to promote bladder emptying, such as running water in the shower or sink, pouring warm water over the perineum, and providing pain medication as needed. *The sound of running water may stimulate the urge to void. Relief of pain may allow the mother to relax enough to void.*
5. Assist Lisa with breastfeeding. Explain the reasons for proper positioning and frequent, adequate feedings. *Poor positioning and short, infrequent feedings may cause nipple trauma, engorgement, and incomplete emptying of the breasts, leading to mastitis.*
6. Offer and encourage Lisa to eat well-balanced meals when she progresses to a regular diet. Emphasize the importance of a diet high in protein and vitamin C. *Adequate protein and vitamin C are necessary for healing damaged tissues.*
7. Organize nursing care to allow periods of rest. *Rest is important to help the body heal and fight infection.*
8. Teach Lisa signs of infection that she should report to her health care provider. Include fever, chills, dysuria, increased incisional tenderness or drainage, lochia with a foul odor, or pain and redness of the breast. *Prompt recognition and reporting of signs of infection ensures early treatment and reduces further complications.*

Evaluation

Lisa is free of signs and symptoms of infection throughout her hospital stay and at her postpartum checkup. She verbalizes measures she will take to reduce her risk for infection when she is discharged from the hospital. She is able to list signs of infection that require treatment.

◆ Evaluation

The interventions can be judged to be successful if the mother does the following:
- Shows no signs of infection
- Explains methods she will use to prevent infection
- Lists signs and symptoms that she should report to her health care provider

If infection occurs, the problem is no longer amenable to independent nursing actions but becomes a collaborative problem requiring medical and nursing interventions.

⚲ KNOWLEDGE CHECK

21. What measures can the woman take to decrease the risk for UTI? How does the treatment for cystitis differ from that for pyelonephritis?
22. How can mastitis be prevented?

SUMMARY CONCEPTS

- Postpartum hemorrhage can sometimes be prevented by careful examination of factors that predispose to excessive bleeding.
- Overstretching of the muscle fibers during pregnancy and repeated stretching during past pregnancies predispose to uterine atony and excessive uterine bleeding.
- Initial management of uterine atony focuses on measures to contract the uterus and provide fluid replacement.
- Soft tissue trauma (lacerations, hematomas) can cause rapid loss of blood even when the uterus is firmly contracted. Management involves repairing the trauma before excessive blood loss occurs.
- Compensatory mechanisms maintain the blood pressure so that vital organs receive adequate oxygen. When these mechanisms fail, hypovolemic shock follows.
- The process of uterine involution may be delayed (subinvolution) when placental fragments are retained or when the uterus is infected.
- Subinvolution of the uterus develops after the mother goes home. The nurse teaches the family the process of normal involution and the signs and symptoms that should be reported to the health care provider.
- Venous stasis that occurs during pregnancy, increased levels of coagulation factors, and decreased levels of thrombolytic factors that persist into the postpartum period increase the risk for thrombus formation during the puerperium.
- Treatment for deep venous thrombosis includes anticoagulants, analgesics, and bed rest with the affected leg elevated.

- Nurses who administer anticoagulant therapy assess the mother to determine whether her laboratory results are within the recommended therapeutic range so that overmedication with anticoagulants does not result in unexpected bleeding.
- Pulmonary embolism occurs when a clot is dislodged from the vein, or amniotic fluid debris is carried by the blood to a pulmonary vessel, which may be completely or partially occluded.
- The risk for infection is increased with childbearing because there is open access to bacteria from the vagina through the fallopian tubes and into the peritoneal cavity. Increased blood supply to the pelvis and the alkalinization of the vagina by the amniotic fluid further increase the risk for infection.
- Any break in the skin or mucous membranes during childbirth provides a portal of entry for pathogenic organisms and increases the risk for puerperal infection. Nurses should assess women with an incision or laceration for signs of localized wound infections.
- Urinary stasis and trauma to the urinary tract increase the risk for urinary tract infection. Nurses should initiate measures to prevent urinary stasis.
- Nurses should provide information about the importance of completely emptying the breasts at each feeding and about measures to avoid nipple trauma to prevent mastitis.

REFERENCES & READINGS

Abdul-Kadir, R., McLintock, C., Ducloy, A., El-Refaey, H., England, A., Federici, A. B., Winikoff, R. (2014). Evaluation and management of postpartum hemorrhage: Consensus from an international expert panel. *Transfusion*, 54(7), 1756–1768.

Adair, F. L. (1935). The American Committee of Maternal Welfare, Inc: Chairman's Address. *American Journal of Obstetrics and Gynecology*, 30(6), 868–871.

American College of Obstetricians and Gynecologists (ACOG). (2014a). *Obstetric data definitions (version 1.0)*. Retrieved from www.acog.org/-/media/Departments/Patient-Safety-and-Quality-Improvement/2014reVITALizeObstetricDataDefinitionsV10.pdf.

American College of Obstetricians and Gynecologists (ACOG). (2014b). Thromboembolism in pregnancy. *Practice bulletin*. no. 123, 2011, reaffirmed 2014. Retrieved from www.acog.org/Resources-And-Publications/Practice-Bulletins-List.

American College of Obstetricians and Gynecologists (ACOG). (2015). Postpartum hemorrhage. *Practice Bulletin*. No. 76, October 2006, Reaffirmed 2015. Retrieved from www.acog.org/Resources-And-Publications/Practice-Bulletins-List.

Association of Women's Health, Obstetric and Neonatal Nurses. (2015a). Guidelines for Oxytocin Administration after Birth: AWHONN Practice Brief Number 2. *JOGNN: Journal of Obstetric, Gynecologic & Neonatal Nursing*, 44(1), 161–163.

Association of Women's Health, Obstetric and Neonatal Nurses (AWHONN). (2015b). Quantification of Blood Loss: AWHONN

Practice Brief Number 1. *JOGNN: Journal of Obstetric, Gynecologic & Neonatal Nursing*, 44(1), 158–160.

Blackburn, S. T. (2013). *Maternal, fetal, and neonatal physiology: A clinical perspective* (4th ed.). St. Louis, MO: Saunders.

California Maternal Quality Care Collaborative. (2015). *Obstetric hemorrhage toolkit version 2.0*. Stanford: California Department of Public Health. Retrieved from www.cmqcc.org/ob_hemorrhage.

Cekmez, Y., Ozkaya, E., Ocal, F., & Kucukozkan, T. (2015). Experience with different techniques for the management of postpartum hemorrhage due to uterine atony: Compression sutures, artery ligation and Bakri balloon. *Irish Journal of Medical Science [serial online]*, 184(2), 399–402.

Council on Patient Safety in Women' Health. (2015). Obstetric Hemorrhage Bundle. Retrieved from www.safehealthcareforeverywoman.org.

Cunningham, F. G., Leveno, K. J., Bloom, S. L., Spong, C. Y., Dashe, J. S., Hoffman, B. L., Casey, B. M., & Sheffield, J. S. (Eds.). (2014). *Williams obstetrics* (24th ed.). New York: McGraw-Hill.

Debost-Legrand, A., Riviere, O., Dossou, M., & Vendittelli, F. (2015). Risk factors for severe secondary postpartum hemorrhages: A historical cohort study. *Birth (Berkeley, Calif.)*, 42(3), 235–241.

Doussou, M., Debost-Legrand, A., Dechelotte, P., Lemery, D., & Venditelli, F. (2015). Severe secondary postpartum hemorrhage: A historical cohort. *Birth (Berkeley, Calif.)*, 42(2), 149–155.

Duff, P. (2014). Maternal and fetal infections. In R. K. Creasy, R. Resnik, J. D. Iams, C. Lockwood, T. Moore, & M. Greene (Eds.), *Creasy & Resnik's maternal-fetal medicine: Principles and practice* (7th ed.) (pp. 802–851). Philadelphia: Saunders.

Duff, P., & Birsner, N. (2017). Maternal and perinatal infection in pregnancy: Bacterial. In S. G. Gabbe, J. R. Niebyl, J. L. Simpson, M. B. Landon, H. L. Galan, E. R. M. Jauniaux, D. A.... & W. A. Grobman (Eds.), *Obstetrics: Normal and problem pregnancies* (7th ed.) (pp. 1130–1146). Philadelphia: Elsevier.

Lawrence, R. A., & Lawrence, R. M. (2016). *Breastfeeding: A guide for the medical profession* (8th ed.). Philadelphia: Mosby.

Leung, A. N., & Lockwood, C. J. (2014). Thromboembolic disease in pregnancy. In R. K. Creasy, R. Resnik, J. D. Iams, C. J. Lockwood, T. R. Moore, & M. F. Greene (Eds.), *Creasy & Resnik's maternal-fetal medicine: Principles and practice* (7th ed.) (pp. 906–917). Philadelphia: Saunders.

Mackeen, A. D., Packard, R. E., Ota, E., & Speer, L. (2015). Antibiotic regimens for postpartum endometritis. *The Cochrane Database of Systemic Reviews*, (2), CD001067.

Main, E. K., Goffman, D., Scavone, B. M., Low, L. K., Bingham, D., Fontaine, P. L., Gorlin, J. B., Lagrew, D. C., & Levy, B. S. (2015). National Partnership for Maternal Safety: Consensus Bundle on Obstetric Hemorrhage. *Obstetrics and Gynecology*, 126(1), 155–162.

Martin, E., Legendre, G., Bouet, P., Cheve, M., Multon, O., & Sentilhes, L. (2015). Maternal outcomes after uterine balloon tamponade for postpartum hemorrhage. *Acta Obstetrica Et Gynecologica Scandinavica*, 94(4), 399–404.

Pettker, C. M., & Lockwood, C. J. (2017). Thromboembolic disorders. In S. G. Gabbe, J. R. Niebyl, J. L. Simpson, M. B. Landon, H. L. Galan, E. R. M. Jauniaux, & W. A. Grobman (Eds.), *Obstetrics: Normal and problem pregnancies* (7th ed.) (pp. 965–980). Philadelphia: Elsevier.

Rhode, M. A. (2016). Postpartum complications. In S. Mattson & J. E. Smith (Eds.), *Core curriculum for maternal-newborn nursing* (5th ed.) (pp. 645–661). St. Louis, MO: Elsevier.

Robbins, K. S., Martin, S. R., & Wilson, W. C. (2014). Intensive care considerations for the critically ill parturient. In R. K. Creasy, R. Resnik, J. D. Iams, C. Lockwood, T. Moore, & M. Greene (Eds.), *Creasy & Resnik's maternal-fetal medicine: Principles and practice* (7th ed.) (pp. 1182–1211). St. Louis, MO: Elsevier.

Wetta, L. A., Szychowski, J. M., Seals, S., Mancuso, M. S., Biggio, J. R., & Tita, A. N. (2013). Risk factors for uterine atony/postpartum hemorrhage requiring treatment after vaginal delivery. *American Journal of Obstetrics & Gynecology*, 209(1), 51.e1-6.

Whitmer, T. (2016). Physical and psychologic changes after birth. In S. Mattson & J. E. Smith (Eds.), *Core curriculum for maternal-newborn nursing* (5th ed.) (pp. 297–313). St. Louis, MO: Elsevier.

Normal Newborn: Processes of Adaptation

Vanessa Flannery

OBJECTIVES

After studying this chapter, you should be able to:

1. Explain the physiologic changes that occur in the respiratory and cardiovascular systems during the transition from fetal to neonatal life.
2. Describe thermoregulation in the newborn.
3. Compare gastrointestinal functioning in the newborn and adult.
4. Explain the causes and effects of hypoglycemia.
5. Describe the steps in normal bilirubin excretion and the development of physiologic, nonphysiologic, breastfeeding, and true breast milk jaundice.
6. Describe kidney functioning in the newborn.
7. Explain the functioning of the newborn's immune system.
8. Describe the periods of reactivity and the six behavioral states of the newborn.

At birth neonates must make profound physiologic changes to adapt to extrauterine life and meet their own respiratory, digestive, and regulatory needs. This chapter focuses on these changes and will assist nurses in identification of behaviors that signify problems or abnormalities. It provides a foundation for discussion of nursing assessment and care related to those changes, detailed in Chapters 20 and 21.

INITIATION OF RESPIRATIONS

The first vital task the newborn must accomplish is the initiation of respirations. Forces occurring throughout pregnancy and during birth bring about this change.

Development of the Lungs

During fetal life the alveoli produce **fetal lung fluid** that expands the alveoli and is essential for normal development of the lungs. Some of the fluid empties from the lungs into the amniotic fluid. The lung fluid is continuously produced at a rate of 4 to 5 mL/kg/hr (Jobe, 2014). As the fetus nears term, the amount of fetal lung fluid produced decreases in preparation for birth, when the fluid must be cleared for the infant to breathe air. Absorption of lung fluid begins during early labor, and by the time of birth only approximately 35% of the original amount remains (Jobe, 2014).

During labor, the fluid begins to move into the interstitial spaces, where it is absorbed. Absorption is accelerated by secretion of fetal epinephrine and corticosteroids but may be delayed by cesarean birth without labor. The removal of the fluid helps reduce pulmonary resistance to blood flow that is present before birth and enhances the advent of air breathing.

Surfactant, a slippery, detergent-like combination of lipoproteins, is detectable by 24 to 25 weeks of gestation (Blackburn, 2013). Surfactant lines the inside of the alveoli and reduces surface tension within alveoli, allowing the alveoli to remain partially open when the infant begins to breathe at birth. Without surfactant the alveoli collapse as the infant exhales. The alveoli must be reexpanded with each breath, greatly increasing the work of breathing and possibly resulting in atelectasis. By 34 to 36 weeks of gestation, sufficient surfactant is usually produced to prevent respiratory distress syndrome (Gardner, Enzman-Hines, & Nyp, 2015a). Surfactant secretion increases during labor and immediately after birth to enhance the transition from fetal to neonatal life.

Steroids given to a woman in preterm labor help increase surfactant production and speed maturation of the lungs. The fetus with intrauterine growth restriction or stressed by conditions such as maternal hypertension, heroin addiction, preeclampsia, infection, placental insufficiency, or premature rupture of membranes greater than 48 hours also may have accelerated lung maturation. Infants of mothers with diabetes have slower lung maturation (Gardner et al., 2015a).

Causes of Respirations

At birth, the infant's first breath must force the remaining fetal lung fluid out of the alveoli and into the interstitial spaces around the alveoli to allow air to enter the lungs.

This requires a much larger negative pressure (suction) than subsequent breathing. Breathing is initiated by chemical, mechanical, thermal, and sensory factors that stimulate the respiratory center in the medulla and trigger respirations (Fig. 19.1).

Chemical Factors

Chemoreceptors in the carotid arteries and the aorta respond to changes in blood chemistry caused by the hypoxemia that occurs with normal birth. A decrease in the partial pressure of oxygen (Po_2) and pH and an increase in the partial pressure of carbon dioxide (Pco_2) in the blood cause impulses from these receptors to stimulate the respiratory center in the medulla. However, stimulation of the respiratory center and breathing do not occur if prolonged hypoxia causes central nervous system depression.

Mechanical Factors

During a vaginal birth the fetal chest is compressed by the narrow birth canal. Approximately one-third of the fetal lung fluid is forced out of the lungs into the upper air passages during birth. The fluid passes out of the mouth or nose as the head emerges from the vagina. When the pressure against the chest is released at birth, recoil of the chest draws a small amount of air into the lungs and helps remove some of the viscous fluid in the airways. This reduces the amount of negative pressure needed for the first breath after birth (Fraser, 2014).

Thermal Factors

The temperature change that occurs with birth also stimulates the initiation of respirations. At birth, the infant moves from the warm, fluid-filled uterus into an environment where the temperature may be much cooler. Sensors in the skin respond to this sudden change in temperature by sending impulses to the medulla that stimulate the respiratory center and breathing.

Sensory Factors

Tactile, visual, auditory, and olfactory stimuli occur during and after birth to stimulate sensors. Nurses hold, dry, and place infants skin-to-skin with the mother or wrap them in blankets, providing further stimulation to skin sensors. The stimulation of the light, sound, smell, and pain at delivery also may aid in initiating respirations.

Continuation of Respirations

As the alveoli expand, surfactant allows them to remain partially open between respirations. Approximately 20 to 30 mL of air from the first breaths remains in the lungs to become the functional residual capacity (FRC) (Carlo, 2016c). Within the first hour after birth 80% to 90% of the FRC is established (Blackburn, 2013). Because the alveoli remain partially expanded with this residual air, subsequent breaths require much less effort than the first one.

As the infant cries, pressure within the lungs increases, causing remaining fetal lung fluid to move into the interstitial spaces, where it is absorbed by the pulmonary circulatory and lymphatic systems. Complete absorption may take several hours. This explains why the lungs may sound moist when first auscultated but become clear a short time later.

KNOWLEDGE CHECK

1. How do hypoxia during birth, a cool delivery room, and handling at birth stimulate the newborn to breathe?
2. Why is surfactant important to the newborn's ability to breathe easily?
3. How is fetal lung fluid removed before and after birth?

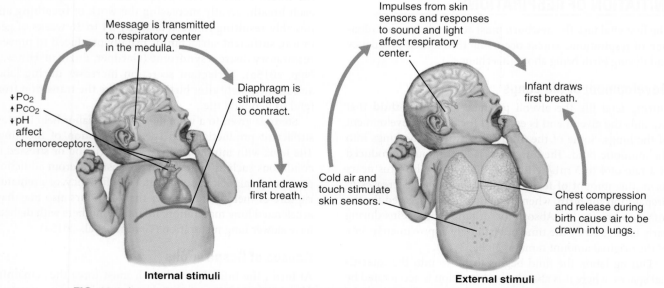

Internal stimuli

Message is transmitted to respiratory center in the medulla.

↓Po_2
↑Pco_2
↓pH
affect chemoreceptors.

Diaphragm is stimulated to contract.

Infant draws first breath.

External stimuli

Impulses from skin sensors and responses to sound and light affect respiratory center.

Infant draws first breath.

Cold air and touch stimulate skin sensors.

Chest compression and release during birth cause air to be drawn into lungs.

FIG. 19.1 Internal causes of the initiation of respirations are the chemical changes that take place at birth. External causes of respirations include thermal, sensory, and mechanical factors.

CARDIOVASCULAR ADAPTATION: TRANSITION FROM FETAL TO NEONATAL CIRCULATION

During fetal life, three shunts—the ductus venosus, foramen ovale, and ductus arteriosus—carry much of the blood away from the lungs and some blood away from the liver. High pressures within the collapsed, fluid-filled lungs permit only a small amount of blood flow into the narrow pulmonary vessels.

At birth, the shunts close and the pulmonary vessels dilate. These changes occur in response to increases in blood oxygen and shifts in pressure within the heart, pulmonary, and systemic circulations, as well as clamping of the umbilical cord. The alterations necessary for transition from fetal to neonatal circulation occur simultaneously within the first few minutes after birth. They are discussed separately here (Table 19.1; see also Fig. 5.9).

As the newborn takes the first breaths at birth, the rise in oxygen concentration causes the ductus arteriosus to constrict, preventing entry of blood from the pulmonary artery. The pulmonary blood vessels respond to the increased oxygenation by dilating. At the same time, fetal lung fluid shifts into the interstitial spaces and is removed by blood and lymph vessels. These changes decrease pulmonary vascular resistance by 80% and allow the vessels to expand to hold the suddenly increased blood flow from the pulmonary artery.

At birth, pressures between the right and left sides of the heart are reversed. The sudden dilation of the vessels of the lungs allows blood to enter freely from the right ventricle and decreases pressure in the right side of the heart. Clamping of the umbilical cord closes the ductus venosus and further decreases pressure in the right side of the heart. Increased blood flow from the pulmonary veins into the left atrium causes pressure in the left side of the heart to build. Systemic resistance increases as blood flow to the placenta ends with clamping of the cord, and this also elevates pressure in the left heart.

The foramen ovale's flap valve closes when the pressure in the left atrium is higher than that in the right atrium. This

TABLE 19.1 Circulatory Changes at Birth

Structure	Purpose in Fetal Life	Change at Birth	Cause of Change at Birth	Results of Change at Birth	Time of Functional and Permanent Change
Umbilical vessels	Carry blood from placenta to fetus and back.	Obstruction of blood flow through vessels.	Clamping of cord.	Decreased pressure in RA and increased systemic resistance occur.	*Functional:* Immediately when clamped. *Permanent:* 1-2 wk.
Ductus venosus	Shunts one-third of blood from umbilical vein to inferior vena cava and away from immature liver.	Blood flow occluded with end of umbilical circulation.	Occlusion of cord stops flow of blood from placenta through umbilical vein to ductus venosus.	Blood travels through liver to be filtered as in adult circulation.	*Functional:* When cord is clamped, becomes ligamentum venosum.
Foramen ovale	Provides flap valve between RA and LA so blood can bypass nonfunctioning lungs and go directly to LV and aorta; opens in R-to-L direction because of high RA pressure and low LA pressure.	Closes when pressure in LA becomes higher than pressure in RA.	Cord occlusion elevates systemic resistance; blood returns from PV to LA; both increase L heart pressure. Decreased pulmonary resistance allows free flow of blood into lungs and decreased pressure in RA.	Blood entering RA can no longer pass through to LA; instead it goes to RV and through PA to lungs.	Closes at birth because of pressure changes. *Functional:* 3 mo, but may be longer; becomes fossa ovale.
Pulmonary blood vessels	Narrowed vessels increase resistance to blood flow to lungs.	Dilation of all vessels in lungs.	Elevated blood oxygen and removal of fetal lung fluid.	Decreased pulmonary resistance allows blood to enter freely to be oxygenated.	Beginning with first breath.
Ductus arteriosus	Is widely dilated to carry blood from PA to aorta and avoid nonfunctioning lungs.	Constriction preventing entrance of blood from PA.	Increase of oxygen level in blood.	Blood in PA is directed to lungs for oxygenation.	*Functional:* Beginning within minutes after birth; complete constriction 1-8 days. *Permanent:* 1-4 mo; becomes ligamentum arteriosum.

L, Left; *LA,* left atrium; *LV,* left ventricle; *PA,* pulmonary artery; *PV,* pulmonary veins; *R,* right; *RA,* right atrium; *RV,* right ventricle.

change forces the blood from the right atrium into the right ventricle and pulmonary artery. Because the ductus arteriosus is also closing, the blood continues into the lungs for oxygenation and returns to the left atrium through the pulmonary veins. Blood from the left atrium enters the left ventricle and leaves through the aorta to circulate to the rest of the body. Thus blood flow through the heart and lungs changes from fetal to neonatal circulation and is similar to that in the normal adult (see Fig. 5.9).

Conditions such as **asphyxia** (insufficient oxygen and excess carbon dioxide in the blood and tissues) and persistent pulmonary hypertension (Chapter 24) may reverse the pressures in the heart and cause the foramen ovale to reopen.

The ductus arteriosus closes gradually as oxygenation improves and prostaglandins, which helped keep it open, are metabolized. Until closure is complete, a small amount of blood may shunt through the ductus arteriosus from the aorta to the pulmonary artery (Rozance & Rosenberg, 2017). This sequence occurs because pressure in the aorta has become higher than that in the pulmonary artery. A murmur may be heard as a result of blood flow through the partially open vessel.

Low levels of oxygen in the blood may cause the ductus arteriosus to dilate and the pulmonary vessels to constrict, increasing resistance to blood flow to the lungs. The result may be opening of the foramen ovale to allow a right-to-left shunt of blood and flow from the pulmonary artery through the ductus arteriosus and into the aorta. A patent ductus arteriosus may occur in the infant who experiences asphyxia at birth, becomes hypoxic, or is preterm.

⚲ KNOWLEDGE CHECK

4. What causes the closure of the ductus arteriosus, foramen ovale, and ductus venosus at birth?
5. What causes the pulmonary blood vessels to dilate and the ductus arteriosus to constrict?

⚲ CRITICAL THINKING EXERCISE 19.1

Understanding the changes that occur during the transition from fetal to neonatal circulation helps in predicting the effect on blood flow of various defects in the heart.

Question
1. What would be the effect on neonatal blood flow of an opening in the septum of the atria of the heart?

NEUROLOGIC ADAPTATION: THERMOREGULATION

At birth the infant must assume **thermoregulation**, the maintenance of body temperature. Although the fetus produces heat in utero, the consistently warm temperature of the amniotic fluid and the mother's body makes thermoregulation unnecessary. The infant's temperature may drop as much as 0.2° to 1°C (0.5° to 1.7°F) per minute if the infant is not kept warm at birth (Blackburn, 2013). Neonates must produce and maintain enough heat to prevent cold stress, which can have serious and even fatal effects.

Newborn Characteristics That Lead to Heat Loss

Certain characteristics predispose newborns to lose heat. The skin is thin, and blood vessels are close to the surface. Little subcutaneous or white fat is present to provide a barrier to heat loss. Heat is readily transferred from the warmer internal areas of the body to the cooler skin surfaces and then to the surrounding air. Newborns have three times more surface area to body mass than adults, which provides more area for heat loss. Newborns lose heat at a rate four times greater than that of adults (Carlo, 2016b).

The healthy full-term infant remains in a position of flexion, reducing the amount of skin surface exposed to the surrounding temperatures and decreasing heat loss. Sick or preterm infants have decreased muscle tone and are unable to maintain a flexed position. Preterm infants also have thinner skin and even less white subcutaneous fat than full-term infants. Therefore they are at increased risk for cold stress.

Methods of Heat Loss

Heat is lost in four ways: evaporation, conduction, convection, and radiation (Fig. 19.2). The nurse can prevent heat loss by each method and must be watchful for situations in which intervention is needed.

Evaporation

Evaporation is air-drying of the skin that results in cooling. Drying the infant, especially the head, as quickly as possible helps prevent loss of heat by evaporation. Insensible water loss from the skin and respiratory tract increases heat loss from evaporation.

Conduction

Movement of heat away from the body occurs when newborns have direct contact with objects that are cooler than their skin. Placing infants on cold surfaces or touching them with cool objects causes this type of heat loss. The reverse is also true: Contact with warm objects increases body heat by conduction. Warming objects that will touch the infant or placing the unclothed infant against the mother's skin ("skin to skin") helps prevent conductive heat loss.

Convection

Transfer of heat from the infant to cooler surrounding air occurs in convection. When infants are in incubators, the circulating warm air helps keep them warm by convection. Providing a warm, draft-free environment avoids convective heat loss.

Radiation

Radiation is the transfer of heat to cooler objects that are not in direct contact with the infant. Infants in incubators

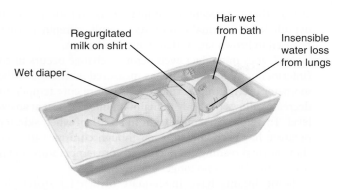

Wet diaper · Regurgitated milk on shirt · Hair wet from bath · Insensible water loss from lungs

Evaporation can occur during birth or bathing from moisture on skin, as a result of wet linens or clothes, and from insensible water loss.

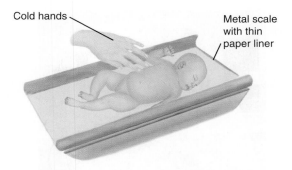

Cold hands · Metal scale with thin paper liner

Conduction occurs when the infant comes in contact with cold objects or surfaces such as a scale, a circumcision restraint board, cold hands, or a stethoscope.

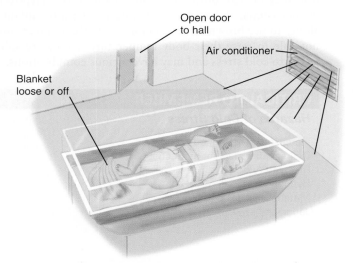

Open door to hall · Air conditioner · Blanket loose or off

Convection occurs when drafts come from open doors, air conditioning, or even air currents created by people moving about.

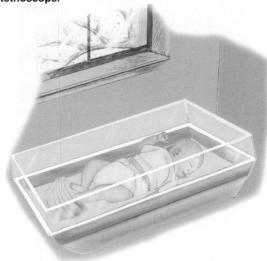

Heat is lost by radiation when the infant is near cold surfaces. Thus heat is lost from the infant's body to the sides of the crib or incubator and to the outside walls and windows.

FIG. 19.2 Methods of Heat Loss.

transfer heat to the walls of the incubator. If the walls of the incubator are cold, the infant is cooled, even when the temperature of the air inside the incubator is warm. To combat this problem, incubators have double walls. Placing cribs and incubators away from windows and outside walls minimizes radiant heat loss. Newborns can gain heat by radiation, too. Using a radiant warmer transfers heat from the warmer to the cooler infant (Fig. 19.3).

CRITICAL THINKING EXERCISE 19.2

Look at a newborn's environment and the care given over a day.

Question
1. What are possible causes of each method of heat loss for the infant?

Nonshivering Thermogenesis

When adults are cold, they shiver, increasing muscle activity to produce heat. Shivering is not an important method of **thermogenesis** (heat production) for newborns, who rarely shiver except during prolonged exposure to low temperatures (Blackburn, 2013). Instead, they become restless and cry. Their increased activity and flexion help generate some warmth and reduce the loss of heat from exposed surface areas of the body.

Exposure to cool temperatures also results in peripheral vasoconstriction, decreasing flow of warm blood to the skin. This helps prevent heat loss from the skin and causes the skin to feel cool to the touch. In addition, a drop in temperature increases the metabolic rate as much a 200% to 300%, causing above-normal oxygen and glucose use (Blackburn, 2013).

The primary method of heat production in infants is **nonshivering thermogenesis** (NST), the metabolism of brown fat to produce heat. Newborns can increase heat production

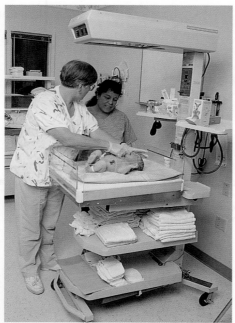

FIG. 19.3 Radiant warmers allow easy access to the infant without increasing heat loss resulting from exposure. The nurse is careful not to come between the infant and the overhead source of heat when caring for the infant.

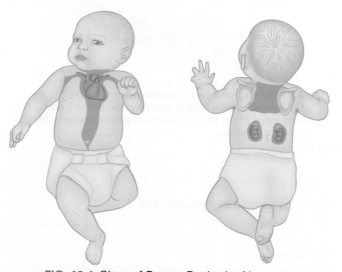

FIG. 19.4 Sites of Brown Fat in the Neonate.

by 100% using NST (Blackburn, 2013). **Brown fat** (also called *brown adipose tissue [BAT]*) contains an abundant supply of blood vessels that causes the brown color. Brown fat is located primarily around the back of the neck; in the axillae; around the heart, kidneys, and adrenals; between the scapulae; and along the abdominal aorta (Fig. 19.4). As brown fat is metabolized, it generates more heat than white subcutaneous fat. Blood passing through brown fat is warmed and carries heat to the rest of the body.

NST begins when thermal receptors in the skin detect a skin temperature of 35° to 36°C (95° to 96.8°F) (Blackburn,

2013). Thermal receptor stimulation is transmitted to the hypothalamic thermal center. As a result, norepinephrine is released in brown fat, initiating its metabolism.

NST goes into effect even before a change occurs in core (interior) body temperature, as measured with a rectal thermometer. Activating thermogenesis before core temperature decreases allows the body to maintain internal heat at an even level. Therefore NST may begin in an infant when skin temperature has been cooled, even though core measurements show normal readings. A decreased core temperature will not occur until NST is no longer effective.

Some infants have inadequate brown fat stores. It is accumulated mainly during the third trimester, so preterm infants may be born before adequate stores of brown fat have accumulated (Wood, 2016). Intrauterine growth restriction may deplete brown fat stores before birth. Hypoxia, hypoglycemia, and acidosis may interfere with the infant's ability to use brown fat to generate heat. These infants are not able to raise their body temperature if they are subjected to cold stress and may have serious complications.

CRITICAL TO REMEMBER

Hazards of Cold Stress

Increased oxygen need
Decreased surfactant production
Respiratory distress
Hypoglycemia
Metabolic acidosis
Jaundice

Effects of Cold Stress

Cold stress causes many body changes (Fig. 19.5). The increased metabolic rate and metabolism of brown fat that result from cold stress can cause a significant rise in the need for oxygen. If an infant is having even mild respiratory distress, the problem may be exacerbated if added oxygen is used for heat production. Cold stress also causes a diminished production of surfactant, impeding lung expansion and leading to more respiratory distress.

Glucose is also necessary in larger amounts when the metabolic rate rises to produce heat. When glycogen stores are converted to glucose, they may be quickly depleted, causing hypoglycemia. Continued use of glucose for temperature maintenance leaves less available for growth.

Metabolism of glucose in the presence of insufficient oxygen causes increased production of acids. Metabolism of brown fat also releases fatty acids. The result can be metabolic acidosis, which can be a life-threatening condition. Elevated fatty acids in the blood can interfere with transport of **bilirubin** to the liver, increasing the risk for **jaundice** (yellow discoloration of the skin and sclera caused by excessive bilirubin in the blood).

As the infant's body attempts to conserve heat, vasoconstriction of the peripheral blood vessels occurs to reduce

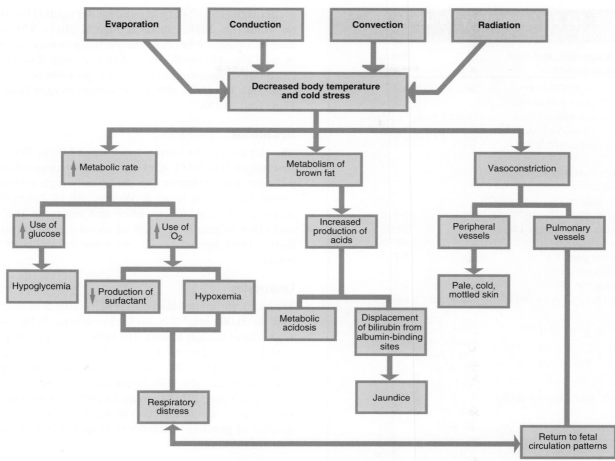

FIG. 19.5 Effects of Cold Stress.

heat loss from the skin surface. Decreased oxygen concentration in the blood, however, also may cause vasoconstriction of the pulmonary vessels, leading to further respiratory distress.

Neutral Thermal Environment

A **neutral thermal environment** is one in which the infant can maintain a stable body temperature with minimal oxygen need and without an increase in metabolic rate. The range of environmental temperature that allows this stability is called the *thermoneutral zone.* In healthy, unclothed, full-term newborns, an environmental temperature of 32° to 33.5°C (89.6° to 92.3°F) provides a thermoneutral zone. When the infant is dressed, the thermoneutral range is 24° to 27°C (75.2° to 80.6°F) (Blackburn, 2013). The thermoneutral zone for each infant varies according to the infant's gestational age, size, and postnatal age.

Hyperthermia

Infants also respond poorly to hyperthermia. With an elevated temperature the metabolic rate rises, causing an increased need for oxygen and glucose and possible metabolic acidosis. In addition, peripheral vasodilation leads to increased insensible fluid losses. Sweating may occur but is often delayed because sweat glands are immature.

Newborns may be overheated by poorly regulated equipment designed to keep them warm. When radiant warmers, warming lights, or warmed incubators are used, the temperature mechanism must be set to vary the heat according to the infant's skin temperature and thus prevent heat that is too high or too low. Alarms to signal that the infant's temperature is too high or too low should be functioning properly.

> **❓ KNOWLEDGE CHECK**
>
> 6. Why are neonates more prone to heat loss than older children or adults?
> 7. What are the effects of low temperature in newborns?

HEMATOLOGIC ADAPTATION

Factors That Affect the Blood

The blood volume of the term newborn is 80 to 100 mL/kg, but this varies according to the time of cord clamping, the gestational age of the infant, and the position of the infant when the cord is clamped (Diehl-Jones & Fraser, 2014). Preterm infants have a greater blood volume per kilogram

TABLE 19.2   Laboratory Values in the Newborn

Test, Specimen, and Unit of Measurement	Age	Normal Ranges
Erythrocyte (red blood cell [RBC]) count, whole blood	Newborn	4.8-7.1 (million/mcL)
Hemoglobin, whole blood	Newborn	15-24 g/dL
Hematocrit, whole blood (%)	Newborn	44-70
Leukocytes, whole blood	Birth	9.1-34 (thousand/mm^3)
Leukocyte differential count, whole blood		
Myelocytes (%)		0
Neutrophils ("bands") (%)		3-5
Neutrophils ("segs") (%)		54-62
Lymphocytes (%)		25-33
Monocytes (%)		3-7
Eosinophils (%)		1-3
Basophils (%)		0-0.75
Platelet count, whole blood	Newborn	84-478 (thousand/mm^3)
Glucose, serum (mg/dL)	Cord	45-96
	Newborn at 1 day	40-60
	Newborn >1 day	50-90
Calcium, total serum (mg/dL)	Cord	9-11.5
	3-24 hr	9-10.6
	24-48 hr	7-12
	4-7 days	9-10.9
Magnesium, plasma (mg/dL)	0-6 days	1.2-2.6
Bilirubin (mg/dL)	Cord	<2
	0-1 day	1.4-8.7
	1-2 days	3.4-11.5
	3-5 days	1.5-12
	>5 days to adult	0.3

Modified from Lo, S. F. (2016). Reference intervals for laboratory tests and procedures. In R. M. Kliegman, B. E. Stanton, J. W. St. Geme, & N. F. Schor. (Eds.), *Nelson textbook of pediatrics* (20th ed., p. 3464). Philadelphia, PA: Saunders; Pagana, K. D., & Pagana, T. J. (2014). *Mosby's diagnostic and laboratory test reference* (12th ed.). St. Louis, MO: Mosby; Blackburn, S. T. (2013). *Maternal, fetal, and neonatal physiology: A clinical perspective* (4th ed.). St. Louis, MO: Saunders; and Malarkey, L. M., & McMorrow, M. E. (2012). *Saunders nursing guide to laboratory and diagnostic tests* (2nd ed.). St. Louis, MO: Saunders.

than term infants. Blood samples drawn from the heel, where the circulation is sluggish, show higher hemoglobin (Hgb), hematocrit (Hct), and erythrocyte values than samples taken from central areas (Blackburn, 2013). Venous blood samples are more accurate and are taken when precise measurement is essential. (See Table 19.2 for specific newborn laboratory values.)

Blood Values
Erythrocytes and Hemoglobin
At birth, the infant has comparatively more erythrocytes (4.8 million/microliter [mcL] to 7.1 million/mcL) and

higher Hgb (15 to 24 grams per deciliter [g/dL]) levels than the adult (Lo, 2016; Pagana & Pagana, 2014). This difference is necessary because the partial pressure of oxygen in fetal blood is much lower than the normal adult level. Adequate oxygenation of the cells is possible because fetal Hgb (Hgb F) carries 20% to 50% more oxygen than adult Hgb (Hall, 2015).

Hematocrit
The Hct level in the normal newborn is 44% to 70% for the first month (Lo, 2016). A level above 65% from a central site indicates **polycythemia** (an abnormally high erythrocyte count) (Luchtman-Jones & Wilson, 2014). Polycythemia increases the risk for jaundice and injury to the brain and other organs as a result of blood stasis. Respiratory distress and hypoglycemia are more common in these infants.

Leukocytes
The leukocyte (white blood cell [WBC]) count at birth is 9100/mm^3 to 34,000/mm^3 (Lo, 2016). The average WBC count is 15,000/mm^3 in term infants. The WBC count falls to 12,000/mm^3 by 4 to 5 days after birth (Blackburn, 2013). In newborns an elevated WBC count does not necessarily indicate infection. In fact, the WBC count may decrease in infections (Wilson & Tyner, 2014). Increased numbers of immature leukocytes are a sign of infection or sepsis in the neonate. The number of platelets (thrombocytes) also may decrease as a result of infections.

Risk for Clotting Deficiency
Newborns are at risk for clotting deficiency during the first few days of life because they have low levels of vitamin K, which is necessary to activate several of the clotting factors (factors II [prothrombin], VII, IX, and X). Vitamin K is synthesized in the intestines, but food and normal intestinal flora are necessary for this process. At birth the intestines are sterile and therefore unable to produce vitamin K (Luchtman-Jones & Wilson, 2014). To decrease the risk for hemorrhagic disease of the newborn, vitamin K is administered intramuscularly to most newborns in the United States during initial care. Drugs such as phenytoin (Dilantin), phenobarbital, and antituberculosis drugs taken by the mother during pregnancy interfere with clotting ability in the infant after birth (Blackburn, 2013).

The platelet (thrombocyte) count ranges from 84,000/mm^3 to 478,000/mm^3 at birth. After the first week, platelet levels are the same as in the adult—150,000/mm^3 to 400,000/mm^3 (Lo, 2016). Although platelet counts in term newborns are near adult levels, platelet response to stimuli is decreased during the first few days of life.

GASTROINTESTINAL SYSTEM

Newborns must begin to take in, digest, and absorb food after birth because the placenta no longer performs these functions for them.

Stomach

The newborn's stomach capacity is about 6 mL/kg at birth. Gastric emptying may be delayed at first. It is twice as rapid after ingestion of human milk than after formula and slower if the infant has swallowed mucus (Blackburn, 2013). The gastrocolic reflex is stimulated when the stomach fills, causing increased intestinal peristalsis. Infants frequently pass a stool during or after a feeding. The cardiac sphincter between the esophagus and the stomach is relaxed, which explains the tendency to regurgitate feedings easily.

Intestines

The intestines of the newborn are long in proportion to the infant's size and compared with those of the adult. The added length allows more surface area for absorption but makes infants more prone to water loss should diarrhea develop. Air enters the gastrointestinal tract soon after birth, and bowel sounds may be heard beginning at 15 minutes after birth (Goodwin, 2014).

The digestive tract is sterile at birth. Once the infant is exposed to the external environment and begins to take in fluids, bacteria enter the gastrointestinal tract. Normal intestinal flora are established within the first few days of life.

Digestive Enzymes

Maturation of the ability to digest and absorb occurs at different rates for various nutrients. Pancreatic amylase, needed to digest complex carbohydrates, is deficient for the first 4 to 6 months after birth (Blackburn, 2013). Amylase is also produced by the salivary glands, but in low amounts until about the third month of life. Amylase is present in breast milk.

The newborn is also deficient in pancreatic lipase, limiting fat absorption significantly. Lipase present in the mouth and stomach helps with some digestion of fat. Lipase is present in breast milk, which may make it more digestible for the newborn than formula. Protein and lactose, the major carbohydrate in the infant's milk diet, are both well digested.

Stools

Meconium is the first stool excreted by the newborn. It consists of particles from amniotic fluid such as vernix, skin cells, and hair, along with cells shed from the intestinal tract, bile, and other intestinal secretions. Meconium is greenish black with a thick, sticky, tarlike consistency. The first meconium stool is usually passed within 12 hours of life, and 99% of neonates pass meconium within 48 hours (Carlo, 2016a). If meconium is not passed within that time, obstruction is suspected.

Meconium stools are followed by transitional stools, a combination of meconium and milk stools. They are greenish-brown and of a looser consistency than meconium. Milk stools characteristic of the type of feeding given to the infant occur next.

The stools of infants fed with breast milk are seedy and the color and consistency of mustard, with a sweet-sour odor. The breastfed infant generally has more frequent stools than the infant who is formula fed. A stool may be passed with each feeding. The normal breastfed newborn should have at least four or more stools daily, after the fourth day of life (Rozance & Rosenberg, 2017).

The formula-fed infant has pale yellow to light brown stools. They are firmer in consistency than those of the breast-fed infant. The infant may excrete several stools daily, or only one or two. The stools have the characteristic odor of feces.

HEPATIC SYSTEM

The liver assumes many different functions after birth. Some of the most important include maintenance of blood glucose levels, conjugation of bilirubin, production of factors necessary for blood coagulation, storage of iron, and metabolism of drugs.

Blood Glucose Maintenance

Throughout gestation, glucose is supplied to the fetus by the placenta. During the third trimester, glucose is stored as glycogen primarily in the fetal liver and skeletal muscles for use after birth. These stores are almost completely depleted within 12 hours after birth (Rozance & Rosenberg, 2017). They are used for energy during the stress of delivery and for breathing, heat production, movement against gravity, and activation of all the functions that the neonate must assume at birth.

Until newborns begin regular feedings and their intake is adequate to meet energy requirements, the glucose present in the body is used. As the blood glucose level falls, stored glycogen in the liver is converted to glucose for use. Although the brain can use alternative fuels such as ketones and fatty acids if necessary, glucose is the primary source of energy. Glucose concentration in the blood commonly falls to the lowest levels by 60 to 90 minutes after birth but rises and stabilizes in 2 to 3 hours after birth (Blackburn, 2013).

In the term infant, glucose levels should be 40 to 60 mg/dL on the first day and 50 to 90 mg/dL thereafter (Lo, 2016). There is no general consensus about the level of blood glucose that defines hypoglycemia, but a level below 40 to 45 mg/dL in the term infant is often used (Blackburn, 2013; Kubicka & Little, 2016; Rozance et al., 2015).

Many newborns are at increased risk for hypoglycemia. In the preterm, late preterm (born between 34 weeks and 36 6/7 weeks of gestation), and small-for-gestational-age infant, adequate stores of glycogen or even fat for metabolism may not have accumulated. Stores may be used up before birth in the postterm infant because of poor intrauterine nourishment from a deteriorating placenta. Infants who are large for gestational age and those with diabetic mothers may produce excessive insulin that consumes available glucose quickly.

Infants exposed to stressors such as asphyxia or infection may exhaust their stores of glycogen. The cold-stressed infant may deplete glycogen to increase metabolism and raise body temperature.

Conjugation of Bilirubin

A major function of the liver is the conjugation of bilirubin (Fig. 19.6). The newborn's liver may not be mature enough to prevent jaundice during the first week of life. Jaundice results from **hyperbilirubinemia**, excessive bilirubin in the blood. It occurs in 60% of term newborns and 80% of preterm infants (Ambalavanan & Carlo, 2016).

Source and Effect of Bilirubin

The principal source of bilirubin is the hemolysis of erythrocytes. This is a normal occurrence after birth, when fewer erythrocytes are needed than during fetal life. The breakdown of red blood cells (RBCs) releases their components into the bloodstream to be reused by the body. Bilirubin remains as an unusable residue in the blood. This substance is toxic to the body and must be excreted.

Bilirubin is released in an unconjugated form. Unconjugated bilirubin, also called *indirect bilirubin,* is soluble in fat but not in water. Before excretion can occur, the liver must change it to a water-soluble form by a process called *conjugation.* The bilirubin is then known as *conjugated* or *direct bilirubin.* Conjugated bilirubin is not toxic to the body and can be excreted.

Because unconjugated bilirubin is fat soluble, it may be absorbed by the subcutaneous fat, causing the yellowish discoloration of the skin called *jaundice.* If enough unconjugated bilirubin accumulates in the blood, staining of the tissues in the brain may occur. This may cause acute **bilirubin encephalopathy**, a neurologic condition resulting from bilirubin toxicity. If this condition becomes chronic, it causes permanent neurologic injury known as **kernicterus**. The level of bilirubin necessary to cause injury to the central nervous system is unknown and may be different for various infants.

Normal Conjugation

When unconjugated bilirubin is released into the bloodstream, it attaches to binding sites on albumin in the plasma and is carried to the liver. If an adequate number of albumin-binding sites are not available, bilirubin circulates as unbound or free unconjugated bilirubin. Bilirubin can be displaced from albumin by some medications. Free fatty acids, acidosis, and infection also decrease albumin binding of bilirubin

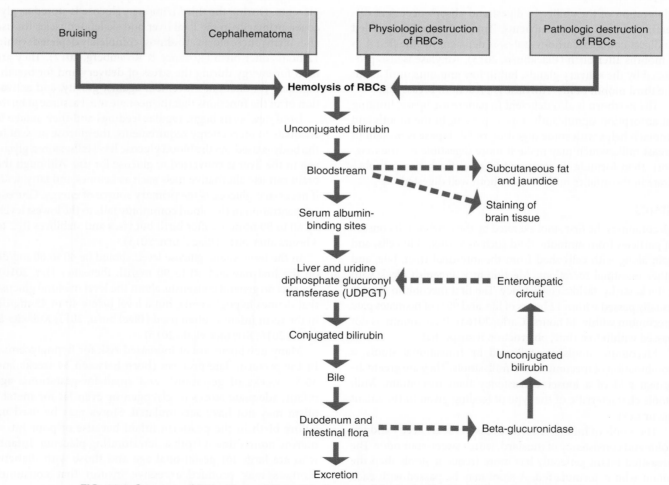

FIG. 19.6 Sources of Bilirubin and How It Is Removed from the Body. *RBCs,* Red blood cells.

(Kamuth, Thilo, Deacon, & Hernandez, 2015). It is the free, unbound unconjugated bilirubin that can move into the tissues and cross the blood-brain barrier.

When the albumin-bound bilirubin reaches the liver, it is changed to the conjugated form of bilirubin by the enzyme uridine diphosphate glucuronyl transferase (UDPGT). Conjugated bilirubin is excreted into the bile and then into the duodenum. In the intestines the normal flora act to reduce bilirubin to urobilinogen and stercobilin, which are excreted in the stools. Some urobilinogen is excreted by the kidneys.

A small percentage of conjugated bilirubin may be deconjugated, or converted back to the unconjugated state, by the intestinal enzyme beta-glucuronidase. This enzyme is important in fetal life because only unconjugated bilirubin can be cleared by the placenta for conjugation by the mother's liver. In the newborn, deconjugated bilirubin in the intestines is reabsorbed into the portal circulation and carried back to the liver, where it again undergoes the conjugation process. This recirculation of bilirubin is called the *enterohepatic circuit,* and it creates additional work for the liver.

Blood tests for bilirubin measure total serum bilirubin (TSB) and direct (conjugated) bilirubin in the serum. TSB is a combination of indirect (unconjugated) and direct bilirubin.

Factors in Increased Bilirubin

A number of factors lead to the production of excessive amounts of bilirubin or interfere with the normal process of conjugation. These increase the incidence of jaundice during the first week of life.

Excess Production. Approximately 8 to 10 milligrams per kilogram (mg/kg) of bilirubin is produced in newborns each day, a rate twice that in adults. The rate of production remains higher for 3 to 6 weeks (Blackburn, 2013). Newborns have more RBCs per kilogram than do adults.

Red Blood Cell Life. Fetal RBCs break down more quickly than adult erythrocytes. They last 80 to 100 days in term infants and 60 to 80 days in preterm infants, compared with RBCs in adults, which have a typical life span of 120 days (Blackburn, 2013). In addition, neonate erythrocytes are more fragile and susceptible to injury than those in the adult. Compared with adults, for their size neonates have more RBCs breaking down faster and producing greater amounts of bilirubin to excrete.

Albumin. Newborns have less albumin, decreased albumin-binding capacity, and decreased albumin affinity for bilirubin than adults (Kaplan, Wong, Sibley, & Stevenson, 2014).

Liver Immaturity. The newborn's immature liver may not produce adequate amounts of UDPGT and other substances during the first few days of life. This limits the amount of bilirubin that can be conjugated.

Blood Incompatibility. Rh, ABO, or other incompatible blood between the mother and the infant may increase RBC breakdown.

Gestation. Preterm and late preterm infants have immature conjugation abilities.

Intestinal Factors. At birth the intestines of the newborn are sterile. Conjugated bilirubin cannot be reduced to urobilinogen or stercobilin for excretion without the action of intestinal flora. In addition, the newborn intestines have a large amount of the enzyme beta-glucuronidase, which changes bilirubin back to the unconjugated state. Intestinal motility is decreased, allowing more time for the enzyme to act. These factors may result in high levels of unconjugated bilirubin, which is reabsorbed into the blood circulation.

Delayed Feeding. Feeding the newborn helps establish the normal intestinal flora and promotes passage of meconium, which is high in bilirubin. When feedings are delayed or taken poorly, normal flora are not established, and passage of meconium, which is high in bilirubin, is delayed. Delayed passage of stools allows more time for exposure to beta-glucuronidase, increasing the chance that conjugated bilirubin will be converted to the unconjugated state and absorbed into the blood.

Trauma. Trauma during birth, such as bruising or a cephalhematoma, causes increased hemolysis of RBCs. As the RBCs in the traumatized areas break down, they add to the bilirubin load.

Fatty Acids. Fatty acids have a greater affinity than bilirubin for the binding sites on albumin and bind to albumin in place of bilirubin. Fatty acids are released when brown fat is used to increase heat during cold stress. During asphyxia, anaerobic metabolism also produces free fatty acids. Therefore the level of unbound unconjugated bilirubin is increased in these infants, and jaundice may develop.

Family Background. Infants who are Asian, American Indian, or Native Alaskan or have a sibling who had jaundice are more likely to be affected. Infants of diabetic mothers are also at increased risk for jaundice.

Other Factors. Some drugs (such as sulfisoxazole) given to the mother during pregnancy or to the infant increase jaundice. Blood swallowed during birth, hypoglycemia, infection, and hemolytic anemias also increase jaundice.

CRITICAL TO REMEMBER

Factors That Increase Risk for Hyperbilirubinemia

Hemolysis of excessive erythrocytes
Short red blood cell life span
Lack of albumin-binding sites
Liver immaturity
Lack of intestinal flora
Breastfeeding
Delayed or inadequate feedings
Blood incompatibility
Preterm or late preterm birth
Trauma resulting in bruising or cephalhematoma
Polycythemia
Fatty acids from cold stress or asphyxia
Sibling with jaundice
Male gender
Asian, American Indian, Native Alaskan heritage
Maternal diabetes or preeclampsia

Hyperbilirubinemia

Physiologic Jaundice

Physiologic jaundice, also called *nonpathologic* or *developmental jaundice,* is a transient hyperbilirubinemia (excess bilirubin in the blood) and is considered normal. The jaundice is not present during the first 24 hours of life in term infants but appears on the second or third day after birth. Jaundice becomes visible when the bilirubin level is greater than 5 mg/dL (Pan & Rivas, 2016). The rate at which the bilirubin level in the blood rises and falls is important because it helps determine whether the rate for a particular infant is following the expected curve for age and birth weight. In physiologic jaundice, the bilirubin peaks between the second and fourth days of life and falls to normal levels by 5 to 7 days (Ambalavanan & Carlo, 2016). The bilirubin level rises higher and falls more slowly in Asian infants.

Nonphysiologic Jaundice

Jaundice that is physiologic or normal must be differentiated from nonphysiologic or pathologic jaundice. One of the most important differences is the time at which jaundice appears. Pathologic jaundice may occur in the first 24 hours. When bilirubin rises higher or more rapidly than expected or stays elevated for longer than expected, earlier treatment is needed to prevent severe hyperbilirubinemia.

Nonphysiologic jaundice is a result of abnormalities causing excessive destruction of RBCs or problems in bilirubin conjugation. These include incompatibilities between the mother's and the infant's blood types, infection, and metabolic disorders. Nonphysiologic jaundice is often treated with phototherapy.

Charts are available that show the rise and fall of bilirubin and the degree of risk at various levels of TSB according to the age of the infant in hours. For example, a full-term infant with no complications who is 24 hours old is considered at low risk if the TSB is 5 mg/dL or less and at high risk if the TSB is greater than 8 mg/dL. At 48 hours of age, that infant would be at low risk if the TSB were 8.5 mg/dL but high risk if the TSB were that high before 48 hours. Infants who are preterm or late preterm or who have other risk factors may receive treatment for hyperbilirubinemia at lower TSB levels than full-term infants.

Jaundice Associated with Breastfeeding

The breastfed infant has a higher risk for developing jaundice, which may begin early or late.

Breastfeeding or Early Onset Jaundice. Bilirubin levels greater than 12 mg/dL develop in 13% of breastfed infants by 1 week of age (Ambalavanan & Carlo, 2016). The most common cause of jaundice in breastfed infants is insufficient intake. Jaundice begins within the first week of life, and serum bilirubin may reach dangerous levels if intake is not increased.

Infants who are sleepy, have a poor suck, or nurse infrequently may not receive enough colostrum—the substance that precedes true breast milk—to benefit from its normal laxative effect in eliminating bilirubin-rich meconium. When meconium is not eliminated, the bilirubin may be deconjugated by beta-glucuronidase in the intestine, absorbed, and recirculated to the liver for conjugation again.

Lack of adequate suckling depresses production of breast milk and increases the problem further. Helping the mother with breastfeeding to increase the infant's intake and stimulate milk production may be the most important treatment. Supplementing with formula interferes with the mother's milk production. However, if breastfeeding is inadequate and the infant is dehydrated or losing excessive weight, supplements of expressed breast milk or formula may be necessary. Glucose-water will not reduce bilirubin levels and should be avoided.

True Breast Milk Jaundice. True breast milk jaundice, also called *late-onset breast milk jaundice,* occurs after the first 3 to 5 days of life. It lasts 3 weeks to as long as 3 months for some infants. The TSB usually peaks at 5 to 10 mg/dL and falls gradually over several months. However, some infants reach levels of 20 to 30 mg/dL (Kaplan et al., 2014).

The exact cause of true breast milk jaundice is unknown. Substances in the breast milk may increase absorption of bilirubin from the intestine or interfere with conjugation. Infants have no signs of illness.

Treatment of breast milk jaundice includes close monitoring of TSB and at least 8 to 12 feedings each 24 hours. If bilirubin levels become too high, phototherapy is begun while the mother continues frequent breastfeeding. Interruption of breastfeeding is generally not recommended. However, if the TSB levels are dangerously high, the health care provider may order formula feeding be given for 1 to 3 days while the mother uses a breast pump to maintain milk supply. Temporarily switching to formula causes a rapid drop in bilirubin level. If the level rises while breastfeeding is interrupted, jaundice from another cause should be investigated. The level may rise again when breastfeeding is resumed but generally not high enough to interfere with further breastfeeding.

Blood Coagulation

Prothrombin and coagulation factors II, VII, IX, and X are produced by the liver and activated by vitamin K, which is deficient in the newborn.

Iron Storage

Iron is stored in the fetal liver and spleen during the last weeks of pregnancy. Full-term infants who are breastfeeding usually do not need added iron until 6 months of age (Lawrence & Lawrence, 2015). At that time, they should begin iron-containing foods or iron supplements. All infants who are not breastfeeding should be given iron-fortified formula (American Academy of Pediatrics & American College of Obstetricians and Gynecologists [AAP & ACOG], 2012).

Metabolism of Drugs

The liver metabolizes drugs inefficiently in the newborn. This must be considered when drugs are given to the neonate. In addition, a breastfeeding mother should alert her primary caregiver before taking medications, because harmful amounts may be transferred to the infant via the breast milk.

URINARY SYSTEM

Kidney Development

By 34 to 36 weeks of gestation, the fetal kidneys have as many nephrons as adult kidneys (Cadnapaphornchai, Schoenbein, Woloschuk, Soranno, & Hernandez, 2015). Blood flow to the kidneys increases after birth, and resistance in the renal vessels decreases. The improved perfusion results in a steady improvement in kidney function during the first few days of life.

Kidney Function

The newborn's kidney function is immature compared with that of the adult. The ability of the glomeruli to filter and the renal tubules to reabsorb is considerably less than in adults. The glomerular filtration rate doubles or triples during the first weeks of life but does not reach adult levels until 1 to 2 years of age (Cadnapaphornchai et al., 2015). Therefore infants have a decreased ability to remove waste products from the blood.

Small amounts of substances such as glucose and amino acids may escape into the urine of the neonate (Blackburn, 2013; Cadnapaphornchai et al., 2015). They disappear within the first few days of life as kidney function improves. Uric acid crystals may give a reddish color to the urine that is sometimes mistaken for blood.

Voiding occurs within 12 hours for 50% of newborns; 92% void within 24 hours, and 99% void within 48 hours of life (Cadnapaphornchai et al., 2015). Failure to void within that time may be a result of hypovolemia from inadequate intake of fluids. Absence of kidneys or anomalies that interfere with excretion of urine are usually discovered before birth because they cause oligohydramnios (low amniotic fluid volume). This generally prompts investigation into the cause during pregnancy. Only one or two voidings may occur during the first 2 days of life, although a higher number is common. The infant voids six times a day by the fourth day.

Fluid Balance

Newborns have a lower tolerance for changes in total volume of body fluid than do older infants. This is because of the location of water within the newborn's body and the inability of the kidneys to adapt to large changes in fluid volume. In addition, the fluid turnover rate is greater than that in adults. To maintain fluid balance, full-term infants need 60 to 100 mL/kg (27 to 45 mL/lb) daily during the first 3 to 5 days of life and 150 to 175 mL/kg (68 to 80 mL/lb) a day by 7 days of age (Halbardier, 2014) (Box 19.1).

BOX 19.1   Daily Intake and Output in the Newborn

First 3 to 5 Days of Life
Intake: 60 to 100 mL/kg (27 to 45 mL/lb)
Output: At least 1 or 2 voidings

After the First 3 to 5 Days
Intake: 150 to 175 mL/kg (68 to 80 mL/lb)
Output: At least 6 voidings by the fourth day

Water Distribution

Seventy-eight percent of the newborn's body is composed of water. Intracellular water constitutes 34% of the body, and extracellular water makes up 44% of the body. Interstitial water volume is three times greater than in adults (Blackburn, 2013).

Although fluid within the cells is relatively stable, extracellular water is easily lost from the body. Because infants have more fluid for their size than adults, and because a larger proportion of it is located outside the cells, total body water is easily depleted. Conditions such as vomiting and diarrhea can quickly result in life-threatening dehydration. At birth, normal diuresis causes a 5% to 10% weight loss as excess extracellular water is lost (Halbardier, 2014; Nyp, Brunkhorst, & Reavey, 2015).

Insensible Water Loss

Water lost from the skin and respiratory tract contributes to insensible water loss. Insensible water losses are increased in the newborn because of the large surface area of the body and the rapid respiratory rate. Fluid losses increase greatly when infants are placed under radiant warmers or phototherapy lights, which accelerate evaporation from the skin. An elevated respiratory rate or low humidity in the air surrounding the infant raises insensible water losses even further.

Urine Dilution and Concentration

The ability of a newborn's kidneys to dilute urine is similar to that of adults, but they have only half the adult's ability to concentrate urine (Blackburn, 2013). However, a newborn's kidneys cannot handle large increases in fluids, which result in fluid overload. This is most likely to happen if infants receive too much intravenous fluid. Normal urine output is 2 to 5 mL/kg/hr, and urine specific gravity is 1.002 to 1.01 (Nyp et al., 2015). When abnormal conditions such as diarrhea cause excessive loss of fluid, the newborn's limited ability to conserve water may result in dehydration more quickly than in the older infant or child.

Acid-Base and Electrolyte Balance

The maintenance of acid-base and electrolyte balance is a primary function of the kidneys and may be precarious in neonates. Newborns tend to lose bicarbonate at lower levels than adults, increasing their risk for metabolic acidosis. The excretion of solutes also is less efficient in newborns. Although newborns conserve needed sodium well, they are limited in excretion of sodium (Blackburn, 2013). This is especially a problem if they receive excessive amounts.

IMMUNE SYSTEM

The neonate is less effective in fighting infection than the older infant or child. Leukocytes are delayed in moving to the site of invasion and are inefficient in destroying the invader. The infant's decreased ability to localize infection leads to a tendency toward generalized sepsis.

Fever and leukocytosis, which occur during infection of the older child, are often not present in the newborn with infection. This lack of response occurs because the hypothalamus and inflammatory responses are immature. Nonspecific signs such as changes in activity, color, tone, or feeding may be the only signs of sepsis.

Because of their immature immune system, infants are susceptible to some pathogens that do not usually affect older children. Full-term newborns receive antibodies from their mothers during the last trimester of pregnancy. The mother continues to provide passive antibodies to the infant in her milk if she chooses to breastfeed. Immunoglobulins (serum globulins with antibody activity) help protect the newborn from infection. The major immunoglobulins are IgG, IgM, and IgA, each of which performs a different function. At birth the infant's total immunoglobulin levels range from 55% to 80% of the adult levels (Blackburn, 2013).

Immunoglobulin G

Only immunoglobulin G (IgG) crosses the placenta, with passage beginning in the first trimester. Preterm infants have less IgG because transfer is greatest during the third trimester. IgG provides the fetus with passive temporary immunity to bacteria, bacterial toxins, and viruses to which the mother has developed immunity. The full-term infant has IgG levels that are as high as or higher than those of the mother (Stoll & Shane, 2016).

Although the fetus makes some IgG, significant production of IgG is delayed until after 6 months of age (Blackburn, 2013). The infant gradually produces larger quantities of the immunoglobulin to replace IgG from the mother, which is being catabolized. The passive immunity gradually disappears, reaching the lowest level at 2 to 4 months of age (Empey & Kolls, 2014).

Immunoglobulin M

Immunoglobulin M (IgM) is the first immunoglobulin produced by the body when the newborn is challenged. This immunoglobulin helps protect against gram-negative bacteria. Rapid production of IgM begins a few days after birth as a result of exposure to environmental antigens. IgM cannot cross the placenta because the molecules are too large. If IgM is found in cord blood, exposure to infection in utero has occurred.

Immunoglobulin A

Immunoglobulin A (IgA) also does not cross the placenta and must be produced by the infant. IgA is important in protection of the gastrointestinal and respiratory systems, and newborns are particularly susceptible to infections of those systems. Secretory IgA is present in colostrum and breast milk (Kapur, Yoder, & Polin, 2014). Therefore breastfed infants may receive protection that formula-fed infants do not.

? KNOWLEDGE CHECK

13. How does the distribution of fluid in the newborn compare with that in the adult?
14. Why are IgG, IgM, and IgA important to the newborn?

PSYCHOSOCIAL ADAPTATION

Periods of Reactivity

In the early hours after birth, the infant goes through changes called *periods of reactivity*. The two periods of reactivity are separated by a period of sleep or decreased activity (Gardner & Hernandez, 2015).

First Period of Reactivity

The **first period of reactivity** begins at birth and lasts for 30 minutes. Infants are active at this time and appear wide awake, alert, and interested in their surroundings. Parents enjoy watching the infant gaze directly at them when held in the en face (face-to-face) position. Infants move their arms and legs energetically, root, and appear hungry. If allowed to nurse, many infants latch on to the nipple and suck well.

The temperature may be decreased during this period. Respirations may be as high as 80 breaths per minute. The heart rate may be elevated to 180 beats per minute. Crackles, grunting, retractions, and nasal flaring may be present. The pulse and respiratory rates gradually slow, and the infant becomes sleepy.

Period of Sleep or Decreased Activity

After the first period of reactivity, infants become quieter or fall into a deep sleep. During this time the pulse and respirations drop into the normal range. Bowel sounds are audible, and meconium may be passed.

Second Period of Reactivity

The **second period of reactivity** lasts 4 to 6 hours. Infants have alert periods, and parents may enjoy the opportunity to get to know their infant at this time. Infants become interested in feeding and may pass meconium. There may be tachycardia and rapid respirations. Mucous secretions increase, and infants may gag or regurgitate.

Behavioral States

Six gradations in the behavioral state of the infant have been identified, ranging from quiet sleep to crying (Blackburn, 2013; Gardner, Goldson, & Hernandez, 2015b). The amount of time infants spend in the different sleep-wake states varies and is a key to their individuality.

Deep or Quiet Sleep State

During the quiet sleep state the infant is in a deep sleep with closed eyes and no eye movements. Respirations are quiet, regular, and slower than in the other states. Although startles occur at intervals, the infant's body is quiet. The infant is very difficult to arouse and will not feed.

Light or Active Sleep State

The active sleep state is a lighter sleep in which the infants' eyes are closed. They move their extremities, stretch, change facial expressions, make sucking movements, and may fuss briefly. During this period, respirations tend to be more rapid and irregular and rapid eye movements occur. Infants are more likely to startle from noise or disturbances and may return to sleep or move to an awake state.

Drowsy State

The drowsy state is a transitional period between sleep and waking similar to that experienced by adults as they awaken. The eyes may remain closed or, if open, appear glazed and unfocused. Infants startle and move their extremities slowly. They may go back to sleep or, with gentle stimulation, gradually awaken.

Quiet Alert State

The quiet alert state (also called *alert inactivity*) should be pointed out to parents because it is an excellent time to increase bonding. Infants focus on objects or people, respond to the parents with intense gazing, and seem bright and interested in their surroundings. They respond to stimuli and interaction with others. Body movements are minimal as infants seem to concentrate on the environment.

Active Alert State

In the active alert state, infants seem restless, have increased motor movements, and may be fussy. Infants have faster and more irregular respirations, may hiccup or regurgitate, and seem more aware of feelings of discomfort from hunger or cold. Although their eyes may be open, infants seem less focused on visual stimuli than during the quiet alert state.

Crying State

The crying state may quickly follow the active alert state if no intervention occurs to comfort the infant. The cries are continuous and lusty, active body movement occurs, and the infant does not respond positively to stimulation. Respirations are irregular and rapid. It may take a period of comforting to move the infant to a state in which feeding or other activities can be accomplished.

KNOWLEDGE CHECK

15. Describe the behaviors of newborns during the first and second periods of reactivity.
16. How do infant behavioral states vary?

SUMMARY CONCEPTS

- Chemical, mechanical, thermal, and sensory factors combine to stimulate the respiratory center in the brain and initiate respirations at birth.
- Surfactant lines the alveoli and reduces surface tension to keep the alveoli open. Fetal lung fluid moves into the interstitial spaces before, during, and after birth and is absorbed by the lymphatic and vascular systems.
- Increases in blood oxygen levels, shifts in pressure in the heart and lungs, and clamping of the umbilical vessels cause closure of the ductus arteriosus, foramen ovale, and ductus venosus at birth.
- Neonates must produce and maintain heat (thermogenesis) to prevent the effects of cold stress.
- Infants are predisposed to heat loss because they have thin skin with little subcutaneous (white) fat, blood vessels close to the surface, and a large skin surface area. They lose heat by evaporation, conduction, convection, and radiation.
- Heat is produced in newborns by increased activity, flexion, and metabolism, vasoconstriction, and nonshivering thermogenesis. These factors increase oxygen and glucose consumption and may cause respiratory distress, hypoglycemia, acidosis, and jaundice.
- Laboratory values for erythrocytes, hemoglobin, and hematocrit are higher for newborns than for adults because less oxygen is available in fetal life than after birth.

- The stools progress from thick, greenish-black meconium to loose, greenish-brown transitional stools to milk stools. Stools of breastfed infants are frequent, soft, seedy, and mustard-colored. Those of formula-fed infants are pale yellow to light brown, firmer, and less frequent.
- The neonate uses glucose rapidly and is at risk for hypoglycemia. Infants at risk for hypoglycemia include those who are preterm, late preterm, small for gestational age, large for gestational age, born to diabetic mothers, or exposed to stressors.
- Physiologic jaundice occurs in normal newborns after the first 24 hours of life as a result of hemolysis of red blood cells and immaturity of the liver. Nonphysiologic (pathologic) jaundice begins within the first 24 hours and often requires treatment with phototherapy. Breastfeeding jaundice is often caused by insufficient intake. True breast milk jaundice begins later than physiologic jaundice and may be caused by substances in the milk.
- The newborn's kidneys filter, reabsorb, and maintain fluid and electrolyte balance less efficiently than the adult's kidneys. The newborn's body is composed of a greater percentage of water, with more located in the extracellular compartment, and fluid is more easily lost.
- Newborns receive passive immunity when immunoglobulin G crosses the placenta in utero. After birth, immunoglobulins M and A are produced to protect against infection.

- During the first and second periods of reactivity, newborns are active and alert and may be interested in feeding. They may have a low temperature, elevated pulse and respiratory rates, and excessive secretions.
- Newborns progress through six behavioral states: quiet sleep, active sleep, drowsy, quiet alert, active alert, and crying.

REFERENCES & READINGS

Ambalavanan, N., & Carlo, W. (2016). Jaundice and hyperbilirubinemia in the newborn. In R. M. Kliegman, B. E. Stanton, J. W. St. Geme, & N. F. Schor (Eds.), *Nelson textbook of pediatrics* (20th ed.) (pp. 871–875). Philadelphia: Saunders.

American Academy of Pediatrics & American College of Obstetricians and Gynecologists (AAP & ACOG). (2012). *Guidelines for perinatal care* (7th ed.). Elk Grove Village, IL: Authors.

Blackburn, S. T. (2013). *Maternal, fetal, and neonatal physiology: A clinical perspective* (4th ed.). St. Louis, MO: Saunders.

Cadnapaphornchai, M. A., Schoenbein, M. B., Woloschuk, R., Soranno, D. E., & Hernandez, J. A. (2015). Neonatal nephrology. In S. L. Gardner, B. S. Carter, M. Enzman-Hines, et al. (Eds.), *Merenstein & Gardner's handbook of neonatal intensive care* (8th ed.) (pp. 689–726). St. Louis, MO: Mosby.

Carlo, W. A. (2016a). Physical examination of the newborn infant. In R. M. Kliegman, B. E. Stanton, J. W. St. Geme, & N. F. Schor (Eds.), *Nelson textbook of pediatrics* (20th ed.) (pp. 794–797). Philadelphia: Saunders.

Carlo, W. A. (2016b). Routine delivery room and initial care. In R. M. Kliegman, B. E. Stanton, J. W. St. Geme, & N. F. Shor (Eds.), *Nelson textbook of pediatrics* (20th ed.) (pp. 798–799). Philadelphia: Saunders.

Carlo, W. A. (2016c). Transition to pulmonary respiration. In R. M. Kliegman, B. E. Stanton, J. W. St. Geme, & N. F. Shor (Eds.), *Nelson textbook of pediatrics* (20th ed.) (pp. 848–849). Philadelphia: Saunders.

Diehl-Jones, W., & Fraser, D. (2014). Hematologic disorders. In *Core curriculum for neonatal intensive care nursing* (5th ed.) (pp. 662–686). St. Louis, MO: Saunders.

Empey, K. M., & Kolls, J. K. (2014). Neonatal pulmonary host defense. In R. J. Martin, A. A. Fanaroff, & M. C. Walsh (Eds.), *Fanaroff and Martin's neonatal-perinatal medicine: Diseases of the fetus and infant* (10th ed) Vol. 2. (pp. 1711–1744). St. Louis, MO: Mosby.

Fraser, D. (2014). Newborn adaptation to extrauterine life. In K. R. Simpson & P. A. Creehan (Eds.), *AWHONN perinatal nursing* (4th ed.) (pp. 581–595). Philadelphia: Lippincott Williams & Wilkins.

Gardner, S. L., Enzman-Hines, M., & Nyp, M. (2015a). Respiratory diseases. In S. L. Gardner, B. S. Carter, M. Enzman-Hines, et al. (Eds.), *Merenstein & Gardner's handbook of neonatal intensive care* (8th ed.) (pp. 565–643). St. Louis, MO: Mosby.

Gardner, S. L., Goldson, E., & Hernandez, J. A. (2015b). The neonate and the environment: impact on development. In S. L. Gardner, B. S. Carter, M. Enzman-Hines, et al. (Eds.), *Merenstein & Gardner's handbook of neonatal intensive care* (8th ed.) (pp. 262–314). St. Louis, MO: Mosby.

Gardner, S. L., & Hernandez, J. A. (2015). Initial nursery care. In S. L. Gardner, B. S. Carter, M. Enzman-Hines, et al. (Eds.), *Merenstein & Gardner's handbook of neonatal intensive care* (8th ed.) (pp. 71–104). St. Louis, MO: Mosby.

Goodwin, M. (2014). Abdomen assessment. In E. P. Tappero, & M. E. Honeyfield (Eds.), *Physical assessment of the newborn: A comprehensive approach to the art of physical examination* (5th ed.) (pp. 105–114). Santa Rosa, CA: NICU Ink.

Halbardier, B. H. (2014). Fluid and electrolyte management. In *Core curriculum for neonatal intensive care nursing* (5th ed.) (pp. 156–171). St. Louis, MO: Saunders.

Hall, J. E. (2015). *Guyton and Hall textbook of medical physiology* (13th ed.). Philadelphia: Saunders.

Jobe, A. H. (2014). Lung development and maturation. In R. J. Martin, A. A. Fanaroff, & M. C. Walsh (Eds.), *Fanaroff and Martin's neonatal-perinatal medicine: Diseases of the fetus and infant* (10th ed.) Vol. 2. (pp. 1075–1092). St. Louis, MO: Mosby.

Kamuth, B. D., Thilo, E. H., Deacon, J., & Hernandez, J. S. (2015). Neonatal hyperbilirubinemia. In S. L. Gardner, B. S. Carter, M. Enzman-Hines, et al. (Eds.), *Merenstein & Gardner's handbook of neonatal intensive care* (8th ed.) (pp. 531–552). St. Louis, MO: Mosby.

Kaplan, M., Wong, R. J., Sibley, E., et al. (2014). Neonatal jaundice and liver disease. In R. J. Martin, A. A. Fanaroff, & M. C. Walsh (Eds.), *Fanaroff and Martin's neonatal-perinatal medicine: Diseases of the fetus and infant* (10th ed) Vol. 2. (pp. 1443–1496). St. Louis, MO: Mosby.

Kapur, R., Yoder, M. C., & Polin, R. A. (2014). The immune system. In R. J. Martin, A. A. Fanaroff, & M. C. Walsh (Eds.), *Fanaroff and Martin's neonatal-perinatal medicine: Diseases of the fetus and infant* (10th ed) Vol. 2. (pp. 761–885). St. Louis, MO: Mosby.

Kubicka, Z., & Little, G. (2016). Common metabolic disturbances in the newborn. In T. K. McInery, H. M. Adam, D. E. Campbell, et al. (Eds.), *Textbook of pediatric care* (2nd ed.) (pp. 960–969). Elk Grove Village, IL: American Academy of Pediatrics.

Lawrence, R. A., & Lawrence, R. M. (2015). *Breastfeeding: A guide for the medical profession* (8th ed.). St. Louis, MO: Mosby.

Lo, S. F. (2016). Reference intervals for laboratory tests and procedures. In R. M. Kliegman, B. E. Stanton, J. W. St. Geme, & N. F. Schor (Eds.), *Nelson textbook of pediatrics* (20th ed.) (p. 3464). Philadelphia: Saunders.

Luchtman-Jones, L., & Wilson, D. B. (2014). The blood and hematopoietic system. In R. J. Martin, A. A. Fanaroff, & M. C. Walsh (Eds.), *Fanaroff and Martin's neonatal-perinatal medicine: Diseases of the fetus and infant* (10th ed.) Vol. 2. (pp. 1303–1373). St. Louis, MO: Mosby.

Malarkey, L. M., & McMorrow, M. E. (2012). *Saunders nursing guide to laboratory and diagnostic tests* (2nd ed.). St. Louis, MO: Saunders.

Nyp, M., Brunkhorst, J. L., Reavey, D., et al. (2015). Fluid and electrolyte management. In S. L. Gardner, B. S. Carter, M. Enzman-Hines, et al. (Eds.), *Merenstein & Gardner's handbook of neonatal intensive care* (8th ed.) (pp. 315–336). St. Louis, MO: Mosby.

Pagana, K. D., & Pagana, T. J. (2014). *Diagnostic and laboratory test reference* (12th ed.). St. Louis, MO: Mosby.

Pan, D. H., & Rivas, Y. (2016). Jaundice. In T. K. McInery, H. M. Adam, D. E. Campbell, et al. (Eds.), *Textbook of pediatric care* (2nd ed.) (pp. 1615–1625). Elk Grove Village, IL: American Academy of Pediatrics.

Rozance, P. J., & Rosenberg, A. A. (2017). The neonate. In S. G. Gabbe, J. R. Niebyl, J. L. Simpson, Landon, H. L. Galan, E. R. M. Jauniaux, & W. A. Grobman (Eds.), *Obstetrics: Normal and problem pregnancies* (7th ed.) (pp. 468–498). Philadelphia: Saunders.

Rozance, P. J., McGowan, J. E., Price-Douglas, W., et al. (2015). Glucose homeostasis. In S. L. Gardner, B. S. Carter, M. Enzman-Hines, et al. (Eds.), *Merenstein & Gardner's handbook of neonatal intensive care* (8th ed.) (pp. 337–359). St. Louis, MO: Mosby.

Stoll, B. J., & Shane, A. L. (2016). The T lymphocytes, B lymphocytes, and natural killer cells. In R. M. Kliegman, B. E. Stanton, J. W. St. Geme, & N. F. Shor (Eds.), *Nelson textbook of pediatrics* (20th ed.) (pp. 911–912). Philadelphia: Saunders.

Wilson, D. J., & Tyner, C. I. (2014). Immunology and infectious disease. In M. T. Verklan, & M. Walden (Eds.), *Core curriculum for neonatal intensive care nursing* (5th ed.) (pp. 689–718). St. Louis, MO: Saunders.

Wood, K. S. (2016). Care of the sick or premature infant before transport. In T. K. McInery, H. M. Adam, D. E. Campbell, et al. (Eds.), *Textbook of pediatric care* (2nd ed.) (pp. 674–682). Elk Grove Village, IL: American Academy of Pediatrics.

20

Assessment of the Normal Newborn

Vanessa Flannery

OBJECTIVES

After studying this chapter, you should be able to:
1. Describe the initial assessments of the newborn.
2. Explain the nurse's responsibilities in cardiorespiratory and thermoregulatory assessments.
3. Describe nursing assessments of newborn body systems.
4. Explain the importance and components of gestational age assessment.

A very important role of the nurse is assessing the newborn to identify abnormalities and problems in adapting to life outside the uterus. The first complete assessment of the newborn is often called an *admission assessment*. Subsequent assessments are less detailed.

EARLY FOCUSED ASSESSMENTS

As soon as the infant is born, the nurse performs assessments that are most immediately crucial to determining the neonate's health status. These include the cardiorespiratory status, muscle tone, thermoregulation, estimation of the gestational age, and presence of anomalies. The nurse determines whether resuscitation or other immediate interventions are necessary. If no anomalies are present and the newborn is adapting to extrauterine life without difficulty, the nurse should facilitate parent-infant attachment and initiation of breastfeeding while continuing ongoing assessments of breathing, activity, and color. Completion of a more thorough admission assessment follows. If possible, this assessment should be performed in the mother's room to provide an opportunity for parent teaching and continued parent-infant attachment.

History

Information about the pregnancy, labor, and birth is important in assessing the likelihood of problems. The gestational

! SAFETY CHECK

After newborns are dried at birth, it is easy to forget that their skin is contaminated with blood and amniotic fluid. The nurse should wear gloves when handling newborns until they are bathed and all blood is removed from the skin and hair. Wearing gloves helps protect the nurse from bloodborne pathogens.

age, maternal age, health problems, and any complications during the pregnancy or birth may affect the neonate's adaptation. For example, if the mother received narcotic analgesics late in labor, depression of the fetal central nervous system (CNS) may interfere with initiation of respirations in the neonate. Preterm infants may not produce adequate amounts of surfactant, and atelectasis may occur because the alveoli do not remain open.

Assessment of Cardiorespiratory Status

Assessments of respiratory and cardiovascular status are performed together because transitional changes take place simultaneously in both systems. Problems of adaptation in one system are likely to result in problems in the other system.

Airway

During birth, some fetal lung fluid is forced into the upper airway and expelled. Excessive fluid and mucus in the infant's respiratory passages may cause respiratory difficulty for several hours after birth.

Respiratory Rate. The nurse assesses respirations at least once every 30 minutes until the infant has been stable for 2 hours after birth (American Academy of Pediatrics & American College of Obstetricians and Gynecologists [AAP & ACOG], 2012). If abnormalities are noted, respirations are assessed more often.

The normal respiratory rate is 30 to 60 breaths per minute (Verklan, 2015). The average rate is 40 to 49 breaths per minute. The infant may breathe faster immediately after birth, during crying, and during the first and second periods of reactivity. Respirations should not be labored, and the chest movements should be symmetric. Because the pattern and depth of respirations are irregular, they must be counted for a full minute for accuracy (Procedure 20.1).

Counting the rapid, shallow, irregular respirations of a newborn can be a challenge at first. Differentiating between the respirations and other movements while observing the infant's chest may be difficult. Observation, auscultation, or palpation, alone or in combination, may be used to obtain an accurate respiratory rate.

The nurse observes for periodic breathing, pauses in breathing lasting 5 to 10 seconds without other changes followed by rapid respirations for 10 to 15 seconds. This occurs in some full-term infants during the first few days but is more common in preterm infants. Apnea is a pause in breathing lasting 20 seconds or more or accompanied by cyanosis, pallor, bradycardia, or decreased muscle tone (Goodwin, 2016). Apnea is abnormal and requires prompt intervention.

Breath Sounds. The anterior and posterior lung fields are auscultated for breath sounds, which should be present equally throughout. Breath sounds should be clear over most areas. However, hearing crackles in the lungs during the first hour or two after birth is not unusual because fetal lung fluid has not been completely absorbed. Infants born by cesarean not preceded by labor do not experience the changes that occur in the lungs during labor and birth and are more likely to have coarse breath sounds for a short time. Wheezes, crackles, rhonchi, or stridor that persists should be reported.

PROCEDURE 20.1 Assessing Vital Signs in the Newborn

PURPOSE: To obtain an accurate measurement of newborn vital signs.

Respirations

1. Assess respirations when the infant is quiet or sleeping and before disturbing the infant for other assessments, if possible. *Allows the lung sounds to be heard more clearly.*
2. Observe, auscultate, and palpate the chest and abdomen. *The rapid, shallow, irregular respirations can be confused with other movements in an active infant. A combination of methods increases accuracy of the assessment.*
3. Lift the infant's blanket and shirt to see the chest and abdomen. Observe the pattern of respirations before beginning to count. *Respirations are often irregular, but a basic pattern is present. Observation of the pattern makes it easier to count the rate.*
4. If desired, place a hand lightly to the side of the infant's chest or abdomen to feel the movement. Avoid covering the chest completely so chest excursions can be watched as well as palpated. *Palpation helps keep track of the rate.*
5. To auscultate respirations, move a stethoscope over the chest until the respirations are easily heard. This is often toward the right side of the infant's chest. After counting, move the stethoscope to listen to breath sounds in all areas. *Allows the sounds of the lungs to be heard with less interference from heart sounds.*
6. Count for a full minute. *Respirations are normally irregular in the newborn. Counting for a full minute increases accuracy.*
7. If the infant is crying, allow the infant to suck on a pacifier or gloved finger. If crying continues, count the respirations and make a note on the chart that the infant was crying. Recheck later when the infant is calm. Sucking may quiet the infant. *Although respirations are most easily assessed on a quiet infant, they can be counted when the infant is crying. Respirations may be faster on a crying infant.*
8. Expect the respiratory rate to be 30 to 60 breaths per minute, with an average rate of 40 to 49 breaths per minute when the infant is at rest. Report signs of respiratory distress, including tachypnea, retractions, flaring, cyanosis, grunting, seesawing, apneic periods, and asymmetry of chest movements. Continue to watch infants whose respiratory rate is near the extremes of the normal range. *Allows early identification and follow-up of abnormalities. Rates near abnormal may become abnormal in a short time.*

Pulse

1. Listen to the apical pulse while the infant is quiet and before disturbing the infant for other assessments, if possible. *The heart sounds are heard more clearly in a quiet or sleeping infant.*
2. Use a stethoscope with a pediatric head, if available, to listen to the apical pulse. *Although a larger head may be used, the small head allows better contact between the stethoscope and the chest wall and eliminates some of the sounds from the lungs and intestines.*
3. If the infant is crying, insert a pacifier or a gloved finger into the infant's mouth. *Sucking often quiets infants.*
4. If the infant cannot be quieted, increase concentration and time spent listening. *Concentration helps separate the sounds heard and focus on the heart sounds.*
5. Listen briefly before beginning to count. Tapping a finger in rhythm with the beat may be helpful. Count for a full minute. Expect the heart rate to be 120 to 160 bpm at rest. *Listening to the pattern allows time to become accustomed to the rapid heartbeat before counting. Counting for a full minute increases chances of identifying abnormalities.*
6. Move the stethoscope to listen over the entire heart area. Assess for arrhythmias, murmurs, or other abnormal sounds. Refer any abnormalities. *Listening over the entire area increases chances of hearing abnormal sounds. Reporting abnormalities to the pediatrician allows further investigation.*

Temperature
Axillary

1. Place the thermometer vertically along the chest wall with the tip of the thermometer against the skin in the center of the axillary space and the infant's arm held firmly against the body over the probe. *If the thermometer is held horizontally, it may protrude behind the axilla and give an inaccurate reading. Holding the arm keeps the thermometer positioned correctly and prevents accidental injury if the infant moves unexpectedly.*
2. Read the thermometer at the proper time: electronic or digital, when indicator sounds; other types according to manufacturer's directions. Normal range: 36.5° to 37.5°C (97.7° to 99.5°F). *Ensures an accurate reading.*

Abnormal and diminished sounds should be reported to the primary care provider if they continue. They may indicate a pneumothorax. Bowel sounds in the chest may be a sign of diaphragmatic hernia.

Signs of Respiratory Distress. Throughout the assessment, the nurse must be alert for signs of respiratory distress, which may be present at birth or develop later. Whenever one sign of labored breathing is present, the assessment must be carefully expanded to identify others.

Tachypnea. Tachypnea, a respiratory rate of more than 60 breaths per minute, is the most common sign of respiratory distress. It is not unusual during the first hour after birth and during the periods of reactivity, but continued tachypnea is abnormal.

Retractions. Retractions occur when the soft tissue around the bones of the chest is drawn in with the effort of pulling air into the lungs. Xiphoid (substernal) retractions occur when the area under the sternum retracts each time the infant inhales. When the muscles between the ribs are drawn in so that each rib is outlined, intercostal retractions are present. The muscles above the sternum and around the clavicles also may be used to aid in respirations (supraclavicular retractions). Retractions may be mild or severe, depending on the degree of respiratory difficulty. Occasional mild retractions are common immediately after birth but should not continue after the first hour.

Flaring of the Nares. A reflex widening of the nostrils occurs when the infant is receiving insufficient oxygen. Nasal flaring helps decrease airway resistance and increase the amount of air entering the lungs. Intermittent flaring may occur in the first hour after birth. Continued flaring indicates a more serious respiratory problem.

Cyanosis. Cyanosis is a purplish-blue discoloration indicating the infant is not getting enough oxygen. It may be preceded by a dusky or gray hue to the skin. Central cyanosis involves the lips, tongue, mucous membranes, and trunk and indicates true hypoxia. This means that not enough oxygen is reaching the vital organs and requires immediate attention.

Bruising of the face may occur from a tight nuchal cord or pressure during birth and may look like central cyanosis. To differentiate cyanosis from bruising, apply pressure to the area. A cyanotic area will blanch, but a bruised area remains blue. Central cyanosis in infants with dark skin tones can be checked by looking at the color of the mucous membranes. A pulse oximeter is used to determine oxygen saturation in infants with cyanosis.

Central cyanosis must be differentiated from acrocyanosis, which is peripheral cyanosis involving only the extremities. Acrocyanosis is normal during the first day after birth and if the infant becomes cold. It results from poor perfusion of blood to the periphery of the body (Fig. 20.1).

Cyanosis may be present at birth or may become apparent later. It is normal to see a cyanotic infant at birth whose color quickly turns pink as the infant begins to breathe. Cyanosis occurs whenever the infant's breathing is impaired. It may occur during feedings because of difficulty in coordinating sucking, swallowing, and breathing. Infants who become

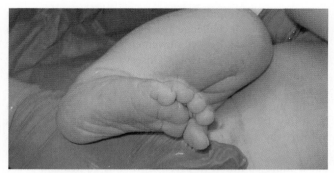

FIG. 20.1 Acrocyanosis. (Courtesy Todd Shires.)

cyanotic on exertion or when crying may have a congenital heart defect.

Grunting. Grunting describes a noise made on expiration when air crosses partially closed vocal cords. This increases the pressure within the alveoli, which keeps the alveoli open and enhances the exchange of gases in the lungs. Grunting may be very mild and heard only with a stethoscope or loud enough to be heard unaided in an infant having severe respiratory difficulty. Persistent grunting is a common sign of respiratory distress syndrome and necessitates expanded assessment and referral for treatment.

Seesaw or Paradoxical Respirations. Normally the chest and abdomen rise and fall together during respiration. In the infant with severe respiratory difficulty, the chest falls when the abdomen rises and the chest rises when the abdomen falls, causing a seesaw effect.

Asymmetry. Chest expansion should be equal on both sides. Asymmetry or decreased movement on one side may indicate the collapse of a lung (pneumothorax).

Choanal Atresia. Choanal atresia is blockage or narrowing of one or both nasal passages by bone or tissue. Assessment for choanal atresia is important because newborns are preferential nose breathers for approximately the first 4 to 6 weeks of life (Sprecher & Arnold, 2016). This means they breathe mostly through the nose except when crying. Bilateral choanal atresia causes severe respiratory distress and requires surgery. Blockage of one side puts the infant at risk for respiratory distress if the other side becomes occluded by mucus or edema.

The nurse can assess for choanal atresia by closing the infant's mouth and occluding one nostril at a time. The infant is observed for breathing, and breath sounds are auscultated while each nostril is occluded. Another method of assessment is to pass a catheter through each nostril to check for patency. Infants with choanal atresia may become cyanotic when quiet but pink when crying because air is then drawn in through the mouth.

Color

In addition to cyanosis, the nurse assesses for pallor and ruddiness.

Pallor. Pallor can indicate that the infant is slightly hypoxic or anemic. A laboratory examination of hemoglobin (Hgb) and hematocrit (Hct) or a complete blood count may be ordered.

Ruddy Color. A ruddy or reddish skin color (plethora) may indicate polycythemia, an excessive number of red blood cells (RBCs). Hct value above 65% confirms polycythemia. Infants with elevated Hct levels are at increased risk for jaundice from the normal destruction of excessive RBCs that occurs after birth.

Heart Sounds

The heart is auscultated for rate, rhythm, and the presence of murmurs or abnormal sounds. The nurse should count the apical heart rate for a full minute for accuracy and listen for abnormalities. The rate should range between 120 and 160 beats per minute (bpm) with normal activity. It may elevate to 180 bpm when infants are crying or drop to as low as 100 bpm when they are in deep sleep.

If there are no problems present at birth, the heart rate should be recorded at least once every 30 minutes until the infant has been stable for 2 hours after birth (AAP & ACOG, 2012). Monitoring is more frequent if abnormalities are present. Once stable, the heart rate is checked once every 8 to 12 hours or according to hospital policy unless a reason for more frequent assessment develops.

Position. The apex of the heart is located at the point of maximum impulse, where the pulse is most easily felt and the sound is loudest. This is at the third or fourth intercostal space, lateral to the midclavicular line. Conditions that affect the position of the heart include pneumothorax and dextrocardia (a right-to-left reversal from the normal heart position).

Rhythm and Murmurs. The rhythm of the heart should be regular, and the first and second sounds should be heard clearly. Abnormalities in rhythm and sounds such as murmurs should be noted. Murmurs are sounds of abnormal blood flow through the heart and may indicate openings in the septum of the heart or problems with blood flow through the valves. They occur in approximately 10% of newborns (Gardner & Hernandez, 2016b). Most murmurs in the newborn are temporary and result from incomplete transition from fetal to neonatal circulation. A murmur is common until the ductus arteriosus is functionally closed. Although it may be a normal or functional murmur, any abnormal sounds of the heart are investigated because they may be signs of cardiac defects. Pulse oximetry screening for cardiac defects is often performed before discharge.

Brachial and Femoral Pulses

The brachial and femoral pulses should be present and equal bilaterally. The brachial pulse is located over the antecubital space, and the femoral pulse is located at the groin. Pulses should be equal bilaterally, and the brachial and femoral pulse rates should be the same. Femoral pulses that are weaker than the brachial pulses may result from impaired blood flow in coarctation of the aorta, a congenital heart defect. In this condition, a narrowed area of the aorta impedes blood flow to the lower part of the body and causes weaker pulses in the lower extremities.

Blood Pressure

Measurement of blood pressure (BP) is not a necessary part of a routine assessment of the newborn. However, the BP is taken on all extremities if the infant has unequal pulses, murmurs, or other signs of cardiac complications. Doppler ultrasonography or other electronic measurement techniques are used. For accurate measurement, the infant should be quiet when the BP is taken because crying elevates it. The width of the BP cuff should be 40% to 50% of the circumference of the arm or leg or 25% to 50% wider than the diameter of the limb (Vargo, 2014a).

The average BP for full-term newborns is 65 to 95 mm Hg systolic and 30 to 60 mm Hg diastolic (Gardner & Hernandez, 2016b). BP varies according to the infant's age, weight, and gestational age. Hypotension may occur in the sick infant.

The BP of the lower extremities should be the same or slightly higher than that of the upper extremities. A systolic BP in the upper extremities that is greater than 20 mm Hg higher than that in the lower extremities may indicate coarctation of the aorta (Vargo, 2014a).

Capillary Refill

Capillary refill is assessed to help determine whether perfusion is adequate. It is checked by depressing the skin over the chest, abdomen, or an extremity until the area blanches. The color should return within less than 3 to 4 seconds (Vargo, 2014b).

Assessment of Thermoregulation

The neonate's temperature is taken soon after birth while the infant is being held by the mother or in a radiant warmer with a skin probe attached to the abdomen. The probe, which should not be attached over bony prominences or areas of brown fat, allows the warmer to measure and display the infant's skin temperature continuously. The temperature control is set to regulate the amount of heat produced according to the infant's skin temperature. The temperature should be assessed at least once every 30 minutes until the infant has been stable for 2 hours after birth (AAP & ACOG, 2012). It is often checked again at 4 hours and then once every 8 to 12 hours or according to facility policy as long as it remains stable (see Procedure 20.1).

The most common method of taking the neonate's temperature is axillary measurement (Fig. 20.2). The normal range for axillary temperature is 36.5° to 37.5°C (97.7° to 99.5°F) (Gardner & Hernandez, 2016a) (Box 20.1). Taking axillary temperatures is safer than taking rectal temperatures because it avoids the possibility of irritation or injury to the rectum, which turns at a right angle approximately 3 cm (1.2 inches) from the anal sphincter (Gardner & Hernandez, 2016b). The location always should be charted along with the temperature measurement.

If a rectal temperature is necessary, the nurse should use great caution because inserting the thermometer too far could cause potentially fatal perforation of the intestinal wall. A thermometer should never be forced into the

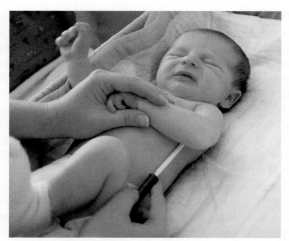

FIG. 20.2 The infant is held securely to prevent injury and obtain an accurate reading when taking the temperature.

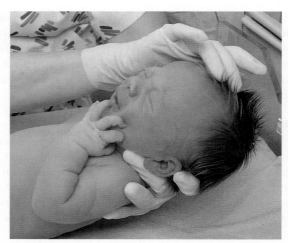

FIG. 20.3 Palpation of the anterior fontanel. Note elevation of the head.

BOX 20.1   Normal Vital Signs in the Newborn

Temperature: 36.5° to 37.5°C (97.7° to 99.5°F) axillary
Apical pulse: 120 to 160 bpm (100 sleeping, 180 crying)
Respirations: 30 to 60 breaths per minute

---

rectum because of the possible presence of an imperforate (closed) anus.

Temperatures are usually measured with an electronic digital thermometer. Inexpensive digital thermometers used while the infant is in the hospital are often given to the parents for home use. Tympanic thermometers, used in some facilities for older infants and children, are not recommended for newborns (Gardner & Hernandez, 2016b). Some agencies use temporal artery thermometers.

⸮ KNOWLEDGE CHECK

1. What is the purpose of the early focused assessments of the infant after birth?
2. What is included in assessment of the newborn's cardiovascular status?
3. Why is taking a rectal temperature dangerous in an infant?

General Assessment

If major abnormalities are present at birth, the nurse must maintain a calm, quiet demeanor to avoid frightening the parents. The provider should be alerted quietly and will explain the condition and possible plan of treatment to the parents.

Head

The newborn's head and neck constitute one fourth of the body surface (Gardner & Hernandez, 2016b). It is much larger in proportion to the rest of the body than that of the adult. The head is palpated to assess the shape and identify abnormalities. The newborn who was delivered by cesarean

not preceded by labor usually has a round head, whereas the infant born vaginally usually has some molding. The head of infants who were in a breech position may be flattened on the top. The degree of molding, size of the fontanels, and presence of the caput succedaneum or later development of a cephalo-hematoma are noted.

The hair should be fine, with a consistent pattern. Abnormal hair growth patterns may indicate genetic abnormalities. The nurse separates the hair, if necessary, to display bruises, rashes, or other marks on the scalp. A small, red mark is apparent if a fetal monitor electrode was inserted into the skin of the scalp. Later, a small scab forms. Occasionally this area becomes infected, and a topical antibiotic is applied.

Molding. Molding refers to changes in the shape of the head that allow it to pass through the birth canal. It is caused by overriding of the cranial bones at the sutures and is common, especially after a vaginal delivery. The parietal bones often override the occipital and frontal bones, and a ridge can be felt at those areas. The condition generally resolves within a few days to 1 week after birth. Often, dramatic improvement is seen by the end of the first day of life. Parents may need reassurance that the infant's head is normal.

All sutures should be palpated. Separation may be the temporary result of molding or, if it persists or widens, may indicate increased intracranial pressure. If no space is found between suture lines, it may be the result of molding and overriding of the bones. However, a hard, ridged area not resulting from molding may indicate premature closure of the sutures. This condition, called *craniosynostosis,* may impair brain growth and the shape of the head and requires surgery.

Fontanels. The fontanels are the areas of the head where sutures between the bones meet. In the newborn the areas are not calcified, but are covered by membrane to allow space for the brain to grow.

The nurse palpates the fontanels and notes the position in relation to the other bones of the skull (Fig. 20.3). The infant's head is elevated during palpation for accurate assessment.

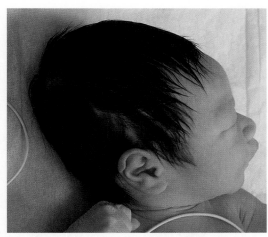

FIG. 20.4 Caput succedaneum is an edematous area on the head from pressure against the cervix. It may cross suture lines.

The infant may be placed in a semisitting position or held in an upright position. The fontanel should be palpated when the infant is quiet because vigorous crying may cause it to protrude.

The anterior fontanel is a diamond-shaped area where the frontal and parietal bones meet. It measures 4 to 6 cm from bone to bone, although this varies because of molding and individual differences. The fontanel closes by 18 months of age (Benjamin & Furdon, 2015).

The anterior fontanel should be soft and flat (level with the surrounding bones) or only slightly sunken. After molding resolves, a depressed fontanel may be a sign of dehydration. Although the anterior fontanel may bulge slightly when the infant cries, bulging at rest may indicate increased intracranial pressure. A fontanel that is between flat and bulging is termed full. A larger-than-normal fontanel may be a sign of increased pressure within the skull. Abnormal signs are reported to the primary care provider.

The posterior fontanel is a triangular area where the occipital and parietal bones meet. It is much smaller than the anterior fontanel, measuring 0.5 to 1 cm, and feels like a dimple at the juncture of the occipital and parietal bones. This fontanel closes by the time the infant is 2 months of age (Benjamin & Furdon, 2015).

Caput Succedaneum. A caput succedaneum is an area of localized edema that appears over the vertex of the newborn's head as a result of pressure against the mother's cervix during labor (Fig. 20.4). The pressure interferes with blood flow from the area, causing localized edema at birth. The edematous area crosses suture lines, is soft, and varies in size. It resolves quickly and generally disappears within 12 to 48 hours after birth (Benjamin & Furdon, 2015). Caput also may occur when a vacuum extractor is used to assist birth. When a vacuum is used, the caput corresponds to the area where the extractor was placed on the skull. The amount of edema and presence of bruising are assessed.

Cephalohematoma. A cephalohematoma, bleeding between the periosteum and the skull, is the result of pressure during birth (Fig. 20.5). It occurs on one or both sides of the head, usually over the parietal bones. The swelling may not be present at birth but may develop within the first 24 to 48 hours.

The area is carefully palpated to determine whether the swelling crosses suture lines. A cephalohematoma has clear edges that end at the suture lines. It does not cross the suture lines, unlike a caput succedaneum, because the bleeding is held between the bone and its covering, the periosteum. A cephalohematoma reabsorbs slowly and may take 2 to 3 months to completely resolve (Mangurten & Puppala, 2016). Because of the breakdown of the RBCs within the hematoma, affected infants are at greater risk for jaundice. Bruising also increases the risk for jaundice.

Both caput succedaneum and cephalohematoma may be frightening to parents. They need reassurance that the conditions are not harmful to the infant. Even if parents do not ask, they need information about the causes and length of time required for the areas to resolve.

Face. The face is examined for symmetry, positioning of the facial features, movement, and expression. A transient asymmetry from intrauterine pressure may occur, lasting a few weeks or months. Drooping of the mouth appears as a one-sided cry and may be caused by facial nerve trauma. Irregularities of the facial features should be reported.

Neck and Clavicles

The nurse assesses the infant's neck visually and notes the ease and extent with which the head turns from side to side. The neck should have full range of motion. It is very short. Webbing or an unusually large fat pad between the occiput and the shoulders may indicate a chromosomal anomaly. No masses should be present. When lying in a prone position, the term newborn should be able to raise the head briefly and turn it to the other side.

Fractures of the clavicle are more likely to occur in large infants, especially when shoulder dystocia occurred. Sliding the fingers along each clavicle while moving the infant's arm helps identify a fractured clavicle. If a fracture is present, a lump, swelling, or tenderness over the bone may be observed. Crepitus (grating of the bone) and movement of the bone may be felt during palpation. Decreased movement of the affected arm also may occur. A difference in the movement of the arms is especially noticeable when the Moro reflex is elicited.

Injury to the brachial plexus may cause paralysis of the arm on the side of the fracture. Treatment of a fractured clavicle includes immobilization of the affected arm for a short time. The fracture heals quickly (Fig. 20.6).

Umbilical Cord

The umbilical cord should contain three vessels. The two arteries are small and may stand up at the cut end. The single vein is larger than the arteries and resembles a slit because its walls are more easily compressed. If only one artery is present, the infant is carefully assessed for other anomalies. A two-vessel cord may be an isolated abnormality or associated with chromosomal and renal defects. The amount of Wharton's jelly

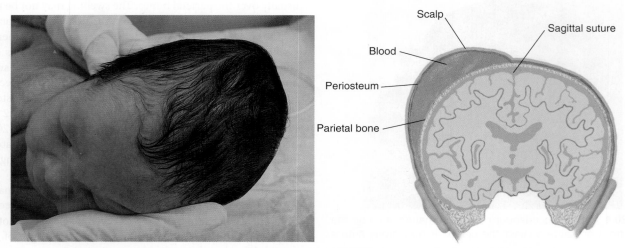

FIG. 20.5 A cephalohematoma is characterized by bleeding between the bone and its covering, the periosteum. It may occur on one or both sides and does not cross suture lines.

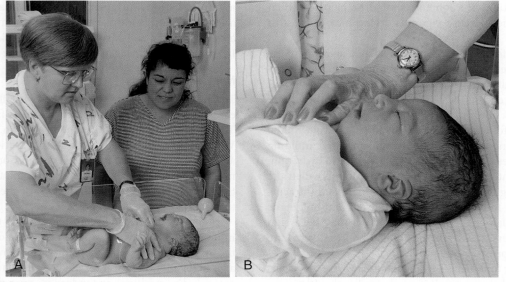

FIG. 20.6 **A,** The nurse palpates the clavicles to identify fractures. A fracture of the left clavicle is present. **B,** The arm on the side of the fractured clavicle is immobilized by pinning the sleeve to the shirt.

in the cord is noted. If the cord appears thin, the infant may have been poorly nourished in utero. A yellow-brown or green tinge to the cord indicates that meconium was released at some time before birth, perhaps as a result of fetal compromise. No redness or discharge from the cord should be present.

Extremities

The infant should actively move the extremities equally in a random manner. The extremities of a term infant should remain sharply flexed and resist extension during examination. Poor muscle tone results in a limp or "floppy" infant, which may occur from inadequate oxygen during birth but should resolve within a few minutes as oxygen intake increases. Continued poor muscle tone may result from prematurity or neurologic injury. Infants with previously good

muscle tone may show decreased flexion if they become hypoglycemic or experience respiratory difficulty.

All extremities are examined for signs of fractures such as crepitus, redness, lumps, or swelling. Lack of use of an extremity may indicate nerve injury that may occur with or without fractures.

Injury to the brachial nerve plexus may result in Erb's palsy (Erb-Duchenne paralysis), paralysis of the shoulder and arm muscles. Instead of the usual flexed position, the affected arm is extended at the infant's side with the forearm prone. Movement of this arm is diminished during the Moro reflex. The condition is treated by splinting, exercise, or both.

Hands and Feet. The fingers and toes are examined for extra digits (polydactyly) and webbing between digits (syndactyly). Extra digits are often small and may not have bones. Tying

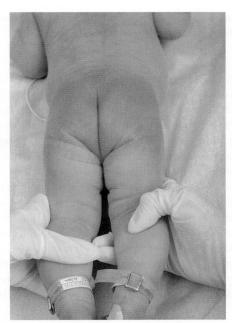

FIG. 20.7 Note the symmetry of gluteal and thigh creases.

the extra digits with sutures causes them to atrophy and fall off. The presence of a bone in the extra digit requires surgical removal. Webbed fingers or toes may be corrected by surgery. Nails in a term infant should extend to the end of the fingers or slightly beyond.

The creases in the hands also are examined. Normally, two long transverse creases extend most of the way across the palm. A single crease parallel with the base of the fingers that crosses the palm without a break is called a *simian crease* or *line*. It may be seen with incurving of the little finger in Down's syndrome (trisomy 21). The simian line alone is not diagnostic of trisomy 21, however, and may occur in 5% to 10% of normal infants (Kaur & Campbell, 2016).

The feet are assessed for talipes equinovarus, or clubfoot, a common malformation of the feet. If a foot looks abnormal, it should be gently manipulated. If it moves to a normal position, the abnormality is probably temporary, resulting from the position of the infant in the uterus. In true clubfoot, the foot turns inward and cannot be moved to a midline position. Casting and manipulation are the usual treatment, but in some cases surgery is necessary.

Hips. The hips are examined for signs of developmental dysplasia. In this condition, instability of the hip joint occurs and the head of the femur can be moved in and out of the acetabulum. Partial dislocation and inadequate development of the acetabulum may occur. Identifying a hip problem early is important to prevent permanent damage to the joint.

The infant's knees should be bent with the feet flat on the bed to compare the height of the knees. If the hip is dislocated, the knee on the affected side is lower. The legs are extended with the infant in the prone position to determine whether they are equal in length and if the thigh and gluteal creases are symmetric (Fig. 20.7). If the hip is dislocated, the leg on the affected side is shorter and the creases are asymmetric. Because the hip may be unstable but not yet dislocated, these signs may not be present at birth.

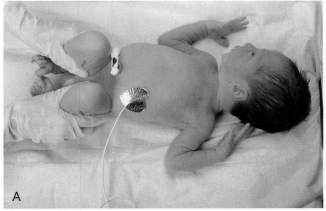

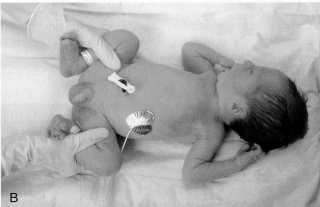

FIG. 20.8 Assessment of the Hips. The physician or advanced practice nurse examining the infant places their fingers over the infant's greater trochanter and thumbs over the femur. The knees and hips are flexed. **A,** Barlow test. The provider adducts the hips, and applies gentle pressure down and back with the thumbs. In hip dysplasia the examiner can feel the femoral head move out of the acetabulum. **B,** Ortolani test. The provider abducts the thighs, and applies gentle pressure forward over the greater trochanter. A "clunking" sensation indicates a dislocated femoral head moving into the acetabulum. A hip click is from ligament movement and is not a problem.

Barlow and Ortolani tests are methods of assessing for hip instability in the newborn period (Fig. 20.8). These maneuvers are performed by the physician or advanced practice nurse. Both legs should abduct equally in normal infants. Abducting the affected hip may be difficult. A hip click may be felt or heard but is usually normal and is different from the "clunk" of hip dysplasia when the femoral head moves in the hip socket (Schwend, Shaw, & Segal, 2014).

Treatment of developmental dysplasia of the hip involves immobilizing the leg in a flexed, abducted position, usually with a harness. Early identification and treatment are essential to provide the best results in correcting the problem. Treatment may involve casting or surgery if the condition is not discovered early.

Vertebral Column

The nurse palpates the entire length of the newborn's vertebral column to discover any defects in the vertebrae.

An indentation is a sign of spina bifida occulta (failure of a vertebra to close). The defect is not obvious on visual inspection because it is covered with skin, but sometimes a tuft of hair grows over the area. Other more obvious neural tube defects include a meningocele (protrusion of spinal fluid and meninges) or a myelomeningocele (protrusion of spinal fluid, meninges, and the spinal cord) through the defect in the vertebrae. They appear as a sack on the back and may be covered by skin or only the meninges. The tissue should be covered with moist sterile saline dressings immediately after birth. A pilonidal dimple may be present at the base of the spine. It should be examined for a sinus and the depth noted.

Measurements

Measurements provide information about the infant's growth in utero. The weight, length, and head and chest circumferences are part of the initial assessment (Procedure 20.2). The measurements are compared with the norms for the infant's gestational age. When a difference is noted between the expected and actual values, expanded assessments are necessary.

Weight

The weight of the term newborn ranges between 2500 and 4000 grams (g) (5 pounds [lb], 8 ounces [oz] and 8 lb, 13 oz) (Cheffer & Rannalli, 2015). If the infant's weight is outside the normal range, possible causes are assessed. Factors affecting weight include gestational age, placental functioning, genetic factors such as race and parental size, and maternal diabetes, hypertension, and substance abuse.

Infants are weighed each day they are in the birth facility and at follow-up visits. They can be expected to lose up to 10% of their birth weight during the first week of life (Feigelman, 2015). The loss results from excretion of meconium, normal loss of extracellular fluid, and inadequate intake of calories during the first few days. Infants normally regain or exceed their birth weight by 14 days of life. Thereafter they gain approximately 30 g per day during the early months (Feigelman, 2016).

PROCEDURE 20.2 Weighing and Measuring the Newborn

PURPOSE: To obtain accurate measurements of the newborn

Weight

1. Cover the scale with a warm blanket. Place a paper cover over the blanket if desired. *Prevents conductive heat loss from contact between the infant and a cold surface, helps prevent cross-contamination and makes cleaning easier.*

2. Balance or adjust the scale to 0 after the covering is placed. Electronic scale: Push the "on" button and check to see that the digital readout is at 0. The electronic scale is usually self-adjusting. Balance scale: Adjust until the balance arm is horizontal. *Results in accurate weighing of the infant without including weight of the scale covering.*

3. Remove clothing and blankets from the infant and place the infant in the supine position on the scale. Keep one hand just above the infant and watch him or her carefully throughout the procedure. *Infants often are upset when first placed on the scale, and the startle or Moro reflex may occur. They may be in danger of sliding off the scale.*

Some electronic scales display an indicator when an accurate weight has been obtained. For a balance scale, move weights slowly until the arm is level. *Waiting until the infant is quiet increases accuracy.*

5. Record the numbers immediately. If the scale is covered with paper, the weight can be written on the paper. Enter the infant's weight in the nurses' notes when the infant is safely settled. *Prevents forgetting the weight.*

6. Compare weight with the normal range for term infants: 2500 to 4000 g (5 lb, 8 oz to 8 lb, 13 oz). *Shows whether the infant is within expected range.*

Length

Ruler Printed on Scale or Crib

1. Place the infant in the supine position with his or her head at the upper edge of the ruler. *Places the infant in the proper position.*

2. While holding the infant with one hand so that the head does not move, use the other hand to fully extend the infant's leg along the ruler. Note the length at the bottom of the heel. *Holding the infant firmly ensures safety and allows an accurate measurement.*

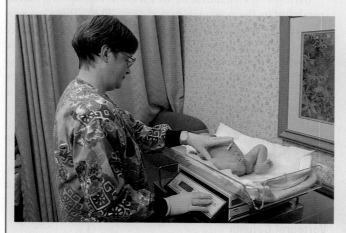

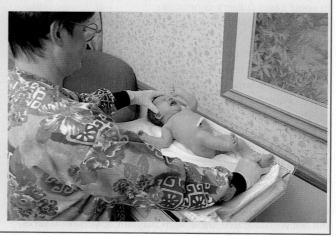

4. Wait until the infant is somewhat quiet. The electronic scale displays weight in pounds and ounces or in grams.

PROCEDURE 20.2   Weighing and Measuring the Newborn—cont'd

Tape Measure

1. Check that a paper tape has no partial tears in it. *A torn measuring tape would give an inaccurate measurement.*
2. Place tape beside the infant, with the upper end at the top of the head. Tuck it beneath the shoulder, and extend it down to the feet. *Helps prevent movement of the tape and ensures accurate measurements.*
3. Hold the tape straight along the side of the infant's body while extending one of the infant's legs to its full length. Be sure that the tape has not moved from the top of the head. *Careful attention to tape placement ensures accurate measurement.*

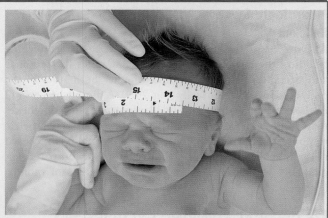

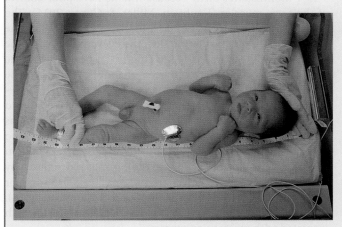

2. Move tape down to measure the chest at the level of the nipples. Keep the tape even and taut. *Ensures accurate measurement.*

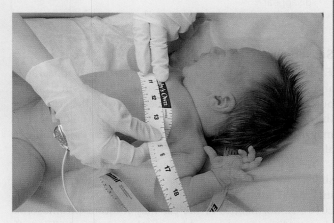

4. Another method is to mark the paper on which the infant is lying at the top of the head and the heel. Then measure the distance between the two marks. *Makes measuring more accurate when the infant is very active.*
5. Compare with the normal range of 48 to 53 cm (19 to 21 inches). *Helps determine abnormalities.*

Head and Chest Circumference

1. Measure around the fullest part of the head, with the tape placed around the occiput and just above the eyebrows. *Allows measurement of the largest diameter of the head.*

3. Remove the tape by lifting or rolling the infant instead of pulling the tape. *Pulling the tape could cut the infant's skin.*
4. Compare measurements with normal range. Head: 32 to 38 cm (13 to 15 inches). Chest: 30 to 36 cm (12 to 14 inches). *Determines whether the infant's measurements are normal.*

Length

The infant's length is measured from the top of the head to the heel of the outstretched leg. The average length of a full-term newborn is 48 to 53 cm (19 to 21 inches) (Cheffer & Rannalli, 2015). Some agencies also record the crown-to-rump measurement, which is approximately equal to the head circumference.

Head and Chest Circumference

The diameter of the head is measured around the occiput just above the eyebrows. The normal range of head circumference for the term newborn is 32 to 38 cm (13 to 15 inches) (Benjamin & Furdon, 2015). The measurement may be affected by molding of the skull during the birth process. If a large amount of molding occurred, the head is remeasured when it regains its normal shape. An abnormally small head may indicate poor brain growth and microcephaly. A very large head may be a sign of hydrocephalus.

The chest is measured at the level of the nipples. It usually is 2 to 3 cm smaller than the head. The normal circumference of the chest is 30 to 36 cm (12 to 14 inches) (Vargo, 2014b). If molding of the head is present, the head and chest measurements may be equal at birth.

? KNOWLEDGE CHECK

4. What are the differences among molding, caput succedaneum, and cephalohematoma?
5. Why are measurements of the neonate important?

ASSESSMENT OF BODY SYSTEMS

Neurologic System

Reflexes

Assessment of the reflexes is important to determine the health of the newborn's CNS. The nurse notes the presence and strength of the reflexes and whether both sides of the body respond symmetrically (Fig. 20.9). A diminished overall response occurs in preterm and ill infants. Absence of reflexes may indicate a serious neurologic problem. Asymmetric responses may indicate that trauma during birth caused nerve injury, paralysis, or fracture. Some newborn reflexes gradually weaken and disappear over a period of months (Table 20.1).

 CRITICAL THINKING EXERCISE 20.1

1. What might be the effect on normal development if reflexes are retained beyond the age when they should disappear?

Sensory Assessment

Ears. The ears are assessed for placement, overall appearance, and maturity. An imaginary horizontal line drawn from the outer canthus of the eye should be even with the area where the upper ear (helix) joins the head (Fig. 20.10). Low-set ears may indicate chromosomal abnormalities. The ears should be almost vertical in placement on the head.

The nurse examines the ears for skin tags and preauricular sinuses and dimples. If they occur with any other abnormalities, renal ultrasound is often performed (Kaur & Campbell, 2016). Abnormalities of the ear may indicate chromosomal abnormalities, hearing problems, or kidney defects. The stiffness of the cartilage and degree of incurving of the pinna are checked as part of the gestational age assessment.

Hearing begins to develop by 23 to 24 weeks of gestation (Blackburn, 2013). Infants can hear by the last trimester of pregnancy, and their hearing is very good after birth. Hearing is assessed by noting the infant's reaction to sudden loud noises, which should cause a startle response. Infants should respond to the sound of voices and prefer a high-pitched tone of voice and rhythmic sounds. They will turn toward the sound of the mother's voice or another interesting sound. A hearing screening is performed before discharge from most birth facilities.

Eyes. The eyes are examined for abnormalities and signs of inflammation. They should be symmetric and of the same size. The iris is dark gray, blue, or brown but may change color by 6 months of age (Johnson, 2014). Slanting epicanthal folds in a non-Asian infant may be a sign of trisomy 21 or other abnormal conditions.

Edema of the eyelids and subconjunctival hemorrhages (reddened areas of the sclera) result from pressure on the head during birth, which causes capillary rupture in the sclera. The edema diminishes in a few days, and the hemorrhages resolve in 7 to 10 days (Johnson, 2014). The sclera should be white or bluish white. A yellow color indicates jaundice. A blue color occurs in osteogenesis imperfecta, a congenital bone condition.

Conjunctivitis may result from infection or a chemical reaction to medications. *Staphylococcus, Chlamydia,* and *Neisseria gonorrhoeae* are common organisms that cause infection. Maternal gonorrhea can cause infection of the infant during birth. The resulting ophthalmia neonatorum may cause blindness. To prevent this condition, all newborns are treated prophylactically with antibiotics to the eyes. Any discharge from the eyes is reported for possible culture and treatment.

Transient strabismus (crossed eyes) is common for the first 3 to 4 months after birth because infants have poor control of their eye muscles (Kaufman, Miller, & Gupta, 2015). The doll's-eye sign is a normal finding in the newborn: When the head is turned quickly to one side, the eyes move toward the other side. The setting-sun sign (the iris appears low in the eye and part of the sclera can be seen above the iris) may be an indication of hydrocephalus.

The pupils should be equal in size and react equally to light. Cataracts (opacities of the lens) appear as white areas over the pupils. They may develop in infants of mothers who had rubella or other infections during the pregnancy. When a light is directed into the eyes, the normal red reflex may not be seen if large cataracts are present. Tears are scant or absent for the first 2 months of life (Kaur & Campbell, 2016). Excessive tearing may indicate a plugged lacrimal duct, which is treated with massage or surgery.

Visual acuity is approximately 20/400 (Olitsky et al., 2016). The eyes cannot accommodate well, but newborns should show a visual response to the environment. They should make eye contact when held in a cradle position during a period of alertness. Although they focus best on objects that are 20 to 30 cm (8 to 12 inches) away, they can see objects to a distance of 76 cm (2.5 feet) (Blackburn, 2013). They should respond well to human faces and geometric patterns of black and white or medium bright colors but show little interest in pastel colors.

Newborns should blink or close their eyes in response to bright lights. Any infant who does not respond to visual stimuli should be reported to the physician or nurse practitioner for further investigation.

Sense of Smell and Taste. The sense of smell is demonstrated when infants recognize breast pads soaked with their mother's milk and differentiate them from pads soaked in water. Their ability to distinguish taste is shown by their preference for sweet liquids and aversion to sour or bitter tastes (Blackburn, 2013).

Other Neurologic Signs

The newborn is assessed for tremors or jitteriness. If tremors are present, the blood glucose should be checked because hypoglycemia is the most common cause. If blood glucose is within normal range, the cause may be low calcium or prenatal exposure to drugs. Tremors increase each time the infant is touched or moved but stop briefly if the extremity is flexed and held firmly.

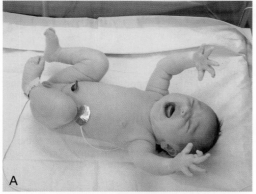

Moro reflex

The Moro reflex is the most dramatic reflex. It occurs when the infant's head and trunk are allowed to drop back 30 degrees when the infant is in a slightly raised position. The infant's arms and legs extend and abduct, with the fingers fanning open and thumbs and forefingers forming a C position. The arms then return to their normally flexed state with an embracing motion. The legs may also extend and then flex.

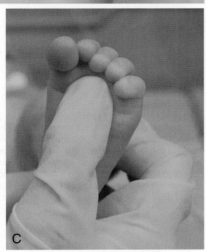

Palmar grasp reflex

The palmar grasp reflex occurs when the infant's palm is touched near the base of the fingers. The hand closes into a tight fist. The grasp reflex may be weak or absent if the infant has injury to the nerves of the arms.

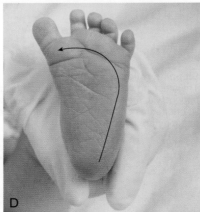

Plantar grasp reflex

The plantar grasp reflex is similar to the palmar grasp reflex. When the area below the toes is touched, the infant's toes curl over the nurse's finger.

Babinski reflex

The Babinski reflex is elicited by stroking the lateral sole of the infant's foot from the heel forward and across the ball of the foot. This causes the toes to flare outward and the big toe to dorsiflex.

FIG. 20.9 Reflexes

Continued

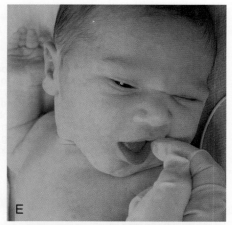

Rooting reflex

The rooting reflex is important in feeding and is most often demonstrated when the infant is hungry. When the infant's cheek is touched near the mouth, the head turns toward the side that has been stroked. This response helps the infant find the nipple for feeding. The reflex occurs when either side of the mouth is touched. Touching the cheeks on both sides at the same time confuses the infant.

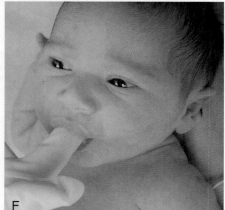

Sucking reflex

The sucking reflex is essential to normal life. When the mouth or palate is touched by the nipple or a finger, the infant begins to suck. The sucking reflex is assessed for its presence and strength. Feeding difficulties may be related to problems in the infant's ability to suck and to coordinate sucking with swallowing and breathing.

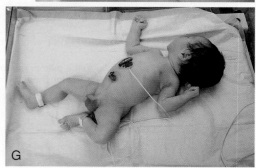

Tonic neck reflex

The tonic neck reflex refers to the posture assumed by newborns when in a supine position. The infant extends the arm and leg on the side to which the head is turned and flexes the extremities on the other side. This response is sometimes referred to as the "fencing reflex" because the infant's position is similar to that of a person engaged in a fencing match.

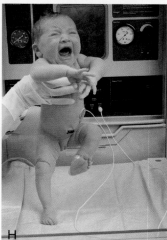

Stepping reflex

The stepping reflex occurs when infants are held upright with their feet touching a solid surface. They lift one foot and then the other, giving the appearance that they are trying to walk.

FIG. 20.9, cont'd

TABLE 20.1   Summary of Neonatal Reflexes

Reflex	Method of Testing	Expected Response	Abnormal Response/Possible Cause	Time Reflex Disappears
Babinski	Stroke lateral sole of foot from heel to across base of toes.	Toes flare with dorsiflexion of the big toe.	No response. Bilateral: CNS deficit. Unilateral: Local nerve injury.	8–9 mo
Gallant (trunk incurvation)	With infant prone, lightly stroke along the side of the vertebral column.	Entire trunk flexes toward side stimulated.	No response: CNS deficit.	4 mo
Grasp reflex (palmar and plantar)	Press finger against base of infant's fingers or toes.	Fingers curl tightly; toes curl forward.	Weak or absent: Neurologic deficit or muscle injury.	Palmar grasp: 2–3 mo Plantar grasp: 8–9 mo
Moro	Let infant's head drop back approximately 30 degrees.	Sharp extension and abduction of arms followed by flexion and adduction to "embrace" position.	Absent: CNS dysfunction. Asymmetry: Brachial plexus injury, paralysis, or fractured bone of extremity. Exaggerated: Maternal drug use.	5–6 mo
Rooting	Touch or stroke from side of mouth toward cheek.	Infant turns head to side touched. Difficult to elicit if infant is sleeping or just fed.	Weak or absent: Prematurity, neurologic deficit, depression from maternal drug use.	3–4 mo
Stepping	Hold infant so feet touch solid surface.	Infant lifts alternate feet as if walking.	Asymmetry: Fracture of extremity, neurologic deficit.	3–4 mo
Sucking	Place nipple or gloved finger in mouth, rub against palate.	Infant begins to suck. May be weak if recently fed.	Weak or absent: Prematurity, neurologic deficit, maternal drug use.	1 yr
Swallowing	Place fluid on the back of the tongue.	Infant swallows fluid. Should be coordinated with sucking.	Coughing, gagging, choking, cyanosis: Prematurity, tracheoesophageal fistula, esophageal atresia, neurologic deficit.	Present throughout life
Tonic neck reflex	Gently turn head to one side while infant is supine.	Infant extends extremities on side to which head is turned, with flexion on opposite side.	Prolonged period in position: Neurologic deficit.	May be weak at birth; disappears 4 mo

CNS, Central nervous system.

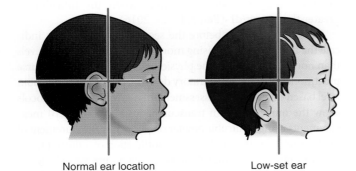

Normal ear location   Low-set ear

FIG. 20.10 An imaginary line is drawn from the outer canthus of the eye to the ear. The line should intersect with the area where the upper ear joins the head.

Seizures indicate CNS or metabolic abnormality. To differentiate between tremors and seizures, the infant's extremities are held in a flexed position. This causes tremors to stop, but a seizure continues. Seizure activity also may include abnormal movements of the eyes and mouth and other subtle signs. Any infant thought to be having seizures is referred for further assessment and treatment.

! SAFETY CHECK

Jitteriness or Tremors
Stop when the extremities are held firmly in a flexed position
Are commonly caused by low glucose or calcium levels

Seizures
Continue even if extremities are held
May include abnormal mouth or eye movements
Indicate central nervous system or metabolic abnormality

The pitch of the cry is important. Cries that are shrill, high-pitched, hoarse, and catlike (mewing) are abnormal. These cries may indicate a neurologic disorder or other problem.

Normal infants respond to holding and are quiet and appear content when their needs are met. Rocking motions are often effective in quieting an irritable infant. Most infants nestle or mold their bodies to that of the people holding them, making them easy to hold and cuddle. Neonates who stiffen the body, pull away from contact, or arch the back when held may be showing signs of CNS injury.

BOX 20.2 Risk Factors for Neonatal Hypoglycemia

Prematurity
Postmaturity
Late preterm infant
Intrauterine growth restriction
Large or small for gestational age
Asphyxia
Problems at birth
Cold stress
Maternal diabetes
Maternal intake of terbutaline

Infants should react to painful stimuli with crying and an increase in vital signs. Excessive irritability also may be a sign of injury to the CNS. All such abnormal signs are reported for further neurologic assessment.

Hepatic System

The major early assessments of the hepatic system are related to blood glucose and bilirubin conjugation.

Blood Glucose

The nurse must be alert for newborns at increased risk for hypoglycemia, which can cause brain damage. Factors that might have caused the infant to deplete available glucose are noted (Box 20.2). A quick estimate to determine whether the newborn appears to be near term and of appropriate size for gestational age is performed at birth.

Observing for signs of hypoglycemia is necessary throughout routine assessment and care. Early signs include jitteriness and other CNS signs and signs of respiratory difficulty, a decrease in temperature, and poor feeding. Some infants with hypoglycemia show no signs at all.

CRITICAL TO REMEMBER

Signs of Neonatal Hypoglycemia

Jitteriness, tremors
Poor muscle tone
Diaphoresis (sweating)
Poor suck
Tachypnea
Tachycardia
Dyspnea
Grunting
Cyanosis
Apnea
Low temperature
High-pitched cry
Irritability
Lethargy
Seizures, coma
No signs (some infants may be asymptomatic)

Screening for blood glucose is not necessary for normal term infants (AAP & ACOG, 2012; Bloomfield, Dinolfo, & Kokotos, 2016). Those in risk categories or showing early signs should be screened. Normal blood glucose for the term infant during the first day of life is 40 to 60 mg/dL and 50 to 90 mg/dL thereafter (Lo, 2016). Because capillary blood is used in screening tests, these tests are less accurate than laboratory tests using venous blood. Therefore a laboratory analysis (per agency policy) should be used to verify readings of 40 to 45 mg/dL or below.

Avoiding injuries to the infant's foot is important when taking blood from the heel (Procedure 20.3). If the lancet goes into the calcaneus bone, osteomyelitis may result. Commercial devices for heel puncture are designed to puncture the heel to the proper depth. They are available for full-term and preterm infants. The site chosen must avoid injury to major nerves and arteries in the area. Other complications include cellulitis, abscess, scarring, bruising, and pain.

Infants are often fed if the reading is 40 to 45 mg/dL or less to prevent a further decrease in glucose, especially if the infant shows signs of hypoglycemia. The blood glucose is rechecked 30 to 60 minutes after the feeding and again before feedings until the results are acceptable or according to hospital policy. Infants who are in risk categories are usually monitored for 12 to 24 hours after birth (AAP & ACOG, 2012).

Bilirubin

The nurse assesses for jaundice at least every 8 to 12 hours and is particularly watchful when infants are at increased risk for hyperbilirubinemia. Jaundice is identified by pressing the infant's skin over a firm surface, such as the end of the nose or the sternum. The skin blanches as the blood is pressed out of the tissues, making it easier to see the yellow color that remains. Jaundice is more obvious when the nurse assesses in natural light. Jaundice begins at the head and moves down the body, and the areas of the body involved should be documented. Jaundice becomes visible when the bilirubin is greater than 5 mg/dL (Pan & Rivas, 2016).

Jaundice appearing before the second day of life may indicate the bilirubin level is rising more quickly and to higher levels than normal and may not be physiologic. The physician or nurse practitioner may order laboratory determinations of the bilirubin level based on the nurse's assessment. In many facilities, protocols allow the nurse to obtain transcutaneous bilirubin (TcB) measurements using a bilirubinometer or laboratory measurement of total serum bilirubin (TSB) before notification of a nurse practitioner or physician. A bilirubinometer is a noninvasive device to measure bilirubin in the infant's skin, thus avoiding repeated skin punctures to obtain blood samples. Obtain TSB or TcB measurements on all infants jaundiced within the first 24 hours.

If serial bilirubin assays are ordered, the nurse notes changes from one reading to the next and correlates the results with the infant's age. Abnormal results of TcB should be confirmed by measurement of TSB. Charts are available that show the degree of risk for infants at different ages (in hours) by the level of TSB.

The AAP and ACOG (2012) recommend obtaining TSB or TcB measurements on every infant before discharge. This

PROCEDURE 20.3   Obtaining Blood Samples from the Newborn by Heel Puncture

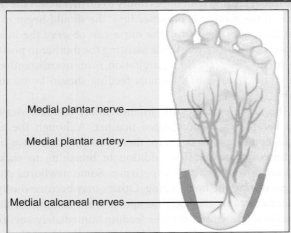

Medial plantar nerve

Medial plantar artery

Medial calcaneal nerves

PURPOSE: To obtain a sample of an infant's blood by heel puncture for analysis of blood glucose level, newborn screening, or other tests. (Instructions are given here for measuring the infant's blood glucose level using a glucometer, but the same method applies to other testing.)

1. Wash hands. *Helps prevent spread of infection.*
2. Gather supplies needed. Supplies vary with different glucose meters and for different tests. Common supplies include gloves, alcohol wipes, 2 × 2 inch gauze, glucometer, commercial lancing device, adhesive bandage, cotton balls, and blood-collecting devices (glucose screening reagent strips, blotting paper for metabolic screening tests, capillary tubes). *Having all supplies ready allows efficient performance of the procedure.*
3. If the infant has not received a bath after birth, bathe the infant or thoroughly wash the puncture site before puncturing the skin. *Avoids contamination of the puncture site with maternal blood on the infant's skin. This is especially important should the mother have a known or unknown infection such as hepatitis B or human immunodeficiency virus.*
4. Calibrate or program the glucose meter and use quality control measures according to the manufacturer's guidelines. *Ensures proper functioning of the machine.*
5. Warm the heel with a commercial heel warmer or a warm wet cloth according to agency policy. Take care not to burn the infant. *Warming helps dilate the vessels.*
6. Provide comforting measures (according to hospital policy) such as swaddling, providing a pacifier, allowing the mother to hold the infant or breastfeed, or giving the

infant oral sucrose (unless testing blood glucose level). Rate the infant's pain level before, during, and after the procedure using an infant pain scale. *Comfort measures help decrease the infant's pain. Rating the pain before the procedure helps determine the effectiveness of pain relief measures during and after the procedure.*

7. Apply gloves. *Prevents contamination of the hands with blood.*
8. Hold the heel in one hand and locate the site. Palpate the bone of the heel and place the thumb or finger over the walking surface of the foot. *Stabilizes the heel to prevent movement and inadvertent injury from the lancet. Locating the bone helps avoid puncturing the calcaneus bone, which could result in osteomyelitis. Covering the walking surface avoids damage to nerves and arteries of this area.*
9. Choose a puncture site on the lateral heel that has not been used previously. *Avoiding a site that was punctured previously decreases the chance of infection and scarring.*
10. Clean the lateral heel with alcohol and wipe dry with sterile gauze or allow to air dry. *Alcohol reduces contaminants. Drying prevents irritation to the tissues and dilution of the specimen with alcohol.*
11. Puncture the side of the heel with a lancet that punctures to the appropriate depth. Place the device in a sharps container. *Insertion to the proper depth avoids injury to the infant and ensures blood flow so further punctures are unnecessary. Proper disposal prevents injury to the infant and injury or unnecessary exposure of others to the infant's blood.*
12. Follow agency policy or manufacturer's directions regarding using or discarding the first drop of blood, collecting the sample, determining the amount of blood to collect, handling the specimen properly, and reading the results. *Correct procedure promotes accuracy of test results.*
13. Avoid excessive squeezing of the foot. *Excessive squeezing causes bruising and dilution of the sample with fluid from the tissues.*
14. Obtain blood sample. Apply adhesive bandage. Check site frequently and remove the bandage when the bleeding stops. *A bandage helps stop bleeding. Checking the site ensures no further bleeding has occurred.*
15. Document the procedure and the results. Send specimens to the laboratory as appropriate. Report abnormal readings and follow up according to agency policy. *Confirm abnormal results by laboratory measurement according to agency policy. Helps ensure proper handling of specimens and proper care of the infant if results are abnormal.*

---

helps determine whether discharge should be delayed or early follow-up arranged. All abnormal results should be documented and reported to the nurse practitioner or physician. Application of the nursing process in the care of infants at risk for hyperbilirubinemia is covered in Chapter 21, and a discussion of phototherapy is in Chapter 24.

KNOWLEDGE CHECK

6. What are some signs of hypoglycemia?
7. Why is it important to use the correct site for heel punctures when obtaining blood samples?

Gastrointestinal System

The initial assessment of the gastrointestinal tract occurs during the first hours after birth, when the nurse observes the parts that can be seen and the infant takes the initial feeding.

Mouth

The mouth is inspected visually and by palpation. Some infants are born with precocious teeth, usually lower incisors (Fig. 20.11). If the teeth are loose, the physician usually removes them to prevent aspiration. Epstein's pearls may be present on the hard palate or gums. These small, white, hard inclusion cysts are accumulations of epithelial cells and

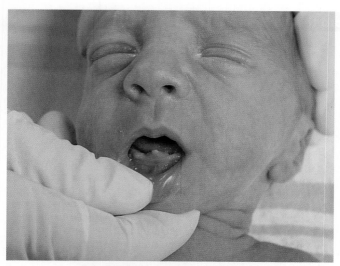

FIG. 20.11 A Precocious Tooth.

disappear without treatment within a few weeks. They are a form of milia.

The nurse examines the tongue for size and movement. A large, protruding tongue is present in hypothyroidism and some chromosomal disorders. Paralysis of the facial nerve affects the movement of the tongue and causes unilateral drooping of the mouth noticeable during crying or sucking. The tongue may appear to be tongue-tied because of the short frenulum, but this is normal and usually has no effect on the infant's ability to feed. In a true tongue-tie, there is limited tongue movement. Clipping of the frenulum seldom is practiced because of the potential for infection.

Although candidiasis (thrush) is not apparent in the mouth immediately after birth, it may appear 1 or 2 days later. The lesions resemble milk curds on the tongue and cheeks that bleed if attempts are made to wipe them away. Newborns may become infected with *Candida albicans* during passage through the birth canal if the mother has a candidal vaginal infection. The infant is treated with antifungal medication such as nystatin suspension.

A cleft lip or palate results if the lip or palate fails to close. Cleft palate may involve the hard or soft palate or both and may appear alone or with a cleft lip. The palate is inspected when the infant cries. A gloved finger is inserted into the mouth to palpate the hard and soft palate. A very small cleft of the soft palate may be missed if only a visual examination is done.

Suck

The normal full-term infant should have a strong suck reflex, which is elicited when the lips or palate are stimulated. The reflex is weaker in the neonate who is preterm, is ill, or has just been fed. The newborn's cheeks have well-developed muscles and sucking pads that enhance the ability to suck. These fatty sucking pads last until late in infancy, when sucking is no longer essential. Blisters may be present on the newborn's hands or arms from strong sucking before birth.

Initial Feeding

The initial feeding is an opportunity to further assess the newborn. If the mother is breastfeeding, she should begin in the first hour after the birth. The nurse can observe the infant's response unobtrusively while assisting the mother to position the infant. To decrease regurgitation from overdistention of the stomach, an initial formula feeding should be no more than 1 oz.

The nurse evaluates the infant's ability to suck, swallow, and breathe in a coordinated manner. Although the fetus sucks and swallows in utero, these acts may not have been performed together. The addition of breathing to sucking and swallowing is a new experience. Some newborns choke or gag during the first feeding. Others may become dusky or cyanotic because they become apneic while feeding. In either case the nurse should stop the feeding immediately, suction if necessary, and stimulate the infant to cry by rubbing the back. Most full-term infants learn to coordinate sucking, swallowing, and breathing very quickly.

Choking, coughing, cyanosis, or excessive oral secretions may indicate closure of the esophagus (esophageal atresia) or a connection between the trachea and esophagus (tracheoesophageal fistula). Neonates who continue to have difficulty with cyanosis during feedings may have a cardiac anomaly. Further assessment and referral are necessary.

Abdomen

The abdomen should be soft and rounded and should protrude slightly, but should not be distended. The stomach may be distended by mucus, blood, and amniotic fluid swallowed during birth. An abdomen so distended that the skin is stretched and shiny may indicate obstruction. If the abdomen is distended, the nurse should measure the abdominal circumference periodically to note changes. The measurements should be recorded and reported to the health care provider. Loops of bowel should not be visible through the abdominal wall. Visible loops could indicate that air and meconium are not passing through the intestines normally.

A sunken or scaphoid appearance of the abdomen occurs in diaphragmatic hernia, in which intestines are located in the chest cavity instead of the abdomen. This condition interferes with development of the lungs, resulting in respiratory difficulty at birth. The nurse listens over the abdomen for bowel sounds, which usually appear about 15 minutes after birth (Goodwin, 2016). Bowel sounds heard in the chest may indicate diaphragmatic hernia.

An umbilical hernia occurs when the intestinal muscles fail to close around the umbilicus, allowing the intestines to protrude through the weak area. The condition is more common in low-birth-weight, male, and African-American infants. By the time the infant is walking well, the muscles are usually strong enough that the hernia is no longer present. Some umbilical hernias require surgical repair.

Palpating the abdomen is easiest when the infant is relaxed and quiet. The abdomen should feel soft because the muscles are not yet well developed. Masses may indicate tumors of the kidneys. Palpation of the liver and kidneys usually is not part of routine nursing assessment of the abdomen, but is performed by the primary care provider. The liver is normally 1 to 2 cm below the right costal margin. If the organ seems large, it should be reported to the physician or nurse practitioner because it may be a sign of congestive heart failure or congenital infection.

Stools

Stools should be assessed for type, color, and consistency. By the third to fourth day, stools reflect the type of feeding the infant receives. A "water ring" should never be present around the solid part of any stool. A water ring is a wet, stained area on the diaper where watery stool has been absorbed. There may be an area of more solid stool in addition, or all stool may have soaked into the diaper. A water ring indicates diarrhea and may be caused by formula intolerance or infection.

The first stool should be passed within 12 to 48 hours after birth. The nurse should be aware of whether any stools have been passed since birth and, if so, when the infant's last stool occurred. If there is a question about whether the infant has had a stool, the nurse must investigate further. Feeding may cause the infant to pass a stool. Although rectal temperatures are not recommended, the provider may gently insert a thermometer into the rectum to determine patency and stimulate stool passage.

? CRITICAL THINKING EXERCISE 20.2

You are caring for an infant who was born 20 hours ago, and you hear on report that the infant has not passed meconium yet.

Question
1. What should you do?

KNOWLEDGE CHECK

8. Why is assessment of newborn reflexes important?
9. Why is it important for the nurse to observe the first feeding carefully?

Genitourinary System
Kidney Palpation

Palpation of the kidneys is not usually performed as part of the routine nursing assessment. The health care provider palpates the kidneys just above the level of the umbilicus on each side of the abdomen during the first hours after birth. Abdominal masses may indicate enlargement or tumors of the kidneys.

Kidney anomalies may accompany other defects because a problem early in fetal development may affect several organs vulnerable at that time. For example, infants with only one umbilical artery or defects involving the ears may have renal anomalies. The nurse should observe carefully for urinary output in these infants to determine whether the kidneys are functioning adequately.

Urine

Most newborns void within 12 to 24 hours of birth and a few within 48 hours of birth. Because absence of urine output during this time may indicate anomalies, the first void should be carefully noted on the chart. The newborn's bladder empties as little as once or twice during the first 2 days, although more frequent voiding is common. Because of the small amount, the first void may be missed. Sometimes it occurs at birth but goes unnoticed because attention is focused on the infant's overall condition.

If there is a concern about whether the newborn has urinated, the delivery notes should be carefully read to see if the infant voided at birth. The nurse should ask the mother if she has changed a wet diaper. Increasing the infant's fluid intake often can initiate urination. If no void occurs in the expected time, the infant's fluid intake should be increased and the physician or nurse practitioner alerted.

By the fourth day of life, at least six wet diapers can be expected daily. Each void is recorded in the infant's chart, including the number of diapers changed by the mother. The total number is correlated with that appropriate for the age of the infant. Mothers should be taught that at least six wet diapers by the fourth day indicates the infant is taking adequate fluid.

If an infant is having feeding difficulties, noting the number of wet diapers is especially important. Disposable diapers are very absorbent, and the pale color of the newborn's urine may cause very little color change on the diaper. Wet diapers generally feel heavier than dry ones. If necessary, the nurse can put on gloves and take the diaper apart to examine it. The absorbent inner lining is damp if urine is present. Cotton balls or tissue placed in the diaper also may be used to increase visibility of small amounts of urine.

The newborn's urine may contain uric acid crystals that cause a reddish or pink stain on the diaper. This is known as *brick dust staining* and may be frightening to parents, who may think the infant is bleeding. It does not continue beyond the first few days as the kidneys mature.

Genitalia

The nurse examines the newborn's genitalia for size, maturation, and presence of any abnormalities.

Female. In the full-term female infant, the labia majora should be large and completely cover the clitoris and labia minora. The labia may be darker than the surrounding skin, a normal response to exposure to the mother's hormones before birth. Edema of the labia and white mucous vaginal discharge are normal. A small amount of vaginal bleeding, known as *pseudomenstruation,* may occur from the sudden withdrawal of the mother's hormones at birth. Hymenal (vaginal) tags are small pieces of tissue at the vaginal orifice. These are normal and disappear in a few weeks. The urinary meatus and vagina should be present.

Male. The scrotum should be pendulous at term and may be dark brown from maternal hormones. Pressure during a breech delivery may cause it to be edematous. Rugae (creases in the scrotum) are deep and cover the entire scrotum in the full-term infant.

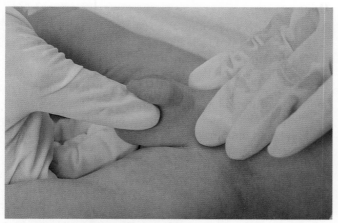

FIG. 20.12 The testes are palpated from front to back with the thumb and forefinger. Placing a finger over the inguinal canal holds the testes in place for palpation.

Enlargement of one or both sides of the scrotum may result from a hydrocele. This collection of fluid around the testes may make palpating the testes difficult. Placing a flashlight against the sac may outline the testes. Parents should be told that hydroceles are not painful and often reabsorb within 1 year. Some require later surgery.

Palpation of the scrotum determines whether the testes have descended (Fig. 20.12). Testes feel like small, round, movable objects that "slip" between the fingers. If the testes are not present in the scrotal sac, they may be felt in the inguinal canal. An empty scrotal sac appears smaller than one with testes.

Undescended testes (cryptorchidism) occurs on one or both sides. Approximately 50% to 70% of undescended testes in full-term infants will descend within 3 months. If the testes do not descend within 12 months, surgery is performed to preserve fertility (North & Gearhart, 2016).

The meatus should be at the tip of the glans penis. It may be abnormally located on the underside of the penis (hypospadias), on the upper side (epispadias), or on the perineum. The prepuce or foreskin of the penis covers the glans and is adherent to it. Attempts to retract it in the newborn are unnecessary and can cause injury. Abnormal placement of the meatus may not be visible because it is covered by the prepuce, but often the prepuce in these infants is incompletely formed. Hypospadias may be accompanied by chordee, a condition in which fibrotic tissue causes the penis to curve downward. These conditions are later corrected by surgery.

Parents are very concerned about any abnormalities of the genitalia. If the meatus is abnormally positioned, they need an explanation of the condition and why the infant should not be circumcised. The foreskin may be needed for later plastic surgery to repair the defect.

Integumentary System
Skin

The newborn's skin is fragile and shows marks easily, especially in infants with fair coloring. Because the skin is so sensitive, reddened areas and rashes may develop during the early days of life. The nurse should examine every inch of skin surface carefully during the initial assessment and at the beginning of each shift. Marks should be documented and explained to parents, who may be worried and need emotional support.

Color. The skin color should be pink or tan. Red, thin skin occurs in preterm infants. Redness (ruddy color or plethora) in the full-term infant may indicate polycythemia. Acrocyanosis is common during the first day as a result of poor peripheral circulation. The infant's mouth and central body areas should not be cyanotic at any time. Blanching the skin over the nose or chest shows the presence of jaundice. Jaundice is abnormal during the first day of life but common during the first week.

A greenish-brown discoloration of the skin, nails, and cord results if meconium was passed in utero. The discoloration may indicate that the infant was compromised at some time before birth, and it is more common in the postterm infant. These infants must be watched for other complications such as respiratory difficulty.

Harlequin Color Change. Harlequin coloration is a clear color division over the body with one side deep pink or red and the other half pale or of normal color. The cause is vasomotor instability, and it is usually transient and benign.

Mottling (Cutis Marmorata). Mottling is a lacy, red or blue pattern from dilated blood vessels under the skin. It is usually normal from vasomotor instability, occurring when the infant is exposed to cold, stressed, or overstimulated. If persistent, it may indicate a chromosomal abnormality.

Vernix Caseosa. Vernix caseosa, a thick white substance that resembles cream cheese, provides a protective covering for the fetal skin in utero. The full-term infant has little vernix left on the body except small amounts in the creases. A thick covering of vernix may indicate a preterm infant, and a postterm infant may have none at all. Yellow-tinged vernix may result from elevated bilirubin in utero, and green-tinged vernix is caused by meconium staining.

Lanugo. Lanugo is fine, soft hair that covers the fetus during intrauterine life (Fig. 20.13). As the fetus nears term, the lanugo becomes thinner. The term infant may have a small amount of lanugo on the shoulders, forehead, sides of the face, and upper back. Dark-skinned infants often have more lanugo than infants with lighter coloring, and their darker hair is more visible. Lanugo is assessed as part of the gestational age assessment.

Milia. Milia are white cysts, 1 to 2 mm in size, that disappear without treatment (Morelli, 2016). They occur on the face over the forehead, nose, cheeks, and chin (Fig. 20.14).

Erythema Toxicum. The nurse notes the presence of erythema toxicum—red, blotchy areas with white or yellow papules or vesicles in the center (Fig. 20.15). It is commonly called *flea bite rash* or *newborn rash* and resembles small bites or acne. The rash occurs in as many as 70% of newborns. It appears during the first 24 to 48 hours after birth and can continue for several days to several months (Witt, 2014). It is most common over the face, back, shoulders, and chest. The condition does not result from infection, but should be differentiated from a pustular rash caused by staphylococcal infection or vesicles from herpes simplex.

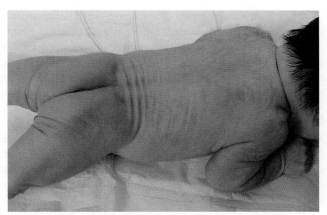

FIG. 20.13 Lanugo is abundant on this slightly preterm infant.

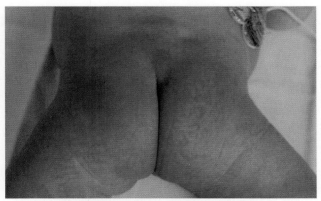

FIG. 20.16 Mongolian Spots.

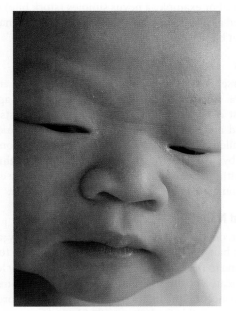

FIG. 20.14 Milia.

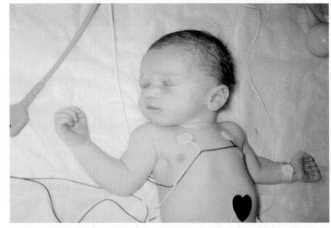

FIG. 20.17 Nevus Simplex, Salmon Patch, or Stork Bite.

Birthmarks. The nurse inspects all areas of the skin for birthmarks or other changes. The size, color, location, elevation, and texture of all birthmarks should be carefully documented. All marks should be explained, as follows, to parents, who are often concerned:

- Mongolian spots are bluish-gray marks that resemble bruises on the sacrum, buttocks, arms, shoulders, and other areas (Fig. 20.16). Mongolian spots occur most frequently in newborns with dark skin: they are seen in 96% of African-Americans, 85% of Asians, and 46% of Hispanics (Trevino, Bakos, & Janik, 2016). Although they usually disappear after the first few years of life, some continue into adulthood.
- A nevus simplex is also called *salmon patch, stork bite,* or *telangiectatic nevus* (Fig. 20.17). It is a flat, pink discoloration from dilated capillaries that occurs on the eyelids, just above the bridge of the nose, or at the nape of the neck. The color blanches when the area is pressed and is more prominent during crying. The lesions disappear by 2 years of age, although those at the nape of the neck may persist.
- Nevus flammeus (port-wine stain) is a permanent, flat, pink to dark reddish-purple mark that varies in size and location and does not blanch with pressure (Fig. 20.18). The lesion may darken and may become nodular as the child gets older.

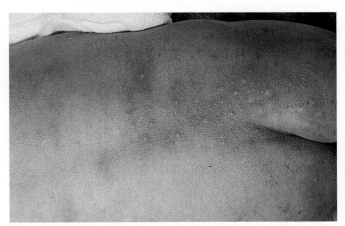

FIG. 20.15 Erythema toxicum. (From Hurwitz, S. [1993]. *Clinical pediatric dermatology* [2nd ed., p. 13]. Philadelphia: Saunders.)

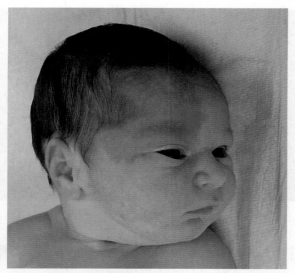

FIG. 20.18 Port-Wine Stain (Nevus Flammeus).

If it is large and in a visible area, it can be lightened by laser surgery, which is often begun in infancy. Lesions located over the forehead and upper eyelid may be associated with Sturge-Weber syndrome, a serious neurologic condition.

- Nevus vasculosus (strawberry hemangioma) consists of enlarged capillaries in the outer layers of skin. It is dark red and raised with a rough surface, giving a strawberry-like appearance. The hemangioma usually is located on the head. It may be present at birth or develop by 6 months of age. After growing larger for 6 months, the hemangioma regresses over several years and disappears. No treatment is necessary unless it becomes infected or ulcerated.
- Café-au-lait spots are permanent, light-brown areas that may occur anywhere on the body. Although they are harmless, the number and size are important. Six or more spots or spots larger than 0.5 cm are associated with neurofibromatosis, a genetic condition of neural tissue.

Marks from Delivery. The nurse inspects the infant for marks, as follows, that may have occurred from injury or pressure during labor or birth.

- Bruises may appear on any part of the body where pressure occurred during birth. Bruising or petechiae of the face may be present if the cord was wrapped tightly around the neck during birth (nuchal cord). Bruising on the head may result from use of a vacuum extractor.
- Petechiae, pinpoint bruises that resemble a rash, may appear on the back, face, and groin. They result from increased intravascular pressure during the birth process. Widespread or continued formation of petechiae may indicate infection or a low platelet count.
- A small puncture mark is present on the newborn's head if a fetal monitor scalp electrode was attached. The area should scab and heal normally but is observed for signs of infection.
- Forceps marks occur over the cheeks and ears where the instruments were applied. Their size, color, and location are carefully documented. Asymmetry or lack of movement of the face may indicate injury of the facial nerve.

Other Skin Assessments. The nurse records other aspects of the skin that may indicate abnormalities. Localized edema may be caused by trauma from birth. Generalized edema shows a more serious condition such as heart failure. Peeling of the skin is normal in full-term newborns. Excessive amounts of peeling may indicate a postterm infant.

Documentation

All marks, bruises, rashes, and other abnormalities of the skin must be recorded in the nurses' notes. The location, size, color, elevation, and texture of each mark are described. Subsequent changes in appearance from previous descriptions also are noted on the chart.

The nurse may not always know the proper name for each type of mark on the infant's skin. Most agencies have books with pictures of the common skin variations.

When in doubt about the name of a mark, a description is sufficient. For example, a nevus simplex (stork bite) might be described as a "flat, pink area 1 × 2 cm in size over nape of the neck that blanches with pressure."

Breasts

The nurse notes the placement of the nipples and looks for extra (supernumerary) nipples, which may appear on the chest or in the axilla. Occasionally, the breasts become engorged and secrete a small amount of white fluid (sometimes called *witch's milk*) a few days later. This condition is caused by maternal hormones and resolves within a few weeks without treatment. The breasts should not be expressed or manipulated, because this could cause infection.

Hair and Nails

The hair on the full-term infant should be silky and soft, whereas hair on the preterm infant is woolly or fuzzy. The nails come to the end of the fingers or beyond. Very long nails may indicate a postterm infant. A green-brown staining of the nails may occur if the infant passed meconium before birth. It is a sign of possible fetal distress (Table 20.2).

ASSESSMENT OF GESTATIONAL AGE

The gestational age assessment is an examination of the newborn's physical and neurologic characteristics to determine the number of weeks from conception to birth. It is important because neonates born before or after term and those whose size is not appropriate for gestational age are at increased risk for complications. Although the gestational age may be calculated from the mother's last menstrual period and by ultrasonography during the pregnancy, the date of the last menstrual period is not always accurate, and ultrasonography is not always performed.

Because the times of development for various fetal characteristics are known, the presence or absence of these characteristics can help estimate gestational age. The estimated age then can be compared with the newborn's weight, length, and head circumference to determine whether the neonate is large, appropriate (average), or small in size for gestational age.

TABLE 20.2 Summary of Newborn Assessment		
Normal	**Abnormal (Possible Causes)**	**Nursing Considerations**
Initial Assessment		
Assess for obvious problems first. If infant is stable and has no problems that require immediate attention, continue with complete assessment.		
Vital Signs		
Temperature		
Axillary: 36.5°-37.5°C (97.7°-99.5°F). Axilla is preferred site.	Decreased (cold environment, hypoglycemia, infection, CNS problem). Increased (infection, environment too warm).	Decreased: Institute warming measures and check in 30 min. Check blood glucose. Increased: Remove excessive clothing. Check for dehydration. Decreased or increased: Look for signs of infection. Check radiant warmer or incubator temperature setting. Check thermometer for accuracy if skin is warm or cool to touch. Report abnormal temperatures to provider.
Pulses		
Heart rate 120-160 bpm (100 sleeping, 180 crying). Rhythm regular. PMI at third to fourth intercostal space lateral to the midclavicular line. Brachial, femoral, and pedal pulses present and equal bilaterally.	Tachycardia (respiratory problems, anemia, infection, cardiac conditions). Bradycardia (asphyxia, increased intracranial pressure). PMI to right (dextrocardia, pneumothorax). Murmurs (normal or congenital heart defects). Dysrhythmias. Absent or unequal pulses (coarctation of the aorta).	Note location of murmurs. Report abnormal rates, rhythms and sounds, pulses.
Respirations		
Rate 30-60 (average 40-49) per min. Respirations irregular, shallow, unlabored. Chest movements symmetric. Breath sounds present and clear bilaterally.	Tachypnea, especially after the first hour (respiratory distress). Slow respirations (maternal medications). Nasal flaring (respiratory distress). Grunting (respiratory distress syndrome). Gasping (respiratory depression). Periods of apnea more than 20 seconds or with change in heart rate or color (respiratory depression, sepsis, cold stress). Asymmetry or decreased chest expansion (pneumothorax). Intercostal, xiphoid, or supraclavicular retractions or seesaw (paradoxical) respirations (respiratory distress). Moist, coarse breath sounds (crackles, rhonchi) (fluid in lungs). Bowel sounds in chest (diaphragmatic hernia).	Mild variations require continued monitoring and usually clear in early hours after birth. If persistent or more than mild, suction, give oxygen, call physician, and initiate more intensive care.
Blood Pressure		
Varies with age, weight, activity, and gestational age. Average systolic 65-95 mm Hg, average diastolic 30-60 mm Hg.	Hypotension (hypovolemia, shock, sepsis). BP ≥20 mm Hg higher in arms than legs (coarctation of the aorta).	Report abnormal BP readings. Prepare for intensive care if BP is very low.
Measurements		
Weight		
Weight 2500-4000 g (5 lb, 8 oz to 8 lb, 13 oz). Weight loss up to 10% in early days.	High (LGA, maternal diabetes). Low (SGA, preterm, multifetal pregnancy, medical conditions in mother that affected fetal growth). Weight loss above 10% (dehydration, feeding problems).	Determine cause. Monitor for complications common to cause.

Continued

TABLE 20.2 Summary of Newborn Assessment—cont'd

Normal	Abnormal (Possible Causes)	Nursing Considerations
Length		
48-53 cm (19-21 inches).	Below normal (SGA, congenital dwarfism).	Determine cause.
	Above normal (LGA, maternal diabetes).	Monitor for complications common to cause.
Head Circumference		
32-38 cm (13-15 inches).	Small (SGA, microcephaly, anencephaly).	Determine cause.
Head and neck are approximately one fourth of infant's body surface.	Large (LGA, hydrocephalus, increased intracranial pressure).	Monitor for complications common to cause.
Chest Circumference		
30-36 cm (12-14 in).	Small (SGA).	Determine cause.
Is 2 cm less than head circumference.	Large (LGA).	Monitor for complications common to cause.
Posture		
Flexed extremities move freely, resist extension, return quickly to flexed state.	Limp, flaccid, "floppy," or rigid extremities (preterm, hypoxia, medications, CNS trauma).	Seek cause, report abnormalities.
Hands usually clenched.	Hypertonic (neonatal abstinence syndrome, CNS injury).	
Movements symmetric.	Jitteriness or tremors (low glucose or calcium).	
Slight tremors on crying.	Opisthotonos, seizures, stiff when held (CNS injury).	
"Molds" body to caretaker's body when held, responds by quieting when needs met.		
Breech: Extended, stiff legs.		
Cry		
Lusty, strong.	High-pitched (increased intracranial pressure).	Observe for changes, report abnormalities.
	Weak, absent, irritable, catlike "mewing" (neurologic problems).	
	Hoarse or crowing (laryngeal irritation).	
Skin		
Color pink or tan with acrocyanosis.	**Color:** Cyanosis of mouth and central areas (hypoxia).	Differentiate facial bruising from cyanosis.
Vernix caseosa in the creases.	Facial bruising (nuchal cord).	Central cyanosis requires suction, oxygen, and further treatment.
Small amounts of lanugo over shoulders, sides of face, forehead, upper back.	Pallor (anemia, hypoxia).	Report jaundice in first 24 hr or more extensive than expected for age.
	Gray (hypoxia, hypotension).	
	Red, sticky, transparent skin (very preterm).	
Skin turgor good with quick recoil.	Ruddy (polycythemia).	
Some cracking and peeling of skin.	Greenish-brown discoloration of skin, nails, cord (possible fetal compromise, postterm).	Watch for respiratory problems in infants with meconium staining.
Normal variations: Milia.	Harlequin color (normal transient autonomic imbalance).	Look for signs and complications of preterm or postterm birth.
Skin tags.	Mottling (normal or cold stress, hypovolemia, sepsis).	Record location, size, shape, color, type of rashes and marks.
Erythema toxicum ("flea bite" rash).	Jaundice (pathologic if first 24 hr).	
Puncture on scalp (from electrode).	Yellow vernix.	Differentiate mongolian spots from bruises.
Mongolian spots.	Thick vernix (preterm).	
	Delivery marks: Bruises on body (pressure), scalp (vacuum extractor), or face (cord around neck).	Check for facial movement with forceps marks.
	Petechiae (pressure, low platelet count, infection).	Watch for jaundice with bruising.
	Forceps marks.	Point out and explain normal skin variations to parents.
	Birthmarks: Mongolian spots.	
	Nevus simplex (salmon patch, stork bite). Nevus flammeus (port-wine stain). Nevus vasculosus (strawberry hemangioma). Café-au-lait spots (≥6 larger than 0.5 cm (neurofibromatosis).	
	Other: Excessive lanugo (preterm). Excessive peeling, cracking (postterm). Pustules or other rashes (infection).	
	"Tenting" of skin (dehydration).	

TABLE 20.2 Summary of Newborn Assessment—cont'd

Normal	Abnormal (Possible Causes)	Nursing Considerations
Head		
Sutures palpable with small separation between each. Anterior fontanel diamond-shaped, 4-6 cm, soft, and flat. May bulge slightly with crying. Posterior fontanel triangular, 0.5-1 cm. Hair silky and soft with individual hair strands. Normal variations: Overriding sutures (molding). Caput succedaneum or cephalohematoma (pressure during birth).	Head large (hydrocephalus, increased intracranial pressure) or small (microcephaly). Widely separated sutures (hydrocephalus) or hard, ridged area at sutures (craniosynostosis). Anterior fontanel depressed (dehydration, molding), full or bulging at rest (increased intracranial pressure). Woolly, bunchy hair (preterm). Unusual hair growth (genetic abnormalities).	Seek cause of variations. Observe for signs of dehydration with depressed fontanel; increased intracranial pressure with bulging of fontanel and wide separation of sutures. Refer for treatment. Differentiate caput succedaneum from cephalohematoma, and reassure parents of normal outcome. Observe for jaundice with cephalohematoma.
Ears		
Ears well formed and complete. Area where upper ear meets head even with imaginary line drawn from outer canthus of eye. Startle response to loud noises. Alerts to high-pitched voices.	Low-set ears (chromosomal disorders). Skin tags, preauricular sinuses, dimples (may be associated with kidney or other abnormalities). No response to sound (deafness).	Check voiding if ears abnormal. Look for signs of chromosomal abnormality if position abnormal. Refer for evaluation if no response to sound.
Face		
Symmetric in appearance and movement. Parts proportional and appropriately placed.	Asymmetry (pressure and position in utero). Drooping of mouth or one side of face, "one-sided cry" (facial nerve injury). Abnormal appearance (chromosomal abnormalities).	Seek cause of variations. Check delivery history for possible cause of injury to facial nerve.
Eyes		
Symmetric. Eyes clear. Transient strabismus. Scant or absent tears. Pupils equal, react to light. Alerts to interesting sights. Doll's-eye sign, red reflex present. Normal variations: May have subconjunctival hemorrhage or edema of eyelids from pressure during birth.	Inflammation or drainage (chemical or infectious conjunctivitis). Constant tearing (plugged lacrimal duct). Unequal pupils. Failure to follow objects (blindness). White areas over pupils (cataracts). Setting-sun sign (hydrocephalus). Yellow sclera (jaundice). Blue sclera (osteogenesis imperfecta).	Clean and monitor any drainage; seek cause. Reassure parents that subconjunctival hemorrhage and edema will clear. Report other abnormalities.
Nose		
Both nostrils open to air flow. May have slight flattening from pressure during birth.	Blockage of one or both nasal passages (choanal atresia). Malformations (congenital conditions). Flaring, mucus (respiratory distress).	Observe for respiratory distress. Report malformations.
Mouth		
Mouth, gums, tongue pink. Tongue normal in size and movement. Lips and palate intact. Sucking pads. Sucking, rooting, swallowing, gag reflexes present. Normal variations: Precocious teeth, Epstein's pearls.	Cyanosis (hypoxia). White patches on cheeks or tongue (candidiasis). Protruding tongue (Down's syndrome). Diminished movement of tongue, drooping mouth (facial nerve paralysis). Cleft lip or palate, or both. Absent or weak reflexes (preterm, neurologic problem). Excessive drooling (tracheoesophageal fistula, esophageal atresia).	Oxygen for cyanosis. Expect loose teeth to be removed. Obtain order for antifungal medication for candidiasis. Check mother for vaginal or breast candidiasis infection Report anomalies.

Continued

TABLE 20.2   Summary of Newborn Assessment—cont'd

Normal	Abnormal (Possible Causes)	Nursing Considerations
Feeding		
Good suck/swallow coordination. Retains feedings.	Poorly coordinated suck and swallow (prematurity). Duskiness or cyanosis during feeding (cardiac defects). Choking, gagging, excessive drooling (tracheoesophageal fistula, esophageal atresia).	Feed slowly. Stop frequently if difficulty occurs. Suction and stimulate if necessary. Refer infants with continued difficulty.
Neck and Clavicles		
Short neck, turns head easily side to side. Infant raises head when prone. Clavicles intact.	Weakness, contractures, or rigidity (muscle abnormalities). Webbing of neck, large fat pad at back of neck (chromosomal disorders). Crepitus, lump, or crying when clavicle or other bones palpated, diminished or absent arm movement (fractures).	Fracture of clavicle more frequent in large infants with shoulder dystocia at birth. Immobilize arm. Look for other injuries. Refer abnormalities.
Chest		
Cylinder shape. Xiphoid process may be prominent. Symmetric. Nipples present and located properly. Normal variation: May have engorgement, white nipple discharge (maternal hormone withdrawal).	Asymmetry (diaphragmatic hernia, pneumothorax). Supernumerary nipples. Redness (infection).	Report abnormalities.
Abdomen		
Rounded, soft. Bowel sounds present within 15 min after birth. Liver palpable 1-2 cm below right costal margin. Skin intact. Three vessels in cord. Clamp tight and cord drying. Meconium passed within 12-48 hr. Urine generally passed within 12-24 hr. Normal variation: "Brick dust" staining of diaper (uric acid crystals).	Sunken abdomen (diaphragmatic hernia). Distended abdomen or loops of bowel visible (obstruction, infection, enlarged organs). Absent bowel sounds after first hour (paralytic ileus). Masses palpated (kidney tumors, distended bladder). Enlarged liver (infection, heart failure, hemolytic disease). Abdominal wall defects (umbilical or inguinal hernia, omphalocele, gastroschisis, exstrophy of bladder). Two vessels in cord (other anomalies). Bleeding (loose clamp). Redness, drainage from cord (infection). No passage of meconium (imperforate anus, obstruction). Lack of urinary output (kidney anomalies) or inadequate amounts (dehydration).	Report abnormalities. Assess for other anomalies if only two vessels in cord. Tighten or replace loose cord clamp. If stool and urine output abnormal, look for missed recording, increase feedings, report.
Genitals *Female*		
Labia majora dark, cover clitoris and labia minora. Small amount of white mucous vaginal discharge. Urinary meatus and vagina present. Normal variations: Vaginal bleeding (pseudomenstruation). Hymenal tags.	Clitoris and labia minora larger than labia majora (preterm). Large clitoris (ambiguous genitalia). Edematous labia (breech birth).	Check gestational age for immature genitalia. Report anomalies.

TABLE 20.2 Summary of Newborn Assessment—cont'd

Normal	Abnormal (Possible Causes)	Nursing Considerations
Male		
Testes within scrotal sac, rugae on scrotum, prepuce nonretractable. Meatus at tip of penis.	Empty scrotal sac (cryptorchidism). Testes in inguinal canal or abdomen (preterm, cryptorchidism). Lack of rugae on scrotum (preterm). Edema of scrotum (pressure in breech birth). Enlarged scrotal sac (hydrocele). Small penis, scrotum (preterm, ambiguous genitalia). Urinary meatus located on upper side of penis (epispadias), underside of penis (hypospadias), or perineum. Ventral curvature of the penis (chordee).	Check gestational age for immature genitalia. Report anomalies. Explain to parents why no circumcision can be performed with abnormal placement of meatus.
Extremities		
Upper and Lower Extremities		
Equal and bilateral movement of extremities. Correct number and formation of fingers and toes. Nails to ends of digits or slightly beyond. Flexion, good muscle tone.	Crepitus, redness, lumps, swelling (fracture). Diminished or absent movement, especially during Moro reflex (fracture, nerve injury, paralysis). Polydactyly (extra digits). Syndactyly (webbing). Fused or absent digits. Poor muscle tone (preterm, neurologic injury, hypoglycemia, hypoxia).	Report all anomalies, look for others.
Upper Extremities		
Two transverse palm creases.	Simian crease (normal or Down's syndrome). Diminished movement (injury). Diminished movement of arm with extension and forearm prone (Erb-Duchenne paralysis).	Report all anomalies, look for others.
Lower Extremities		
Legs equal in length, abduct equally, gluteal and thigh creases and knee height equal, no hip "clunk." Normal position of feet.	Ortolani and Barlow tests abnormal, unequal leg length, unequal thigh or gluteal creases (developmental dysplasia of the hip). Malposition of feet (position in utero, talipes equinovarus).	Report all anomalies, look for others. Check malpositioned feet to see if they can be gently manipulated back to normal position.
Back		
No openings observed or felt in vertebral column. Anus patent. Sphincter tightly closed.	Failure of one or more vertebrae to close (spina bifida), with or without sac with spinal fluid and meninges (meningocele) or spinal fluid, meninges, and cord (myelomeningocele) enclosed. Tuft of hair over spina bifida occulta. Pilonidal dimple or sinus. Imperforate anus.	Report abnormalities. Observe for movement below level of defect. If sac is present, cover with sterile dressing wet with sterile saline. Protect from injury.
Reflexes		
See Table 20.1.	Absent, asymmetric, or weak reflexes.	Observe for signs of fractures, nerve injury, or injury to CNS.

BP, Blood pressure; *bpm,* beats per minute; *CNS,* central nervous system; *LGA,* large for gestational age; *PMI,* point of maximum impulse; *SGA,* small for gestational age.

NEWBORN MATURITY RATING & CLASSIFICATION

ESTIMATION OF GESTATIONAL AGE BY MATURITY RATING
Symbols: X - 1st Exam 0 - 2nd Exam

NEUROMUSCULAR MATURITY

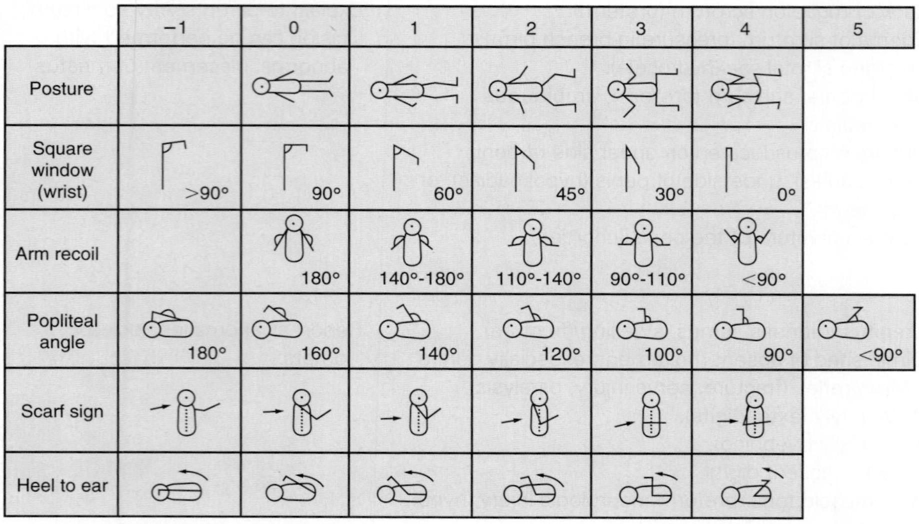

	−1	0	1	2	3	4	5
Posture							
Square window (wrist)	>90°	90°	60°	45°	30°	0°	
Arm recoil		180°	140°-180°	110°-140°	90°-110°	<90°	
Popliteal angle	180°	160°	140°	120°	100°	90°	<90°
Scarf sign							
Heel to ear							

Gestation by Dates _____ wks

Birth Date _____ Hour _____ am/pm

Apgar _____ 1 min _____ 5 min

MATURITY RATING

score	weeks
−10	20
−5	22
0	24
5	26
10	28
15	30
20	32
25	34
30	36
35	38
40	40
45	42
50	44

PHYSICAL MATURITY

Skin	Sticky friable transparent	Gelatinous red, translucent	Smooth pink, visible veins	Superficial peeling &/or rash, few veins	Cracking pale areas rare veins	Parchment deep cracking no vessels	Leathery cracked wrinkled
Lanugo	None	Sparse	Abundant	Thinning	Bald areas	Mostly bald	
Plantar surface	Heel-toe 40-50 mm:−1 <40 mm:−2	>50 mm no crease	Faint red marks	Anterior transverse crease only	Creases ant. 2/3	Creases over entire sole	
Breast	Imperceptible	Barely perceptible	Flat areola no bud	Stippled areola 1-2 mm bud	Raised areola 3-4 mm bud	Full areola 5-10 mm bud	
Eye/Ear	Lids fused loosely:−1 tightly:−2	Lids open pinna flat stays folded	Sl. curved pinna; soft; slow recoil	Well-curved pinna; soft but ready recoil	Formed & firm instant recoil	Thick cartilage ear stiff	
Genitals (male)	Scrotum flat, smooth	Scrotum empty faint rugae	Testes in upper canal rare rugae	Testes descending few rugae	Testes down good rugae	Testes pendulous deep rugae	
Genitals (female)	Clitoris prominent labia flat	Prominent clitoris small labia minora	Prominent clitoris enlarging minora	Majora & minora equally prominent	Majora large minora small	Majora cover clitoris & minora	

SCORING SECTION

	1st Exam=X	2nd Exam=O
Estimating Gest Age by Maturity Rating	_____ Weeks	_____ Weeks
Time of Exam	Date _____ Hour _____ am/pm	Date _____ Hour _____ am/pm
Age of Exam	_____ Hours	_____ Hours
Signature of Examiner	_____ M.D.	_____ M.D.

FIG. 20.19 New Ballard Score. (Courtesy Bristol-Myers Co., Evansville, IN. From Ballard, J. L., Khoury, J. C., Wedig, K., Wang, L., Eilers-Walsman, B. L., & Lipp, R. [1991]. New Ballard Score, expanded to include extremely premature infants. *Journal of Pediatrics, 19*[3], 417–423.)

Assessment Tools

The New Ballard Score (Fig. 20.19) is often used to assess gestational age based on neuromuscular and physical characteristics. It is designed to assess gestational age from 20 to 44 weeks and provides accurate information within 2 weeks. It is most accurate when performed within 12 hours of birth (Benjamin & Furdon, 2015). A score is given to each assessment, and the total score is used to determine the gestational age of the infant. The New Ballard Score is described in the following section.

Neuromuscular Characteristics
Posture

The posture and degree of flexion of the extremities are scored before disturbing the quiet infant (Fig. 20.20). Preterm

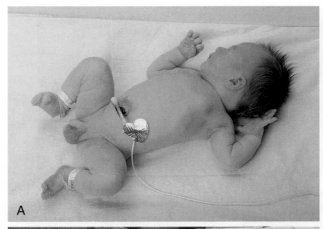

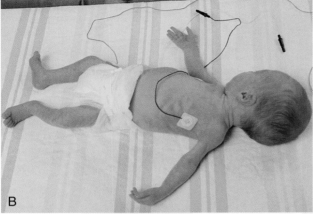

FIG. 20.20 **Posture in Newborns. A,** The healthy full-term infant remains in a strongly flexed position. **B,** The preterm infant's extremities are extended.

neonates have immature flexor muscles and little energy or muscle tone. Therefore they have extended, limp arms and legs that offer little resistance to movement by the examiner. Flexor tone improves as the gestational age increases, and it moves in a cephalocaudal manner down the infant's body. Full-term infants hold their arms close to the body with the elbows sharply flexed. The legs should be flexed at the hips, knees, and ankles. Posture is scored from 0 for a limp, flaccid posture to 4 if the newborn demonstrates good flexion of all extremities. The legs of infants who were in a frank breech position may be more extended than flexed even when they are full term.

Square Window

The square window sign is elicited by flexing the hand at the wrist until the palm is as flat against the forearm as possible with gentle pressure (Fig. 20.21). The angle between the palm and forearm is measured. If the palm bends only 90 degrees (which is the extent of flexion in the adult wrist and looks like a square window), the score is 0. The gestational age of the infant is probably 32 weeks or less. The more mature the neonate, the smaller the angle until the palm folds flat against the forearm at term, the result of maternal hormones at the end of pregnancy.

Arm Recoil

Full-term infants resist extension of the arms. In testing for arm recoil, the nurse holds the neonate's arms fully flexed at the elbows for 5 seconds, then pulls the hands straight down to the sides (Fig. 20.22). The hands are quickly released, and the degree of flexion is measured as the arms return to their normally flexed position. Preterm infants may move the arms slowly or not at all and receive a score of zero. Somewhat older infants have a sluggish recoil, with only partial return

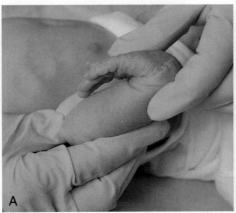

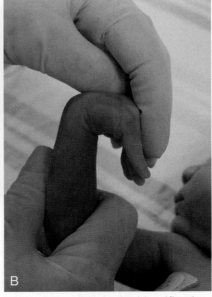

FIG. 20.21 The square window sign is performed on the arm without the identification bracelet. The nurse flexes the wrist and measures the angle. **A,** Infant near full term. **B,** Preterm infant.

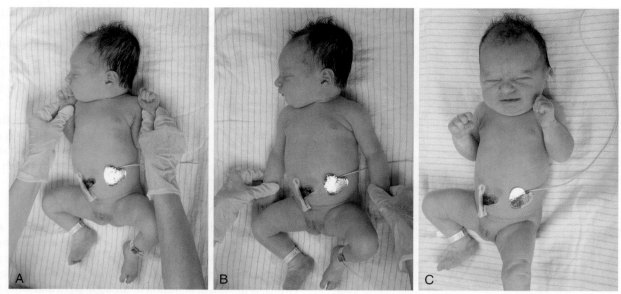

FIG. 20.22 **Arm Recoil. A,** Arms flexed. **B,** Arms extended. **C,** Recoil for the full-term infant.

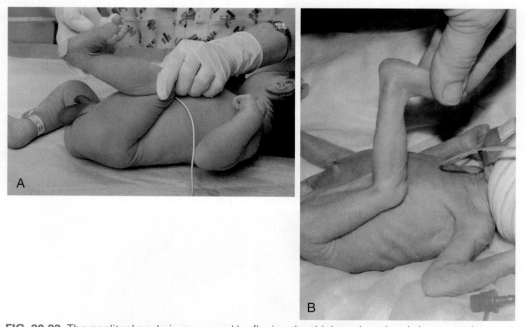

FIG. 20.23 The popliteal angle is measured by flexing the thigh against the abdomen and extending the lower leg to the point of resistance. **A,** Full-term infant. **B,** Preterm infant.

to flexion. If the arms move briskly to an angle of less than 90 degrees at the elbows, the score is 4.

Popliteal Angle

To measure the popliteal angle, the newborn's lower leg is folded against the thigh, with the thigh on the abdomen (Fig. 20.23). With the thigh still flexed on the abdomen, the lower leg is straightened just until resistance is met. Continued pressure causes the infant to further extend the leg and results in an inaccurate score. The angle at the popliteal space when resistance is first felt is scored on a scale of 0 (if the leg can be

fully extended) to 5 (if the angle at the popliteal space is less than 90 degrees). The preterm infant extends the leg farther than the full-term infant. The leg may extend with little resistance if the infant was in a frank breech position at birth.

Scarf Sign

For the scarf sign, the nurse grasps the infant's hand and brings the arm across the body to the opposite side, keeping the shoulder flat on the bed and the head in the middle of the body (Fig. 20.24). The position of the elbow in relation to the midline of the infant's body is noted. The infant receives a score of 0 if

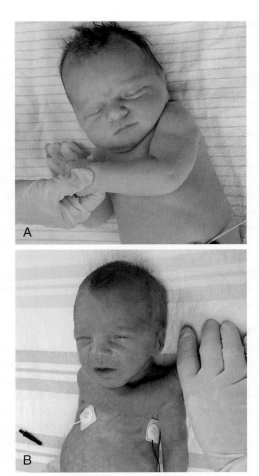

FIG. 20.24 Scarf Sign. The nurse determines how far the arm will move across the chest and observes the position of the elbow when resistance is felt. **A,** Full-term infant. **B,** Preterm infant. (Note the many visible veins in the preterm infant and the absence of visible veins in the full-term infant.)

muscle tone is so poor that the arm wraps across the body like a scarf, with the elbow beyond the edge of the body. A top score (4) shows that the elbow fails to reach the midline.

Heel to Ear

The heel-to-ear assessment is similar to the measurement of the popliteal angle. However, in this case, the nurse grasps the infant's foot and pulls it straight up alongside the body toward the ears while the hips remain flat on the surface of the bed (Fig. 20.25). When resistance is felt, the position of the foot in relation to the head and the amount of flexion of the leg are compared with the diagrams. Increasing maturity is identified by the level of resistance and flexion. Record the position when resistance is first felt because the neonate may relax the leg if pressure continues. This assessment also may be inaccurate in infants who were in a breech position at birth.

Physical Characteristics
Skin

The skin is assessed for color, visibility of veins, peeling, and cracking. The very preterm infant's skin is translucent because

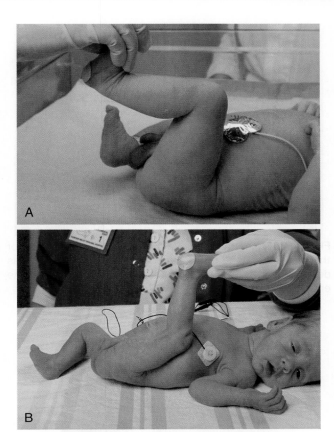

FIG. 20.25 Heel-to-Ear Assessment. The nurse grasps the foot and brings it up toward the ear. The score is recorded when resistance is felt. **A,** Full-term infant. **B,** Preterm infant.

it is thin and has little subcutaneous fat beneath the surface. The skin is red, sticky, and fragile, with easily visible veins. In the mature newborn, the skin is thicker and the color is paler. Few veins are visible, usually over the chest and abdomen (see Fig. 20.24). At term, vernix is present only in the creases.

The full-term infant exhibits some peeling and cracking of the skin, especially around areas with creases, such as the ankles and feet. The postmature infant has deeply cracked skin that appears as dry and thick as leather. Peeling becomes even more apparent during the hours after birth as the skin loses moisture.

Lanugo

Lanugo appears at 20 weeks of gestation and increases in amount until 28 weeks (see Fig. 20.13), when it begins to disappear. Most is shed by 32 to 36 weeks (Gardner & Hernandez, 2016b). A small amount may remain over the upper back and shoulders, on the ears, or on the sides of the forehead. The infant receives a score based on the amount of lanugo present on the back.

Plantar Surface

Plantar creases begin to appear at 28 to 32 weeks of gestation and cover the entire foot by term (Trotter, 2014) (Fig. 20.26). Although the creases are only red lines near the toes at first, they gradually spread down toward the heel and become deeper. The

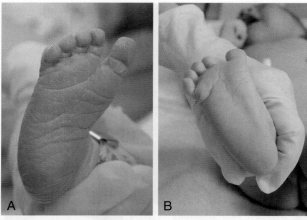

FIG. 20.26 Plantar creases begin to develop at the base of the toes and extend to the heel. **A,** The postterm infant has deep creases. **B,** The preterm infant has few creases on the entire foot.

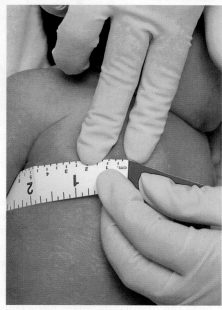

FIG. 20.27 The nurse places a finger on either side of the breast bud and measures the size. In the full-term infant, breast tissue is raised and the nipple is easily distinguished from surrounding skin. (Note the peeling skin.)

plantar creases must be assessed during the early hours after birth because creases appear more prominent as the infant's skin begins to dry. For the very preterm infant, the length of the foot is measured to help determine gestational age.

Breasts

The nipples, areolae, and size of the breast buds are assessed and scored. In very preterm infants, the structures are not visible. Gradually they grow larger and the areolae become raised above the chest wall. The breast buds enlarge until they are approximately 1 cm at term. To determine their size, the nurse places a finger on each side and measures the diameter (Fig. 20.27). Use of the thumb and forefinger may cause excess tissue to be drawn together, resulting in an inaccurate score.

Eyes and Ears

The eyelids are fused until 26 to 28 weeks of gestation (Trotter, 2014). When the ear is assessed, the incurving and thickness of each pinna are rated (Fig. 20.28). At about 34 weeks of gestation, the upper pinnae, which have been flat, begin to curve over. The incurving continues around the ear until it reaches near the earlobe at 40 weeks of gestation (Benjamin & Furdon, 2015).

The amount of cartilage present in the ears is a more accurate guide to gestational age than the incurving of the pinnae because of individual differences in ear shape. As cartilage is deposited in the pinnae, the ears become stiff and stand away from the head. The ear is folded longitudinally and horizontally to assess the resistance and speed with which the ear returns to its original state. In newborns less than 34 weeks of gestation, the ear has little cartilage to keep it stiff. When folded, it remains folded over or returns slowly. In the term neonate, the ear springs back to its original position immediately.

Genitals

In the female infant, the relationship in size of the clitoris, labia minora, and labia majora is noted (Fig. 20.29). In the preterm infant, the labia majora are small and separated, and the clitoris and labia minora are large by comparison. As the infant nears term, the labia majora enlarge until the clitoris and labia minora are completely covered. Because the size of the labia majora is affected by the amount of fat deposited, the infant who is malnourished in utero may have genitalia with an immature appearance.

In the male infant, the location of the testes and the rugae on the scrotum are assessed (Fig. 20.30). The testes originate in the abdominal cavity and begin to descend at 28 weeks of gestation. By 37 weeks of gestation, they are located high in the scrotal sac, and they are generally completely descended by term. Rugae cover the surface of the scrotum by 40 weeks of gestation (Benjamin & Furdon, 2015). Once the testes are completely down into the scrotum, the scrotum appears large and pendulous.

Scoring

As each part of the gestational age assessment is performed, the infant's response is matched with the diagrams and descriptions on the assessment tool. The total score is compared with the corresponding gestational age. It is important to understand that one or two characteristics alone are not enough to assign a gestational age. It is the total score of all assessed characteristics that determines the gestational age.

A difference of 2.5 points is necessary to change the gestational age by 1 week. Therefore slight differences in the scores of different examiners are not likely to cause significant differences in the outcome of the examination.

Gestational Age and Infant Size

The appropriateness of the neonate's size for gestational age is determined by plotting the weight, length, head circumference, and gestational age on a graph of intrauterine

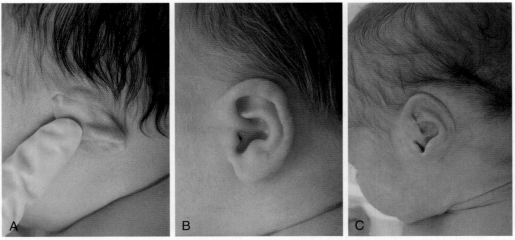

FIG. 20.28 Ear Maturation. A, The nurse folds the ears and notes how quickly they return to position. **B,** Ears in the full-term infant are well formed and have instant recoil. **C,** In the preterm infant, ears show less incurving of the pinna and recoil slowly or not at all.

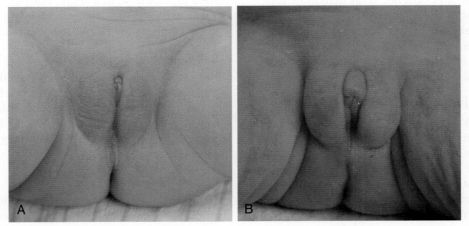

FIG. 20.29 Female Genitals. As the female matures, the labia majora cover the labia minora and clitoris completely; in the preterm infant, these structures are not covered. **A,** Near-term infant. **B,** Preterm infant.

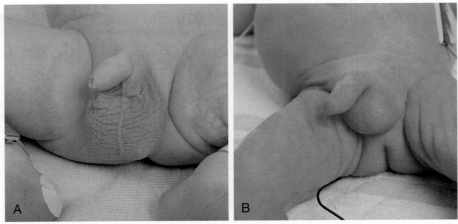

FIG. 20.30 Male Genitals. A, The full-term infant has a pendulous scrotum with deep rugae. **B,** In the preterm infant, the testes may not be descended and rugae are few.

development. This score determines how well the infant has grown for the amount of time spent in the uterus. An infant may be small, large, or of appropriate size for gestational age. The infant whose size is appropriate for gestational age falls between the 10th and 90th percentiles on the graph. The large-for-gestational-age (LGA) infant is above the 90th percentile, and the small-for-gestational-age (SGA) infant is below the 10th percentile.

Further Assessments

When an infant's gestational age or measurements fall outside the expected range, the nurse monitors for complications. Specific complications are common to preterm, postterm, SGA, and LGA infants. For example, pregnancy complications may cause a poorly functioning placenta and an SGA infant. LGA infants are also prone to complications.

ASSESSMENT OF BEHAVIOR

Assessment of the infant's behavior helps determine intactness of the CNS and provides information about the ability to respond to caretaking activities. Because behavior differs at various times after birth, the nurse should be aware of the periods of reactivity and the six different states of behavior so that nursing care can be adapted appropriately.

Periods of Reactivity

During the first and second periods of reactivity, newborns may have elevated pulse and respiratory rates, low temperatures, and excessive respiratory secretions. Careful observation is important at this time but usually can be done unobtrusively so that parents can continue to enjoy the newborn. During the time between the first and second periods of reactivity, newborns cannot be awakened easily and are not interested in feeding.

Behavioral Changes

Nurses assess the infant's behavior and alert the physician to abnormalities. Assessment includes the six different behavioral states: quiet sleep, active sleep, drowsy, quiet alert, active alert, and crying. Movement between states should be smooth and not abrupt. The Brazelton Neonatal Behavioral Assessment Scale is often used when detailed knowledge about the infant is needed. In addition to assessing behavioral states, the scale analyzes other aspects of the newborn's behavior, such as orientation, habituation, self-consoling behaviors, social behaviors, and the appropriateness of the amount of time in each of these activities.

Orientation

The nurse notes the infant's orientation (ability to pay attention) to interesting visual or auditory stimuli. It is most prominent during the quiet alert state. Infants focus their eyes and turn their heads toward a stimulus in an attempt to prolong contact with it. Preterm and ill neonates have less ability to orient to stimuli.

Habituation

The infant's response to a visual, auditory, or tactile stimulus is an important assessment. Generally, the first response of a healthy newborn to an interesting stimulus, such as a brightly colored object or bell, is a period of alertness. If the stimulus is disturbing, such as a bright light flashed in the eyes, the infant startles and attempts to escape by averting the eyes.

Infants gradually stop responding to continued unpleasant stimuli. This gradual habituation allows them to ignore the stimuli and save energy for physiologic needs. Newborns may display a dull, drowsy state or fall into a deep sleep. Those who seem unresponsive in a bright, noisy environment may be in a state of habituation. The preterm infant or one with damage to the CNS may not be able to habituate.

Self-Consoling Activities

Normal newborns are able to console themselves for short periods. Self-consoling activities include bringing their hands to their mouth, sucking on their fists, listening to voices, and watching objects in the environment. Infants who are ill, preterm, or exposed to drugs prenatally have less ability to console themselves.

Parents' Response

The parents' growing ability to respond to the infant's behavioral cues should be noted. The nurse can point out the infant's behavioral changes to facilitate attachment and help the parents learn to interpret the infant's cues. The methods the parents use to meet the infant's needs during different behavior states also are noted.

> ### ❓ KNOWLEDGE CHECK
>
> 10. When should the first voiding occur? How often do infants void?
> 11. What is the nurse's responsibility regarding marks on the newborn's skin?
> 12. Why is the gestational age assessment important?
> 13. How do the periods of reactivity affect nursing care?

▌ SUMMARY CONCEPTS

- Nurses assess newborns immediately after birth to detect serious abnormalities. If no problems are detected with a quick assessment, a more comprehensive examination is performed after parent-infant attachment and initiation of breastfeeding.

- Assessment of cardiorespiratory status includes history, airway, color, heart sounds, pulses, and blood pressure.
- Because they are safer, axillary temperatures are preferred to rectal temperatures.

- Molding of the head is normal during birth and may cause the head to appear misshapen. Caput succedaneum (localized swelling from pressure against the cervix) or a cephalohematoma (bleeding between the periosteum and the bone) may be present.
- Measurements are an important way to learn about growth before birth. Abnormal measurements alert the nurse that complications may occur.
- Reflexes are an indication of the health of the central nervous system. Asymmetry or retention of reflexes beyond the time when they should disappear is abnormal.
- Early signs of hypoglycemia include jitteriness, poor muscle tone, respiratory distress, sweating, low temperature, and poor suck.
- In performing heel sticks to obtain blood samples, the nurse must choose the site carefully to avoid injury to the bone, nerves, or blood vessels of the heel.

- The initial feeding provides information about the neonate's ability to coordinate sucking, swallowing, and breathing and tolerance to feeding.
- Newborns pass the first stool within 12 to 48 hours of birth. Absence of stool for 48 hours may indicate an obstruction.
- The newborn's first void occurs within 12 to 48 hours. Infants may void only one or two times during the first 2 days and at least six times daily by the fourth day.
- Marks on the skin should be documented, including location, size, color, elevation, and texture. Because marks can be upsetting, they should be explained to the parents.
- The gestational age assessment provides an estimate of the infant's age from conception. It alerts the nurse to possible complications related to age and size.

REFERENCES & READINGS

American Academy of Pediatrics & American College of Obstetricians and Gynecologists (AAP & ACOG). (2012). *Guidelines for perinatal care* (7th ed.). Elk, Grove Village, IL: Author.

Ballard, J. L., Khoury, J. C., Wedig, K., Wang, L., Eilers-Walsman, B. L., & Lip, R. (1991). New Ballard Score, expanded to include extremely premature infants. *Journal of Pediatrics, 19*(3), 417–423.

Benjamin, K., & Furdon, S. A. (2015). Physical assessment. In *Core curriculum for neonatal intensive care nursing* (5th ed.) (pp. 110–145). St. Louis, MO: Elsevier Saunders.

Blackburn, S. T. (2013). *Maternal, fetal, and neonatal physiology: A clinical perspective* (4th ed.). St. Louis, MO: Saunders.

Bloomfield, D., Dinolfo, E. A., & Kokotos, F. (2016). Care of the newborn after delivery. In T. K. McInerny, H. M. Adam, D. E. Campbell, et al. (Eds.), *Textbook of pediatric care* (2nd ed.) (pp. 800–809). Elk Grove Village, IL: American Academy of Pediatrics.

Cheffer, N. D., & Rannalli, D. A. (2015). Transitional care of the newborn. In S. Mattson & J. E. Smith (Eds.), *Core curriculum for maternal-newborn nursing* (5th ed.) (pp. 345–361). St. Louis, MO: Saunders.

Feigelman, S. (2015). The first year. In R. M. Kliegman, B. E. Stanton, J. W. St. Geme, & N. E. Schor (Eds.), *Nelson textbook of pediatrics* (20th ed.) (pp. 65–69). Philadelphia: Saunders.

Feigelman, S. (2016). Assessment of growth. In R. M. Kliegman, B. E. Stanton, J. W. St. Geme, & N. E. Schor (Eds.), *Nelson textbook of pediatrics* (20th ed.) (pp. 60–61). Philadelphia: Saunders.

Gardner, S. L., & Hernandez, J. A. (2016a). Heat balance. In S. L. Gardner, B. S. Carter, M. Enzman-Hines, & J. A. Hernandez (Eds.), *Merenstein & Gardner's handbook of neonatal intensive care* (8th ed.) (pp. 105–125). St. Louis, MO: Mosby.

Gardner, S. L., & Hernandez, J. A. (2016b). Initial nursery care. In S. L. Gardner, B. S. Carter, M. Enzman-Hines, & J. A. Hernandez (Eds.), *Merenstein & Gardner's Handbook of neonatal intensive care* (8th ed.) (pp. 71–104). St. Louis, MO: Mosby.

Goodwin, M. (2015). Apnea. In *Core curriculum for neonatal intensive care nursing* (5th ed.) (pp. 474–483). St. Louis: MO Saunders.

Goodwin, M. (2016). Abdomen assessment. In E. P. Tappero, & M. E. Honeyfield (Eds.), *Physical assessment of the newborn: A comprehensive approach to the art of physical examination* (5th ed.) (pp. 105–114). Santa Rosa, CA: NICU Ink.

Hurwitz, S. (1993). *Clinical pediatric dermatology* (2nd ed.) (p. 13). Philadelphia: Saunders.

Johnson, P. J. (2014). Head, eyes, ears, nose, mouth, and neck assessment. In E. P. Tappero & M. E. Honeyfield (Eds.), *Physical assessment of the newborn: A comprehensive approach to the art of physical examination* (5th ed.) (pp. 57–74). Santa Rosa, CA: NICU Ink.

Kaufman, L. M., Miller, M. T., & Gupta, B. K. (2015). The eye: Examination and common problems. In R. J. Martin, A. A. Fanaroff, & M. C. Walsh (Eds.), *Fanaroff and Martin's neonatal-perinatal medicine: Diseases of the fetus and infant* (Vol. 2, 10th ed.) (pp. 1737–1763). St. Louis, MO: Mosby.

Kaur, H., & Campbell, D. (2016). Physical examination of the newborn. In T. K. McInerny, H. M. Adam, D. E. Campbell, D. M. Kamat, & K. J. Kelleher (Eds.), *Textbook of pediatric care* (2nd ed.) (pp. 757–774). Elk Grove Village, IL: American Academy of Pediatrics.

Lo, S. F. (2016). Reference intervals for laboratory tests and procedures. In R. M. Kliegman, B. E. Stanton, J. W. St. Geme, & N. E. Schor (Eds.), *Nelson textbook of pediatrics* (20th ed.) (p. 3460). Philadelphia: Saunders.

Mangurten, H. H., & Puppala, B. L. (2016). Birth injuries. In R. J. Martin, A. A. Fanaroff, & M. C. Walsh (Eds.), *Fanaroff and Martin's neonatal-perinatal medicine: Diseases of the fetus and infant* (Vol. 1, 10th ed.) (pp. 501–529). St. Louis, MO: Mosby.

Morelli, J. G. (2016). Diseases of the neonate. In R. M. Kliegman, B. E. Stanton, J. W. St. Geme, & N. E. Schor (Eds.), *Nelson textbook of pediatrics* (20th ed.) (pp. 2218–2220). Philadelphia: Saunders.

North, A. C., & Gearhart, J. P. (2016). Hypospadias, epispadias, and cryptorchism. In T. K. McInerny, H. M. Adam, D. E. Campbell, D. M. Kamat, & K. J. Kelleher (Eds.), *Textbook of pediatric care* (2nd ed.) (pp. 2157–2161). Elk Grove Village, IL: American Academy of Pediatrics.

Olitsky, S. E., Hug, D., Plummer, L. S., Stahl, E. D., Ariss, M. M., & Lindquist, T. D. (2016). Disorders of the eye: Growth and development. In R. M. Kliegman, B. E. Stanton, J. W. St. Geme, & N. E. Schor (Eds.), *Nelson textbook of pediatrics* (20th ed.) (p. 3016). Philadelphia: Saunders.

Pan, D. H., & Rivas, Y. (2016). Jaundice. In T. K. McInery, H. M. Adam, D. E. Campbell, D. M. Kamat, & K. J. Kelleher (Eds.), *Textbook of pediatric care* (2nd ed.) (pp. 1615–1625). Elk Grove Village, IL: American Academy of Pediatrics.

Parikh, A. S., & Wiesner, G. L. (2016). Congenital anomalies. In R. J. Martin, A. A. Fanaroff, & M. C. Walsh (Eds.), *Fanaroff and Martin's neonatal-perinatal medicine: Diseases of the fetus and infant* (Vol. 1, 10th ed.) (pp. 531–552). St. Louis, MO: Mosby.

Schwend, R. M., Shaw, B. A., & Segal, L. S. (2014). Evaluation and treatment of developmental hip dysplasia in the newborn and infant. *Pediatric Clinics of North America, 61*(6), 1095–1107.

Sprecher, R. C., & Arnold, J. E. (2016). Upper airway lesions. In R. J. Martin, A. A. Fanaroff, & M. C. Walsh (Eds.), *Fanaroff and Martin's neonatal-perinatal medicine: Diseases of the fetus and infant* (Vol. 2, 10th ed.) (pp. 1170–1179). St. Louis, MO: Mosby.

Trevino, J. J., Bakos, M. A., & Janik, M. P. (2016). Neonatal skin. In T. K. McInerny, H. M. Adam, D. E. Campbell, D. M. Kamat, & K. J. Kelleher (Eds.), *Textbook of pediatric care* (2nd ed.) (pp. 778–788). Elk Grove Village, IL: American Academy of Pediatrics.

Trotter, C. W. (2014). Gestational age assessment. In E. P. Tappero & M. E. Honeyfield (Eds.), *Physical assessment of the newborn: A comprehensive approach to the art of physical examination* (5th ed.) (pp. 21–39). Santa Rosa, CA: NICU Ink.

Vargo, L. (2014a). Cardiovascular assessment. In E. P. Tappero & M. E. Honeyfield (Eds.), *Physical assessment of the newborn: A comprehensive approach to the art of physical examination* (4th ed.) (pp. 87–103). Santa Rosa, CA: NICU Ink.

Vargo, L. (2014b). Newborn physical assessment. In K. R. Simpson & P. A. Creehan (Eds.), *AWHONN perinatal nursing* (5th ed.) (pp. 597–620). Philadelphia: Lippincott Williams & Wilkins.

Verklan, M. T. (2015). Adaptation to extrauterine life. In S. Mattson & J. E. Smith (Eds.), *Core curriculum for maternal-newborn nursing* (5th ed.) (pp. 72–90). St. Louis, MO: Saunders.

Witt, C. (2014). Skin assessment. In E. P. Tappero & M. E. Honeyfield (Eds.), *Physical assessment of the newborn: A comprehensive approach to the art of physical examination* (5th ed.) (pp. 41–55). Santa Rosa, CA: NICU Ink.

Care of the Normal Newborn

Vanessa Flannery

The role of the nurse in ongoing assessments and care of the newborn in the birth facility is to help the newborn and parents have a successful transition after birth. The nurse identifies and responds to changes in the condition of newborns as they adapt to life outside the uterus, keeps infants safe, and teaches parents how to provide care. Nurses often receive questions from parents about care of infants after discharge. Infant home care for the first 12 weeks of life is discussed. Detailed information about ill or older infants can be found in pediatrics textbooks.

INPATIENT CARE

EARLY CARE

Early care after birth involves assignment of Apgar scores and assessment and stabilization of the infant as necessary. Once the infant's condition is stable, and he or she has had the opportunity to bond with the parents, prophylactic medications are given. Ongoing assessments continue during this time, including temperature, heart rate, respiratory rate and character, skin color, muscle tone, level of consciousness, and activity level. These assessments should be documented every 30 minutes until the newborn is stable for 2 hours (American Academy of Pediatrics & American College of Obstetricians and Gynecologists [AAP & ACOG], 2012).

Because of blood and amniotic fluid on the infant's skin from birth, the nurse wears gloves during all contact with the infant until the bath is completed. After the bath, gloves are necessary only when contact with body fluids may occur.

Administering Vitamin K

Vitamin K is given to neonates because they cannot synthesize it in the intestines without bacterial flora. This places them at risk for hemorrhagic disease of the newborn. One dose of vitamin K intramuscularly after birth prevents bleeding problems until the infant is able to produce vitamin K in sufficient amounts. Although the injection is usually given within the first hour after birth, it can be delayed until the infant has finished breastfeeding at birth (AAP & ACOG, 2012) (Procedure 21.1; Drug Guide: Vitamin K_1 [Phytonadione]).

PURPOSE: To place medication into the muscle without injury.

1. Wash the infant's thigh if the bath has not yet been given. *Blood from the mother is present on the infant's skin. Washing prevents that blood from being carried into the infant's tissues during the needle insertion.*

2. Prepare medication for injection. Use a 1-mL syringe and a ⅝-in, 25-gauge needle. If the medication is in a glass ampule, use a filter needle to draw it up. Remove the filter needle, and place a 25-gauge needle on the syringe to give the injection. *Use of a filter needle prevents particles of glass from being drawn into the syringe. A small needle reaches the newborn's muscle but avoids the bone.*

3. Put on gloves. *Gloves protect the nurse from contamination by blood.*

4. Locate the correct site. The best site for newborn intramuscular injections is the vastus lateralis muscle. Divide the area between the greater trochanter of the femur and the knee into thirds. Give the injection in the middle third of the muscle, lateral to the midline of the anterior thigh. *The large vastus lateralis is located away from the sciatic nerve and the femoral artery and vein. The rectus femoris muscle is nearer to these structures and poses more of a danger. (Note: The gluteal muscles are not used until a child has been walking for at least a year. These muscles are poorly developed and dangerously near the sciatic nerve.)*

5. Cleanse the area with an alcohol wipe. *Cleansing removes organisms and prevents infection.*

6. Stabilize the leg firmly while grasping the thigh between the thumb and fingers. *Holding the leg prevents sudden movement by the infant and possible injury.*

7. Insert the needle at a 90-degree angle. Inject the medication. *This places the medication into the muscle rather than into the subcutaneous tissue.*

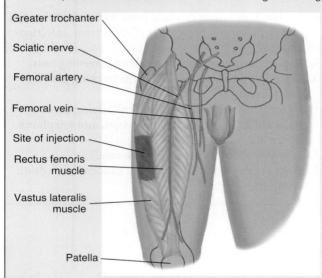

Greater trochanter
Sciatic nerve
Femoral artery
Femoral vein
Site of injection
Rectus femoris muscle
Vastus lateralis muscle
Patella

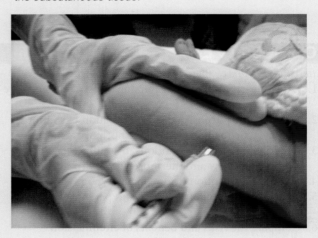

8. Withdraw the needle and apply gentle pressure to the site with small gauze pad. *Massaging promotes absorption of the medication.*

9. Discard the needle and syringe in the appropriate place and comfort the infant. *The needle and syringe should be placed in the proper container to prevent injury or contamination to others. Infants should be comforted after painful procedures.*

DRUG GUIDE

Vitamin K₁ (Phytonadione)

Classification
Fat-soluble vitamin, antihemorrhagic.

Other Names
AquaMEPHYTON, Konakion, Mephyton.

Action
Promotes the formation of factors II (prothrombin), VII, IX, and X by the liver for clotting; provides vitamin K, which is not synthesized in the intestines until intestinal flora necessary for vitamin K production are established.

Indication
Prevention or treatment of vitamin K–deficiency bleeding (hemorrhagic disease of the newborn).

Neonatal Dosage and Route
0.5 to 1 mg (0.25 to 0.5 mL of solution containing 1 mg/0.5 mL) given once intramuscularly within 1 hour of birth for prophylaxis. May be delayed for breastfeeding at birth.

Absorption
Readily absorbed after intramuscular injection; effective within 1 to 2 hours; metabolized in the liver.

Adverse Reactions
Erythema, pain, and edema at injection site; anaphylaxis; hemolysis; or hyperbilirubinemia, especially in a preterm infant or when a large dose is used.

Nursing Considerations
Protect the drug from light until just before administration to prevent decomposition and loss of potency. Observe all infants for signs of vitamin K deficiency (ecchymoses or bleeding from any site). Check that the infant has had vitamin K before a circumcision is performed.

Providing Eye Treatment

Infants also receive prophylactic treatment to prevent ophthalmia neonatorum, conjunctivitis that is most often caused by *Neisseria gonorrhoeae* acquired from the mother's birth canal. Because this infection can cause blindness if not treated promptly, most states mandate prophylactic treatment within 1 to 2 hours of birth, regardless of mode of birth (Fig. 21.1; Drug Guide: Erythromycin Ophthalmic Ointment). Erythromycin 0.5% is most commonly used. Tetracycline 1% ophthalmic ointment also may be used. Topical antibiotics are not effective against chlamydia, which often occurs with gonorrhea (AAP & ACOG, 2012).

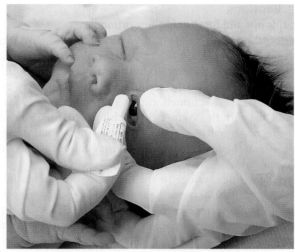

FIG. 21.1 Administration of Ophthalmic Ointment. The nurse wears gloves and gently cleans the eyes of blood or vernix. Then, placing a finger and thumb near the edge of each lid, the nurse gently presses against the periorbital ridges to open the eyes, avoiding pressure on the eye itself. The tube is held horizontally as a ribbon of ointment is squeezed into each conjunctival sac from the inner canthus to the outer canthus. The tube should not touch any part of the eye. Use a new tube for each infant.

 DRUG GUIDE

Erythromycin Ophthalmic Ointment
Classification:
Antibiotic.

Other Name
Ilotycin ophthalmic ointment.

Action:
Inhibits protein synthesis in bacteria; bacteriostatic.

Indications
Prophylaxis against the organism *Neisseria gonorrhoeae*; helps prevent ophthalmia neonatorum in infants of mothers infected with gonorrhea; required by law for all infants, even if the mother is not known to be infected.

Neonatal Dosage and Route
A "ribbon" of 0.5% erythromycin ointment, 1 cm (0.4 inch) long, is applied to the lower conjunctival sac of each eye within 1 to 2 hours after birth.

Adverse Reactions
Burning, itching; irritation may result in chemical conjunctivitis lasting 24 to 48 hours; ointment may cause temporary blurred vision.

Nursing Considerations
Do not rinse. Ointment may be wiped from the outer eye after 1 minute. Observe for irritation.

Because the ointment may temporarily blur the infant's vision, parents may wish to delay treatment for a short time during initial bonding. It may be delayed until the end of the first hour after birth or after the first breastfeeding (AAP & ACOG, 2012).

Some infants develop a mild inflammation a few hours after prophylactic treatment. Any discharge from the eyes, especially if purulent, should alert the nurse to the possibility of infection. A culture may be ordered, and the drainage should be removed with sterile saline and a cotton ball. If the mother is infected, the infant needs additional antibiotics because routine prophylactic treatment may not completely prevent infection.

◆ APPLICATION OF THE NURSING PROCESS: CARDIORESPIRATORY STATUS

The transition from fetal life to neonatal life may include temporary problems in cardiorespiratory status.

◆ Assessment

Assess the newborn for signs of difficult transition. Note the rate and character of the heart rate, pulses, respirations, and breath sounds. Look for signs of respiratory distress, including tachypnea, retractions, flaring of the nares, pallor or cyanosis, grunting, seesaw respirations, and asymmetry of chest movements. Check blood pressure, if indicated.

◆ Identification of Patient Problems

Fluid from the lungs must be removed by absorption or drainage from the respiratory passages after birth. This does not happen immediately and may cause a temporary problem during the early hours after birth. A common patient problem is difficulty clearing the airway because of excessive secretions.

◆ Planning: Expected Outcomes

The expected outcomes for this patient problem are that the newborn will do the following:
1. Maintain a patent airway as evidenced by a respiratory rate within the normal range of 30 to 60 breaths per minute.
2. Show no signs of respiratory distress (retractions, grunting, nasal flaring).

◆ Interventions

Positioning and Suctioning Secretions

Position the infant on the back with the head in a neutral position or to the side. Use the bulb syringe, if necessary, to suction secretions as they drain into the infant's mouth or nose. Suction the mouth first because the infant may gasp when the nose is suctioned, causing aspiration of mucus or fluid in the mouth (Weiner & Zaichikin, 2016). Then suction the nose gently and only if necessary. Suctioning is traumatic to the delicate tissues and may cause edema of the nasal passages.

Keep the bulb syringe in the crib near the infant's head, where it is available if needed quickly. Teach both parents how to use the bulb syringe correctly (Procedure 21.2). Send the syringe home with the infant so the parents can use it if the infant experiences a problem.

If mechanical suctioning is necessary to remove deeper secretions, choose a small catheter to avoid damaging the tissues of the respiratory tract. Suction for no more than 5 seconds at a time, using minimal negative pressure to avoid trauma, laryngospasm, and bradycardia. Apply suction only as the catheter is being withdrawn.

Providing Continuing Care

Continue monitoring the infant for problems throughout the stay in the birth facility. By the second period of reactivity, the infant may be alone with the mother. Although nurses know that regurgitation, gagging, and brief episodes of cyanosis are normal during this time, these may be very frightening to the mother.

Teach the appropriate responses to the behaviors common to this phase. Assess the parents' ability to use the bulb syringe and their comfort with its use. Remind the mother to use the bulb syringe and call for help, if needed. Check frequently to see if the infant is having difficulty.

◆ Evaluation

The normal newborn has little difficulty clearing the airway after the first few hours of life. The expected outcomes are met if the following occur:

- The respiratory rate is between 30 and 60 breaths per minute.
- The infant shows no signs of respiratory distress.

◆ APPLICATION OF THE NURSING PROCESS: THERMOREGULATION

Because any neonate may have difficulty with thermoregulation, the nurse should identify problems and intervene to prevent complications related to this vital function.

◆ Assessment

Assess the newborn's temperature shortly after birth and then according to agency policy. Generally, the temperature is assessed every half hour until it has been stable for 2 hours. It is checked again at 4 hours and then every 8 to 12 hours or according to agency policy. Assess the temperature more often if it is abnormal.

◆ Identification of Patient Problems

Ineffective temperature maintenance is a common problem for newborns because of their immature compensation for changes in environmental temperature.

NURSING PROCEDURE 21.2   Using a Bulb Syringe

PURPOSE: To provide an open airway by removing secretions or regurgitated feeding from the infant's mouth and nose.

1. Position the infant's head to the side. *Positioning allows fluids to pool in the lower cheek.*

2. Compress the bulb before inserting it into the mouth. *This removes air from the syringe so it will suction. (Do not compress the bulb while it is in the infant's mouth, or secretions in the bulb will be expelled back into the mouth.)*

3. Gently insert the tip of the syringe into the side of the infant's mouth between the gums and the cheek. Do not insert it straight to the back of the throat. *Inserting the bulb to the back of the throat could stimulate the gag reflex, causing regurgitation, or could cause a vagal response that results in bradycardia or apnea.*

4. Release the bulb slowly while it is in the infant's mouth. Remove and empty it by compressing several times before using again. *Releasing the bulb draws secretions into the bulb. Emptying it prepares it for use again.*

5. Suction the nose, only if necessary, after the mouth is suctioned. *Infants often gasp when the nose is suctioned and might aspirate secretions in the mouth if it is not cleared first.*

6. Suction the nose gently, and avoid unnecessary suction. *Trauma could cause edema and obstruction of delicate nasal passages. Infants have respiratory difficulty if nasal passages are blocked.*

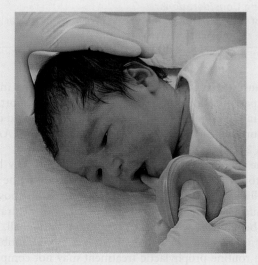

◆ Planning: Expected Outcome

The expected outcome for this problem is that the infant will maintain an axillary temperature within the normal range of 97.7° to 99.5°F (36.5° to 37.5°C).

◆ Interventions

Preventing Heat Loss

Preparing the Environment before Birth. Begin preventive measures before the infant is born. Prepare a neutral thermal environment with a radiant warmer to use during initial assessments. This ensures that excess oxygen and glucose are not used to maintain body temperature. Check the radiant warmer to ensure it is functioning properly. Turn it on early enough to warm the bed before the birth.

Providing Immediate Care. Immediately after birth, place the infant on the mother's abdomen to provide warmth from skin-to-skin contact or under a radiant warmer to counteract the cool temperature of the birth environment. Routine

---

EVIDENCE-BASED PRACTICE

Recognizing the Importance of Immediate Skin-to-Skin Contact Following Birth

The ability of a stable newborn to adjust to life outside the womb is facilitated with skin-to-skin contact with mom immediately after delivery. The first hour after birth can be a sacred hour in which a family is shaped. One may consider the first hour of life as a once-in-a lifetime chance, and unless the mother and/or infant are unstable, this opportunity should not be interrupted. Phillips (2013), reviewed studies regarding the benefits of early skin-to-skin contact between the mother and newborn.

1. Skin-to-Skin Contact Provides Physiological Stability
   The opportunity to provide skin-to-skin contact immediately after delivery stabilizes the newborn's respiration and oxygenation, will increase glucose levels of the infant, thus reducing hypoglycemia and allows for optimal maintenance of the newborn's temperature. In addition, skin-to-skin regulates blood pressure, decreases crying, and intensifies the quiet alert state.

2. Skin-to-Skin Promotes Maternal Attachment Behaviors
   Attachment is vital for the survival of the newborn. Hormones that are known to influence attachment behaviors are increased through the process of skin-to-skin contact. The hormone Oxytocin increases attraction, facial recognition, relaxation, and maternal caregiving behaviors. Mothers who engage in early skin-to-skin contact with their newborn demonstrate more confidence in caring for their baby.

3. Skin-to-Skin Contact Protects From Negative Effects of Separation
   Phillips indicates that a newborn's separation from his/her mom is life threatening. The baby will first protest and then despair. The newborn's behavior during separation of protesting is indicated with loud crying due to being away from the natural environment of warmth, nutrition and safety. In comparison of crying infants who are separated from their mothers to those who are skin-to-skin with their mothers, the separated infants have "10 times the number of cries and 40 times the duration of crying" (Phillips, R., 2013, p. 68). Continued, loud crying for an extended period of time leads to hypothermia, hypoglycemia, and bradycardia of the newborn.

4. Skin-to-Skin Contact Supports Optimal Brain Development
   The brain of a newborn is approximately 25% the size it will be in adulthood. The amygdala is located in the center of the brain. The amygdala is in a critical period of maturation the first two months after birth. The amygdala is involved in emotional learning, memory, and activation of the sympathetic nervous system. The process of skin-to-skin activates the amygdala and influences the maturation of the brain. Through research at the National Institute of Child Health and Human Development from 1966 to 1980, it was noted that touch and motion are critical for normal brain development.

5. Skin-to-Skin Contact Increases Breastfeeding Rates and Duration
   The newborn actually initiates breastfeeding rather than the mother. Babies are born knowing how to breastfeed. Skin-to-skin contact allows the infant to have a purposeful motor activity of crawling to the breast to feed.

   Protocols are necessary to implement in hospitals that will delay the list of "tasks" a nurse feels she must accomplish the first hour of the newborn's life. To achieve the benefits of early skin-to-skin contact, any intervention not necessary for the immediate well-being of the newborn and mother should be delayed the first 1-2 hours of life and after the first breastfeeding.

   Additionally, protocols are necessary for implementation of skin-to-skin in the operating room after cesarean births. The benefits to the newborn following a cesarean delivery equate to the benefits following a vaginal delivery. The practice of skin-to-skin in the operating room improves maternal satisfaction, especially for those who strongly desired a vaginal delivery.

   In conclusion, the most suitable avenue for a baby to adjust to life outside of the womb is skin-to-skin contact. This concept is supported by many organizations who are accountable for the care of newborns. Such organizations include The World Health Organization and the American Academy of Pediatrics.

Questions

1. Some mothers are resistant to skin-to-skin contact. What are some of the reasons?
2. Do the benefits of skin-to-skin contact differ for bottle-fed infants? If so, how?
3. What are some factors in which hospitals may be resistant to providing skin-to-skin in the operating room?

Reference

Phillips, R. (2013). The sacred hour: Uninterrupted skin-to-skin contact immediately after birth. *Science & Infant Nursing Reviews, 13,* 67–72.

assessment and care can be performed while the infant is on the mother's abdomen, and breastfeeding can begin if the mother so desires and both mother and infant are stable. Infants placed skin-to-skin with the mother immediately after birth are more likely to have stable temperatures (Brockman, 2015).

Dry the wet infant quickly with warm towels to prevent heat loss by evaporation. Pay particular attention to drying the hair because the head has a large surface area and hair that remains damp increases heat loss. Remove towels or blankets as soon as they become wet and replace them with dry, warmed linens. Cover the head with a pre-warmed cap when the infant is not under a radiant warmer. Do not use a hat when the infant is under the warmer because it interferes with transfer of heat to the infant's head.

When the infant is placed under a radiant warmer, set the **servocontrol** (the mechanism that regulates the amount of heat produced) to 36.5°C (Gardner & Hernandez, 2016). This setting regulates the heat from the warmer to maintain the infant's skin temperature at the normal level. Attach the skin probe to the infant's abdomen to allow the warmer to monitor and display the infant's temperature continuously. Check frequently to see if the infant's skin temperature is increasing as expected.

Providing Ongoing Prevention. Warm objects that will come in contact with the infant to avoid conduction of heat away from the infant's body. Pad cool surfaces such as scales or circumcision restraint boards with warm blankets before placing infants on them. Warm stethoscopes and clothing before using them. Before touching the infant, run warm water over your hands if they are cold.

To prevent heat loss by radiation in cold weather, position the newborn's crib or incubator away from exterior walls or windows of the building. These sources of heat loss are easily overlooked when the objects and air around the infant seem warm, but infants may lose heat to objects not in close contact with them. Keep this possibility in mind when positioning cribs in mothers' rooms, which are often short of space. Place the crib away from windows or doors, if possible. Avoid areas with drafts such as those near hall doors or air conditioners. Keep traffic low around radiant warmers because movement increases air currents, causing heat loss by convection. When assessing or caring for newborns, avoid exposing more of their bodies than necessary. Remove clothing and blankets only from areas being assessed. Keep the upper part of the infant's body covered when changing diapers. Wrap newborns in blankets, and place a stockinette or insulated hat on the infant to prevent heat loss from the large surface area of the head.

Restoring Thermoregulation

If an infant with a previously normal temperature develops a low temperature, institute nursing measures to assist thermoregulation immediately. First, look for obvious causes. The blankets around the infant may have come loose or the infant's diapers or clothing may have become wet. The mother's room may be too cold, or the crib may have been placed near the air conditioner. These causes can be corrected easily.

A slight drop in temperature may only require placing the infant, dressed in just a diaper and hat, next to the mother's bare skin. This skin-to-skin contact is very effective in using the mother's body heat to warm the infant. Place a warm blanket over both mother and infant.

If skin-to-skin contact is not possible, add extra clothing. Use two blankets, each wrapped separately around the infant, to increase insulation of heat by trapping air between the layers. Place another blanket over the infant in the crib and a hat on the infant's head. Warm linens in a warmer before use if more warmth is desired.

A greater drop in the infant's body temperature or a temperature that has not improved within an hour of using skin-to-skin contact requires additional measures. Place the infant under a radiant warmer for a short time. For an infant with a markedly decreased temperature, set the temperature control on the warmer to warm the infant slowly. Gradually increase the temperature until the infant's temperature is within the normal range. Warming the infant too rapidly can cause complications such as apnea (Gardner & Hernandez, 2016).

Performing Expanded Assessments

Expanded assessments are necessary whenever the body temperature decreases in a newborn. Assess the respiratory rate and observe for signs of respiratory distress because nonshivering thermogenesis increases the need for oxygen. Because the cold infant uses more glucose to produce heat, test the blood glucose when the temperature is abnormal, following agency protocol.

Ingestion of warm colostrum or breast milk helps warm the infant. Notify the physician or nurse practitioner if the infant does not respond to these measures. Place the infant under a radiant warmer or in an incubator for close observation until the temperature stabilizes.

◆ Evaluation

When the infant's body temperature has been maintained within the normal range for several hours, the infant can be considered stable. Continue to monitor thermoregulation throughout the stay.

❓ KNOWLEDGE CHECK

1. Why are prophylactic medications given to all newborns?
2. How can nurses prevent heat loss in newborns?

◆ APPLICATION OF THE NURSING PROCESS: HEPATIC FUNCTION

The major early assessments and care of the hepatic system are related to blood glucose and bilirubin conjugation.

BLOOD GLUCOSE

◆ Assessment

Assess all infants for risk factors and signs of hypoglycemia. Perform screening tests for blood glucose according to the symptoms and agency policy.

◆ Identification of Patient Problems

The infant is considered hypoglycemic when the glucose level is below 40 to 45 milligrams per deciliter (mg/dL) (or the value according to agency policy). These infants have the potential for injury because of decreased blood sugar levels.

◆ Planning: Expected Outcomes

Hypoglycemia requires an interprofessional approach between the nurse and the provider. The nursing plan of care will reflect both dependent and independent nursing functions. Agency protocols usually allow the nurse to intervene for hypoglycemia and then notify the provider of the infant's response. Planning revolves around the nurse's role, including the following:

1. Assessing for signs of hypoglycemia
2. Notifying the provider of signs of hypoglycemia or following hospital protocol for infants with hypoglycemia and then notifying the provider
3. Intervening to minimize hypoglycemia

◆ Interventions

Maintaining Safe Glucose Levels

Follow agency policy and physician orders regarding feeding infants with low glucose levels. A common practice is to feed the newborn if the glucose screening shows 40 to 45 mg/dL or less to prevent further depletion of glucose. Infants with severe hypoglycemia may need intravenous feedings to provide glucose rapidly.

For most infants, breastfeeding or giving formula is sufficient. Glucose water alone is not recommended for newborns because the rapid rise in glucose results in increased insulin production, causing a further drop in blood glucose. Milk provides a longer-lasting supply of glucose.

Assist the breastfeeding mother with the feeding. Help formula-feeding mothers with positioning the infant and the bottle. Explain the need for prompt feeding in infants with hypoglycemia.

Repeating Glucose Tests

Until blood glucose is stable, closely observe newborns who have shown signs of hypoglycemia. Repeat glucose screenings may be performed according to agency policy. Keep the physician or nurse practitioner aware of the newborn's status. If the blood glucose does not remain at an adequate level, other causative factors are investigated. The infant may be transferred to an intensive care nursery for more treatment, including intravenous feedings, until the blood glucose is stabilized.

Providing Other Care

Watch for signs of other complications. Infants who do not have enough glucose may experience a drop in temperature that could lead to respiratory distress as oxygen is used for nonshivering thermogenesis. The parents will be distressed over the multiple heel sticks their infant must endure. Explain the importance of maintaining adequate blood glucose and why the tests and frequent feedings are necessary. Discuss the plans for blood testing and criteria for discontinuing it.

◆ Evaluation

In evaluating collaborative interventions for hypoglycemia, note the infant's response to interventions and the presence or absence of continued signs of hypoglycemia. The blood glucose should remain above 40 to 45 mg/dL.

BILIRUBIN

Because elevated bilirubin is common in newborns, be alert to situations that require intervention.

◆ Assessment

Assess for jaundice by blanching the infant's skin on the nose or sternum. Assess for jaundice every 8 to 12 hours along with vital signs. Determine how far down the body the jaundice extends. Because visual assessment of jaundice is unreliable to determine the degree of hyperbilirubinemia accurately, obtain transcutaneous or serum bilirubin measurements in any jaundiced infant. Compare the results with what is expected for the infant's age and previous results.

◆ Identification of Patient Problems

Hyperbilirubinemia may not occur until after discharge, especially if discharge was early. The newborn has a potential for jaundice because of the parents' lack of knowledge about hyperbilirubinemia.

◆ Planning: Expected Outcomes

The expected outcomes for this problem are as follows:

1. Parents will identify methods for preventing or reducing jaundice.
2. Parents will seek treatment if jaundice develops or worsens after discharge.

◆ Interventions

Determine which infants are at increased risk for hyperbilirubinemia. Explain the significance of jaundice to parents and show them how to assess for color changes in the skin. Answer parents' questions about blood tests, phototherapy, and other care.

Discuss the importance of adequate feedings to stimulate passage of stools and prevent high levels of bilirubin. If a newborn is feeding poorly, determine the reasons and intervene appropriately. Help mothers wake sleeping infants to feed, encourage them to spend extra time with the infant with a poor suck, and explain the appropriate amount to give at each feeding. Explain that giving water to jaundiced infants does not stimulate stool excretion and should be avoided.

If the infant is breastfeeding, evaluate the infant's suck and the mother's understanding of positioning and other techniques. Instruct mothers to nurse at least 8 to 12 times each 24 hours for adequate lengths of time. Assist mothers having difficulty to ensure infants are feeding well before discharge. Refer to a lactation consultant if needed.

Instruct parents to contact their care provider if they see an increase in jaundice if the infant is not eating well, not voiding at least six times daily by the sixth day, or not producing stools appropriately (at least one stool per day for formula-fed infants and at least four stools daily for breast-feeding infants).

Stress the importance of making and keeping follow-up appointments with the infant's health care provider. Offer written materials about jaundice for the parents to take home.

Continue to check the infant for jaundice during early clinic or home visits. Transcutaneous or serum bilirubin levels may be used to determine the degree of jaundice. Reinforce teaching about identification of jaundice and importance of feedings and stooling. Answer questions that have occurred to parents since discharge from the birth facility.

If an infant develops true breast milk jaundice, explain it to the parents. The mother who must discontinue breastfeeding for 1 or 2 days will be very concerned. Reassure her that her milk is adequate and not harmful to the infant. Help her maintain her milk supply by using a breast pump during the time the infant is taking formula.

◆ Evaluation

With proper nursing observation and parent teaching, infants with hyperbilirubinemia are identified early to allow for appropriate treatment and prevention of injury. Parents are able to discuss signs, prevention, and management of jaundice at home.

> **? KNOWLEDGE CHECK**
>
> 3. What should the nurse do when an infant shows signs of hypoglycemia?
> 4. What are some interventions for preventing jaundice in newborns?

ONGOING ASSESSMENTS AND CARE

A complete assessment is necessary every 8 hours or according to birth facility policy, but the nurse should always watch for signs of change in the newborn's condition. Vital signs are assessed more often if they are abnormal. The infant is weighed once daily, and weight loss or gain is documented.

Providing Skin Care

The skin should be assessed for new marks or changes in old ones. To assess skin turgor, the nurse pinches a small area of skin over the chest or abdomen and notes how quickly it returns to its normal position. The return should be immediate in the normal newborn, with no "tenting." Skin that remains "tented" is an indication of dehydration.

Bathing

The newborn receives a bath to remove blood and amniotic fluid as soon after birth as the temperature is stable. A temperature of 36.7°C (98°F) or higher is often used to determine when to bathe the infant. Removal of all vernix is unnecessary. Early bathing decreases exposure to maternal blood and possible bloodborne organisms on the infant's skin. The bath is given before any invasive procedures such as injections or heel sticks that might draw organisms on the skin into the infant's tissues or bloodstream. If the skin must be punctured before the bath is given, the area is washed well first.

The infant may be bathed by immersion in a tub. Studies have shown that tub bathing does not increase infection or decrease cord healing. Infants maintain their temperatures better during tub bathing than during sponge bathing. To be kept warm, infants should be immersed in water that covers their shoulders. Water temperature should be approximately 38° to 40°C (100°F to less than 104°F) (Association of Women's Health, Obstetric and Neonatal Nurses [AWHONN], 2013).

If a sponge bath is given, it can be done with the infant under the radiant warmer to help maintain the infant's temperature. The bath should be performed quickly and the infant thoroughly dried to prevent heat loss by evaporation. While shampooing the hair, the nurse combs through it to remove dried blood. Combing the infant's hair hastens drying.

The infant remains under the radiant warmer until the hair is dry and the temperature returns to the previous level. The infant is dressed and wrapped in two warm blankets, and a warm cap is placed on the infant's head before he or she is removed from the radiant warmer. The temperature should be rechecked within 1 hour to ensure that the infant is maintaining thermoregulation adequately.

Bathing the infant in the presence of the parents allows the nurse to point out infant characteristics in addition to demonstrating the bath procedure. It is also a good time to teach parents about safety precautions.

After the initial bath, the infant may not receive another full bath during the stay in the birth facility. The skin is cleansed at diaper changes and to remove regurgitated milk. Clear water or a mild soap solution is used, according to agency policy.

Providing Cord Care

The cord should be checked for bleeding or oozing during the early hours after birth. The cord clamp should be securely fastened with no skin caught in it. Purulent drainage or redness or edema at the base indicates infection. The cord begins to dry shortly after birth. It becomes brownish black within 2 to 3 days and falls off within approximately 10 to 14 days.

Evidence-based practice guidelines show that cleaning the cord with water when necessary and keeping it clean and dry is the best method of cord care. This natural treatment of cords may shorten the time to cord separation and does not lead to increased infections (AWHONN, 2013). The diaper is folded below the cord to keep the cord dry and free from contamination by urine. The cord clamp is removed about 24 hours after birth if the end of the cord is dry (Fig. 21.2). Although the base of the cord is still moist, there is no danger of bleeding if the end is dry and crisp.

Cleansing the Diaper Area

Because contact with body fluids is likely, it is important to wear clean gloves while changing diapers. Meconium is very thick and sticky and can be difficult to remove from the skin. Plain water or mild soap solutions may be used for cleaning

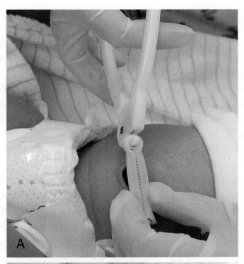

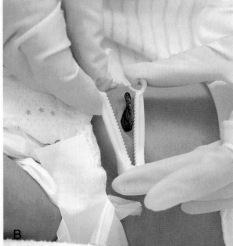

FIG. 21.2 The cord clamp is removed when the end of the cord is dry and crisp. The clamp is cut **(A)** and separated **(B)**.

the diaper area. If commercial diaper wipes are used, they should be free of detergent and alcohol (AWHONN, 2013).

Assisting with Feedings

The nurse should ensure the infant is eating well and that parents understand their chosen feeding method. This is particularly important for breastfeeding infants. A short period of observation at the start of feedings followed by another check during the feedings will help the nurse identify any problems that may have developed.

Positioning for Sleep

Parents need to understand how to position infants properly. Placing infants in the prone position for sleep is associated with an increased risk for sudden infant death syndrome (SIDS). The AAP Task Force on Sudden Infant Death Syndrome (2016) recommends that mothers be taught to place infants on their back for sleep, because this position is associated with the lowest rate of SIDS. It is important for nurses to model correct positioning for sleep for parents by positioning the newborn on his or her back to sleep at the birth facility.

Parents should also be taught to use a firm sleep surface without bumper pads and avoid loose or soft bedding that might interfere with breathing. Sack-like sleepers that take the place of blankets are available. The infant should not sleep in a bed or on a couch with another person (Fig. 21.3). However, placing the infant's bed in the parents' room is recommended. Giving a pacifier when putting the infant to sleep is also recommended, but this may be delayed for 1 month in infants who are breastfeeding to help establish breastfeeding. Overheating during sleep should be avoided (AAP Task Force on Sudden Infant Death, 2016; Jana & Shu, 2015).

Positioning and Head Shape

Infants who spend long periods in the supine position may develop flattening or asymmetry of the back of the head (positional **plagiocephaly**). This occurs because the bones are not fully developed and can be molded by positioning.

To prevent flattening of the head, infants should be placed on the abdomen several times each day while they are awake. This "tummy time" is an opportunity for play and interaction with the parents. It is essential that infants be supervised at all times when in the prone position, and they should be moved to the supine position if they fall asleep.

Protecting the Infant

Safeguarding the infant is a major nursing role. Primary ways nurses protect newborns are by (1) ensuring that infants always go to the correct parents, (2) taking precautions to prevent infant abductions, (3) preventing infections or recognizing early signs, and (4) preventing infant falls.

Identifying the Infant

Methods to identify the infant, mother, and a support person are used to ensure that an infant is never given to the wrong person.

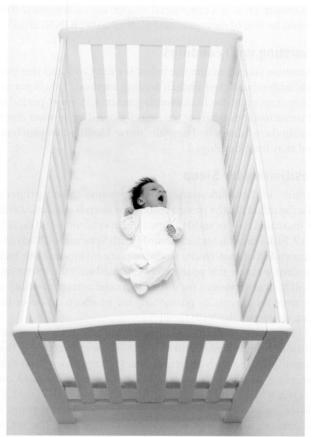

FIG. 21.3 A safe crib has a firm mattress without pillows, blankets, sheep skins, bumper pads, or stuffed toys. The infant is placed on his or her back and is dressed in a sleeper, not covered with blankets, quilts, or comforters. The baby should not sleep on an adult bed, a couch or chair, or with another person. (From Monkey Business Images/thinkstock.com.)

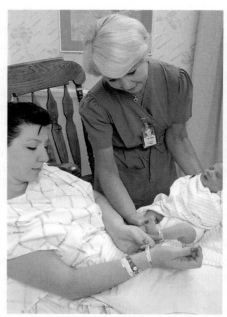

FIG. 21.4 The nurse unwraps the infant to compare the infant's identification band with the mother's band.

Electronic devices or identification bands with imprinted numbers are used. The electronic device is designed to set off an alarm if removed or the infant is taken beyond a certain area of the facility. The devices or bands are used to identify the mother and the infant at any time the infant is brought to the mother after a period of separation, however brief (Fig. 21.4). All staff should follow the facility protocol for identification of infants.

Other methods to identify infants include taking footprints of the infant and a fingerprint of the mother or photographs of the infant. Birthmarks or other distinguishing features are carefully documented in the nurses' notes.

Preventing Infant Abduction

An essential nursing role is protecting the infant from abduction (kidnapping). Between 1983 and 2014, 132 infants were abducted from health care facilities, 119 were abducted from homes, and 41 were abducted from other places. Many of the abductions from health care facilities (58%) were from the mother's room. Infants have been safely returned to their

parents in 96% of hospital abductions (National Center for Missing & Exploited Children, 2014).

Newborns are usually abducted by women who are familiar with the birth facility and its routines. They usually visit more than one agency several times to learn the routines so they can impersonate birth facility staff to gain access to a newborn. They often know the layout of the facility and the locations of exits well.

The profile of the abductor is a woman of childbearing age, often overweight, who may want an infant to solidify her relationship with her husband or boyfriend. She may be pretending to be pregnant, have had a previous pregnancy loss, or be unable to have a child of her own. Although the woman plans the kidnapping, she waits for an appropriate opportunity to take any infant available. She may wear a uniform to impersonate hospital staff and tell the parents she is taking the baby to have a test performed (Rabun, 2014). Many precautions are necessary to protect infants from abduction (Box 21.1). Additional information about abduction is available for parents and professionals at the National Center for Missing and Exploited Children website, www.missingkids.com.

Preventing Infection

Because the newborn has a limited ability to combat infection, prevention is of utmost importance and constitutes a major part of parent teaching.

Many nursing actions help prevent infection. At the beginning of their shift, nurses wash their hands and arms thoroughly. Throughout the day, hand hygiene according to agency policy is important before and after touching any infant.

BOX 21.1   Precautions to Prevent Infant Abductions

All personnel should wear picture identification that is easily visible at all times. No one without appropriate identification should handle or transport infants.

Enlist parents' help in preventing kidnapping. Teach them to allow only hospital staff with proper identification to take their infants from them.

Teach parents and staff to transport infants only in their cribs and never by carrying them. Question anyone carrying an infant outside the mother's room.

Question anyone with a newborn near an exit or in an unusual part of the facility.

Be suspicious of anyone who does not seem to be visiting a specific mother, asks detailed questions about maternity or discharge routines, asks to hold infants, or behaves in an unusual manner.

Be suspicious of unknown people carrying large bags or packages that could contain an infant.

Respond immediately when an alarm signals that a remote exit has been opened or an infant has been taken into an unauthorized area.

Never leave infants unattended. Teach parents that infants should be observed at all times. Infants may be taken into the bathroom with the mother, if necessary. Suggest that mothers have the nursing staff take care of the infant if the mother wants to nap or feels unwell and no family members are present.

If infants need to be moved to another area, take one infant at a time. Never leave an infant in the hall while the nurse is in a room with another mother. Never leave an infant unsupervised.

When infants are in mothers' rooms, position the crib away from the doorways, preferably on the side of the mother's bed opposite the door.

Protect codes, card keys, and identification badges that allow entrance to maternity units or nurseries so unauthorized people cannot use them. Report lost access devices to security immediately.

When a parent or family member comes to a nursery to take their infant, always match the infant and adult identification. Never give an infant to anyone who does not have the correct identification.

Alert hospital security immediately of any suspicious activity.

Suggest that parents do not place announcements in the paper or signs in their yard that might alert an abductor that a new baby is in the home.

To avoid cross-contamination, each infant's supplies are kept separate from those used for other infants. Supplies in drawers or cupboards of each crib unit should be used only for that infant.

The nurse should instruct parents and visitors to wash their hands before touching infants. Parents should be instructed to discourage visitors with colds or other infections from visiting the mother and the newborn at the birth facility or during the early weeks at home.

Nurses should be vigilant for signs of infection during assessment and care of the infant. These signs are often different from those in the older infant or child and may be subtle. Instead of a fever, the infant's temperature may decrease. The infant may feed poorly, be lethargic, or have periods of apnea without obvious cause. Any change in behavior that is unexplained should be recorded and investigated. The same holds true, of course, for the more obvious signs of infection such as drainage from the eyes, cord, or circumcision site.

Preventing Infant Falls

Infant falls are another concern. They are most likely to happen when mothers are feeding infants during the night. Because the mothers are often exhausted, they may fall asleep, loosening their hold on the infant who then slips from the bed. Nurses should offer to help mothers who are very tired and encourage them to put infants into their cribs when they become sleepy. Checking frequently on mothers who are feeding during the night can reinforce this.

 KNOWLEDGE CHECK

5. How can the nurse prevent a baby being given to the wrong parent?
6. What can nurses and parents do to prevent infant abductions?
7. What is the most important method of preventing infection in newborns?

Circumcision

In the United States, circumcision is the most common surgical procedure performed on males (Swanson, 2016). It is the removal of the prepuce (foreskin), a fold of skin that covers the glans penis. Although it can be retracted easily for cleaning in the older child, the prepuce may not be fully retractable until 3 to 6 years of age (Eze & Smith, 2015). The prepuce should never be forcibly retracted in any infant because trauma and adhesions can result.

Circumcision is a controversial issue, and parents may have questions about choosing it for their son. The AAP recently stated that the health benefits of circumcision outweigh the risks of the procedure, but that the benefits are not so great that it should be recommended as a routine for all newborns. Parents should have access to circumcision if they choose it for their infants (AAP Task Force, 2012a).

Reasons for Choosing Circumcision

The major benefits of circumcision are that it reduces penile cancer, urinary tract infections in the first year of life, human immunodeficiency virus (HIV) infection, and transmission of other sexually transmitted diseases (AAP Task Force, 2012b). Some parents choose circumcision for religious, cultural, or social reasons. Some parents want their son to look like his circumcised father or peers. Others think circumcision is an expected part of newborn care, and some do not realize they have a choice in the matter.

Lack of knowledge about care of the prepuce leads to some circumcisions. Poor hygiene may increase the risk for infections and other problems. Teaching parents and children about proper care of the uncircumcised penis can prevent complications related to inadequate cleanliness.

Reasons for Rejecting Circumcision

Parents decide against circumcision for various reasons. Some parents believe that the incidence of conditions more common in uncircumcised males is too low to warrant the pain and risks associated with surgery. Others believe that having the infant circumcised to look like the father or peers is cosmetic surgery and therefore unnecessary. These parents especially object to subjecting their son to pain during and after surgery. Circumcision is less often practiced by families from Asian, Hispanic, and Native American cultures. It is less common in Europe, Asia, South and Central America, Canada, and Australia (Swanson, 2016).

Parents may be concerned about removing the prepuce, which serves to protect the glans. The glans is more prone to irritation from constant exposure to urine and rubbing against diapers when unprotected by the prepuce.

Complications of circumcision are rare but include hemorrhage and infection. Removal of too much or too little of the prepuce, an unsatisfactory cosmetic result, urinary retention, stenosis or fistulas of the urethra, adhesions, necrosis, or other injury to the glans penis also may occur.

Only healthy newborns should undergo circumcision. The preterm or sick infant should not be circumcised until he is healthy enough to tolerate the procedure. For the repair of anatomic abnormalities of the penis such as hypospadias or epispadias, an intact prepuce may be needed for use in plastic surgery.

Pain Relief

The AAP recommends that adequate pharmacologic pain relief be given to newborns during circumcision (AAP Task Force, 2012b). A dorsal penile nerve block (anesthetic injected into the dorsal penile nerve) is a safe method to eliminate pain during circumcision. It has been found to be more effective than other methods of pain relief. EMLA (eutectic mixture of local anesthetics) cream may be applied to anesthetize the skin before the procedure, but it is less effective than anesthetic injection and requires a longer waiting period before it is effective. Acetaminophen may be given throughout the first day for postprocedure pain (Gardner, Enzman-Hines & Agarwal, 2016).

Nonpharmacologic pain relief methods include pacifiers, oral sucrose, soothing music, recordings of intrauterine sounds, decreased lights, and talking softly to the infant. All have shown some success in reducing an infant's pain responses to circumcision but are not as effective as anesthetics. Pain and pain management in newborns is discussed further in Chapter 23.

Methods

The Gomco (Yellen) clamp (Fig. 21.5) and the PlastiBell (Fig. 21.6) are two devices used for performing circumcisions. In both methods, the prepuce is first separated from the glans

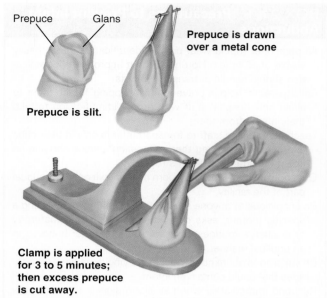

FIG. 21.5 Circumcision Using the Gomco (Yellen) Clamp. The physician pulls the prepuce over a cone-shaped device that rests against the glans. A clamp is placed around the cone and the prepuce and tightened to provide enough pressure to crush the blood vessels. This prevents bleeding when the prepuce is removed after 3 to 5 minutes.

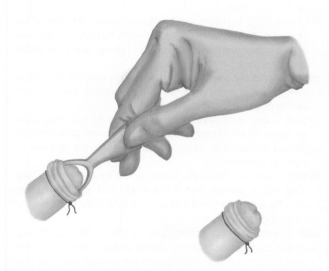

FIG. 21.6 Circumcision Using the PlastiBell Ring. The physician places the PlastiBell, a plastic ring, over the glans, draws the prepuce over it, and ties a suture around the prepuce and the PlastiBell ring. This prevents bleeding when the excess prepuce is removed. The handle is removed, leaving only the ring in place over the glans.

with a probe and incised to expose the glans. A Mogen clamp may also be used for circumcisions, especially for ritual circumcisions of Jewish infants.

Nursing Considerations

Assisting in Decision Making. Ideally, parents decide about circumcision early in pregnancy on the basis of a careful consideration of risks and benefits. Although the physician is responsible for explaining the risks and benefits of circumcision to parents, the nurse may be asked to answer questions or clarify misconceptions.

Although nurses generally teach parents of circumcised infants how to care for the penis, they may not think about providing teaching for parents who decide against circumcision. Proper care of the intact penis should be included in the teaching plan for these parents and should be discussed with parents who are undecided about the procedure as well.

PATIENT TEACHING

How to Care for the Uncircumcised Penis

Wash your baby's penis daily and when soiled diapers are changed. Do not retract the foreskin because it does not separate from the glans (or end of the penis) for 3 to 6 years.

Occasionally, gently pull back on the foreskin to see how much separation has occurred. However, *never* force the foreskin to retract because it would be painful and might cause bleeding, infection, and adhesions.

As your son gets older and is able to take care of himself, teach him to wash under the foreskin by gently pulling it back as far as it retracts easily. This should become a part of his daily bath.

Providing Care during Circumcision. As with any surgical procedure, informed consent from parents is necessary before a circumcision is performed. The nurse sees that the consent has been signed, the infant is stable, and vitamin K has been given to prevent excessive bleeding. The physician is informed of any problems that might impair the infant's ability to withstand circumcision.

The nurse gathers equipment and supplies before the procedure. To prevent regurgitation and possible aspiration while the infant is restrained in the supine position, feedings may be withheld for 2 to 4 hours before the procedure. A bulb syringe should be placed nearby in case suction is necessary.

When the physician and equipment are ready, the infant is placed on the circumcision board. (Fig. 21.7). A warm blanket is placed under the infant, and a surgical drape provides warmth and maintains sterility. A heat lamp or radiant warmer helps prevent cold stress.

The nurse should comfort the infant during the procedure. The physician administers the anesthesia. The nurse may provide a pacifier or sucrose, talk to the infant, or play soft music or recordings of intrauterine sounds to help distract the infant from pain.

Evaluating Pain. Nurses should evaluate the infant's pain with one of the pain scales available for use with newborns. An example is the Neonatal Inventory Pain Scale (NIPS) (Lawrence et al., 1993). This scale measures facial expression, crying, breathing pattern, muscle tone

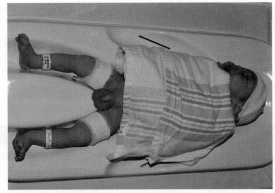

FIG. 21.7 The infant is placed on the circumcision board just before the procedure is begun.

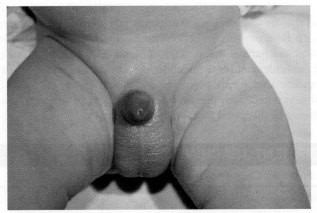

FIG. 21.8 An infant with a recently circumcised penis. (Courtesy Cheryl Briggs, RNC, Annapolis, MD.)

of the extremities, and state of arousal. The infant's pain responses should be measured before, during, and after the procedure.

Providing Postprocedure Care. The infant should be removed from the restraints immediately after the circumcision is completed. If a Gomco clamp was used, the nurse squeezes petroleum jelly on the circumcision site to prevent the diaper from sticking to it. A small piece of gauze may be placed over the area. Petroleum jelly should not be used with a PlastiBell because it may cause the ring to be displaced. The diaper is attached loosely to prevent pressure. The infant should be comforted and returned to his mother, who may be anxious about her son. Breastfeeding will provide comfort to both the baby and his mother.

The nurse watches carefully for signs of complications after the circumcision (Fig. 21.8). The wound is checked frequently for bleeding during the first few hours after the procedure. If the infant is to be discharged after the circumcision, he should be observed for at least 2 hours before release (AAP & ACOG, 2012).

If excessive bleeding occurs, pressure is applied to the site. The nurse notifies the physician, who may apply Gelfoam or epinephrine or may suture the small blood vessels. Even a small amount of blood loss may be significant in an infant, who has a small total blood volume.

Noting the first urination after circumcision is important because edema could cause obstruction. If the infant goes home before voiding, the mother is instructed to call the physician if the baby does not urinate within 6 to 8 hours.

! SAFETY CHECK

Signs of complications of circumcision include the following:
Bleeding more than a few drops with first diaper changes
Failure to urinate
Signs of infection: Fever or low temperature, purulent or foul-smelling drainage
Displacement of the PlastiBell ring

Teaching Parents. Because circumcision is often performed on the day of discharge, the parents take over care of the site. Each time the site is checked for bleeding, the nurse should show the parents the amount of blood on the diaper to help them understand how much to expect. The normal yellowish exudate that forms over the site should be described and differentiated from purulent drainage. Signs of complications should be discussed thoroughly with parents.

PATIENT TEACHING

How to Care for the Circumcision Site

Observe the circumcision site at each diaper change and check the amount of bleeding. Call the physician if more than a few drops of blood are present with diaper changes on the first day or any bleeding thereafter.
Continue to apply petroleum jelly to the penis with each diaper change for the first 4 to 7 days or as directed by your pediatrician. If a PlastiBell ring was used, do not use petroleum jelly because it might make the ring fall off too soon.
Keeping the circumcision site clean is important for healing. Squeeze warm water from a clean washcloth over the penis to wash it. Pat gently to dry the area. Fasten the diaper loosely to prevent rubbing or pressure on the incision site.
Expect a yellow crust or scab to form over the circumcision site. This is a normal part of healing and should not be removed. The scab will fall off within 7 to 10 days. If a PlastiBell ring was used, the plastic rim will fall off in 10 to 14 days (AAP, 2017). If it does not fall off by that time or falls off sooner, notify your physician. Watch for signs of infection such as fever or drainage that smells bad or has pus in it. *Call your physician if you suspect any abnormalities.* The circumcision site should be fully healed in approximately 10 days.

? KNOWLEDGE CHECK

8. What are the reasons parents decide for or against circumcision?
9. What information do parents need about care of the intact and circumcised penis?

◆ APPLICATION OF THE NURSING PROCESS: PARENTS' KNOWLEDGE OF NEWBORN CARE

Parents often feel anxious about taking over total care of their newborn. Mothers dealing with exhaustion and physiologic changes from childbirth may have difficulty remembering the extensive information they are given. Therefore finding creative teaching methods is especially important. The nurse should use every contact with the parents as an opportunity for further teaching.

◆ Assessment

Assess parents' changing learning needs throughout the birth facility stay. Consider the mother's and infant's physical conditions and any special concerns the mother may have.

Determine the learning needs of experienced mothers. They may be unaware of information that has changed since the birth of the last infant. Concerns about helping other children adjust to the newborn may be especially important.

Assess the father's learning needs and his plans for involvement in infant care. Determine whether there are cultural dictates about the father's participation in infant care. They often have many questions and are eager to learn about care of their infant.

◆ Identification of Patient Problems

In general, newborns are healthy; nursing care is wellness oriented. Patient problems center around parent education. Most parents are ready to improve their knowledge of infant care in anticipation of discharge.

◆ Planning: Expected Outcomes

The primary expected outcomes for this teaching opportunity are that before discharge the parents will do the following:

1. Identify their own information needs and seek assistance from nurses to meet those needs.
2. Correctly demonstrate infant care.
3. Express confidence in their ability to meet their infant's needs.

◆ Interventions
Setting Priorities

Because of the short time available for teaching, set priorities in determining what to teach. After assessing the parents' learning needs, make a teaching plan with them. Use a topic list to help them point out major concerns regarding infant care to ensure effective use of the teaching time. Begin by discussing their most pressing concerns to decrease anxiety so they can concentrate on the information. Then proceed to other subjects.

Using Various Teaching Methods

Use a variety of teaching methods to increase effectiveness, make the subject more interesting, and increase retention of the material. Use verbal and written methods, demonstrations, and return demonstrations. Parents often learn best by seeing skills performed correctly and then practicing them while the nurse gives suggestions. To increase the likelihood that parents will follow instructions, explain the rationale for each point made during teaching sessions.

Use audiovisual materials, including pamphlets, magazines, television programs, and Internet sites. Highlight the most important areas in written material, discuss the programs with the new mother, and clarify information, as necessary, to reinforce learning.

Many parents use the Internet to obtain information about child care. Suggest that they look for websites provided by well-known organizations such as the American Academy of Pediatrics (www.healthychildren.org). Warn them to be wary of sites with unclear sources or information that seems contrary to generally accepted knowledge. Suggest they have their health care provider confirm the validity of the information if they are unsure about it. Commend parents for their interest in obtaining information to increase their parenting skills.

Texts to cell phones are another source of information. One source that provides tips for infant care during the first year is Text4baby from the National Healthy Mothers Healthy Babies Coalition.

Modeling Behavior

Mothers watch closely when nurses handle infants. Nurses model mothering behavior by the way they hold, care for, and talk to infants. Modeling is particularly important for the mother with no experience in infant care.

Use every opportunity during general care of the infant to point out infant characteristics and behavior states and to model how to calm crying infants. Teach mothers to use progressive consoling interventions such as talking to the infant, folding the infant's arms across the chest, holding, swaddling, and facilitating sucking of the infant's finger or a pacifier. Point out the different behavior states and how to help infants move to a more awake state for feeding. Instruct parents to intervene before infants reach the point of frantic crying.

Teaching Intermittently

Plan teaching in small segments that are interspersed with infant care. Check the parents' understanding often. Encourage them to take over various tasks until they are performing all of the infant's routine care. Use a checklist of major teaching topics to ensure that all important areas are covered (Box 21.2).

Including the Partner

Identify partners who would like to participate in the care of their infants but hesitate because they lack experience. Offer them the same teaching given to the inexperienced mother. Give praise liberally to increase confidence when the partners practice their new infant care skills.

BOX 21.2 Major Teaching Topics

Newborn characteristics and behavior
Use of bulb syringe
Breastfeeding
- Frequency, length, positioning, latch on, supply and demand, supplementing, potential problems
Formula feeding
- Frequency, amount, positioning, avoiding propping, types of formula, formula preparation
Burping
Cord care
Care of the penis, uncircumcised or circumcised
Holding and positioning
Sleep pattern and position
Elimination patterns
Bathing and skin care
Clothing
Signs of problems
Taking a temperature
Infant safety
Abusive head trauma (shaken baby syndrome)
Car seat use

Documenting Teaching

Document all teaching performed and the evaluation of the parents' abilities to carry out infant care. This information shows other nurses what teaching has been completed and what is still needed. It also provides legal proof that teaching was completed before discharge.

Providing for Follow-Up Care

If the mother and infant will be seen by a clinic or home visit nurse, provide information about unmet learning needs. Reinforcement then can be provided at a time when the mother's memory has improved after the stress of birth.

Give as much information as possible in written form so that parents can refer to it later if they have concerns. Also, provide telephone numbers they can call for further help. Offer written information in the parents' primary language, if possible. Even if they speak English as a second language, they may prefer to read the information in their native language.

Remind parents about timing of follow-up care. Suggest that they schedule the appointment before they leave the birth facility.

Incorporating Cultural Considerations

Consider the family's cultural beliefs about child care when teaching. Asian parents may be uneasy when caregivers are too complimentary about the baby or casually touch the infant's head. Mexican parents, however, may prefer that a person who compliments the infant touch the infant to ward off the *mal ojo* or "evil eye" (Owen, Gonzalez, & Esperat, 2017).

Some cultures may delay naming of the baby or choose "ugly" names to decrease the envy of evil spirits (Galanti, 2015). Care of the cord differs in various cultures, too. Women from Mexico may strap a coin to the navel to keep it attractive (Galanti, 2015). Other women may use a binder or belly band or put a raisin or oil on the cord (Callister, 2013).

Ask the parents who will be helping them care for the baby to determine family members who should be included in the teaching. This varies according to the culture and availability of the traditional caregiver. In addition to the father of the infant, the woman's mother is often the major support person. However, in the Korean culture the husband's mother is the primary caregiver for both the infant and the mother in the early weeks (Callister, 2013).

Elicit questions during the discussions. However, be aware that women from some cultures will not ask questions. For many Native Americans, asking questions is considered rude (Spector, 2017). Other women may be too shy or uneasy about their limited English. When questions are not asked, discuss questions often asked by other parents.

◆ Evaluation

Ongoing evaluation of parents' learning is necessary throughout the birth facility stay and during the follow-up home, clinic, or office visits. Determine whether the parents think their questions have been answered and if they can demonstrate important aspects of infant care safely and correctly. As

they learn more caregiving skills, they should verbalize more confidence in their abilities.

CRITICAL THINKING EXERCISE 21.1

Sue, an RN on the mother-baby unit, is caring for Vicki and Nicholas. Both mother and baby have been doing well. As Sue enters the room after lunch, Vicki says, "My baby's hands and feet are so cold! His hands are shaky, too. Is he all right? Am I doing something wrong? I keep him covered up."

Questions
1. What are the nursing priorities in this situation?
2. What expanded assessments are necessary?
3. What interventions are necessary?
4. How should Sue respond to Vicki?
Vicki's mother-in-law comes to visit. When Sue enters the room to assess Nicholas, the grandmother says, "I always put my babies on their tummies to sleep, and they did just fine. Are you sure he should sleep on his back? Some babies get a flat head because they sleep on their back. I don't want that to happen to my grandson."

Question
5. How should Sue respond to the grandmother?

PATIENT TEACHING

Techniques of Infant Care

This guide is written in language the nurse might use when teaching parents about infant care. Adapt the subjects to meet the needs of individual parents.

Handling the Infant
Head Support
An infant's head is the heaviest part of the body. Infants are unable to support the head when held in an upright position for the first few months of life. You should place one hand behind the infant's head to support it when you pick up or carry the baby.

Positions
Most mothers hold the infant in the cradle position. For the "football" position, support the baby's head in the palm of your hand with the body held along your arm and supported against your side (see Fig. 22.4). This position allows one hand to be free when washing the baby's hair or breastfeeding.
The shoulder hold is good for burping the baby. Or sit the baby on your lap, and support the head and chest with one hand while gently patting or rubbing the infant's back with the other hand. This allows you to see the baby's face in case of spit-ups.

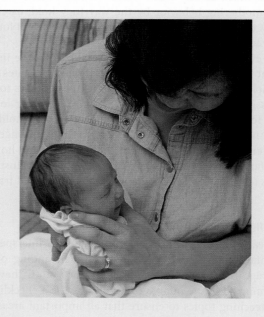

PATIENT TEACHING—cont'd

Techniques of Infant Care

Always place your baby on the back for sleep. This position is recommended by the American Academy of Pediatrics because it helps prevent sudden infant death syndrome (SIDS), the sudden unexplained death of an infant. The baby should sleep on a firm mattress and have no loose blankets or pillows in the bed. The baby should not sleep with anyone else. Use a pacifier when you put the baby down to sleep. If you are breastfeeding, you can wait 1 month to fully establish breastfeeding and then give the baby a pacifier.

Place your baby on the abdomen for play when the infant is awake and will be observed. This "tummy time" helps the infant develop muscles in the back and neck and prevents flattening of the back of the head. If the infant becomes sleepy, change the position to lying on the back for safety during sleep.

Wrapping

Young infants seem to feel secure when wrapped firmly in a blanket (swaddled). Fussy babies often respond well to swaddling. To swaddle the infant, turn down one corner of a blanket and position the baby's head over the edge. Fold one side of the blanket over the body and arm. Bring the lower corner up, and fold it over the chest. Then bring the other side around the infant, and tuck it underneath snugly.

Normal Body Processes
Breathing

Newborns normally breathe about 30 to 60 times a minute. Their breathing is irregular and may vary from loud to very soft. Sneezing is normal and not likely to be from a cold unless there are other signs.

Using a Bulb Syringe

Use the bulb syringe if the infant has excessive mucus in the mouth or nose or spits up milk. Be very gentle, and use the bulb only if necessary. Squeeze the bulb before you gently insert the tip into the side of the mouth. Do not aim it to the back of the mouth because the baby might gag. Always suction the mouth before the nose. Extra mucus is common in the first days of life but is usually not a problem thereafter.

Clean the bulb with soap and water. Rinse and dry well before using again. Call your physician if the baby's skin becomes blue or the baby stops breathing for more than 15 seconds, has difficulty breathing, or has yellow or green drainage from the nose.

Regulating Temperature

Newborns have difficulty regulating their body temperature. If they become cold, they need more calories and oxygen than when they are warm. Dress your baby as you would like to be dressed. Add a light receiving blanket, except in very hot weather.

Using a Thermometer

Check your baby's temperature during illness. Place the thermometer in the pit of the arm so that the bulb does not stick out the other side of the arm. Hold the arm firmly over the thermometer. Read it according to the manufacturer's directions. Call your physician if the baby has a temperature higher than 37.8°C (100°F) or lower than 36.5°C (97.7°F).

Urine Output

Your baby will have at least one or two wet diapers a day during the first day or two and at least six wet diapers a day by the sixth day. Counting the number of wet diapers helps you know if the baby is getting enough milk. *Call your baby's doctor if the baby has no wet diapers for more than 12 hours.*

Stool Output

Breastfed infants pass at least four soft, seedy stools that have a sweet-sour odor and are mustard yellow each day. Formula-fed infants pass one to several stools each day that are pale yellow to light brown and formed. Babies are not constipated when they turn red and seem to strain when passing a stool. Constipated stools are dry with small, hard pieces like marbles.

Diarrhea

Babies with diarrhea pass more frequent stools that are greener and more liquid than usual. There may be a *water ring,* an area in the diaper where the watery stool has been absorbed, sometimes around an area of more solid stool. Call your physician if the infant passes more than two diarrhea stools because serious dehydration can occur very quickly in infants.

Skin Care

A number of normal marks occur on the newborn's skin. A normal newborn rash called *erythema toxicum* resembles small insect bites or pimples. Small whiteheads called *milia* are normal and disappear without treatment. Do not squeeze them, or they may become infected. Newborns have dry, peeling skin that will be soft after peeling. Lotions or creams are unnecessary and may cause irritation.

Cord

Clean the cord with plain water, if necessary, and keep it dry. Fold the diaper below it so it is not wet by urine. The cord generally falls off in about 10 to 14 days. Some care providers suggest waiting for the cord to fall off before tub bathing, but others allow tub baths. Check with your health care provider. When the cord detaches, there may be a few drops of blood or a slight odor, which is normal. Notify your physician if you see more bleeding or signs of infection, such as redness, drainage, or a foul odor.

Diaper Area

Clean the diaper area with each diaper change. For girls, separate the labia (folds) and remove all stool. Wipe the diaper area from front to back. Wiping back and forth may move stool into the vagina or urethra and cause an infection. For boys, wash under the scrotum to help prevent rashes. Changing the diaper frequently, avoiding commercial diaper wipes, and using absorbent diapers may help prevent diaper rash. If the diaper area becomes red, change the diaper more often. Leaving the diaper off to expose the area to air is also helpful. Petroleum jelly or a barrier-type zinc oxide ointment may be used. If redness persists, ask your baby's doctor for suggestions.

Continued

PATIENT TEACHING—cont'd

Techniques of Infant Care

Bathing

Because infants are washed as needed after they spit up and with diaper changes, baths are not necessary every day. Partners often enjoy giving the infant a bath and make this their special time with the baby.

Sponge Baths

Before the bath, gather all the supplies: a container or sink for warm water, washcloth, towel, baby shampoo, and clean clothes. Soap is not necessary for the young infant, but, if used, it should be gentle and nonalkaline to protect the natural acids of the infant's skin.

Give the bath in a room that is warm and free of drafts. Bathe the baby on a safe surface at a comfortable height for you. If you use a counter, pad it with blankets or towels.

Never leave the infant alone on an unprotected surface, even for a moment. Keep one hand on the infant at all times to prevent falls. Avoid answering the phone during bath time to avoid distractions. If you must leave the room, take the baby along or place the baby in the crib.

Before fully undressing the baby, use the football position to shampoo the baby's head. Although the fontanel or "soft spot" may seem delicate, it is covered with a tough membrane and is not injured by washing. Pulse movements in the fontanel are normal. Dry the hair well to prevent heat loss.

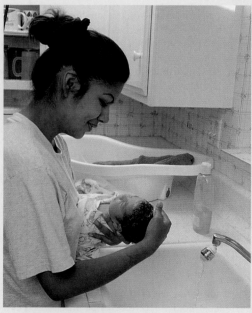

Keep the baby warm by uncovering only the area you are washing. Wash and dry one part of the baby's body at a time. Wash the face with clear water. Use a separate clean area of the washcloth to wipe across each eyelid and around each eye. Use a washcloth to clean in and around the ears, where milk may accumulate. Do not use cotton-tipped swabs in the infant's ears or nose, because injury may occur if the baby moves suddenly.

To clean the neck folds, put one hand under the baby's shoulders and lift slightly to cause the head to drop back enough that the creases in the neck can be washed. Clean the diaper area last.

Tub Bath

For a tub bath, use a plastic tub or a clean sink. Pad the bottom with a towel or foam pad to make it more comfortable and prevent the infant from slipping. Place enough warm water in the tub to cover the shoulders to prevent chilling. Wash the baby's face and hair before placing the baby in the tub. Keep the infant dressed until after the hair is washed to prevent chilling.

It may be easier, at first, to lather the infant's body and then immerse the baby in the tub for rinsing. It is not unusual for infants to be frightened when they are first put into the water. To help your baby adjust to this new experience, talk softly and calmly while holding the baby securely.

Keep the bath short so the baby does not get cold. Dry quickly, dress, and wrap the infant in two blankets for a short while to help the baby maintain heat.

Feeding

See Chapter 22 for information on breastfeeding and formula feeding.

Behavior

Knowing infants' different behavioral states helps you learn about your baby's individual characteristics.

Sleep Phases

During quiet sleep the infant sleeps soundly with quiet breathing and little movement. Your baby will not be disturbed by noises from appliances or other children at this time. In active sleep, the baby moves or fusses while still asleep. During the drowsy state, the baby is beginning to wake but may go back to sleep if not disturbed. However, if it is time for feeding or other activities, talk softly to help the baby awaken.

Awake Phases

The quiet alert state is a good time for infant stimulation and "play time." The quiet alert state lasts only a short time, and infants often need a break from interaction. Signs of overstimulation are present if the infant turns the head away; begins to cough, sneeze, hiccup, or spit up; or becomes fussy. They show the infant needs a short quiet time.

The active alert or "fussy" phase is a time when the infant may show hunger, discomfort, or fatigue. With intervention the baby may move back to the quiet alert state or eat and then go to sleep. If you do not intervene, the baby soon moves to the crying state.

The baby may use self-consoling measures such as sucking on a finger. However, if these efforts are not effective, parents should comfort the infant quickly. Babies who cry too long may not respond at first to care activities. A few minutes of rocking and holding close may be necessary before the infant settles down.

Socialization

Infants are social beings who enjoy contact with people. The baby should be part of family life. Use an infant seat or carrier to keep the baby near you and the rest of the family. Infants enjoy watching the human face. Hold your baby close, and talk to your baby to provide social stimulation.

PATIENT TEACHING—cont'd

Techniques of Infant Care

Stimulation

Babies respond best to gentle stimulation and enjoy a variety of types. They enjoy music that is not too loud. They focus their eyes best at a distance of 8 to 12 inches. Items such as mobiles should be placed within this range. Newborns especially like black and white geometric figures and bright colors. Infants respond to gentle stimulation when they are in the quiet alert state. Do not try to use stimulation techniques with a fussy infant. Overstimulation causes the baby to be irritable and have difficulty going to sleep.

Immunization

Immunization for hepatitis B is now included with other routine childhood vaccinations. Newborns of mothers with acute or chronic hepatitis B infection (hepatitis B surface antigen [HBsAg] positive) may become infected from exposure to the mother's blood at birth. Infected infants have a very high chance of developing chronic infection, which may later cause cancer or other serious liver disease.

These infants should receive both the vaccine and hepatitis B immune globulin (HBIG). HBIG provides passive immunity against hepatitis to protect infants until they develop their own antibodies and should be given within 12 hours of birth. The vaccine promotes antibody formation to protect infants from further exposure to the disease. The rest of the vaccine series is given in the health care provider's office or in a clinic.

Newborns of uninfected mothers also receive hepatitis B vaccine. It is often given during the stay in the birth facility but may also be given later in the pediatrician's office. A national voluntary standard for perinatal care is that all infants receive the appropriate hepatitis prophylaxis before discharge (National Quality Forum, 2012). Parents should be referred to their pediatrician for two more doses of the vaccine after discharge (see Drug Guide: Hepatitis B Vaccine and Drug Guide: Hepatitis Immune Globulin [HBIG]).

Newborn Screening Tests

Prompt identification and treatment of infants with conditions that can affect their survival or long-term health is essential. Newborns may be screened for critical congenital heart defects, hearing, metabolic, hematologic, and genetic disorders. Each state determines which specific tests are performed before discharge from the birth facility. Infants identified by these tests may need repeat screening or more complex diagnostic testing.

DRUG GUIDE

Hepatitis B Vaccine
Classification
Vaccine.

Other Names
Engerix-B, Recombivax HB.

Action
Immunization against hepatitis B infection.

Indications:
Prevention of hepatitis B in exposed and unexposed infants.

Neonatal Dosage and Route
Recombivax HB
5 mcg.

Engerix-B
10 mcg.

The first dose of hepatitis B vaccine is given to newborns before hospital discharge. The second dose of vaccine is given at age 1 to 2 months. The third dose is given at 6 to 18 months (at least 16 weeks after the first dose)

Infants of HBsAg-Negative Mothers
The usual routine is followed.

Infants of HBsAg-Positive Mothers
The vaccine is given within 12 hours of birth along with hepatitis B immune globulin (HBIG), which is given at a different site. The usual routine is followed for the rest of the series. The infant should be tested for HBsAg and antibody to HBsAg after completing three doses of vaccine.

Infants of Mothers Whose HBsAg Status Is Unknown
The vaccine is given within 12 hours of birth, and the mother is tested. If the HBsAg test is positive, the infant should receive HBIG as soon as possible and no later than 1 week of age. The usual routine is followed for the rest of the series. Give intramuscularly in the anterolateral thigh.

Absorption
Absorbed slowly; not affected by maternal antibodies.

Contraindications:
Hypersensitivity to yeast.

Adverse Reactions
Pain or redness at site, fever, fatigue, headache.

Nursing Considerations
If the solution is in a vial, shake well before preparing. Give vaccine within 12 hours of birth to infants of infected mothers. Do not inject intravenously or intradermally. Obtain parental consent before administering.

DRUG GUIDE

Hepatitis B Immune Globulin (Hbig)

Classification
Immune globulin.

Other Names
HBIG, Hep-B-Gammagee, HyperHEP.

Action
Provides antibodies and passive immunity to hepatitis B.

Indications
Prophylaxis for infants of hepatitis B surface antigen–positive mothers.

Neonatal Dosage and Route
0.5 mL within 12 hours of birth if possible but no later than 1 week of age; given intramuscularly in the anterolateral thigh; should not be given intravenously.

Absorption
Absorbed slowly.

Contraindications
None known.

Adverse Reactions
Pain and tenderness at the site, urticaria, anaphylaxis.

Nursing Considerations
Do not shake or give intravenously. Hepatitis vaccine series should begin within 12 hours of birth. Give injections of vaccine and immune globulin at separate sites.

Critical Congenital Heart Defect Screening

It is essential that critical congenital heart defects (CCHDs) be identified early after birth to prevent injury or death to infants. The AAP recommends pulse oximetry as a part of normal screening for all infants before discharge from the birth facility (Mahle et al., 2012). The screening should be done on the right hand and either foot with motion-tolerant oximeters after the first 24 hours of life. An oximetry reading of 95% or less in either extremity or 3% or more absolute difference between the upper and lower extremity requires further testing.

Hearing Screening

Approximately 12,000 infants are born in the United States each year with hearing impairment (CDC, 2014). It is the most common congenital abnormality in newborns (Cunningham & Sydlowski, 2016).

Because early detection and treatment can prevent or reduce developmental delays and help the child communicate better, auditory screening of all newborns within the first month is recommended. Infants who do not pass the screening should be rescreened, and if they still do not pass, they should have audiologic and medical evaluations by no later than 3 months of age (AAP Joint Committee on Infant Hearing, 2013).

A goal of *Healthy People 2020* is to increase the proportion of newborns who are screened for hearing impairment by age 1 month, have audiologic evaluation by age 3 months, and are enrolled in appropriate intervention services by age 6 months (U.S. Department of Health and Human Services [DHHS], 2010). To accomplish this goal, a screening test is usually given to infants before discharge from the birth facility.

Otoacoustic emissions and acoustic brainstem response tests are used for screening. The tests can be done while the infant sleeps. The nurse ensures that infants receive screening and explains the testing to the parents. An infant who fails the first screening is often retested in the birth facility. Parents of infants referred for further testing after discharge need more explanation and emotional support.

Other Screening Tests

Blood tests to screen for metabolic, hematologic, or genetic disorders are also performed. With early identification and treatment, infants with these conditions may avoid severe intellectual disability or other serious problems. Common disorders often included are phenylketonuria (PKU), hypothyroidism, galactosemia, hemoglobinopathies such as sickle cell disease and thalassemia, and congenital adrenal hyperplasia.

Screening tests are easy and inexpensive. They require a blood sample taken from the infant's heel, and only one blood sample is needed for all of the tests. The tests are performed at 24 to 48 hours after birth. Further testing is necessary to confirm any abnormal test results.

Parents may have questions for the nurse about the purpose of the tests. A pamphlet with information about the tests may be given to parents. Nurses often refer to the tests as "PKU tests," but they should call them "screening tests" instead to emphasize that a number of conditions are included.

Tests performed within the first 24 hours of life are less sensitive than those performed after 24 hours. Infants tested before age 12 to 24 hours should have repeat tests at age 1 to 2 weeks so disorders are not missed because testing was done too early (Botkin et al., 2016).

Commonly Screened Conditions

Phenylketonuria. PKU is a genetic condition in which the infant cannot metabolize the amino acid phenylalanine, which is common in protein foods such as milk. Although some phenylalanine is essential to growth, accumulations of it can result in severe intellectual disability. Treatment should be started by the third week of life (Braverman & Hamosh, 2016).

PKU is treated with a special low-phenylalanine diet, in which the amount of the amino acid is carefully regulated.

Congenital Hypothyroidism. Congenital hypothyroidism occurs when the thyroid does not produce enough thyroid hormones, which affect the entire body. Symptoms in an untreated infant include a hoarse cry, large fontanel and tongue, slow reflexes, abdominal distention, lethargy, and feeding problems and can lead to intellectual disability. Infants may have no signs in the early weeks, but early treatment with thyroid hormones is necessary to ensure normal growth and intellectual function.

Galactosemia. Absence of the enzyme necessary for the conversion of the milk sugar galactose to glucose causes galactosemia. The condition results in damage to the liver, increased susceptibility to infection, intellectual disability, and other developmental problems. Treatment includes a diet free of lactose and galactose. Long-term complications such as delayed growth and neurologic impairment may occur even with treatment.

Hemoglobinopathies. Hemoglobinopathies include sickle cell anemia, thalassemia, and other disorders. The conditions are most often found in infants of African, Mediterranean, Indian, or South and Central American background. The hemoglobinopathies cause chronic anemias, sepsis, and other serious conditions.

Congenital Adrenal Hyperplasia. The term *congenital adrenal hyperplasia* refers to a group of disorders with an enzyme defect that prevents adequate adrenal corticosteroid and aldosterone production and increases production of androgens. Infants may have ambiguous genitalia or masculinization of female infants at birth. Salt-wasting crisis with low sodium and glucose and high potassium levels may occur within the first week of life. Treatment is administration of corticosteroids and mineralocorticoids for the remainder of the child's life.

Other Conditions. Screening also may be performed for maple syrup urine disease, biotinidase deficiency, homocystinuria, cystic fibrosis, and other conditions. Each of these conditions can be accurately diagnosed in newborns so treatment can begin early. Knowing that many conditions are included in testing allows the nurse to explain its importance to the parents.

KNOWLEDGE CHECK

10. What are some important considerations in planning parent teaching?
11. What immunization may be performed at the birth facility?
12. Why is it important to perform screening tests on infants' blood as close to discharge as possible? For which infants is retesting important?

DISCHARGE AND NEWBORN FOLLOW-UP CARE

Discharge

Although state and federal legislation allows women and infants to stay in the birth facility for 48 hours after vaginal birth and 96 hours after cesarean birth, some women choose to go home earlier. The time of discharge varies according to the wishes and needs of the mother and the primary caregiver's assessment of conditions of the mother and baby.

Discharge is considered when term newborns who are appropriate for gestational age have normal physical examination results and show that they are making the transition from fetal to neonatal life without difficulty. Infants should have normal stable vital signs for the 12 hours before discharge, have fed successfully at least twice, passed urine and stool, and have no excessive bleeding at the circumcision site for at least 2 hours. Newborn laboratory and screening tests and evaluation for sepsis should have been completed. Hepatitis B vaccine should have been given or plans for administration made.

If infants have significant jaundice, plans for follow-up after discharge should be made or the infant's discharge may be delayed. The mother should have received teaching about infant care and should demonstrate knowledge, ability, and confidence to provide adequate care to the newborn. An appropriate infant car seat should be available at discharge. Family, environmental, and social risk factors should have been assessed and plans made to safeguard the infant as necessary. The family should have an adequate support system and have plans for continued care from a health care provider (AAP & ACOG, 2012).

Follow-Up Care

Care after discharge from the birth facility is very important. The AAP recommends that follow-up by a health care professional be provided within 48 hours for all newborns who are taken home from the birth facility less than 48 hours after birth. This care can be provided in the home, clinic, or office (AAP & ACOG, 2012). Any infant who is breastfeeding or has risk factors should be seen within the first week and usually within 2 to 3 days of discharge (Sullivan & Dela Cruz-Rivera, 2016).

HOME CARE OF THE INFANT

In the birth facility, parents often receive more information about care of the newborn than they can absorb. This may leave them inadequately prepared to cope with the multiple demands of early parenting. Family members, once the primary source of support for new parents, frequently live far away, and parents must rely on friends, health care personnel, child care classes, television, books, magazines and the Internet for information. Nurses are ideal sources of assistance in these situations and can also help parents evaluate the validity of information they receive from nonprofessional sources.

CARE AFTER DISCHARGE

Various programs have been instituted to provide after-discharge care for mothers and infants. They may include parenting and childbirth classes or nursing contact with the family in the home, in the clinic, or by telephone.

Home Visits

The home visit is ideally scheduled during the first 24 to 72 hours after discharge. This timing allows early assessment and

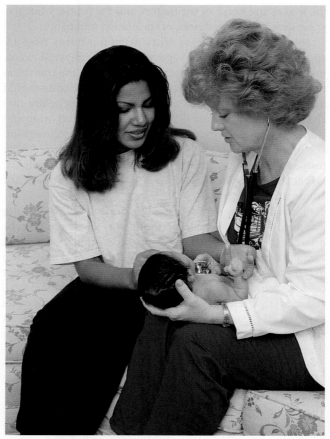

FIG. 21.9 During the home visit, the nurse performs a complete assessment of the infant. Here, she is checking the apical pulse and listening to breath sounds.

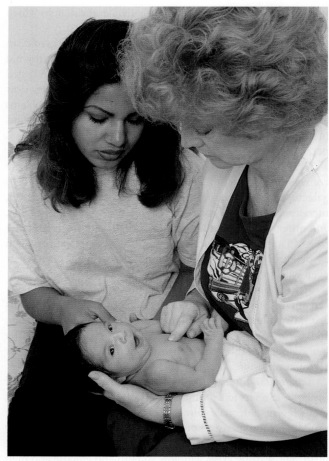

FIG. 21.10 Jaundice is especially of concern when infants are discharged early after birth. The nurse shows the mother how to blanch the skin to check for jaundice and discusses what the mother should do if she sees jaundice in her baby.

intervention for problems in nutrition, jaundice, newborn adaptation, and parent–infant interaction. Nurses may visit low-risk mothers and infants or may follow high-risk infants after discharge from the neonatal intensive care nursery (Figs. 21.9 to 21.12). Visits usually are 60 to 90 minutes to allow enough time for assessment and teaching. Home visits are expensive and are not available in all areas, but they do provide the most comprehensive care.

Visits to Low-Risk Families

During the home visit, the nurse performs a physical examination of the mother and the infant. Family adaptation to the addition of a new member and the adequacy of the mother's support system is also assessed. Reinforcement of the teaching that was begun at the birth facility is important. A feeding session should be observed, especially if the mother is breastfeeding. The nurse may take blood for metabolic screening if the infant went home too early to have had reliable testing in the birth facility. Safety in the home is often discussed, and questions about infant care and general parenting are answered.

Home visits provide reassurance for parents and may increase a woman's confidence and competence in caring for herself and her infant. The visits are especially valuable in recognizing jaundice and intervening before bilirubin levels become dangerously high. When jaundice is found, the nurse

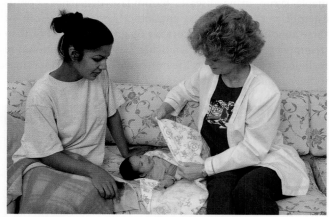

FIG. 21.11 The nurse discusses thermoregulation with the mother and demonstrates swaddling.

can discuss the implications and check the transcutaneous bilirubin level or draw blood for testing serum bilirubin levels. Appropriate care, including hydration and phototherapy, is discussed, as necessary.

Feeding is an area of concern for many mothers, especially if they are breastfeeding. When the nurse helps a woman cope with problems, the infant's intake may increase. Increased

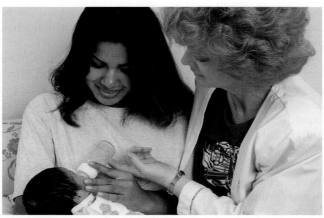

FIG. 21.12 The nurse observes a feeding during the visit to assess feeding techniques and provide a chance for parents to ask questions about feeding. This is a good time to assess parent–infant interaction. The infant is weighed to help determine adequacy of intake.

intake leads to greater bilirubin excretion, which may help avoid the need for phototherapy.

Visits to Families with High-Risk Infants

High-risk infants often need special care after discharge. Parents may be very anxious about assuming the care of an infant who has had a prolonged hospitalization. Many hospitals have programs that enable parents to take over their infant's care gradually before discharge.

A nurse may visit the home before the infant's discharge to help the family plan for accommodating the equipment and the type of care the infant needs. The home is checked for the availability of electricity, heat, and a telephone. If the family has a technology-dependent infant, the nurse checks that they have notified the utility companies and have battery backup to ensure that no disruption of services occurs.

After the infant is discharged, nursing visits can help the family maintain the infant's health and decrease the need for rehospitalization. Components of each visit vary according to the infant's needs. The nurse provides assessment of the infant and the parents' caregiving ability in addition to necessary teaching and nursing care.

Medically fragile infants may require home treatment with mechanical ventilation, oxygen therapy, or apnea monitors. Parents may have to perform such nursing skills as tracheostomy care, tube feedings, suctioning, and care of intravenous sites. Mothers often have concerns about feeding the infant, which may differ greatly from feeding a healthy full-term infant. Follow-up telephone calls from nurses between visits help families adapt to the needs of these infants and may also decrease the need for rehospitalization.

Infants with complications often need more frequent visits to the pediatrician or nurse practitioner or are rehospitalized during the early months after birth. Common problems include respiratory illness, infections (gastroenteritis, sepsis, urinary tract infections, otitis media), and need for surgery. These parents need information on preventive measures and care of the infant with an acute illness.

General Considerations in Home Visits

The nurse making a home visit is a guest of the family and should adapt nursing care to the home setting. The needs of other family members should be considered.

Careful planning before the visit is essential. The nurse calls to schedule the visit at a time convenient for the family. Setting priorities based on the needs identified by the nurse and the family is important. Strong communication skills and the ability to quickly develop rapport facilitates accomplishment of mutual goals. A brief social interaction may be beneficial at the beginning of the visit to develop a trusting relationship. The purpose of the visit should be explained and the family's expectations and desires discussed.

The nurse should be aware of any cultural practices affecting the family's view of care. In patriarchal cultures, the father is the head of the family and teaching should be performed through him. In some cultures, one or both grandmothers are important influences in the care of the mother and the infant.

After the visit, additional visits may be planned or the family may be given a telephone number to call to receive further help, if needed. The results of the assessments, teaching, nursing care, referrals, and plans for follow-up should be recorded. Copies of the record usually are sent to the primary caregiver. If problems are identified that need to be discussed with the primary care provider, a report is made by telephone.

Outpatient Visits

Outpatient visits may be provided in a pediatrician's office or in a birth facility clinic. Assessment and care are essentially the same as those provided for home visits. A feeding session is often observed for the lactating mother so the nurse may offer assistance.

The advantage of outpatient visits is that the nurse does not have to travel to the home and can see more patients each day, thereby reducing the cost of the service. Assessment of the home setting and family interaction, however, is not possible. Clinic visits usually last 30 to 45 minutes.

Telephone Counseling

Telephone counseling may be provided during follow-up calls to discharged patients or when parents call "warm lines" for help with problems or questions. The major disadvantage is that the nurse cannot perform an in-person assessment of the mother, baby, or home environment and must rely on the caller to present an accurate picture of the situation.

Follow-Up Calls

Follow-up calls are placed by nurses in the first few days after discharge. The nurse asks a series of questions to assess the physical condition of the mother and infant and to identify any needs or problems. All mothers may receive calls or only those considered at risk for problems. If problems are discovered, the nurse may schedule another call or a home visit or refer the woman to her primary care provider.

Warm Lines

Warm lines, also called *help lines* or *information lines,* provide parents with an opportunity to ask a nurse questions arising from the daily challenges of parenting. Warm lines are used for troubling, but not emergency, situations. The service should be available 24 hours a day and should be staffed by qualified nurses. Parents often call about infant feeding, breastfeeding concerns, postpartum blues, and basic care of the mother and infant. Calls last about 15 to 20 minutes. The nurse answers the caller's questions and assesses for other problems. The nurse may call back later to find out if the issue has been resolved.

Telephone Techniques

Nurses caring for patients by telephone should understand telephone counseling techniques. They need special education in telephone communication and triage.

Telephone triage involves determining the existence of and solution to a serious problem. The nurse should be skilled at soliciting information to identify problems and determining the priority of the problems identified.

The nurse should help the caller describe the major concerns, which may not be those discussed first. "What worries you most?" may help the caller focus on the most important problems. Although most problems discussed are concerns about normal infants, the nurse should be alert for "red flags" that signal serious situations needing immediate referral.

The patient should be allowed enough time to avoid feeling hurried. Lay terminology should be used and questions asked to elicit detailed description of the problems. Parents should be reassured that their questions are valued so they do not feel hesitant to ask what they may see as a "silly" question.

CRITICAL TO REMEMBER

Red Flags of Telephone Triage

An emergency situation (such as respiratory difficulty, bleeding). Tell the parent to call 9-1-1 or take the infant to a hospital emergency department immediately. Call back in 5 minutes to ensure that parents did seek help.

Illness (fever, dehydration, change in feeding or behavior, unusual rashes).

Severe feeding problems (infant may become dehydrated or jaundiced or may fail to thrive).

Problem has been present for longer than usual or usual remedies are ineffective (e.g., prolonged crying or sleeping, rash is spreading).

Parent's affect seems inappropriate for situation (extremely emotional with apparently minor situation or unconcerned when situation could be serious).

Note: Callers should be referred to the primary health care provider or the hospital emergency department, if necessary, when a serious problem may be present. Being overcautious is preferable. Refer parents to the primary care provider early rather than miss a serious situation.

Guidelines and Documentation

When nurses give care by telephone, they should have written protocols and policies that provide guidelines for care to ensure that all who perform this service provide patients with similar information. A list of common questions can be compiled to help nurses give appropriate information when parents call about a problem.

Parents should always be told when and how to seek more care if problems are not resolved. If the infant seems ill, referral to the pediatrician or hospital emergency department is most appropriate. The nurse's judgment, based on education, expertise, and experience, determines how helpful the service is to patients.

All calls should be documented so that accurate records are available for future reference. The nurse may use a checklist or a simple written description of the call. Documentation should include identifying information for the caller, reason for the call, problems described, advice given, and any referrals given. A copy of the information is sent to the primary caregiver to provide continuity of care.

? KNOWLEDGE CHECK

13. Where do parents obtain information about caring for their infant during the early weeks after birth?
14. What are some ways in which nurses offer follow-up services to new parents?

INFANT EQUIPMENT

Generally, parents obtain most of their baby equipment before the infant is born, but nurses may receive questions in the weeks after the birth. Although nurses should not recommend specific brand names of equipment, their guidance about features and safety is helpful.

Safety Considerations

Parents, especially those of limited means, need to understand that few, if any, pieces of equipment are absolutely essential for newborns. Infants sleep in padded dresser drawers and designer cribs with equal comfort. Safety is the most important consideration.

New equipment sold in the United States is generally safe because manufacturers are required to follow certain governmental standards for safety. A ruling by the U.S. Consumer Protection Safety Commission (2011) banned the sale of cribs with a side rail that drops down. Other changes included in the ruling have made cribs more durable and safer for infants.

Hand-me-down equipment may have been recalled by the manufacturer for safety defects. Parents can check with the Consumer Product Safety Commission (CPSC) for a list of recalled products at www.cpsc.gov. Older equipment should be checked carefully to ensure all parts are strong and working properly (Box 21.3). All nuts, screws, bolts, and hooks should be checked periodically to ensure that they are tight.

Car Safety Seats

Child safety seats for cars are essential to reduce injury and death to infants and children when accidents occur. An infant carried by an adult while in a car is never safe. Legislation

BOX 21.3   Safety Considerations for Infant Equipment

Cribs

Cribs that meet the new Consumer Protection Safety Commission guidelines should be used for infants.

If parents choose to use an older crib, an immobilizer should be added to prevent drop sides from moving. The crib should be checked frequently to be sure hardware is secured tightly and no loose, missing, or broken parts are present.

The crib mattress should fit snugly with only one finger able to fit into the space between the mattress and the sides of the crib. More room could allow the infant to become wedged in that space and possibly suffocate. The mattress should be firm. The crib should contain no loose bedding, pillows, or stuffed animals because they increase the risk for suffocation.

Crib toys or mobiles should be firmly attached, with no straps or strings within the infant's reach. Mobiles should be removed when the infant can reach them.

Cribs should be placed away from hanging cords of blinds or drapes, which could become wrapped around an active infant.

Cribs should be placed away from windows.

Other Equipment

Paint used to refurbish infant equipment should be marked "lead-free" and "safe for children's equipment" to prevent lead poisoning.

All parts should function properly: Highchair trays should stay firmly in place, latches should remain fastened, and so on. The frame and basic construction of all equipment should be sturdy.

All moving parts should be examined carefully to see whether little fingers could get caught or whether the infant could trigger a catch that would cause the equipment to become unsafe.

Safety straps for infant seats, swings, changing tables, high chairs, or other equipment must be in good condition. Straps should fit around the infant but not be long enough that the infant could become entangled.

Automatic swings should have legs that are stable so the swing does not tip over. Note how difficult it is to put the infant into the swing and remove the infant from the swing safely.

All toys should be examined carefully for parts that can be removed and swallowed. Small toys should have a diameter of more than 3.5 cm (1⅜ inches) and be at least 6.35 cm (2½ inches) long to prevent the infant from choking on them.

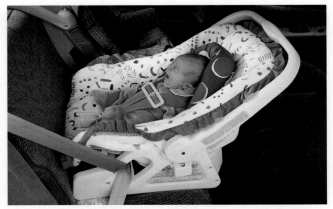

FIG. 21.13 A car seat for an infant under 2 years should face the rear of the car. Note the clip that holds the straps together for a snug fit.

Discharge teaching should include information about state car seat laws and the change in the age at which infants can move to a forward-facing seat. Infants should be placed in a rear-facing car seat when they are discharged from the hospital. The seat should recline at approximately a 45-degree angle (Fig. 21.13).

Car seats should be installed per vehicle and car seat manufacturer instructions (Box 21.4). Helpful information from the AAP is available at www.healthychildren.org.

Preterm and small infants may need special adaptations. Blankets or bolsters placed at the head, along the sides, and between the legs may improve the fit. Blankets and bolsters should not be placed under the infant. Some infants have low oxygen levels, bradycardia, or apnea when in a car seat. Facilities often have parents of infants who are less than 37 weeks of gestation or low birth weight bring their car seat to the hospital to test the infant's response to being placed in the seat. During testing, the infant's vital signs and oxygen level are monitored. Infants who have respiratory compromise in car seats may need to use special seats or beds designed specifically for preterm or low-birth-weight infants (Carter, Granty, & Carter, 2016).

In many agencies, nurses are not allowed to install car seats for parents. Some agencies have technicians on site who have special training to help parents determine whether car seats are correctly installed. Car seat fitting stations are available in some areas to determine whether car seats are used properly and to provide teaching for parents. A list of such stations is available at www.nhtsa.dot.gov/cps/cpsfitting/index.cfm. Further information about proper use of car seats, recall of seats, and a rating system of car seat brands is available on the Internet from sources such as the National Transportation Safety Board at www.nhtsa.gov.

has been passed in all 50 U.S. states requiring restraint of infants and young children in car seats when they are riding in automobiles.

Laws vary with regard to when and at what weight or height an infant or child can move from one type of car seat to another. The AAP had earlier recommended that infants be placed in a rear-facing seat until 12 months of age. The current recommendation is that rear-facing seats be used for infants until they are 2 years of age or have reached the highest weight or height allowed by the car seat manufacturer (AAP, 2016).

KNOWLEDGE CHECK

15. What advice can the nurse offer to parents about the safety features of equipment used for infants?
16. What should the nurse teach parents about buying and using a car seat?

BOX 21.4 Safety Considerations for Infant Car Seats

Use only car seats that are approved for use in automobiles. Seats designed for use in the home do not provide adequate protection in a car.

Use car seats that are appropriate for the infant's age and size. Place the seat in the center of the back seat of the car, never where an air bag is installed.

Use a rear-facing car seat placed in the back seat until your baby is at least 2 years old or reaches the highest height and weight recommended by the manufacturer. Never place the baby in the front seat of a car if there are passenger-side air bags.

Follow the manufacturer's directions for fastening the seat in the car and the infant in the car seat. Recheck the restraint straps each time the seat is used.

Be certain that the straps are tight enough to prevent the infant from getting out of the restraints or turning over in the seat. Infants who turn over can suffocate in the padding of the seat.

Be certain the infant cannot become caught with the straps tightly around the neck.

Use car seats only in an automobile. Do not place them on a soft surface such as a bed, where they might turn over and suffocate the infant.

Do not place car seats on surfaces from which they might fall, for example, grocery carts.

Never leave infants alone in a car, even for a few minutes. They could be kidnapped or injured in an accident involving the car even though it is parked. Cars quickly become very warm, and the infant could become dangerously overheated. To avoid "forgetting" that the infant is in the car, use available cell phone apps or simple reminders, like putting one shoe or your purse in the back seat with the infant.

EARLY PROBLEMS

Crying

Crying is a major parental concern during the early weeks after birth. Crying peaks at approximately 6 weeks of age at up to 3 hours a day. It usually decreases to 1 hour or less each day by 3 months (Feigelman, 2016). Crying is most frustrating to parents when they cannot find the cause for it. Infants cry for many reasons, including hunger, discomfort, fatigue, overstimulation, and boredom. Parents often can identify the problem on the basis of the type of sound made during crying. Sometimes no specific cause can be determined.

When the cause for crying is not obvious, some parents are afraid that responding may spoil the infant. If the infant stops crying when picked up, their concern may increase. However, changing the infant's position may help gas move in the intestines, relieve tired muscles, or distract the infant by changing the scenery, bringing about a temporary end of crying.

Infants cannot signal that they have unmet needs in any other way but by crying and are not spoiled when parents meet their needs. In fact, their needs should be met in a consistent, warm, and prompt manner for the development of trust to occur. Infants who are consistently held when in distress cry less at 1 year and are less aggressive at 2 years of age (Feigelman, 2016). Therefore parents should be taught the importance of consistently and quickly answering infant cries.

PATIENT TEACHING

Techniques to Relieve Crying in Infants

Treating Common Causes

Hunger—Try feeding the infant if it has been more than 30 minutes since the last feeding. A bubble of air may have caused a feeling of fullness too soon during the last feeding. The infant may be experiencing a "growth spurt" and need more frequent feedings for a day or two to provide necessary nutrients for rapid growth. However, avoid overfeeding the baby, because that may cause discomfort.

Air bubbles—Fussy infants may need more frequent burping during and after feedings compared with other infants. Try burping during crying spells because the infant may swallow air.

Diapers—Although most infants do not mind wet or soiled diapers, they may become cold or their skin may be irritated when diapers are not changed frequently enough.

Clothing—Check the infant's clothing for anything that could cause discomfort. Look for stiff seams, tags that are scratchy, or elastic that is too tight.

Warmth—Be sure that the infant is warm enough, but not too warm. The abdomen should feel warm even if the hands and feet are slightly cool. Dress a newborn as warmly as an adult would want to be dressed, but add a receiving blanket.

Infants who are overdressed rarely perspire but often cry because of their discomfort.

Overstimulation—Too many visitors handling the infant or too much noise and commotion in the household may be overstimulating the infant. Holding the infant in a quiet environment, rocking, or walking with the infant may be helpful.

Quieting Techniques

Rocking—The gentle motion of rocking, reminiscent of intrauterine life, is often soothing for infants.

Automatic swings—The continued motion of automatic swings may be helpful. Be sure they move smoothly and are not noisy. Getting the baby into and out of the swing should be easy to avoid awakening the infant. All parts of the body should be supported. Small infants may need padding with blankets for safety and comfort. Observe the baby throughout the time in the swing.

Walking, jiggling, swaying—Sometimes, newborns prefer a particular style of motion. Rocking sideways with the infant held in an upright position is helpful for some infants, whereas others prefer vertical rocking. Taking a walk outside with new sights and sounds may provide distraction.

PATIENT TEACHING—cont'd

Techniques to Relieve Crying in Infants

Skin-to-skin contact—Remove the baby's clothes and leave just the diaper. Place the baby against the parent's bare skin and cover both with a blanket. This skin-to-skin contact is often soothing to a young infant.

Swaddling—Wrap the infant snugly. This is comforting because infants are used to restricted activity in the uterus. Swaddling is especially helpful during the first few weeks after birth.

5Ss Technique—A combination of soothing techniques that includes *swaddling* with the infant in the *side* or stomach position, making *shushing* sounds while *swinging* the baby in the arms, and having the baby *suck* on a pacifier has been found to be calming for babies (Grover, 2014a; Harrington et al., 2012).

Stroller rides—The motion of a stroller may be soothing to some infants. The ride can be inside or outside the house. A parent can move a stroller back and forth with one foot while eating meals. The stroller should allow the infant to lie down rather than sit. Padding the stroller may increase comfort.

Car rides—Some infants go to sleep in a moving car. A short ride may put the infant to sleep. The infant may stay asleep when carried into the house.

Music—The sound of a parent singing or humming may be reassuring to the infant. Some newborns respond well to a music box, radio, or CD. Soft music with a steady beat or classical music may be particularly effective.

White noise—Background noise sometimes puts infants to sleep by diffusing other noises. A radio set on low volume, a clock ticking, an indoor fountain, a fan, or the sound of a dishwasher, dryer, vacuum cleaner, or shower may be effective. Tapes of sounds heard in utero are available.

Heat—A blanket warmed in the clothes dryer for a few minutes held against the infant's skin may be soothing. (Take care not to burn the infant's skin.) Do not use a heating pad. Placing the newborn in an infant seat on top of a dishwasher or clothes dryer provides heat and background noise. Be sure that the infant is well secured and watched at all times.

Bathing—Although older infants love baths, young infants may not yet have reached that stage. However, giving a bath may be a distraction for both parent and infant, and the infant may fall asleep after the bath.

Infant carriers or packs—Front carriers are designed for the young infant and may be especially helpful during crying episodes. A parent's warm body, soothing voice, and gentle swaying motion can often put an infant to sleep. At the same time, the parent can accomplish other tasks. Backpacks should be used only for older infants who are able to support the head well.

Pacifiers—Parents may find pacifiers useful for an irritable infant. The infant may be comforted by sucking even though not hungry.

Position changes—Try varying the infant's position. Laying the infant prone across a parent's lap (or over a warmed blanket) may help expel gas. Placing the infant in the supine position and gently flexing the knees on the abdomen may also help.

Massage—Gentle massage may be soothing for some infants. Massage of the abdomen may help infants with colic.

Taking turns—Ask your partner to take turns comforting the baby. This provides each partner with a chance to rest, and sometimes a different approach is effective.

Some families develop creative methods for dealing with crying infants. Others benefit from a nurse's suggestions about appropriate techniques to use.

Colic

Description

Colic is characterized by irritable crying for no obvious reason for 3 hours or more a day. It usually takes place during the late afternoon or evening on at least 3 days a week, lasting at least 3 weeks. It occurs in 10% to 20% of infants under 3 months of age. Colic begins at 2 to 3 weeks, peaks at 6 to 8 weeks, and ends at 3 to 4 months of age (Grover, 2014a). Some infants continue to have colic until 6 months of age. The infant is in good health, eats well, and gains weight appropriately despite the daily crying episodes. Both breastfed and formula-fed infants have colic.

Infants with colic cry as though in pain, draw their knees onto the abdomen or rigidly extend the legs, and may pass flatus. The crying is intense and may last until the infant falls asleep, exhausted. Because crying causes so much parental distress and may interfere with bonding or be a factor in parenting disorders or child abuse, nurses should find ways to provide support to parents of infants with colic.

Although many theories have been investigated, the cause of colic remains unknown. Allergies to cow's milk or to substances in the breastfeeding mother's diet, abnormal intestinal peristalsis, gastrointestinal tract or nervous system immaturity, feeding techniques such as overfeeding, and parental stress have all been considered. The cause is probably a combination of factors. Actual disease states should be ruled out before a diagnosis of colic can be made.

Interventions

Nursing interventions include using therapeutic communication to help parents express their frustrations and teaching techniques for coping with the problem. Parents should be encouraged to talk about their feelings and should be reassured that colic is temporary and does not indicate poor parenting. They often feel inadequate because of their failure to manage the problem and guilty if their frustration develops into anger.

The nurse should explain that it is not abnormal to have ambivalent feelings or even anger toward the infant. It is essential to take time away from infant care to rest and recoup energy needed to cope with the demands of a crying infant. Parents should leave the infant with a babysitter for short periods or take turns consoling the infant to provide breaks from the crying.

The techniques listed in "Patient Teaching: Methods to Relieve Crying in Infants" may temporarily alleviate crying caused by colic, but generally no technique gives prolonged relief. Feeding the infant in an upright position and burping frequently may help relieve discomfort caused by swallowed air. Use of the "5Ss" technique may be helpful (Grover, 2014a). Chamomile tea is often given to infants, because it has an antispasmodic effect. Any herbs the parents are using should be checked with the health care provider to ensure they are safe. Simethicone, an antiflatulent, has not been found effective, although some parents have reported that it helps (Baum, 2016; Grover 2014a).

A quiet environment, a calm approach, and a fairly regular schedule may help some infants with colic. Increasing the time spent carrying the infant often results in some improvement. Parents should be assured that spoiling does not result from responding to the infant's cries.

THERAPEUTIC COMMUNICATIONS
Coping with Crying

Linda tells her nurse, Daniel, about her daughter, Rebecca, who has been having crying spells every day lasting 4 hours or longer. Linda looks tired and worried. Rebecca, age 4 weeks, eats well, shows good weight gain, and is developing appropriately for her age.

Linda: It seems like all I do is try to stop Rebecca's crying. I can't get anything else done.

Daniel: You spend a lot of time trying to find ways to comfort her. *(Paraphrasing to encourage the mother to continue.)*

Linda: I've tried everything! I rock her, walk with her, feed her, and change her. We go for car rides and put her in her swing, but nothing works for long. She just starts crying again.

Daniel: It's so frustrating when nothing seems to work! *(Reflecting mother's feelings shows that the nurse is trying to understand them.)*

Linda: Sometimes I wonder if I was cut out to be a mother. I never thought it would be like this.

Daniel: Being a mother is so much harder than you expected that sometimes you aren't sure you made the right choice. *(Reflecting the content of what the mother said helps her focus and shows acceptance.)*

Linda: But I really do love her. I just don't know how to help her. I must be a terrible mother *(becomes teary).*

Daniel: Parents often feel guilty when they can't find a way to help an upset baby. Yet we really don't know all the reasons why babies cry. You've tried very hard to help Rebecca. Maybe we can work together to think of some other techniques to use. *(Gives reassurance that what the mother is feeling is normal, then offers information and further help.)*

Linda: I'd love that. It worries me to have Rebecca so unhappy. What else can I do for her?

One possible result of crying in infants is abusive head trauma (AHT), formerly known as *shaken baby syndrome*. AHT results from blunt trauma or shaking an infant vigorously enough to cause the soft tissue of the brain to bounce against the skull. Subdural or subarachnoid hemorrhage, retinal hemorrhage or detachment, skull and other fractures, and damage to the spinal cord may result. The infant may show little sign of external trauma.

AHT is the leading cause of deaths from child abuse in the United States. It causes death in 25% of babies who are shaken violently. The primary cause of AHT is inconsolable crying in an infant, usually 4 months of age of less (CDC, 2016).

Nurses can help prevent AHT by making parents aware of the danger in shaking infants and by helping parents learn methods to cope with infant crying and their own anger that may result from it. Parents are encouraged to share information about the dangers of AHT with other caregivers.

Birth facilities often include pamphlets and other information on AHT with discharge teaching. Various educational programs have been held in hospitals, middle and high schools, daycare facilities, and other community centers to increase the public awareness of the problem. Further information on AHT may be found at Internet sites such as the National Center on Shaken Baby Syndrome at www.dontshake.org.

❓ KNOWLEDGE CHECK

17. Why should parents respond to crying without fear of spoiling the infant?
18. How can nurses help parents of crying infants?

Sleep
Parents

During the early months after birth, parents often wonder whether they will ever get a full night's sleep again. Because they are so often up during the night, they should try to make up for lost sleep at other times. If the mother is not employed, she may be able to sleep during the day when the infant naps. If she is working, parents can alternate responsibility for night or early morning feedings. When mothers are breastfeeding, fathers can change the diaper, bring the infant to the mother for night feedings, and settle the infant back in bed when the feeding is finished. This allows the mother more time to sleep and lets the father share the middle-of-the-night care.

Infant Sleep Patterns

Although many newborns sleep 16 to 17 hours per day, there is wide variation in the amount of time infants spend sleeping. Infants sleep less deeply than adults and spend 50% of their sleep time in rapid eye movement (REM) sleep (Grover, 2014c). During this type of sleep, they sometimes make noises loud enough to wake parents in the same room, and they move about as if awakening. Going to them at this time is likely to wake them, but they may return to quiet sleep if left alone.

Infants should be positioned on the back for sleep. The nurse should explain that the prone position has been associated with SIDS. No pillows or soft stuffed animals should be placed in the crib because they could cause suffocation (see Fig. 21.3)

Sleeping through the Night

Parents are often confused about when infants should sleep through the night. Newborns are not ready to sleep through the night during the early weeks of life because of their neurologic immaturity. By 12 weeks of age, many infants sleep at least 5 hours at night and most infants sleep that long by 4 months. By 12 months of age, infants take two naps during the day and sleep about 10 hours at night (Grover, 2014c).

Once infants establish longer sleep patterns, they often awaken at night again when they are teething or ill. Therefore parents can expect to be awakened frequently during the early years. Parents should be taught methods of helping their infants achieve longer sleep periods at night.

PATIENT TEACHING

How to Help Infants Sleep through the Night

Allow infants to fall asleep at bedtime on their own instead of always rocking or feeding the infant. If rocking is used, place the infant into the bed when the infant is drowsy but not fully asleep. This may help the infant go back to sleep after awakening in the night even when alone.

Allow the infant who wakes during the night to cry for a few minutes before responding. The infant may not be completely awake and often returns to sleep if left undisturbed. However, once the infant is awake, respond quickly to meet the infant's needs.

Keep night feedings for feeding only. Avoid unnecessary activity, or the infant may learn to think of this as a playtime.

Use a soft light that provides only the amount of light essential for care.

Give night feedings in the infant's room to further avoid stimulation.

Keep sounds subdued. Soft music or humming may help the infant return to sleep, but talking should be kept to a minimum.

Keep night feedings short, and put the infant back to bed immediately.

Change diapers before beginning the feeding to avoid awakening the infant after feeding.

As infants near 12 weeks, when sleeping 5 or more hours is more likely, try patting them on the back instead of feeding.

Concerns of Working Mothers

Although it has been traditional for women who work to have at least 6 weeks of maternity leave, this is not always possible. Some women must return to work as early as 3 weeks after childbirth. The problems of working mothers are different from those of mothers who remain at home. They must find adequate child care, identify methods of managing the household, and try to find enough time and energy to meet the needs of the infant, other family members, and themselves.

Working mothers should not become so involved in their many responsibilities that they have little time for their own needs. Some mothers regularly schedule time for themselves and for family activities. Many working mothers find that the time they can spend with their infant is particularly precious.

Concerns of Adoptive Parents

Although adoptive parents have not experienced pregnancy and childbirth, they must make many of the same adjustments made by biologic parents. In some cases, adoptive parents meet the biologic mother during pregnancy and may even be with her during the birth. Other adoptive parents receive a call after months of waiting to be told that their new infant is ready for them. In both cases, the lives of the adoptive parents change abruptly.

In some agencies, adoptive parents receive the same teaching given to biologic parents. However, their ability to absorb information may be impaired by the excitement of the situation. Although adoptive mothers have not been pregnant or undergone childbirth, they are still tired from the loss of sleep and sudden changes they experience. This may be surprising and worrisome to some. They may have many questions that nurses can answer.

These parents need reassurance and emotional support as they experience this happy but exhausting time in their lives.

❓ CRITICAL THINKING EXERCISE 21.2

Mary and Skip received their adopted daughter, Susan, 3 days ago. They bring the 5-day-old infant to the pediatrician's office and discuss their concerns with the nurse. They received basic discharge teaching at the hospital where Susan was born but have many questions about infant care. The last two nights Susan slept very little, and both parents are exhausted. "We've waited so long to get Susan," Mary says, "but I'm beginning to wonder if she's all right and if I'll be a good mother."

Questions
1. What are the priorities in this situation?
2. How should the nurse support Mary and Skip?
3. What information should the nurse include in teaching these parents?
4. How should the nurse address Susan's nighttime wakefulness?

COMMON QUESTIONS AND CONCERNS

Dressing and Warmth

The infant should be dressed as the parents would like to be dressed, with a receiving blanket added. The abdomen should be checked to see if the infant is warm enough. The infant's hands and feet may be slightly cooler than the rest of the body but should not be mottled or blue. The infant's head should be kept warm because many thermal skin sensors are located in the scalp. A hat is appropriate if the infant is outside when it is cold or windy.

Stool and Voiding Patterns

Formula-fed infants generally pass at least one stool each day. Breastfed infants may pass a stool after every feeding or, occasionally in the older infant, only one stool every 2 to 3 days. Infants may get red in the face and appear to be straining when having a bowel movement, but this is normal behavior and does not indicate constipation. Stools that are dry, hard, and marble-like indicate constipation.

Watery stools indicate diarrhea. A watery stool is absorbed into the diaper with little or no solid material left at the surface. A "water ring" remains on the diaper, showing where the liquid was absorbed. Diarrheal stools occur more frequently compared with the infant's normal stool pattern and are greenish from bile moving quickly through the intestines. Diarrhea can be serious because life-threatening dehydration develops rapidly. Infants should be taken to the pediatrician or nurse practitioner for treatment.

The infant should have at least six wet diapers by the sixth day of life. If there are fewer voidings, feedings should be assessed. The mother should be nursing 8 to 12 times daily, and the formula-fed infant should be fed 6 to 8 times each day.

Smoking

Many mothers quit smoking before or during pregnancy but may not realize that preventing infant exposure to smoke is just as important after birth as before. Infants exposed to smoke from parents' cigarettes are more likely to develop frequent respiratory tract problems. Parental smoking is a risk factor in SIDS. Smoke absorption by infants occurs even when smoking is done in another room. Parents who continue to smoke should do so outside the house and away from the infant.

Eyes

Parents can remove small amounts of mucus that accumulate in the corners of the eyes with a damp, clean washcloth, using a separate section for each eye. A large amount of mucus, redness, or excessive tearing indicates an infection or a blocked lacrimal duct. The infant should be seen by the pediatrician or nurse practitioner.

Transient **strabismus**—misalignment or deviation of one or both eyes—is sometimes called "crossing" of the eyes. Although the condition is normal for the first 2 to 3 months, it can be frightening to parents. The nurse should reassure them that it will end after the first few months, when the infant gains control of the small muscles of the eye. It does not indicate that the infant will have later problems. Strabismus that continues after 4 months should be evaluated by an ophthalmologist (Rosales, 2014).

Baths

Bathing, cord care, and care of the circumcision site are discussed earlier. If the infant is washed well at diaper changes and when milk is regurgitated, bathing the child every day is not necessary. Bathing should be a time for infant stimulation and parent–infant interaction. It can be done at any time of the day that is convenient for parents.

Nails

Nails should be cut straight across with either blunt-ended scissors or clippers. Pressing down on the skin at the fingertip makes it easier to avoid cutting the skin. Nail edges can be carefully smoothed with an emery board. Some mothers prefer to cut nails while the infant is sleeping. Others have someone else hold the baby's hand steady while cutting nails. Nails grow rapidly and may need trimming once a week.

Sucking Needs

Parents often have questions about pacifiers and thumb sucking or finger sucking. All infants have an urge to suck, although the amount of sucking needed varies with individual infants. Some infants seem satisfied by feedings, but others suck their fingers or a pacifier even when not hungry. The AAP recommends the use of pacifiers for sleep and to help prevent SIDS. Use may be delayed until 1 month in breastfeeding infants (AAP Task Force on Sudden Infant Death Syndrome, 2016).

Parents may be concerned that sucking on a pacifier or thumb will cause the teeth to become maloccluded. The nurse should reassure them that sucking that is not all day long, or on an upside down pacifier, and that ends before the secondary teeth begin to erupt is unlikely to cause malocclusion (Berkowitz, 2014).

In some infants, nonnutritive sucking increases because the time they spend sucking during feedings is too short. Breastfed infants should be allowed to continue sucking at the breast long enough to meet basic sucking needs. A short time of sucking after the end of feeding generally satisfies the infant's sucking needs and increases production of milk. For formula-fed infants, bottle nipples should have small holes and be replaced every couple of months before they get soft.

When infants use a pacifier, parents should be instructed to examine it often to see if it is in good condition. Cracked, torn, or sticky nipples or nipples that can be pulled away from the shield should be discarded. Pacifiers should be replaced every month or two because they may come apart as they deteriorate and cause aspiration of parts. The shield on the pacifier should be large enough that it cannot be pulled into the mouth. Pacifiers should not have any decorations that might come off and cause a choking hazard.

Pacifiers should be kept clean by frequent washing, and parents should buy several so that a clean one is always available when needed. Pacifiers should never be placed on a string around the infant's neck. The string could become tangled tightly around the neck and cause strangulation. Clips with a short band to attach pacifiers to the infant's clothing without danger are available, or several pacifiers can be placed in the bed for the infant to find.

Some parents find that one advantage of pacifier use is that the infant gives it up more quickly than a thumb or finger because it is not so easily accessible. Parents who resort to the use of a pacifier as the first response when the infant is fussy are likely to reinforce its use and increase dependence on it. Pacifiers used only after other causes of distress are ruled out may be given up sooner by the infant. Because the need for nonnutritive sucking begins to diminish between 4 and 6 months of age, pacifier use may begin to decrease at that time with parents' help.

Common Rashes

Diaper Rash (Diaper Dermatitis)

Diaper rash occurs as a result of prolonged exposure of skin to wetness, urine, feces, and friction against the diaper. A rash is more likely to develop when infants begin to sleep for longer periods and the time between diaper changes increases. Another cause may be sensitivity to commercial disposable wipes or components of paper diapers.

Diaper rash is primarily treated by keeping the diaper area clean and dry. The nurse should instruct the parents to change diapers as soon as they are wet or soiled. They should gently wash the perineum with mild soap and warm water but should avoid excessive washing or scrubbing. If commercial wipes are used, they should be free of alcohol, perfumes, or preservatives. Removing the diapers and exposing the perineum to warm air helps healing.

Applying a thin layer of zinc oxide or petrolatum may speed healing and help prevent recurrence. Vigorous rubbing to remove the skin barrier product is not necessary. Gentle cleansing to remove the soiled layer of barrier in the skin folds is adequate (AWHONN, 2013). Low-potency corticosteroid preparations may be necessary for severe cases. Talc-based powders should not be used because they can cause pneumonia if they get into the infant's lungs.

Secondary infection of diaper rash with organisms such as *Candida albicans* or *Staphylococcus* is common. When infection occurs, severe rash, pustules, or crusted areas may appear. The infant should be taken to a pediatrician or nurse practitioner for treatment. Antifungal or antibiotic creams may be necessary for infections.

Miliaria (Prickly Heat)

Although most common during hot weather, **miliaria**, or prickly heat, develops in infants who are too warmly dressed in any weather. It may also occur in infants with a fever. This rash results from occlusion and inflammation of the sweat (eccrine) glands. It has a red base with papules or clear vesicles in the center.

Treatment involves cooling the infant by removing excess clothing or by giving a soothing lukewarm bath. The condition clears quickly with removal of the cause, and ointments or other skin preparations should be avoided. The nurse should discuss the appropriate amount of clothing with parents when infants develop prickly heat.

Seborrheic Dermatitis (Cradle Cap)

Seborrheic dermatitis is a chronic inflammation of the scalp or other areas of the skin characterized by yellow, scaly, oily lesions. It sometimes results when parents do not wash the anterior fontanel for fear that they will hurt the infant.

Treatment is application of oil or shampoo to the area to help the lesions soften and then removal with a comb or soft brush before shampooing the head. The nurse should teach parents how to shampoo the scalp and explain that they will not injure the fontanel by normal gentle shampooing. The scalp should be rinsed well to remove all soap, which otherwise may cause irritation. A persistent problem may be treated with hydrocortisone cream or special shampoos recommended by the pediatrician or nurse practitioner.

Feeding Concerns

Breastfeeding, formula feeding, and weaning are discussed in Chapter 22. This section addresses only regurgitation and introduction of solid foods.

Regurgitation

Infants often regurgitate ("spit up") because they may eat more than the stomach can easily hold and because the immature lower esophageal sphincter allows the stomach contents to flow into the esophagus easily. "Wet burps" result when air is trapped under the stomach contents. As the air is expelled, a small amount of milk comes with it.

The nurse should teach parents to differentiate normal spitting up from vomiting, which is a sign of illness. Regurgitation may occur frequently but is usually only a small amount at a time. Vomiting may involve the entire feeding, and it is expelled forcefully. Parents should always seek treatment for the infant with projectile vomiting, in which the vomitus is expelled with such force that it travels some distance.

If an infant has frequent regurgitation, place the infant in a more upright position during and for a short time after feedings. Small, more frequent feedings also may help. Some infants swallow excessive air because they feed rapidly. Nurses can instruct parents to feed infants before they get too hungry and to stop often for burping. If the hole in a bottle nipple is too small, an infant may swallow the air around the nipple. Enlarging the nipple hole slightly with a hot needle may prevent this. The hole should not be too big or the flow of milk may be too fast and cause choking.

The infant who has excessive regurgitation or vomiting should be referred for follow-up with the pediatrician or nurse practitioner.

Introduction of Solid Foods

Infants do not need solid foods until 6 months of age. It is recommended that infants should have only breast milk for the first 6 months (AAP & ACOG, 2012). Some mothers introduce solids earlier in the hope that the infant will sleep longer at night. This is seldom successful because the infant receives no more calories from the small amounts of solids taken than from breast milk or formula. When infants are started on solids, they drink less milk, thus replacing a food that meets their nutrient needs well with a food that is poorly digested.

The **extrusion reflex**, in which infants push the tongue out against anything that touches it, continues until approximately 4 to 6 months of age (Eiger, 2016). This makes feeding a younger infant difficult because the infant pushes almost all of every spoonful out of the mouth. The nurse should explain the problems involved with early introduction of solid foods and encourage parents to wait until the infant is physiologically ready, at 6 months of age. The concerns that made the parents consider changing the feeding routine should also be discussed.

Growth and Development
Anticipatory Guidance

Parents often have questions about normal patterns of growth and stages of development. Nurses provide anticipatory guidance about these areas to help parents develop realistic expectations about infants' abilities at various ages.

Growth and Developmental Milestones

A brief summary of the changes that can be expected during the infant's first 12 weeks is included here. More in-depth information is found in pediatrics textbooks. The nurse should emphasize to parents that guidelines are only averages, the range of normal is often broad, and individual differences are expected.

Growth proceeds at a predictable rate in normal infants. The weight lost after birth is usually regained by 14 days of age. In the first 3 months, the average infant gains approximately 1 oz (30 g) each day and 2 lb (0.9 kg) per month. Each month they grow 1.4 inches (3.5 cm) and have an increase in head circumference of 0.8 inch (2 cm) (Keane, 2016). The posterior fontanel closes by 2 months and the anterior fontanel by 18 months of age (Benjamin & Furdon, 2015). Tears are scant or absent for the first 2 months of life (Kaur & Campbell, 2016).

Parents are especially interested in the Moro, grasp, and rooting reflexes. The nurse should point out that their gradual disappearance helps prepare the infant to learn new skills such as voluntary grasping or turning over, which are impossible if the reflexes continue. The infant gradually develops more control of the heavy head and has less bobbing or head lag by the end of the third month.

Infants are social beings. They stare at objects of interest and focus best within a range of 8 to 12 inches (20 to 30 cm) as newborns (Blackburn, 2013). By 3 months, infants can follow interesting objects horizontally across the midline (Gundy, 2016). A social smile begins at 1 to 3 months. Infants start making vowel sounds ("cooing") at 1 to 4 months and laugh at 3 to 6 months (Grover, 2014b).

Accident Prevention

Knowing what infants can do helps prevent accidents. In the first 3 months after birth, they are totally helpless. Although they can communicate their needs through crying, someone must be available at all times to care for them. Parents should be taught the dangers of leaving the infant on any unprotected surface, even for seconds. In a short time, an infant can wiggle from the middle to the edge of a large bed and fall.

If parents must turn away, they should keep one hand on an infant lying on an unprotected surface. Infants should never be left, even for an instant, in even 1 inch of water because of the danger of drowning. Parents should turn the telephone off or take it with them and ignore the doorbell while bathing the infant. If they must leave the room, parents should take the infant out of the water and with them.

As infants learn to grasp objects with increasing accuracy (4 months), parents should be certain that nothing that could be swallowed or otherwise cause harm is within the infant's reach. Help parents think ahead to the time when the infant will be crawling and walking and make plans for how they will "child-proof" their home.

Well-Baby Care
Well-Baby Checkups

Well-baby checkups are an opportunity for the pediatrician or nurse practitioner to assess the infant's growth and development, answer questions about feeding and infant care, observe for abnormalities, and give immunizations. These checkups may be provided by a private practitioner or in a well-baby clinic where examinations and immunizations are free or at reduced cost. Infants are usually taken to their first checkup between 48 hours to 2 weeks after discharge from the birth facility. They generally receive well-baby checkups at 1, 2, 4, 6, 9, and 12 months of age (Hagan & Duncan, 2016). Anticipatory guidance is a major part of well-baby visits. Safety is discussed as parents are taught about skills infants will soon develop that might place them in danger.

Immunizations

Nurses often receive questions about the need for immunizations for uncommon diseases, such as diphtheria, that parents have never seen. Parents may consider a condition such as varicella (chickenpox) to be a harmless childhood illness. When they do not understand the need for immunizations, parents may be reluctant to have their infants undergo painful procedures.

The nurse should explain to parents the importance of immunizations, briefly describing the serious illnesses that are prevented by immunizations. Discuss the age at which each immunization is given and when boosters are needed. Because recommendations for immunizations change from time to time, parents should be referred to their pediatrician for the latest information. Another source is the AAP website (www.aap.org), which offers information for parents as well as professionals.

In the United States, national health objectives for the year 2020 include achieving and maintaining effective vaccination coverage levels for universally recommended vaccines among young children with targets of 85% to 90% depending on the vaccine (DHHS, 2010). Maintaining a high level of immunization is important to prevent the rise of communicable diseases, as has happened in the past when a resurgence of measles occurred in many U.S. communities.

Illness

Parents have many questions about illnesses in the infants. They have concerns about how to recognize an illness and when to call the pediatrician or nurse practitioner.

Recognizing Signs

Parents may need help in recognizing signs of illness in infants (Box 21.5). The nurse should explain that any time the infant appears sick or parents think something is wrong with the infant, they should call the pediatrician or nurse practitioner. Office staff is usually educated to help parents determine whether the infant is sick enough to need an appointment.

Calling the Pediatrician or Nurse Practitioner

When calling the health care provider about an illness, parents should prepare by writing down the information about the illness to avoid forgetting something. They should have the name and telephone number of a pharmacy available in case a prescription drug is needed, and they should be ready to write down instructions (Box 21.6).

Office staff members are usually able to answer questions on the telephone about common concerns and simple illnesses. They can help determine whether an infant should be seen by the health care provider, but parents should be assertive in asking for an appointment if they believe that one is needed. Parents should immediately identify emergencies so that the staff can act accordingly.

Knowing When to Seek Immediate Help

Parents should take the infant to the pediatrician or to a hospital if signs of dyspnea are present. An infant from birth to 3 months of age should not have a sustained respiratory rate above 60 breaths per minute. If retractions, cyanosis, or extreme pallor is present, parents should get immediate help. If respiratory difficulty occurs suddenly in an infant who is well, the infant may have aspirated a feeding or small object. Parents should call the emergency medical services (EMS). Nurses should encourage all parents to take classes in cardiopulmonary resuscitation.

If an infant's respiratory rate is below 30 breaths per minute, parents should stimulate the infant and see if the respirations increase and stay within the normal range of 30 to 60 breaths per minute. If the respiratory rate continues to be below normal, the infant should be seen by a pediatrician, by a nurse practitioner, or at a hospital.

Parents should call the pediatrician if the infant is hard to arouse and keep awake. The infant could be semicomatose and showing signs of a central nervous system disease such as meningitis or encephalitis.

Learning about Sudden Infant Death Syndrome

Sudden infant death syndrome (SIDS) is the abrupt death of an infant younger than 1 year of age that is unexplained by history, autopsy, or examination of the scene of death. In the United States approximately 2250 infants die of SIDS each year. It is the third leading cause of death in infants from birth to 1 year of age and the most common cause of death in infants from 1 month to 1 year of age (CDC, 2014c).

SIDS occurs in apparently healthy infants during sleep and more often in male infants. It peaks in infants who are 2 to 3 months of age, and 90% of SIDS cases occur before 6 months of age (Smith, 2014). African-American, American Indian, and Alaska Native infants are two to three times more likely to have SIDS. The incidence is lower in Asian, Pacific Islander, and Hispanic infants (Keys & Rankin, 2015).

There have been many studies, but the cause of SIDS remains unknown. Sleeping in the prone position; sleeping on a soft surface; overheating; maternal smoking or drug use during or after pregnancy; young maternal age; low socioeconomic status; late or no prenatal care; prematurity, low birth weight, and male gender; and prenatal exposure to nicotine, alcohol, and illicit drugs have been associated with SIDS. Risk for SIDS is increased when infants sleep in the same bed with another person; on adult beds or sofas; or with pillows, stuffed toys, or loose bedding; or become overheated during sleep. Bed-sharing with a parent is controversial and not recommended at this time (AAP Task Force on Sudden Infant Death Syndrome, 2016; Keys & Rankin, 2015).

The current AAP Task Force (2016) recommendation is that a healthy infant be placed in the supine position for sleep because the prone position may increase the risk for upper airway obstruction, rebreathing of expired air, and hyperthermia. A national goal for the year 2020 is to reduce the number of SIDS deaths by increasing to at least 75.9% the number of infants who are put to sleep on their backs (DHHS, 2010). Approximately 20% of SIDS cases occur when the caregiver is not the parent (Smith, 2014). Parents should ensure that all caregivers of their child are aware of the risk associated with the prone position and follow the guidelines.

Nurses should teach parents about the AAP recommendations for the supine position for sleep and give parents educational material about the position. It is important for nurses to model this behavior in addition to teaching about it. For suggestions on modifying some risk factors, see "Patient Teaching: How to Help Prevent Sudden Infant Death Syndrome"?

Parents may be concerned about abnormalities in head shape that may occur in some infants from sleeping on the back. Flattening of the head may result from prolonged lying in the supine position. This can be prevented by the parents placing the infant in the prone position on a firm surface during awake periods several times a day while watching the infant.

Parents should be taught the importance of "tummy time" to help develop the shoulder muscles as well as prevent plagiocephaly. The prone position helps the infant develop neck, shoulder, and arm muscles. Toys placed within reach can help infants focus and begin to reach for objects. The position also helps the infant attain developmental milestones such as rolling over and crawling.

Infants tend to look toward the center of the room or the door when in their beds. Placing the infant at alternating ends of the crib often influences the direction of turning the head and distributes pressure more evenly. Avoiding prolonged time in car seats or other seats and holding the baby in an upright position some of the time may also help. Infants who develop flattening of the head should spend very little time in infant seats, swings, or car seats because these put pressure on the back of the head.

Because parents often have many concerns about SIDS, therapeutic communication techniques may assist them to talk about their fears. They may need reassurance that the chance that any one infant will experience SIDS is small. When parents have experienced loss of an infant from SIDS, they need appropriate counseling. One organization that provides this is First Candle, which can be reached at 1-800-221-SIDS or www.firstcandle.org.

> **? KNOWLEDGE CHECK**
>
> 25. When should immediate help be sought for an infant?
> 26. What should nurses teach parents about SIDS?

PATIENT TEACHING

How to Help Prevent Sudden Infant Death Syndrome

The following are suggestions that may help prevent sudden infant death syndrome (SIDS):

Always place the baby on his or her back for sleep, whether for naps or at night. Never allow the infant to be placed on the abdomen or side for sleep.

Ensure all other caregivers (babysitters, daycare workers, relatives) position the baby properly for sleep.

The infant's sleep surface should be firm. Do not put the baby to sleep on a couch, armchair, soft mattress, or waterbed.

Do not let the baby sleep with any other person, whether an adult or a child.

If you feed your infant while you are in bed, put the baby back into the infant's bed when you are ready to sleep.

The infant's bed should be placed in the parent's room.

Do not put any loose bedding, comforters, quilts, pillows, bumper pads, sheepskins, positioning devices, stuffed toys, or any soft items in the baby's bed.

Dress the baby in pajamas, sleepers, or a sleep sack instead of using blankets.

If blankets are used, place them no higher than the baby's waist and tuck the edges under the mattress to prevent blankets from covering the infant's face.

Do not let the infant get overheated. Dress the baby appropriately.

Consider giving the baby a pacifier for sleep. If you are breastfeeding, wait until the baby is 1 month old and breastfeeding is well established before giving the pacifier for sleep, if you wish. If the pacifier falls out during sleep, it is not necessary to reinsert it.

Do not smoke during or after birth or let anyone smoke around your baby.

Avoid alcohol and illicit drug use during pregnancy or after birth.

If possible, breastfeed your baby, because breastfeeding has been found to protect infants from SIDS.

To prevent flattening of the head, several times each day place your baby on his or her abdomen for "tummy time" when the baby is awake and you can watch the baby. This also helps develop the muscles of the baby's upper body.

Do not let infants sleep routinely in sitting devices such as car seats, strollers, and swings because infants may slump enough to obstruct the airway.

SUMMARY CONCEPTS

- Prophylaxis against vitamin K–deficiency bleeding (hemorrhagic disease of the newborn) and ophthalmia neonatorum is necessary shortly after birth. It is provided by an injection of vitamin K and use of erythromycin ophthalmic ointment.

- Newborns may need help with clearing the airway. Positioning, wiping secretions from the nose and mouth or suctioning, and close observation may be necessary.

- Nurses can prevent heat loss in newborns by keeping them dry and covered, avoiding contact between newborns and cold objects or surfaces, and keeping newborns away from drafts and exterior windows and walls.

- The nurse should identify actual or potential hypoglycemia and intervene appropriately.

- Important interventions for jaundice are to assess for its presence, ensure the infant is feeding well, and explain the condition to the parents.

- Parents should be taught to place infants supine for sleep to prevent sudden infant death syndrome. Infants should have supervised periods of lying prone while awake each day.

- The nurse should prevent mistaken identification of infants by checking the mother's and infant's identification whenever they have been separated.

- Parents and nurses should work together to prevent infant abductions. Parents should know how to identify hospital staff. Nurses should be alert for suspicious behavior.

- Infection can be best prevented by scrupulous handwashing by staff and all who come in contact with newborns.

- Reasons parents may choose circumcision are to decrease the risk of certain conditions, for religious reasons, parental preference, or lack of knowledge about care of the foreskin.

- Parents reject circumcision because of belief that uncommon conditions do not necessitate surgery and pain in infants and concerns about the complications that can occur.

- Risks of circumcision include hemorrhage, infection, unsatisfactory cosmetic effect, urinary retention, urethral stenosis or fistulas, adhesions, necrosis, injury to the glans, and pain during and after surgery.

- Infants who are circumcised should have pain relief provided. Dorsal penile nerve block along with non-pharmacologic methods of pain relief such as oral sucrose are often used.

- Parents of uncircumcised infants should be taught not to retract the foreskin until it becomes separated from the glans later in childhood.

- Parents of circumcised infants should be taught signs of complications and how to care for the area.

- Every nursing contact with parents should be used as an opportunity to teach.

- Screening tests are commonly performed to rule out cardiac and hearing abnormalities, phenylketonuria, hypothyroidism, galactosemia, congenital adrenal hyperplasia, and hemoglobinopathies.

- Nurses assist parents after discharge by way of home or clinic visits and telephone calls.

- Careful planning, good communication skills, and knowledge of cultural practices are necessary during home visits.

- Outpatient visits include the same assessment and teaching as home visits but do not allow the nurse to assess the home. They are, however, more cost-effective.

- Telephone calls after discharge from the birth facility are less expensive than home or clinic visits but do not allow the nurse to assess the patient or home environment in person.

- All equipment, particularly older, used articles, should be checked by parents for safety.

- Infants should use a rear-facing car seat until they are 2 years old or have reached the greatest weight and height recommended by the manufacturer. Older children need car seats that face forward. All should be placed in the back seat of the car.

- Crying is a major source of concern for parents. They should be reassured that infants are not spoiled by prompt attention to their needs.

- Colic—crying without obvious cause that lasts 3 or more hours a day—usually occurs in the afternoon or evening and often disappears after 3 to 4 months. The cause is unknown, and infants with colic grow and develop normally.

- The nurse can help prevent abusive head trauma (shaken baby syndrome) by teaching parents not to shake their baby and helping them cope with crying.

- Infants may sleep 5 or more hours at night by about 12 weeks.

- Diaper rash may be caused by prolonged exposure to wet and soiled diapers or sensitivity to substances in diapers or disposable wipes. The rash can become infected.

- Solid foods should be started at 6 months of age when the extrusion reflex is gone and solids can be digested by infants.

- Well-baby checkups are important for assessment of growth and development and to provide guidance and immunizations. Immunizations safeguard infants and communities from spread of communicable diseases.

- Parents should learn signs of illness in the infant and when immediate medical care is necessary. They should seek immediate medical attention if infants have respiratory difficulty or are difficult to arouse from sleep.

- The nurse should teach parents about current knowledge about SIDS and the fact that the cause remains unknown. Parents should be taught to place their infants in the supine position for sleep in their own beds.

REFERENCES & READINGS

American Academy of Pediatrics Joint Committee on Infant Hearing. (2013). Supplement to the JCIH 2007 position statement: Principles and guidelines for early hearing detection and intervention programs. *Pediatrics, 131*(4), e1324–e1349.

American Academy of Pediatrics (AAP). (2016). *Car safety seats: a guide for families 2016*. Elk Grove Village, IL: Author.

American Academy of Pediatrics (AAP). (2017). *Circumcision problems*. Retrieved from www.healthychildren.org.

American Academy of Pediatrics & American College of Obstetricians and Gynecologists (AAP & ACOG). (2012). *Guidelines for perinatal care* (7th ed.). Elk Grove, IL: American Academy of Pediatrics.

American Academy of Pediatrics (AAP) Joint Committee on Infant Hearing. (2013). Supplement to the JCIH 2007 position statement: Principles and guidelines for early hearing detection and intervention programs. *Pediatrics, 131*(4), e1324–e1349.

American Academy of Pediatrics (AAP) Task Force on Circumcision. (2012a). Circumcision policy statement. *Pediatrics, 130*(3), 585–586.

American Academy of Pediatrics (AAP) Task Force on Circumcision. (2012b). Male circumcision. *Pediatrics, 130*(3), e757–e785.

American Academy of Pediatrics (AAP) Task Force on Sudden Infant Death Syndrome. (2016). SIDS and other sleep-related infant deaths: updated 2016 recommendations for a safe infant sleeping environment. *Pediatrics, 138*(5), 1–12.

Association of Women's Health, Obstetric and Neonatal Nurses (AWHONN). (2013). *Evidence-based clinical practice guideline: Neonatal skin care* (2nd ed.). Washington, DC: Author.

Baum, R. A. (2016). Colic. In T. K. McInerny, H. M. Adam, D. E. Campbell, T. G. DeWitt, J. M. Foy, & D. M. Kamat (Eds.), *Textbook of pediatric care* (2nd ed.) (pp. 1931–1934). Elk Grove Village, IL: American Academy of Pediatrics.

Benjamin, K., & Furdon, S. A. (2015). Physical assessment. In M. T. Verklan & M. Walden (Eds.), *Core curriculum for neonatal intensive care nursing* (5th ed.) (pp. 110–145). St. Louis, MO: Saunders.

Berkowitz, C. D. (2014). Thumbsucking and other habits. In C. D. Berkowitz (Ed.), *Pediatrics: A primary care approach* (5th ed.) (pp. 291–295). Elk Grove Village, IL: American Academy of Pediatrics.

Blackburn, S. T. (2013). *Maternal, fetal, and neonatal physiology: A clinical perspective* (4th ed.). Philadelphia: Saunders.

Botkin, J. R., Rothwell, E., Anderson, R. A., Rose, N. C., Dolan, S. M., Kuppermann, M., Wong, B. (2016). Prenatal education of parents about newborn screening and residual dried blood spots. *JAMA Pediatrics, 170*(6), 543–549.

Braverman, N. E., & Hamosh, A. (2016). Recognition of genetic-metabolic diseases by clinical diagnosis and screening. In T. K. McInerny, H. M. Adam, D. E. Campbell, T. G. DeWitt, J. M. Foy, & D. M. Kamat (Eds.), *Textbook of pediatric care* (2nd ed.) (pp. 364–384). Elk Grove Village, IL: American Academy of Pediatrics.

Brockman, V. (2015). Implementing the mother-baby model of nursing care using models and quality improvement tools. *Nursing for Women's Health, 19*(6), 490–503.

Callister, L. C. (2013). Integrating cultural beliefs and practices when caring for childbearing women and families. In K. R. Simpson & P. A. Creehan (Eds.), *AWHONN perinatal nursing* (4th ed.) (pp. 41–64). Philadelphia: Lippincott.

Carter, A., Granty, L., & Carter, B. S. (2016). Discharge planning and follow-up of the neonatal intensive care unit infant. In S. L. Gardner, B. S. Carter, M. Enzman-Hines, et al. (Eds.), *Merenstein & Gardner's handbook of neonatal intensive care* (8th ed.) (pp. 903–923). St. Louis, MO: Mosby.

Centers for Disease Control and Prevention (CDC). (2014). *Summary of 2014 National CDC EHDI Data*. Retrieved from www.cdc.gov.

Centers for Disease Control and Prevention (CDC). (2014c). *New Classification System Could Improve Tracking of Sudden Unexplained Infant Death*. Retrieved from www.healthychildren.org/English/news/Pages/New-Classification-System-Could-Improve-Tracking-of-Sudden-Unexplained-Infant-Death.aspx.

Centers for Disease Control and Prevention (CDC). (2016). *Preventing Abusive Head Trauma in Children*. Retrieved from www.cdc.gov/violenceprevention/childmaltreatment/abusive-head-trauma.html.

Cunningham, D. R., & Sydlowski, S. A. (2016). Auditory screening. In T. K. McInerny, H. M. Adam, D. E. Campbell, T. G. DeWitt, J. M. Foy, & D. M. Kamat (Eds.), *Textbook of pediatric care* (2nd ed.) (pp. 314–322). Elk Grove Village, IL: American Academy of Pediatrics.

Eiger, M. S. (2016). Feeding of infants and children. In T. K. McInerny, H. M. Adam, D. E. Campbell, T. G. DeWitt, J. M. Foy, & D. M. Kamat (Eds.), *Textbook of pediatric care* (2nd ed.) (pp. 212–219). Elk Grove Village, IL: American Academy of Pediatrics.

Eze, N., & Smith, L. M. (2015). Circumcision. In C. D. Berkowitz (Ed.), *Pediatrics: A primary care approach* (5th ed.) (pp. 120–123). Elk Grove, IL: American Academy of Pediatrics.

Feigelman, S. (2016). The first year. In R. M. Kliegman, B. E. Stanton, J. W. St. Geme, & N. E. Schor (Eds.), *Nelson textbook of pediatrics* (20th ed.) (pp. 65–69). Philadelphia: Saunders.

Galanti, G. (2015). Birth. In *Caring for patients from different cultures* (pp. 173–193). University of Pennsylvania Press. Retrieved from www.jstor.org/stable/j.ctt13x1n1q.13.

Gardner, S. L., & Hernandez, J. A. (2016). Heat balance. In S. L. Gardner, B. S. Carter, M. Enzman-Hines, & J. A. Hernandez (Eds.), *Merenstein & Gardner's handbook of neonatal intensive care* (8th ed.) (pp. 105–125). St. Louis, MO: Elsevier.

Gardner, S. L., Enzman-Hines, M., & Agarwal, R. (2016). Pain and pain relief. In S. L. Gardner, B. S. Carter, M. Enzman-Hines, & J. A. Hernandez (Eds.), *Merenstein & Gardner's handbook of neonatal intensive care* (8th ed.) (pp. 218–261). St. Louis, MO: Elsevier.

Grover, G. (2014a). Crying and colic. In C. D. Berkowitz (Ed.), *Pediatrics: A primary care approach* (5th ed.) (pp. 267–270). Elk Grove Village, IL: American Academy of Pediatrics.

Grover, G. (2014b). Normal development and developmental surveillance, screening, and evaluation. In C. D. Berkowitz (Ed.), *Pediatrics: A primary care approach* (5th ed.) (pp. 151–158). Elk Grove Village, IL: American Academy of Pediatrics.

Grover, G. (2014c). Sleep: Normal patterns and common disorders. In C. D. Berkowitz (Ed.), *Pediatrics: A primary care approach* (5th ed.) (pp. 137–144). Elk Grove Village, IL: American Academy of Pediatrics.

Gundy, J. H. (2016). Pediatric physical examination. In T. K. McInerny, H. M. Adam, D. E. Campbell, T. G. DeWitt, J. M. Foy, & D. M. Kamat (Eds.), *Textbook of pediatric care* (2nd ed.) (pp. 101–146). Elk Grove Village, IL: American Academy of Pediatrics.

Hagan, J. F., & Duncan, P. M. (2016). Maximizing children's health: Screening, anticipatory guidance, and counseling. In R. M. Kliegman, B. E. Stanton, J. W. St. Geme, & N. E. Schor (Eds.),

Nelson textbook of pediatrics (20th ed.) (pp. 37–47). Philadelphia: Saunders.

Harrington, J. W., Logan, S., Harwell, C., Gardner, J., Swingle, J., McGuire, E., & Santos, R. (2012). Effective analgesia using physical interventions for immunizations. *Pediatrics, 129*(5), 815–822.

Jana, L. A., & Shu, J. (2015). *Heading home with your newborn: From birth to reality* (3rd ed.). Elk Grove Village, IL: American Academy of Pediatrics.

Kaur, H., & Campbell, D. (2016). Physical examination of the newborn. In T. K. McInerny, H. M. Adam, D. E. Campbell, T. G. DeWitt, J. M. Foy, & D. M. Kamat (Eds.), *Textbook of pediatric care* (2nd ed.) (pp. 757–774). Elk Grove Village, IL: American Academy of Pediatrics.

Keane, V. (2016). Assessment of growth. In R. M. Kliegman, B. E. Stanton, J. W. St. Geme, & N. E. Schor (Eds.), *Nelson textbook of pediatrics* (20th ed.) (p. 39). Philadelphia: Saunders.

Keys, E. M., & Rankin, J. A. (2015). Bed sharing, SIDS research, and the concept of confounding: a review for public health nurses. *Public Health Nursing, 32*(6), 731–737.

Lawrence, J., Alcock, D., McGrath, P., Kay, J., MacMurray, S. B., & Dulberg, C. (1993). The development of a tool to assess neonatal pain. *Neonatal Network, 14*(5), 59–62.

Mahle, W. T., Martin, G. R., Beekman, R. H., III, Morrow, W. R., Rosenthal, G. L., Synder, C. S., & Tweddell, J. S. (2012). Endorsement of Health and Human Services recommendation for pulse oximetry screening for critical congenital heart disease. *Pediatrics, 129*(1), 190–192.

National Center for Missing & Exploited Children. (2014). *Guidelines on prevention of and response to infant abductions.* Retrieved from www.missingkids.com.

National Quality Forum. (2012). *National voluntary consensus standards for perinatal care, 2008: A consensus report.* Washington, DC: Author.

Owen, D. C., Gonzalez, E. W., & Esperat, C. R. (2017). Mexican Americans. In J. N. Giger (Ed.), *Transcultural nursing: Assessment and intervention* (7th ed.) (pp. 208–240). St. Louis, MO: Mosby.

Rabun, J. B. (2014). *For healthcare professionals: Guidelines on prevention of and response to infant abductions* (10th ed.). Alexandria, VA: National Center for Missing & Exploited Children.

Rosales, T. (2014). Strabismus. In C. D. Berkowitz (Ed.), *Pediatrics: A primary care approach* (5th ed.) (pp. 459–463). Elk Grove Village, IL: American Academy of Pediatrics.

Smith, L. M. (2014). Sudden infant death syndrome and apparent life-threatening events. In C. D. Berkowitz (Ed.), *Pediatrics: A primary care approach* (5th ed.) (pp. 341–346). Elk Grove Village, IL: American Academy of Pediatrics.

Spector, R. E. (2017). *Cultural diversity in health and illness* (9th ed.). Upper Saddle River, NJ: Pearson Prentice Hall.

Sullivan, C. K., & Dela Cruz-Rivera, S. (2016). Discharge planning and follow-up care. In T. K. McInerny, H. M. Adam, D. E. Campbell, T. G. DeWitt, J. M. Foy, & D. M. Kamat (Eds.), *Textbook of pediatric care* (2nd ed.) (pp. 830–838). Elk Grove Village, IL: American Academy of Pediatrics.

Swanson, J. T. (2016). Circumcision. In T. K. McInerny, H. M. Adam, D. E. Campbell, T. G. DeWitt, J. M. Foy, & D. M. Kamat (Eds.), *Textbook of pediatric care* (2nd ed.) (pp. 818–820). Elk Grove Village, IL: American Academy of Pediatrics.

U.S. Consumer Product Safety Commission. (2011). *News from COSC: Safer cribs for babies available starting today.* Retrieved from www.cpsc.gov.

U.S. Department of Health and Human Services. (2010). *Healthy People 2020.* Washington, DC: Author.

Winer, G., & Zaichikin, J. (2016). *Textbook of neonatal resuscitation.* Elk Grove, IL: American Academy of Pediatrics and American Heart Association.

Infant Feeding

Karen Stanzo

Nurses should support and promote breastfeeding as the normal way to feed babies and as the reference against which infant nutrition is considered (American Academy of Pediatrics [AAP] 2012; Association of Women's Health, Obstetric and Neonatal Nurses [AWHONN], 2015). Nurses should also partner with other health care workers and advocates to ensure that any social, cultural, economic, or educational barriers to breastfeeding are removed (AWHONN, 2015). Given the numerous documented health and developmental disadvantages to infants who are not breastfed, breastfeeding support should be viewed as an important health promotion activity and not merely a lifestyle choice (AAP, 2012). Helping women choose and feel comfortable with a feeding method is an important nursing contribution that requires knowledge of the newborn's nutritional needs and the techniques to meet those needs.

NUTRITIONAL NEEDS OF THE NEWBORN

Calories

The full-term newborn needs 85 to 100 kilocalories per kilogram of body weight (kcal/k) (39 to 45 kilocalories per pound of body weight [kcal/lb] each day if breastfed and 100 to 110 kcal/kg (45 to 50 kcal/lb) if formula fed (Box 22.1) (Blackburn, 2013). The infant must consume sufficient calories to meet energy needs, prevent the use of body stores, and provide for growth.

Breast milk and formulas used for the normal newborn contain 20 kilocalories per ounce (kcal/oz). During the early days after birth, infants may lose up to 10% of their birth weight (Fonseca, Severo, Barros, & Santos, 2014). This loss is a result of normal excretion of extracellular water and meconium and newborns consuming fewer calories than needed. Newborns have a small stomach capacity and may fall asleep before feeding adequately or may sleep through feeding times in the early days of life. Nurses and other health care providers should consider weight loss in their feeding assessment, but should also consider the quality of a directly observed breastfeeding session, the infant's output, and other clinical factors such as prematurity and jaundice risk.

Infants should be evaluated for feeding problems if weight loss exceeds 7% of birth weight, if weight loss continues beyond 3 days of age, or if the birth weight is not regained by 10 days of age in the term infant (American Academy of Pediatrics & American College of Obstetricians and Gynecologists [AAP & ACOG], 2012). This information should be explained to parents.

Nutrients

Nutrients needed by the newborn are provided by carbohydrates, proteins, and fats in breast milk or formula. Full-term neonates digest simple carbohydrates and proteins well. Complex carbohydrates and fats are less well digested because of the lack of pancreatic amylase and lipase in the newborn. Vitamins and minerals are provided by both breast milk and formula.

Water

The newborn needs larger amounts of fluid in relationship to size than the adult because infants lose water more easily from the skin, kidneys, and intestines. Breast milk or formula supplies the infant's fluid needs. Additional water is unnecessary.

BREAST MILK AND FORMULA COMPOSITION

Breast Milk

Breast milk is species specific (made for human infants) and is the reference point on which to compare necessary infant nutrition. The nutrients in breast milk are proportioned appropriately for the neonate and vary to meet the newborn's changing needs. Breast milk provides protection against infection and is easily digested. Maternal immunoglobulins, leukocytes, antioxidants, enzymes, and hormones important for growth are present in breast milk but are not available in formula.

Changes in Composition

The composition of breast milk changes in three phases: **lactogenesis** (the production of milk) stages I, II, and III.

Lactogenesis I. Lactogenesis I begins during pregnancy and continues during the early days after giving birth. At this time, the breasts secrete **colostrum**—a thick, yellow substance. Colostrum is higher in protein and some vitamins and minerals than mature milk. It is lower in carbohydrates, fat, lactose, and some vitamins. It is rich in immunoglobulins, especially secretory immunoglobulin A (IgA), which helps protect the infant's gastrointestinal (GI) tract from infection. Colostrum helps establish the normal flora in the intestines, and its laxative effect speeds the passage of meconium. Colostrum is sometimes referred to as "liquid gold" because of its many benefits (Pletsch, Ulrich, Angelini, Fernandes, & Lee, 2013).

Lactogenesis II. Lactogenesis II begins 2 to 3 days after birth. **Transitional milk**, milk that gradually changes from colostrum to mature milk, appears over about 10 days (Lawrence & Lawrence, 2016). The amount of milk increases rapidly as the milk "comes in." Immunoglobulins and proteins decrease and lactose, fat, and calories increase. The vitamin content is approximately the same as that of mature milk.

Lactogenesis III. **Mature milk** replaces transitional milk during lactogenesis III. Because breast milk is bluish and not as thick as colostrum, some mothers think their milk is not "rich" enough for their infants. Nurses should explain the normal appearance of breast milk to mothers. Mature milk contains approximately 20 kcal/oz and nutrients sufficient to meet the infant's needs. It continues to provide immunoglobulins and other antibacterial components. Discussions of breast milk and its contents refer to mature milk unless otherwise stated.

Nutrients

The nutrients provided in breast milk are present in the amounts and proportions needed by the infant.

Protein. The concentrations of amino acids in breast milk are suited to the infant's needs and ability to metabolize them. Breast milk is high in taurine, which is important for bile conjugation and brain development. Tyrosine and phenylalanine levels are low in breast milk to correspond to the infant's low levels of enzymes to digest them (Lawrence & Lawrence, 2016). Milk proteins produce a lower solute load (the amount of nitrogenous waste and minerals excreted by the kidneys) for the infant's immature kidneys.

Casein and whey are the proteins in milk, but their ratio differs significantly in cow's milk and in human milk. Casein forms a large, insoluble curd that is harder to digest than the curd from whey, which is very soft (Riordan, 2016). Breast milk is easily digested because it has a high ratio of whey to casein, especially in early lactation. By contrast, formula has a higher ratio of casein to whey, which results in formula-fed babies having firmer stools with a large amount of the protein in formula not digested (Riordan, 2016).

Cow's milk is one the most common allergens; the body's immune system recognizes and may react to the cow's milk protein found in formula. Because breast milk is made for the human infant, it is unlikely to cause allergies. However, antigens in foods the mother has eaten may pass into her milk. If the infant reacts to the mother's diet, the offending food should be identified and eliminated. Foods in the mother's diet that are most likely to trigger an allergic response in an infant are those from dairy sources, shellfish, peanuts, and tree nuts (Prescott et al., 2013). Studies have been unable to determine whether infants whose mothers avoid eating common allergens are less likely to develop food allergies. Therefore current recommendations are for mothers to eat a regular, unrestricted diet during pregnancy and while breastfeeding (Muraro et al., 2014). Only after a food allergy is suspected in a breastfeeding infant might a mother be encouraged to modify her diet.

Carbohydrate. Lactose is the major carbohydrate in breast milk. It improves absorption of calcium and provides energy for brain growth. Other carbohydrates in breast milk increase intestinal acidity and impede growth of pathogens (Riordan, 2016).

Fat. Fat provides 50% of the calories in breast milk (Riordan, 2016). The fat in breast milk is more easily digested by the newborn than that in cow's milk. The amount of fat in breast milk varies during the feeding, between feedings, and on the same or different days. Hindmilk, the milk produced at the end of the feeding is higher in fat than foremilk, the milk produced at the beginning of the feeding. Hindmilk produces satiety and helps the infant gain weight.

Triglycerides form the majority of fat content. Cholesterol and essential fatty acids such as the long-chain polyunsaturated fatty acids docosahexaenoic acid and arachidonic acid are also present. These nutrients are important for vision and for the growth of the brain and the nervous system.

Vitamins. Levels of vitamins A, E, and C are high in breast milk. The vitamin D content of breast milk is low, and daily supplementation with 400 international units (IU) is recommended within the first few days of life (AAP & ACOG, 2012). Breastfeeding infants who are not exposed to the sun and those with dark skin are particularly at risk for insufficient vitamin D. Infants receiving adequate amounts of formula do not need added vitamin D because it is present in formula.

The presence of water-soluble vitamins in breast milk varies according to the mother's intake. The infant of a vegan mother may need supplementation with vitamin B$_{12}$.

Minerals. The casein protein in cow's milk interferes with iron absorption. Although the level of iron in breast milk is lower than that in formula, it is absorbed five times as well and breastfed infants are rarely deficient in iron (Riordan, 2016).

The full-term infant who is breastfed exclusively maintains iron stores for the first 6 months of life (Lawrence & Lawrence, 2016). Generally, iron is added when the infant begins eating solids. Preterm infants need iron supplements earlier. All formula-fed infants should receive iron-fortified formula (AAP & ACOG, 2012).

Sodium, calcium, and phosphorus levels are higher in cow's milk than in human milk. This difference could cause an excessively high renal solute load if formula is not diluted properly. Fluoride supplements may be given starting at 6 months of age to improve dental health, depending on fluoridation of water in the area (AAP & ACOG, 2012).

Enzymes. Breast milk contains enzymes that aid in digestion. The amount of pancreatic amylase necessary for digestion of carbohydrates is low in the newborn but present in breast milk. Breast milk also contains lipase to increase fat digestion.

❓ KNOWLEDGE CHECK

1. Why do most newborns lose weight after birth?
2. What are the differences among colostrum, transitional breast milk, and mature breast milk?
3. How does breast milk compare with commercial formulas?

Infection-Preventing Components

Other factors present in human milk help prevent infection in the newborn. Bifidus factor promotes the growth of *Lactobacillus bifidus,* an important part of the intestinal flora that helps produce an acidic environment in the GI tract. This protects the infant against infection from common intestinal pathogens.

Leukocytes present in breast milk also help protect against infection. Macrophages are the most abundant and secrete lysozyme and lactoferrin. Lysozyme is a bacteriolytic enzyme that acts against gram-positive and enteric bacteria. Lactoferrin is a protein that binds iron in iron-dependent bacteria, preventing their growth. It also makes the iron in milk absorbed more easily. Giving infants supplementary iron may interfere with the effectiveness of lactoferrin (Riordan, 2016).

Immunoglobulins are present in highest amounts in colostrum but also are present throughout lactation. Higher levels occur when the infant is born prematurely. Lymphocytes in the milk produce secretory IgA, which helps prevent viral

or bacterial invasion of the intestinal mucosa, resulting in fewer intestinal infections. Infants who are not breastfed have an increased incidence of respiratory, GI, and urinary tract infections, otitis media, asthma, diabetes, some cancers, obesity, sudden infant death syndrome (SIDS), and necrotizing enterocolitis (Lawrence & Lawrence, 2016).

Effect of Maternal Diet

Although the fatty acid content of breast milk is influenced by the mother's diet, malnourished mothers' milk has about the same proportions of total fat, protein, carbohydrates, and most minerals as milk from those who are well nourished. Levels of water-soluble vitamins in breast milk, however, are affected by the mother's intake and stores (Lawrence & Lawrence, 2016). It is important for breastfeeding women to eat a well-balanced diet to maintain their own health and energy levels.

Formulas

Commercial formulas are produced to replace or supplement breast milk. They are sometimes called "breast milk substitutes" or "artificial breast milk" because manufacturers must adapt them to correspond to the components in breast milk as much as possible. However, an exact match is impossible and although formula provides adequate nutrition, it cannot provide the important immunologic components of breastmilk. A variety of formulas, which differ in price and ingredients, are available.

Cow's Milk

Unmodified cow's milk (whole milk, low-fat milk, or fat-free milk) is not recommended for infants under 12 months of age. It contains too much protein and sodium and lacks essential fatty acids, vitamin C, iron, zinc, and other nutrients (Grodner, Escott-Stump & Dorner, 2016).

Modified cow's milk is the source of most commercial formulas. Manufacturers specifically formulate it for infants by reducing protein content to decrease renal solute load. Saturated fat is removed and replaced with vegetable fats. Vitamins and other nutrients are added to simulate the contents of breast milk. Formula with added iron should be used for all infants receiving formula (AAP & ACOG, 2012).

Formulas for Infants with Special Needs

Soy formula may be given to infants with galactosemia or lactase deficiency and to those whose families are vegetarians. Soy milk is derived from the protein of soybeans and supplemented with amino acids. Protein hydrolysate formulas are better tolerated by infants with allergies. The protein is treated to make it less allergenic. The formulas are also used for infants with malabsorption disorders. Amino acid formulas are used for allergic infants who do not thrive on hydrolyzed protein formulas.

The preterm infant may require a more concentrated formula with more calories in less liquid. Modifications of other nutrients are also made. Human milk fortifiers can be added to breast milk to adapt it for preterm infants. Lactose-free formula uses primarily glucose instead of lactose for infants who do not tolerate lactose. Low-phenylalanine formulas are needed for infants with phenylketonuria (PKU), a deficiency in the enzyme to digest phenylalanine found in standard formulas.

CONSIDERATIONS IN CHOOSING A FEEDING METHOD

Nurses should encourage breastfeeding as the best method of feeding most infants. Unless there is a rare circumstance that contraindicates breastfeeding, nurses should provide patient and family education on the risks of formula feeding as well as on the benefits of breastfeeding. This patient education should begin early in pregnancy. However, nurses should be supportive of the mother's chosen method once a fully informed decision has been made.

Breastfeeding

Mothers choose breastfeeding because, in almost all cases, it is the best choice for the health of the mother and the infant (Box 22.2 presents the risks of not breastfeeding). It has been increasingly recognized that formula feeding can never fully equal breastfeeding in terms of providing for the infant's optimal health, growth, and development.

The American Academy of Pediatrics (AAP) recommends that infants receive only breast milk for the first 6 months after birth. Breastfeeding should continue until the infant is at least 12 months old, with the addition of complementary foods (AAP, 2012). Breastfeeding and support to help mothers achieve it are also recommended by the World Health Organization (WHO, 2015) and the U.S. Surgeon General (U.S. Department of Health and Human Services [DHHS], 2011).

A goal set by the DHHS for the year 2020 is for 81.9% of all infants to be breastfed at some time, for at least 60.5% to be breastfeeding at 6 months, and 34.1% at 1 year of life. Additional goals are to increase the number of mothers who exclusively breastfeed their infants through 3 months to 44.3% and through 6 months to 23.7% (DHHS, 2010). One study found that if 90% of women breastfed exclusively for 6 months, the United States would prevent 721 infant deaths annually (mostly the result of SIDS and necrotizing enterocolitis) and 2619 deaths of women (mostly due to increase lifetime risks for heart attacks, breast cancer, and diabetes in women who do not optimally breastfeed) (Bartick et al., 2016). In addition, the United States would save $3 billion per year in health care costs (Bartick et al., 2016).

The Centers for Disease Control and Prevention (CDC, 2016a) reports that in 2013, 81.1% of infants were ever breastfed. At 6 months, 51.8% of mothers were breastfeeding, and at 12 months the rate was 30.7% breastfeeding. These statistics show a gradual but steady increase over previous years, but continued improvement is needed.

In an effort to promote breastfeeding, the United Nations Children's Fund (UNICEF), the WHO, and the U.S. Surgeon General advocate that birth facilities become designated through the Baby Friendly Hospital Initiative. Guidelines to becoming certified as a baby-friendly hospital emphasize education of staff and parents about breastfeeding, early initiation

---

BOX 22.2 Risks of Not Breastfeeding

For the Infant

Allergies are more likely to develop.

Not receiving the immunologic properties of breast milk increases the risk for infections.

Increased incidence of necrotizing enterocolitis and respiratory tract, ear, urinary tract, and gastrointestinal tract infections.

Increased incidence of diabetes, asthma, obesity, some cancers, sudden infant death syndrome.

Formula's nutritional and immunologic properties do not change according to the infant's needs.

Formula is not as easily digested and nutrients are not as well absorbed.

Protein, fat, and carbohydrate do not occur in the most suitable proportions in formula.

Formula can be improperly and potentially dangerously diluted.

Formula can be contaminated and can be affected by water supply.

Formula is more easily overfed.

Constipation is more common.

For the Mother

Formula feeding does not release oxytocin. Oxytocin enhances uterine involution.

Mother loses more blood because of earlier return of menses.

Mother resumes ovulation earlier.

Increased incidence of some cancers.

Mother receives less rest while feeding.

A balanced maternal diet that improves healing is less likely.

Less frequent skin-to-skin contact can be detrimental to bonding.

Inconvenient—Bottles to wash and formula to buy, prepare, or heat.

Expensive—Cost of formula and bottles and time spent in preparation.

Infant is more likely to be ill, increasing medical care costs.

Working mothers miss more days of work to care for sick infants.

Travel more difficult—Bottles to prepare, carry, refrigerate, and warm.

---

of breastfeeding, demand feedings, rooming-in, no pacifiers, and avoidance of formula unless medically indicated. In 2016, 17.9% of U.S. hospitals were certified as baby-friendly (Baby Friendly, USA, 2016).

The Joint Commission (2011) has issued a brochure titled "Speak Up" for women who want to breastfeed. They encourage mothers to ask for help with breastfeeding. Skin-to-skin contact, breastfeeding as soon as possible after birth, and avoidance of formula or water unless medically indicated are emphasized. The brochure is available at www.jointcommission.org/assessts/1/18/Breastfeeding_final_7_19_11.pdf.

Formula Feeding

Parents choose formula feeding for many reasons. Some women are embarrassed by breastfeeding, seeing their breasts only in the sexual context. Many mothers have few relatives or friends who have had breastfeeding experiences. A woman may feel a need to maintain a strict feeding schedule and be uneasy not knowing exactly how much milk the infant consumes at each feeding. Her partner or mother may not be supportive of breastfeeding. Rarely, a woman must take medications that might harm the infant. A frequent reason mothers choose formula feeding instead of breastfeeding is lack of understanding and education about the two methods.

Combination Feeding

Some parents prefer a combination of breastfeeding and formula feeding. Unless medically indicated, it is best to delay giving bottles or formula until lactation has been well established when the infant is 3 to 4 weeks of age. Giving formula to breastfeeding infants leads to a decrease in breastfeeding frequency and milk production, making successful breastfeeding less likely (AAP & ACOG, 2012; Newton, 2017). Nurses can inform mothers who wish to combination feed of the option of expressing breast milk so that the baby can bottle feed breast milk instead of formula. If the mother chooses to both breastfeed and formula feed after being fully educated, however, the nurse should be supportive so that the mother and infant receive the benefits of breastfeeding at least part of the time.

Factors Influencing Choice

Many factors influence a woman's choice of feeding method. These factors must be considered when educating women about their choices, because breastfeeding education is an important health promotion activity and not just a lifestyle choice.

Support from Others

Family members and friends may share in the decision-making process. Women with a support system are more likely to begin breastfeeding and continue longer than those without a perceived support system. The woman's partner and the baby's grandmothers are often important influences in determining whether women breastfeed. Advice from friends who have breastfed may also influence the woman's decision. The woman with little support or active discouragement from her family is more likely to have a difficult time breastfeeding. Some women choose not to breastfeed because of their partners' objections.

Involvement of the father in infant care is important in some families, and some may think it is possible mainly with feedings. Nurses can suggest other ways fathers can participate in infant care, for example, holding, rocking, and bathing infants. Educating family members about the importance of breastfeeding and risks of formula feeding may lead to their encouragement and support as well.

Prenatal classes that include breastfeeding information may help a woman decide to breastfeed and may help her develop confidence that she will be successful. Support people, such as fathers or grandmothers, also should attend the classes so they can learn techniques to help cope with any challenges that might arise. Prenatal breastfeeding classes, individual and group breastfeeding support groups, and breastfeeding counseling are all associated with increased breastfeeding initiation and duration (Haroon, Das, Salam, Imdad, & Bhutta, 2013).

Encouragement from the woman's health care provider may be a powerful influence in the woman choosing to breastfeed (Newton, 2017). The support the mother receives from the nursing staff plays a significant part in whether she feels comfortable with her choice of feeding method. The mother who does not feel confident in her ability to breastfeed before she leaves the birth facility is less likely to continue breastfeeding if she encounters difficulties at home.

Culture

Cultural influences may dictate decisions about how a mother feeds her infant. Women who are most likely to breastfeed are Asian, Pacific Islander, or Hispanic. Those with the lowest breastfeeding rates include women who are non-Hispanic black (Callister, 2014; CDC, 2016b).

However, immigrants from countries in which breastfeeding is the norm may breastfeed for shorter durations or not at all because they lack the support system they had in their own country. Hispanic women who are new immigrants are more likely to begin breastfeeding and continue for a longer period than more acculturated immigrants (Wambach, Domain, Page-Goertz, Wurtz, & Hoffman, 2016).

Some women may think formula feeding is the preferred method in the United States because it is available in birth facilities. They also may think breastfeeding is inferior to formula feeding and consider formula a way to help their infants grow larger and become stronger. Nurses must emphasize the normalcy of breastfeeding and the risks of formula feeding and encourage these women to continue their cultural tradition of breastfeeding.

Nurses should be particularly watchful for ways to help mothers from other cultures who wish to breastfeed but fail to do so because of lack of information or support. Nurses should first examine their own cultural attitudes and ideas about breastfeeding. They should then practice culturally competent care by asking families about their cultural practices and beliefs about breastfeeding and helping find ways for the family to both honor their culture and successfully breastfeed.

Employment

The need to return to roles outside the home soon after giving birth may cause concern about feeding methods. Unfortunately, returning to work or school is a major cause of discontinuation of breastfeeding. The mother may choose to directly breastfeed while she is not at work and then express her milk for her baby to be fed while she is at work. She may also feed formula from the beginning, plan a short period of breastfeeding before weaning the infant to formula, or use a combination of breastfeeding and bottle feeding with breast milk or formula.

The nurse should encourage women to continue to breastfeed when they return to work and point out the risks of formula feeding. The increased incidence of illness in formula fed infants means mothers are more likely to miss work to care for a sick infant. This is a disadvantage for the employer as well as the nonbreastfeeding family.

Nurses who provide practical information about breastfeeding and working, use of breast pumps, and storage of breast milk help a mother continue breastfeeding for a longer period. Pamphlets and books for the working breastfeeding mother are particularly helpful. Referral to a lactation consultant can provide a mother with continued education and support after she goes home.

Staff Knowledge

It is important that all birth facility staff members have education about how to help women breastfeed and not provide inaccurate or conflicting information to new mothers. Educational programs are effective in helping ensure all staff have the same basic knowledge and skills to help breastfeeding mothers. Programs may involve formal classes, protocols, and self-paced learning modules (Siggia & Rosenburg, 2014).

Other Factors

Other factors also may influence a woman's decision. Her knowledge and past experience with infant feeding are important. Modesty may be an issue for some women who are concerned about breastfeeding in public situations.

Maternal education level and parity affect breastfeeding (higher levels of education and multiparas are more likely to breastfeed and breastfeed longer) (Whipps, 2017). Mothers who live in rural areas or the southeastern United States have lower breastfeeding rates compared with women in other parts of the United States (CDC, 2016a). Women who are overweight or underweight are less likely to breastfeed than women who begin their pregnancy at a normal weight (Thompson et al., 2013).

> ### ❓ KNOWLEDGE CHECK
>
> 4. What factors that help prevent infection are present in breast milk?
> 5. What types of commercial formulas are available?
> 6. What factors influence a woman's choice of feeding method?

NORMAL BREASTFEEDING

The anatomy and physiology of the breast are discussed in Chapter 3, and breast changes occurring in pregnancy are discussed in Chapter 6 (see Figs. 3.8 and 6.3).

Breast Changes during Pregnancy

Breast changes begin early in pregnancy in preparation for the production of milk. The ducts, lobules, and alveoli develop in response to the hormones estrogen, progesterone, human chorionic somatomammotropin (hCS), and prolactin. Prolactin levels are high, but milk production is prevented by estrogen, progesterone, and hCS, which inhibit breast response to prolactin. Colostrum is present by 16 weeks of gestation (Lawrence & Lawrence, 2016).

Milk Production

Milk is produced in the alveoli of the breasts through a complex process by which substances from the mother's bloodstream are reformulated into breast milk. Thus amino acids, glucose, lipids, enzymes, leukocytes, and other materials are used to manufacture the nutrients needed by the infant. The milk is ejected from the secretory cells of the alveoli into the alveolar lumen by contraction of the myoepithelial cells. From there, it travels through the lactiferous ducts to the nipple. The infant compresses the areola during breastfeeding to move a stream of milk through pores in the nipple (Blackburn, 2013).

Hormonal Changes at Birth
Prolactin

At birth, loss of placental hormones results in increasing levels and effectiveness of prolactin and activates milk production. The tactile stimulation of **suckling** and the removal of colostrum or milk causes continued increased levels of prolactin. Prolactin is secreted at the highest levels with suckling and during the night (Lawrence & Lawrence, 2016). Levels are high during the early months and then gradually decrease until weaning.

Oxytocin

Oxytocin increases in response to nipple stimulation and causes the **milk-ejection reflex** or **let-down reflex**, the release of milk from the alveoli into the ducts. During feeding, the milk-ejection reflex occurs several times. Some mothers have a tingling sensation of the breast when the let-down occurs.

When mothers see, hear, or think about their infants, they often have an increase in oxytocin, resulting in let-down of milk, causing milk to drip or spurt from the breasts (Fig. 22.1). Pain or lack of relaxation can inhibit oxytocin release. Oxytocin also causes the uterine contractions mothers may feel at the beginning of breastfeeding sessions. These contractions are beneficial because they hasten involution of the uterus and can decrease postpartum bleeding.

Continued Milk Production

The amount of milk produced depends primarily on adequate stimulation of the breast and removal of the milk by suckling or a breast pump, which causes production of prolactin. This "supply-and-demand" effect continues throughout lactation. Early and frequent suckling may increase prolactin receptors in the breast and therefore increase the milk-making capacity of the breasts. Therefore increased demand with more frequent and longer breastfeeding results in more milk being available.

If milk (or colostrum) is not removed from the breasts, components in the milk cause a feedback that decreases prolactin secretion and milk production. The milk in the ducts is absorbed, the alveoli become smaller, the cells return to a resting state, and milk production ends.

Preparation of Breasts for Breastfeeding

Little preparation is needed during pregnancy for breastfeeding. The mother should avoid applying soap on her nipples

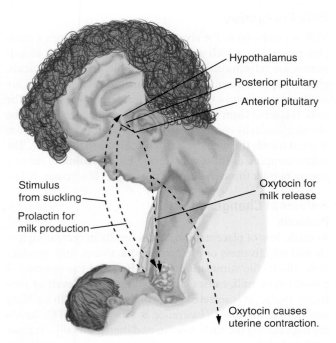

FIG. 22.1 **Effect of Prolactin and Oxytocin on Milk Production.** When the infant begins to suckle at the breast, nerve impulses travel to the hypothalamus, causing the anterior pituitary to secrete prolactin to increase milk production. Suckling causes the posterior pituitary to secrete oxytocin, producing the let-down reflex, which releases milk from the breast. Oxytocin also causes the uterus to contract, which aids in involution.

because it removes the natural protective oils secreted by the Montgomery tubercles of the breasts. The use of creams and nipple rolling, pulling, and rubbing to "toughen" nipples does not decrease nipple pain after birth and may cause irritation or uterine contractions from release of oxytocin.

Breasts should be assessed during pregnancy to identify flat or inverted nipples (Fig. 22.2). Normally, nipples protrude. Flat nipples appear soft, like the areola, and do not stand erect unless stimulated by rolling them between the fingers. Inverted nipples are retracted into the breast tissue. Both conditions make it more difficult for infants to **latch** (attach) onto the nipples.

Some nipples appear normal but draw inward when the areola is compressed in the infant's mouth. Compressing the areola between the thumb and forefinger identifies whether the nipple projects normally or becomes inverted. Nipples that appear inverted early in pregnancy may be improved near the end (Wambach & Genna, 2016).

The helpfulness of breast shells for flat or inverted nipples is debated. Some find them helpful for some women, and others think they decrease motivation to breastfeed and do not improve nipple eversion (Lawrence & Lawrence, 2016; Wambach & Genna, 2016). The dome-shaped devices are worn during the last weeks of pregnancy and between feedings after birth. The shells are placed in the bra with the opening over the nipple. They exert slight pressure against the areola to help the nipples protrude. Pumping the breasts for a few minutes before feeding helps the nipples protrude and may be more effective.

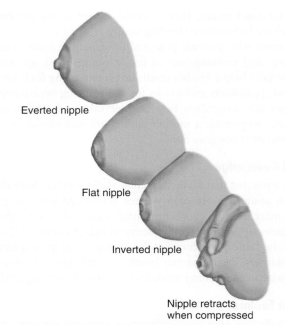

FIG. 22.2 Normal everted nipple and other types of nipples that may cause difficulty in latching on.

◆ **APPLICATION OF THE NURSING PROCESS: BREASTFEEDING**

◆ **Assessment**

Assess both the mother and the infant during the breastfeeding process. Various scoring tools have been developed to assess breastfeeding, but none is completely satisfactory. One method often used is the LATCH breastfeeding assessment tool (Table 22.1).

Maternal Assessment

Breasts and Nipples. Assess the condition of the breasts and nipples and the mother's knowledge about breastfeeding to determine her need for assistance.

Examine the breasts and nipples during late pregnancy to identify problems that might interfere with feeding. If this assessment did not occur before birth, examine the breasts and nipples before the initial feeding. Assess the protrusion of the nipples to identify flat or inverted nipples.

Ongoing assessments after birth include identification of breast fullness and breast engorgement. Fullness is the swelling of the breasts that may occur early in lactation as a result of increased blood and lymph circulation. It may progress to engorgement if feedings are delayed, too short, or not frequent enough. Palpate the breasts to see if they are soft, filling, or engorged.

TABLE 22.1   The Latch Scoring Tool*

	0	1	2
L			
Latch	Infant too sleepy or reluctant No sustained latch achieved	After repeated attempts is able to sustain latch and suck Must hold nipple in infant's mouth Must stimulate infant to suck	Grasps breast Tongue down Lips flanged Rhythmic sucking
A			
Audible swallowing	None	A few with stimulation	Spontaneous and intermittent <24 hr old Spontaneous and frequent >24 hr old
T			
Type of nipple	Inverted	Flat	Everted (with or without stimulation)
C			
Comfort (breast or nipple)	Engorged Cracked, bleeding, large blisters, or bruises Severe discomfort	Filling Reddened or small blisters or bruises Mild to moderate discomfort	Soft Nontender
H			
Hold (positioning)	Full assist (staff holds infant at breast)	Minimal assist (e.g., elevate head of bed; place pillows for support) Teach one side; mother does other Staff holds and then mother takes over	No assist from staff Mother able to position or hold infant

*The nurse can use the LATCH scoring system to assess and document the need for assistance with breastfeeding. Each assessment area is scored 0 to 2. A score of 7 or less indicates the mother needs more assistance in feeding.
Modified from Jensen, D., Wallace, S., & Kelsay, P. (1994). LATCH: A breastfeeding charting system and documentation tool. *Journal of Obstetric, Gynecologic, and Neonatal Nursing, 23*(1), 27–32. Reprinted with permission of Sage Publications.

Soft breasts feel like a cheek. If milk is beginning to fill the breasts or "come in," they may be slightly firmer, which is charted as "filling." **Engorgement** is congestion and increased vascularity, edema from obstruction of lymphatic drainage, and accumulation of milk as lactation is established. Engorged breasts may be hard and tender, with taut, shiny skin. Note any redness, tenderness, and lumps within the breasts. Engorged breasts may not be seen until after discharge from the birth facility.

Assess the nipples, which may be red, bruised, blistered, fissured, or bleeding. Ask about nipple tenderness and when it occurs. Evaluate breastfeeding techniques of the mother having problems with her nipples.

THERAPEUTIC COMMUNICATIONS
Anxiety about Breastfeeding

Brianna gave birth to her second baby, Luis, by cesarean birth. She tells her nurse, Chela, that she breastfed her first infant for a week and then switched to bottle feeding because she did not have enough milk. Luis is a sleepy baby but does nurse at times. Brianna's breasts are engorged, and her nipples are sore.

Brianna: I really wanted to nurse Luis, but I don't know if it's worth the effort. My breasts hurt, and I don't know if he's getting enough milk. I probably should just use the bottle again.

Chela: You sound really discouraged! *(Reflecting the feelings expressed.)*

Brianna: When I couldn't nurse my daughter, I was so disappointed. I had this "Mother Earth" view of the kind of mother I was going to be. But the baby wouldn't stop crying, so I went to the bottle.

Chela: That must have been hard for you! *(Reflecting the feelings expressed.)*

Brianna: It was awful, and now it looks like I'm going to fail again. Luis won't nurse half the time, and I'm going home this afternoon.

Chela: And you're worried about what's going to happen at home. *(Seeking clarification of the mother's concerns.)*

Brianna: What if he won't nurse at home? I don't know what to do!

Chela: Breastfeeding isn't always easy. Mothers and babies both have to learn the process, and that takes time and a lot of patience. Luis seems hungry now—would you like to try again? I'll stay with you, help you find a comfortable latch, and answer your questions. *(Offering realistic encouragement and assistance in techniques.)*

Brianna: That would be great! Maybe I'll get the hang of this yet! *(By allowing Brianna to express her feelings of discouragement and disappointment before beginning to teach, the nurse learns how important breastfeeding is to Brianna and how best to go about teaching her. Brianna feels accepted, even though she is discouraged.)*

BOX 22.3 Hunger Cues in Infants

Licking or sucking movements
Lip smacking
Rooting
Hand to mouth movements
Sucking on the hands
Increased activity
Crying (a late sign)

Knowledge. The mother who is breastfeeding for the first time may have many questions and need substantial guidance during her first attempts. If she has nursed before, she has more knowledge but may have forgotten some aspects and may be unaware of current information that was unavailable when she breastfed her last infant. It is particularly important that all staff give the same instructions to mothers. Conflicting advice is very confusing to mothers trying to learn how to breastfeed.

Infant Feeding Behaviors

Before initiating a breastfeeding session, assess the infant's readiness for feeding (Box 22.3). The infant should be awake and hungry. Trying to feed an infant in a deep sleep period is frustrating to both mother and infant. Sucking on the hands, rooting when the cheek or side of the mouth is touched, smacking the lips, and hand-to-mouth movements are common hunger cues. Feeding should begin before crying, which is a late sign of hunger. Crying infants must be calmed before they are ready to feed. Continue to assess for problems throughout the feeding.

◆ Identification of Patient Problems

Women with and without experience often need information to have a successful breastfeeding experience. A woman's confidence in her ability to breastfeed may be an important determinant of her success. Therefore nurses should help women increase their confidence and help prevent early weaning. Lack of understanding of breastfeeding techniques and confidence in using them are common patient problems that may lead to breastfeeding problems.

◆ Planning: Expected Outcomes

The expected outcomes are:
1. The infant will breastfeed using nutritive suckling and swallowing for at least 8 feedings per day before discharge.
2. The mother will demonstrate breastfeeding techniques (such as positioning and latch) as taught before discharge.
3. The mother will verbalize satisfaction and confidence with the breastfeeding process before discharge.

◆ Interventions

Interventions are focused on the teaching the nurse should provide all breastfeeding mothers and their support persons. Inexperienced mothers may need detailed teaching. Experienced mothers often need only a review or clarification about techniques they have used previously.

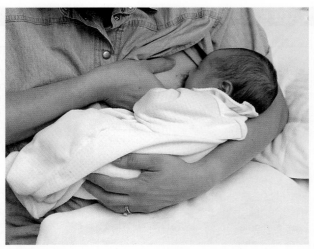

FIG. 22.3 For the cradle hold, the mother positions the infant's head at or near the antecubital space and level with her nipple, with her arm supporting the infant's body. Her other hand is free to hold the breast. Once the infant is positioned, pillows or blankets can be used to support the mother's arm, which may tire from holding the baby.

Assisting with the First Feeding

Nurses are encouraged to keep babies in uninterrupted skin-to-skin contact with their mothers after birth and then help mothers begin breastfeeding when they show feeding cues, usually within the first hour after birth. This assumes that both mother and infant are in stable condition (AAP & ACOG, 2012). During this first hour after birth, infants are in an alert state and many begin to nurse. Others may nuzzle, lick, or suck intermittently at the breast.

Skin-to-skin contact after birth and breastfeeding within the first hour after birth is associated with longer breastfeeding duration (Moore, Anderson, Bergman, & Dowswell, 2013). Early breastfeeding provides stimulation for milk production and improves suckling and maternal confidence. Feeding at this time also helps increase early bonding. The mother may be very gratified to see her infant nurse right after birth.

Teaching Feeding Techniques

Position of the Mother and Infant. Both the mother and the infant must be positioned properly for optimal breastfeeding. Make the mother as comfortable as possible before the feeding begins. Provide pain medications, if necessary. Pain or an awkward position may interfere with the let-down reflex and cause her to tire. Provide privacy and prevent interruptions so that she can concentrate on learning techniques.

The cradle, football (or clutch), and cross-cradle holds and the side-lying position are commonly used (Figs. 22.3 to 22.6). To increase her comfort, use pillows behind the mother's back, over the abdominal incision (if any), and to support her arms. Her shoulders should be relaxed, and she should not be in a hunched position. Arrange folded blankets or

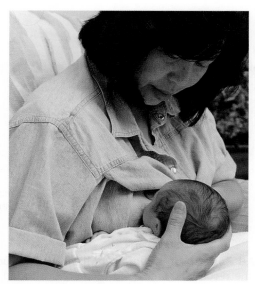

FIG. 22.4 For the football or clutch hold, the mother supports the infant's head and neck in her hand, with the infant's body resting on pillows alongside her hip. This method allows the mother to see the position of the infant's mouth on the breast, helps her control the infant's head, and is especially helpful for mothers with heavy breasts. This hold also avoids pressure against an abdominal incision.

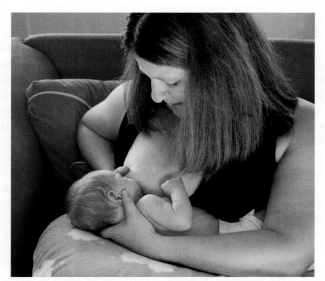

FIG. 22.5 The cross-cradle or modified cradle hold is helpful for infants who are preterm or have a fractured clavicle. The mother holds the infant's head with the hand opposite the side on which the infant will feed and supports the infant's body across her lap with her arm. The other hand holds the breast. The mother can guide the infant's head to the breast and see the mouth on the breast during the feeding.

pillows to elevate the infant to the level of the nipple and to prevent pulling and tension on the nipple.

The infant's head and body should directly face the breast. If the infant must turn the head to reach the breast, swallowing is difficult. The neck should be slightly extended. The

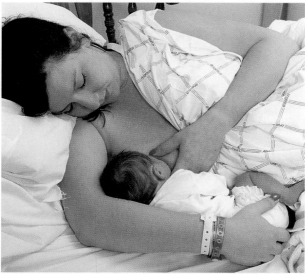

FIG. 22.6 The side-lying position avoids pressure on episiotomy or abdominal incisions and allows the mother to rest while feeding. She lies on her side, with her lower arm supporting her head or placed around the infant. Pillows behind her back and between her legs provide comfort. Her upper hand and arm are used to position the infant on the side at nipple level and hold the breast. When the infant's mouth opens to nurse, the mother draws the infant to her to insert the nipple into the mouth. A small blanket or towel can be placed over an abdominal incision to protect it from infant movement.

infant's body should be aligned so that the ear, shoulder, and hips are in a straight line.

Position of the Mother's Hands. The mother's hand position is also important. She can position her hand in either a "C" position (Fig. 22.7) or a "U" position so her hand gently shapes her breast so her fingers and thumb are parallel to the baby's mouth. Her fingers should be behind the areola so the baby has plenty of room to latch onto as much breast tissue as possible.

The mother should support her breast in place for the first few weeks if the weight of the breast makes it difficult for the infant to hold on to it. As the infant becomes more adept at breastfeeding, the mother no longer needs to hold the breast.

Although mothers worry about the infant's ability to breathe while breastfeeding, indenting the breast tissue near the infant's nostrils is unnecessary. This might cause improper positioning of the nipple in the infant's mouth, interfere with the grasp of the nipple, or interfere with milk flow. Bringing the infant's hips closer to the mother and lifting the body to a more horizontal position are usually sufficient if there is concern about the infant's ability to breathe while breastfeeding.

Latch-On Techniques. Teach the mother techniques to help the infant latch on to the breast. Helping mothers and babies achieve a comfortable latch is a key nursing intervention in the first few days postpartum because correct

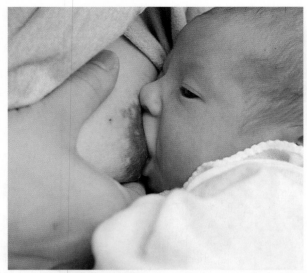

FIG. 22.7 "C" Position of Hand on Breast. The hand is positioned so that the thumb is on top of the breast while the fingers support the breast from below. Note the flaring of the infant's lips.

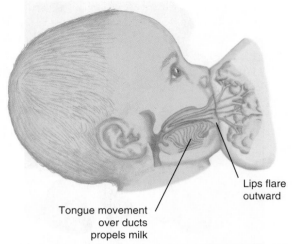

Lips flare outward

Tongue movement over ducts propels milk

FIG. 22.8 Position of the Infant's Mouth While Suckling. When the nipple and areola are properly positioned in the infant's mouth, the gums compress the areola instead of the nipple. The tongue is between the lower gum and breast. The infant's lips are flared outward.

latch is key to preventing nipple trauma and promoting optimal milk transfer. The infant should be awake and hungry. Undressing a baby and placing him skin-to-skin with his mother can help a sleepy infant awaken and calm an upset infant.

Eliciting Latch-On. After positioning the infant to face the breast, instruct the mother to hold her breast so the nipple brushes against the infant's lips. A hungry infant usually opens the mouth, but some need a minute of stroking the area around the mouth. The breast should not be inserted until the infant's mouth is opened widely, or the infant will compress the end of the nipple, causing pain, trauma, and little milk flow.

When the infant's mouth is wide open with the tongue down and forward over the gum, the mother should latch the baby asymmetrically by aiming her nipple toward the roof of the baby's mouth. She will then then quickly bring the infant close to her so that the infant can latch on to the areola with his chin touching the breast first. Suggesting to the mother that during latch-on the infant opens the mouth as though yawning or eating a large sandwich may help her understand what is needed.

Position of the Mouth. Assess the position of the infant's mouth on the breast (Fig. 22.8). The infant's lips should be positioned on the areola about 2.5 to 3.8 cm (1 to 1½ inches) from the base of the nipple to allow the nipple to be drawn toward the back of the mouth (Lawrence & Lawrence, 2016). This prevents the infant from sucking on the nipple only, which leads to sore nipples and insufficient milk production. It also places the infant's gums over the ducts so the milk is released into the mouth as the gums compress the breast. The nurse should note that most of the areola on the underside is covered by the baby's mouth; some of the areola on the top side may be visible.

Assess the position of the infant's tongue by gently pulling down on the lower lip. The tongue should be forward, cupped under the breast and over the top of the lower gums. The lips should be flared outward. Be sure that the lower lip is not turned in, which may result in a friction burn on the lower side of the nipple.

Suckling Pattern. Teach the mother about the infant's suckling pattern. During **nutritive suckling (sucking)**, the infant sucks with smooth, continuous movements with occasional pauses to rest. The infant may swallow after each suck or may suck several times before swallowing. **Nonnutritive sucking**, in which little or no milk flow is obtained, often occurs when the infant is falling asleep. A fluttery or choppy motion of the jaw not accompanied by the sound of swallowing indicates nonnutritive sucking.

Explain the milk-ejection reflex to the mother. After the mature milk increases in volume, many mothers learn to recognize a feeling of tingling in the nipples as the let-down occurs. The reflex occurs several times throughout the feeding. She will see the infant begin to swallow more rapidly each time a new let-down brings more rapid expulsion of milk. Milk may drip from the opposite breast when the reflex occurs.

Mothers often wonder whether their infants are actually receiving milk from the breast. Point out the sound of swallowing when it occurs. A soft "ka" or "ah" sound indicates the infant is swallowing colostrum or milk.

Short pauses are normal during breastfeeding. Gentle breast massage can help the baby transfer more milk with less effort and keep him awake and involved in the feeding. In addition, gently stroking the baby's back or hands and feet may keep a sleepy baby feeding.

Removal from the Breast. Teach the mother to remove the infant from the breast if suckling becomes painful. Show her how to avoid trauma to the breast by inserting her finger into the corner of the infant's mouth between the gums to break the suction. She then removes the breast quickly before the infant begins to suck again.

Frequency of Feedings. Breastfeeding is most successful when babies are not subjected to scheduled feedings, but are instead allowed to feed as frequently and for as long as they show feeding cues. Most babies need to feed 8 to 12 times per day, but these feedings may not be evenly spaced. Frequent feedings are especially important in the early days after birth, while lactation is being established and the infant's stomach capacity is small. Explaining that the hormone prolactin, which is responsible for milk production, is released in increased amounts while the infant is suckling helps the mother understand the relationship between frequent feeding and milk supply. Long periods between feedings increase the likelihood of breast engorgement.

An infant may vary in the length of feedings and time between each feeding. Several feedings close together (sometimes called "cluster feedings") are followed by a longer interval between feedings. Cluster feedings may occur on the second or third night at home or in later weeks when an appetite spurt occurs in the infant (Academy of Breastfeeding Medicine [ABM], 2009). An infant's frequent need to nurse may cause the mother to think that her milk supply is inadequate, when, in fact, it may be normal. Nurses should provide mothers with anticipatory guidance about frequent nighttime feedings and should encourage daytime maternal rest.

Length of Feedings. Early feedings were once limited to only a few minutes per breast to prevent sore nipples; however, improper positioning, rather than time at breast, is the usual cause of nipple trauma. When feedings are too short, infants receive little or no colostrum or milk. It may take as long as 5 minutes for the milk-ejection (let-down) reflex to occur during the early days after birth.

Generally, mothers can allow infants to set the length of feedings. Mothers should be taught to note the quality of a breastfeeding session instead of the length. The infant should suckle vigorously for a certain period with swallowing noted. Gentle breast massage and infant stimulation can help keep a baby in a nutritive sucking pattern. When choppy, nonnutritive suckling without the sound of swallowing occurs, the mother should burp the infant and complete the feeding at the other breast. When the infant is satisfied, the suckling pattern changes and the infant may fall asleep.

Although variations in the length of feedings occur, early feedings that last less than an average of 20 minutes and occur less than eight times in 24 hours may not be enough (Hoover, 2016). Feeding time increases as needed by the infant over the next few days. Teach the mother that longer feedings do not cause sore nipples if the infant is positioned properly.

Explain the differences between **foremilk**, the watery first milk that quenches the infant's thirst, and **hindmilk**, which comes at the end of the feeding. Hindmilk is richer in fat, more satisfying, and leads to weight gain. Feeding for too short a time prevents the infant from getting the hindmilk and decreases weight gain. Therefore the mother should continue feeding on the first side as long as the infant nurses vigorously before burping and continuing on the other breast. Mothers should alternate the breast offered first at each feeding to provide equal stimulation of the breasts.

Preventing Problems. Women who intend to breastfeed but encounter difficulties that cause them to switch to formula feeding may express guilt and disappointment for months or years after the experience. Nurses can help prevent early problems in several ways.

Teaching. Once women leave the birth facility, they often have no one to advise them about breastfeeding. Help prevent problems after discharge by intensive teaching during the short stay at the birth facility. Check the woman frequently as she feeds her infant so that her questions can be answered as she thinks of them.

Include suggestions on how to improve positioning and techniques. Discuss common problems that may occur after discharge and offer solutions. Some facilities hold classes for groups of women during the birth facility stay. Pamphlets and trusted web resources provide another means of teaching. Nurses should teach families about community breastfeeding resources, including classes; telephone support lines; breastfeeding mothers' support groups; Women, Infant, and Children Food and Nutrition Service (WIC) resources; and outpatient lactation consults.

Minimizing Interruptions. While the mother and baby are establishing breastfeeding, keep interruptions to a minimum. Ask her if she would like visitors to wait until she has finished feeding. Hang a "Do Not Disturb" sign on the door to advise staff and visitors that the mother should not be interrupted. Tell the mother to use her call light to notify the nurse if she needs help or when she is ready for interruptions.

Formula Gift Packs. The AAP and ACOG (2012) recommend against giving formula gift packs to mothers at hospital discharge because this practice may lead to an expectation in some mothers that formula will be necessary. This is contrary to the message nurses should give to parents about their ability to exclusively breastfeed.

Formula Supplementation. Avoid use of formula supplementation in the hospital unless there are medical indications. Avoidance of supplements of any kind during the first 72 hours is a nursing care quality measure being introduced by the Association of Women's Health, Obstetric, and Neonatal Nurses (AWHONN, 2013). Supplements may lessen the success of breastfeeding because they decrease feeding from the breast and decrease milk production (AAP & ACOG, 2012). A *Healthy People 2020* goal is to reduce the proportion of breastfed newborns who receive formula in the first 2 days of life to no more than 15.6% (DHHS, 2010). In 2016, 17.1% of breastfed infants received formula before they were 2 days old (CDC, 2016a). Teach mothers that supplementing with formula will not necessarily result in their getting more sleep during the night. Breastfed infants do not need water or glucose water because they will interfere with adequate intake of breast milk.

Insufficient Milk Supply. One of the major reasons for early weaning to formula is parents' perception of insufficient milk supply. Women with positive attitudes toward breastfeeding and confidence that they will produce enough milk are less likely to wean early because of perceived insufficiency of milk. Explain the normal course of breastfeeding and the methods of handling problems to help mothers feel more confident in their abilities.

Teach the parents how to assess swallowing and nutritive suckling. Discuss ways to determine whether the infant is receiving enough milk. Suggest that the mother count the number of wet and soiled diapers to help her determine whether the infant is receiving enough milk. A simple chart can be used to record the quality and total number of feedings per day along with the number of voids and stools each day.

Infants should have at least three wet diapers and three stools a day by the third day (Moran & Kallam, 2015). After that time, the normal breastfed infant should have at least four or more stools daily (Lawrence & Lawrence, 2016). The baby who is breastfeeding well will have copious yellow stools by day 6 (Smith, 2016). There should be at least six wet diapers per day by day 4.

Intake also can be gauged when weight gain is assessed at well-baby checkups. After the initial weight loss following birth, infants generally gain approximately 20 to 30 grams (g) (0.7 to 1 oz) each day during the first 3 months (Keane, 2016).

Common causes of decreased milk supply include ineffective suckling by the infant, feedings that are infrequent or too short, maternal fatigue, low maternal thyroid function, preterm or late preterm infants, and some medications, including oral contraceptives containing estrogen. Intervene appropriately if any common causes are present.

Although women were once taught to drink large quantities of liquids to maintain milk supply, fluid intake sufficient to satisfy the mother's thirst and to keep her urine light yellow is adequate.

Because the breasts are soft and the mother does not see large amounts of milk during the first few days, she may believe that little or none is present. This may lead her to give the infant formula before or after the feeding, decreasing milk production. Teach mothers who need to increase milk supply to feed more often and to hand express or use a breast pump after feedings.

If problems persist, refer the woman to a lactation consultant. Lactation professionals are often available in the birth facility and in the community. They can help with breastfeeding techniques and special problems.

PATIENT TEACHING

Is My Baby Getting Enough Milk?

Your baby is probably getting enough milk if:

You hear the baby swallow frequently during feedings. It sounds like a soft "ka" or "ah" sound.

You see nutritive suckling—a smooth series of suckling and swallowing with occasional rest periods. This is different from short, choppy sucks that occur when the baby is falling asleep and not getting milk. After the first few days, you may feel a tingling of your nipples each time a new let-down reflex occurs. This sensation is followed by more nutritive suckling as the infant swallows the increased milk available.

Once your milk has increased, your breast is getting softer during the feeding. (However, your breasts do not have to be hard [engorged] for you to have enough milk.)

You can see milk in the baby's mouth or dripping from your breast occasionally.

You feed your baby 8 to 12 times every 24 hours. More milk is produced when you nurse more often. (Keep track, at first, by writing down the quality and number of feedings each day.)

Your baby has at least one or two wet diapers per day for the first 2 days after birth, at least three or four wet diapers a day by day 3, and at least six wet diapers per day by day 4. Disposable diapers are very absorbent, and knowing whether they are wet is sometimes hard. If you are unsure, place a tissue or cotton ball inside the diaper to show even small amounts of urine. Urine should be light yellow, not dark yellow.

Your baby has at least three or four bowel movements per day by day 3 and four bowel movements per day after that time. The bowel movements transition in color over the first week from black tarry to brown to green to yellow.

Your baby seems satisfied after feedings. (An occasional fussy time is not unusual and does not mean that the baby is not getting enough to eat.)

Well-baby checkups show that your baby is gaining weight.

Getting Help from Family. Fathers often feel there is nothing they can do to help the mother during breastfeeding. Give suggestions on how the father can be involved. Helping the mother recognize early hunger signs can alert the mother to get ready to feed. Fathers can prepare the infant for feeding by changing the diaper and calming the infant. Assisting the mother to position the infant so both mother and baby are comfortable and burping the infant after feedings are other methods of support. Caring for other children, preparing meals, and helping with housework can help mothers get more rest.

Increasing Confidence. Use every opportunity to offer praise and reinforcement of the woman's ability to breastfeed her infant. Point out the infant's positive response to the mother's handling and feeding. Mention the improvements she makes in recognizing hunger cues, positioning, latch-on, and other aspects of care. The nurse's support and encouragement will help the woman feel more confident with each feeding and may lead to a longer duration of breastfeeding.

Providing Resources. Women who stop breastfeeding before they originally planned often cite nipple pain, problems with latch-on, belief that their milk supply was insufficient, and need to return to work as their reasons. Give them contact information for lactation consultants, the local La Leche League (www.llli.org), and other breastfeeding resources in their area that may help them continue breastfeeding. Providing written material and Internet resources such as www.breastfeeding.com or www.womenshealth.gov/breastfeeding is also helpful.

◆ Evaluation

Evaluation of interventions should be continued throughout the birth facility stay. Before discharge, the infant should be feeding well with nutritive sucking and audible swallowing at least 8 to 12 times per day. Mothers should be taught to evaluate feeding by monitoring for a comfortable latch, listening for the infant to swallow while feeding, and watching the baby for signs of satiety. The woman should correctly demonstrate feeding techniques and voice her satisfaction with breastfeeding and confidence in her ability. Satisfaction and confidence are major determinants of whether she continues breastfeeding at home.

? KNOWLEDGE CHECK

9. How can the nurse help the mother establish breastfeeding during the initial feeding sessions?
10. What should the nurse teach the mother about frequency and quality of feedings?

COMMON BREASTFEEDING CONCERNS

Because mothers may be discharged from the birth facility before problems arise, nurses should teach them how to prevent and treat common concerns. When the mother seeks help for problems that have developed after discharge, the nurse should ask what the mother has tried to solve the problem and whether she has used any complementary or alternative therapies. The safety of any therapy should be determined. The mother may have used other herbs to promote milk production. Research on the use of these therapies is inadequate; therefore she should be referred to a health care provider for information before using any substances, because some may be harmful.

Problems may be divided into those originating with the infant and those pertaining to the mother.

Infant Problems

Infant problems require prompt attention to ensure successful breastfeeding.

⚠ SAFETY CHECK

Signs an infant is having breastfeeding problems include the following:
Falling asleep after feeding for less than 5 minutes
Refusal to breastfeed
Tongue thrusting
Smacking or clicking sounds
Dimpling of the cheeks
Failure to open the mouth widely at latch-on
Lower lip turned in
Short, choppy motions of the jaw
No audible swallowing
Use of formula

Sleepy Infant

During the first few days after birth, infants often sleep longer than expected or fall asleep at the breast after feeding for only a short time. They may be tired from the birth process and may not recognize or respond appropriately to hunger.

The nurse should show mothers how to arouse sleepy infants for breastfeeding (see "Patient Teaching: Solutions to Common Breastfeeding Problems,"). If infants start the feeding fully awake, they are more likely to stay awake to finish the feeding. Pointing out the various behavioral states to the mother helps her develop a greater understanding of her infant and recognize when her attempts to feed will be most successful.

When the infant falls asleep during feedings, the nurse should evaluate whether the infant has fed adequately, should be awakened to feed longer, or should be fed again sooner than usual. Emphasizing that wake-up techniques should be gentle is important. The mother should avoid techniques that are excessively irritating to the infant, because feeding should be associated with pleasurable sensations. Infants who continue to be excessively sleepy or nurse poorly need further evaluation. Poor feeding may be an early sign of a complication such as sepsis (see Chapter 24).

Nipple Confusion

Nipple confusion (or nipple preference) may occur when an infant who has been fed by bottle confuses the tongue movements necessary for bottle feeding with the suckling of breastfeeding. Some infants may refuse to breastfeed or use tongue movements that push the breast out of the mouth.

Movements of the mouth and tongue are different in breastfeeding and bottle feeding. During breastfeeding, the infant uses suction to hold the nipple in place near the soft palate. The tongue cups around the nipple and areola with the tip over the lower gum. With each compression of the lower jaw, the tongue presses against the breast, causing the milk to move forward from the ducts and into the infant's mouth.

To feed from a bottle, infants must push the tongue over the nipple to slow the flow of milk and prevent choking. This constant flow can be demonstrated by noting the steady drip of milk when a bottle is held upside down. The infant's lips are relaxed because there is no need to hold the nipple in place. If the infant uses the same thrusting tongue motion and relaxed lips while breastfeeding, the breast may be pushed out of the mouth.

Nurses should discourage the use of bottles or formula in normal breastfeeding infants. It reduces breastfeeding time, which decreases prolactin secretion and therefore milk production. The increased time between feedings limits breast stimulation and may lead to engorgement.

Early pacifier use may be associated with suckling problems and an earlier weaning from the breast for some infants. Pacifiers are advised as one way to decrease the risk for SIDS, but their use can be delayed for the first month until breastfeeding is well established (AAP, 2015a).

Suckling Problems

Suckling problems may occur when the nipple is poorly positioned in the infant's mouth. Dimpling of the cheeks and smacking or clicking sounds may indicate that the infant is sucking on the tongue or nipple only. Some infants do not open their mouths widely enough and suck on the end of the nipple.

Inserting a gloved finger into the infant's mouth helps assess suckling. The motion of the tongue should be felt as the infant sucks. The infant who is thrusting the tongue may have become confused by the use of artificial nipples, which should be avoided until the problem is resolved.

The tongue should be cupped under the breast and should cover the lower gum. If the infant tends to place the tongue on top of the nipple, inserting a finger in the mouth and pressing the infant's tongue down just before latch-on may be effective. Helping the infant open the mouth wide before attachment may improve suckling. More complicated suckling problems may require assistance from a lactation consultant.

Infant Complications

Infant complications may be minor and cause minimal interference with breastfeeding or may prevent the infant from breastfeeding for a long period.

Jaundice. Jaundice (hyperbilirubinemia) in the infant does not necessarily interfere with breastfeeding. Even when infants receive phototherapy, they usually can be removed from the lights for feedings or may able to breastfeed with a biliblanket in place. Concern about adequate intake may be more prevalent in caring for the infant with jaundice. Insensible water loss from the skin is increased as a result of the heat and lights used in treatment and could lead to dehydration.

Infants receiving phototherapy should not be given water, which may decrease the intake of breast milk. Decreased intestinal motility from insufficient milk intake allows reabsorption of bilirubin through the intestinal wall into the bloodstream, increasing the work of the immature liver.

Frequent breastfeeding increases the number of stools, which aids in bilirubin excretion and provides adequate intake of protein and fluid.

Prematurity. If the preterm infant cannot breastfeed immediately after birth, the mother needs encouragement and instruction on how to express her breast milk. She should be assisted in hand expression within the first 1 to 2 hours after delivery and then in the use of a breast pump to establish and maintain her milk supply. Breast pumping should be initiated within the first 6 hours of separation to maximize long-term milk supply. Breast milk offers immunologic and nutritional benefits and is adapted to the preterm infant's needs. Formula use is associated with necrotizing enterocolitis, a serious complication of prematurity, so providing breastmilk to a preterm infant can be lifesaving. It also helps the mother feel she is providing care for her infant even when she is not able to take the baby home with her.

The woman can express her milk and take it to the nursery for the infant's feedings. The nurse should provide sterile containers for the woman to take home and instruct her in special nursery requirements. The containers should be labeled with the infant's name and the date and time the milk was pumped.

Some preterm infants or those with breastfeeding problems respond well to the use of supplementary feeding devices. These consist of a container of milk with a small plastic feeding tube attached to the breast. When the infant begins to breastfeed, milk is drawn from both the container and the breast, increasing the infant's intake and motivation to continue suckling. As the infant gains weight and feeding ability increases, use of the device is gradually decreased until it can be discontinued completely.

Women who provide breast milk for their preterm infants may feel something is wrong with their milk when additions such as human milk fortifier are used. They should be reassured that their milk is very important in providing nutrition and protection against infection but that the infant needs more of some nutrients during the period of very rapid growth.

Late preterm infants (born between the 34th week and the 37th week of gestation) may have difficulty feeding. Although they may look like full-term infants, they are immature. Coordination of sucking, swallowing, and breathing may be poor, and they may be sleepier than full-term infants.

A lactation consultant should be involved in teaching the mother her late preterm infant's special needs and monitoring the effectiveness of feedings. The infants need to be positioned in such a way that the head is supported, as in a football hold. Infants should be seen by a health care provider within 1 to 2 days after discharge to check the weight, adequacy of feeding, and jaundice. Frequent visits and weight checks should be made for any infants having feeding difficulties. Weekly weight checks should be performed until the infant reaches 40 weeks of postconceptional age (ABM, 2011).

Illness and Congenital Defects

Infant illness and congenital defects such as a cleft palate may cause breastfeeding problems. If the mother is not able to nurse the infant at first, she will need assistance to maintain lactation until breastfeeding is possible. Referral to support groups can be particularly helpful. Some groups focus on particular congenital defects, and others focus on breastfeeding infants with special problems.

Maternal Concerns

Early nursing intervention can help the mother overcome common breast problems.

Common Breast Problems

Engorgement, nipple trauma, flat or inverted nipples, plugged ducts, and **mastitis** (infection of the breast) are common problems involving the breasts.

Engorgement. Many women experience a temporary swelling or fullness of the breasts, which peaks at 72 to 96 hours after giving birth when the production of milk begins to increase or the milk "comes in" (Lawrence & Lawrence, 2016). This normal temporary fullness is the result of congestion, increased vascularity, accumulation of milk, and edema. It should not interfere with breastfeeding.

Engorgement may become a problem if feedings are delayed, too short, or infrequent. Engorged breasts become edematous, hard, and tender, making feeding and even movement painful. The areola may become so hard that the infant cannot compress it for feeding. An engorged areola causes the nipple to become flat, making it more difficult for the infant to draw it into the back of the mouth. Engorgement may lead to nipple trauma, mastitis, and even the discontinuation of breastfeeding.

Nurses help prevent engorgement by assisting women to begin breastfeeding early and to feed frequently. Encouraging mothers to breastfeed with all infant feeding cues, even at night, ensures that the breasts are emptied regularly. The use of water and formula should be discouraged.

> ### ! SAFETY CHECK
>
> Maternal signs of breastfeeding problems are as follows:
> Hard, tender breasts
> Painful, red, cracked, blistered, or bleeding nipples
> Flat or inverted nipples
> Localized edema or pain in either breast
> Fever, generalized aching, or malaise

Nipple Pain. Nipple pain is common during early breastfeeding. Pain for 1 minute or less may occur at the beginning of feedings because of tissue stretching and suction on the ductules before they fill with milk. Nipple pain is common during the first week, usually peaks at the third to sixth day, and resolves soon afterward (Smith, 2016).

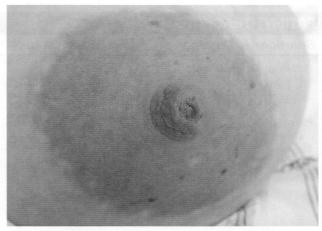

FIG. 22.9 Note the cracked area on this nipple.

Nipple trauma causes more sustained pain. Traumatized nipples appear red, cracked, blistered, or bleeding (Fig. 22.9). Minor nipple trauma can be treated by independent nursing interventions. Redness of breast tissue, purulent drainage, and fever indicate mastitis or breast abscess and require antibiotic treatment.

Improper positioning or latch-on techniques, and exposure to soaps, prolonged moisture from wet breast pads, or irritating creams may cause sore nipples. Using a breast pump too long or with the suction set on high may be traumatic.

Flat and Inverted Nipples. Nipple abnormalities should be identified during pregnancy, if possible, but interventions can begin after birth, if necessary. Nipple rolling just before feeding helps flat nipples become more erect so the infant can grasp them more readily (Fig. 22.10). A breast pump used for a few minutes before feedings or a breast shield may help draw out inverted nipples.

Plugged Ducts. Although the exact cause of occlusion of a lactiferous duct is unknown, engorgement, missed feedings, or a constricting bra may be involved. Localized edema and tenderness are present, and a hard area may be palpated. A tiny, white area may be present on the nipple. Massage of the area (Fig. 22.11), frequent breastfeeding, heat application, and using varied breastfeeding positions are helpful. A plugged duct may progress to mastitis if not treated promptly. Mastitis involves localized pain accompanied by fever, generalized aching, and malaise.

Illness in the Mother

It is rarely necessary for a mother to stop breastfeeding when she is ill. If breastfeeding must be temporarily stopped because of the mother's condition or the drugs she receives, the nurse should help the mother hand express or use a breast pump until she resumes breastfeeding. Abrupt weaning may lead to mastitis.

Drug Transfer to Breast Milk

Most medications taken by the mother are compatible with breastfeeding. Some drugs interfere with milk production.

PATIENT TEACHING

Solutions to Common Breastfeeding Problems

Problem: Sleepy Infant

An infant is sleepy at feeding time or falls asleep shortly after beginning feeding.

Prevention

Look for signs your baby is ready to wake up, such as movement of the eyes through closed eyelids, small twitches of the face, sucking movements, stretching, and increased movements of the entire body.

Gently awaken your baby when you see those signs. Talk, gently move the infant's arms and legs, and play with the infant for a short time before beginning the feeding.

Unwrap the baby's blankets and change the diaper. Swaddling infants by wrapping them tightly with blankets is a calming technique that often helps them sleep. Leave the blanket and shirt off as you begin the feeding with the baby skin-to-skin against your chest. Your body and a blanket draped over both of you after your baby begins to nurse will provide adequate warmth.

Solutions

If your baby goes to sleep during the feeding and has fed for just a few minutes, try the following:

Undress the baby (except for the diaper) and place the infant against your skin (if you have not done this already).

Rub the baby's hair or back gently, stroke around his or her mouth, or shift the baby's position slightly to see if he or she will wake up.

Remove the baby from the breast. Rub the infant's back to bring up bubbles of air that may cause a sensation of stomach fullness. Rubbing the back also stimulates the central nervous system and arouses the baby.

Change the diaper.

Express a few drops of colostrum onto the nipple. The baby tastes the colostrum when the nipple is offered and often resumes suckling.

Wipe the face gently with a lukewarm washcloth to help the infant wake up.

If your baby cannot be aroused with a few of these gentle techniques, a longer sleep period may be needed. Let the infant remain skin-to-skin with you for another half hour, then begin again. Watch for signs the baby is in a lighter phase of sleep and can be awakened more easily.

Problem: Nipple Confusion

An infant who has taken bottles pushes the nipple out of the mouth and sucks poorly during breastfeeding. The infant has become confused about the way to suckle from the breast and is using sucking movements for bottle feeding.

Prevention

Avoid all bottles and pacifiers unless absolutely necessary. If the baby has a medical need for extra breastmilk, consider using a supplemental nursing system, spoon or cup feeding, or an oral syringe.

Do not give the baby formula during the night. The extra sleep is not worth the possibility of later feeding difficulties.

Avoid giving formula before or after breastfeeding because it is unnecessary for healthy newborns. It may cause the infant's stomach to become distended causing more "spitting up." Adding formula will cause the infant to wait longer before breastfeeding again, which decreases milk production.

Solution

Stop all bottle feeding and pacifier use so that the baby becomes accustomed to suckling from the breast instead of the bottle. Nurse more often to stimulate milk production and help the baby learn what to do.

Problem: Latch-On Difficulty

The infant sucks on the end of the nipple or fails to open his or her mouth widely enough.

Prevention

Do not insert the breast into the infant's mouth until the infant opens the mouth widely with the tongue down and forward (like biting into a large sandwich).

Bring the baby to the breast with your nipple pointed toward the roof of the baby's mouth and the baby's chin touching your breast first. The baby should have more breast tissue from underneath the breast than from on top (asymmetric latch).

Solutions

Stop the feeding and start again if the infant is sucking on the end of the nipple, you see dimples in the infant's cheeks, or hear smacking, slurping, or clicking sounds. Short, choppy movement of the jaw means that the infant is going to sleep or has finished feeding.

If you believe the infant should nurse longer, awaken the infant and begin again.

Problem: Engorgement

The mother's breasts are hard and tender from engorgement.

Prevention

Room-in with your baby so you can respond to feeding cues. Breastfeed the infant with all feeding cues, usually at least 8 to 12 times in a 24-hour period. Do not give bottles during the day or night, because this increases the risk for engorgement. Waiting even 4 hours between feedings may increase the risk for engorgement, but frequent breastfeeding often can prevent it.

Solutions

To reduce edema and pain, apply cold packs to the breasts between feedings. Use commercial cold packs or make inexpensive cold packs from frozen washcloths, packages of frozen vegetables, or plastic bags filled with crushed ice. Cover cold packs with a washcloth before applying to the skin. A disposable diaper with crushed ice placed between the layers also may be used.

Some women find application of cool cabbage leaves are helpful. Studies on their use have had mixed results (Lawrence & Lawrence, 2016).

PATIENT TEACHING—cont'd

Solutions to Common Breastfeeding Problems

Although heat to the breasts can increase blood flow to the area and make engorgement worse, some mothers find that breast massage and hand expression in a warm shower immediately before a feeding is helpful (Lawrence & Lawrence, 2016).

Massage the breasts before and during feedings to stimulate the let-down reflex so that the baby can nurse more easily.

If the areola is engorged and hard, making it difficult for the baby to latch on, express a little milk by hand or with a breast pump. Or apply gentle pressure on the areola to move some swelling back into the breast and soften the areola to allow the infant to latch on. As soon as the areolae are soft, begin to feed.

Increase skin-to-skin contact and feed more often, such as every 1.5 to 2 hours.

Wear a well-fitting bra for support during the day and at night for comfort.

Take prescribed pain medication just before feedings to make you more comfortable.

Problem: Sore Nipples
The nipples are sore and may be cracked, blistered, or bleeding.

Prevention
Position the baby at the breast in an asymmetric latch with enough of the breast in the mouth that the nipple is not compressed between the baby's gums during breastfeeding.

Avoid engorgement by breastfeeding frequently. Express enough milk to soften the areola if engorgement makes the areola too hard for the infant to grasp.

Vary the position of the baby to change the areas of pressure on the nipple.

Do not use soap on the nipples because it removes the protective oils and causes drying.

If you use breast pads for leaking milk, remove them when they become wet to prevent irritation of the skin. Avoid pads with plastic linings that retain moisture. Use a handkerchief or pieces of cotton cloth as inexpensive, washable substitutes for commercial breast pads.

Solutions
Using warm compresses before feedings will help the milk flow more quickly. Use them between feedings to soothe nipples.

Express a small amount of milk before feeding to begin the let-down reflex.

Begin each feeding with the less sore breast first. The hungry baby nurses more vigorously at first, which may be painful. The let-down reflex is started, causing milk to flow more quickly from the second breast.

Massage the breasts when the infant pauses during feedings to enhance milk flow.

Vary the position of the infant during feedings. The area of the nipple directly in line with the infant's nose and chin is most stressed during the feeding.

Nipple shields (artificial nipples that fit over your own nipples) may be helpful in some situations, but they also can contribute to breastfeeding difficulties. A lactation consultant should help you determine whether they are appropriate for your situation and help you use them correctly for a short period of time.

Breast creams may cause sensitivity and irritation. If you choose to use lanolin, use only purified lanolin to protect against allergens and pesticides. Creams that have to be removed before each feeding may increase soreness. Hydrogel pads may also be used to soothe nipples.

Apply colostrum or breast milk to the nipples after feedings because they have healing properties. Allow your nipples to air dry.

If you have burning, itching, or stabbing pain throughout your breast, call the health care provider for further evaluation.

Take prescribed pain medication just before feedings to help you relax.

Problem: Flat or Inverted Nipples
The mother's nipples are flat or inverted, and the baby has difficulty drawing them into his or her mouth.

Prevention
None.

Solutions
Some women find wearing breast shells in the bra helps make the nipples protrude.

Just before beginning breastfeeding, roll the nipple between your thumb and forefinger to help it protrude (see Fig. 22.10).

Use a breast pump for a few minutes just before feedings. Put the baby to your breast immediately after the pump causes the nipple to become erect. The normal suckling process usually causes the nipple to stay erect.

In some situations, a nipple shield may be used for a short time with the help of a lactation consultant to help the infant latch onto inverted nipples.

❓ KNOWLEDGE CHECK

11. What wake-up techniques should the nurse teach the mother of a sleepy infant?
12. How does sucking from a bottle differ from suckling from the breast?
13. What help can the nurse offer the mother with engorged breasts?
14. How should the nurse advise the mother with sore nipples?

Therefore both prescription and over-the-counter drugs should be approved by the health care provider. In many cases, another drug can be substituted for one that adversely affects the infant. If a mother must take a drug that will be harmful to her infant, she should pump her breasts and discard the milk while she is taking the medication. Once the drug clears her bloodstream, she may resume breastfeeding. Some drugs may not reach the infant in harmful amounts if taken after a feeding or at night when there is a longer time between feedings. The U.S. National Library of Medicine has a website for information about drugs during lactation at www.toxnet.nlm.nih.gov/newtoxnet/lactmed.htm.

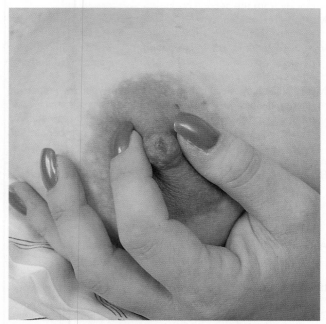

FIG. 22.10 Rolling helps flat nipples become erect in preparation for latch-on.

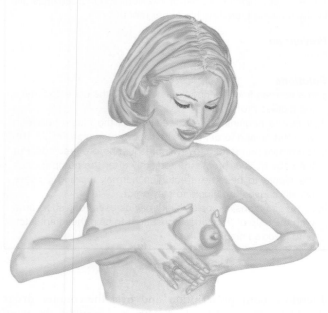

FIG. 22.11 To massage the breasts, the mother places her hands against the chest wall with her fingers encircling the breasts. She gently slides her hands forward until the fingers overlap. The position of the hands is rotated to cover all breast tissue. Massaging with the fingertips in a circular motion over all areas of the breast is also helpful.

Conditions in Which Breastfeeding Should Be Avoided.
In some situations, such as a mother's serious illness that can be transmitted to the infant, breastfeeding is contraindicated. Women who take methadone or buprenorphine for opiate addiction are allowed to breastfeed because only minimal amounts of the drugs pass to breast milk (ACOG, 2016). Other types of drug abuse, active untreated tuberculosis, human immunodeficiency virus (HIV) infection, galactosemia, maternal chemotherapy, and mothers who must take drugs that are unsafe for the infant are situations in which breastfeeding is not advised.

Mothers with hepatitis A, B, or C may breastfeed. Infants of mothers with hepatitis B should receive hepatitis B vaccine and immunoglobulin. Herpes simplex does not preclude breastfeeding if the mother does not have a lesion on her breast and uses thorough handwashing (Lawrence & Lawrence, 2016). Women who smoke can breastfeed but should stop smoking if possible or not smoke around the infant.

Previous Breast Surgery

Women who have had surgery for breast reduction, augmentation, or other conditions may have difficulty with lactation. The ability to produce and transfer milk to the nipple depends on the surgical technique used and the amount of tissue involved. Surgery may disrupt the neural pathways, ducts, and blood supply. Some women can breastfeed without problems. Others may be able to do so by pumping to help build up milk supply or using a supplementation device when the breasts are unable to produce a sufficient amount of milk.

Women with pierced nipples should not have difficulty with breastfeeding. They should remove the rings or studs before feeding the infant.

Employment

Although some women remain at home for 6 or more weeks after giving birth, others must return to work earlier. With some advance planning, breastfeeding can be efficiently combined with working. Breastfeeding classes and support groups are often helpful in providing practical advice on how to merge employment with lactation.

The mother will need to procure a breast pump. The expense of a pump is covered under most insurance plans. A week or two before she returns to work, the mother should use a breast pump once or twice a day to practice pumping her breasts and to build up a small supply of frozen breast milk. The breasts should be pumped after the infant has nursed. Giving the infant breast milk from a bottle occasionally about 2 weeks before returning to work makes the transition smoother.

Most working mothers use a pump two or three times a day during lunch or breaks at work. The woman needs a clean, private place to pump. A national goal is to increase the proportion of employers that have worksite lactation support programs (DHHS, 2010). U.S. law now requires employers to provide reasonable break time for a nursing employee to express milk for 1 year after her child's birth. A place to express milk, other than a bathroom, is also to be provided and must be shielded from view and intrusions (U.S. Department of Labor, 2010).

The milk should be refrigerated or placed in an insulated container with ice to be used for the next day's feedings by the caregiver. Breastfeeding just before the mother leaves for work and again when she returns home keeps the time between feedings at a minimum. Frequent breastfeeding throughout the evenings and on weekends help her maintain her milk supply.

Some mothers choose to use formula during work hours but breastfeed when at home. They should prepare for this by gradually eliminating the feedings that occur during work hours and substituting a bottle. Although the total milk supply is diminished, breastfeeding can continue in the mornings and evenings.

Milk Expression and Storage

When milk expression is needed, the nurse helps the mother use hand expression (Fig. 22.12) or a breast pump (Fig. 22.13).

Hand Expression. Hand expression can be performed without other equipment and is often a more effective way to collect colostrum. It also can be used in emergency situations when a mother is separated from her baby and may be done without electricity or a pump. Hand expression or manual pumps are also useful for the mother who wants to save breast milk for another feeding occasionally or whose areolae are so engorged that the infant cannot grasp them.

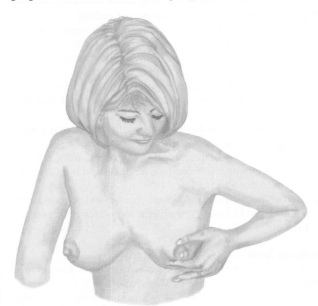

FIG. 22.12 To express milk from the breast, the mother places her hand just behind the areola, with the thumb on top and the fingers supporting the breast. The tissue is pressed back against the chest wall; then the fingers and thumb are brought together and toward the nipple. This compresses the ducts and causes milk to flow. The action is repeated to simulate the suckling of the infant. Moving the hands around the areola allows compression of all areas and increases removal of milk from the breast. Compression should be gentle to avoid trauma. Application of heat and massage before expression increase the flow of milk.

Use of a Breast Pump. The mother who plans to pump her milk for a prolonged period should use an electric breast pump. Battery-operated pumps are small, portable, and relatively inexpensive for short-term use. Large electric hospital-grade pumps can be rented for home use. They are more efficient than hand pumps or battery-operated pumps and are indicated when the mother plans to pump for a long time. A double pump allows the mother to pump both breasts at once, saving time and increasing milk production.

A woman who cannot breastfeed her infant should be instructed in the use of the breast pump as soon as possible after birth, but at least within the first 6 hours (Spatz, 2016). She should pump her breasts as often as the infant would nurse or at least eight times a day if she plans to breastfeed for a prolonged time (Spatz, 2016). Sessions should last approximately 15 to 20 minutes.

The mother should wash her hands before using the pump and before preparing the pumped milk for storage or feeding. Breast massage and application of heat before pumping help initiate the flow of milk. Massaging the breast during pumping may increase the volume of milk obtained at each session. Pumping after the first morning feeding often produces the greatest volume. Relaxation during pumping increases volume, but tension or discomfort may reduce the output. The mother should plan enough time for pumping so she does not feel hurried, because that would increase tension and decrease the output.

The amount of suction should be set at a low level in the beginning and gradually increased, if necessary. Too much negative pressure traumatizes the breast. If the woman needs to increase her milk supply, pumping more often and with breast massage and hand expression is more effective than longer sessions. The pump should be cleaned according to the manufacturer's instructions after each use.

Milk Storage. Milk should be stored in clean (sterile for a hospitalized infant) glass or rigid polypropylene containers with a tight cap (Spatz, 2016). A nipple should not be used to cover the container during storage because the hole allows passage of organisms that can contaminate the milk.

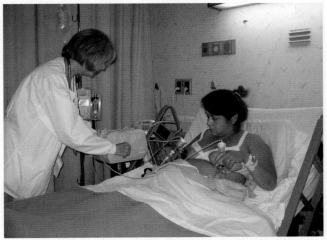

FIG. 22.13 The nurse helps the mother use an electric breast pump.

Fresh unrefrigerated breast milk should generally be used within 3 to 4 hours of pumping. Under very clean conditions using it within 6 to 8 hours is acceptable. It may be stored in a refrigerator at 4°C (39°F) or below for 72 hours in usual circumstances or for 5 to 8 days under very clean situations (ABM, 2010). Milk that is fresh or has been refrigerated rather than frozen should be used as much as possible so the leukocytes are available for the infant (Spatz, 2016).

If the milk is to be frozen, it should be placed in the back of the freezer and kept at −17°C (0°F) or below. It should optimally be used by 6 months, although use within 12 months is acceptable (ABM, 2010). Milk should be frozen in amounts that are likely to be used for one feeding. Containers should be marked with the date and the oldest used first. Newly pumped milk should not be added to containers of previously pumped milk.

Breast milk can be thawed and warmed by holding the container under running water. Cool water should be used first to defrost it; then the milk can be warmed by placing it under warm running water or in a bowl of warm water. It also can be thawed in the refrigerator and used within 24 hours. It should not be refrozen.

Milk should not be heated in a microwave because the microwave heats unevenly. The infant might be burned because the container may be cool but the milk may have hot spots. Thawed breast milk should be gently inverted a few times to mix the foremilk and hindmilk. Milk that is not finished in one feeding should be discarded within 1 hour.

Breastfeeding after Multiple Births

Mothers who have more than one newborn have many questions about breastfeeding and need help and support from nurses and family members to be successful. Explain to the mother that her milk supply adjusts to the demand and that she can produce enough milk for her infants. Breastfeeding each baby 8 to 12 times per day to build up the milk supply is important. If the infants cannot breastfeed at first, the woman will need help hand expressing and using a breast pump.

If the woman decides to feed two infants simultaneously, the nurse helps position them in the football (clutch) hold, cradle hold, or a combination of both. She should be encouraged to eat well, get enough rest, and ask for help from family and friends.

PATIENT TEACHING

Breastfeeding after the Birth of More than One Infant

Ensuring Adequate Milk Production

Because the amount of milk produced depends on the amount of suckling the breasts receive, mothers can produce enough milk for more than one baby. Breastfeeding each baby frequently (8 to 12 times per day) helps build up the milk supply. Production of milk may be more evenly stimulated if you alternate breasts for each infant, especially if one baby has a weaker suck.

Using a Breast Pump

If your infants are not ready for breastfeeding, use hand expression and a breast pump to build up your milk supply and provide milk for them until they are ready to nurse. Use the pump every 2 to 3 hours while you are awake and once or twice during the night. Pump for 15 to 20 minutes during at least 8 to 12 pumping sessions daily. Use a double pump to decrease the time spent pumping and increase the production of milk.

If one baby is ready to breastfeed before the other(s), nurse the baby and pump your breasts after each feeding to stimulate milk production. An alternative is to nurse the infant on one breast and use a breast pump on the other at the same time.

Feeding Simultaneously or Individually

You can feed each baby separately or feed two infants at once. Simultaneous breastfeeding shortens feeding times, but both infants must be awake at once. You may need help positioning the infants at first. Individual feeding can be done without help and on each infant's own schedule, but a larger portion of your day will be spent feeding. If the babies initially need help latching and staying in a nutritive feeding pattern, it may be necessary to feed the infants separately at first and begin simultaneous feedings when each infant is feeding well at the breast.

Positioning Infants for Simultaneous Feeding

Use a variety of positions for breastfeeding two infants at once. Place pillows under both infants to lift them to the right height and keep them in place. Use pillows under your arms and behind your back to make yourself comfortable.

Football (clutch) hold—Support each infant's body on pillows along your side. Place a hand behind each infant's shoulders and bring the infants to the breasts.

Football and cradle hold—Place one infant in a cradle position on pillows across your lap. Place the other infant in a football position with the body supported on pillows alongside you. Once the infants are in position, help one and then the other latch onto the breast.

Crisscross hold—Place pillows on your lap and hold each baby in the cradle position. The infants' legs crisscross over one another.

Keeping Track

Keep track of the frequency and quality of each infant's feedings. Record the number of wet diapers and bowel movements each infant has each day. You can assign each infant one breast without changing to the opposite breast, if you choose. Mothers often alternate the breast each infant nurses from at each feeding to keep stimulation of the breasts similar. Alternating breasts every 24 hours may be easier to remember.

Care for Yourself

Eating well and getting enough rest are important. Ask for help from family and friends. Pamper yourself as much as possible, and leave care of the house and cooking to others if you can. Your major responsibility during this time should be to care for yourself and your new babies!

Weaning

Mothers are sometimes subjected to opinions and pressure from family and friends about weaning. There is no one "right" time to wean the infant. The AAP suggests exclusive breastfeeding for at least 6 months and then to add complementary foods and continue to breastfeed until the baby is at least 1 year old and as long after that as both mother and baby desire (AAP, 2012). Mothers choose to wean their infants for various reasons. The nurse should provide information so women can make informed decisions about weaning and should support the woman once her decision is made. Explaining that even a short period of breastfeeding offers her infant many advantages is reassuring.

Mothers may need help in planning a slow weaning process to help avoid engorgement and allow the infant to become accustomed to a bottle or cup gradually. Mothers who are not in a hurry to wean may allow the infant to take the lead. Omitting one breastfeeding session a day and waiting several days or a week before omitting another will allow the mother and the infant to adjust to the change more easily. Weaning too rapidly increases the risk for plugged ducts or mastitis. Infants who are weaned before 12 months of age should be given iron-fortified formula instead of cow's milk (AAP & ACOG, 2012).

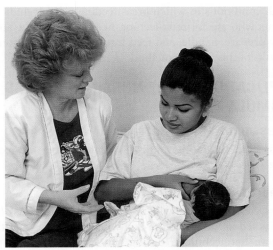

FIG. 22.14 The nurse offers suggestions on hand position during the clinic visit.

Home Care

Some infants have not breastfed well by the time of discharge from the birth facility, placing them at risk for failure to gain weight, dehydration, and hyperbilirubinemia. Problems with engorgement and sore nipples are more likely to occur after discharge. These families need continued support by nurses during home, clinic, or office visits (Fig. 22.14). The infant should be seen by the physician or other health care provider 3 to 5 days after birth or within 48 hours of discharge and again at 2 to 3 weeks of age to assess for any problems that might occur early after discharge (AAP & ACOG, 2012).

A mother may be concerned when her infant suddenly seems to want to nurse much more often. She may assume she is not producing enough milk. Nurses can teach mothers this behavior shows their infants are experiencing growth spurts. These growth spurts occur at approximately 10 days, 2 weeks, 6 weeks, 3 months, and 6 months after birth (Grodner et al., 2016).

Guidance for dealing with breastfeeding problems can be continued after discharge by referring the mother to lactation consultants or organizations such as La Leche League, a support group that gives assistance to breastfeeding mothers. La Leche League groups are available in most communities and are available on their website (www.llli.org). Support groups also may be provided by the birth facility.

PATIENT TEACHING

How to Wean from Breastfeeding

Deciding When to Wean

Breastfeeding protects both your health and the health of your baby and this protection is stronger the longer your baby breastfeeds. You can continue to breastfeed as long as both you and your baby wish. Only you and your baby can make the decision about when to wean. Before you decide to begin weaning, evaluate the reasons for continuing breastfeeding or beginning weaning.

How to Proceed

Gradual weaning is best for both you and your baby. Abrupt weaning can lead to engorgement and mastitis for you and can be upsetting for both you and your baby. You both need to get used to this change slowly.

Eliminate one feeding at a time. Replace it with a bottle for the young infant who needs to continue sucking. Infants generally do not drink as much from a cup as they do from a bottle. They may need a bottle to get enough milk to meet their nutritional requirements. The older infant who has learned to use a cup may not need a bottle at all. Use formula instead of cow's milk until the infant is at least 1 year old because formula is more suited to an infant's needs.

Omit a middle of the day feeding first. Begin with the feeding in which the baby seems least interested, and then gradually eliminate others.

Wait several days before eliminating another feeding. This allows time for your milk production to adjust and the baby to accept the changes.

Eliminate the baby's favorite feedings last. Many infants are particularly fond of morning and bedtime feedings.

Expect your infant to want to nurse again when tired, ill, or hurt during the weaning process. This is sometimes called "comfort breastfeeding." A few minutes of breastfeeding may be all that is necessary to comfort the baby.

? KNOWLEDGE CHECK

15. What teaching should be included for the mother who plans to work and breastfeed?
16. What should the mother know about weaning?

FORMULA FEEDING

According to the AAP (2012), "Breastfeeding and human milk are the normative standards for infant feeding and nutrition" (p.e827). However, some parents make an informed decision to formula feed. In addition, there are some rare health conditions in which breastfeeding is contraindicated. Parents who are formula feeding need to be taught how to safely prepare, handle, and feed formula to mitigate some of the risks of this feeding method.

◆ APPLICATION OF THE NURSING PROCESS: FORMULA FEEDING

◆ Assessment

Assess both the mother and the infant during the feeding process.

Mother's Knowledge

Assess the mother's knowledge of formula feeding. Ask her if she has fed an infant before and whether she has questions. Observe her technique during the initial and subsequent feedings. Note how she holds the infant and the bottle, and evaluate her burping technique to identify areas in which she seems unsure.

Infant Feeding Behaviors

Point out infant feeding cues, which are the same regardless of how infants are fed. Waiting until the infant is frantic may result in a feeding taken too fast, with excess swallowing of air or choking. Assess the way the infant sucks to identify problems.

◆ Identification of Patient Problems

Because improper formula preparation and feeding techniques could harm the infant, the parents' lack of understanding of formula preparation and feeding techniques is a potential patient problem that could lead to a potential for injury to the infant.

◆ Planning: Expected Outcomes

The mother will demonstrate correct techniques in holding the infant and bottle during feedings and will correctly describe how to prepare formula and the frequency of feedings.

◆ Interventions
Teaching about Formula

The parents must learn about types of formula available and how to prepare them.

Types of Formula. The physician or nurse practitioner prescribes the type of formula the mother is to use. Infants should receive iron-fortified formula. Formula may be purchased in three different forms: ready-to-use formula, concentrated liquid formula, and powdered formula.

Ready-to-Use Formula. Ready-to-use formula is available in bottles to which a nipple is added or in cans to be poured directly into a bottle. It should not be diluted. The container should be shaken and the top of the can washed before opening and pouring it into a bottle. Although expensive, it is presterilized and practical when traveling, when there is difficulty in mixing formula, or if the water supply is in question. Refrigeration is not necessary until the container is opened. An open can should be refrigerated and used within 48 hours.

Concentrated Liquid Formula. Explain to the parents how to dilute concentrated liquid formula. Equal parts of concentrated liquid formula and water are mixed together and poured into a bottle to provide the amount desired for each feeding. Once again, the can should be shaken well and the top washed before opening. Opened cans should be stored in the refrigerator and used within 48 hours (AAP, 2015b).

Powdered Formula. Powdered formula is more economical, but because it is not a sterile product, can harbor pathogens that cause significant illness in infants (World Health Organization [WHO], 2007). Therefore it is not recommended for infants who are preterm, less than 2 months of age, or immunocompromised (WHO, 2007).

To help kill pathogens that may be present in the powder, powdered formula should be mixed with boiling water that has not been allowed to cool for more than 30 minutes (WHO, 2007). Usually one level scoop of powder is added to each 60 mL (2 oz) of water in a bottle. Formula should be well mixed to dissolve the powder and make the solution uniform. The bottle should then be rapidly cooled to a temperature safe for feeding by placing the bottle under running cold tap water or placing it in a cup of cold water (WHO, 2007)

Because prepared formula is an ideal growth medium for pathogens, new formula should be prepared for each feeding and used immediately. However, for practical reasons, several feedings can be prepared at once and refrigerated for no more than 24 hours (WHO, 2007). Any prepared formula left at room temperature for more than 2 hours should be discarded (WHO, 2007).

> **! SAFETY CHECK**
>
> Formulas must be properly diluted to prevent serious, possibly fatal, illness (such as fluid and electrolyte imbalance) and promote weight gain and growth in the infant. It is essential that the instructions on the label be followed accurately. Many parents may not read labels because they are unaware of the different types of formula.
> **Ready-to-use preparations:** Use as is without dilution.
> **Concentrated formulas:** Dilute with equal parts of water.
> **Powdered formulas:** Mix one level scoop of powder with 60 mL (2 oz) of water that is at least 70°C (158°F) (WHO, 2007).

Equipment. Many different types of bottles and nipples are available. Mothers may use glass or plastic bottles or a plastic liner that fits into a rigid container. Selection of type of bottles and nipples depends on individual preference. Although bisphenol-A (BPA) was once a concern, it is no longer used in baby bottles in the United States.

Preparation. Discuss preparation of formula with the mother. Instruct the mother to wash her hands as well as the top of the can and the can opener (if needed). Infection may occur if the equipment, milk, or water used for preparation is contaminated. Emphasize the importance of following the directions on the label when mixing the formula. Improper dilution of the formula may cause undernutrition, imbalances of sodium level, and an excessively high renal solute load, which can be dangerous to the infant. If water from a well is used, it should be tested for high levels of nitrates, which can be harmful to infants.

Bottles and nipples can be washed in hot, sudsy water using a brush to clean well, then rinsed and allowed to air-dry. They also may be washed in a dishwasher. The formula and water are poured into the bottles, which then are capped. Emphasize that the proportion of water and liquid or powdered formula must be followed exactly to avoid causing illness in the infant.

Explain that if safety of the water supply is questionable, sterilization is necessary. All equipment is washed and rinsed well before beginning. The equipment needed for the procedure is boiled for 10 to 12 minutes in a sterilizer or deep pan (Nickols-Richardson, 2015). Water for diluting the formula is boiled separately. The bottles are then assembled using sterilized tongs. The formula and boiled water are added, and the bottles are capped and refrigerated until needed. Prepared bottles should be used within 24 hours (AAP, 2015b).

Explaining Feeding Techniques

Positioning. Show the parents how to position the infant in a semiupright position such as the cradle hold. This allows them to hold the infant close in a face-to-face position. The bottle is held with the nipple kept full of formula to prevent excessive swallowing of air (Fig. 22.15). Placing the infant in the opposite arm for each feeding provides varied visual stimulation during feedings.

Burping. For the first few days, the infant should be burped or "bubbled" after every 15 mL (0.5 oz) of formula. Gradually, the infant is able to take more formula before burping and should be burped halfway through feeding. Show the parents how to burp the infant over the shoulder or in a sitting position with the head supported while patting or rubbing the infant's back (Fig. 22.16).

Frequency and Amount. Instruct the parents to feed the infant every 3 to 4 hours but to avoid rigid scheduling and take cues from the infant. Hunger signs are the same as for breastfed infants. Teach the parents to begin feeding 15 to 30 mL (0.5 to 1 oz) at a time during the first 24 hours, then gradually increase by 15 mL (0.5 oz). The baby should not be forced to finish a bottle (Janke, 2014).

Cautions. Instruct the mother not to heat formula in a microwave oven because the heating will be uneven. This may result in some parts of the liquid being very hot even when the outside of the bottle feels only warm. Formula can be heated by placing it in a container of warm water for 5 to 10 minutes. Suggest that the mother test the formula temperature by allowing a few drops from the bottle to fall on her inner arm.

Sometimes, formula flow is too fast for infants. If this occurs, the infant may choke, gag, sputter, drool, or bite the nipple. Some infants suck without stopping to breathe frequently enough. To provide a rest period, the mother should tip the baby forward to stop the flow of milk.

Caution parents not to prop the bottle. Propping increases the likelihood of choking if regurgitation occurs and eliminates the holding and cuddling that should accompany feeding. Some mothers put an infant to bed with a bottle propped. This not only increases the danger of aspiration but also allows milk to pool in the mouth. Prolonged contact of teeth with milk promotes growth of bacteria and leads to cavities once teeth erupt. Otitis media is also more common in infants who sleep with a bottle or feed from a propped bottle.

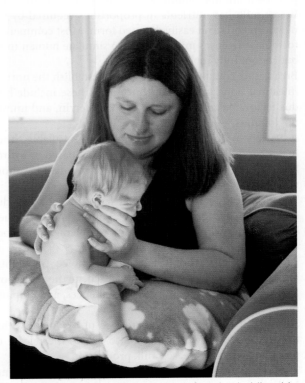

FIG. 22.16 The mother burps the infant by holding him in the sitting position. She supports the infant's head and chest with one hand and gently pats the back with the other hand.

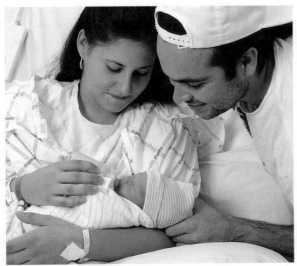

FIG. 22.15 This mother holds her infant close during bottle feeding. The bottle is positioned such that the nipple is filled with milk at all times. The father offers encouragement.

The parents should not try to coax the infant to finish every bottle because it could cause regurgitation and excessive weight gain. The mother should not save formula from one feeding to the next because of the danger of rapidly growing bacteria. Any formula not used within 1 hour should be discarded.

Infant Variations. Infants vary in their feeding preferences. Some infants drink from the bottle reluctantly. Although formula is usually given at room temperature, some infants take heated or cool formula better. The mother of a sleepy infant needs to use the same wake-up techniques described for the breastfeeding mother.

Angling the tip of the nipple so that it rubs the palate triggers the suck reflex in most infants. It may take patience and persistence to find the most effective techniques.

◆ Evaluation

The mother should hold the infant and bottle correctly during feedings. She should be able to correctly describe formula preparation and the amount and frequency of feedings.

> ### ❓ KNOWLEDGE CHECK
> 17. What questions might a mother have about formula feeding?
> 18. Why should mothers avoid propping bottles?

SUMMARY CONCEPTS

- Full-term breastfed infants need 85 to 100 kcal/kg (39 to 45 kcal/lb) and formula-fed infants need 100 to 110 kcal/kg (45 to 50 kcal/lb) daily. They may lose weight in the first few days after birth as a result of insufficient intake and normal loss of extracellular fluid and meconium.
- Lactogenesis I begins during pregnancy and continues after birth with the secretion of colostrum. Lactogenesis II begins 2 to 3 days after birth when transitional milk appears. Lactogenesis III is the time when mature milk replaces transitional milk.
- Colostrum is rich in protein, vitamins, minerals, and immunoglobulins. Transitional milk appears between colostrum and mature milk. Mature milk continues to provide immunoglobulins and antibacterial components.
- Breast milk has nutrients in proportions required by the newborn and in an easily digested form. Most commercial formulas are cow's milk adapted to simulate human milk, but cannot fully replicate breast milk.
- Breast milk contains factors that help establish the normal intestinal flora and prevent infection. These include bifidus factor, leukocytes, lysozymes, lactoferrin, and immunoglobulins.
- A variety of commercial formulas are available. They include modified cow's milk formula, soy-based or hydrolyzed formulas, and formulas for preterm infants or those with special problems.
- The American Academy of Pediatrics recommends exclusive breastfeeding for the first 6 months and continued breastfeeding with the addition of complementary foods until the infant is 12 months old or longer.
- Factors that influence the mother's choice of feeding method include knowledge about each method, support from family and friends, cultural influences, and employment.
- Suckling at the breast causes release of oxytocin, which triggers the let-down reflex. It also causes the release of prolactin, which increases milk production.
- The principle of supply and demand applies to breastfeeding. Milk production increases when the infant feeds frequently. When breastfeeding ceases, prolactin is decreased and eventually the alveoli of the breasts stop producing milk.

- Flat and inverted nipples should be identified during pregnancy. Creams and methods to toughen the nipples are not necessary.
- The nurse should assess the mother's knowledge and the condition of her breasts and nipples. The LATCH score can be used to identify problems.
- The nurse can help the mother establish breastfeeding by initiating early skin-to-skin contact and breastfeeding, assisting her to position the infant at the breast, and showing her how to position her hands. The nurse should teach the mother how to help the infant latch onto the breast, assess the position of the mouth on the breast, and remove the infant from the breast.
- The mother should feed the infant with hunger cues 8 to 12 times per day, watching for nutritive sucking, audible swallowing, and infant satiety.
- Wake-up techniques for sleepy infants include unwrapping the blankets, placing the infant skin to skin with the mother, talking to the infant, changing the diaper, rubbing the infant's back, and expressing colostrum onto the breast.
- When infants suck from a bottle, they must push the tongue against the nipple to slow the flow of milk. When they suckle at the breast, they position the nipple far into the mouth so that the gums compress the areola.
- The nurse can help the woman with engorged breasts by encouraging her to nurse frequently, apply cold compresses, massage the breasts, and express milk to soften the areola.
- The nurse teaches the mother with sore nipples how to check the positioning of the infant at the breast. The mother should vary the position of the infant at the breast and apply breast milk and warm-water compresses to the nipples.
- Teaching for the mother who plans to work and breastfeed includes expression of breast milk by hand or pump and proper storage of the milk.
- Mothers who use formula need information about the types of formula available, correct preparation, and feeding techniques.
- Formula should be diluted exactly according to directions. It should not be heated in a microwave.

REFERENCES & READINGS

Academy of Breastfeeding Medicine (ABM). (2011). ABM Clinical Protocol #10: Breastfeeding the late preterm infant (34 0/7 to 36 6/7 weeks gestation) (First revision June 2011). *Breastfeeding Medicine, 6*(3), 151–156.

Academy of Breastfeeding Medicine (ABM) Protocol Committee. (2009). ABM Clinical Protocol #3: Hospital Guidelines for the Use of Supplementary Feedings in the Healthy Term Breastfed Neonate, Revised 2009. *Breastfeeding Medicine, 4*(3), 175–283.

Academy of Breastfeeding Medicine (ABM) Protocol Committee. (2010). ABM Clinical Protocol #8: human milk storage information for home use for full-term infants (original protocol March 2004; Revision #1 March 2010). *Breastfeeding Medicine, 5*(3), 127–130.

American Academy of Pediatrics. (2015a). AAP publications reaffirmed or retired. *Pediatrics, 135*(4), e1105–e1106. http://dx.doi.org/10.1542/peds.2015-0339.

American Academy of Pediatrics (AAP). (2015b). *Feeding and nutrition: Storing prepared formula.* Retrieved www.healthychildren.org/English/ages-stages/baby/feeding-nutrition/Pages/Sterilizing-and-Warming-Bottles.aspx.

American Academy of Pediatrics & American College of Obstetricians and Gynecologists (AAP & ACOG). (2012). *Guidelines for perinatal care* (7th ed.). Elk Grove Village, IL: Author.

American Academy of Pediatrics (AAP) Section on Breastfeeding. (2012). Policy Statement: Breastfeeding and the use of human milk. *Pediatrics, 129*(3), e827–e841.

American College of Obstetricians and Gynecologists (ACOG). (2016). Published 2012, reaffirmed 2016. Committee opinion number 524: Opioid abuse, dependence, and addiction in pregnancy. *Obstetrics & Gynecology, 119*, 1070–1076.

Association of Women's Health, Obstetric and Neonatal Nurses (AWHONN). (2013). *Women's health and perinatal nursing care quality draft measures specifications.* Washington, DC: Author.

Association of Women's Health, Obstetric and Neonatal Nurses (AWHONN). (2015). Breastfeeding: An official position statement of the Association of Women's Health, Obstetric and Neonatal Nurses. *Journal of Women's Health, Obstetric and Neonatal Nurses, 44*(1), 145–150.

Baby Friendly, USA. (2016). *Find Facilities.* Retrieved from www.babyfriendlyusa.org.

Bartick, M. C., Schwarz, E. B., Green, B. D., Jegier, B. J., Reinhold, A. G., Colaizy, T. T., Stuebe, A. M. (2017). Suboptimal breastfeeding in the United States: Maternal and pediatric health outcomes and costs. *Maternal & Child Nutrition, 13*(1). http://dx.doi.org/10.1111/mcn.12366.

Blackburn, S. T. (2013). *Maternal, fetal, and neonatal physiology* (4th ed.). Philadelphia, PA: Saunders.

Callister, L. C. (2014). Integrating cultural beliefs and practices when caring for childbearing women and families. In K. R. Simpson & P. A. Creehan (Eds.), *AWHONN's Perinatal Nursing* (4th ed.) (pp. 41–70). Philadelphia, PA: Lippincott Williams & Wilkins.

Centers for Disease Control and Prevention (CDC). (2016a). *Breastfeeding report card—United States, 2016.* Retrieved from www.cdc.gov/breastfeeding/pdf/2016breastfeedingreportcard.pdf.

Centers for Disease Control and Prevention (CDC). (2016b). *Progress in increasing breastfeeding and reducing racial/ethnic differences—United States, 2000–2008 births.* Retrieved from www.cdc.gov/breastfeeding/resources/breastfeeding-trends.htm.

Fonseca, M. J., Severo, M., Barros, H., & Santos, A. C. (2014). Determinants of weight change during the first 96 hours of life in full-term newborns. *Birth: Issues in Perinatal Care, 41*(2), 160–168.

Grodner, M., Escott-Stump, S., & Dorner, S. (2016). *Nutritional foundations and clinical applications: A nursing approach* (6th ed.). St. Louis, MO: Mosby.

Haroon, S., Das, J. K., Salam, R. A., Imdad, A., & Bhutta, Z. A. (2013). Breastfeeding promotion interventions and breastfeeding practices: A systematic review. *BMC Public Health, 13*(Suppl. 3), S20. http://dx.doi.org/10.1186/1471-2458-13-S3-S20. Epub 2013 Sept 17.

Hoover, L. (2016). Perinatal and intrapartum care. In K. Wambach & J. Riordan (Eds.), *Breastfeeding and human lactation* (5th ed.) (pp. 227–272). Burlington, MA: Jones and Bartlett.

Janke, J. (2014). Newborn nutrition. In K. R. Simpson & P. A. Creehan (Eds.), *AWHONN's Perinatal Nursing* (4th ed.) (pp. 626–661). Philadelphia, PA: Lippincott Williams & Wilkins.

Jensen, D., Wallace, S., & Kelsay, P. (1994). LATCH: A breastfeeding charting system and documentation tool. *Journal of Obstetric, Gynecologic, and Neonatal Nursing, 23*(1), 27–32.

Joint Commission. (2011). *Speak up: What you need to know about breastfeeding.* Retrieved from www.jointcommission.org/assets/1/18/breastfeeding_final_7_19_11.pdf.

Keane, V. (2016). Assessment of growth. In R. M. Kliegman, R. E. Stanton, J. W. St. Geme, et al. (Eds.), *Nelson textbook of pediatrics* (20th ed.) (p. 87). Philadelphia, PA: Saunders.

Lawrence, R. A., & Lawrence, R. M. (2016). *Breastfeeding: a guide for the medical profession* (8th ed.). Philadelphia, PA: Elsevier.

Moore, E. R., Anderson, G. C., Bergman, N., & Dowswell, T. (2013). Early skin-to-skin contact for mothers and their healthy newborn infants. *Cochrane Database of Systematic Reviews, 16*(5), CD003519. http://dx.doi.org/10.1002/14651858.CD003519.pub3.

Moran, D. E., & Kallam, G. B. (2015). *A new beginning: Your personal guide to postpartum care.* Arlington, TX: Customized Communications, Inc.

Muraro, A., Halken, S., Arshad, S. H., Beyer, K., Dubois, A. E., Du Toit, G., Sheikh, A. (2014). EAACI Food Allergy and Anaphylaxis Guidelines: Primary prevention of food allergy. *Allergy, 69*(5), 590–601.

Newton, E. R. (2017). Breastfeeding. In S. G. Gabbe, J. R. Niebyl, J. L. Simpson, M. B. Landon, H. L. Galan, R. M. Jauniaux, D. A. Driscoll, et al. (Eds.), *Obstetrics, normal and problem pregnancies* (7th ed.) (pp. 518–547). New York: Churchill Livingstone.

Nickols-Richardson, S. M. (2015). Nutrition for normal growth and development. In E. D. Schlenker & J. Gilbert (Eds.), *Williams' essentials of nutrition and diet therapy* (11th ed.) (pp. 274–303). St. Louis, MO: Mosby.

Pletsch, D., Ulrich, C., Angelini, M., Fernandes, G., & Lee, D. S. (2013). Mothers' "liquid gold": A quality improvement initiative to support early colostrum delivery via oral immune therapy to premature and critically ill newborns. *Nursing Leadership, 26*, 34–42.

Prescott, S. L., Pawankar, R., Allen, K. J., Campbell, D. E., Sinn, J. K., Fiocchi, A., Lee, B. (2013). A global survey of changing patterns of food allergy in children. *World Allergy Organization Journal, 6*(1), 21.

Riordan, J. (2016). The biologic specificity of breastmilk. In K. Wambach & J. Riordan (Eds.), *Breastfeeding and human lactation* (5th ed.) (pp. 121–169). Burlington, MA: Jones and Bartlett.

Siggia, G., & Rosenberg, S. (2014). Does breastfeeding education of nurses increase exclusive breastfeeding rates in a large academic medical institution? *JOGNN: Journal of Obstetric Gynecologic & Neonatal Nursing, 43*(1), S38.

Smith, L. (2016). Postpartum care. In K. Wambach & J. Riordan (Eds.), *Breastfeeding and human lactation* (5th ed.). Burlington, MA: Jones and Bartlett. 272–218.

Spatz, D. (2016). The use of human milk and breastfeeding in the neonatal intensive care unit. In K. Wambach & J. Riordan (Eds.), *Breastfeeding and human lactation* (5th ed.) (pp. 469–522). Burlington, MA: Jones & Bartlett.

Thompson, L. A., Zhang, S., Black, E., Das, R., Ryngaert, M., Sullivan, S., & Roth, J. (2013). The association of maternal pre-pregnancy body mass index with breastfeeding initiation. *Maternal and Child Health Journal, 17*(10), 1842–1851.

U.S. Department of Health and Human Services (DHHS). (2010). *Healthy People 2020*. Washington, DC: Author.

U.S. Department of Health and Human Services (DHHS). (2011). *The Surgeon General's call to action to support breastfeeding*. Washington, DC: U.S. Department of Health and Human Services, Office of the Surgeon General.

U.S. Department of Labor. (2010). Break time for nursing mothers. Retrieved from www.dol.gov/whd/nursingmothers/.

Wambach, K., & Genna, C. W. (2016). Anatomy and physiology of lactation. In K. Wambach & J. Riordan (Eds.), *Breastfeeding and human lactation* (5th ed.) (pp. 121–169). Burlington, MA: Jones and Bartlett.

Wambach, K., Domain, E. W., Page-Goertz, S., Wurtz, H., & Hoffman, K. (2016). Exclusive breastfeeding rates among Mexican American Women. *Journal of Human Lactation, 32*(1), 103–111. http://dx.doi.org/10.1177/0890334415599400.

Whipps, M. D. M. (2017). Education attainment and parity explain the relationship between maternal age and breastfeeding duration in U.S. mothers. *Journal of Human Lactation, 33*(1), 220–224.

World Health Organization (WHO). (2007). *Safe preparation, storage and handling of powdered infant formula: Guidelines*. Geneva: Author.

World Health Organization (WHO). (2015). *Breastfeeding advocacy initiative: For the best start in life. WHO reference number: WHO/NMH/NHD/15.1*. Retrieved from www.who.int/nutrition/publications/infantfeeding/breastfeeding_advocacy_initiative/en/.

High-Risk Newborn: Complications Associated with Gestational Age and Development

Della Wrightson

Maternity nurses identify and begin care for the immediate needs of neonates with complications until nurses from the neonatal intensive care unit (NICU) can assume care. NICU nurses often attend births when complications of the newborn are expected.

CARE OF HIGH-RISK NEWBORNS

Nurses care for minor illness or conditions in the mother-baby unit or the normal newborn nursery, but more serious problems require intensive care in NICUs, specialized nurseries designed for that purpose. NICU admission rates across the United States range from 84% of infants born weighing less than 1500 grams (g) (3 lb. 5 oz) to 7.8% of infants born weighing 2500 g (5 lb. 8 oz) or more (Harrison & Goodman, 2015).

Multidisciplinary Approach

The care of infants with problems at birth often involves collaboration among many different professionals. In the hospital setting, such professionals may include nurses, nurse practitioners, physicians with different specialties, respiratory therapists, laboratory personnel, and pharmacists. Care from social workers, physical therapists, feeding specialists, occupational therapists, and infant development experts may begin during the hospital stay and continue after the infant is discharged. Nurses often coordinate this care and explain or clarify it for parents.

LATE PRETERM INFANTS

Infants born between 34 $^{0/7}$ and 36 $^{6/7}$ weeks of gestation are called **late preterm infants** because they have many needs similar to those of preterm infants. They are more stable than preterm infants but are physiologically and metabolically immature and have higher mortality and morbidity rates than full-term infants. In 2005, the Association of Women's Health, Obstetric and Neonatal Nurses (AWHONN) launched a multiyear Late Preterm Infant Initiative to develop evidence-based practice guidelines for care of the late preterm infant. Results of the study showed 46% of late preterm infants spent some time in a special care nursery. Hypothermia, hypoglycemia, feeding difficulties, hyperbilirubinemia, respiratory distress, and/or a need for a septic workup occurred in half of the infants studied (Cooper et al., 2012). More information is available at www.AWHONN.org.

Incidence and Etiology

Late preterm births comprised 8% of births in 2013 (Osterman, Kochaneck, MacDorman, Strobino & Guyer, 2015). Contributing factors in late preterm birth include elective and medically indicated inductions and cesarean births, preterm labor, premature rupture of membranes, preeclampsia, multifetal pregnancies, obesity, assisted reproductive technology, advanced maternal age, and inaccurate estimate of gestational age before birth (Ramachandrappa & Jain, 2015).

Characteristics of Late Preterm Infants

Because late preterm infants often look like full-term infants, they may not be recognized as being preterm. However, they are physiologically immature. They are at risk for respiratory disorders, problems with temperature maintenance, hypoglycemia, hyperbilirubinemia, feeding difficulties, acidosis, and infection (such as respiratory syncytial virus) because of their immaturity (Coffman, 2009; Pappas & Robey, 2015; Ramachandrappa & Jain, 2015). They are also at risk for long-term neurodevelopmental disorders as well as cognitive and behavioral problems (Talge et al., 2010). They are more likely to be admitted to the NICU after birth and are at increased risk for rehospitalization after discharge.

Therapeutic Management

Therapeutic management varies according to the problems presented. Many interventions are similar to those for preterm infants discussed in this chapter.

Nursing Considerations
Assessment and Care of Common Problems

Late preterm infants may receive care similar to that for full-term infants, but, compared with full-term infants, these infants need closer monitoring for complications during the hospital stay. Nursing care is similar to that given to preterm infants in many aspects.

Thermoregulation. Once stable, normal newborns usually have their temperature checked only once every 8 to 12 hours. A late preterm infant may develop cold stress that is not noticed until signs appear or it is time for the next vital sign assessment. Therefore nurses should be more vigilant in watching for thermal instability in these infants. The temperature, as well as other vital signs, should be checked every 3 to 4 hours for the first 24 hours and then every shift, depending on need and agency policy (AWHONN, 2014; Ramachandrappa & Jain, 2015). **Kangaroo care (KC)**, a method of providing skin-to-skin contact between infants and their parents, is often used to keep infants warm. A radiant warmer or an incubator also may be used if the infant cannot maintain normal temperature.

Feedings. Late preterm infants may have immature suck and swallow reflexes, have shorter awake periods, and fall asleep during feedings before they have fed adequately (Cleveland, 2010). They may have difficulty with latch when breastfeeding. Their low tone and weak suck may decrease the amount of milk they obtain with each suck (Walker, 2008). They have an increased caloric need and should be fed every 2 to 3 hours.

Feeding problems are common, and nurses should assess feeding sessions to ensure swallowing is occurring. Breastfeeding mothers need special help to see that infants are feeding well. Two key breastfeeding elements to be assessed and supported are protecting the mother's milk supply and ensuring the infant is adequately gaining weight (Meier, Patel, Wright, & Engstrom, 2013). The football and cross-cradle holds are helpful in positioning these infants at the breast. Urine and stool output are monitored as indications of adequate intake. Late preterm infants are at risk for hypoglycemia, and blood glucose measurements should be performed according to hospital protocol, especially during the first 24 hours. Because late preterm infants are at greater risk for breastfeeding-associated rehospitalization compared with term infants, lactation consultants should be involved in their care (Radtke, 2011) and evaluation of breastfeeding should be documented at least twice daily (American Association of Pediatrics & American College of Obstetricians and Gynecologists [AAP & ACOG], 2012).

Discharge. Late preterm infants often can be discharged at the same time as full-term infants. They should not be discharged earlier than 48 hours after birth. Before discharge, nurses should ensure infants are feeding adequately and have had normal vital signs for at least 24 hours. Bilirubin levels should be assessed before discharge (AWHONN, 2014; Ramachandrappa & Jain, 2015).

Teaching should include the need for keeping the infant warm. The infant should be kept away from drafts and dressed with one more layer than an adult would wear. Late preterm infants are subject to overstimulation. This may occur when parents take the baby home to an environment of many different stimuli. The nurse should teach signs of overstimulation and how to minimize them.

A car seat challenge should be conducted before discharge to ensure the infant can tolerate sitting in a car seat without bradycardia, apnea, or decreased oxygen saturation. The parents bring their own car seat for the test. Preterm and low-birth-weight (LBW) infants should be observed in the car seat for 90 to 120 minutes (or more, if travel time to go home is longer) (AAP & ACOG, 2012).

Parents should be taught signs of common complications such as jaundice or dehydration and what to do if they occur. Because some problems may not be noticeable at discharge, late preterm infants should have a follow-up visit with the health care provider 24 to 48 hours after discharge (AAP & ACOG, 2012; Ramachandrappa & Jain, 2015).

PRETERM INFANTS

Preterm infants (also called *premature infants*) are born before the completion of 37 weeks gestation (WHO, 2016). The word *preterm* is sometimes confused with the term **low birth weight (LBW)**, which refers to infants weighing 2500 g (5 lb, 8 oz) or less at birth and of any gestational age. **Very-low-birth-weight (VLBW)** infants weigh 1500 g (3 lb, 5 oz) or less at birth. **Extremely low-birth-weight (ELBW)** infants weigh 1000 g (2 lb, 3 oz) or less at birth. Although most of these infants are preterm, others are full term and have failed to grow normally while in the uterus, a condition called **fetal growth restriction (FGR)** or intrauterine growth restriction (IUGR).

Incidence and Etiology

Scope of Problem

Advances in technology have resulted in infant survival at much lower birth weights than ever before. The preterm birth rate for 2013 declined for the seventh year in a row to 11.39% of births (Osterman et al., 2015). Disorders related to short gestation and LBW are the second leading cause of infant mortality, surpassed only by those from congenital anomalies and chromosomal abnormalities (Kochanek, Murphy, Xu, & Tejeda-Vera, 2016). In terms of the suffering of infants and their parents, lost potential, and medical expense, preterm birth is extremely costly. Infant mortality and morbidity rates increase as gestational age decreases.

Causes

The exact causes of preterm birth are not known, but all risk factors in pregnancy are potential causes. See "Maternal Risk Factors for Preterm Labor" (Box 16.1).

Prevention

Prevention of preterm birth is best accomplished by provision of adequate prenatal care for every pregnant woman to identify and treat risk factors as early as possible. Teaching women signs of preterm labor will encourage them to seek care early, maximizing treatment outcomes.

Characteristics of Preterm Infants

Characteristics of preterm infants vary, depending on gestational age. For example, the appearance and problems of infants born at 34 weeks of gestation are different from those of infants born at 26 weeks of gestation. Some characteristics, however, are common to all preterm infants.

Appearance

Preterm infants often appear frail and weak, and they have less developed flexor muscles and muscle tone compared with full-term infants. Their extremities are limp and offer little or no resistance when moved. Premature newborns typically lie in an extended position (see Fig. 20.20). The infant's head is large compared with the rest of the body.

Preterm infants lack subcutaneous or white fat, which makes their thin skin appear red and translucent, with blood vessels being clearly visible. The nipples and areola may be barely perceptible, but vernix caseosa and lanugo may be abundant. Plantar creases are absent in infants younger than 32 weeks of gestation (see Fig. 20.26).

The pinnae of the ears are flat and soft and contain little cartilage (see Fig. 20.28). They lack the rolled-over appearance of the pinnae of a full-term infant. In the female infant, the clitoris and labia minora appear large and are not covered by the small, separated labia majora. The male infant may have undescended testes, with a small, smooth scrotal sac (see Figs. 20.29 and 20.30).

Behavior

The behavior of preterm infants varies, depending on gestational age. It often differs from that of full-term infants because of the stress of having to adjust to extrauterine life before they are ready. Premature newborns may have poor development of flexion and little excess energy for maintaining muscle tone. They are easily exhausted by noise and routine activities. Their responses are varied, including lowered oxygenation levels and stress-related behavior changes. The cry may be feeble.

Assessment and Care of Common Problems

Because preterm infants are "unfinished" in their growth and development, they are prone to problems affecting all systems and body processes.

Problems with Respiration

Problems of the respiratory system are a major concern because preterm newborns have immature lungs but must go through the same processes as the full-term infant to begin breathing. The presence of surfactant in adequate amounts is of primary importance. Surfactant reduces surface tension in the alveoli and prevents their collapse with expiration. It allows the lungs to inflate with lower negative pressure, decreasing the work of breathing. Infants born before surfactant production is adequate develop respiratory distress syndrome (RDS). In addition, preterm infants have a poorly developed cough reflex and narrow respiratory passages, which increase the risk for respiratory difficulty.

Assessment. The infant's respiratory status should be observed constantly. The lungs are assessed for adventitious breath sounds or areas of absent breath sounds.

The nurse differentiates periodic breathing from apneic spells. **Periodic breathing** is the cessation of breathing for 5 to 10 seconds without other changes followed by 10 to 15 seconds of rapid respirations (Goodwin, 2015). Changes in color or heart rate do not occur. Although periodic breathing sometimes occurs in term infants, preterm infants experience it more often.

Apneic spells involve absence of breathing lasting more than 20 seconds or less if accompanied by cyanosis, pallor, bradycardia, or hypotonia (Goodwin, 2015). Apneic spells are common in preterm infants, increasing in incidence with lower gestational age. Apnea without an identified cause in a preterm infant is called *idiopathic apnea* or *apnea of prematurity* and generally improves as the infant matures. Episodes may occur along with periodic breathing, and the infant may require gentle tactile stimulation, bag and mask ventilation, medications, or assisted ventilation. Apnea should be investigated because it may be related to other conditions.

The nurse observes the effort required for breathing and the location and severity of retractions. Retractions are particularly noticeable in preterm infants, whose weak chest wall is drawn in with each inspiration. The excessive **compliance** (elasticity) of the chest cage during retractions occurs because the bones of the chest wall are very pliable. This may interfere with full expansion of the lungs.

Grunting may be an early sign of RDS. It closes the glottis and increases the pressure within the alveoli. This keeps the alveoli partially open during expiration and increases the amount of oxygen absorbed.

Nursing Interventions. Interventions focus on collaborating with other team members such as the respiratory therapist to manage technical equipment and facilitate removal of secretions.

Working with Respiratory Equipment. An oxygen hood is often used for infants who can breathe independently but need extra oxygen. The hood is a plastic dome that fits over the infant's head or over the head and upper body. The infant breathes the higher levels of oxygen within the hood, and the device does not interfere with access to the rest of the infant's body for care (Fig. 23.1).

Oxygen also may be given by nasal cannula to the infant who breathes well independently. After discharge, many preterm infants continue to receive oxygen via nasal cannula at home. Oxygen should be warmed to maintain body temperature and humidified to prevent insensible water loss and drying of the delicate mucous membranes.

Continuous positive airway pressure (CPAP) may be necessary to keep the alveoli open and improve expansion of the lungs. CPAP can be delivered via nasal prongs, a mask, or an endotracheal tube. The infant may need conventional mechanical ventilation when respiratory failure, severe apnea, bradycardia, or other conditions are present. High-frequency ventilation may be used to provide very fast respirations with less pressure and volume. This helps decrease lung injury from pressure (barotrauma) and volume (volutrauma).

When oxygen is administered, the level of oxygen in the infant's blood should be monitored. Arterial blood may be drawn for testing oxygen levels. **Pulse oximetry** may also be used. This method is less invasive and provides continuous information about oxygen partial pressure (Po_2) levels through sensors attached to the skin. Nurses and respiratory therapists titrate oxygen, depending on the pulse oximetry or arterial oxygen levels, according to facility policy.

The nurse should observe the infant's increasing or decreasing dependence on breathing assistance and need for oxygen during activity such as handling, feeding, and linen changes. An increase in oxygen and/or other respiratory support settings may be needed during care activities.

Positioning the Infant. The side-lying and prone positions facilitate drainage of respiratory secretions and regurgitated feedings. The prone and side-lying positions are not recommended for normal newborn infants because they are associated with an increased incidence of sudden infant death syndrome (SIDS). In the preterm infant, however, the prone position increases oxygenation, enhances respiratory control, improves lung mechanics and volume, and reduces energy expenditure (Gardner, Goldson, & Hernandez, 2016a).

The reason for prone positioning should be explained to parents. Supine positioning for sleep is begun as soon as the infant can tolerate it and before discharge so that the infant can become accustomed to sleeping on the back before going home. The supine position often can be used at approximately 32 weeks' gestational age (AAP & ACOG, 2012). Before discharge parents should be taught the importance of supine positioning in preventing SIDS. It is important for nurses to model SIDS prevention by placing infants in the supine position as soon as infants are able and removing any soft, loose items from the bed because parents are more likely to mimic the conditions they saw in the hospital (Gelfer, Cameron, Masters, & Kennedy, 2013; Gardner et al., 2016a).

Suctioning Secretions. The weak or absent cough reflex and very small air passages make the preterm infant's airways susceptible to obstruction by mucus. The nurse checks the suction equipment at the beginning of each shift to ensure that it is available and functioning properly at all times.

The infant is suctioned only as necessary. Suction should be gentle to avoid traumatizing the delicate mucous membranes. Trauma could cause edema, decreasing the size of the air passages further and leading to more respiratory difficulty.

Suctioning also provides an entry for organisms and decreases oxygenation. The procedure causes changes in heart rate, blood pressure, and cerebral blood flow. Suction should be applied for only 5 to 10 seconds at a time, and increased oxygen should be provided before and after each suction attempt. The mouth is suctioned before the nose because stimulation of the nares causes reflex inspiration that could cause aspiration of fluids in the infant's mouth (Gardner, Enzman-Hines, & Nyp, 2016d). A rest period should be provided after suctioning.

Maintaining Hydration. Adequate hydration is essential to keep secretions thin so they can be removed by drainage or suction. If infants become dehydrated, secretions will become thick and viscous and could obstruct tiny air passages. Fluid intake should be increased, as ordered by the provider, if secretions seem to indicate even minimal dehydration.

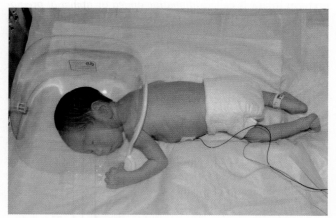

FIG 23.1 The oxygen hood is one way of delivering oxygen to an infant who can breathe unassisted. (Courtesy Cheryl Briggs, RN.)

? KNOWLEDGE CHECK

1. How does the appearance of a preterm infant differ from that of a full-term infant?
2. What factors contribute to respiratory problems in preterm infants?
3. What nursing responsibilities relate to care of preterm respiratory problems?

Problems with Thermoregulation

Although heat loss can be a thermoregulation problem for full-term infants, it is even more significant in preterm infants. Their skin is thin, with blood vessels near the surface, and little subcutaneous white fat for insulation. As a result, heat loss is rapid. The preterm infant's shorter time in the uterus allows less brown fat to accumulate before birth, impairing the infant's ability to produce heat.

Preterm infants have a larger head in proportion to body size compared with full-term infants. The preterm infant's extended extremities increase exposure to air and thus heat loss. Their body surface area in proportion to their body mass is larger than that of adults (Fanaroff & Klaus, 2013). The temperature control center of the brain of preterm infants is less mature and may be further impaired by asphyxia. These conditions all contribute to heat loss.

Complications from heat loss are more likely to develop in preterm infants. These include hypoglycemia, respiratory problems, metabolic acidosis, pulmonary vasoconstriction, impaired surfactant production, and more respiratory difficulty. In addition, calories used for heat production are unavailable for growth and weight gain.

Assessment. The infant's temperature is monitored continuously by a skin probe attached to the heat control mechanism of the radiant warmer or incubator. Common probe placement sites are the abdomen, flank, and axilla (Schafer et al., 2014). The infant should not lie on the probe. The skin temperature is usually maintained at 36°C to 36.5°C (96.8°F to 97.7°F) (Gardner & Hernandez, 2016). The infant's skin temperature as shown on the bed or monitor should be recorded every 30 to 60 minutes initially and every 1 to 3 hours when the infant is stable. The axillary temperature should be compared with the heat control reading to ensure that the equipment is functioning properly.

The axillary temperature for a preterm infant should remain between 36.3°C and 36.9°C (97.3°F and 98.4°F), slightly lower than the temperature for full-term infants (Gardner & Hernandez, 2016). If the infant has accumulated brown fat, a normal axillary temperature when the monitor shows a decreased skin temperature may indicate that heat from brown fat in the axillary space is being used to maintain the infant's core temperature.

Rectal temperatures should not be used in preterm neonates. Checking a core temperature is of little value in a neonate because it may not show a decrease until the infant has completely decompensated (Brand & Boyd, 2015; Gardner & Hernandez, 2016).

Indications of inadequate thermoregulation include poor feeding or intolerance to feedings in an infant who previously had little difficulty, irritability, lethargy, poor muscle tone, cool skin temperature, and mottled skin. Hypoglycemia and respiratory distress may be the first signs that the infant's temperature is low. A decrease in weight gain or weight loss may occur over time. Because temperature instability may be an early sign of infection, the nurse should assess for other evidence that infection may be present.

CRITICAL TO REMEMBER
Signs of Inadequate Thermoregulation

Axillary temperature <36.3°C or >36.9°C (<97.3°F or >98.4°F)
Skin temperature <36°C or >36.5°C (<96.8°F or >97.7°F)
Poor feeding or feeding intolerance
Irritability followed by lethargy
Weak cry or suck
Decreased muscle tone
Cool skin temperature
Mottled, pale, or acrocyanotic skin
Signs of hypoglycemia
Signs of respiratory difficulty (e.g., apnea, retractions)
Poor weight gain, if chronic

Nursing Interventions. Maintenance of heat in preterm infants involves the same basic nursing care principles as for the full-term infant. These principles, however, should be adapted to meet the needs of the preterm infant.

Maintaining a Neutral Thermal Environment. A neutral thermal environment (NTE) is especially important to prevent the need for increased oxygen to maintain the infant's body temperature. The temperature necessary to maintain the NTE varies according to gestational age. Charts are available that indicate the appropriate temperature setting to maintain an NTE according to the infant's size and maturity.

The delivery room should be warm to decrease heat loss at birth. Immediately after birth, the infant is dried and placed on the mother's abdomen or a prewarmed radiant warmer for care and a hat is put on the infant's head. Before infants are dried, place those who are younger than 32 weeks of gestation (or up to 35 weeks if the baby is small for age or the environment is cool) in a polyethylene bag or wrap that covers the body from the shoulders down. This prevents heat loss by evaporation during initial care and transfer to the NICU and is used until the infant's condition is stabilized. It also decreases insensible water loss. The infant should be placed on a chemical thermal mattress, which can provide heat for up to an hour after activation (Weiner, 2016).

Because they produce heat less effectively and lose more heat than larger or older preterm infants, smaller, less-mature infants need more warmth to maintain body heat. Radiant warmers or incubators are used until infants can maintain normal body temperature alone. Some devices convert from a radiant warmer to an incubator and back again to eliminate the need to move the infant from one device to another.

Infants needing many procedures are usually placed under an open radiant warmer to make it easier to see them and work with equipment. However, air currents around an unclothed infant can cause heat loss by convection despite the heat generated by the warmer. Doors near the warmer should be closed and traffic kept to a minimum to decrease convective heat loss. The infant should receive only warmed oxygen because thermal receptors in the face are very sensitive to cold. Cold oxygen could quickly lead to cold stress.

Equipment and caregivers should not come between the infant and the heat source, preventing heat from reaching the infant. A transparent plastic blanket over the infant allows heat from the warmer to pass across to the infant. The blanket decreases convective heat loss from exposure to drafts and insensible water loss while maintaining visibility of the infant's body.

Incubators are used for infants who do not need to be under radiant warmers. They have double walls to minimize radiant heat loss to the cooler outer walls. Warmed air circulating inside the incubator provides heat. Humidity should be added to decrease evaporative heat loss and insensible water loss, especially in very preterm infants. Incubators should be placed away from air-conditioning ducts or windows that may affect the incubator temperature.

When infants are in incubators, the nurse should keep portholes and doors closed as much as possible. A significant amount of heat is lost each time the incubator is opened, and it takes time to build up the heat again. When removed from the incubator for procedures or holding, infants should be wrapped in heated blankets and a hat applied. Incubator doors should be closed while the infant is outside to retain the heat inside. Infants should be placed under a radiant warmer or on a surface padded with warm blankets for procedures that cannot be performed inside the incubator. A heat lamp provides an alternative source of heat.

Although temperature loss is the most common concern, overheating also is a problem for preterm infants. Overheating may occur when heating devices such as radiant warmers are set too high or a skin probe comes loose. Overheating leads to an increase in the metabolic rate, with increased oxygen and glucose needs, and insensible water losses. Alarms to detect high or low temperature should be turned on at all times.

Although temperature regulation in preterm infants is usually provided in incubators until infants can maintain their own temperature, warmth is also provided when parents hold them. Adequate temperature is maintained in stable infants during KC.

Weaning to an Open Crib. Preparation of infants for moving to an open crib should begin early. When stable, infants can be dressed in a shirt, diaper, and hat while in the incubator. Clothing conserves heat and helps infants adjust to a different temperature on the face than the rest of the body. Infants who weigh about 1600 g (3 lb, 8 oz), have a consistent weight gain for 5 days, have no medical complications, and are tolerating feedings can begin gradual weaning from external heat (Gardner & Hernandez, 2016).

Each NICU has its own protocol for the weaning process. The incubator temperature is usually decreased gradually. It is raised if the infant's temperature falls below the normal range. If the temperature remains stable, the process can continue the next day.

When the infant is ready for transfer to an open crib, double-wrapping with warm blankets helps insulate body heat.

Sleep sacks (sleepers made of blanket material and closed at the bottom) are often used when infants are dressed. The temperature is assessed at gradually increasing intervals until the infant's temperature is stable and then may be monitored on a routine schedule. A blanket is added for a low temperature, but if the temperature does not rise to normal, the infant is returned to the incubator.

Nurses should observe infants carefully during the first few days after transfer to an open crib. Signs that may indicate inadequate thermoregulation include decreased weight gain, poor feeding, or increased requirement for oxygen.

Problems with Fluid and Electrolyte Balance

Preterm infants lose fluid very easily, and the loss increases with the degree of prematurity. The rapid respiratory rate and the use of oxygen increase fluid losses from the lungs. Their thin skin has little protective subcutaneous white fat and is more permeable than the skin of term infants. The large surface area in proportion to body weight and lack of flexion further increase transepidermal water losses. Radiant warmers raise insensible water losses by 40% to 50% compared with loss in an incubator (Gardner & Hernandez, 2016). Heat from phototherapy lights causes even more fluid to be lost through the skin.

The ability of the kidneys to concentrate or dilute urine is poor, causing a fragile balance between dehydration and overhydration. Great differences in fluid needs occur, depending on variables such as the infant's size, gestational age, insensible water losses, and medical needs. Normal urinary output is 1 to 3 mL/kg/hr for preterm infants for the first few days. After 24 hours of life, output less than 0.5 mL/kg/hr is considered oliguria (Blackburn, 2013).

Regulation of electrolytes by the kidneys is also a problem. Preterm infants need higher intakes of sodium because the kidneys do not reabsorb it well. If they receive too much sodium, however, they may be unable to increase sodium excretion adequately and are susceptible to sodium and water overload.

Assessment. The nurse should be alert for fluid overload or deficit. Monitoring intake and output of fluids helps determine fluid balance. The infant's intake and output by all routes are carefully calculated. Parenteral fluids, feeding tube intake, medication, and oral fluids are included when measuring intake. Output from regurgitation, drainage tubes, stools, and urine should be measured. The nurse should also keep track of the amount of blood taken for laboratory tests because the loss can be substantial and the infant cannot make new blood fast enough.

Urine Output. There are several methods of measuring urine output. Plastic bags that adhere to the perineum are not suitable for the preterm infant because they may damage the fragile skin. Weighing diapers is less harmful to the infant. The weight of dry diapers is subtracted from the weight of wet diapers to determine the amount of urine excreted. One gram (1 g) is equivalent to 1 mL of urine. However, humidification may add moisture to the diaper and a radiant warmer may cause evaporation of urine on the diaper. When precise measurement is essential, diapers can be fastened instead of being placed open under the infant.

Specific gravity should be checked to determine whether urine is more concentrated or dilute than expected. Urine is collected by placing gauze or a cotton ball at the perineum. The specific gravity should range between 1.005 and 1.012 (Nyp et al., 2016).

Weight. Changes in the infant's weight can give an indication of fluid gain or loss, especially if the changes are sudden or greater than would be expected. The undressed infant should be weighed at the same time each day with the same scale. Very small infants are often placed in a bed with a scale so they are not disturbed for daily weighing. They may be weighed two to three times a day to monitor their fluid status more closely.

Signs of Dehydration or Overhydration. The nurse should observe for signs that indicate the infant has received too little or too much fluid. See the Critical to Remember box for a list of these signs.

CRITICAL TO REMEMBER

Signs of Fluid Imbalance in the Newborn

Dehydration
Urine output <1 mL/kg/hr
Urine specific gravity >1.012
Weight loss greater than expected
Dry skin and mucous membranes
Sunken anterior fontanel
Poor tissue turgor
Blood—Elevated sodium, protein, and hematocrit levels
Hypotension

Overhydration
Urine output >3 mL/kg/hr
Urine specific gravity <1.005
Edema
Weight gain greater than expected
Bulging fontanels
Blood—Decreased sodium, protein, and hematocrit levels
Moist breath sounds
Difficulty breathing

Nursing Interventions. Intravenous (IV) fluids should be carefully regulated using infusion control devices that administer fluid with a precision of 0.01 mL/hr to help prevent fluid volume overload (Nyp et al., 2016). IV medications should be diluted in as little fluid as is consistent with safe administration of the drug and should be considered when intake is measured. Starting IV lines on infants can be a difficult procedure. Once IV access is achieved, care should be taken to prevent infiltration.

IV sites should be assessed at least every hour for signs of infiltration; some solutions, if they infiltrate, cause extensive damage as a result of tissue sloughing. When identified, IV infiltrations require immediate intervention.

Many infants have central venous catheters or umbilical lines that should be assessed for infection and position changes. Small blood transfusions may be necessary to replace blood drawn for frequent laboratory tests.

Problems with the Skin

Preterm infants have fragile, permeable, easily damaged skin. They often have endotracheal tubes, IV lines, electrodes, and other equipment that should be maintained in place, but standard adhesive tape should not be used because it can be very damaging to the skin. Removal of adhesive tape may strip the epidermal layer of the skin, causing pain and increasing transepidermal water loss and the risk for infection. Preparations used to disinfect the skin before invasive procedures can injure fragile skin and may be absorbed. Diaper dermatitis, or diaper rash, is common in infants.

Assessment. The nurse should frequently assess the condition of the infant's skin and record any changes, using a valid and reliable tool. The infant's response to products used for cleansing and disinfection should be noted.

Nursing Interventions. Guidelines for evidence-based practice in care of the neonate's skin have been developed by the AWHONN (2013a). Medical adhesives that effectively secure devices and monitoring equipment but cause the least injury to tissues should be used. Skin can be protected from adhesives by using silicone-based protective films.

Adhesives should be removed slowly and gently by pulling horizontally parallel to the skin. The interface between the adhesive and the skin should be wet with gauze or saline pledgets. Mineral oil, petrolatum, or silicone-based adhesive removers also can be used to wet the area. (AWHONN, 2013a).

All disinfectants have potential risks when used on neonates. Aqueous chlorhexidine gluconate solutions are commonly used at this time. Povidone-iodine may injure the skin and may have toxic effects on the thyroid gland in premature infants. All disinfectants should be removed with sterile water or saline. Alcohol should not be used (AWHONN, 2013a; Lund & Durand, 2016).

Cleansers with a pH of 5.5 to 7 may be used for bathing infants. Preterm infants usually should not be bathed every day. Warm water without soap should be used for infants younger than 32 weeks of gestational age for the first week after birth. Sterile water is not necessary unless there are concerns about the safety of tap water or there is a break in skin integrity (AWHONN, 2013a). Stable preterm infants without umbilical IV lines may be immersed in water that covers the shoulders for bathing if there are no contraindications. Swaddled bathing, in which the infant is wrapped in a blanket and then immersed in water for bathing, also may be used. Tubs should be used by only one infant for the duration of hospital stay or cleaned well if used between infants.

Humidity in incubators should be regulated to reduce the drying effects of heat. Emollients can help reduce fissures in dry skin and transepidermal water loss. They are safe to use under radiant warmers and during phototherapy (AWHONN, 2013a). The infant's skin should be observed for signs of infection.

Infants and their equipment should be positioned to avoid undue pressure on the skin. The most common cause of pressure-related injuries in neonates is from equipment. Skin breakdown may occur over any bony prominence but especially on the head, which has the largest body surface area. Frequent position changes are important but should be based on the infant's ability to tolerate changes. Alcohol-free skin protectant and pressure-reducing devices may help prevent skin breakdown (AWHONN, 2013a).

Problems with Infection

The incidence of infection in preterm infants is 3 to 10 times greater than that in full-term newborns (Stoll & Shane, 2016). Many preterm infants have one or more episodes of sepsis during their hospital stay. Factors that contribute to the high rate of infection include exposure to maternal infection, lack of adequate passive immunity from the transfer of immunoglobulin G (IgG) from the mother during the third trimester, and immature response to infection.

Preterm infants are often exposed to situations that may cause infection. A prolonged stay in the hospital increases the likelihood of acquiring an infection from multiple exposures to organisms.

Infants are subject to invasive procedures such as insertion of IV lines and drawing of blood specimens. Peripherally inserted central catheters (PICCs) are commonly used for IV therapy. However, catheter-related bloodstream infections may occur and special care is necessary when they are used. Infants often have central IV catheters that require sterile dressings. All dressing changes should be done under strict sterile technique.

Assessment. The nurse should be alert for signs of sepsis at all times (see Chapter 24).

Nursing Interventions. Handwashing is one of the most important aspects of preventing hospital-acquired infections. Nursing care involves scrupulous cleanliness and maintenance of the infant's skin integrity. Even normal flora on the hands of caregivers may cause sepsis. Therefore parents and staff members should thoroughly wash their hands and arms before handling infants. No jewelry is worn in many units because of the possibility of it carrying organisms. Exposure to family and staff members who have contagious diseases should be prevented.

Early signs of infections should be identified and reported so treatment may begin immediately. The nurse carefully notes the infant's response to treatment, because some organisms become resistant to antibiotics. Other nursing care for infection is discussed in Chapter 24.

Problems with Pain

Infants in the NICU undergo many painful procedures and treatments such as intubation, heel sticks, chest tube placement, venipuncture, and suctioning each day. Younger and sicker infants tend to need more interventions and suffer more pain-producing procedures compared with older, less-ill infants. It was once thought that newborns, particularly preterm infants, were neurologically too immature to feel pain. It is now recognized that preterm infants do feel pain and that pain stimuli cause physiologic and behavioral changes in infants (National Association of Neonatal Nurses [NANN], 2012).

Pain can have numerous untoward effects. For example, increases in intracranial pressure resulting from pain elevate the risk for intraventricular hemorrhage. Other risks include hypoxia, changes in metabolic rate, and adverse effects on growth and wound healing. Stress and pain in the newborn may alter pain thresholds and cause permanent changes in neural pathways (Ranger, Beggs, & Grunau, 2017). Tissue injury occurring early in development may lead to higher sensitivity to pain at the involved site and the surrounding areas (Gardner, Enzman-Hines, & Agarwal, 2016c).

The long-term effects of pain in the neonate are not yet fully understood. It is possible that repeated painful events may cause emotional, behavioral, and learning disabilities. The American Academy of Pediatrics (AAP), the American College of Obstetricians and Gynecologists (ACOG), and the National Association of Neonatal Nurses (NANN) recommend that pain be routinely assessed, painful procedures be minimized, and nonpharmacologic and pharmacologic therapies be used to prevent pain from minor procedures and eliminate pain from surgeries and major procedures in neonates (AAP & ACOG, 2012; NANN, 2012).

Assessment. Because pain is the fifth vital sign, pain assessment is performed whenever vital signs are taken. In addition, the nurse should assess the infant's response to potentially painful stimuli and pharmacologic and nonpharmacologic interventions.

Assessment tools are available to evaluate physiologic and behavioral responses to pain in term and preterm infants. Some such as the Premature Infant Pain Profile (PIPP) are designed for term or preterm infants. This tool assesses gestational age and behavior states, heart rate, oxygen saturation, brow bulge, eye squeeze, and nasolabial furrow (lines from the edge of the nostrils to beyond the corners of the mouth) to assign a pain score (Gardner et al., 2016c).

CRITICAL TO REMEMBER

Common Signs of Pain in Infants

Increased or decreased heart and respiratory rates, apnea
Increased blood pressure
Decreased oxygen saturation
Color changes—Red, dusky, pale
High-pitched, intense, harsh cry
Whimpering, moaning
"Cry face"
Eyes squeezed shut
Mouth open
Grimacing
Furrowing or bulging of the brow
Tense, rigid muscles or flaccid muscle tone
Rigidity or flailing of extremities
Sleep-wake pattern changes

Both physiologic and behavioral responses to pain occur. However, physiologic changes may be unpredictable and cannot be used alone to assess pain.

Infants who are intubated or too weak to cry have a "cry face," a facial expression of crying without the sound of a cry. Fewer than half of preterm infants experiencing painful stimuli respond with crying (Gardner et al., 2016c). Infants who have been exposed to prolonged or repeated pain may no longer be able to show behavioral changes even though they are experiencing pain. Critically ill or very immature infants also may not show pain responses in the same way that older, less sick infants do. Therefore lack of response to a painful situation should not be perceived as absence of pain.

Parents often spend many hours with their preterm infants in the NICU setting. The nurse should involve them in assessing the infant's pain and encourage them to share their evaluation of the infant's response to relief measures. They may have questions the nurse can answer about the effects of pain and the measures used to treat it.

Nursing Interventions. Nurses should prepare infants for potentially painful procedures by waking them slowly and gently and using containment. **Containment** simulates the enclosed space of the uterus, prevents excessive and disorganized motor activity, and is comforting to infants. It involves keeping the extremities in a flexed position with swaddling, with positioning devices, or with the nurse's hands. The infant is in the supine or side-lying position with at least one of the infant's hands near the mouth for sucking. Containment is also called *facilitated tucking* (Fernandes, Campbell-Yeo, & Johnston, 2011).

KC and breastfeeding also are used to reduce pain. They are a way for mothers to be involved in helping relieve infant pain. The mother's voice and smell, which are familiar to the infant, are added to skin-to-skin contact to increase pain relief (Campbell-Yeo, Fernandes, & Johnston, 2011).

Handling before a painful procedure should be minimized, if possible. Even positioning for procedures can be uncomfortable and upsetting. Therefore other care should be performed at another time to allow the infant to rest before and after the procedure. If several things must be done together, the least traumatic should be performed first. The infant is often hypersensitive after a painful stimulus and may perceive other activities as painful (NANN, 2012).

Comfort measures help the infant cope with short-term, mild pain and reduce agitation. Nonnutritive sucking with a pacifier or the infant's hands is helpful but is effective only as long as the infant continues to suck. Sucrose placed on a pacifier or in the infant's mouth 2 to 3 minutes before a painful stimulus increases pain relief. Combining sucrose with nonnutritive sucking has been found to reduce pain in neonates when used before and during painful procedures (Naughton, 2013). Sucrose may not be appropriate, however, for very young preterm infants.

Talking softly, holding, rocking, and restraining the extremities to prevent flailing are other common methods of pain relief that may be used alone or with sucrose. Measures should be adapted according to the infant's responses. A combination of measures, such as skin-to-skin contact and breastfeeding may increase effectiveness (Academy of Breastfeeding Medicine, 2010).

Comfort measures alone are not enough for moderate to severe pain. The nurse should discuss the infant's pain with the primary care provider to ensure that medications are available for long-term and more severe pain. Opioids such as morphine and fentanyl can be tolerated by preterm infants. Nonnarcotic analgesics such as acetaminophen also may be used. Topical anesthesia can be used to reduce pain during some procedures.

Sedatives may be used for agitation in sick newborns but are not effective for pain and should not be used in place of analgesics. Regional or general anesthesia is given during surgery.

The nurse gives ordered medications before painful procedures and when indicated by pain assessments. The infant's response is carefully noted to determine the need to increase or decrease the dosage. Analgesics may be given continuously or on an as-needed basis. To be most effective, analgesics should be given before pain reaches its peak. To avoid inconsistent pain relief occurring with as-needed (PRN) dosing, pain medications are best given on a regular schedule or by continuous infusion (Gardner et al., 2016c).

EVIDENCE-BASED PRACTICE

Managing pain in the preterm infant is of concern to both nurses and parents. Herrington and Chiodo (2014) conducted a study on gentle human touch (GHT) and the reduction of pain responses in patients in the neonatal intensive care unit (NICU). Eleven premature infants were randomized into control and experimental groups. GHT was provided to the experimental group during a heelstick. Infants who did not receive GHT experienced increased heart rate and cry times and decreased respiratory rates. Conversely, the group who received the GHT did not experience increase heart rates or cry times or any reduction in breathing rates. This study presented evidence that GHT reduces pain in patients in the NICU. GHT is an effective and feasible intervention that bedside nurses can perform to improve patient outcomes.

Reference
Herrington, C. J., & Chiodo, L. M. (2014). Human touch effectively and safely reduces pain in the newborn intensive care unit. *Pain Management Nursing, 15*(1), 107–115.

KNOWLEDGE CHECK

4. How do nurses help infants adjust to the cooler environment of an open crib?
5. How does the nurse keep track of an infant's intake and output?
6. What special problems related to fluid balance, infections, and pain occur in preterm infants?
7. What nonpharmacologic measures can nurses use to manage pain in infants?

◆ APPLICATION OF THE NURSING PROCESS: ENVIRONMENTALLY CAUSED STRESS

Preterm infants commonly have difficulty with stress from the NICU environment. Their parents may have difficulty with bonding. The effects of environmental factors on the preterm infant have led to developmentally supportive care. Developmental care keeps stressors in the environment to a minimum based on the infant's physiologic and behavioral responses.

In the past, the effects of exposing preterm infants to bright lights and a noisy environment were not well understood. Improvements have occurred, but noise continues to be a problem. Although the recommended noise level in NICUs is below 45 decibels, levels may range between 38 and 90 decibels or higher (Gardner, Goldson & Hernandez, 2016a). Noise tends to be loudest during report and caregiver rounds and in areas where staff congregate, such as at entrances, sinks, and computer areas.

The sounds of ventilators, incubators, doors, people, and alarms from equipment and monitors can create a noise level that increases the risk for hearing loss and other complications. In addition, stimulation of any kind can cause increased energy expenditure by the preterm infant. Noise and even routine handling and nursing interventions are often accompanied by changes in heart rate, oxygen saturation levels, and behavior states.

Preterm infants undergo multiple assessments, procedures, and treatments that may cause frequent interruptions of sleep and may interfere with the development of normal sleep-wake cycles. Sleep disruption alters neuronal maturation and secretion of growth hormone and interferes with growth and development (Gardner et al., 2016a). Energy that must be directed toward coping with an overstimulating and stressful environment may be unavailable for normal growth and development.

Although touch is generally thought to be comforting to infants, it is often associated with painful events for preterm infants. This can cause them to develop touch aversion, a negative response to touch of any kind. They may cry, squirm, and recoil when touched, expecting that touch will lead to pain.

◆ Assessment

Assess the amount of noise to which the infant is exposed. Determine how often interruptions occur and how the infant responds to different types of care.

Assess the infant's ability to tolerate activity and noise. Overstimulation results in changes in oxygenation and behavior. Behavioral indications of stress, also called *avoidance cues* or *avoidance behavior*, show the infant is seeking to escape the noxious stimuli. Observe for these signs and determine what situations cause them to occur or increase.

◆ Identification of Patient Problems

Preterm infants may have difficulty with multiple stimuli and have a potential for infant stress resulting from exposure to environmental overstimulation.

CRITICAL TO REMEMBER
Signs of Overstimulation in Preterm Infants

Oxygenation Changes
Blood pressure, pulse, and respiratory instability
Cyanosis, pallor, or mottling
Flaring nares
Decreased oxygen saturation levels
Apnea
Sneezing, coughing

Behavior Changes
Stiff, extended arms and legs
Fisting of the hands or splaying (spreading wide apart) of the fingers
Arching
Alert, worried expression
Turning away from eye contact (gaze aversion)
Regurgitation, gagging, hiccupping
Yawning
Fatigue signs

◆ Planning: Expected Outcomes

The expected outcomes are that the infant will do the following:
1. Show decreasing signs of overstimulation during routine activity as evidenced by fewer respiratory and behavioral changes during handling and increased periods of relaxed behavior or sleep.
2. Gradually show an ability to withstand more activity before signs of overstimulation occur.

◆ Interventions

Interventions are focused on providing developmentally supportive nursing care that meets the preterm infant's ability to tolerate stimulation. Developmental care keeps stressors in the environment to a minimum based on the infant's physiologic and behavioral responses.

Scheduling Care

Schedule periods of undisturbed rest throughout the day to allow the infant to recover from treatments. Avoid waking the infant during the short quiet sleep phase. If the infant must be awakened for care, try to do it during an active period of sleep when the infant can be more easily aroused using quiet talking and gentle touch.

Arrange routine care to correspond with the infant's awake periods, and avoid disturbing rest. Decrease the frequency of taking vital signs and performing other routine care as soon as possible. Even the handling involved in routine sponge bathing may cause stress in small infants.

Routine daily baths are unnecessary and should be avoided. Bathing every fourth day does not increase skin flora or pathogen counts. Bathing should be postponed until infants are physiologically stable (Gardner et al., 2016a).

Cluster or group care so that several tasks are performed at once to allow for more rest between interruptions. However, keep clustered care short and be alert to the infant's signs of stress. Too many activities may be more than the infant can tolerate without rest. Clustered care may not be appropriate for preterm infants younger than 28 weeks of gestational age (Gardner et al., 2016a).

Provide short rest periods or "time out" periods for recovery within grouped activities or during long or painful procedures. Do not include painful procedures in a cluster of other care. Rest is needed before and after painful procedures.

An important nursing responsibility is managing the infant's care by coordinating activities of different health care workers.

Reducing Stimuli

Keep noise around the infant as low as possible. Place incubators away from traffic and congestion areas, and avoid talking near the incubator. Use incubator covers to help lower sound inside the incubator. Set alarms, per facility policy, and respond quickly when they sound. Alarms should be audible, but not disturbing to nearby patients. Open and close portholes and doors on incubators and cabinets quietly.

Do not place objects on top of the incubator or use it as a writing surface because it increases the noise inside. Teach parents and others to avoid tapping on the incubator. Soft classical music is sometimes used to help promote rest.

Lights that are on 24 hours a day in the nursery may interfere with the development of sleep cycles. Position the incubator so the infant is not facing bright lights, and drape a blanket or incubator cover over the top and sides to decrease light and noise further. Use a dimmer switch to vary the intensity of lights, as needed. Reduce lighting at night to as low as possible to help promote rest, conserve energy for growth, and help development of circadian rhythms.

Some NICU have single rooms for each infant. This reduces noise and allows environmental stimuli to be adapted to each infant's individual needs. It also provides more privacy for visiting family members and may reduce hospital-acquired infections.

Promoting Rest

When possible, schedule "quiet periods" when lights and noise in the unit are kept to a minimum to promote rest. Rest periods should be at least an hour long to allow preterm infants to complete a sleep cycle (Gardner et al., 2016a). Only emergency procedures should take place during rest times.

Contain the infant's arms and legs to promote flexion and reduce energy loss from flailing extremities. Containment also promotes quieting, improves physiologic stability, and reduces stress (Gardner et al., 2016a). Provide boundaries with rolled blankets or commercial positioning devices placed around the infant. For the side-lying and supine positions, arrange the infant's arms and legs in a flexed position, with the hands near midline to allow hand-to-mouth activity and sucking.

Stroking and gentle massage may be calming for stable preterm infants. It may help increase weight gain and improve development. It also can help involve parents in care of the infant. Not all types of touch are appropriate for smaller, more fragile infants; however, an appropriate option can be used to facilitate parent-infant interaction (Spruill, 2015).

Promoting Motor Development

Preterm infants may have musculoskeletal and developmental problems from prolonged immobilization and the effects of gravity on their immature neuromuscular system. Because the extensor muscles mature before the flexor muscles, the infant tends to remain in an extended, "frog-leg" position. Shoulder retraction, abduction and external rotation of the lower extremities, lateral flexion of the arms, neck hyperextension, and flattening of the sides of the head may be prevented by using correct positioning.

Reposition the infant every 2 to 3 hours or when other care is given. Change the position slowly, because position changes may be stressful. When possible, position the infant with the extremities flexed and the hands placed in the midline and near the mouth to allow the infant to suck them for comfort. Use swaddling, blanket rolls, and commercial positioning devices to maintain flexion.

Individualizing Care

Although all NICU nurses are competent in caring for preterm infants, they have slightly different styles in approaching infants. When possible, the same nurse or nurses should be assigned to care for the infant. This allows the nurse to learn the infant's unique behavior and response to stress and allows the infant to get accustomed to the nurse's individual caregiving pattern. It is also very helpful to parents to relate with a small number of nurses who know their infant well.

The ability to tolerate stress varies with each infant. Adapt general care according to the infant's ability to tolerate it. Determine the infant's response to various stimuli, particularly those that cause adverse responses. Even positive stimuli such as soft music or talking quietly can cause overstimulation at times.

Infants often require extra energy to adjust to changes in care. Observe how well they tolerate changes such as moving from assisted to more independent breathing or introduction of new feeding methods. Increase rest periods during these times.

Communicating Infants' Needs

Use the nursing care plan and shift reports to inform other caregivers of techniques that are especially effective for certain infants. Tape laminated notes near the bedside as reminders of needs unique to each infant. Doing so also alerts the parents to the methods that nurses use to care for the infant. Explain all techniques to the parents, and solicit their suggestions so they can participate in care appropriately.

◆ Evaluation

As a result of interventions, the infant displays fewer and less frequent signs of overstimulation and shows an increasing tolerance to stimuli before signs appear.

◆ APPLICATION OF THE NURSING PROCESS: NUTRITION

Preterm infants are born before full accumulation of nutrient stores has occurred or digestive capacity is achieved. The problem increases with decreasing gestational age.

Full-term newborns have reservoirs of calcium, iron, and other nutrients, but these are lacking in preterm infants. Fat stores are minimal or absent, and glucose reserves are used soon after birth. Hypoglycemia develops very quickly and should be prevented or treated promptly.

Preterm infants receiving enteral feedings need approximately 105 to 130 kcal/kg/day (Poindexter & Ehrenkranz, 2015). This amount varies according to activity, illness, and other factors that may affect caloric need. These infants need more protein, iron, calcium, and phosphorus. The average healthy preterm infant should gain approximately 15 to 20 g/kg/day (Brown et al., 2016).

The gastrointestinal (GI) tract of preterm infants does not absorb nutrients as well as that of full-term infants. Although they digest protein well, preterm infants have insufficient bile acids and pancreatic lipase to absorb fat adequately. They have some lactase deficiency but rarely have lactose intolerance (Brown et al., 2016). Their smaller stomach capacity limits the volume preterm infants can tolerate at each feeding. They need more of many nutrients per kilogram than do full-term infants, and supplementation is necessary.

◆ Assessment

Changes in feedings are often made according to the nurse's recommendations based on assessment of an infant's tolerance of feedings, readiness for change, and signs indicating complications.

Feeding Tolerance

Assess how well the infant tolerates enteral feedings, whether by gavage (feeding tube) or nipple. Aspirate the stomach contents to measure the residual amount of feeding in the stomach before intermittent gavage feedings or every 2 to 4 hours for continuous feedings or according to hospital policy. This procedure helps determine whether the stomach is emptying and prevents overdistention. Report residuals to the provider if they are more than half the previous feeding for intermittent feedings or more than 2 to 4 mL/kg or a 1-hour volume for continuous feeding (Brown et al., 2016). An excessive residual indicates that the amount, type, or flow rate of formula may need to be changed. It also may be an early sign of a complication such as necrotizing enterocolitis (NEC).

Unless they are bloody, have large amounts of mucus, or are otherwise abnormal, gastric residuals are often replaced to prevent loss of electrolytes. Abnormal residuals are also reported to the provider, and the feeding may be held. The next feeding may be reduced by the amount of the residual. If residuals are not replaced, observe carefully for signs of electrolyte imbalance.

Vomiting or frequent regurgitation may indicate the feedings are too large. Vomitus or residuals containing bile may be a sign of intestinal obstruction and may require surgery. Diarrhea may be caused by too rapid advancement of the feeding or intolerance to the type of formula.

Observe for signs of intestinal complications such as visible loops of bowel. Obtain objective data about abdominal distention by using a tape to measure abdominal girth per facility protocol. Place the tape directly above the umbilicus and record the placement to ensure consistency. Stools may be tested for reducing substances (which indicate malabsorption of carbohydrates) or occult blood if feeding intolerance is suspected. Report signs to the health care provider because they may be early indications of complications such as ileus, sepsis, obstruction, or NEC.

Readiness for Nipple Feeding

Preterm infants often are initially fed parenterally or by gavage. The ability to feed orally and the ability to gain weight are important milestones, as they are often among the criteria for discharge from the hospital. Coordination of sucking, swallowing, and breathing is a complex task for infants.

Preterm infants do not have the well-developed buccal sucking pads in the cheeks that term infants use to form a seal around the nipple for efficient sucking. The jaw is less stable, and the infant tires easily during oral feedings. The gag reflex may function poorly. The infant's respiratory status, other problems, and distractions in the environment can greatly affect feeding ability.

During gavage feedings, watch for signs that nipple feeding may soon be possible. These include rooting, respiratory rate below 60 breaths per minute, and increasing ability to tolerate holding and handling. Although sucking on the gavage tube, a finger, or a pacifier may be a sign of readiness, it is not enough. Infants should also have an intact gag reflex, or they are more likely to aspirate feedings. Note whether the infant gags on the catheter or a gloved finger inserted into the mouth.

Most infants are ready to begin oral feedings when they reach 34 weeks gestational age. Some are ready as early as 30 weeks and others need until 36 weeks (Brown et al., 2016). At this age, many healthy preterm infants are able to coordinate sucking with swallowing and breathing and have a functional gag reflex. In addition, infants must have enough energy to feed orally without compromising oxygenation. Very weak infants expend too much oxygen, glucose, and energy when sucking and must continue to receive gavage feedings.

By 30 to 32 weeks, feeding readiness assessments should be initiated (NANN, 2013). When the infant begins to feed by nipple, assess coordination of suck, swallow, and breathing and observe for aspiration. Frequent choking, gagging, or cyanosis during feedings may indicate that the infant cannot coordinate all feeding movements well enough for nipple feeding. In many infants, signs of aspiration are minimal or absent; this is called *silent aspiration*.

Assess the respiratory rate before and during feedings. When the respiratory rate is more than 60 breaths per minute before feedings, gavage feed to prevent aspiration. During feedings observe for signs that the effort of nipple feeding requires too much energy and oxygen for the infant.

◆ Identification of Patient Problems

When the infant's nutritional needs are met by parenteral methods, the nursing care is collaborative. However, once the infant is able to breast feed or take formula by bottle, many nursing interventions are involved. They include the potential for ineffective feeding because of uncoordinated suck and swallow as well as fatigue during feedings.

◆ Planning: Expected Outcomes

The expected outcomes are that the infant will do the following:

1. Consume adequate amounts of breast milk or formula to meet nutrient needs for age and weight.
2. Gain weight as appropriate for age, generally 15 to 20 g/kg/day.

The actual amount of feedings and weight gain will vary according to the infant's gestational age and other conditions. Discuss what is appropriate for a particular infant with the physician or nurse practitioner.

◆ Interventions

Administering Parenteral Nutrition

The nurse manages the administration of **total parenteral nutrition (TPN)**, the IV infusion of solutions containing major nutrients needed for metabolism and growth. It may be necessary for very immature infants because of respiratory problems, limited gastric capacity, surgery, or reduced peristalsis. It provides calories, amino acids, fatty acids, vitamins, and minerals in amounts adapted to the specific needs of infants. TPN is decreased as enteral feedings are increased, continuing until the infant is able to tolerate full enteral feedings.

Administering Enteral Feedings

Enteral feedings (feeding into the GI tract, orally or by feeding tube) are usually begun within the first few days with minimal enteral feedings, also called *trophic feedings*. These feedings are only a few milliliters of breast milk or formula given at a time. They stimulate development of the GI tract, enhance gut motility, decrease the need for parenteral nutrition, and decrease feeding intolerance (Poindexter & Ehrenkranz, 2015). Bowel sounds should be present, there should be no significant abdominal distention, and infants should be in relatively stable condition. Mother's milk is preferred if it is available. Donor breast milk also may be used. Colostrum is especially high in immune agents to help prevent infection. Feedings are gradually increased according to the infant's tolerance.

Colostrum or breast milk also can be used for oral care of infants. It is applied to the infant's lips and inside of the mouth every 3 hours with a sterile swab. It provides the immunologic benefits of breast milk before the infant can take feedings (Gardner & Lawrence, 2016).

Preterm infants need special formulas or fortified breast milk. These formulas are adapted to meet the need for easily digestible, concentrated nutrients in a smaller volume of fluid. Preterm infants may need formulas that have 24 kcal/oz, or more (instead of 20 kcal/oz used for the full-term infant)

to meet their requirements. Preterm formulas may contain added calories, protein, vitamins, minerals, and complex fatty acids. Other components may be added to meet individual needs. Breast milk fortifiers add needed nutrients to breast milk.

Administering Gavage Feedings

Gavage feedings are usually started before oral feedings for preterm infants (Procedure 23.1). A small, soft catheter is inserted through the nose or mouth every 2 to 3 hours for intermittent (bolus) feedings. An indwelling catheter also may be used to provide for intermittent or continuous feedings. Indwelling catheters stay in place up to 30 days.

Inserting the catheter at each feeding may be more traumatic than leaving it in place. Frequent oral placement may cause vomiting or increase infant aversion to oral stimuli, which may lead to difficulty with oral feedings later. Vagal stimulation during insertion may cause apnea and bradycardia. Nasal placement avoids aversive oral stimulation but may increase airway resistance by interfering with air flow through the infant's small nasal passages.

Intermittent bolus feedings provide a more normal feeding pattern with periodic stimulation of gastric hormones and enzymes. They should be given slowly over 30 to 60 minutes.

Continuous feedings may be better for infants with short-bowel syndrome, congenital heart disease, or intolerance to bolus feedings or those recovering from NEC (Brown et al., 2016). However, continuous feedings carry a higher risk for aspiration because the infant is not observed at all times during the feeding. In addition, bacteria counts in the milk or formula may become too high, and fats tend to adhere to the tubing during continuous feeding.

Feedings are gradually increased according to the infant's tolerance. Carefully observe the infant's response at each feeding to determine when the feeding type or amount can be changed. Parenteral nutrition continues until the infant is able to take adequate enteral feedings.

Pacifiers are often used during gavage feedings. Preterm infants have been exposed to noxious oral stimulation, such as intubation and suctioning. As a result, they may react negatively to any additional oral stimulation, which interferes with feedings. Providing a pacifier during gavage feedings gives positive oral stimulation and helps associate the comfortable feeling of fullness with sucking. Nonnutritive sucking increases later success in oral feedings and decreases behavior changes during feedings.

Nonnutritive sucking also can be provided by having an infant who is not ready for oral feeding suck on the mother's emptied breasts as a way to prepare for feeding from the breast. Gavage feeding can be done at the same time to help infants associate the breast with the feeling of being fed. This may improve breastfeeding ability when the infant is ready to be fed at the breast (Black, 2012).

Administering Oral Feedings

Oral feedings should be cue based (begun when the infants shows signs of physiologic and behavioral readiness to

NURSING PROCEDURE 23.1   Administering Gavage Feeding

Purpose:

To feed infants who are unable to take the full feedings by nipple; may be used alone or along with nipple feedings.

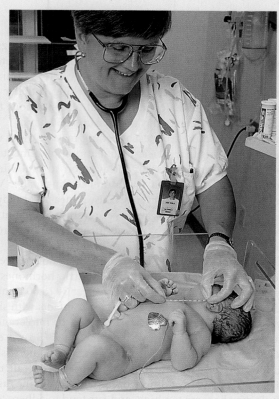

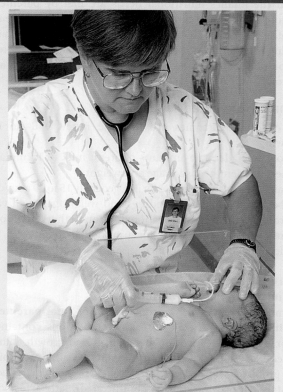

1. Wash hands. Gather equipment, including gavage catheter of proper size (4 to 8 French, depending on the size of the infant); measured container, 20 mL or larger; syringe; stethoscope; syringe pump, if appropriate; and extension tubing, if needed. Warm the breast milk or formula to room or body temperature. Check the chart to determine how previous feedings were tolerated. Add fortifier to breast milk, if ordered. *Having all materials ready helps the procedure go smoothly and avoids disturbing the infant or delaying feedings. Cold milk could interfere with thermoregulation. Information about previous feedings will help meet the infant's needs.*

2. Don gloves. If the parents are present, they may hold the infant in their arms or in kangaroo care once the catheter is inserted. If the infant cannot be held, they may hold the infant's hands. *Feeding is important to the parents, and helping increases their sense of involvement.*

3. Determine the length of catheter to insert. Measure from the tip of the nose to the base of the ear to halfway between the xiphoid process and the umbilicus. Mark the catheter at the proper point with a piece of tape or indelible ink. *The measured distance is equal to the distance from the mouth or nose to the stomach. The mark on the catheter shows whether the tube has moved out of place.*

4. For oral placement, insert the tube gently into the mouth until the mark on the tube is reached. For nasal placement, lubricate the tip with sterile water or lubricant. Gently insert into one nostril until premeasured mark is reached. Remove the catheter immediately if persistent coughing, choking, cyanosis, apnea, or bradycardia occurs. *Moistening or lubricating the tip allows easier passage. Gentle insertion prevents trauma. Signs may indicate that the catheter is entering the trachea instead of the esophagus. Stimulation of the vagus nerve may cause bradycardia or apnea.*

5. Check for placement according to hospital protocol. Attach a syringe to the catheter and gently aspirate stomach contents. Move or rotate the catheter slightly if the plunger does not withdraw easily. Check that the mark on the tube is in the same place whenever care is given and before feeds. *The pH shows if the aspirate is stomach contents. Radiography also may be used to verify placement (usually only if done for another reason). Use of force could traumatize the stomach lining if the end of the catheter is resting against it. Moving the catheter may draw it away from the stomach lining. Checking the tube marking ensures the tube is still in the correct place.*

6. Secure the catheter to the cheek with an adhesive dressing. *Securing ensures the catheter will remain inserted to the proper point during the procedure.*

NURSING PROCEDURE 23.1 Administering Gavage Feeding—cont'd

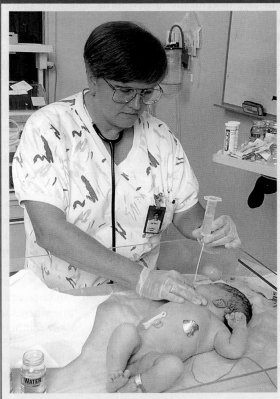

7. Withdraw the stomach contents to check the gastric residual. Observe the amount, color, and consistency of the aspirate. During continuous feedings, check the gastric residual every 2 to 4 hours or according to hospital policy. Do not feed the infant if the aspirate is abnormal. The residual should not be more than half the previous feeding or happen more than once or twice. Report abnormal appearance or amount of stomach contents. *Stomach contents that are red or dark brown may indicate blood. If the aspirate is green with bile or brown with feces, intestinal obstruction may have occurred. An excessive residual may mean the infant is receiving too much or that stomach emptying is delayed.*

8. Return residuals according to hospital protocol. If it is replaced, subtract the amount of gastric residual from the amount of milk to be given. *Replacement of aspirate prevents loss of electrolytes. Overdistention of the stomach is avoided by subtracting the residual from the feeding to be given.*

9. For gravity flow feedings, remove the plunger and attach the syringe to the feeding tube. Pour the correct amount of milk into the syringe. Raise or lower the syringe to increase or decrease the flow rate so the feeding moves slowly into the stomach over 30 minutes. *The higher the syringe, the faster the flow of solution and the greater the pressure. Feedings should be given slowly to prevent sudden distention or trauma from pressure, and from filling the stomach too fast.*

10. For timed or continuous feedings, place no more than a 2- to 4-hour supply of milk in a syringe. Set the pump to deliver the correct rate of flow. Change the equipment according to hospital policy. *Limiting the amount of feeding and changing equipment prevent excessive growth of bacteria in the milk or tubing. Infusion pumps deliver the feeding at a constant, measured rate.*

11. Give the infant a pacifier during the feeding. *The pacifier stimulates the sucking reflex, helps prepare the infant for nippling, is comforting, and helps the infant associate sucking with feeding.*

12. Burp the infant after feeding. *Air may be swallowed around the catheter and can cause the infant to regurgitate and aspirate.*

13. For intermittent feedings with a catheter that remains in place, flush the tube with the smallest amount of sterile water needed to clear the tube (1 to 2 mL) and close off the end when the feeding is completed. *This prevents clogging of the tubing. Closing the end prevents formula from coming back through the catheter.*

14. When the catheter is to be withdrawn, pinch it and remove quickly. *Pinching prevents drops of fluid from entering the trachea as the catheter is removed, and quick removal decreases irritation.*

15. Record time, amount, and characteristics of gastric residual, type and amount of feeding given, and how the infant tolerated it. *Documentation allows monitoring of the infant's ability to tolerate feedings and meet nutritional needs.*

CRITICAL TO REMEMBER

Nipple Feedings

Signs of Readiness for Nipple Feedings
Rooting
Sucking on gavage tube, finger, or pacifier
Ability to tolerate holding/handling
Respiratory rate <60 breaths per minute
Presence of gag reflex
Maintains quiet alert state for at least 10 minutes

Signs of Nonreadiness for Nipple Feedings
Respiratory rate >60 breaths per minute
No rooting or sucking
Absence of gag reflex
Excessive gastric residuals

Adverse Signs during Nipple Feedings
Tachycardia
Bradycardia
Increased or decreased respiratory rate
Nasal flaring
Markedly decreased oxygen saturation level
Cyanosis, pallor
Apnea
Choking, coughing, sneezing, hiccoughs
Finger splaying—"Stop sign" hand
Gagging, regurgitation
Drooling, gulping
Falling asleep early in the feeding
Feeding time longer than 20 to 30 minutes

feed) rather than on a time schedule. Crying is a late hunger sign and may cause the infant to be too tired to eat. The frequency and volume of oral feedings are based on the infant's readiness and ability. Oral feedings may be offered at each feeding time if the infant shows positive feeding readiness signs (Fig. 23.2). Full oral feedings are reached faster using cue-based feedings (Newland, L'Huillier, & Scheans, 2013; NANN, 2013). Cue-based feedings may help infants develop sleep-wake cycles and begin to self-regulate better.

Feedings. Provide for maintenance of heat during feedings. When infants have stable temperature maintenance, wrap them in warm blankets and hold them for feedings. If thermoregulation is a problem, feed the infant in the radiant warmer or incubator.

Nipple feedings involve a greater expenditure of energy by the infant than gavage feedings. Allow for a period of rest before and after feedings. Use of a pacifier before feedings helps bring preterm infants to an alert state that enhances oral feeding success. Infants take feedings better if they are awake. Assess for signs of overstimulation and stress during feedings. If they occur, stop the feeding and let the infant rest. If the infant continues to show signs of stress, the feeding should be completed by gavage.

Choosing a Nipple. A variety of nipples for neonates are available. Soft, high-flow nipples ("preemie" nipples) are more pliable than regular nipples and require less energy for sucking. However, they may deliver milk too rapidly, cause choking, and interfere with breathing between sucking bursts. Standard nipples are firmer and deliver the milk more slowly so the infant can control it more easily. Nipples are available in several sizes, including those for infants with a very small mouth.

Facilitating Breastfeeding

Breast milk is best for almost all infants and especially for preterm infants. The NANN Position Statement (NANN,

2015) states human milk and breastfeeding are essential components in care of critically ill newborns. The AAP (2012) recommends that all preterm infants receive human milk.

Explain to parents that the immunologic benefits of breast milk are particularly important to the preterm infant who did not receive passive immunity during fetal life. Human milk provides protection against infections and decreases the incidence of NEC (Geddes, Hassiotou, Wise, & Hartmann, 2017). Breast milk may stimulate the immune system and GI maturation. It is well tolerated, and the nutrients in it are more available than those in cow's-milk formulas. Nutrients in breast milk are more easily digested, and it provides antimicrobial components, enzymes, hormones, and growth factors important for the preterm infant.

In addition, breastfeeding may be less stressful than bottle feeding for preterm infants. Oxygenation levels are often higher during breastfeeding because the infant can regulate breathing and suckling better than with bottle feeding (Lawrence & Lawrence, 2016).

Offer support and encouragement to mothers who want to breastfeed. Contributing her milk helps the mother realize she has something important to offer at a time when she may believe she can do little to help her baby. Many mothers find this particularly rewarding and worth the effort involved. They may develop a sense of increased control when they are able to breastfeed and may take on more responsibility in infant care (Black, 2012).

The mother who plans to breastfeed needs help with maintaining lactation until the infant is mature enough to nurse. Help her begin to use a breast pump as soon as possible after birth and instruct her to pump at least five times a day for 20 minutes per pumping session or a total of at least 100 minutes per day (Lawrence & Lawrence, 2016). The AWHONN (2013b) considers providing a breast pump and instruction to mothers of preterm infants within 6 hours of birth a nursing care quality measure.

Give the mother sterile containers to store her milk. Show her how to label her milk and where to take it when she brings it to the NICU. When she goes home, tell her to place her milk in a refrigerator if the infant will receive it within 24 hours or in a freezer if it will be more than 24 hours. If fortifiers will be added to the milk, explain the higher needs of the preterm infant so that the mother does not think something is wrong with her milk or that it is inadequate.

In some facilities, healthy preterm infants progress to breastfeeding from gavage feedings without using the bottle at all. This should be encouraged with eligible infants and mothers who desire breastfeeding.

Ongoing support for the mother is important. Encourage her efforts in feeding, which may be difficult at first. Remind her that even full-term infants must learn how to breastfeed. Mothers who have not breastfed previously have to learn the basic techniques and also how to adapt them for the preterm infant.

Relaxation needed for feeding is difficult in the busy NICU. Provide as much privacy as possible, using a separate room or screens. Help the mother feel comfortable holding

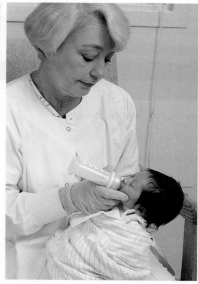

FIG 23.2 The nurse feeds a preterm infant.

the tiny infant and any attached equipment. The presence of a lactation consultant during initial breastfeeding sessions is very helpful.

Adapt breastfeeding teaching to the needs of a very small infant. Show the mother how to use the football and cross-cradle holds, which allow her to see the infant's face well during latching on and throughout the feeding (see Figs. 22.4 and 22.5). A supplemental nursing system, a device that holds expressed breast milk in a bag with a small tube attached to the mother's nipple, may be used to help infants receive more milk with less effort during early feedings. Feedings should begin gradually and progress similar to initial bottle feedings.

Make the same observations of the infant during breastfeeding as during bottle feeding. Signs of fatigue, bradycardia, tachypnea, or apnea may show lack of readiness for breastfeeding. Be sure the infant stays warm. The mother's body heat will help maintain the infant's temperature during feedings. KC is often started before the infant is able to breastfeed. As the infant becomes ready to breastfeed, KC can be continued during the feeding.

Thin nipple shields may be used in the first few days of breastfeeding to help the infant latch onto the breast and remain latched. Instruct the mother to pump her breasts at the end of each feeding because preterm infants may not suckle well enough to extract all milk from the breasts at first (Gardner & Lawrence, 2016).

Making Ongoing Assessments

Continually assess the infant for feeding readiness cues and the infant's responses to all feeding methods. Watch for signs of distress, especially when feedings are first initiated. Record the amount of breast milk or the amount of formula the infant takes by gavage or bottle and compare it with the amount needed to meet nutrient needs for the infant's age and weight.

Because accurate estimation of milk intake is difficult during breastfeeding, infants may be weighed on an electronic scale before and after feedings to determine intake. Both weights should be taken with the infant wearing the same clothing and before the diaper is changed after the feeding. The difference in the weights in grams equals the milliliters taken. This allows supplementary gavage feeding amounts to be calculated on the basis of the infant's oral intake of breast milk.

Note the infant's response to other stimuli during feedings. Some infants respond well to being talked to and rocked during feedings. Others become distracted by any noise, motion, or nearby activities.

Weigh the infant daily at the same time with the same scale. Record the length and head circumference each week. Plot measurements on a growth chart for preterm infants and compare results with expected ranges. Weight increase not accompanied by increased length may be caused by edema and may be a sign of a complication such as congestive heart failure.

Observe changes in the infant's ability to take feedings. The suck and swallow coordination should gradually improve with maturity and practice. As the infant becomes more mature, less energy should be expended during the feeding sessions.

The infant will take the feedings more quickly and show fewer signs of fatigue such as falling asleep during feedings.

Explain to the mother that she may need to continue to pump her breasts after feedings several times a day after the infant goes home. The infant's suck may still be too weak to adequately stimulate milk production. Pumping helps maintain the milk supply. The need to pump will lessen gradually as the infant nurses more vigorously.

◆ Evaluation

If the expected outcomes have been met, the infant will consume adequate amounts of breast milk or formula to meet nutrient needs for age and weight and will gain weight as appropriate for age.

> **? CRITICAL THINKING EXERCISE 23.1**
>
> Giovanni was born 2 weeks ago at 30 weeks of gestation. His mother, Katherine, asks the nurse if there are any differences between how to give her baby a bottle and feeding her sister's baby who was not premature.
>
> **Question**
> 1. How should the nurse answer her?

> **? KNOWLEDGE CHECK**
>
> 8. What can the nurse do for the infant at risk for stress from overstimulation?
> 9. How does the nurse assess feeding tolerance?
> 10. Why should the nurse allow the infant to set the pace of feedings instead of urging continuous sucking?
> 11. How can the nurse help the mother who wants to breastfeed her preterm infant?

◆ APPLICATION OF THE NURSING PROCESS: PARENTING

The birth of a preterm infant is generally unexpected and always emotionally traumatic to parents. Infants are often hurried to the NICU shortly after birth. Later, when parents go to the NICU, the infant is attached to an array of machines.

Parents cannot hold or feed the infant at first, or offer any of the usual care that parents expect to give their infants. The infant may not be capable of common newborn behaviors such as making eye contact and grasping the parent's finger. When the infant's appearance and behavior are different from the parents' expectations, attachment may be delayed.

The extended hospitalization of the preterm infant causes separation of the parents from their newborn, produces emotional trauma, and disrupts family life. Parents must relinquish the role of primary caregiver during their infant's hospitalization. They may feel they are in the nurse's way and may state they do not feel like parents at all. Loss of the parental role is a major stressor for these parents.

Being unable to participate fully in the infant's care for a prolonged period hampers the parents' ability to learn their baby's unique characteristics, such as the way the infant responds to stress and the methods of consolation that work best. Separation delays the development of the parent–infant relationship and may impair bonding.

In addition, parents worry about the infant's condition and outcome. They need help in understanding the infant's condition and what can be expected to occur throughout the hospital stay. Nurses should evaluate the progress of attachment to assist parents to feel important in caring for their infant.

◆ Assessment

Assess for signs of parental attachment on the first and subsequent visits to the NICU nursery. Expect parents to be fearful at first but more able to focus on the infant as they recover from the initial shock of preterm birth. Assess for common behaviors that show normal progression of attachment. These include talking about the infant in positive terms, making eye contact, pointing out physical characteristics, naming the infant, and calling the infant by name.

Parents should ask questions about the infant. When they are able to hold and participate in the care of the infant, observe for gradual increase in comfort and skill. The parents should smile and talk to the infant and verbalize increasing confidence in their caregiving abilities.

Watch for signs that bonding is not occurring as expected. These include failure to show usual attachment behaviors or a decrease in behaviors that were previously present. Parents who seem as interested in other infants in the NICU as in their own infant or talk about the infant in an impersonal way may be having difficulty. Note how often the parents make visits or calls to the NICU and changes that may indicate their need for support.

Determine whether there are other stressors in the parents' lives that may interfere with their ability to visit and form attachment to the infant. The financial need to return to work, lack of transportation, long distances, or the need to care for other children may prevent parents from visiting as often as they would like.

After the critical period in the early days after birth, healthy preterm infants become more stable. They still require specialized nursing care and hospitalization but gradually need fewer technologic interventions. They are sometimes called

---

CRITICAL TO REMEMBER

Signs That Bonding May Be Delayed

Using negative terms to describe the infant
Discussing the infant in impersonal or technical terms
Failing to give the infant a name or to use the name
Visiting or calling infrequently or not at all
Decreasing the number and length of visits
Showing interest in other infants equal to that in their own infant
Refusing offers to hold and learn to care for the infant
Showing a decrease in or lack of eye contact
Spending less time talking to or smiling at the infant

"growers" at this time. This is a time when parental participation in the infant's care should increase in preparation for discharge.

◆ Identification of Patient Problems

For parents of preterm infants, an important patient problem is the potential for inadequate development of parent–infant relationship resulting from lack of understanding of the infant's condition and separation from the infant.

◆ Planning: Expected Outcomes

The expected outcomes are that the parents will do the following:
1. Demonstrate bonding behaviors, including visiting or calling frequently and interacting as appropriate for the infant's condition throughout the hospital stay.
2. Verbalize understanding of the preterm infant's condition and characteristics within 2 days.
3. Express gradually increasing comfort in participating in infant care throughout the hospital stay.

◆ Interventions
Making Advance Preparations

Preparing for stressful situations such as preterm birth helps parents cope with the actual event. Parents at higher risk for a preterm birth should visit the NICU before delivery. If the mother is confined to bed, arrange for a nurse from the NICU to visit her so that she feels a link with the nursery. The father or another support person should tour the nursery so that he can discuss the nursery environment with the mother. Encourage the parents to ask questions.

Assisting Parents after Birth

After the birth, allow the parents to see and touch the newborn in the delivery room, even if only for a few moments, so they have a realistic idea of the infant's appearance and condition. This helps the bonding process that began in pregnancy to continue.

If possible, allow the father or primary support person to watch the initial care in the NICU. Explain what is happening and why. This attention allows him to see the intense efforts made on behalf of his infant, increases his confidence in the staff, and enables him to give the mother a full description later. Support the father as well as the mother by using therapeutic communication during this difficult time.

If the infant must be transported to another facility, ask the transport team to visit the parents before leaving, if possible. The visit helps parents feel connected to their infant and to the staff providing care. Leaving photographs with the mother is another way of helping her bond even though the infant is not with her.

Supporting Parents during Early Visits

Take the parents to the NICU as soon as possible. If the mother is too ill to be with her infant, bring her photographs. Before parents first visit the infant, prepare them for what they will see. Describe the equipment, the various attachments to the infant, and the purposes (Fig. 23.3). Explain how the infant will look and behave. Box 23.1 provides specific steps that

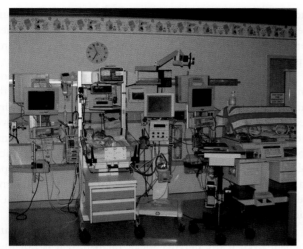

FIG 23.3 An infant in the neonatal intensive care unit is surrounded by highly technologic equipment. This can be very frightening to parents at first. Preparation of parents before they visit is an important nursing responsibility.

BOX 23.1 Introducing Parents to the Neonatal Intensive Care Unit Setting

Before Parents Visit the Neonatal Intensive Care Unit

If possible, provide the parents with a tour of the NICU before the birth.

If a tour is not possible, describe the NICU environment. Include the noise of alarms, the busyness of the staff, and the number of people and sick infants.

Describe the equipment. Include ventilators, intravenous lines, feeding tubes, and monitors. Explain how they look and how they are attached to the infant. Keep the explanations simple, without technical details.

Show the parents photographs of their infant. This helps prepare them, but seeing photographs is not as overwhelming as seeing the infant in person.

Describe the infant. Include the size, lack of fat, breathing problems, and weak cry. Explain that no sound of crying can be heard if the infant is intubated. Include some personal aspects: "He's a real fighter" or "She makes the funniest faces during her feedings."

When Parents Visit the Neonatal Intensive Care Unit

Help the parents perform thorough handwashing, and explain the importance.

Stay with the parents during their visit. Having a familiar person nearby will help them feel more comfortable while they adjust to this unfamiliar environment.

Introduce them to their infant's nurse. Ask the NICU nurse to explain some of the care being provided for the infant.

Give parents printed information about the NICU so that they can take it home to read later. This includes visiting hours, telephone updates, availability of classes on preterm infant care, and support groups.

Tell the parents they will receive instruction on how to care for their infant in time. Encourage them to visit the infant as much as they can. Emphasize how important they are to their infant.

Offer realistic encouragement based on the infant's condition.

Provide an opportunity for the parents to express their concerns and feelings and ask questions.

NICU, Neonatal intensive care unit.

---

the nurse can follow to help parents become familiar with the NICU setting.

At first, stay with the parents during visits. When they are comfortable, allow them time alone with the infant so they can interact in private. Answer questions and explain changes in the infant's condition and treatment. Expect to repeat explanations because stressed parents may not understand or remember what was said. Parents often do not know what questions to ask at first or are too overwhelmed to ask questions. In this situation, discuss questions that are common when parents first visit the NICU. Use therapeutic communication as the parents cope with their grief, guilt, and emotional turmoil.

Parents should touch the infant as soon as possible because touching helps promote attachment. They may be hesitant initially because of fear they will interfere with equipment. The smaller the infant, the more reluctant the parents may be. Some parents may hesitate to touch because they are afraid of becoming attached to an infant who may not live. They need sensitive support from the nurse until they are ready to progress in their relationship with the infant.

THERAPEUTIC COMMUNICATIONS

Reassuring Parents during Visits to the Neonatal Intensive Care Unit

Shareen gave birth to a preterm infant, Valerie, at 28 weeks of gestation. Shareen is visiting the NICU for the first time the day after the birth. Andy, the nurse, has talked to her about what to expect and stays with her during the visit.

Shareen: Oh, she looks so tiny! I saw her for only a minute after she was born, and I didn't really get a good look. How can she ever survive when she's so small and covered with tubes?

Andy: So far, Valerie's doing very well. Her vital signs are stable, and she's holding her own. But it's frightening when she looks so small and vulnerable, isn't it? *(Offering realistic reassurance and reflecting Shareen's fearful feelings. Using infant's name to promote bonding.)*

Shareen: I stayed in bed like they told me to do to help my blood pressure. I thought she wouldn't be born so soon if I stayed in bed.

Andy: It must have been a shock, especially when you tried so hard to prevent it. *(Reflecting feelings and acknowledging that Shareen did what she could to prevent early birth.)*

Shareen: Now she's so tiny and so sick! She looks very different from what I expected.

Andy: Valerie's small, but babies her size grow very quickly. Would you like to touch her? *(Offering realistic reassurance and attempting to bring Shareen closer to her infant.)*

Shareen: Oh, I might hurt her. Maybe I should wait until she's bigger.

Andy: Even tiny babies like to have their mothers touch them and talk to them. She listened to your voice all through your pregnancy, so it's familiar to her. Why don't you talk softly to her while I work with her? And I can tell you about all this equipment and what we are doing for Valerie. *(Emphasizing the mother's importance, involving her in care being given, and offering information about the infant's equipment and care.)*

Show parents how to touch in ways appropriate for the infant, such as holding the infant's hand through the portholes of the incubator or touching the small areas of skin not encumbered by equipment. Explain that handling is kept to a minimum for physiologically unstable infants because it is too stressful to them. As the infant becomes more stable and mature, show parents which forms of touch work best with their infant. This helps parents feel more a part of the infant's plan of care.

Help the parents hold the baby as soon as possible. Parents often look forward to the opportunity to hold the baby as a positive sign of the infant's condition. Yet it is frightening, too, especially if the infant is attached to various kinds of equipment. Help the parents find a comfortable position for themselves and the infant and point out positive responses from the infant.

Supporting the Father

Nurses often concentrate on the mother in providing support. However, fathers also must deal with the shock of having a preterm infant in the NICU. They need support in learning about their infant and how to parent. One study showed fathers of NICU infants had elevated levels of stress and symptoms of depression throughout the 7 weeks of the study (Mackley, Locke, Spear, & Joseph, 2010).

In addition, fathers may have work responsibilities, are expected to provide emotional support for the mother and explain the condition of the mother and infant to friends and family, and may take on other family responsibilities as the mother focuses on care of the newborn. Fathers may spend less time in the NICU because of other responsibilities but may have many questions and concerns. If their time for visiting is limited, fathers may be less comfortable than the mother with caregiving activities. Encourage them to participate in hands-on care whenever possible. Compliment both parents as they care for the infant so they are encouraged to participate even more.

Providing Information

An important role of the nurse is providing accurate information to parents. Allow parents to express their concerns before beginning to teach. Encourage them to ask questions about all aspects of their infant's condition and care. Although some parents are not hesitant to ask questions, others may avoid asking for explanations or advocating for their need to care for their infants because they are afraid they might be seen as difficult or "demanding parents" (Gardner, Voos, & Hills, 2016b). Let the parents know their questions are welcome, and do everything possible to give them the answers when they do ask questions. Give information about common concerns if the parents do not ask questions.

Explain the equipment used to care for the infant. Interpret the information obtained from monitors and the meanings of alarms. Clarify all nursing care, its purpose, and the expected response. Point out how preterm infants are similar to and different from full-term infants to help parents develop an accurate understanding of the infant's capabilities.

Offer realistic reassurance about the infant's condition, emphasizing positive aspects while being truthful. If the parents have misconceptions or did not understand a physician's explanations, clarify or ask the physician to go over specific information again. Translate medical terms into words the parents can understand. Avoid using medical abbreviations and acronyms. Repeat explanations, especially at first. Because of their emotional distress, parents are often unable to fully comprehend or remember what is said to them.

Use an interpreter if the parents do not understand English. Even if the parents speak English, if it is not their primary language, they may have difficulty understanding the information. Provide an interpreter as needed. Offer written information about NICU policies and procedures in the parents' language. Explanations about visiting hours, who can visit, routines for handwashing, and the role of parents can be reinforced in writing so they are available for later reading by overwhelmed parents.

❓ CRITICAL THINKING EXERCISE 23.2

A woman delivered a 23-week preterm infant 3 days ago. She comes to see her baby infant each day, but refuses to touch the infant, in spite of frequent offers from the nurses.

Questions
1. What might explain her behavior?
2. How might the nurse help her?

Instituting Kangaroo Care

Parents need to feel they can contribute to the care their infants receive. One way to do this is KC. Begin KC as soon as possible, if the parents are interested. KC is a method of providing skin-to-skin contact between stable preterm infants and their parents.

During KC, the infant, wearing only a diaper and hat, is placed upright under the mother's clothes between her breasts. A blanket is placed over them both (Fig. 23.4). Mothers may breastfeed if they wish and if the infant is able. Fathers are encouraged to participate in KC (Fig. 23.5). The infant is monitored for changes in vital signs and behavior.

Explain the advantages of KC to parents, and elicit their participation. This method of care has been found safe for stable infants, even if intubated. It provides an opportunity for parents to participate in the infant's care and increases parental attachment. KC provides developmental care that is so important for the preterm infant. It is associated with stability of vital signs, increased weight gain, shorter length of stay, more quiet sleep, and less crying (Spruill, 2015). It also

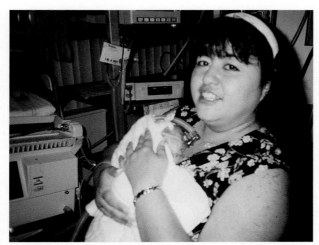

FIG 23.4 This mother has her 27-week-gestation preterm infant tucked under her clothes against her skin as she gives kangaroo care. Such care enhances bonding and has many other benefits for infants and parents.

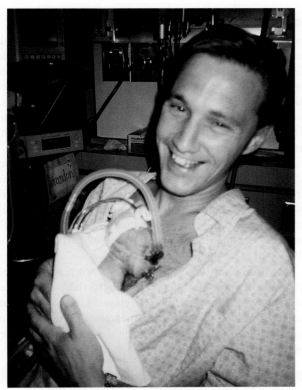

FIG 23.5 Even though he is intubated, this 1 lb, 8 oz preterm infant goes to sleep against his father's chest.

promotes thermoregulation and bonding, and it helps relieve pain (Hardy, 2011).

The upright position of the infant against the parent's chest makes breathing easier. The containment of the extremities decreases purposeless movements that use valuable oxygen and calories. Breastfeeding is facilitated, and the infant has more alert periods and increased deep sleep. The contact with the parent's skin maintains the infant's body temperature.

In addition, KC enhances early and long-term maternal–infant interaction and maternal confidence and competence (Gardner et al., 2016a).

KC also provides gentle stimulation. This includes tactile stimulation against the parent's skin, auditory stimulation as the infant listens to the parent's heartbeat and voice, and the vestibular stimulation of moving with the parent's breathing or rocking.

Provide privacy for parents interested in KC. Assist them, following facility protocol, in transferring the infant from the bed, managing the attachments, and making the infant comfortable. Also, check to see that they are comfortable. KC should last at least an hour to improve the infant's sleep (Hardy, 2011).

Facilitating Interaction

Preterm infants often have little facial expression and seldom make eye contact. Parents may feel rejected by the infant's lack of response or by negative responses during interactions. Explain that the interaction that is so effective with full-term infants may be too stimulating for very young or sick preterm infants. Suggest forms of touch and interaction based on the individual infant's capacity. Quiet holding may be better until the infant is able to tolerate more stimulation.

Help parents understand the infant's behavior and cues. Teach them signs of overstimulation to help them adapt their interaction to meet the infant's needs. Explain that these signs help protect the infant from overstimulation and show that the infant needs a quiet rest period without added stimulation. Discuss methods to avoid too much stimulation and to calm the infant. If several types of simultaneous stimulation (such as rocking, eye contact, and talking) cause signs of distress, suggest they stop one or more activities until the infant has had a rest period.

In learning to provide comfort care, parents may go through stages. At first they are afraid to touch the infant. They spend time just observing the infant before they feel comfortable enough to touch the infant. When they begin to participate in caregiving such as changing a diaper, their confidence grows. Parents become more confident in their ability to recognize when the infant is uncomfortable and their skill in comforting their infant (Skene, Franck, Curtis, & Gerrish, 2012).

Teach parents how to soothe infants when they show signs of stress. Explain containment and demonstrate how to do it. Placing the palm of the hand over the infant's chest or holding the infant's arms on the chest may help quiet the infant (Gardner et al., 2016a). Show the parents how to position the infant with the hands near the mouth so the infant can suck on them as a self-comforting measure. As the infant is ready for more interaction, suggest appropriate types of stimulation.

Point out small signs of improvement and even minor strengths. Talk about normal preterm characteristics and emphasize individual traits that make this infant different

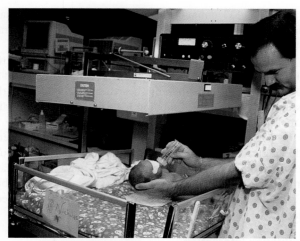

FIG 23.6 To promote family bonding with the infant, parents are involved as much as possible in the care of their infant. This father bottle feeds his infant who is in a radiant warmer.

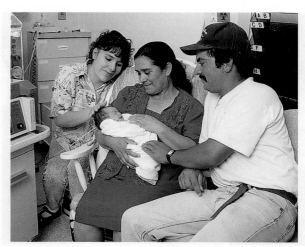

FIG 23.7 The parents look on while the grandmother holds the infant in the neonatal intensive care unit.

from all others. The way the infant eats, reacts to sounds, or seems to get tangled in the monitor leads may help parents feel closer to their newborn.

Involve the parents in care of the infant as soon as possible to help them gain a sense of control (Fig. 23.6). Plan to change the linens in the incubator or radiant warmer when the parents are there so they can hold their infant, even if for only a few moments. Save baths and other routine caregiving for times when parents can be present and participate. Taking an axillary temperature is something that a parent can be taught to do for even a critically ill infant that does not disturb the infant but fosters a feeling of contribution in the parent. As the infant's condition improves, parents can develop skill in caring for the tiny infant by changing diapers, feeding, and bathing.

In some NICUs, infants who are stable, who weigh more than 1000 g, and who do not need phototherapy, an umbilical catheter, or chest tubes are dressed in normal baby clothes. This helps them appear more normal to parents and assists in attachment. Parents use hospital-supplied clothing or bring their own and enjoy the opportunity to dress their infants (Bosque & Haverman, 2009).

Include other family members by allowing them to visit with the parents (Fig. 23.7). Being able to see the infant in the hospital setting allows family members to provide the parents with more realistic emotional support. Involve family members in learning how to feed and care for the infant if they will be helping the parents after discharge.

In some facilities, parents and, in some cases, grandparents are allowed to visit at any time of the day or night. They might be asked to leave during reporting or be invited to stay and participate to help them feel more a part of the infant's care.

Web cameras are used in some NICUs to allow parents to see their infants from their homes or from the hospital room. A web camera is placed over the infant's bed, and parents use a computer to access a secure website to see their infant. The camera may be on continuously or only on at certain times. Parents can share the website with family and friends so they

can see the infant as well. Families report being very satisfied with this opportunity (Rhoads, Green, Lewis, & Rakes, 2012).

Increasing Parental Decision Making

Parents should be considered an essential part of the health care team, rather than visitors. Give them the information they need to take an active part in decisions made about the infant's treatment plan (Thomson-Salo, 2015). This is true even for decisions that seem insignificant to the staff (Baker, 2009). This knowledge will increase their feelings of control over a situation in which many parents feel they have little power.

As parents get to know the infant better, they become experts on the infant's response to various situations and caregiving activities. Their expertise should be recognized and respectfully considered in planning infant care. Although parents often feel like outsiders when first visiting the NICU, they can, in time, move into the role of partners with the NICU staff in caring for the infant.

Look for opportunities to praise parenting abilities. Point out positive ways the infant responds to the parents' touch and caregiving. Model methods to respond to behavioral cues and acknowledge parents when they respond to the infant's signals appropriately. Listen to their ideas about what works best for the infant, and incorporate them if at all possible.

Alleviating Concerns

Invite parents to call the NICU at any time for information about their infant. This helps allay worry when parents wake up at night and wonder how the infant is doing. Phone calls are especially beneficial for parents unable to visit the infant because of distance or other reasons.

Parents also need support from others besides nursing staff. Put them in touch with parents of other preterm infants, and refer them to support groups, parent-to-parent groups with veteran NICU parents, telephone support, educational offerings, or counseling sessions. Tell them about Internet sources such as www.preemiecare.org and www.preemiepa rentalliance.org. Talking with others who have faced the same problems can be very comforting as parents compare notes and get practical suggestions from an experienced parent's point of view. Some agencies pair parents with a "buddy," who has had a similar experience and is from the same culture. Special programs may be available after discharge to provide parents with ongoing support and education. It is important to consider language and culture during this process.

Cultural practices should be incorporated into the care of the infant. Determine who in the family will make the decisions and who will be managing the infant's care. In some cultures, the father makes decisions, and the grandmother, rather than the mother, is the major caregiver. In these cases, it is essential that the right persons be included in appropriate teaching (Gardner et al., 2016b). In many cultures, the mother is expected to stay at home to recover after giving birth. This interferes with her ability to spend time in the NICU. Another family member may be enlisted to be with the infant in these cases (Moore, Moos, & Callister, 2010).

Helping with Ongoing Problems

Parents may be unprepared for the inconsistent progress infants often make after surviving the risks of the early days. They expect steady progress once the infant can breathe independently and take feedings. However, complications such as NEC or sepsis can cause major setbacks at this time. To cope with a new crisis, parents need extensive support from the nurse. Use therapeutic communication techniques such as reflecting feelings to help them express and cope with their extreme disappointment. Give information about the infant's changing condition and what to expect in the days ahead.

Having a hospitalized child can be exhausting for the parents. Remind them to take breaks away from the infant, whether to go to the cafeteria for a meal or to go home and rest. As the infant's condition improves, parents may take more time away as they begin to prepare for discharge. Encourage them to do this, while making sure they feel welcome to stay with the infant as much as they desire (Discenza, 2009).

Mothers with infants in a NICU may have problems with sleep disturbances and depressive symptoms. Be alert for signs of postpartum depression because fatigue and having an ill infant are factors that may lead to this condition (Gardner et al., 2016b). One study found a 20% rate of depression in mothers during the 18 months after their high-risk infants' discharge from a NICU (Northrup, Evans, & Stotts, 2013).

Preparing for Discharge

In the past, preterm infants often were discharged about the time of their expected birth. However, many infants now go home before their due date. It is important that the parents understand the expected hospital course.

Begin early to teach parents and other caregivers any special procedures, treatments, and medications that the infant will need after discharge. Observe the parents as they perform care until they are comfortable and can do it safely. Praise their efforts, and provide hints to make the care easier. Provide written information about home care of the preterm infant.

Help the parents learn what is normal for their infant and how to recognize and respond to abnormal signs. Some hospitals have the parents spend a night or two "rooming-in" in a special parent room, where they assume full 24-hour care of the infant and still have help when they need it. This helps increase parents' confidence that they can care for the infant by themselves. It also allows staff to evaluate the parents' abilities to care for the infant.

In one study, the parents reported that they felt more confident in activities such as recognizing changes in the infant's condition, giving medications, and working with cardiorespiratory monitoring when they were in the NICU than when they were home with the infant (Raines & Brustad, 2012). Help them practice more with these "medical" care activities so they know how to handle problems that might occur at home.

Help the parents determine what adaptations they will need to make at home before discharge. Utility companies should be notified if the infant is considered medically fragile to ensure the family receives priority service in case of a power failure. Provision for emergency electricity such as batteries also should be arranged. Organize home nursing services, purchase of supplies, and delivery of special equipment before discharge, if needed.

Discuss what to expect with regard to care of the infant after discharge. Infants may require oxygen, cardiorespiratory monitoring, suctioning, gavage or gastrostomy (tube) feedings, or other treatments that parents will have to learn to perform. Many infants need feedings every 3 hours, day and night, to help them gain weight adequately. Feedings may be time consuming, and parental fatigue resulting from sleep interruptions may be more than they expected, especially if they are parents of multiples.

Infants are accustomed to the noises of a nursery 24 hours a day and may not sleep well at first in a quiet home environment. Suggest parents play soft music and use a night light for the first week. They should gradually eliminate these aids to avoid conditioning the infant to their use. Visitors and noise or activity may be too much for the infant at first and should be limited.

Explore with parents what kind of help they might need to meet the everyday requirements of the infant and the rest of the family. Help them identify where they might find assistance from family and friends. Reassure them that friends and family often welcome opportunities to help.

The AAP and ACOG (2012) recommend the following in determining the time of discharge:

- Signs of readiness for discharge include a sustained pattern of weight gain, adequate maintenance of body temperature in an open bed, feeding without cardiorespiratory compromise, and stable cardiorespiratory function.
- Appropriate immunizations should have been given; car seat evaluation completed; metabolic screening performed; assessment of hearing, the eyes, hematologic status, and nutritional risks performed; and appropriate treatment plans completed before discharge.
- The family and home should have been evaluated. The family must have at least two members who demonstrate

the ability to feed and provide all needed care, perform cardiopulmonary resuscitation, give medications, operate equipment, and show understanding of signs of problems and what to do about them.

- A primary care physician and other appropriate follow-up care should have been arranged.

Help parents form realistic expectations about the infant. For example, they should know that the infant will accomplish developmental tasks such as crawling and walking later compared with full-term infants. Parents should base their expectations on the infant's **corrected age** (corrected or developmental age is the chronologic age minus the number of weeks the infant was born early) rather than on chronologic age.

Assist the parents in planning how to integrate the new infant into the family. Meeting the needs of their other children, in addition to the new responsibilities of caring for the preterm infant, is a major source of worry. Listen to their concerns about their other children, and encourage siblings who do not have infections to visit, if possible.

Help parents prepare siblings for what they will see and do when visiting. Siblings should touch or hold the infant, if possible, to help them bond. Taking photographs of the siblings with the infant will help them remember the visit.

Before discharge, a car seat challenge is often performed. Proper positioning with blanket rolls may be necessary because the infants may slump over, interfering with chest expansion. Some infants need car beds to allow them to ride in the recumbent position.

◆ Evaluation

Expected outcomes are met if parents visit often and interact appropriately with the infant, express their understanding of and comfort with the infant's needs, and take an increasingly active role in the care of the infant. Parents and designated caregivers should be able to independently provide care before discharge.

? CRITICAL THINKING EXERCISE 23.3

A preterm infant, born at 30 weeks gestation, was discharged from the hospital at 8 weeks of age. She was seen by the pediatrician at 48 hours after discharge and again at 2 weeks. At a well-baby checkup 6 weeks after discharge, her mother asks many questions about infant development. One question is when will her baby begin to roll over from her abdomen to the back. The nurse knows that most full-term infants reach this developmental milestone at 4 to 5 months of age.

Question
1. How should the nurse answer this mother?

? KNOWLEDGE CHECK

12. How can the nurse help parents be comfortable with their preterm infant?
13. How should the nurse prepare parents for the discharge of their preterm infant?

COMMON COMPLICATIONS OF PRETERM INFANTS

Complications of prematurity increase as the infant's gestational age and birth weight decrease. Some complications that occur in full-term and preterm infants, such as hyperbilirubinemia, are discussed in Chapter 24. Complications most often associated with preterm birth are discussed here. Further information about each condition can be found in pediatric texts.

Respiratory Distress Syndrome

Respiratory distress syndrome (RDS) is a condition caused by insufficient production of surfactant in the lungs. It occurs most often in preterm infants under 28 weeks of gestation and increases as the gestational age decreases. Other risk factors for RDS include birth asphyxia, cesarean birth, multiple births, male gender, cold stress, and maternal diabetes because these conditions interfere with surfactant production. It is less frequent, however, when antenatal corticosteroids or chronic fetal stress, such as in heroin addiction, maternal hypertension, or prolonged rupture of membranes, causes the lungs to mature more quickly (Carlo & Ambalavanan, 2016a).

Pathophysiology

Surfactant is a phospholipid that lines the alveoli. Surfactant decreases surface tension to allow the alveoli to remain open when air is exhaled. It must be continuously produced as it is used. Sufficient surfactant is usually produced beginning at 34 to 36 weeks of gestation to prevent RDS (Gardner et al., 2016d).

When too little surfactant is present, the alveoli collapse each time the infant exhales. The lungs become **noncompliant** or "stiff" and resist expansion. Noncompliant lungs require a much higher negative pressure for the alveoli to open with each inhalation. This results in severe retractions with each breath because the chest wall is very compliant. The weak muscles of the chest are drawn inward, placing pressure on the lungs that further interferes with expansion. Seesaw respirations also may occur.

As fewer alveoli expand, atelectasis, hypoxia, and hypercapnia occur. This causes pulmonary vasoconstriction and decreased blood flow to the lungs because of the high resistance within the pulmonary blood vessels. Persistent pulmonary hypertension can result in a return to fetal circulation patterns, with opening of the ductus arteriosus. Acidosis and alveolar ischemic injury further complicate the condition by interfering with surfactant synthesis.

Tests of amniotic fluid can detect lecithin, sphingomyelin, phosphatidylglycerol, and phosphatidylinositol, which are components of surfactant. These tests can predict whether the fetal lungs are mature enough for survival outside of the uterus. They are done before an elective induction or cesarean birth is performed on an infant younger than 38 weeks of gestation. The incidence and severity of RDS may be reduced by giving the mother corticosteroids before birth.

Manifestations

Signs of RDS begin during the first hours after birth. They include tachypnea, tachycardia, nasal flaring, and cyanosis. Retractions of accessory muscles are common. They may be above or below the sternum and/or between or below the ribs. Audible grunting on expiration is characteristic. It results from air moving past a partially closed glottis, which helps maintain lung expansion; gas exchange during exhalation; and functional residual capacity. Breath sounds may be decreased, and crackles may be present.

Acidosis develops as a result of hypoxemia. Blood gases show increased carbon dioxide levels and decreased oxygen levels. Chest radiographs show the "ground glass" reticulogranular appearance of the lungs that is characteristic of RDS. Areas of atelectasis are present. Signs become worse, peak within 3 days, and then begin to improve gradually (Carlo & Ambalavanan, 2016a).

Therapeutic Management

Surfactant is instilled into the infant's trachea shortly after birth or as soon as signs of RDS become apparent. Doses are repeated, if necessary. Infants treated with surfactant have higher survival rates, although the incidence of other complications of prematurity such as bronchopulmonary dysplasia (BPD) is unchanged (Carlo & Ambalavanan, 2016a; Gardner et al., 2016d).

Other treatment is supportive, including oxygen, continuous CPAP or mechanical ventilation, inhaled nitric oxide, correction of acidosis, IV fluids, and care of other complications. Antibiotics may be given because signs of neonatal pneumonia are similar to those of RDS (Wambach & Hamvas, 2015). Low temperature and low glucose level may occur and should be treated promptly.

Nursing Considerations

The nurse observes for signs of developing RDS at birth and during the early hours after birth. Changes in the infant's condition are constantly assessed. Changes in ventilator settings may be necessary as the infant's ability to oxygenate increases. Observation for signs of common complications such as patent ductus arteriosus and BPD is important. The nurse should monitor the results of laboratory tests for abnormalities in blood gases and acid-base balance. Early signs of sepsis should be identified and reported. Other care is similar to general care for the preterm infant.

Bronchopulmonary Dysplasia (Chronic Lung Disease)

Bronchopulmonary dysplasia (BPD), also known as *chronic lung disease,* is a chronic condition in which damage to the infant's lungs requires prolonged dependence on supplemental oxygen. It occurs most often in infants younger than 32 weeks of gestational age and in one-third of VLBW infants. The diagnostic criteria for BPD include gestational age, the length of time on oxygen, and the amount of oxygen needed. The common definition of BPD is when an infant requires oxygen 28 days after birth (Bancalari & Walsh, 2017).

Pathophysiology

BPD results from a combination of factors such as mechanical ventilation, high levels of oxygen, a symptomatic PDA, and infections that injure bronchial epithelium and interfere with alveolar development. The result is inflammation, atelectasis, edema, and airway hyperreactivity with loss of cilia, thickening of the walls of the alveoli, and fibrotic changes (Bancalari & Jain, 2017).

Manifestations

The major sign of BPD is an increased need for or an inability to be weaned from respiratory support and oxygen. Other signs include tachycardia, tachypnea, retractions, crackles, wheezing, respiratory acidosis, cyanosis, increased secretions, bronchospasm, and characteristic changes in the lungs on chest radiographs. Pulmonary edema may occur (Gardner et al., 2016d).

Therapeutic Management

Prevention includes use of maternal steroids to reduce prematurity and RDS, minimizing exposure to oxygen and pressure with ventilation as much as possible, avoidance of fluid overload, and increased nutrition. Treatment is supportive, with antibiotics and bronchodilators as necessary, and gradual decreases in the amount of oxygen. Diuretics are given and fluids are restricted because infants are prone to fluid overload. Increased calories and protein are important. The infant may be discharged home with long-term oxygen therapy, and some need frequent rehospitalization during the first 2 years of life because of respiratory tract infections.

Intraventricular Hemorrhage

Intraventricular hemorrhage (IVH) is also called *germinal matrix hemorrhage* and *periventricular-intraventricular hemorrhage.* It is bleeding into and around the ventricles of the brain. Approximately 30% of preterm infants weighing less than 1500 g (3 lb 5 oz) develop intraventricular hemorrhage (Carlo & Ambalavanan, 2016b). The first few days of life are the most common times for hemorrhage to occur. It may also occur in approximately 3.5% of term infants (Parsons, Seay, & Jacobson, 2016).

Pathophysiology

IVH results from rupture of the fragile blood vessels in the germinal matrix, located around the ventricles of the brain. It is associated with increased or decreased blood pressure, asphyxia or respiratory distress requiring mechanical ventilation, and increased or fluctuating cerebral blood flow. Rapid blood volume expansion, hypercarbia, anemia, and hypoglycemia are other causes.

Hemorrhage is graded 1 through 4, according to the amount of bleeding. Grade 1 is a very small bleed at the germinal matrix. Grade 2 hemorrhage extends into the lateral ventricles without distention, and grade 3 causes distention of ventricles. Grade 4 hemorrhage causes ventricular dilation and extends into surrounding brain tissue. The condition is diagnosed by cranial ultrasound through the anterior fontanel.

Manifestations

Signs of IVH are determined by the severity of the hemorrhage. They may be subtle or remarkable, including lethargy, poor muscle tone, bradycardia, deterioration of respiratory status with cyanosis or apnea, drop in hematocrit, acidosis, hyperglycemia, tense fontanel, and seizures.

Therapeutic Management

Most hemorrhages take place in the first week. Ultrasonography performed at 7 days of age for preterm infants at risk for IVH shows 90% of hemorrhages (de Vries, 2015). If bleeding is found, serial ultrasonography may be performed to determine progression of the problem.

Treatment is supportive and focuses on maintaining respiratory function and dealing with other complications. Outcomes vary depending on the severity of the hemorrhage. Of preterm infants with an IVH, 50% have no neurologic complications (Verklan, 2015). Hydrocephalus may develop from blockage of cerebrospinal fluid flow. A ventriculoperitoneal shunt (catheter leading from the ventricles of the brain to the peritoneal cavity) may be necessary to drain the fluid.

Nursing Considerations

Many aspects of care may increase cerebral blood flow and blood pressure. These include mechanical ventilation, suctioning, and excessive handling. Even crying and changing diapers may produce changes in cerebral blood flow. Therefore the nurse should avoid situations that may increase the risk for IVH as much as possible. Handling is kept to a minimum, and pain and environmental stressors are reduced as much as possible. Developmental care has been found helpful. Nurses are alert for early signs of IVH. Nursing care includes daily measurement of the head circumference and observation for changes in neurologic status, which may be subtle.

Parents need assistance to cope with the diagnosis and their concerns regarding long-term implications. They should learn how to assess for signs of increasing intracranial pressure if their infant has IVH-induced hydrocephalus and understand that follow-up care may include periodic ultrasound examinations.

Retinopathy of Prematurity

Retinopathy of prematurity (ROP) is a condition in which injury to the blood vessels in the eye leads to growth of new blood vessels that abnormally develop and may result in visual impairment or blindness in preterm infants. It occurs in up to 67% of infants weighing 1250 g (2 lb. 12 oz) or less (Fraser & Diehl-Jones, 2015).

Pathophysiology

The exact cause of ROP is unknown, but high levels of oxygen in the blood are a risk factor. However, ROP develops in some infants who have never received supplementary oxygen. Prolonged ventilation, acidosis, sepsis, shock, IVH, and fluctuating blood oxygen levels have been associated with ROP (AAP & ACOG, 2012; Pollan, 2009).

In ROP, immature blood vessels in the eye are injured. After a period, new vessels proliferate, extending throughout the retina and into the vitreous humor of the eye in some infants. Fluid leakage and hemorrhages from the fragile vessels may cause scarring, traction on the retina, and retinal detachment. However, the progress of pathologic processes stops in more than 90% of infants and there is little visual loss (Olitsky, Hug, Plummer et al., 2016).

Therapeutic Management

Infants with a birth weight of 1500 g (3 lb. 5 oz) or less or gestational age of 32 weeks or less and selected infants with a birth weight of 1500 to 2000 g (4 lb 6.6 oz) or gestational age of more than 32 weeks with an unstable clinical course should be screened to detect changes of the eye. The frequency of repeat examinations is determined by the results of screenings.

Laser surgery to destroy abnormal blood vessels is the current treatment of choice. Intravitreal bevacizumab has been used in some cases and will have more study to determine its use in the future. Cryosurgery or reattachment of the retina also may be necessary (Olitsky et al., 2016).

Nursing Considerations

The nurse should check the pulse oximetry readings frequently for any infant receiving oxygen. Oxygen should be titrated to keep oxygen saturation levels within prescribed limits. Extremes of high or low saturations should be avoided. Parents should be informed about ophthalmologic tests and receive an explanation of the results. Eye examinations can be very stressful to the infant, and swaddling and rest periods should be provided as appropriate. Mydriatic eye drops given to dilate the eyes may cause hypertension, bradycardia, and apnea (Fraser & Diehl-Jones, 2015). If surgery is performed, the eye is assessed for drainage. Ice packs may be used for edema, and pain medication should be given. Support for parents is essential throughout the examinations and especially if damage to the eye is found.

Necrotizing Enterocolitis

Necrotizing enterocolitis (NEC) is a serious inflammatory condition of the intestinal tract that may lead to cellular death of areas of intestinal mucosa. It occurs in 1% to 5% of infants admitted to NICUs (Greenberg et al., 2014). The mortality rate is approximately 40%, and survivors may have long-term GI problems (Caplan, 2015). The ileum and proximal colon are the areas most often affected.

Pathophysiology

Although the exact causes are unknown, immaturity of the intestines is a major factor in preterm infants. The rate of NEC increases with decreasing gestational age. Previous hypoxia of the intestines may be a causative factor. The incidence of NEC is much higher after infants have received feedings.

Although minimal enteric feedings are thought to increase maturation of the intestines, feedings that are too early or increased too fast may cause NEC. When infants are fed, bacteria proliferate, and gas-forming organisms may invade the intestinal wall in some infants. Eventually, necrosis, perforation, and peritonitis may occur. Breast milk, which contains immunoglobulins, leukocytes, and antibacterial agents, may have a preventive effect on the development of NEC. Studies about using prenatal steroids to prevent NEC are mixed, with some showing less and others showing greater incidence (Gephart, McGrath, Efken, & Halpern, 2012).

Manifestations

Signs include increased abdominal girth caused by distention, increased gastric residuals, decreased or absent bowel sounds, loops of bowel seen through the abdominal wall, vomiting, bile-stained residuals or emesis, abdominal tenderness and discoloration, signs of infection, and occult blood in the stools. Respiratory difficulty may occur because of pressure from the distended abdomen on the diaphragm. Apnea, bradycardia, temperature instability, lethargy, hypotension, and shock also may be present. On radiographs, there may be loops of bowel dilated with air. The presence of air within the intestinal wall is characteristic of the condition. Free air in the peritoneum indicates that perforation has occurred, although perforation may occur without this sign.

Therapeutic Management

An increasing number of studies are showing encouraging results using probiotics as a means of establishing normal intestinal flora and preventing NEC (Caplan, 2015). Mothers should be encouraged to breastfeed, especially if the infant has risk factors for NEC. If maternal breast milk is not available, donor milk can be used.

Treatment of NEC includes antibiotics, discontinuation of oral feedings, continuous or intermittent gastric suction, and use of parenteral nutrition to rest the intestines. Surgery may be necessary if perforation or continued lack of improvement occurs. The necrotic area is removed, and an ostomy may be performed. Infants who have had large areas of bowel removed may develop short-bowel syndrome with malabsorption and malnutrition.

Nursing Considerations

Nurses should encourage interested mothers to provide breast milk for their infants because NEC is less likely to occur in breastfed infants. Early recognition of signs of NEC is essential to decrease mortality. Because nurses are constantly observing the infant, they often are able to detect the early, subtle signs that lead to prompt diagnosis. If one or more signs are noted, the nurse withholds the next feeding and notifies the provider.

Abdominal girth is measured, and IV fluids and parenteral nutrition must be managed. Intake and output are important because third-space fluid loss occurs when fluid moves from the intravascular spaces to the extracellular spaces. The infant should be positioned on the side to minimize the effects of pressure on the diaphragm from the distended intestines. During recovery, the nurse must should observe for signs of feeding intolerance when feedings are resumed. Scar tissue may cause partial or complete bowel obstruction.

Short Bowel Syndrome

Short bowel syndrome (SBS) is a condition caused by a bowel that is shorter than normal. It is caused by congenital malformations of the GI tract or surgical resection that decreases the length of the small intestines.

Pathophysiology

When the bowel is too short, decreased mucosal surface area causes inadequate absorption of fluids, electrolytes, and nutrients. A loss of more than 50% of the small bowel may result in symptoms of generalized malabsorption or deficiencies of certain nutrients related to the region of bowel that has been removed (Branski, 2016).

Manifestations

The most common symptoms of SBS are malabsorption, diarrhea, and failure to thrive. If the small bowel is 40 cm or more, the malabsorption may improve in time because the remaining bowel continues to grow and adapt in function.

Therapeutic Management

During surgery, every effort is made to preserve as much of the small bowel length as possible. After surgery, the child's fluid and electrolyte balance must be restored and stabilized. The mainstay of treatment for infants and children is nutritional support.

TPN is begun as the primary source of nutrition. It is formulated to meet the child's nutritional needs as well as promote weight gain and growth. Enteral nutrition is begun as soon as possible after surgery to allow the intestines to adapt to food.

Nursing Considerations

The nurse manages the infant's TPN and enteral feedings. TPN is generally infused through a central venous access device. Strict asepsis should be used when performing central line dressing changes and when administering TPN to prevent central line–associated bloodstream infections. Enteral nutrition is advanced slowly while corresponding adjustments are made to the composition of the TPN. The nurse carefully assesses and documents tolerance of enteral feedings noting any signs of dehydration, electrolyte imbalances, and nutritional deficits. Nonnutritive sucking is provided as well.

POSTTERM INFANTS

Postterm infants are those who are born after the 42nd week of gestation. Their longer-than-normal gestation places them at risk for a number of complications.

Scope of the Problem

Less than 10% of all pregnancies are considered postterm (Rampersand & Macones, 2017). In some cases, the fetus continues to be well supported by the placenta and is of normal size or is large for gestational age. Some grow to more than 4000 g (8 lb, 13 oz), placing them at risk for birth injuries or cesarean birth.

In other cases, placental functioning decreases when pregnancy is prolonged. If placental insufficiency is present, decreased amniotic fluid volume (oligohydramnios) and compression of the umbilical cord may occur. The fetus may not receive the appropriate amount of oxygen and nutrients and may be small for gestational age. This condition results in hypoxia and malnourishment in the fetus and is called **postmaturity syndrome** or *dysmaturity syndrome*. Postmaturity syndrome occurs in about 20% of postterm pregnancies (Rampersand & Macones, 2017).

When labor begins, poor oxygen reserves may cause fetal compromise. The fetus may pass meconium as a result of hypoxia before or during labor, increasing the risk for meconium aspiration at delivery (see Chapter 24). These infants are also at higher risk for asphyxia than are other infants. Postterm infants have a higher perinatal mortality rate than infants born at term.

Assessment

Most infants will be normal at birth. If the infant is large, the nurse should observe for injury and hypoglycemia. The infant with postmaturity syndrome may have an apprehensive look associated with hypoxia (Hardy, D'Agata, & McGrath, 2016). The infant may be thin with loose skin and little subcutaneous fat. The umbilical cord is thin with little Wharton's jelly. There is little or no vernix caseosa, but the infant generally has abundant hair on the head and long nails. The skin is wrinkled, cracked, and peeling (Fig. 23.8). If meconium was present in the amniotic fluid, the cord, skin, and nails may be stained yellow green, indicating that meconium was present for some time.

Postterm infants should be assessed for hypoglycemia because of rapid use of glycogen stores. If loss of subcutaneous fat has occurred, the infant is at risk for low temperature.

Therapeutic Management

Therapeutic management focuses on prevention and symptomatic treatment. Expectant mothers who are "overdue" are scheduled for tests of placental functioning, and labor is induced if signs of placental deterioration are discovered during fetal diagnostic testing. If the fetus cannot tolerate labor, a cesarean birth is necessary. Apgar scores less than 7 are more likely in postterm infants. In cases of asphyxia or meconium aspiration, respiratory support is needed at birth (see Chapter 24).

Nursing Considerations

The nurse's role is primarily one of prevention of complications, where possible, and monitoring of changes in status. During labor and delivery, the nurse responds appropriately to fetal heart rate decelerations, prepares for and assists in emergency delivery, and cares for respiratory problems at birth.

Signs of postmaturity syndrome in infants are noted during the initial assessment. Respiratory problems may necessitate continued assessment and care. Infants with any indications of postmaturity should be tested for hypoglycemia soon after birth and again an hour later or according to hospital policy. They need early and more frequent feedings to help compensate for the period of poor nutrition before birth.

Temperature regulation may be poor because fat stores were used for nourishment in utero. Providing extra blankets, assessing temperature frequently, and teaching parents about prevention of cold stress are important throughout the hospital stay. Polycythemia, resulting from hypoxia before birth, increases the risk for hyperbilirubinemia.

SMALL-FOR-GESTATIONAL-AGE INFANTS

Small-for-gestational-age (SGA) infants are those who fall below the tenth percentile in size on growth charts. They have failed to grow in the uterus as expected and have FGR. Some infants who do not meet the definition for SGA may have FGR and fail to grow to full potential before birth for a variety of reasons. However, the terms SGA and FGR often are used interchangeably.

SGA infants may be preterm, full-term, or postterm. Infant mortality and morbidity increase steadily as growth restriction increases. Approximately one-third of all LBW infants are SGA (Resnik & Creasy, 2014).

Causes

Many risk factors may cause an infant to be SGA. Congenital malformations, chromosomal anomalies, genetic factors, multiple gestations, and fetal infections such as rubella or cytomegalovirus may cause FGR. Poor placental function resulting from aging of the placenta, small size, separation, or malformation may interfere with fetal growth. Illness in the expectant mother, such as preeclampsia or severe diabetes, restricts uteroplacental blood flow and decreases fetal growth. Smoking, drug or alcohol abuse, and severe maternal malnutrition also impair fetal growth.

Scope of the Problem

Infants affected with FGR have higher perinatal morbidity and a mortality rate that is 10 to 20 times that of infants who are not growth restricted (Calkins & Devaskar, 2015). Death may occur from asphyxia before or during labor because of poor placental functioning or from complications of congenital anomalies or prematurity.

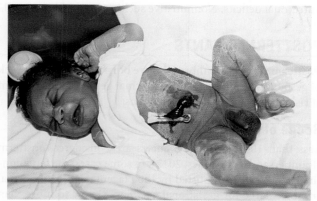

FIG 23.8 The postmature infant has no vernix and dry, cracked, peeling skin.

Full-term SGA infants are subject to many of the same complications as those who are preterm or postterm. Problems tend to be greatest in infants who are preterm in addition to being SGA.

Low Apgar scores, meconium aspiration, and polycythemia are increased in the SGA infant. Hypoglycemia is common because of inadequate storage of glycogen in the liver. Although mature muscle tone enables the SGA infant to maintain better flexion than the preterm infant, SGA infants are prone to inadequate thermoregulation because subcutaneous white fat and brown fat stores have been used to survive in utero. If hypoglycemia develops, inadequate glucose is available for increased metabolism to produce heat, increasing the problem.

Characteristics of Small-for-Gestational-Age Infants

The appearance of the SGA infant varies, depending on whether the cause of growth restriction began early or late in the pregnancy. Variation occurs because growth restriction affects the weight first. If it continues, the length and then the head size eventually will be affected.

Symmetric growth restriction involves the entire body. It may be caused by congenital anomalies, genetic disorders, exposure to infections or drugs early in pregnancy, or normal genetic predisposition. Although the infant's weight, length, and head circumference are all below the 10th percentile, the body is proportionate and appears normally developed for size. The total number of cells as well as the cell size are decreased, and the infant may have long-term complications. These infants are often small throughout their lives. They have a higher rate of neonatal mortality. Approximately 20% to 30% of SGA infants have symmetric growth restriction (Calkins & Devaskar, 2015).

Asymmetric growth restriction is caused by complications such as preeclampsia that begin in the third trimester and interfere with uteroplacental function. In asymmetric restriction, the head is normal in size but seems large for the rest of the body. Brain growth and heart size are normal. The length is normal, but the weight is below the 10th percentile for gestational age. The abdominal circumference is decreased because the liver, spleen, and adrenals are smaller than normal (Calkins & Devaskar, 2015).

The infant appears long, thin, and wasted. The dry, loose skin has longitudinal thigh creases from loss of subcutaneous fat. The infant has a sunken abdomen, sparse hair, a thin cord, and the facial appearance of being elderly. The anterior fontanel may be large with wide or overlapping cranial sutures. These infants generally "catch up" in growth, particularly in the first 2 years, if they are adequately nourished after birth (Mandy, 2016).

Therapeutic Management

Therapeutic management is focused on prevention, with good prenatal care to identify and treat problems early. When growth restriction cannot be prevented, ultrasound examination may permit early discovery of the condition. Serial nonstress tests and biophysical profiles help determine whether the infant should be delivered early, and preparation can be made for the expected complications at birth. Problems during and after birth are treated as they occur. They may include asphyxia, meconium aspiration, hypoglycemia, and polycythemia (Calkins & Devaskar, 2015). SGA infants have a greater surface area and higher metabolic rate than infants who are appropriate for gestational age. This increases their risk for problems with temperature stability (Gardner & Hernandez, 2016).

Nursing Considerations

Because the causes of growth restriction are so varied, care of the SGA infant should be adapted to meet the specific problems presented. When signs of growth restriction are present, the nurse should observe for complications that commonly accompany it. The general appearance and measurements give an indication of the type of growth restriction that has occurred. Measurements of the head, chest, length, and weight are below normal in the infant with symmetric growth restriction. If the restriction is asymmetric, the head circumference and length are normal, but the abdominal circumference and weight are low.

The nurse should assess for hypoglycemia, especially in asymmetric, growth-restricted infants. The brain of the infant is normal and needs large amounts of glucose, but the liver is small and has inadequate stores of glycogen. Caloric needs are greater than for a normal infant, making early and more frequent feedings important. Temperature regulation and respiratory support are additional nursing concerns. Observation for jaundice is important in infants with polycythemia because a large amount of bilirubin may be released when the red blood cells break down.

LARGE-FOR-GESTATIONAL-AGE INFANTS

Large-for-gestational-age (LGA) infants are those who are above the 90th percentile for gestational age on intrauterine growth charts. They may have **macrosomia** (weigh more than 4000 to 4500 g [8 lb, 13 oz to 9 lb, 15 oz]) and are usually born at term, although they may be preterm or postterm. The preterm LGA infant may be mistaken for a full-term infant but has the same problems as other preterm infants.

Causes

Infants who are LGA may be born to multiparas, large parents, mothers who are obese, and members of certain ethnic groups (Asian, Black, and Hispanic [Tutlam, Liu, Nelson, Flick & Chang, 2017]). Diabetes in the mother also may cause increased size, as may erythroblastosis fetalis (see Chapter 24).

Scope of the Problem

The LGA infant is more likely to go through a longer labor, suffer injury during birth, or need a cesarean birth. Shoulder dystocia may occur because the shoulders are too large to fit through the pelvis. Fractures of the clavicle or skull, injury to the brachial plexus or the facial nerve, cephalhematoma, subdural hematoma, and bruising occur more often in these infants than those of normal size. Congenital heart defects and a higher mortality rate also are more common (Carlo, 2016b).

Therapeutic Management

Therapeutic management is based on identification of increased size during pregnancy by measurements of fundal height and ultrasound examination. Delivery problems may lead to use of vacuum extraction, forceps, or cesarean birth. Birth injuries and complications are treated as they arise.

Nursing Considerations

The nurse assists in a difficult delivery or cesarean birth resulting from dystocia when the infant is LGA. After birth the infant is carefully assessed for injuries or other complications such as hypoglycemia or polycythemia (Chapter 24). Nursing care is geared to the problems presented.

❓ KNOWLEDGE CHECK

14. What is the typical appearance of the infant with postmaturity syndrome?
15. What special problems might a postmature infant have?
16. How are symmetric and asymmetric FGR different?
17. What problems may occur in infants who are LGA?

SUMMARY CONCEPTS

- Late preterm infants, born between 34 $^{0/7}$ and 36 $^{6/7}$ weeks, are at risk for respiratory, thermoregulation, and feeding problems, as well as hypoglycemia, hyperbilirubinemia, acidosis, and sepsis.
- Preterm infants differ in appearance from full-term infants. Some differences include small size, limp posture, red skin, abundant vernix and lanugo, and immature ears and genitals.
- The lungs of preterm infants may lack adequate surfactant, which interferes with expansion of the lungs, increasing the amount of energy necessary for breathing and leading to atelectasis.
- Other factors that may increase respiratory problems are poor cough reflex, narrow respiratory passages, and weak muscles.
- The prone position is used for preterm infants because it decreases breathing effort and increases oxygenation.
- Preterm infants are subject to cold stress because they have thin skin with blood vessels near the surface, little subcutaneous white fat or brown fat, a large surface area, a limp position, and an immature temperature control center.
- Maintaining a neutral thermal environment at all times for infants is important. The nurse should prevent drafts, use warmed oxygen, and keep incubator doors and portholes closed. When taken out of heating devices, the infant should be wrapped in warmed blankets and should wear a hat.
- Preterm infants are subject to increased insensible water losses and have difficulty maintaining fluid balance. Their kidneys do not concentrate or dilute urine as well as those of full-term infants. Intake and output should be carefully measured.
- The fragile skin of a preterm infant is easily damaged. Adhesives or chemicals that could injure the skin should be avoided. Special products designed to prevent injury to the skin should be used.
- Preterm infants are subject to infections because they lack passive antibodies from the mother, have an immature immune system, have fragile skin, and are subjected to many invasive procedures.
- The nurse should watch carefully for signs of pain and use comfort measures, containment, pacifiers, sucrose, breastfeeding, kangaroo care, and medications to alleviate it.
- Infants demonstrate they are receiving too much stimulation by changes in oxygenation and behavior. The nurse should schedule care to allow rest periods, keep noise to a minimum, and teach parents how to interact with the infant appropriately.
- Preterm infants lack nutrient stores and need more nutrients but do not absorb them well. They lack coordination in sucking and swallowing and become fatigued easily.
- Signs indicating an infant may be ready for nipple feeding include rooting, sucking on a gavage catheter or pacifier, presence of gag reflex, and respiratory rate less than 60 breaths per minute.
- The nurse should teach mothers who wish to breastfeed their preterm infants how to use a breast pump and store breast milk. Nurses provide privacy, give support and encouragement, explain the infant's behavior, and answer questions about breastfeeding.
- Nurses can increase parents' comfort with their preterm infant by providing information about the infant's condition and characteristics, the neonatal intensive care unit, equipment, and infant care. Spending time with parents during visits, offering therapeutic communication and realistic encouragement, and involving parents in care of the infant also help with bonding.
- Preparation for discharge should be started early in the infant's hospital stay. This allows parents to learn gradually and assume increasing responsibility in the care of the infant until they are comfortable with complete care.
- Common complications of preterm birth are respiratory distress syndrome, bronchopulmonary dysplasia, intraventricular hemorrhage, retinopathy of prematurity, necrotizing enterocolitis, and short bowel syndrome.
- Infants with postmaturity syndrome may appear thin, with loose skin folds, cracked and peeling skin, and meconium staining. They may have respiratory difficulties at birth and suffer from hypoglycemia and inadequate temperature regulation.
- Infants with fetal growth restriction may be small for gestational age at birth. In symmetric growth restriction, the infant is proportionately small; in asymmetric growth restriction, the head and length are normal and the body is thin.
- Large-for-gestational-age infants may have birth injuries such as fractures, nerve damage, or bruising as a result of their size. They may have hypoglycemia or polycythemia.

REFERENCES & READINGS

Aagaard, H., Uhrenfeldt, L., Spliid, M., & Fegran, L. (2015). Parents' experiences of transition when their infants are discharged from the Neonatal Intensive Care Unit: A systematic review protocol. *JBI Database of Systematic Reviews and Implementation Reports*, *13*(10), 123–132.

Academy of Breastfeeding Medicine (ABM) Protocol Committee. (2010). ABM clinical protocol #23: Non-pharmacologic management of procedure-related pain in the breastfeeding infant. *Breastfeeding Medicine*, *5*(6), 315–319.

Almadhoob, A., & Ohlsson, A. (2015). Sound reduction management in the neonatal intensive care unit for preterm or very low birth weight infants. *The Cochrane Library of Systematic Reviews* (1), CD010333.

American Academy of Pediatrics (AAP). (2012). Policy statement: Breastfeeding and the use of human milk. *Pediatrics*, *129*(3), e827–e841 Reaffirmed 2015.

American Academy of Pediatrics (AAP) & American College of Obstetricians and Gynecologists (ACOG). (2012). *Guidelines for perinatal care* (7th ed.). Elk Grove Village, IL, and Washington, DC: Authors.

Association of Women's Health, Obstetric and Neonatal Nurses (AWHONN). (2013a). *Neonatal skin care: Evidence based clinical practice guideline* (3rd ed.). Washington, DC: Author.

Association of Women's Health, Obstetric, and Neonatal Nurses (AWHONN). (2013b). *Women's health and perinatal nursing care quality draft measures specifications*. Washington, DC: Author.

Association of Women's Health, Obstetric and Neonatal Nurses (AWHONN). (2014). *Assessment and care of the late preterm infant: Evidence-based clinical practice guideline*. Washington, DC: Author.

Baker, B. (2009). Supporting the maternal experience in the neonatal NICU. *Newborn and Infant Nursing Reviews*, *9*(2), 81–82.

Bancalari, E. H., & Jain, D. (2017). Pathophysiology of bronchopulmonary distress syndrome. In R. A. Polin, S. H. Abman, D. H. Rowitch, & W. E. Benitz (Eds.), *Fetal and neonatal physiology* (5th ed.) (pp. 273–280). Philadelphia, PA: Elsevier.

Bancalari, E. H., & Walsh, M. C. (2017). Bronchopulmonary dysplasia in the neonate. In R. J. Martin, A. A. Fanaroff, & M. C. Walsh (Eds.), *Fanaroff and Martin's neonatal-perinatal medicine: Diseases of the fetus and infant* (10th ed.) (pp. 1157–1169). Philadelphia, PA: Saunders.

Barkemeyer, B. M. (2015). Discharge planning. *Pediatric Clinics of North America*, *62*(2), 545–556.

Black, A. (2012). Breastfeeding the premature infant and nursing implications. *Advances in Neonatal Care*, *12*(1), 10–14.

Blackburn, S. T. (2013). Renal systems and fluid and electrolyte homeostasis. In *Maternal, fetal and neonatal physiology: A clinical perspective* (4th ed.) (pp. 356–392). St. Louis, MO: Saunders.

Bosque, E. M., & Haverman, C. (2009). Making babies real: Dressing infants in the NICU. *Neonatal Network*, *28*(2), 85–92.

Brand, M. C., & Boyd, H. A. (2015). Thermoregulation. In M. T. Verklan & M. Walden (Eds.), *Core curriculum for neonatal intensive care nursing* (5th ed.) (pp. 95–109). St. Louis, MO: Saunders.

Branski, D. (2016). Disorders of malabsorption. In R. Kliegman, B. Stanton, J. St. Geme, & N. Schor (Eds.), *Nelson textbook of pediatrics* (20th ed.) (pp. 1831–1850). Philadelphia, PA: Elsevier.

Brown, L. D., Hendrickson, K., Evans, R., Davis, J., Anderson, M. S., & Hay, W. W. (2016). Enteral nutrition. In S. L. Gardner, B. S. Carter, M. Enzman-Hines, et al. (Eds.), *Merenstein & Gardner's handbook of neonatal intensive care* (8th ed.) (pp. 377–418). St. Louis, MO: Elsevier.

Calkins, K. L., & Devaskar, S. U. (2015). Intrauterine growth restriction. In R. J. Martin, A. A. Fanaroff, & M. C. Walsh (Eds.), *Fanaroff and Martin's neonatal-perinatal medicine: Diseases of the fetus and infant* (10th ed.) (pp. 227–235). St. Louis, MO: Elsevier.

Campbell-Yeo, M., Fernandes, A., & Johnston, C. (2011). Procedural pain management for neonates using nonpharmacological strategies. Part 2: Mother-driven interventions. *Advances in Neonatal Care*, *11*(5), 312–318.

Caplan, M. S. (2015). Neonatal necrotizing enterocolitis. In R. J. Martin, A. A. Fanaroff, & M. C. Walsh (Eds.), *Fanaroff and Martin's neonatal-perinatal medicine: Diseases of the fetus and infant* (10th ed.) (pp. 1423–1432). St. Louis, MO: Saunders.

Carlo, W. A. (2016). The high-risk infant. In R. M. Kliegman, B. E. Stanton, J. W. St. Geme, & N. Schor (Eds.), *Nelson textbook of pediatrics* (20th ed.) (pp. 818–831). Philadelphia, PA: Elsevier.

Carlo, W. A., & Ambalavanan, N. (2016ba). Nervous system disorders. In R. M. Kliegman, B. E. Stanton, J. W. St. Geme, & N. Schor (Eds.), *Nelson textbook of pediatrics* (20th ed.) (pp. 834–844). Philadelphia, PA: Elsevier.

Carlo, W. A., & Ambalavanan, N. (2016ba). Respiratory tract disorders. In R. M. Kliegman, B. E. Stanton, J. W. St. Geme, & N. Schor (Eds.), *Nelson textbook of pediatrics* (20th ed.) (pp. 848–867). Philadelphia, PA: Elsevier.

Cleveland, K. (2010). Feeding challenges in the late preterm infant. *Neonatal Network*, *29*(1), 37–41.

Cleveland, L. M., & Horner, S. D. (2012). Normative cultural values and the experiences of Mexican-American mothers in the neonatal intensive care unit. *Advances in Neonatal Care*, *12*(2), 120–125.

Coffman, S. (2009). Late preterm infants and risk for RSV. *MCN: The American Journal of Maternal/Child Nursing*, *34*(6), 378–384.

Cooper, B. M., Holditch-Davis, D., Verklan, M. T., Fraser-Askin, D., Lamp, J., Santa-Donato, A., Bingham, D. (2012). Newborn clinical outcomes of the AHWONN infant research-based practice project. *Journal of Obstetric, Gynecologic, & Neonatal Nursing*, *41*(6), 774–785.

Cosimano, A., & Sandhurst, H. (2011). Strategies for successful breastfeeding in the NICU. *Neonatal Network*, *30*(5), 340–343.

Craighead, D. V. (2012). Early term birth: Understanding the health risks for infants. *Nursing for Women's Health*, *16*(2), 136–144.

De Vries, L. S. (2015). Intracranial hemorrhage and vascular lesions in the neonate. In R. J. Martin, A. A. Fanaroff, & M. C. Walsh (Eds.), *Fanaroff and Martin's neonatal-perinatal medicine: Diseases of the fetus and infant* (10th ed.) (pp. 886–903). St. Louis, MO: Saunders.

Discenza, D. (2009). Taking care of the NICU mom. *Neonatal Network*, *28*(5), 351–352.

Discenza, D. (2012). Premie parent frustration: Dealing with insensitive comments. *Neonatal Network*, *31*(1), 52–53.

Embleton, N. D., Zalewski, S., & Berrington, J. E. (2016). Probiotics for prevention of necrotizing enterocolitis and sepsis in preterm infants. *Current Opinion in Infectious Diseases*, *29*(3), 256–261.

Fanaroff, A. A., & Klaus, M. H. (2013). The physical environment. In A. A. Fanaroff & J. M. Fanaroff (Eds.), *Klaus and Fanaroff's care of the high-risk neonate* (6th ed.) (pp. 132–150). Philadelphia, PA: Saunders.

Fernandes, A., Campbell-Yeo, M., & Johnston, C. C. (2011). Procedural pain management for neonates using nonpharmacological strategies. *Advances in Neonatal Care*, *11*(4), 235–241.

Fraser, D., & Diehl-Jones, W. (2015). Ophthalmologic and auditory disorders. In M. T. Verklan, & M. Walden (Eds.), *Core curriculum for neonatal intensive care nursing* (5th ed.) (pp. 813–831). St. Louis, MO: Elsevier.

Gardner, S. L., & Hernandez, J. A. (2016). Heat balance. In S. L. Gardner, B. S. Carter, M. Enzman-Hines, et al. (Eds.), *Merenstein & Gardner's handbook of neonatal intensive care* (8th ed.) (pp. 105–125). St. Louis, MO: Elsevier.

Gardner, S. L., & Lawrence, R. A. (2016). Breastfeeding the neonate with special needs. In S. L. Gardner, B. S. Carter, M. Enzman-Hines, et al. (Eds.), *Merenstein & Gardner's handbook of neonatal intensive care* (8th ed.) (pp. 419–463). St. Louis, MO: Elsevier.

Gardner, S. L., Enzman-Hines, M., & Agarwal, R. (2016a). Pain and pain relief. In S. L. Gardner, B. S. Carter, M. Enzman-Hines, et al. (Eds.), *Merenstein & Gardner's handbook of neonatal intensive care* (8th ed.) (pp. 218–261). St. Louis, MO: Elsevier.

Gardner, S. L., Enzman-Hines, M., & Nyp, M. (2016b). Respiratory diseases. In S. L. Gardner, B. S. Carter, M. Enzman-Hines, et al. (Eds.), *Merenstein & Gardner's handbook of neonatal intensive care* (8th ed.) (pp. 565–643). St. Louis, MO: Elsevier.

Gardner, S. L., Goldson, E., & Hernandez, J. A. (2016c). The neonate and the environment: Impact on development. In S. L. Gardner, B. S. Carter, M. Enzman-Hines, et al. (Eds.), *Merenstein & Gardner's handbook of neonatal intensive care* (8th ed.) (pp. 262–314). St. Louis, MO: Elsevier.

Gardner, S. L., Voos, K., & Hills, P. (2016d). Families in crisis: Theoretical and practical considerations. In S. L. Gardner, B. S. Carter, M. Enzman-Hines, et al. (Eds.), *Merenstein & Gardner's handbook of neonatal intensive care* (8th ed.) (pp. 821–864). St. Louis, MO: Elsevier.

Geddes, D., Hassiotou, F., Wise, M., & Hartmann, P. (2017). Human milk composition and function in the infant. In R. A. Polin, S. H. Abman, D. H. Rowitch, & W. E. Benitz (Eds.), *Fetal and neonatal physiology* (5th ed.) (pp. 273–280). Philadelphia, PA: Elsevier.

Gelfer, P., Cameron, R., Masters, K., & Kennedy, K. A. (2013). Integrating "Back to Sleep" recommendations into neonatal ICU practice. *Pediatrics, 131*(4), e1264–e1270.

Gephart, S. M., McGrath, J. M., Efken, J. A., & Halpern, M. D. (2012). Necrotizing enterocolitis risk. *Advances in Neonatal Care, 12*(2), 77–87.

Goodwin, M. (2015). Apnea. In M. T. Verklan & M. Walden (Eds.), *Core curriculum for neonatal intensive care nursing* (5th ed.) (pp. 478–486). St. Louis, MO: Saunders.

Greenberg, J. M., Narendran, V., Schibler, K. R., Warner, B. B., Haberman, B., & Donovan, E. F. (2014). Neonatal morbidities of prenatal and perinatal origin. In R. K. Creasy, R. Resnik, J. D. Iams, C. J. Lockwood, & T. R. Moore (Eds.), *Creasy & Resnik's maternal-fetal medicine: Principles and practice* (7th ed.) (pp. 1215–1239). Philadelphia, PA: Saunders.

Hall, R. W., & Anand, K. J. (2014). Pain management in newborns. *Clinics in Perinatology, 41*(4), 895–924.

Hardy, W. (2011). Integration of kangaroo care into routine caregiving in the NICU. *Advances in Neonatal Care, 11*(2), 119–121.

Hardy, W., D'Agata, A., & McGrath, J. M. (2016). The infant at risk. In S. Mattson & J. E. Smith (Eds.), *Core curriculum for maternal-newborn nursing* (5th ed.) (pp. 363–416). St. Louis, MO: Elsevier.

Harrison, W., & Goodman, D. (2015). Epidemiologic trends in neonatal intensive care, 2007-2012. *JAMA Pediatrics, 169*(9), 855–862.

Hendson, L., Reis, M. D., & Nicholas, D. B. (2015). Health care providers' perspectives of providing culturally competent care in the NICU. *Journal of Obstetric, Gynecologic, & Neonatal Nursing, 44*(1), 17–27.

Klaus, M. H., Kennell, J. H., & Fanaroff, J. M. (2013). Care of the parents. In A. A. Fanaroff & J. M. Fanaroff (Eds.), *Klaus and Fanaroff''s care of the high-risk neonate* (6th ed.) (pp. 201–224). Philadelphia, PA: Saunders.

Kochanek, K. D., Murphy, S. L., Xu, J., & Tejeda-Vera, B. (2016). Deaths: Final data for 2014. *National Vital Statistics Reports, 65*(4). Hyattsville, MD: National Center for Health Statistics.

Krueger, C., Horesh, E., & Crossland, A. (2012). Safe sound exposure in the fetus and preterm infant. *Journal of Obstetric, Gynecologic, & Neonatal Nursing, 41*(2), 166–170.

Lawrence, R. A., & Lawrence, R. M. (2016). Premature infants and breastfeeding. In *Breastfeeding: A guide for the medical profession* (8th ed.) (pp. 524–562). Philadelphia, PA: Elsevier.

Lopez, G. L., Anderson, K. H., & Feutchinger, J. (2012). Transition of premature infants from hospital to home life. *Neonatal Network, 31*(4), 207–214.

Lund, C. H., & Durand, D. J. (2016). Skin and skin care. In S. L. Gardner, B. S. Carter, M. Enzman-Hines, et al. (Eds.), *Merenstein & Gardner's handbook of neonatal intensive care* (8th ed.) (pp. 464–478). St. Louis, MO: Elsevier.

Mackley, A. B., Locke, R. G., Spear, M. L., & Joseph, R. (2010). Forgotten parent: NICU paternal emotional response. *Advances in Neonatal Care, 10*(4), 200–203.

Mandy, G. T. (2016). Infants with fetal (intrauterine) growth restriction. In L. E. Weisman (Ed.), *UpToDate*. Waltham, MA: Wolters Kluwer. Retriever from www.uptodate.com.

McMullen, S. L. (2013). Transitioning premature infants supine: State of the science. *MCN The American Journal of Maternal/Child Nursing, 38*(1), 8–12.

Meier, P. P., Patel, A. L., Wright, K., & Engstrom, J. L. (2013). Management of breastfeeding during and after the maternity hospitalization for late preterm infants. *Clinical Perinatology, 40*(4), 689–705.

Moore, M. L., Moos, M., & Callister, L. C. (2010). *Cultural competence: An essential journey for perinatal nurses.* White Plains, NY: March of Dimes.

National Association of Neonatal Nurses (NANN). (2012). *Pain assessment and management: Guideline for practice.* Chicago: Author.

National Association of Neonatal Nurses (NANN). (2013). *Infant-directed oral feeding for premature and critically ill hospitalized infants: Guidelines for practice.* Chicago: Author.

National Association of Neonatal Nurses (NANN). (2015). *The use of human milk and breastfeeding in the neonatal intensive care unit. Position Statement #3065.* Chicago: Author.

Naughton, K. A. (2013). The combined use of sucrose and nonnutritive sucking for procedural pain in both term and preterm neonates. *Advances in Neonatal Care, 13*(1), 9–19.

Newland, L., L'Huillier, M. W., & Scheans, P. (2013). Implementation of cue-based feeding in a Level III NICU. *Neonatal Network, 32*(2), 132–137.

Northrup, T. F., Evans, P. W., & Stotts, A. L. (2013). Depression among mothers of high-risk infants discharged from a neonatal intensive care unit. *MCN American Journal of Maternal/Child Nursing, 38*(2), 89–94.

Nyp, M., Brunkhorst, J. L., Reavey, D., et al. (2016). Fluid and electrolyte management. In S. L. Gardner, B. S. Carter, M. Enzman-Hines, & J. Hernandez (Eds.), *Merenstein & Gardner's handbook of neonatal intensive care* (8th ed.) (pp. 315–336). St. Louis, MO: Elsevier.

Olitsky, S. E., Hug, D., Plummer, L. S., & Stahl, E. D. (2016). Disorders of the retina and vitreous. In R. M. Kliegman, B. E. Stanton, J. W. St. Geme, & N. Schor (Eds.), *Nelson textbook of pediatrics* (20th ed.) (pp. 3049–3057). Philadelphia, PA: Elsevier.

Osterman, M. J. K., Kochanek, K. D., MacDorman, M. F., Strobino, D. M., & Guyer, B. (2015). Annual summary of vital statistics: 2012-2013. *Pediatrics, 135*(6), 1115–1125.

Pappas, B. E., & Robey, D. L. (2015). Care of the late preterm infant. In M. T. Verklan & M. Walden (Eds.), *Core curriculum for neonatal intensive care nursing* (5th ed.) (pp. 439–446). St. Louis, MO: Saunders.

Parsons, J. A., Seay, A. R., & Jacobson, M. (2016). Neurologic disorders. In S. L. Gardner, B. S. Carter, M. Enzman-Hines, et al. (Eds.), *Merenstein & Gardner's handbook of neonatal intensive care* (8th ed.) (pp. 727–762). St. Louis, MO: Elsevier.

Patton, C., Stiltner, D., Wright, K. B., Kautz, D. D., Ikuta, L., & Zukowsky, K. (2015). Do nurses provide a safe sleep environment for infants in the hospital setting? An integrative review. *Advances in Neonatal Care, 15*(1), 8–22.

Poindexter, B. B., & Ehrenkranz, R. A. (2015). Nutrient requirements and provision of nutritional support in the premature neonate. In R. J. Martin, A. A. Fanaroff, & M. C. Walsh (Eds.), *Fanaroff and Martin's neonatal-perinatal medicine: Diseases of the fetus and infant* (10th ed.) (pp. 592–612). Philadelphia, PA: Saunders.

Poindexter, B. B., & Martin, C. R. (2015). Impact of nutrition on bronchopulmonary dysplasia. *Clinics in Perinatology, 42*(4), 797–806.

Pollan, C. (2009). Retinopathy of prematurity: An eye toward better outcomes. *Neonatal Network, 28*(2), 93–101.

Purdy, I. B., Craig, J. W., & Zeanah, P. (2015). NICU discharge planning and beyond: Recommendations for parent psychosocial support. *Journal of Perinatology, 35*, S24–S28.

Radtke, J. V. (2011). The paradox of breastfeeding-associated morbidity among late preterm infants. *Journal of Obstetric, Gynecologic, and Neonatal Nursing, 40*(1), 9–24.

Raines, D. A., & Brustad, J. (2012). Parent's confidence as a caregiver. *Advances in Neonatal Care, 12*(3), 183–187.

Ramachandrappa, A., & Jain, L. (2015). The late preterm infant. In R. J. Martin, A. A. Fanaroff, & M. C. Walsh (Eds.), *Fanaroff and Martin's neonatal-perinatal medicine: Diseases of the fetus and infant* (Vol. 1) (10th ed.) (pp. 577–591). Philadelphia, PA: Saunders.

Rampersand, R., & Macones, G. A. (2017). Prolonged and postterm pregnancy. In S. G. Gabbe, J. R. Niebyl, J. L. Simpson, M. B. Landon, H. L. Galan, R. M. Jauniaux, D. A. Driscoll, et al. (Eds.), *Obstetrics: Normal and problem pregnancies* (7th ed.) (pp. 796–802). Philadelphia, PA: Elsevier.

Ranger, M., Beggs, S., & Grunau, R. E. (2017). Developmental aspects of pain. In R. A. Polin, S. H. Abman, D. H. Rowitch, & W. E. Benitz (Eds.), *Fetal and neonatal physiology* (5th ed.) (pp. 1390–1395). Philadelphia, PA: Elsevier.

Resnik, R., & Creasy, R. K. (2014). Intrauterine growth restriction. In R. K. Creasy, R. Resnik, J. D. Iams, C. J. Lockwood, & T. R. Moore (Eds.), *Resnik & Creasy's maternal-fetal medicine: Principles and practice* (7th ed.) (pp. 743–775). Philadelphia, PA: Elsevier.

Rhoads, S. J., Green, A. L., Lewis, S. D., & Rakes, L. (2012). Challenges of implementation of a web-camera system in the neonatal intensive care unit. *Neonatal Network, 31*(4), 223–228.

Schafer, D., Boogaart, S., Johnson, L., Keezel, C., Ruperts, L., & Vander Laan, K. J. (2014). Comparison of neonatal skin sensor temperatures with axillary temperature: Does skin sensor placement really matter? *Advances in Neonatal Care, 14*(1), 52–60.

Shapiro, N., Rios, A., Bogdanffy, H., & Caprio, M. (2016). The effect of breastfeeding education in the NICU on post-discharge breastfeeding duration. *Pediatrics, 137*(Suppl. 3) 442A–442A.

Skene, C., Franck, L., Curtis, P., & Gerrish, K. (2012). Parental involvement in neonatal comfort care. *Journal of Obstetric, Gynecologic, & Neonatal Nursing, 41*(6), 786–797.

Spatz, D. L. (2011). Innovations in the provision of human milk and breastfeeding for infants requiring intensive care. *Journal of Obstetric, Gynecologic, & Neonatal Nursing, 41*(1), 139–143.

Spruill, C. T. (2015). Developmental support. In M. T. Verklan & M. Walden (Eds.), *Core curriculum for neonatal intensive care nursing* (5th ed.) (pp. 197–215). St. Louis, MO: Elsevier.

Stoll, B. J., & Shane, A. L. (2016). Infections of the neonatal infant. In R. M. Kliegman, B. F. Stanton, J. W. St. Geme, & N. Schor (Eds.), *Nelson textbook of pediatrics* (20th ed.) (pp. 909–925). Philadelphia, PA: Elsevier.

Talge, N. M., Holzman, C., Wang, J., Lucia, V., Gardiner, J., & Breslau, N. (2010). Late-preterm birth and its association with cognitive and socioemotional outcomes at 6 years. *Pediatrics, 126*(6), 1124–1131.

Thomson-Salo, F. (2015). Care of the long stay infant and parents. In R. J. Martin, A. A. Fanaroff, & M. C. Walsh (Eds.), *Fanaroff and Martin's neonatal-perinatal medicine: Diseases of the fetus and infant* (10th ed.) (pp. 642–646). Philadelphia, PA: Saunders.

Tutlam, N., Liu, Y., Nelson, E., Flick, L., & Chang, J. (2017). The Effects of race and ethnicity on the risk of large-for-gestational-age newborns in women without gestational diabetes by prepregnancy Body Mass Index categories. *Maternal & Child Health Journal, 21*(8), 1643–1654.

Tymann, H. (2015). Increasing breastfeeding rates in the NICU. *Journal of the Academy of Nutrition and Dietetics, 115*(9), A97.

Verklan, M. T. (2015). Neurologic disorders. In M. T. Verklan & M. Walden (Eds.), *Core curriculum for neonatal intensive care nursing* (5th ed.) (pp. 734–766). St. Louis, MO: Elsevier.

Walker, M. (2008). Breastfeeding the late preterm infant. *Journal of Obstetric, Gynecologic, & Neonatal Nursing, 37*(6), 692–701.

Wambach, J. A., & Hamvas, A. (2015). Respiratory distress syndrome in the neonate. In R. J. Martin, A. A. Fanaroff, & M. C. Walsh (Eds.), *Fanaroff and Martin's neonatal-perinatal medicine: Diseases of the fetus and infant* (Vol. 2) (10th ed.) (pp. 1074–1086). St. Louis, MO: Saunders.

Weiner, G. M. (Ed.). (2016). *Textbook of neonatal resuscitation* (7th ed.) Elk Grove Village, IL: American Academy of Pediatrics and American Heart Association

World Health Organization (2016). Preterm Birth Fact Sheet. Geneva Switzerland. Retrieved from: http://www.who.int/mediacentre/factsheets/fs363/en/

High-Risk Newborn: Acquired and Congenital Conditions

Della Wrightson

In addition to the high-risk conditions related to gestational age discussed in Chapter 23, the newborn at risk may have acquired or congenital complications. Acquired conditions may be associated with prenatal complications or may occur at birth or shortly thereafter

RESPIRATORY COMPLICATIONS

Respiratory distress is one of the most common problems of the neonate. It may be caused by asphyxia before or during birth, disease of the respiratory system, and other conditions that affect the infant's ability to breathe. The nurse is responsible for identification and evaluation of respiratory status at birth and throughout the hospital stay.

Asphyxia

Asphyxia is insufficient oxygen and excess carbon dioxide in the blood and tissues. It may occur in utero, at birth, or later and results in ischemia to major organs. When asphyxia occurs at birth, it may be a continuation of asphyxia that began before birth or the result of other factors such as preterm lungs with insufficient surfactant to function adequately. Maternal, placental, or fetal factors may be involved.

Maternal factors include complications such as hypertension, infection, and drug use. Asphyxia in utero may be caused by placental conditions such as placenta previa, placental abruption, or postmaturity. Cord problems, infection, premature birth, and multifetal gestation are among the fetal causes of asphyxia.

Lack of oxygen transported to the cells leads to anaerobic metabolism and the production of lactic acid. Metabolic acidosis develops when inadequate bicarbonate is available to buffer the accumulating acids. Respiratory acidosis occurs as carbon dioxide accumulates. A high partial pressure of carbon dioxide occurs in arterial blood ($Paco_2$), and the partial pressure of oxygen (Po_2), the pH, and bicarbonate are low.

Vasoconstriction caused by low oxygen decreases blood flow to all organs except the brain, myocardium, and adrenal glands. The ductus arteriosus and foramen ovale may remain open because of the low oxygen in the blood, high resistance to blood flow through constricted pulmonary vessels, and elevated pressure on the right side of the heart. Therefore even circulating blood remains low in oxygen concentration. Progression toward brain injury and death is rapid unless intervention is prompt.

Problems may continue even if the infant survives. Pulmonary ischemia interferes with the ability to produce surfactant, increasing the risk for respiratory distress syndrome (RDS). Intrauterine stress may lead to passage of meconium and meconium aspiration syndrome (MAS).

Manifestations

When asphyxia occurs after birth, rapid respirations are followed by cessation of respirations (primary apnea) and a rapid fall in heart rate. Stimulation, alone or with oxygen, may restart respirations. If asphyxia continues without intervention, gasping respirations may resume weakly until the infant enters a period of secondary apnea. In secondary apnea, the oxygen levels in blood continue to decrease, the infant loses consciousness, and stimulation is ineffective. Resuscitative measures should be initiated immediately to prevent permanent injury to the brain or death. Asphyxia seen at birth may be a continuation of asphyxia that began before or during birth. Therefore it is essential to begin resuscitation without delay.

Infants at Risk

Complications that occur during pregnancy, labor, or birth increase the infant's risk for asphyxia. In addition, if the expectant mother receives narcotics for analgesia shortly before birth, the infant's central nervous system (CNS) may be too depressed at birth to allow adequate spontaneous breathing.

Neonatal Resuscitation

Although most newborns have no difficulty with breathing at birth, up to 10% require some help to begin respirations and 1% require extensive resuscitative measures (Weiner, 2016). Therefore all personnel involved in deliveries should know how to perform resuscitative measures. Courses in neonatal resuscitation are usually required of all staff members working with newborns, and many agencies expect these skills to be updated every 1 to 2 years.

Chest compressions and medications are rarely needed during resuscitation. Nurses should be prepared for situations in which asphyxia may develop. Effective ventilation is the most important element in resuscitation (Weiner, 2016). Equipment should be readily available and functioning properly at all times so there is no delay in starting resuscitation. Nurses begin resuscitation measures as necessary and assist the physician or nurse practitioner with intubation, insertion of umbilical vein catheters, and administration of medications.

Maintenance of thermoregulation is very important throughout care. A warming pad may be placed under linens in the radiant warmer to provide extra heat. Infants less than 29 weeks of gestation may be placed in a polyethylene bag up to the neck before they are dried to reduce heat loss from evaporation. The bag also reduces stress from handling during drying. It is important to prevent hyperthermia when the bag is used with a chemical warming pad (Weiner, 2016).

Some infants develop hypoxic-ischemic encephalopathy after asphyxia. Therapeutic hypothermia has been used to improve neurologic outcomes for these infants. Infants should be 36 or more weeks of gestation, have evidence of an acute perinatal hypoxic-ischemic event, and be in a facility where the treatment can be initiated within 6 hours of birth (Weiner, 2016).

Once the infant is stabilized, the nurse continues to assess for changes. Infants with asphyxia often have other complications such as hypoglycemia, feeding and thermoregulation problems, seizures, hypotension, pulmonary hypertension, metabolic acidosis, renal problems, and fluid and electrolyte imbalances. They need close monitoring and often need intensive nursing care.

Communication with the parents is a vital nursing function. They will be confused and frightened and will need explanation and realistic reassurance. Parents often need continued support after the crisis to talk about their fears and concerns.

Transient Tachypnea of the Newborn (Retained Lung Fluid)

Infants who experience **transient tachypnea of the newborn (TTN)** develop rapid respirations soon after birth from inadequate absorption of fetal lung fluid. Although the condition usually resolves within 24 to 48 hours, it is the most common respiratory cause of admission to a neonatal intensive care nursery (NICU) (Greenberg et al., 2014).

Risk factors include cesarean birth with or without labor, macrosomia, multiple gestation, excessive maternal sedation, prolonged or precipitous labor, male gender, and maternal diabetes or asthma. Mild immaturity of surfactant production also may be a factor. Infants are usually term or late preterm, although some may be preterm (Fraser, 2015; Greenberg et al., 2014).

Cause

Although the exact cause of TTN is unknown, it is thought to result from a delay in absorption of fetal lung fluid by the pulmonary capillaries and lymph vessels. This leads to decreased lung compliance and air trapping and produces signs similar to those of RDS.

Manifestations

In TTN, tachypnea develops within 6 hours of birth. Grunting, retractions, nasal flaring, and mild cyanosis also are present. Chest radiography demonstrates hyperinflation, perihilar streaking that shows engorged lymphatics, and the presence of fluid in the fissures between the lobes and in the pleural space.

Therapeutic Management

Treatment is supportive and may include oxygen for cyanosis. Gavage feeding may be given when the respiratory rate is high to prevent aspiration and conserve energy. Because the signs are similar to those of RDS and sepsis, the infant is observed for those complications. Antibiotics may be given until sepsis is ruled out. Continuous positive airway pressure is rarely needed.

Nursing Considerations

The nurse may be the first person to see signs of TTN, especially if they are not apparent at birth. After identifying these signs, the nurse notifies the provider and carries out treatment. General nursing care is similar to that of the respiratory care of the preterm infant (see Chapter 23).

> ### ❓ KNOWLEDGE CHECK
> 1. What is the most important element in resuscitation?
> 2. What is the role of the nurse in care of the infant with asphyxia?
> 3. How is TTN different from RDS?

Meconium Aspiration Syndrome

Meconium staining of amniotic fluid occurs in 10% to 15% of births. **Meconium aspiration syndrome (MAS)** is a condition in which there is obstruction, chemical pneumonitis, and air trapping caused by meconium in the lungs. It develops in 5% of those infants (Ambalavanan & Carlo, 2016) (Fig. 24.1). The condition occurs most often in infants who are postterm, small for gestational age (SGA), and compromised before birth by placental insufficiency with decreased amniotic fluid and cord compression (Crowley, 2015).

Causes

Although a normal fetus may pass meconium, MAS occurs most often when hypoxia causes increased peristalsis of the intestines and relaxation of the anal sphincter before or during labor. MAS develops when meconium in the amniotic fluid enters the lungs during fetal life or at birth. It may be drawn into the lungs if gasping movements occur in utero as a result of asphyxia and acidosis, or the meconium in the upper airways may be pulled deep into the respiratory passages when the infant takes the first breaths after birth.

Obstruction of the airways may be complete or partial. Atelectasis may result if small airways are completely obstructed. In partial obstruction, air can enter but not escape from the alveoli. During inhalation, the bronchioles expand slightly as air flows into them past the meconium. During exhalation, the passages constrict and meconium blocks the movement of air out of the lungs.

This ball-valve mechanism results in air trapping. The overdistended alveoli may develop an air leak, with escape of air into the pleural cavity (pneumothorax) or mediastinum (pneumomediastinum). Surfactant production may be inhibited, increasing respiratory distress. In addition, meconium is irritating to lung tissue and causes an inflammatory reaction and chemical pneumonitis.

Severe MAS develops in only a small number of newborns with meconium below the vocal cords. The addition of meconium to lungs injured by asphyxia may increase the severity of the condition. Injury from asphyxia interferes with clearing of

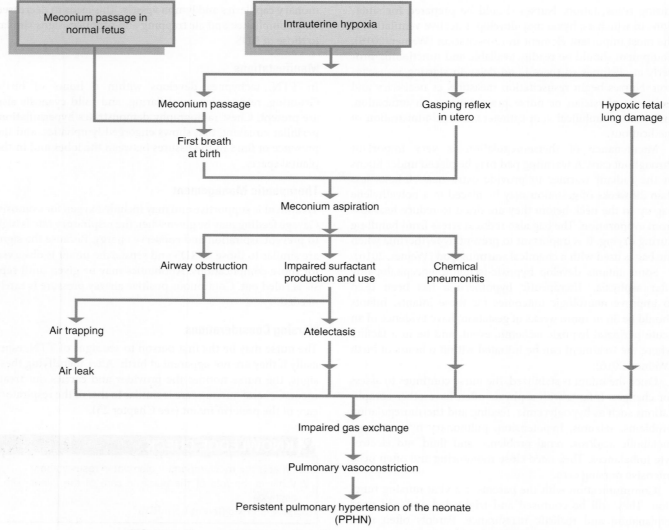

FIG. 24.1 Flow chart showing the effects of meconium aspiration syndrome.

lung fluid and production of surfactant and causes pulmonary vasoconstriction that can result in return to fetal circulation patterns. MAS may lead to persistent pulmonary hypertension.

Manifestations

If meconium in the amniotic fluid is minimal, respiratory problems usually do not develop. However, more meconium may cause serious respiratory pathologic issues. Signs of mild to severe respiratory distress are present at birth, with tachypnea, cyanosis, retractions, nasal flaring, grunting, crackles, and, in severe cases, a barrel-shaped chest from hyperinflation. Radiography shows patchy infiltrates, atelectasis, consolidation, and hyperexpansion from air trapping. The infant's nails, skin, and umbilical cord may be stained yellow-green.

Therapeutic Management

Suctioning the infant's secretions as soon as the head is born has not been found to reduce the incidence of MAS. At birth, the vigorous infant (who has a heart rate more than 100 beats per minute [bpm], spontaneous respirations, and good muscle tone) does not need special suctioning and receives routine care. Infants with depressed respirations and muscle tone should be moved to a radiant warmer and suctioned with a bulb syringe. If the infant is not breathing or has a heart rate below 100 bpm after opening the airway, suctioning, and being dried and stimulated, positive pressure ventilation is required (Weiner, 2016).

Infants may need only warmed, humidified oxygen, or extensive respiratory support with mechanical ventilation may be required. High-frequency ventilation may be used. Surfactant lavage has been used in severe cases but is controversial (Gardner, Enzman-Hines, & Nyp, 2016).

Ongoing management consists of supportive care to meet the problems presented. Infants with severe MAS who do not respond to conventional treatment may benefit from extracorporeal membrane oxygenation (ECMO). ECMO, which is available in some hospitals, oxygenates blood while bypassing the lungs, much like heart-lung machines used during heart surgery. It allows the infant's lungs to rest temporarily and recover.

Nursing Considerations

When meconium is noted in the amniotic fluid during labor, the nurse notifies the primary provider so that delivery care can be adapted as necessary. Nurses from the NICU and a neonatologist may be present for the birth. The nurse ensures that equipment such as oxygen and suction devices are functioning properly and assists with care at birth. After the infant's birth, nursing care is adapted to the problems presented. Although meconium is sterile, lung injury promotes the growth of bacteria. Infants should be closely observed for infection, which may further complicate the condition. Nursing attention to thermoregulation and decreased stimulation is important.

Persistent Pulmonary Hypertension of the Newborn

Persistent pulmonary hypertension of the newborn (PPHN) is a condition in which pulmonary vasoconstriction occurs after birth and elevates vascular resistance of the lungs. Normal changes to neonatal circulation are impaired as a result. For this reason, the condition is also called *persistent fetal circulation.*

Causes

PPHN occurs most often in infants who are term or postterm. The cause may be abnormal lung development or maternal use of nonsteroidal, antiinflammatory drugs (NSAIDs) or selective serotonin reuptake inhibitors (SSRIs), or it may be unknown. It is often associated with hypoxemia and acidosis from conditions such as asphyxia, MAS, sepsis, polycythemia, diaphragmatic hernia, and RDS (Ambalavanan & Carlo, 2016).

Inadequate oxygenation results in vasoconstriction, instead of the normal dilation, of the pulmonary artery and small pulmonary vessels, which causes increased vascular resistance in the lungs. The elevated pulmonary vascular resistance causes a rise in pressure on the right side of the heart. This results in a right-to-left shunt of unoxygenated blood that flows through the foramen ovale. In addition, unoxygenated blood from the pulmonary artery flows through the ductus arteriosus to the aorta. Thus, blood bypasses the lungs, as occurs during fetal circulation. Metabolic acidosis causes more pulmonary vasoconstriction, making the condition even worse.

Manifestations

Infants with PPHN develop signs within the first 12 hours after birth. Tachypnea, respiratory distress, and progressive cyanosis often become worse with handling. Oxygen saturation and partial pressure of oxygen in arterial blood (PaO_2) are decreased, $PaCO_2$ is increased, and acidosis is present. Other signs may result from associated conditions. An echocardiogram demonstrates right-to-left shunting through the foramen ovale and ductus arteriosus.

Therapeutic Management

Management involves treating the underlying cause of poor oxygenation and relieving pulmonary vasoconstriction. Arterial pH may be increased with respiratory therapy and drug therapy to cause pulmonary vasodilation. Sedation, high-frequency ventilation, and surfactant therapy may be necessary. Inhaled nitric oxide may be given to dilate pulmonary vessels. ECMO therapy may be lifesaving if conventional therapies are unsuccessful.

Nursing Considerations

Nursing care is similar to care of other infants with severe respiratory disease. Because infants become hypoxic with activity and other stimuli, handling and noise are kept to a minimum. Cold stress increases the metabolic rate and need for oxygen and causes additional pulmonary vasoconstriction. Therefore the nurse should pay particular attention to maintaining the infant's temperature. Assessment for hypoglycemia, hypocalcemia, anemia, and metabolic acidosis is important.

Hyperbilirubinemia (Pathologic Jaundice)

Jaundice is a common concern in the care for neonates. Conjugation of bilirubin and physiologic jaundice are discussed in Chapter 19 and Chapter 20. This discussion focuses on nonphysiologic or pathologic jaundice.

When the total serum bilirubin (TSB) level is greater than 5 to 6 milligrams per deciliter (mg/dL), jaundice appears (Kaplan, Wong, Sibley, & Stevenson, 2015). Jaundice is considered abnormal or nonphysiologic when the TSB rises more rapidly and to a higher level than is expected or stays elevated for longer than normal. Charts showing the expected rise and fall of bilirubin according to the age of the infant in hours are used to determine the degree of risk and which infants need treatment for rising TSB level.

Nonphysiologic jaundice may be seen in the first 24 hours of life. It is a concern because it may lead to **bilirubin encephalopathy**, the acute manifestation of bilirubin toxicity. This may lead to **kernicterus**, the chronic and permanent result of bilirubin toxicity. In this condition, bilirubin deposits cause yellowish staining of the brain, especially the basal ganglia, cerebellum, brainstem, and hippocampus. It is more likely to occur in infants who have suffered hypoxemia, respiratory acidosis, infection, dehydration, or other injury that impairs the blood-brain barrier and allows unconjugated bilirubin to enter the brain (Blackburn, 2013).

Although bilirubin encephalopathy and kernicterus are rare today because of improved treatment measures, the mortality and morbidity rates among affected infants are high. Those who survive may suffer from cerebral palsy, cognitive impairment, hearing loss, or more subtle long-term neurologic and developmental problems. The exact level at which bilirubin encephalopathy develops is not known. The toxic level may not be the same for all infants. It occurs at lower TSB levels and is more severe in infants who have complications, who are preterm or late preterm, or who have low birth weight than in full-term healthy infants.

Causes

The most common cause of pathologic jaundice is hemolytic disease of the newborn from incompatibility between the blood of the mother and that of the fetus. The best known cause is Rh incompatibility, in which the Rh-negative mother forms antibodies when blood from an Rh-positive fetus enters her circulation (see Chapter 10). Antibodies may have developed during a previous pregnancy or after injury, abortion, amniocentesis, or a transfusion of Rh-positive blood. The antibodies cross the placenta, attach to fetal red blood cells (RBCs), and destroy them. The result is **erythroblastosis fetalis**, agglutination and hemolysis of fetal erythrocytes from maternal-fetal blood incompatibility.

Infants with erythroblastosis fetalis are anemic from destruction of RBCs. Severely affected infants may develop **hydrops fetalis**, a severe anemia that results in heart failure and generalized edema. Intrauterine fetal transfusions may be given. After birth, phototherapy and exchange transfusions are used to prevent kernicterus. Use of Rho(D) immune globulin (RhoGAM) to prevent the mother from forming antibodies against Rh-positive blood has greatly decreased the incidence of erythroblastosis fetalis.

ABO incompatibility also causes pathologic jaundice. Mothers with type O blood have natural antibodies to type A and B blood. The antibodies cross the placenta and cause hemolysis of fetal RBCs. However, the destruction is much less severe than with Rh incompatibility and causes milder signs. This is because most of the antibodies are immunoglobulin M (IgM), which does not cross the placenta. Some of the antibodies are immunoglobulin G (IgG), which does cross the placenta and can cause RBC destruction, but usually at a lower rate (Dahlke & Magnann, 2015).

Other causes of nonphysiologic jaundice include infection, hypothyroidism, glucuronyl transferase deficiency, polycythemia, glucose-6-phosphate dehydrogenase deficiency, and biliary atresia. Infants of diabetic mothers are more likely to develop nonphysiologic jaundice, especially if they have macrosomia. Any condition that causes destruction of erythrocytes or impairment of the liver may result in elevated bilirubin levels.

Therapeutic Management

The focus of therapeutic management is prevention of bilirubin encephalopathy and kernicterus. The cause is determined by history and diagnostic tests to identify infections or blood abnormalities. During pregnancy, an Rh-negative mother will have blood drawn for an indirect Coombs' test to identify the presence of antibodies against fetal blood. If the antibodies are present, additional testing may be performed to evaluate fetal status (see Chapter 10).

When an infant is jaundiced, the infant's blood type and a direct Coombs' test are performed. A positive Coombs' test indicates that antibodies from the mother have attached to the infant's RBCs. TSB levels are monitored closely to detect changes that indicate treatment should be initiated or changed. The health care provider considers the bilirubin level as well as other factors such as gestational age and presence of other risk factors to determine whether therapy is appropriate for an individual infant.

Nurses assess infants for changes in jaundice. However, visual inspection for jaundice is not an accurate way of determining actual bilirubin levels. Because taking blood samples for TSB measurement is painful and expensive, other noninvasive tests may be used. Transcutaneous bilirubinometers are hand-held devices that allow screening of transcutaneous bilirubin (TcB) level. When the sensor on the device is placed against the infant's skin, the amount of bilirubin in the tissues is measured. This noninvasive test allows frequent estimates of the TSB level without discomfort to the infant. However, it may not be accurate in preterm infants, in infants receiving phototherapy, or if TSB levels are above 15 mg/dL (Kamath-Rayne, Thilo, Deacon, & Hernandez, 2016).

Phototherapy

Phototherapy is the most common treatment for jaundice and involves placing the infant under special fluorescent lights. During phototherapy, bilirubin in the skin absorbs the light and changes into water-soluble products, the most important of which is lumirubin. These products do not require conjugation by the liver and can be excreted in bile and urine. Because preterm infants are more vulnerable to bilirubin toxicity, phototherapy is begun at lower TSB levels than for full-term infants.

Phototherapy can be delivered in several ways. A bank of fluorescent lamps or "bili" lights can be placed over the infant who is in an incubator or under a radiant warmer to maintain heat or in an open crib. The infant wears only a diaper to ensure maximal exposure of the skin to the lights. The diaper is removed if the TSB is becoming dangerously high. The eyes are closed and patches placed over them to protect them from injury (Fig. 24.2). The lights are placed above the infant at a distance determined by the type of bulb used. More than one bank of lights may be used if the bilirubin level is very high. Bilirubin levels are checked frequently to determine the effectiveness of treatment and when it can be discontinued.

Other options for phototherapy include light-emitting diodes (LEDs), halogen lamps, and fiberoptic phototherapy blankets. As with fluorescent lights, the LED device is placed over the infant. It is long lasting, does not generate excessive heat, and decreases insensible water loss. The halogen spotlight is used alone or with other lamps. The infant can be swaddled with the fiberoptic phototherapy blanket against the skin and does not require patches over the eyes. With the blanket, the mother may hold the infant without interfering with therapy. However, the blanket is not as effective alone as the other methods. To increase its effectiveness, the blanket may be placed under the infant when phototherapy lights are used. A "bilibed" is also available with the phototherapy device built into the part of the bed that lies under the infant.

The side effects of phototherapy include frequent, loose, green stools that result from increased bile flow and peristalsis. This causes more rapid excretion of the bilirubin but may be damaging to the skin and result in fluid loss. A 25% increase in fluid intake is needed during phototherapy (Kaplan et al., 2015). A macular skin rash may occur in some infants. *Bronze baby syndrome,* a grayish brown discoloration of the skin and urine, occurs in some infants with cholestatic jaundice. The rash and color changes disappear gradually when phototherapy is completed.

When phototherapy is discontinued, a rebound TSB level increase of 1 to 2 mg/dL is normal. Therefore the TSB should be monitored for at least 24 hours to see that it does not become excessively high. Explain the expected elevation to parents and that the health care provider may order additional blood tests after discharge.

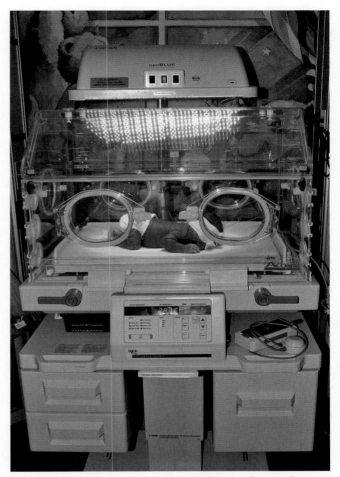

FIG. 24.2 An infant receiving phototherapy is wearing eye patches to protect the eyes.

Exchange Transfusions

Exchange transfusions are seldom necessary but are performed when phototherapy cannot reduce dangerously high bilirubin levels quickly enough. This treatment removes maternal antibodies, unconjugated bilirubin, and antibody-coated (sensitized) RBCs. It provides fresh albumin with binding sites for bilirubin and helps correct severe anemia. When an immediate transfusion is needed for Rh incompatibility, type O, Rh-negative blood cross-matched against the mother and infant is used. In ABO incompatibility, packed RBCs with type AB plasma are used so there are no anti-A or anti-B antibodies present to destroy the erythrocytes (Kamath-Rayne et al., 2016).

Procedure. During the exchange transfusion, small portions of blood are removed from the infant and replaced with an equal amount of donor blood. Because the donor blood mixes with the infant's blood, approximately twice the infant's blood volume is administered. At the end of the transfusion, approximately 85% to 90% of the infant's RBCs will have been replaced and the bilirubin level reduced by 50% or less (Fasano, Said, & Luban, 2015).

When the bilirubin level in blood decreases, bilirubin from tissues moves into plasma. This may increase the level of bilirubin in the blood to 60% of the preexchange level (Kamath-Rayne et al., 2016). This rebound elevation of bilirubin level may necessitate repeat transfusions, but phototherapy is generally adequate to resolve it.

Complications. Complications that may occur from exchange transfusions include electrolyte and acid-base imbalance, hypocalcemia, hypomagnesemia, hypoglycemia, hyperkalemia, infection, cardiac dysrhythmias, necrotizing enterocolitis, bleeding, thrombosis, thrombocytopenia, and air embolism. Samples of blood are analyzed for a complete blood cell (CBC) count, bilirubin and calcium levels, and other tests as needed before and after the exchange.

Role of the Nurse. The nurse's role during exchange transfusion is to prepare equipment, assess the infant during and after the procedure, and keep accurate records. A cardiac monitor is attached to the infant, and warmth is provided by a radiant heater. The nurse also should clarify any misunderstandings that the parents may have about the treatment and help allay their anxiety.

◆ APPLICATION OF THE NURSING PROCESS: HYPERBILIRUBINEMIA

◆ Assessment

Assess the level of jaundice at least every 8 hours by blanching the skin (pressing the skin over a bony prominence) to see the color in the area before blood returns. Evaluate the skin color in good light with phototherapy lights turned off because they distort the skin color. In infants with dark skin, assess the color of the palate and mucous membranes of the mouth and the conjunctivae. Determine the areas of the body affected by jaundice, and document carefully to use for comparison during future assessments. Jaundice begins at the head and moves down the body as the bilirubin level rises. Monitor the TSB and TcB levels for change because visualization of jaundice is a subjective assessment and the color in the skin may be affected by phototherapy.

Assess for risk factors that might further increase bilirubin levels. Note temperature fluctuations, hypoglycemia, and infection. Determine the infant's oral intake and number of stools.

◆ Identification of Patient Problems

In addition to the possibility of increasing bilirubin levels, the infant receiving phototherapy is at risk for associated problems. These potential problems include injury caused by the light, temperature instability, changes in fluid and nutrition status and damage to the retina.

◆ Planning: Expected Outcomes

Nurses can do many things to prevent situations that might cause further rises in bilirubin. They should also protect the infant from injury caused by the light during phototherapy. The expected outcome for this diagnosis is that the infant will have no injury resulting from increased bilirubin levels or exposure of the skin or eyes to phototherapy lights.

◆ Interventions

Interventions are designed to prevent situations that might cause injury to the infant from rising bilirubin levels or effects of treatment.

Maintaining a Neutral Thermal Environment

Prevent situations such as cold stress or hypoglycemia, which could result in increased fatty acids in blood caused by acidosis. Acidosis would decrease the availability of albumin-binding sites for unconjugated bilirubin. Prevent cold stress at birth and during all care by maintaining the infant in a neutral thermal environment. Check the infant's axillary temperature every 2 to 4 hours to identify an early decrease before it becomes a problem. Dress the infant in warmed clothes and blankets on removal from phototherapy lights.

Prevent elevation of the infant's temperature from exposure to the heat of the "bili" lights. Position the lights according to the manufacturer's guidelines to prevent overheating. Use a skin probe when the infant is in an incubator or radiant warmer to maintain the appropriate environmental temperature, and monitor the settings to be sure they are correct for the infant's needs.

Providing Optimal Nutrition

Ensure the infant receives feedings as prescribed. Breastfeeding should not be stopped because the infant is receiving phototherapy. Provide extra support and teaching to breastfeeding mothers having difficulty. Frequent feedings prevent hypoglycemia, provide protein to maintain the albumin level in the blood, and promote gastrointestinal (GI) motility and prompt removal of bilirubin from the intestines.

Avoid offering water because the infant may take less milk, which is more effective in promoting stooling and removal of bilirubin from the intestines. If breastfeeding must be supplemented, use formula instead of water. Weigh the infant at least daily, and monitor intake and output to identify dehydration early and intervene appropriately.

Protecting the Eyes

Provide patches to protect the eyes from retinal damage from the phototherapy lights. Close the infant's eyes before placing the patches to avoid abrasions to the cornea. Check the position of the patches at least every hour. Infants often wiggle enough to push the patches above or below the eyes, leaving them exposed. The edges of the patches can press too hard on the eyes or compress the nose and interfere with breathing. Turn off the lights, and observe for skin irritation around or under the patches at least every 4 hours. Explain to the parents that it is normal for the yellow color under the patches to be deeper than in areas that have been exposed to the lights.

⍰ CRITICAL THINKING EXERCISE 24.1

1. Why is it important to remove the patches from the eyes each time the infant is taken from phototherapy for feeding or when parents visit?

Enhancing Response to Therapy

Position the lights the proper distance from the infant. Lights that are too close may burn the skin. Lights too far away from the infant will not be effective in reducing jaundice. Halogen lights should be placed farther away from the infant than other lights to prevent burning. Follow the manufacturer's instructions about light placement. Although phototherapy increases insensible water loss from the skin, avoid the use of creams or lotions on the infant's skin that might cause burning.

Use a light meter to check the level of irradiance (energy output) to be sure the apparatus is functioning appropriately and to determine whether the bulbs need to be replaced. Check laboratory reports of TSB levels to determine the effectiveness of treatment and when it can be discontinued.

Expose as much skin as possible to the light. Remove all of the infant's clothing except a diaper. Turn the infant frequently to expose all areas evenly and prevent irritation of the skin from lack of position change. If a fiberoptic blanket is used, check the position of the blanket frequently. Infants sometimes need to be repositioned so that the blanket remains in contact with the skin.

Detecting Complications

Observe for other complications. Although bilirubin encephalopathy is rare today, monitor for signs that indicate its presence. These include lethargy, increased or decreased muscle tone, poor feeding, decreased or absent Moro reflex, high-pitched cry, opisthotonos, and seizures (Kamath-Rayne et al., 2016). Note the presence of rashes or changes in the color of the skin. Inform parents that they are not harmful and will disappear when phototherapy is discontinued.

Teaching Parents

Explain care to parents, who may be frightened to see their infant in an incubator with the infant's eyes covered. Explaining the causes of jaundice and the purpose of phototherapy will decrease their worry. Removing the infant from phototherapy for feeding and interaction with the parents for periods up to an hour at a time does not significantly decrease the effectiveness of phototherapy (Kamath-Rayne et al., 2016). In addition, allowing the parents to hold their baby increases their opportunity for attachment. Explain the importance of minimizing further interruptions to phototherapy.

When the infant is discharged, give the parents written and verbal information about jaundice. Teach them how to assess for further jaundice, signs of complications, and when to call the health care provider. Emphasize the need to keep follow-up laboratory work and visits to the health care provider so any increases in jaundice or other problems can be identified and treated early. Explain that most infants have no further problem with jaundice.

Although sunlight is known to reduce bilirubin level, caution the parents against putting the infant in direct sunlight. The infant might be sunburned or have temperature instability and is exposed to unnecessary ultraviolet light from the sun.

◆ Evaluation

No signs of injury should be present. The infant's eyes will not have been exposed to the phototherapy lights, and the skin should not be harmed. Laboratory reports should show a steady decrease of serum bilirubin level.

 KNOWLEDGE CHECK

6. How can kernicterus be prevented?
7. How can the nurse help reduce bilirubin levels in infants receiving phototherapy?

INFECTION

Nurses should be constantly alert for signs of infection in newborns. As many as 10% of infants develop infections during the first month of life (Stoll & Shane 2016).

Transmission of Infection

Newborns can acquire infections before, during, or after birth. Vertical infection is acquired before or during birth from the mother. Organisms such as those causing rubella, cytomegalovirus infection, syphilis, human immunodeficiency virus (HIV) infection, and toxoplasmosis may pass across the placenta and cause infection during pregnancy. During labor and birth, organisms in the vagina such as group B *Streptococcus* (GBS), herpes, and hepatitis may enter the uterus after rupture of membranes or infect the infant during passage through the birth canal.

Horizontal infection occurs after birth, acquired from hospital staff members or from contaminated equipment (health care–associated infections), or from family members or visitors. An example is staphylococcal infections associated with central venous catheters. Some of the most common infections and their effects on the neonate are listed in Table 24.1. Other infections are discussed in Chapter 10.

Sepsis Neonatorum

Infection that occurs during or after birth may result in sepsis neonatorum, a systemic infection from bacteria in the bloodstream. Newborns are particularly susceptible to sepsis because their immune systems are immature and they react more slowly to invasion by organisms. Newborns and especially preterm infants have fewer antibodies and are unable to localize infection as well as older children. This inability allows the infection to spread easily from one organ to another. In addition, the blood-brain barrier is less effective in preventing the entrance of organisms, and CNS infection may result.

Causes

Common causative agents of neonatal sepsis include bacteria such as GBS, *Escherichia coli*, coagulase-negative *Staphylococcus*, *Staphylococcus aureus*, and *Haemophilus influenzae* and fungi such as *Candida albicans* (Wilson & Tyner, 2015). Sepsis may be divided into early-onset and late-onset sepsis, according to when

TABLE 24.1 Common Infections in the Newborn*

Transmission	Effect on Newborn	Nursing Considerations
Viral Infections		
Cytomegalovirus		
Transplacental, during birth, in breast milk	Most asymptomatic at birth. SGA, FGR, enlarged liver, CNS abnormalities, jaundice, learning impairment, hearing loss, purpura, chorioretinitis, microcephaly, seizures. May have no signs for months or years.	Diagnosed by urine or pharyngeal culture. May shed virus in saliva and urine for months or years. Antiviral drug therapy may be used but has toxic effects and is not recommended routinely. Treatment supportive.
Hepatitis B		
Usually during birth through contact with maternal blood. Also transplacental and from breast milk	Asymptomatic at birth. LBW, prematurity. Most become chronic carriers. Risk for later liver cancer.	Wash well to remove all blood before skin is punctured for any reason. After cleaning, administer HBIG and hepatitis B vaccine to prevent infection. May breastfeed if infant receives vaccine and HBIG.
Herpes		
Usually during birth through infected vagina or ascending infection after rupture of membranes. Transplacental rarely. Transmission highest with primary infection	Clusters of vesicles, temperature instability, lethargy, poor suck, seizures, encephalitis, jaundice, purpura. Death or severe neurologic impairment is high with disseminated infection. High mortality rate if untreated.	Contact precautions. Obtain specimens of lesions for culture. Antiviral drugs given to mother during pregnancy and to infant after birth. May breastfeed if no lesions on the breasts.
Human Immunodeficiency Virus and Acquired Immunodeficiency Syndrome		
Transplacental, during birth from infected blood and secretions, or from breast milk. Transmission rate much lower if mother receives antiretroviral drugs during pregnancy and labor, and birth is by cesarean before rupture of membranes	Asymptomatic at birth; signs usually apparent at 12–24 mo. Enlarged liver and spleen, lymphadenopathy, failure to thrive, pneumonia, persistent *Candida* and bacterial infections, diarrhea, meningitis, septic joints.	Diagnosis may be delayed because of maternal antibodies. Some early tests available. Wash early to remove blood before skin is punctured. Treat with antiretroviral drugs and prophylaxis against other infections. Advise against breastfeeding.
Rubella		
Transplacental	Spontaneous abortion, asymptomatic or FGR, cataracts, cardiac defects, deafness, microcephaly, cognitive impairment. Injury greatest if infected in first trimester.	Contact precautions. Infant may shed virus for 1 year after birth. Diagnosed by presence of antibody and virus. Treatment supportive.
Varicella-Zoster Virus (Chickenpox)		
Transplacental	Congenital varicella syndrome (skin scarring, limb hypoplasia, CNS and eye abnormalities, death), rash. Highest incidence between 13 and 20 wk of gestation. Severe effects with maternal infection between 5 days before and 2 days after birth.	Varicella immune globulin for pregnant woman exposed in pregnancy or for infants of mothers infected just before or after delivery. It modifies but does not prevent infection. Acyclovir to treat. Strict isolation precautions for mothers and infants with lesions.
Other Infections		
Group B Streptococcal Infection		
During birth or ascending after rupture of membranes	Sudden onset of respiratory distress in infant usually well at birth, temperature instability, pneumonia, shock, meningitis. May have early or late onset.	Early identification essential to prevent death. Antibiotic treatment of infected mothers during labor has decreased neonatal infection. IV antibiotics given to infected infants.

TABLE 24.1 Common Infections in the Newborn*—cont'd

Transmission	Effect on Newborn	Nursing Considerations
Gonorrhea Usually during birth	Conjunctivitis (ophthalmia neonatorum), with red, edematous lids and purulent eye drainage. May result in blindness if untreated.	All infants receive prophylactic treatment. Erythromycin eye ointment is most common. Infected infants are treated with IV antibiotics.
Chlamydia During birth	Conjunctivitis 1–2 wk after birth, pneumonia at 4–11 wk, otitis media, bronchiolitis.	Treated with oral azithromycin or erythromycin. Topical treatment of conjunctivitis is not effective.
Candidiasis During birth	White patches in mouth (thrush) that bleed if removed. Rash on perineum. May be systemic in preterm or LBW.	Administer nystatin drops or cream and teach parents how to administer them. Assess mother for vaginal or breast infection. IV medications for systemic infection.
Toxoplasmosis Transplacental	Asymptomatic or FGR, LBW, preterm, thrombocytopenia, enlarged liver and spleen, jaundice, cerebral calcifications, encephalitis, seizures, microcephaly, hydrocephalus, chorioretinitis. Signs may not develop for years.	Consider in infants with FGR. Confirmed by serum tests. Treatment: Spiramycin during pregnancy, pyrimethamine, sulfadiazine, and folinic acid for 1 yr for infant.
Syphilis Transplacental	Asymptomatic or spontaneous abortion, stillbirth, enlarged liver and spleen, jaundice, hepatitis, anemia, rhinitis, pink or copper-colored peeling rash, pneumonitis, osteochondritis, CNS involvement.	Diagnosed by blood and CSF testing. Treated with penicillin.

*Standard precautions for infection control apply to all patients and are not listed in this table. *CNS,* Central nervous system; *CSF,* cerebrospinal fluid; *FGR,* fetal growth restriction; *HBIG,* hepatitis B immune globulin; *IV,* intravenous; *LBW,* low birth weight; *SGA* small-for-gestational-age.

signs of disease begin. Early-onset sepsis is acquired during birth, often from complications of labor such as prolonged rupture of membranes, prolonged labor, or chorioamnionitis (Triple I). Infants show signs within the first 3 days of life (Pammi, Brand, & Weisman, 2016). It is a rapidly progressive multisystem illness with high mortality and morbidity rates. Pneumonia and meningitis are commonly present.

Late-onset sepsis is most common after the first week of life (Pammi et al., 2016). It is acquired during or after birth, before or after hospital discharge. It usually is a localized infection such as meningitis, and serious long-term effects are common.

Therapeutic Management

Diagnostic Testing. Neonatal sepsis may be confused with other illnesses. For example, GBS pneumonia has the same initial symptoms as RDS. Diagnostic testing helps identify sepsis and the organisms responsible.

A CBC count with differential may show decreased total neutrophils, increased bands (a form of immature neutrophils), an increased ratio of immature neutrophils to total neutrophils, and decreased platelets. Elevated levels of leukocytes are normal in newborns. However, a sudden rise or fall in leukocyte levels compared with previous results is abnormal. The presence of elevated IgM levels in cord blood or shortly after birth indicates that infection was acquired in utero because this immunoglobulin does not cross the placenta. It often indicates transplacental infection.

The C-reactive protein (CRP) level, a sign of an inflammatory process, may be elevated. Serial tests of CRP are often performed to check for rise and then fall as infection improves. Cultures of blood, urine, any skin lesions, and cerebrospinal fluid may be obtained. Cultures of the nasopharynx, umbilical cord, and gastric aspirate usually show colonization with organisms but not infection. Chest radiography helps differentiate between RDS and sepsis. Blood glucose levels should be checked because they may be unstable (high or low) in sepsis.

Treatment. Infants who develop signs of infection are treated with broad-spectrum antibiotics, given intravenously, until culture and sensitivity results are available. Continued antibiotic therapy is based on culture results. Commonly used antibiotics include ampicillin, aminoglycoside, and cephalosporins. Vancomycin also may be used (Pammi et al., 2016).

Other care is supportive to meet the infant's specific needs. The infant may require oxygen or mechanical ventilation. Fluid balance maintenance and monitoring of the blood pressure and hourly urine output are important. Shock, hypoglycemia or hyperglycemia, electrolyte imbalances, and problems in temperature regulation are potential complications.

Nursing Considerations

Assessment

Risk Factors. The nurse should identify infants at risk for infection. Prematurity and low birth weight are the most important risk factors. Infants of mothers who have rupture of membranes longer than 12 to 18 hours also have an increased risk for infection. Other risk factors for sepsis include prolonged or precipitous labor, signs of maternal infection before or during labor, chorioamnionitis (also known as "Triple I"), and foul-smelling amniotic fluid (Wilson & Tyner, 2015). The nurse should identify women known to be GBS positive and those who show signs of infection so they can be treated with antibiotics during labor to reduce risk to the infant.

Every infant in the NICU is at risk for health care–associated infections. These infants have complications or conditions such as prematurity that make them more susceptible to infection. The risk for infection increases as gestational age and birth weight decrease. Preterm infants have not received maternal antibodies that help protect them from infection. In addition, they sometimes spend prolonged periods in the NICU, where they are exposed to many invasive procedures such as use of IV catheters and endotracheal tubes, which increase their risk for infection. NICU patients may develop abnormal flora that may be carried by personnel from one infant to another and may be resistant to usual drug therapy. Catheter-related bloodstream infections are a significant problem in NICUs (Taylor, McDonald, & Tan, 2015).

Signs of Infection. In the newborn, early signs of infection are not as specific or obvious as those in the older infant or child. Instead, they tend to be subtle and could indicate other conditions. Temperature instability may occur. Only 50% of infected newborns have an axillary temperature above 37.8°C (100°F) (Stoll & Shane, 2016).

Respiratory problems are common, and changes may occur in feeding habits or behavior. The nurse may identify the early, subtle changes in behavior that could indicate sepsis. Experienced nurses may have a feeling that the infant is not doing well even before specific signs of infection are present. When this occurs, the nurse expands the assessment and watches carefully for the development of other signs. Early identification and treatment are important because infants can develop septic shock with little warning.

CRITICAL TO REMEMBER
Signs of Sepsis in the Newborn

General Signs
Temperature instability (usually low)
Nurse's or parents' feeling that the infant is not doing well
Rash

Respiratory Signs
Tachypnea
Respiratory distress (nasal flaring, retractions, grunting)
Apnea

Cardiovascular Signs
Color changes (cyanosis, pallor, mottling)
Tachycardia
Hypotension
Decreased peripheral perfusion
Edema

Gastrointestinal Signs
Decreased oral intake
Vomiting
Excessive gastric residuals
Diarrhea
Abdominal distention
Hypoglycemia or hyperglycemia

Neurologic Signs
Decreased or increased muscle tone
Lethargy
Jitteriness
Irritability
Full fontanel
High-pitched cry

Signs That May Indicate Advanced Infection
Jaundice
Evidence of hemorrhage (petechiae, purpura, pulmonary bleeding)
Anemia
Enlarged liver and spleen
Respiratory failure
Shock
Seizures

Nursing Interventions

Preventing Infection. Although it is not always possible to prevent infection, every effort should be made. Careful and frequent hand hygiene is the most important aspect of infection prevention. The nurse should practice and teach parents to perform good handwashing or to use hospital-provided hand disinfectants before and after touching any infant. Equipment should be disinfected according to hospital protocols. Meticulous sterile technique should be used during invasive procedures. Invasive procedures should be kept to the lowest number possible.

The skin is delicate in the newborn, particularly so in preterm infants. Handling and trauma to the skin should be minimized as much as possible to prevent skin breakdown and infection.

Precautions should be taken to avoid transmission of infection to other infants. This is accomplished with hand hygiene, separation of each infant's supplies, and standard precautions for infection control. These techniques should be conscientiously performed by all who come in contact with the infant. Parents should be taught about all infection control measures so that they can help protect their infants.

Placing the infant in an incubator provides a physical separation between infected and well infants, similar to placing adults in isolation in private rooms. In addition, the nurse can observe the infant in an incubator more easily.

Providing Antibiotics. The nurse is responsible for obtaining or helping obtain specimens for laboratory analysis and checking that other tests ordered by the provider are completed. Laboratory tests will help determine the type and duration of antibiotics prescribed.

Because the signs of infection are nonspecific and the disease can be fatal, physicians may order antibiotics before an actual diagnosis is made for infants who are at high risk or show early signs. Broad-spectrum IV antibiotics are given after samples for culture and sensitivity are taken and before the results are available. Continued antibiotic therapy is specific to organisms found on culture. The nurse should be knowledgeable about the antibiotics used and possible side effects.

The nurse starts IV fluids and ensures that medications are administered as scheduled. If more than one antibiotic is ordered, the timing of administration should be coordinated to increase effectiveness. Antibiotics usually are continued for 10 to 14 days for sepsis and 21 days for meningitis (Wilson & Tyner, 2015).

Providing Other Supportive Care. Infants may be critically ill and need intensive nursing care. Care includes giving oxygen or other respiratory support, as needed. Fluid balance maintenance, monitoring of vital signs, and hourly urine output measurements are important. IV or gavage feeding may be necessary if the infant is unable to take oral feedings.

Infants with sepsis may have additional problems. They may be premature or have other transplacentally acquired infections. In addition, the nurse should be alert for signs of complications such as disseminated intravascular coagulopathy (DIC).

Supporting Parents. Nurses provide support to parents of newborns with sepsis and help them understand their infant's illness and treatment. The infant with sepsis often appears healthy at birth but suddenly becomes critically ill. Parents experience feelings of shock, fear, and disappointment when their apparently healthy newborn is suddenly moved to the NICU or the preterm infant they thought was making good progress may suddenly develop a life-threatening illness. Parents benefit from a chance to talk about their feelings with an understanding nurse who can explain the infant's treatment and care. Keeping the parents informed and involving them in care are essential.

INFANT OF A DIABETIC MOTHER

Scope of the Problem

The infant of a diabetic mother (IDM) faces many risks that depend on the type of diabetes the mother has and how well it is controlled. The neonatal mortality rate is greater than five times that of infants born to mothers without diabetes, and congenital anomalies are three times more likely in IDMs (Carlo & Ambalavanan, 2016). Cardiac, urinary tract, and gastrointestinal anomalies, neural tube anomalies, and sacral agenesis are most frequent. Cardiomegaly is common and may lead to heart failure. The incidence of anomalies is decreased with good control of diabetes before conception and during the early weeks of gestation when fetal organs are being formed. It is not increased in women with gestational diabetes (Blickstein, Perlman, Hazan, Topf-Olivestone, & Shinwell, 2015).

Insulin acts as a growth hormone. The accelerated protein synthesis and the deposit of fat and glycogen in fetal tissues result in macrosomia (Fig. 24.3). Strict control of the mother's blood glucose level, especially during the third trimester, reduces the risk for macrosomia (Blickstein et al., 2015). Infants with macrosomia are at risk for trauma during birth, including fracture of the clavicles from shoulder dystocia, cephalohematoma, and facial nerve and brachial plexus injury.

When the mother is hyperglycemic, large amounts of amino acids, free fatty acids, and glucose are transferred to the fetus. Insulin does not cross the placenta because the molecules are too large. The excessive glucose received by the fetus causes the fetal pancreas to secrete large amounts of insulin and leads to hypertrophy of the islet cells. Hypoglycemia may occur after birth when the supply of glucose from the mother is no longer available but the infant's high insulin production continues.

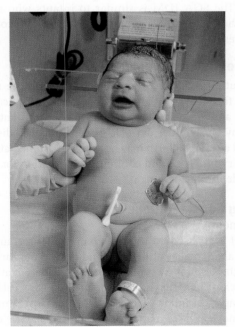

FIG. 24.3 Macrosomia is common in infants of mothers with diabetes.

Infants of mothers with long-term diabetes and vascular changes may have fetal growth restriction (FGR), which is also known as intrauterine growth restriction (IUGR), instead of macrosomia because of decreased placental blood flow. Hypertension occurs more often in women with diabetes and further compromises uteroplacental blood flow.

The IDM has a higher risk for asphyxia and RDS. RDS occurs because increased levels of insulin block the effect of cortisol on stimulation of lung maturation (Devaskar & Garg, 2015). Other complications for which the IDM is at risk include hypocalcemia as a result of decreased parathyroid hormone production. Magnesium levels may also be low.

Polycythemia may occur as a response to chronic hypoxia in utero. It may cause hyperbilirubinemia when the large number of RBCs break down after birth. In addition, IDMs are more likely to be born prematurely.

Characteristics of Infants of Diabetic Mothers

The IDM with macrosomia is different from other large-for-gestational-age (LGA) infants. The infant's size results from fat deposits and hypertrophy of the liver, spleen, and heart. The brain and kidneys are normal in size (Devaskar & Garg, 2015). The length and head circumference are also generally within the normal range for gestational age. Other LGA infants do not have enlargement of the organs and tend to be long, with large heads to match the rest of their bodies. IDMs have a characteristic appearance. The face is round, the skin is often red (plethoric), and the body is obese. The infant has poor muscle tone at rest but becomes irritable and may have tremors when disturbed. The SGA IDM is similar to infants who are SGA from other causes but is more likely to have congenital anomalies.

Therapeutic Management

Therapeutic management includes controlling the mother's diabetes throughout pregnancy to decrease complications in the fetus and newborn (see Chapter 10). If the infant is large, there may be shoulder dystocia or cephalopelvic disproportion, and a cesarean birth may be required. Immediate care of respiratory problems and continued observation for complications determine treatment.

Nursing Considerations
Assessment

The IDM is assessed for signs of complications, trauma, and congenital anomalies at delivery and during the early hours after birth. Respiratory problems may be apparent at birth or may develop later. The initial assessment may reveal injuries. For example, an infant who cries when an arm is moved or fails to move an arm may have a fractured clavicle or nerve injury.

Hypoglycemia occurs in 25% to 50% of infants of mothers with pregestational diabetes and 15% to 25% of those with gestational diabetes (Carlo & Ambalavanan, 2016).

It may be present without observable signs. The most frequent sign of low blood glucose is jitteriness or tremors. Diaphoresis is uncommon in newborns but may occur with hypoglycemia. Rapid respirations, low temperature, and poor muscle tone are also common. Because these signs are not specific for hypoglycemia, the nurse should be alert for other complications, particularly if signs continue after feeding.

Nursing Interventions

The nurse assesses glucose levels according to hospital policy. Because these infants are at risk for hypoglycemia, they should have a blood glucose screen done shortly after birth and be monitored more frequently than other infants. Glucose levels reach the lowest point at 1 to 3 hours after birth and begin to improve by 4 to 6 hours. Glucose levels of less than 40 to 45 mg/dL measured with a bedside glucometer should be reported and verified by laboratory analysis (Carlo & Ambalavanan, 2016). Infants should be fed early to prevent hypoglycemia and immediately if low blood glucose occurs to prevent further decreases. Gavage feeding may be used if the infant does not suck well or if respirations are rapid. The glucose level is rechecked in 30 to 45 minutes. Infants whose glucose levels are not maintained with feedings or whose condition does not allow enteral feedings need IV glucose to maintain glucose balance and prevent injury to the brain.

The nurse should be alert for signs of other complications that occur in IDMs. RDS or other respiratory complications may develop. Cold stress, which increases the need for oxygen and glucose, could increase respiratory problems and exacerbate hypoglycemia. Infants with polycythemia need adequate hydration to prevent sluggish blood flow to vital organs and ischemia. Hypocalcemia may be suspected if tremors continue and the blood glucose concentration is normal.

Providing support to parents is important. Greater than one-third of IDMs may have neurologic or developmental complications (Rozance, McGowan, Price-Douglas, & Hay, 2016). The nurse should work with the infant and the parents to ensure feedings are adequate. Parents may have many questions for the nurse. They may not understand why their infant, who appears fat and healthy to them, needs close observation and frequent blood tests. The mother may have had a difficult pregnancy and may feel guilty, even if she followed a program of good diabetic control. Ample opportunity for discussion of feelings as well as information about the care of the infant is important.

? KNOWLEDGE CHECK

8. What is the role of the nurse in caring for the infant with sepsis?
9. Why are IDMs more likely to develop macrosomia?
10. Why are IDMs at risk for hypoglycemia after birth?

POLYCYTHEMIA

In polycythemia, infants have a venous hematocrit greater than 65% (Gallagher, 2015). The increased viscosity of the blood causes resistance in the blood vessels and decreases blood flow. Blood flow to all organs is impaired. Organ damage from ischemia and venous thrombosis may result along with neurologic and developmental problems (Diehl-Jones & Fraser, 2015). Polycythemia also may result in hyperbilirubinemia as the excessive RBCs break down after birth.

Causes

Polycythemia may occur when poor intrauterine oxygenation causes the fetus to compensate by producing more erythrocytes than normal. It is more common in infants who are postterm, LGA, or SGA or have FGR. It also occurs in infants of mothers who smoke or have hypertension or diabetes. Delayed cord clamping or a transfusion from one twin to another also may cause the condition.

Manifestations

Most infants have minimal or no signs of polycythemia. Symptomatic infants may have a plethoric color, lethargy, irritability, poor tone, and tremors. Abdominal distention, decreased bowel sounds, poor feeding, hypoglycemia, and respiratory distress also may be present. Hyperbilirubinemia occurs as RBCs are broken down.

Therapeutic Management

Treatment is primarily supportive. Infants who are asymptomatic are observed and receive increased hydration. A partial exchange transfusion may be performed if the hematocrit is above 70% to 75% in asymptomatic infants and 65% in infants with symptoms (Gallagher, 2015). Blood is replaced with normal saline to decrease the total number of RBCs. Phototherapy is used to treat the jaundice.

Nursing Considerations

Monitoring of bilirubin levels is important to determine whether phototherapy is necessary. Infants should be hydrated adequately to prevent dehydration that would slow already sluggish blood flow and increase ischemia to vital organs. If an exchange transfusion is performed, the nurse assists and watches for complications.

HYPOCALCEMIA

Hypocalcemia is a total serum calcium concentration of less than 7 mg/dL. It is divided into early-onset (in the first 72 hours of age) and late-onset (1 week of age) forms (Nyp, Brunkhorst, Reavey, & Pallotto, 2016).

Causes

Early-onset hypocalcemia occurs most often in IDMs and in infants with asphyxia, prematurity, and delayed nutrition. Late-onset hypocalcemia is caused by hypoparathyroidism, malabsorption, low magnesium levels, extensive diuretic therapy, and rickets (Nyp et al., 2016).

Manifestations

Signs of hypocalcemia include irritability, jitteriness, poor feeding, high-pitched cry, muscle twitching, apnea, seizures, and electrocardiographic changes. It is often asymptomatic.

Therapeutic Management

Laboratory testing of serum calcium level determines the presence of the problem. IV calcium gluconate is given if feeding alone does not raise the calcium level. A cardiac monitor is necessary when IV calcium is given because bradycardia can occur.

Nursing Considerations

The nurse should be alert for signs of hypocalcemia. IV calcium should be administered slowly and stopped immediately if bradycardia or dysrhythmia develops. The IV site should be assessed frequently because infiltration can cause necrosis and ulceration.

PRENATAL DRUG EXPOSURE

Substance abuse affects the fetus at any time during pregnancy. Most drugs readily cross the placenta and cause a variety of problems. The effects of substance abuse on pregnancy, the fetus, and the neonate are discussed in Chapter 11. This section includes nursing care for infants with **neonatal abstinence syndrome (NAS)**, a disorder in which infants exposed to maternal drugs before birth demonstrate signs of drug withdrawal.

Identification of Drug-Exposed Infants

Maternal substance abuse may be identified before an infant is born, but some infants are born to women whose substance use is not known to the health care professionals caring for them. A history of minimal or no prenatal care or the mother's behavior during labor may cause nurses to suspect substance abuse. When there is any reason to suspect drug use, the infant is observed closely for signs of prenatal drug exposure.

NAS occurs in infants who have suffered prenatal opiate exposure sufficient to cause withdrawal signs after birth. Women who use heroin are generally switched to methadone or buprenorphine during pregnancy to decrease the incidence of wide variations in the drug dosage, which is harmful to the fetus. These women usually receive better prenatal care, and their infants have a higher birth weight than those exposed to heroin. However, infants may still undergo withdrawal after birth.

NAS is also seen in some infants exposed to other drugs such as amphetamines and antidepressants. Methamphetamine exposure results in lethargy, irritability, high-pitched cry, and hypertonicity in infants.

SSRIs and other antidepressants taken during pregnancy also result in NAS behaviors (Wiener & Finnegan, 2016). Signs of drug exposure usually begin during the first 24 to 72 hours after birth but may not occur for up to 2 weeks depending on the specific drug, the dose, and the time of the mother's last use (Wiener & Finnegan, 2016). Use near the time of delivery causes a later onset but more severe signs of withdrawal.

NURSING PROCEDURE 24.1 Applying a Pediatric Urine Collection Bag

PURPOSE: To collect a nonsterile urine specimen from an infant.

1. Wash hands and obtain needed equipment. Include pediatric urine collector, washcloth and towel, diaper, sterile specimen cup, and clean gloves. *Gathering equipment allows the procedure to be completed efficiently.*

2. Apply gloves. Wash and dry the genitalia. Dry the skin completely. *Removal of gross contaminants prevents contamination of the specimen. The bag adheres to a clean, dry surface best.*

3. Remove the paper covering on the posterior adhesive tabs of the bag first. To apply to female infants, gently hold the skin taut at the perineum. Fold the bag in half and apply smoothly over the perineum, extending the tabs to the side. For male infants, place the penis and scrotum (if small enough) inside the bag and apply the posterior adhesive tabs to the perineum. If the scrotum will not fit in the bag easily, apply the tabs smoothly over the scrotum. *Covering the perineum with the posterior tabs first helps ensure a smooth fit at this area, where leakage of urine may occur in the female infant especially, and prevents contamination with feces. Care in application prevents losing the specimen.*

4. Remove the paper covering on the anterior adhesive tabs, and apply to cover the genitalia. Be sure that there are no wrinkles in the tabs. *Wrinkles allow openings for urine to leak out of the bag.*

5. Cut a slit in the diaper, and gently pull the bag through the slit. Apply the diaper loosely. *Cutting a slit in the diaper allows visualization of the bag. Placing the diaper too tightly over the bag might pull against the adhesive, causing trauma to the skin and providing an opening through which the specimen is lost.*

6. Check the bag for urine frequently and gently remove the bag as soon as urine is present. Transfer the urine to a specimen cup by removing the tab over the hole in the bottom and pouring. The specimen also can be aspirated with a syringe after cleaning the puncture site with alcohol. *This step ensures removal of the bag before urine loosens the adhesive and prepares the specimen to be sent to the laboratory for analysis.*

7. Clean the genitalia and observe for irritation. *This removes urine and adhesive from the skin.*

8. Place the specimen in a biohazard bag and label it. Transport the specimen to the laboratory or refrigerate it, if necessary. Record the date and time of urine collection, and the amount, color, and appearance of urine in the infant's chart. *This ensures proper disposition of the specimen.*

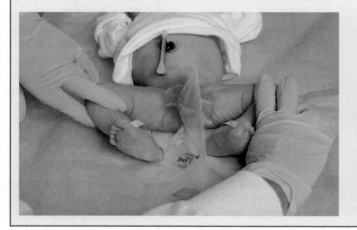 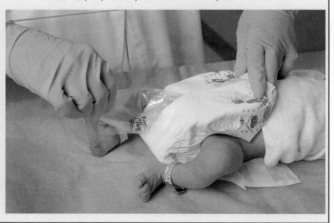

Polydrug use along with use of alcohol and cigarettes is common. This makes it difficult to determine which substance led to individual effects. Signs differ according to the drug or combination of drugs used but often include neurologic and GI abnormalities. Some infants with prenatal drug exposure show no abnormal signs at all.

Infants with NAS may be irritable and have hyperactive muscle tone and a high-pitched cry. Although they have tremors, the blood glucose level is normal. Infants appear hungry and suck vigorously on their fists but have poor coordination of suck and swallow. Frequent regurgitation, vomiting, and diarrhea are common. Infants are restless, and their excessive activity coupled with poor feeding ability results in failure to gain weight. Seizures may occur.

Various scoring systems are available to determine the number, frequency, and severity of behaviors that indicate NAS. The score is used when considering whether drug therapy to alleviate withdrawal signs is needed and to determine dosage. Behaviors are generally scored every 2 to 4 hours until low scores are obtained consistently. It is important that all nurses are able to use the scoring tool consistently to provide for optimal treatment of the infant.

Congenital anomalies and other effects of prenatal drug exposure may be apparent at birth. FGR and prematurity are common. Infants are more likely to have respiratory problems at birth, jaundice, or sudden infant death syndrome. Infants with fetal alcohol syndrome have a characteristic appearance.

When drug exposure is suspected, a urine specimen is collected for analysis. Drugs or their metabolites are present in the newborn's urine for various lengths of time after the mother has used them. Some drugs last several days because the infant's immature liver and kidneys delay excreting them, whereas others disappear very soon. Therefore it is important to obtain the first urine output from the infant, if possible (Procedure 24.1). Meconium analysis may detect drug exposure as far back as the second trimester (Sherman, 2015). A hair sample or a segment of umbilical cord is tested in some facilities.

EVIDENCE-BASED PRACTICE

Nurses who care for infants with neonatal abstinence syndrome (NAS) face multiple challenges in caring for the infants and their families. Murphy-Oikomen, Brownlee, Montelpare, and Gerlachet al. conducted a qualitative study to learn about the experiences of nurses dealing with these families in the neonatal intensive care unit (NICU). They asked open-ended questions of 14 nurses using computer-assisted confidential interviews. The questions asked about what caring for babies with NAS had been like for the nurses, what their experiences with the families had been, how these experiences affected their lives outside of work, and what suggestions they would make to improve nurses' experiences caring for these infants.

The results showed that nurses had a strong commitment to caring for infants. Although they expected to use their advanced skills as NICU nurses most of the time, they found that caring for NAS infants was demanding in different ways. The infants were often inconsolable, difficult to feed, and required much time that interfered with their ability to care for other infants. The nurses felt a disconnect between their expectations and those of families. They had difficulty feeling empathy for mothers who would continue to be addicted to drugs and worried about what life would be like for the infants after discharge. They felt stressed, frustrated, and burned out by caring for NAS infants. They also had an increased awareness of the problems of drug use in their community.

The authors concluded that nurses who care for infants with NAS need more education and specialized training about addictions to better understand the difficulties of addicted mothers and how to deal with them. Nurses also need support within their organization that recognizes the strain of caring for NAS infants. Scheduling that allows nurses to take breaks from caring for these difficult infants may lessen the frustration and increase positive nurse-family interaction.

Ask nurses in your facility about their experiences with caring for infants with NAS. What education and training do they need to provide evidence-based care to infants with NAS?

Reference
Murphy-Oikonen, J., Brownlee, K., Montelpare, W., & Gerlach, K., et al. (2010). The experiences of NICU nurses in caring for infants with neonatal abstinence syndrome. *Neonatal Network, 29*(5), 307–312.

CRITICAL TO REMEMBER
Signs of Intrauterine Drug Exposure*

Behavioral Signs
  Irritability
  Jitteriness, tremors, seizures
  Muscular rigidity, increased muscle tone
  Restless, excessive activity
  Exaggerated Moro reflex
  Prolonged high-pitched cry
  Difficult to console
  Poor sleeping patterns
  Yawning

Signs Relating to Feeding
  Exaggerated rooting reflex
  Excessive sucking
  Uncoordinated sucking and swallowing

  Frequent regurgitation or vomiting
  Diarrhea
  Weight loss

Cardiovascular and Respiratory Signs
  Nasal stuffiness, sneezing
  Tachypnea, apnea
  Retractions
  Tachycardia

Other Signs
  Hypertension
  Fever
  Diaphoresis
  Excoriation
  Mottling

*Some infants with prenatal drug exposure have no abnormal signs at all, or signs may be delayed.

Therapeutic Management

Because many signs of drug exposure are similar to those for other conditions, testing may be performed to rule out other causes. Sepsis, hypoglycemia, hypocalcemia, and neurologic disorders are possible causes for the infant's problems. In addition, the infant may have been exposed to infections from the mother, such as hepatitis or sexually transmitted diseases.

Therapeutic management includes dealing with the complications common to drug-exposed infants during and after birth. Respiratory problems and those related to prematurity are treated as for other infants. Drug therapy may be necessary for approximately 50% to 60% of infants because of high scores on abstinence scales (Weiner & Finnegan, 2016). Medications commonly used include oral morphine and methadone. Phenobarbital may be used for polydrug exposure. Buprenorphine and clonidine also have been used, but further studies are needed (Kraft, Stover & Davis, 2016). Medication dosage is gradually tapered until the infant no longer needs it. Although these drugs help relieve the signs of withdrawal, all have side effects that may be undesirable.

Because the infant's suck and swallow are uncoordinated, gavage or IV feeding may be required. Some infants need more than the normal caloric requirements because of their excessive activity. The specific calories needed for each infant will be prescribed by the health care provider.

Involvement by social services in and out of the hospital is important to deal with the long-term effects of the drugs, placement of the infant after hospitalization, and follow-up of the mother or other caregiver to help provide for the infant's needs.

Nursing Considerations

The infant who has been exposed to drugs prenatally needs special care to cope with drug withdrawal. Care is focused on minimizing withdrawal symptoms, encouraging feeding, promoting rest, and, if possible, enhancing parental attachment.

Feeding

Feeding can be difficult and time consuming. The poor suck and swallow coordination of drug-exposed infants interferes with caloric intake, yet their excessive activity increases their caloric needs.

Assessment. Infants often suck frantically on their fists or a nipple but are unable to coordinate feeding behaviors well. The nurse should assess the infant's ability to suck and swallow with breathing. Changes in the frequency and amount of regurgitation, vomiting, or the length of time it takes infants to finish feedings should be noted.

Nursing Interventions. Gavage feedings may be necessary to conserve the infant's energy and prevent aspiration if the infant is excessively agitated, is unable to suck and swallow adequately, or has rapid respirations. The infant's excessive activity, poor sleeping, vomiting, and diarrhea increase the caloric need. The infant may need as many as 150 to 250 calories per kilogram (cal/kg) each day (Sherman, 2015). Formula with 24 calories or more per ounce instead of the usual 20 calories per ounce may be used. More frequent feedings may be needed, as well.

Distractions during feedings can be prevented by choosing a quiet, low-activity area of the nursery for feedings. Infants should be swaddled to prevent the startling that occurs when drug-exposed infants are handled. Stimuli such as rocking and talking should be kept to a minimum during feedings. After feedings, infants should be positioned on the right side with the head of the bed elevated 30 to 45 degrees. Some infants respond better to the prone position. If possible, the infant should be positioned in the supine position for sleep.

Rest

The excessive activity and poor sleep patterns of drug-exposed neonates interfere with their ability to rest.

Assessment. The infant's muscle tone, tremors, and tendency for excessive activity with and without being disturbed should be assessed. The degree of tremors and stimuli that increase or decrease irritability are important. The nurse also keeps track of the number of hours the infant sleeps after each feeding.

Nursing Interventions. Keep stimulation of the drug-exposed infant to a minimum, especially at first when the infant is excessively irritable. Position the crib in the quietest area of the nursery or, ideally, a private room. Place a sign nearby to remind others of the need for quiet near the infant. The number of different types of stimulation should be kept to a minimum and adapted to each infant's needs. Reduce noise and bright lights as much as possible. If the infant shows signs of overstimulation, stop all activity briefly to allow a rest.

Swaddling the infant in a flexed position helps prevent startling and agitation. Placing the excessively agitated infant

in a dark, quiet room may be necessary. As the infant shows the ability to withstand stimulation, add new types of stimuli gradually, one at a time. Some infants respond well to soft music, which has the added advantage of masking other environmental sounds.

Organize nursing care to reduce handling and disturbances. Cluster care activities to avoid unnecessary interruptions, yet provide rest periods if signs of stress occur. A calm approach and slow, smooth movements during care help avoid startling the infant. A pacifier for nonnutritive sucking also helps quiet the infant.

Skin abrasions from excessive activity and rubbing of the face, elbows, and knees may increase discomfort and agitation. Cover the infant's hands with mittens or the end of the shirtsleeves to help prevent facial scratching. Diaper rash from frequent diarrhea also may occur. Skin breakdown should be prevented, if possible, and treated promptly if it occurs. Placing the infant in the prone position promotes better sleep for some infants, but supine positioning should be used as soon as possible.

Bonding

When maternal drug use is known or suspected, many hospitals require a 3- to 5-day observation period to monitor for appearance of withdrawal symptoms. If the infant is transferred to another unit for observation and the mother is discharged from the hospital without her baby, bonding is jeopardized. Many mothers do not understand the need for this observation period because they mistakenly think that if they are using prescription medication, or switched from heroin to methadone or buprenorphine, their infant will not suffer from withdrawal.

When an infant tests positive for drugs, child protective services become involved. The infant may not be released to the mother until her ability to care for her infant safely has been assessed by social services or a court. She may be required to enter a drug rehabilitation program before she can obtain custody of the infant. After hospital discharge, the infant may be cared for by family members approved by the court, in a foster home, or in an institution. The mother will most likely gain custody of the infant eventually if she complies with court-ordered treatment, and attachment to the infant should be encouraged.

Assessment. The frequency of the mother's visits and her response to the infant may give an indication of her apparent interest in the infant. Although some substance-abusing mothers are uninterested in their infants, for others the infant provides a reason to attempt to overcome their addiction. Bonding behaviors such as calling the infant by name and smiling at the infant should be noted.

Nursing Interventions. Child neglect, abuse, and failure to respond appropriately to infant signals and cues are associated with alcohol and drug abuse. Because the mother may become the infant's primary caregiver, it is essential that nurses do whatever they can to enhance mother–infant bonding. Helping the mother feel welcome when she visits the infant poses a challenge. It is sometimes easy to be judgmental and difficult to be accepting of the mother whose behavior has been harmful to her infant. Yet a friendly approach will make the mother more likely to visit the infant and accept teaching from the nurse.

Promote bonding by encouraging mothers to participate actively in infant care during visits. If the mother thinks the nurses trust her to care for the infant, her confidence may increase. This may encourage her efforts to go through rehabilitation to regain custody of her newborn.

The mother's participation also provides a chance to assess her infant care skills and areas in which further discussion of the newborn's needs will be helpful. In addition, it gives the nurse an opportunity to demonstrate parenting skills. Many mothers who use drugs have not had good parenting role models and do not know how to care for an infant. Frequent positive feedback about the mother's participation is also important.

Provide the mother the same teaching given to all new parents, as well as special techniques necessary to meet the needs of drug-exposed infants. Teach her about her newborn's unique characteristics and help her assume more of the infant's care as she demonstrates readiness.

Teach the mother that infants are easily overstimulated. These infants cannot tolerate simultaneous visual and tactile stimulation. Signs of overstimulation in drug-exposed infants have some similarities with those for the preterm infant. In addition, some infants cannot tolerate more than brief periods of interaction. They may not make eye contact, or they may avert their eyes after 30 to 60 seconds of social interaction. Cuddling and soothing to console the infant may not elicit the same response in these infants as in other infants. Teach the mother that the infant responds poorly to everyone, so she does not think that only she is being rejected.

Parents of a drug-exposed infant may experience feelings of rejection, frustration, and even hostility when the infant stiffens while being held, cries after being fed, or looks away. Explain that drug-exposed infants are easily stressed because of the decreased stability of their CNS. Emphasize that the infant needs gentle handling. Also explain that crying indicates a need, not a spoiled infant.

Show the mother comfort measures that work best for her infant. These infants are often comforted when they are snugly swaddled in a flexed position with their hands brought to midline. Holding the swaddled infant close to the mother's body may increase comfort. Some infants are consoled with slow, rhythmic, vertical or horizontal rocking movements. Placing them in a front pack as the nurse or mother moves around may also be comforting.

When the infant is nearing discharge explain that sleep problems will probably continue at home. The infant should sleep in a quiet room because normal household noises will disturb the drug-exposed infant more than other infants (Weiner & Finnegan, 2016).

Cocaine, amphetamines, heroin, and other drugs pass into breast milk. Trying to breastfeed an infant with poorly developed feeding skills may be too much stress for the mother who is trying to recover from addiction. Therefore mothers who are likely to continue drug use after delivery should be discouraged from breastfeeding.

Women taking methadone may be allowed to breastfeed if they are not taking other drugs that are contraindicated. Methadone and buprenorphine have been found to be at very low levels in breast milk and may result in lower pharmacologic treatment doses and duration (Wiener & Finnegan, 2016). Breastfeeding assistance should be given to women who are interested because of the advantages of breast milk over formula and because it may help the mother with bonding.

Provide information and referral to any special programs available to help parents learn stimulation techniques appropriate for drug-exposed infants. Some withdrawal signs may continue for 4 to 6 months, and the mother needs to know how to cope with them (Weiner & Finnegan, 2016). If the mother is unable or not allowed to care for the newborn after discharge, the same interventions can be used to help the person who will take over care of the infant.

PATIENT TEACHING

Measures to Prevent Frantic Crying in a Drug-Exposed Infant

Swaddle the infant with the hands brought to the midline.
Provide a pacifier.
Slowly and smoothly rock in a vertical or horizontal motion with the infant held upright.
Coo softly and gently.
Place the infant over your shoulder, and gently stroke the back.
Keep the room fairly dark because some infants are particularly sensitive to light.
Avoid simultaneous auditory and visual stimuli.
Curtail stimulation if the infant shows signs of stress (yawning, sneezing, jerky movements, or spitting up).

 ### KNOWLEDGE CHECK

11. How can the nurse deal with the inability to rest in infants with prenatal exposure to drugs?
12. How can the nurse promote bonding when there has been prenatal drug abuse?

PHENYLKETONURIA

Phenylketonuria (PKU) is a genetic disorder that causes CNS injury from toxic levels of the amino acid phenylalanine in blood. The incidence is 1 in 10,000 (Zinn, 2015). Severe cognitive impairment occurs in untreated infants and children. In the United States all newborns are screened for this condition before or shortly after discharge from the birth facility. Positive screening tests are followed by other testing to confirm the diagnosis.

Causes

PKU is caused by a deficiency of the liver enzyme phenylalanine hydrolase, which is necessary to convert phenylalanine to tyrosine for use. It is an autosomal recessive disorder.

Manifestations

Signs of untreated disease may begin with digestive problems and vomiting and later progress to seizures, musty odor of the urine, and severe cognitive impairment. Older children have eczema, hypertonia, hyperactive behavior, cognitive impairment, and hypopigmentation of the hair, skin, and irises.

Therapeutic Management

Treatment is a low-phenylalanine diet that should start immediately after the diagnosis is made and continue throughout life to avoid irreversible neurologic damage (Rezvani & Ficicioglu, 2016). Women with PKU who are not following the diet closely need to return to it before they conceive and throughout pregnancy to prevent abnormalities in the fetus. Infants with PKU receive a special formula low in phenylalanine, and low-protein foods are introduced when solids are started. Small amounts of phenylalanine are allowed because it is a necessary amino acid. Early and continued treatment is necessary to prevent or minimize cognitive impairment.

Nursing Considerations

The nurse should be sure that all newborns are screened for PKU at the appropriate time in the birth facility. Screening performed before 24 hours of age should be repeated because the infant may not yet have consumed enough protein for the test to be accurate.

The nurse assists parents in regulating the diet to meet the infant's changing phenylalanine needs. Parents may need to talk about their feelings regarding the difficulty of following the diet for their children. They can be reassured that good control helps avoid long-term neurologic problems. However, mild decrease in intelligence and behavioral difficulties may occur (Zinn, 2015).

CONGENITAL ANOMALIES

Approximately 2% of newborns have a major malformation at birth (Parikh & Mitchell, 2015). Congenital anomalies are the leading cause of deaths in the first year of life. Some infants have more than one anomaly, which may be part of a syndrome or result from unrelated causes. Although congenital anomalies generally are treated in the pediatric setting, they are often identified soon after birth. Common congenital anomalies are noted in Box 24.1. Congenital cardiac conditions are discussed in this section. (See a pediatric nursing textbook for more detailed information.)

BOX 24.1   Common Congenital Anomalies

Gastrointestinal Tract

Cleft Lip and Palate

These are among the most common congenital anomalies. They occur together or separately on one or both sides.

  Lip—Minor notching of the lip or complete separation through the lip and into floor of nose.

  Palate—Only the soft palate or division of the entire hard and soft palate. Both genetic and environmental factors are included in the causes.

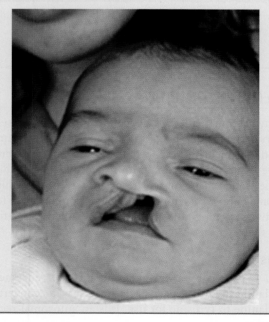

Assessment

Severe clefts are obvious at birth.

Palpate the hard and soft palate of all neonates during initial assessment.

Therapeutic Management

Lip surgery is usually performed by 3 months to enhance appearance and parental bonding.

Further surgery may be needed at 4 to 5 years.

Palate surgery is usually done by 1 year to minimize speech problems.

Long-term follow-up is necessary for orthodontia, speech therapy, and treatment of possible hearing problems.

Nursing Considerations

The degree of the cleft determines the approach to feeding.

Experiment to find methods that work best for individual infants. Try:

  1. Breastfeeding (soft breast tissue fills in a small cleft of the lip or palate)
  2. Nipples with enlarged hole
  3. Compressible bottles
  4. Special longer nipples
  5. Special assistive devices

Feed the infant in the upright position because milk enters nasal passages through the palate, causing an increased tendency to aspirate.

Feed slowly with frequent stops to burp because infants tend to swallow excessive air.

Wash away milk curds with water after feeding.

BOX 24.1   Common Congenital Anomalies—cont'd

Help the parents deal with their disappointment over the infant with an obvious anomaly. Show them before and after pictures of plastic surgery.

Reinforce the physician's explanation of plans for surgery.

Teach parents feeding techniques. Let them observe at first, then then take over gradually.

Prevent infections. Infants are especially susceptible to respiratory tract and ear infections, which can delay surgery. Ear infections may lead to hearing loss.

Emphasize the need for long-term follow-up. Refer to agencies that help with the expense of long-term care and to support groups for help and emotional support from other parents.

Esophageal Atresia and Tracheoesophageal Fistula

In **esophageal atresia (EA)** the esophagus is most commonly divided into two unconnected segments (atresia) with a blind pouch at the proximal end. If the distal end is connected to the trachea, it causes **tracheoesophageal fistula (TEF)**. The cause is a failure of normal development during the fourth week of pregnancy.

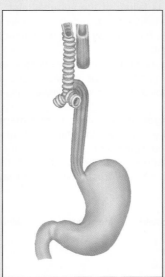

Assessment

Watch for EA when polyhydramnios occurs because the excessive fluid may be caused by fetal inability to swallow amniotic fluid.

Observe for other defects that may occur.

Signs vary by the type of defect.

Suspect EA in infants with excessive frothy drooling and needing suction more often than usual, when regurgitation occurs from secretions that pool in a blind pouch, and when a catheter will not pass into the stomach.

If a fistula connects the distal esophagus and the trachea, the stomach becomes distended with air from the trachea. Gastric secretions may be aspirated into the lungs, causing a severe inflammatory reaction.

Therapeutic Management

Diagnosis is confirmed by symptoms and radiography.

Esophageal suctioning should be used for the upper pouch, and a gastrostomy tube is placed.

Surgery involves ligation of the fistula and anastomosis of the esophageal segments. If the separation is large, surgery may be done in stages to allow growth.

Long-term follow-up is needed for esophageal reflux and dilation of strictures that may form at the surgical site.

Nursing Considerations

Observe all infants carefully during the first feeding for respiratory difficulty or other signs.

Prevent aspiration by maintaining the infant in a semiupright position to prevent reflux of gastric fluids.

Maintain suction equipment.

Care after surgery involves low-pressure ventilation, chest tubes, parenteral nutrition, and gastrostomy feedings.

Omphalocele and Gastroschisis

Both of these anomalies are caused by congenital defects in the abdominal wall. In **omphalocele**, the intestines protrude into the base of the umbilical cord. Other anomalies often occur with omphalocele.

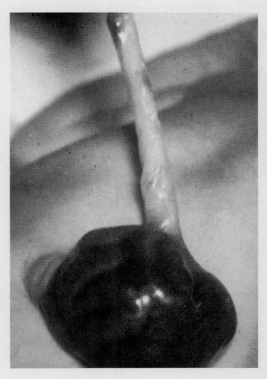

Gastroschisis is a defect to the side of the abdomen, through which the intestines protrude. They are not covered by peritoneum or skin and float freely in the amniotic fluid.

Assessment

Diagnosis is made by prenatal measurement of elevated alpha-fetoprotein level and by prenatal ultrasound and is obvious at birth.

Therapeutic Management

A gastric tube is placed to decrease air in the stomach. Gastric suction, parenteral nutrition, and antibiotics are necessary.

Continued

BOX 24.1   Common Congenital Anomalies—cont'd

Surgery is performed as soon as the infant is stable. A Silastic silo (pouch) may be used to replace the intestines gradually over a period of days to prevent pressure on the other organs. The abdomen is closed when the contents have been replaced in the abdominal cavity.

Nursing Considerations

Place the infant's torso into a sterile plastic bag or cover the intestines with Silastic or warm sterile saline dressings wrapped with plastic immediately after birth to reduce heat and water loss.

Observe for respiratory distress from increased intraabdominal pressure.

Prevent infection and trauma.

Position to avoid pressure on the intestines.

Diaphragmatic Hernia

The diaphragm fails to fuse during gestation. A large or small part of the abdominal contents moves into the chest cavity, usually on the left side.

If the herniation is large enough, the lungs may fail to develop (hypoplastic lungs). When gas fills the bowel, further pressure on the heart and lungs results.

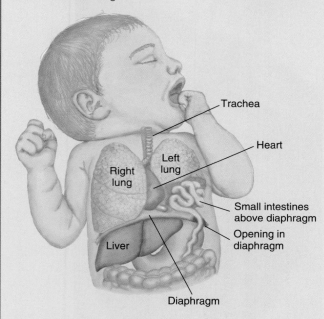

Trachea
Heart
Left lung
Right lung
Small intestines above diaphragm
Opening in diaphragm
Liver
Diaphragm

Assessment

Mild to severe respiratory distress may occur at birth, with breath sounds diminished or absent over the affected area, and barrel chest. The heartbeat may be displaced to the right. Bowel sounds are heard in the chest.

The abdomen may be scaphoid (concave).

The condition may be diagnosed prenatally by ultrasound or by radiography after birth.

Therapeutic Management

Fetal surgery may be performed.

An endotracheal tube is placed for mechanical ventilation and a gastric tube for decompression of the stomach.

Surgery to replace the intestines and repair the defect is performed when the infant is stable.

Extracorporeal membrane oxygenation (ECMO) or inhaled nitric oxide may be used.

Nursing Considerations

Avoid bag and mask ventilation to minimize distention of the stomach and bowels.

Position the infant on the affected side to allow the unaffected lung to expand. Elevate the head to decrease pressure on the heart and lungs. Assist with ventilation and monitor respiratory status.

Continue to monitor respiratory status after surgery to determine whether lung function will be adequate.

Central Nervous System
Neural Tube Defects

Folic acid supplements in pregnancy help prevent neural tube defects, especially if they are taken before conception and in early pregnancy.

Spina bifida is failure of the vertebral arch to close. *Spina bifida occulta* is failure of the vertebra to close, usually without other anomalies. It is seen by a dimple on the back, which may have a tuft of hair over it.

Meningocele is protrusion of meninges and spinal fluid through the spina bifida, covered by skin or a thin membrane. Because the spinal cord is not involved, paralysis does not occur.

Myelomeningocele is protrusion of a membrane-covered sac through the spina bifida. The sac contains meninges, nerve roots, the spinal cord, and spinal fluid. The degree of paralysis depends on the location of the defect. The infant also may have hydrocephalus, or it may develop after surgery.

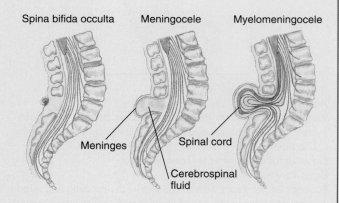

Spina bifida occulta   Meningocele   Myelomeningocele

Meninges   Spinal cord   Cerebrospinal fluid

Assessment

Prenatal diagnosis by elevated alpha-fetoprotein level or ultrasound.

Note the position and covering of the defect at birth.

Observe movement below the defect to determine the degree of paralysis.

Examine for a relaxed anus and dribbling of stool and urine.

Check for other anomalies.

BOX 24.1   Common Congenital Anomalies—cont'd

Therapeutic Management

Fetal surgery may be performed.

Surgery is performed for meningocele and myelomeningocele as soon as possible to prevent infection.

A shunt is placed to divert cerebrospinal fluid if hydrocephalus develops.

Antibiotics are given to prevent infection.

Long-term follow-up is necessary, with physical therapy and other care as needed.

Nursing Considerations

Place the infant's torso in a sterile plastic bag or cover the defect with a sterile saline dressing and plastic to prevent drying.

Handle the infant carefully, and position prone or to the side to prevent trauma to the sac.

Observe for signs of infection. Keep free of contamination from urine and feces.

Inspect the sac for intactness before surgery.

Every shift, check for increasing head circumference, bulging fontanels, separation of sutures, intermittent apnea, and other signs of increased intracranial pressure to identify early hydrocephalus.

The mother should take increased folic acid before and during future pregnancies to reduce the risk for a recurrence.

Congenital Hydrocephalus

This is a problem with absorption or obstruction to the flow of cerebrospinal fluid in the ventricles of the brain, causing compression of the brain and enlargement of the head.

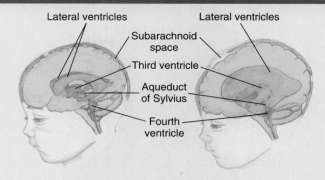

Assessment

The fontanel is full or bulging, and sutures may be separated.

The head is enlarged, especially in the frontal area.

Irritability and poor feeding occur.

The setting-sun sign is apparent (sclera visible above the pupils of the eyes).

Therapeutic Management

Surgery, most often with a ventriculoperitoneal shunt to drain fluid into the peritoneal cavity.

Will need revision as the child grows.

Nursing Considerations

Measure head circumference daily.

Prevent pressure areas.

Observe for signs of infection and intracranial pressure.

Teach parents how to care for the shunt and to observe for signs of increased intracranial pressure.

CONGENITAL CARDIAC DEFECTS

Approximately 0.8% of newborns have congenital heart defects. The defects are discovered by 1 week of age in 40% to 50% of infants and by 1 month of age in 50% to 60% of infants. Congenital heart defects are the leading cause of death from congenital anomalies (Bernstein, 2016). Genetics, teratogens, maternal diabetes, and rubella are known to be possible factors.

Classification of Cardiac Defects

Cardiac defects are generally categorized according to whether cyanosis results from the defect and by the pattern of blood flow. Some of the most common defects are illustrated in Fig. 24.4.

Acyanotic Defects

In acyanotic conditions, an obstruction of blood flow from the ventricles or a defect that causes increased flow of blood to the lungs occurs. Both increase the work of the heart. In addition, congestion in the lungs may eventually cause increased resistance of the pulmonary vessels and pulmonary hypertension. Infants are prone to respiratory tract infections because of the pulmonary congestion and increased work of the heart and lungs. Growth is slowed, and the infant fatigues easily. The heart may fail from overwork. Patent ductus arteriosus is an example of this group.

Cyanotic Defects

In cyanotic defects, blood flow to the lungs decreases, or venous blood and oxygenated blood are mixed in the systemic circulation, or both, decreasing the oxygen carried to the tissues and resulting in cyanosis. When venous blood from the right side of the heart flows through an abnormal opening to the left side of the heart, it is called a *right-to-left shunt*. Although the heart and lungs work harder, adequate oxygenation may be impossible, resulting in hypoxia of the major organs. Infants usually have serious problems from birth. They grow poorly, have frequent infections, and are easily fatigued. Heart failure may be an early complication. Transposition of the great vessels is an example of a cyanotic heart defect.

The presence of cyanosis depends on the severity and combination of defects and the child's ability to compensate. Some infants with cyanotic heart disease may be pink, and some with acyanotic heart defects may develop cyanosis. Because of this potential change in classification, further classification by blood flow is helpful.

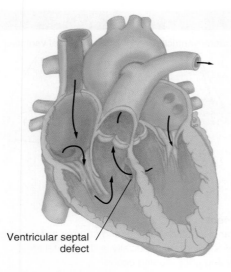

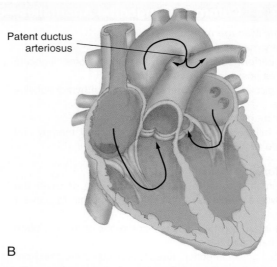

A

B

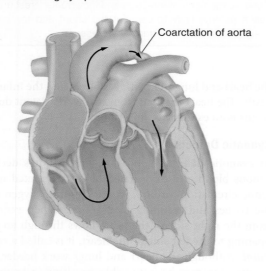

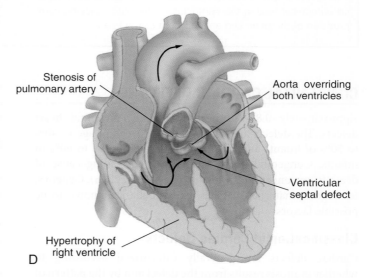

C

D

Ventricular septal defect is the most common type of congenital heart defect. It occurs alone or with other defects. The opening in the septum ranges from the size of a pin to very large. Many small defects close spontaneously. When the pressure in the left ventricle increases after birth, oxygenated blood is shunted through a large ventricular septal defect into the right ventricle and then recirculated to the lungs (a left-to-right shunt). Increased pulmonary resistance may cause pulmonary hypertension, hypertrophy of the right ventricle, and heart failure. Surgery is necessary for a large ventricular septal defect and increasing symptoms.

Patent ductus arteriosus is a failure of the ductus arteriosus to close after birth. Blood flows from the higher pressure of the aorta to the pulmonary artery and the lungs (left-to-right shunt). It is most common in the preterm infant. Symptoms vary from none to early congestive heart failure. Prostaglandins cause vasodilation and may interfere with closure of the ductus arteriosus. Indomethacin or ibuprofen lysine, prostaglandin inhibitors, may be effective in causing closure. Surgical ligation is used when necessary. Devices to close the defect nonsurgically are also used.

In *coarctation of the aorta,* blood flow is impeded through a constricted area of the aorta near the ductus arteriosus, increasing pressure behind the defect. The blood pressure is higher in the upper extremities than in the lower extremities. Carotid, brachial, and radial pulses are bounding, but pulses in the legs are weak or absent. The increased pressure in the left ventricle causes hypertrophy from the added workload. Congestive heart failure may result.

Tetralogy of Fallot has four characteristics: a ventricular septal defect, aorta positioned over the ventricular defect, pulmonary stenosis, and hypertrophy of the right ventricle. Cyanosis occurs if venous blood from the right ventricle flows through the septal defect and into the overriding aorta and blood flow to the lungs is diminished because of the narrowed pulmonary valve. The amount of right-to-left shunting and cyanosis varies according to the degree and position of each defect.

FIG. 24.4 Common Congenital Heart Defects. **A,** Ventricular septal defect. **B,** Patent ductus arteriosus. **C,** Coarctation of the aorta. **D,** Tetralogy of Fallot.

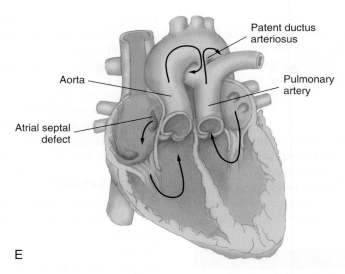

E

In *transposition of the great arteries*, the positions of the aorta and the pulmonary artery are reversed. The aorta carries venous blood from the right ventricle back to the general circulation. The pulmonary artery returns oxygenated blood from the left ventricle to the lungs. Unless there is another source for mixing oxygenated and venous blood, the infant cannot survive. A septal defect, open foramen ovale, or patent ductus arteriosus may be present. Prostaglandins may be given to keep the ductus open, and surgical correction is performed.

FIG. 24.4, cont'd E, Transposition of the great arteries.

Left-to-Right Shunting Defects

These heart defects allow blood to flow from the higher pressure of the left side of the heart to the right side or from the aorta to the pulmonary artery. This increases blood flow to the lungs and is called a *left-to-right shunt*. It causes some oxygenated blood to be sent to the lungs instead of to the rest of the body, increasing the work of the right side of the heart and the lungs. Congestive heart failure and pulmonary hypertension may result. Examples are ventricular septal defects and patent foramen ovale.

Defects with Obstruction of Blood Outflow

In defects with obstruction of blood flow, a decrease in the blood flow through a vessel or valve occurs because of stenosis (narrowing). This adds to the work of the heart, causes hypertrophy of the heart or major blood vessels, and may lead to heart failure. Coarctation of the aorta and stenosis of the pulmonary or aortic valves fit into this classification.

Defects with Decreased Pulmonary Blood Flow

An impairment in the flow of blood from the right side of the heart to the lungs, combined with abnormal openings between pulmonary and systemic circulations, occurs in defects with decreased pulmonary blood flow. Systemic hypoxemia causes cyanosis. An example is Tetralogy of Fallot.

Cyanotic Defects with Increased Pulmonary Blood Flow

These defects allow survival only if a mixing of venous and oxygenated blood in the heart occurs. There is increased blood flow to the lungs and mixing of venous and oxygenated blood in the systemic circulation. Transposition of the great vessels is an example of this type of defect.

Manifestations

Congenital heart defects may present obvious signs at birth or may not become apparent until later, when changes from fetal to neonatal circulation are completed. Some infants have no difficulty for months or years, but others experience early heart failure. The most common indications of cardiac problems are cyanosis, heart murmurs, tachycardia, and tachypnea.

Cyanosis

Cyanosis is a major sign of cardiac anomaly when it is not a result of respiratory disease. If the cyanosis is caused by mixing of oxygenated and unoxygenated blood, giving oxygen will not improve the infant's color. Cyanosis increases with crying, feeding, or other activity. Pallor, mottling, or a gray color may be present in infants who do not have cyanosis.

Heart Murmurs

Murmurs may sound like clicks, machinery, rumbling, swishing, or other muffled noises. It takes much practice to detect heart murmurs accurately. Although many infants have a temporary murmur until the fetal structures are closed, all abnormal sounds should be referred to the provider.

Tachycardia and Tachypnea

Tachycardia and tachypnea may occur any time the heart and lungs must work harder to provide sufficient oxygen to the body. Therefore they are present in both respiratory conditions and cardiac conditions. They increase in congestive heart failure.

Other Signs

Fatigue and tachypnea may interfere with the infant's ability to eat. Infants may feed slowly and take small amounts. They may fall asleep before the feeding is finished because of the effort required for sucking. As a result, weight gain may be slow. Although diaphoresis is uncommon in the newborn, it may appear during feedings in the infant with a heart defect.

CRITICAL TO REMEMBER

Common Signs of Cardiac Anomalies

Cyanosis increasing with crying
Pallor
Murmurs
Tachycardia
Tachypnea
Dyspnea
Choking spells
Poor intake, falling asleep during feedings
Diaphoresis

Therapeutic Management

Therapeutic management involves diagnosis of the specific defect and supportive and surgical treatment, as indicated. Various tests such as echocardiograms and cardiac catheterizations confirm the diagnosis. The decision for surgery depends on the status of the infant and whether surgery can be delayed safely. Palliative surgery may be performed to partially correct a defect or make another defect to allow greater amounts of oxygenated blood to get to the systemic circulation.

Oxygen and drugs such as digitalis, diuretics, potassium supplements, and sedatives may be prescribed for the infant. Prostaglandins may be given to prevent the ductus arteriosus from closing in those cases in which keeping it open will increase the flow of oxygenated blood in the infant's body.

Nursing Considerations

Nursing care is focused on assessing for changes in condition and reducing the infant's need for oxygen. The need for rest is especially important, and the infant's response to all activity is evaluated. Infants with rapid respirations are at risk for aspiration and may need feeding by gavage. Oxygen may be increased during feedings or other exertion, but only enough oxygen to maintain saturation levels adequately should be used. Frequent rest periods are provided by clustering small amounts of nursing care.

Feedings with increased calories may be used to promote nutrition and weight gain. Accurate intake and output measurement are necessary. Maintaining a neutral thermal environment is important to avoid increasing oxygen need.

Support of the parents and education about the infant's condition and expected treatment are essential. The physician may use drawings to help parents understand the defect and plans for surgery. The nurse verifies the parents' understanding and provides additional teaching, as necessary. The parents are taught techniques for accurate administration of medications because the range between the therapeutic and toxic dosage of the drugs is narrow. Parents may be referred to support groups for families of children with heart anomalies.

SUMMARY CONCEPTS

- Asphyxia before or during birth may cause apnea, acidosis, pulmonary hypertension, and possible death. Neonatal resuscitation should be initiated immediately.
- Nurses should identify conditions that increase the risk for asphyxia, begin resuscitation promptly, and assist other members of the team during treatment. Continued follow-up of the infant and parental support are important.
- In transient tachypnea of the newborn, respiratory difficulty in infants is caused by failure of fetal lung fluid to be absorbed completely. It usually resolves spontaneously with supportive care.
- In meconium aspiration syndrome, meconium in amniotic fluid enters the lungs before birth during gasping movements or is drawn in during the first breaths after birth, causing obstruction, air trapping, and inflammation.
- The nurse's role in meconium aspiration is to notify caregivers when meconium is discovered in amniotic fluid, prepare equipment, assist with intubation if necessary, and observe for further respiratory difficulty, infection, and other problems.

- Persistent pulmonary hypertension is a condition in which pulmonary vascular resistance remains high after birth and right-to-left shunting of blood occurs, causing severe respiratory difficulty.
- Nonphysiologic jaundice appears in the first 24 hours of life. Bilirubin levels rise faster and to higher levels than in physiologic jaundice. If untreated, it may result in injury to the brain.
- The nurse's role in phototherapy is to decrease situations such as cold stress or hypoglycemia that might further elevate bilirubin levels, ensure that lights are used properly, protect the eyes, observe for excessive fluid loss or skin impairment, ensure adequate oral intake, and teach parents.
- Infection can be transmitted to the neonate from the mother during pregnancy or birth or from the mother, family members, visitors, or agency staff after birth.
- Infection in neonates is a problem because their immune system is immature, infection spreads easily, and the blood-brain barrier is less effective.

- The infant of a diabetic mother may have congenital anomalies, may be large or small for gestational age, and may suffer from respiratory distress syndrome, hypoglycemia, hypocalcemia, and polycythemia.
- Nursing responsibilities in caring for the infant with a diabetic mother include early identification and follow-up of complications, monitoring of blood glucose levels, ensuring early and adequate feedings, and support of the parents.
- Infants with polycythemia have increased viscosity of blood that may cause thromboemboli, stroke, hyperbilirubinemia, and other complications.
- Infants with prenatal exposure to drugs may have behavioral and feeding abnormalities. They may have difficulty interacting or bonding with their parents or caregivers, and fail to gain weight.
- Nursing care for infants with neonatal abstinence syndrome includes obtaining accurate neonatal abstinence syndrome scores; decreasing stimuli from lights, noise, and handling; increasing feeding abilities; and fostering the mother's attachment to and ability to care for her infant.
- Infants with phenylketonuria should be on a low-phenylalanine diet to prevent severe intellectual disability.
- Congenital heart defects include left-to-right shunting defects, defects with obstruction of blood outflow, defects with decreased pulmonary blood flow, and cyanotic defects with increased pulmonary blood flow.

REFERENCES & READINGS

Ambalavanan, N., & Carlo, W. (2016). Respiratory disorders. In R. M. Kliegman, B. E. Stanton, J. W. St. Geme, & N. Schor (Eds.), *Nelson textbook of pediatrics* (20th ed.) (pp. 848–867). Philadelphia, PA: Elsevier.

American Academy of Pediatrics (AAP) & American College of Obstetricians and Gynecologists. (2012). *(ACOG). Guidelines for perinatal care* (7th ed.). Elk Grove Village, IL: American Academy of Pediatrics.

Bernstein, D. (2016). Epidemiology and genetic basis of congenital heart disease. In R. M. Kliegman, B. F. Stanton, J. W. St. Geme, & N. Schor (Eds.), *Nelson textbook of pediatrics* (20th ed.) (pp. 2182–2187). Philadelphia, PA: Elsevier.

Blackburn, S. T. (2013). *Maternal, fetal, and neonatal physiology: a clinical perspective* (4th ed.). St. Louis, MO: Saunders.

Blickstein, I., Perlman, S., Hazan, Y., Topf-Olivestone, C., & Shinwell, E. S. (2015). Diabetes mellitus in pregnancy. In R. J. Martin, A. A. Fanaroff, & M. C. Walsh (Eds.), *Fanaroff and Martin's neonatal-perinatal medicine: Diseases of the fetus and infant* (10th ed.) (pp. 265–270). St. Louis, MO: Saunders.

Carlo, W. A., & Ambalavanan, N. (2016). The endocrine system. In R. M. Kliegman, B. E. Stanton, J. W. St. Geme, & N. Schor (Eds.), *Nelson textbook of pediatrics* (20th ed.) (pp. 896–899). Philadelphia, PA: Elsevier.

Cleveland, L. M. (2016). Breastfeeding recommendations for women who receive medication-assisted treatment for opioid use disorders: AWHONN Practice Brief Number 4. *Nursing for Women's Health*, 20(4), 432–434.

Cowley, M. A. (2015). Neonatal respiratory disorders. In R. J. Martin, A. A. Fanaroff, & M. C. Walsh (Eds.), *Fanaroff and Martin's neonatal-perinatal medicine: Diseases of the fetus and infant* (10th ed.) (pp. 1113–1136). St. Louis, MO: Saunders.

D'Apolito, K. (2010). Assessing signs and symptoms of neonatal abstinence using the Finnegan scoring tool: An inter-observer reliability program. *Neo Advances*. Retrieved from www.neoadvances.com.

Dahlke, J. D., & Magann, E. F. (2015). Immune and nonimmune hydrops fetalis. In R. J. Martin, A. A. Fanaroff, & M. C. Walsh (Eds.), *Fanaroff and Martin's neonatal-perinatal medicine: Diseases of the fetus and infant* (10th ed.) (pp. 327–339). St. Loui, MO: Saunders.

Devaskar, S. U., & Garg, M. (2015). Disorders of carbohydrate metabolism. In R. J. Martin, A. A. Fanaroff, & M. C. Walsh (Eds.), *Fanaroff and Martin's neonatal-perinatal medicine: Diseases of the fetus and infant* (10th ed.) (pp. 1434–1459). St. Louis, MO: Saunders.

Diehl-Jones, W., & Fraser, D. (2015). Hematologic disorders. In M. T. Verklan, & M. Walden (Eds.), *Core curriculum for neonatal intensive care nursing* (5th ed.) (pp. 662–688). St. Louis, MO: Elsevier.

Edwards, L., & Brown, L. F. (2016). Nonpharmacologic management of neonatal abstinence syndrome: An integrative review. *Neonatal Network*, 35(5), 305–313.

Fasano, R. M., Said, M., & Luban, N. L. C. (2015). Blood component therapy for the neonate. In R. J. Martin, A. A. Fanaroff, & M. C. Walsh (Eds.), *Fanaroff and Martin's neonatal-perinatal medicine: Diseases of the fetus and infant* (10th ed.) (pp. 1344–1361). St. Louis, MO: Saunders.

Fraser, D. (2015). Respiratory distress. In M. T. Verklan, & M. Walden (Eds.), *Core curriculum of neonatal intensive care nursing* (5th ed.) (pp. 447–477). St. Louis, MO: Elsevier.

Gallacher, D. J., Hart, K., & Kotecha, S. (2016). Common respiratory conditions of the newborn. *Breathe*, 12(1), 30–42.

Gallagher, P. G. (2015). The neonatal erythrocyte and its disorders. In S. H. Orkin, D. G. Nathan, D. Ginsberg, et al. (Eds.), *Nathan and Oski's hematology and oncology of infancy and childhood* (8th ed.) (pp. 52–75). Philadelphia, PA: Saunders.

Gardner, S. L., Enzman-Hines, M., & Nyp, M. (2016). Respiratory diseases. In S. L. Gardner, B. S. Carter, M. Enzman-Hines, et al. (Eds.), *Merenstein & Gardner's handbook of neonatal intensive care* (8th ed.) (pp. 565–643). St. Louis, MO: Elsevier.

Greenberg, J. M., Narendran, V., Schibler, K. R., et al. (2014). Neonatal morbidities of prenatal and perinatal origin. In R. K. Creasy, R. Resnik, J. D. Iams, C. J. Lockwood, T. Moore, & M. F. Greene (Eds.), *Creasy & Resnick's maternal-fetal medicine: Principles and practice* (7th ed.) (pp. 1215–1239). Philadelphia, PA: Saunders.

Kamath-Rayne, B. D., Thilo, E. H., Deacon, J., & Hernandez, J. A. (2016). Neonatal hyperbilirubinemia. In S. L. Gardner, B. S. Carter, M. Enzman-Hines, et al. (Eds.), *Merenstein & Gardner's handbook of neonatal intensive care* (8th ed.) (pp. 511–536). St. Louis, MO: Elsevier.

Kaplan, M., Wong, R. J., Sibley, E., & Stevenson, D. K. (2015). Neonatal jaundice and liver disease. In R. J. Martin, A. A. Fanaroff, & M. C. Walsh (Eds.), *Fanaroff and Martin's neonatal-perinatal medicine: Diseases of the fetus and infant* (10th ed.) (pp. 1618–1673). St. Louis, MO: Saunders.

Kraft, K. W., Stover, M. W., & Davis, J. M. (2016). Neonatal abstinence syndrome: Pharmacologic strategies for the mother and infant. *Seminars in Perinatology*, 40(3), 203–212.

Nyp, M., Brunkhorst, J. L., Reavey, D., & Pallotto, E. K. (2016). Fluid and electrolyte management. In S. L. Gardner, B. S. Carter, M. Enzman-Hines, et al. (Eds.), *Merenstein & Gardner's handbook of neonatal intensive care* (8th ed.) (pp. 315–336). St. Louis, MO: Elsevier.

Oster, M. E., Aucott, S. W., Glidewell, J., Hackell, J., Kochilas, L., Martin, Kemperet, A. R. (2016). Lessons learned from newborn screening for critical congenital heart defects. *Pediatrics, 137*(5), e20154573.

Pammi, N., Brand, M. C., & Weisman, L. E. (2016). Infection in the neonate. In S. L. Gardner, B. S. Carter, M. Enzman-Hines, et al. (Eds.), *Merenstein & Gardner's handbook of neonatal intensive care* (8th ed.) (pp. 537–563). St. Louis, MO: Elsevier.

Parikh, A. S., & Mitchell, A. L. (2015). Congenital anomalies. In R. J. Martin, A. A. Fanaroff, & M. C. Walsh (Eds.), *Fanaroff and Martin's neonatal-perinatal medicine: Diseases of the fetus and infant* (10th ed.) (pp. 436–457). St. Louis, MO: Saunders.

Patrick, S. W., Schumacher, R. E., Horbar, J. D., et al. (2016). Improving care for neonatal abstinence syndrome. *Pediatrics,* e20153835.

Rezvani, I., & Ficicioglu, C. H. (2016). Defects in metabolism of amino acids. In R. M. Kliegman, B. E. Stanton, J. W. St. Geme, & N. Schor (Eds.), *Nelson textbook of pediatrics* (20th ed.) (pp. 636–678). Philadelphia, PA: Elsevier.

Rozance, P. J., McGowan, J. E., Price-Douglas, W., & Hay, W. W., Jr. (2016). Glucose homeostasis. In S. L. Gardner, B. S. Carter, M. Enzman-Hines, et al. (Eds.), *Merenstein & Gardner's handbook of neonatal intensive care* (8th ed.) (pp. 337–359). St. Louis, MO: Elsevier.

Sherman, J. (2015). Perinatal substance abuse. In M. T. Verklan & M. Walden (Eds.), *Core curriculum for neonatal intensive care nursing* (5th ed.) (pp. 43–57). St. Louis, MO: Elsevier.

Slavotinek, A. (2016). Dysmorphology. In R. M. Kliegman, B. E. Stanton, J. W. St. Geme, & N. Schor (Eds.), *Nelson textbook of pediatrics* (20th ed.) (pp. 899–909). Philadelphia, PA: Elsevier.

Srinivas, G. L., Cuff, C. D., Ebeling, M. D., & Mcelligott, J. T. (2016). Transcutaneous bilirubinometry is a reliably conservative method of assessing neonatal jaundice. *The Journal of Maternal-Fetal & Neonatal Medicine, 29*(16), 2635–2639.

Steinhorn, R. H. (2016). Treatment of hypoxemic respiratory failure in neonates: Past, present and future. *Journal of Perinatology, 36,* S1–S2.

Stoll, B. J., & Shane, A. L. (2016). Infections of the neonatal infant. In R. M. Kliegman, B. E. Stanton, J. W. St. Geme, & N. Schor (Eds.), *Nelson textbook of pediatrics* (20th ed.) (pp. 909–925). Philadelphia, PA: Elsevier.

Taylor, J. E., McDonald, S. J., & Tan, K. (2015). Prevention of central venous catheter-related infection in the neonatal unit: A literature review. *The Journal of Maternal-Fetal & Neonatal Medicine, 28*(10), 1224–1230.

Weiner, G. M. (Ed.). (2016). *Textbook of neonatal resuscitation* (7th ed.). Elk Grove Village, IL: American Academy of Pediatrics and American Heart Association.

Weiner, S. M., & Finnegan, L. P. (2011). Drug withdrawal in the neonate. In S. L. Gardner, B. S. Carter, M. Enzman-Hines, et al. (Eds.), *Merenstein & Gardner's handbook of neonatal intensive care* (8th ed.) (pp. 199–217). St. Louis, MO: Elsevier.

Wilson, D. J., & Tyner, C. I. (2015). Infectious diseases in the neonate. In M. T. Verklan, & M. Walden (Eds.), *Core curriculum for neonatal intensive care nursing* (5th ed.) (pp. 689–718). St. Louis, MO: Elsevier.

Zinn, A. B. (2015). Inborn errors of metabolism. In R. M. Kliegman, B. E. Stanton, J. W. St. Geme, & N. Schor (Eds.), *Nelson textbook of pediatrics* (20th ed.) (pp. 1553–1615). Philadelphia, PA: Elsevier.

25

Family Planning

Susan Peck

OBJECTIVES

After studying this chapter, you should be able to:

1. Discuss the nurse's role in contraceptive counseling and education.
2. Explain factors a couple should consider when choosing a method of contraception.
3. Explain the mechanism of action, advantages, disadvantages, side effects, and teaching needed for methods of family planning.
4. Explain why informed consent is important for contraception.
5. Compare and contrast contraceptive needs at both ends of the reproductive spectrum, in adolescence and perimenopause.

Family planning involves choosing if and when to become pregnant. It includes **contraception**—the prevention of pregnancy—as well as methods to achieve pregnancy. Thinking about goals for having or not having children and how to achieve those goals is called a *reproductive life plan*. There are various reproductive life plans, and each is unique to a woman's own personal goals and dreams (www.cdc.gov/preconception/reproductiveplan.html). Chapter 26 describes methods used by couples having difficulty attaining pregnancy. This chapter focuses on techniques used to avoid pregnancy.

If both partners are fertile, approximately 85% will become pregnant over the course of a year without using contraception (Trussell, 2011). Therefore those who wish to avoid or control the timing of pregnancies should practice effective contraception.

Approximately 61 million women in the United States are fertile, sexually active, and do not currently desire a pregnancy. Of those women, 62% are practicing contraception (Alan Guttmacher Institute [AGI], 2016b). However, they may not be using contraception consistently.

Unintended pregnancies are those that are unwanted or are mistimed, occurring in women who may wish to become pregnant at a time in the future but not at the time their pregnancies occur. The ability to delay and space childbearing is crucial to women's social and economic advancement. Women's ability to obtain and effectively use contraceptives has a positive impact on their education and workforce participation, as well as on

subsequent outcomes related to income, family stability, mental health and happiness, and children's well-being (Sonfield et al., 2013).

In the United States in 2011, 45% of pregnancies were unintended. Although this is an improvement from the previous 51%, it is still much higher than most industrialized nations. (Finer & Zolna, 2016). A *Healthy People 2020* goal is to increase the number of intended pregnancies to 56% (U.S. Department of Health and Human Services [DHHS], 2010).

Because most contraceptive methods available are the responsibility of women, they often choose the type of contraception used. During a woman's reproductive lifetime, her needs for contraception evolve. Most women use a variety of methods before they reach menopause. Because the average woman in the United States bears only two children, she must make contraceptive decisions for more than 30 years. Many of those years occur after she has completed childbearing and is highly motivated to avoid further pregnancy.

INFORMATION ABOUT CONTRACEPTION

Common Sources

Women often obtain information about contraception from friends, relatives, the Internet, television, and magazines. They seek answers to practical questions about side effects, effectiveness, comfort, and partners' responses. The information they receive, however, is often incomplete or incorrect when their source is not a qualified health care professional. Women frequently turn to nurses in outpatient ambulatory office settings, birth settings, and even social settings for accurate information about family planning.

Role of the Nurse

The nurse's role in family planning is that of counselor and educator. To fulfill this role, nurses need current, correct information about contraceptive methods and should share this information with women who seek their advice.

Unintended pregnancies may occur less often if women had adequate ongoing education and reevaluation regarding their chosen method. The initial teaching that accompanies selection of the contraceptive technique may be insufficient to meet the woman's needs. Reinforcing teaching and providing an opportunity to ask questions after initial use can help ensure that the woman is using the method correctly and is satisfied with the method. A woman is more likely to use contraception if she has received counseling that is directed to her own needs instead of general information about contraception. Therefore the nurse should provide individualized family planning information to women in every situation in which it would be appropriate.

Nurses should feel comfortable discussing contraception and be sensitive to the woman's concerns, feelings, and culture. When discussing family planning, the woman's preferences take priority. Care should be taken that nurses do not introduce their own biases toward or against specific methods. The focus of counseling should be tailored to the reproductive life plan goals of the woman and her partner (Fig. 25.1).

Counseling about contraception should include the following:

- Types of contraception available, both reversible and permanent
- Risks and benefits of each and determination of which methods may not be safe based on health status or concurrent medication use

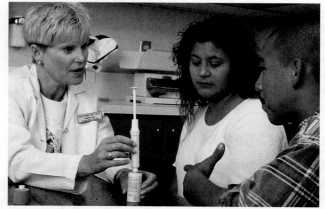

FIG 25.1 Success of contraception is more likely when both the woman and her partner are involved in discussions. The nurse demonstrates filling a foam applicator.

- How to ensure proper use of each method to maximize effectiveness
- What to do if an error is made
- Emergency contraception (EC)— specifically access and instruction
- Backup methods and when they should be used
- What to do if the woman wants to change methods
- Questions and concerns

CONSIDERATIONS WHEN CHOOSING A CONTRACEPTIVE METHOD

The perfect contraceptive method does not exist. Each has advantages and disadvantages (Table 25.1). Women change contraceptive methods as circumstances in their lives change and in response to dissatisfaction with side effects or other traits of their current contraceptive (Table 25.2). Women often try several methods before finding one that is satisfactory. Some women have an interval of using no contraception before beginning a new method, even though they do not wish to become pregnant.

Of women who practice contraception, 67% currently use reversible methods, primarily oral contraceptives (OCs), the patch, the injectable and the vaginal ring, long-acting reversible contraceptives (LARC) such as an intrauterine device (IUD) or the implant, and condoms. The most popular methods of contraception in the United States since 1982 are OCs and female sterilization (Daniels, Daugherty & Jones, 2015; Jones, Mosher, & Daniels, 2012). However, the most popular methods are often not right for every woman. Nurses can help women weigh the factors involved in choosing a family planning method. Careful consideration of all factors can help a woman choose the safest method that best meets her current needs.

Safety

The safety of a contraceptive method is a primary consideration and is unique to each woman's health status. Medical conditions or social practices such as tobacco use may make certain methods unsafe. For example, OCs should not be used by women who have had a thromboembolic event such as deep vein thrombosis or stroke, because the hormones in the contraceptives increase the risk for recurrence and mortality. It is imperative for nurses who provide contraceptive counseling to be well versed in the Centers for Disease Control and Prevention's (CDC, 2016b) *US Medical Eligibility Criteria for Contraceptive Use* (US MEC) and *US Selected Practice Recommendations for Contraceptive Use* (US SPR), most recently published in July 2016; however, it is important to understand that the use of contraceptives, even hormonal contraception, is generally safer than pregnancy (Trussell & Guthrie, 2011).

Protection from Sexually Transmitted Diseases

No contraceptive (other than abstinence practiced perfectly) is 100% effective in preventing sexually transmitted infections (STDs). The risk for exposure to STDs should be discussed

TABLE 25.1 Advantages and Disadvantages of the Most Common Contraceptive Methods

Method	Advantages	Disadvantages
Sterilization	• Ends concern about contraception. • Tubal sterilization performed during or right after childbirth or between pregnancies. • Vasectomy performed in physician's office with local anesthesia. • Low long-term cost.	• No protection against STDs. • Reversal is difficult and expensive, and it may be unsuccessful. • Potential complications as in any surgery. • Vasectomy requires another contraceptive method until semen is free of sperm.
Intrauterine device or intrauterine system	• Unrelated to coitus. • In place at all times. • Low long-term cost. • Effective for 5-10 yr. • Decreases dysmenorrhea and menstrual blood loss. • Some women become amenorrheic. • Copper IUD may also be used for EC.	• No protection against STDs. • Can be expelled without woman's knowledge; must check for threads. • Potential side effects or complications: Menorrhagia, infection near time of insertion, ectopic pregnancy, spontaneous abortion if pregnancy occurs, perforation.
Progestin implant	• Unrelated to coitus. • Provides 3-yr protection. • Safe during lactation. • Body weight has no effect.	• No protection against STDs. • Major side effect is irregular bleeding.
Progestin injections (Depo-Provera)	• Unrelated to coitus. • Avoids need for daily use. • May cause amenorrhea with continued use. • Requires use only every 12 wk.	• No protection against STDs. • Must remember to repeat every 12 wk. • Causes temporary decrease in bone density. • Effect on peak bone mass and osteoporosis unknown. • Side effects similar to those of other progestin contraceptives.
Oral contraceptives	• Taken at a time unrelated to coitus. (See Table 25.4.)	• No protection against STDs. • Must be taken daily at or near same time. • May cause side effects and complications. (See Table 25.4.)
Emergency contraception	• Helps prevent pregnancy after unprotected coitus. • Some available without prescription	• No protection against STDs. • Must be taken within 120 hr of unprotected intercourse. • May cause nausea.
Transdermal contraceptive patch	• Unrelated to coitus. • Requires only weekly application. • Regulates menstrual cycles.	• No protection against STDs. • Must apply on the right day. • Less effective for women over 90 kg (198 lb). • May cause skin irritation. • Other side effects similar to those of OCs. • Higher risk for clot formation.
Vaginal contraceptive ring	• Unrelated to coitus. • In place for 3 wk at a time. • No fitting required.	• No protection against STDs. • Must remember when to remove and when to insert. • Side effects include headache, expulsion, vaginitis, vaginal discomfort or discharge, and others similar to those of OCs.
Barrier		
All methods	• Avoid use of systemic hormones. • Offer some protection against STDs.	• Most coitus-related (must be used just before coitus). • May interfere with sensation. • Contraindicated for allergies to components of spermicide or latex.
Chemical (spermicide)	• Quick and easy. • No prescription needed. • Inexpensive per single use. • Provides lubrication.	• Films and suppositories must melt to be effective. • Effective time less than 1 hour. • No douching for 6 hr. • May be messy. • May cause irritation. • New application needed for repeated intercourse.
Condom	• Quick and easy. • No prescription needed. • Best protection available for STDs. • Low cost per single use. • Can be carried discreetly. • Vaginal condoms increase women's control over contraceptive use and protection from STDs.	• Interferes with spontaneity. • Must be checked for expiration date and holes. • Can break or slip off. • Can be used only once. • Female condoms may seem unattractive.

Continued

TABLE 25.1   Advantages and Disadvantages of the Most Common Contraceptive Methods—cont'd

Method	Advantages	Disadvantages
Sponge	• Available over the counter. • Can be inserted several hours before coitus. • Effective for repeated intercourse. • No prescription needed.	• No protection against STDs. • Must remain in place for 6 hr but no more than 30 hr total. • May cause irritation. • Risk for toxic shock syndrome if used too long or during menstruation.
Diaphragm	• Can be inserted several hours before coitus. • Provides some protection from STDs. • Can remain in place up to 24 hr.	• Requires education on proper use. • Difficult to insert or remove for some women. • Added spermicide necessary for repeat coitus. • Possibility of toxic shock syndrome with prolonged use or use during menses. • Bladder infection may occur. • Must remain in place at least 6 hours after coitus. • Should be checked for fit annually and after pregnancy or weight change of more than 4.5 kg (10 lb).
Cervical cap	• Smaller than diaphragm and may fit women who cannot use a diaphragm. • No pressure against bladder. • Less noticeable and requires less spermicide than diaphragm. • Provides some protection from STDs. • Can remain in place 48 hr.	• Initially expensive. • Requires health care provider to fit. • Requires education on proper use. • Added spermicide needed for repeat coitus. • Possibility of toxic shock syndrome. • Must remain in place at least 6 hr after coitus.
Natural Family Planning		
All methods	• Inexpensive. • No drugs or hormones. • Help woman learn about her body. • Can be combined with barrier methods to increase effectiveness. • Acceptable in most religions. • May be used to help achieve pregnancy.	• No protection from STDs. • Requires high motivation and extensive education. • Abstinence necessary for large part of each cycle. • High risk for pregnancy from error. • Many factors may change ovulation time.

EC, Emergency contraception; *IUD,* intrauterine device; *OCs,* oral contraceptives; *STD,* sexually transmitted disease.

TABLE 25.2   Discontinuation of Various Types of Contraception

Method	Women Who Discontinue Use at 1 Year (%)
Implant (Implanon)	16
Intrauterine devices	
LNG-IUS (Mirena)	20
Copper T 380A (ParaGard)	22
Depo-Provera	44
Oral contraceptives	33
Contraceptive patch	33
Vaginal ring	33
Condoms	
Male	57
Female	59
Diaphragm	43
Sponge	64
Spermicides, gel, foam, films, suppositories (used alone)	58
Natural family planning (all types)	53
Withdrawal	54

Data from Trussell, J., & Guthrie, K. A. (2011). Choosing a contraceptive: Efficacy, safety, and personal considerations. In R. A. Hatcher, J. Trussell, A. L. Nelson, et al. (Eds), *Contraceptive technology* (20th ed., pp. 45–74). New York: Ardent Media.

when counseling women about contraceptive choices. The male condom is inexpensive and offers the best protection available. It should be used whenever there is a risk for STD exposure, when a woman engages in high-risk sexual behaviors or if one partner may have an STD, and even when another form of contraception is practiced or during pregnancy.

Effectiveness

The importance of avoiding pregnancy must be considered when choosing a contraceptive method. A woman may wish to delay pregnancy for a time but may not mind if pregnancy occurs earlier. Other women may be extremely upset about an accidental pregnancy.

Efficacy is determined by how well the method prevents pregnancy (Table 25.3). Effectiveness rates reflect the following two types of contraceptive failure:

1. The ideal, perfect, or theoretic effectiveness rate refers to *perfect, consistent* use of the method with every act of intercourse. Failures are caused by a problem with the method itself rather than with the use of the method.
2. The typical, actual, or user effectiveness rate is most useful because it refers to the occurrence of pregnancy under *typical* use of the method. Failure is presumably the result of incorrect or inconsistent use of the technique.

TABLE 25.3 Comparison of Pregnancy Rates among Common Contraceptive Methods

Method	Pregnancies during First Year of Typical Use (%)
Sterilization	
Male	0.15
Female	0.5
Contraceptive implant (Nexplanon)	0.05
Intrauterine devices	
Copper T 380A (ParaGard)	0.8
LNG-IUS	0.2
Depo-Provera	6
Transdermal contraceptive patch (NuvaRing)	9
Vaginal contraceptive ring (Evra)	9
Oral contraceptives	9
Condoms	
Male	18
Female	21
Diaphragm with spermicide	12
Sponge	
Nulliparous women	12
Parous women	24
Natural family planning (all types)	24
Coitus interruptus (withdrawal)	22
Spermicides, gel, foam, films, suppositories (used alone)	28
No contraceptive use	85

Data from Trussell, J., & Guthrie, K. A. (2011). Choosing a contraceptive: Efficacy, safety, and personal considerations. In R. A. Hatcher, J. Trussell, A. L. Nelson, et al. (Eds.), *Contraceptive technology* (20th ed., pp. 45–74). New York: Ardent Media; and Speroff, L., & Darney, P. D. (2011). *A clinical guide for contraception* (5th ed.). Philadelphia, PA: Lippincott Williams & Wilkins.

The difference between the two rates of effectiveness shows how forgiving a method is—that is, how likely pregnancy is to occur if the use is occasionally imperfect. For example, in 100 women using OCs in 1 year, perfect use results in 0.3 pregnancies but typical use results in 9 pregnancies. The typical failure rate is more meaningful when counseling women and their partners. When comparing different methods, the same method of analysis should be used.

Efficacy is highly correlated to accuracy of use. It drops greatly when the user does not understand how to use the method. The failure rate commonly decreases after the first year of use as experience with the method leads to more accurate use. Combining two less reliable methods, for example, a condom and a spermicide, increases effectiveness. LARCs, IUDs, and the contraceptive implant are the most effective reversible methods and do not require intervention by a woman or her partner to achieve this efficacy (American Association of Pediatrics [AAP], 2012; American College of Obstetricians and Gynecologists [ACOG], 2015b, 2015c).

Other factors that affect the number of unintended pregnancies that occur with contraceptive use include frequency of intercourse and age of the woman. Women who have more frequent intercourse have more opportunities for failure. As women progress into perimenopause, fertility rates decline.

Acceptability

The effectiveness of a method should be balanced against its acceptability to the couple. For example, permanent sterilization is an extremely effective method but is unacceptable to couples planning to have children at a later time. Side effects or religious/cultural objections may cause some women to choose less effective methods. A woman or her partner may be concerned about certain contraceptives because of perceived or suspected side effects such as weight gain.

A chemical contraceptive such as a spermicide or the sponge may appear "messy" and unacceptable because it is "unattractive" or may cause vaginal irritation. Women of any age who are not comfortable touching their bodies may be unlikely to accept methods that involve inserting a device into the vagina or assessing the cervical mucus.

Convenience

Convenience is another important factor in choosing a contraceptive method. If the woman perceives her contraceptive as difficult to obtain or use, time consuming, or too much "bother," she is less likely to use it consistently even if her level of motivation is very high. The education she receives about the method may affect her perception of its convenience. Women who are knowledgeable about their family planning method are less likely to think the contraceptive is difficult to use.

Methods that can be used monthly or weekly instead of daily or with each act of intercourse are more convenient and likely to lead to better compliance. Other inconveniences include breakthrough bleeding (spotting between periods) common with some methods or needing to visit the health care provider's office for a prescription or injection may be viewed as very inconvenient.

The desire to avoid monthly menstruation also should be considered. Some women prefer extended cycles with several months between menses or to avoid menstrual periods altogether. Extended or continuous use of OCs, the patch, and the ring may be used. Hormone implants or injections and IUDs may also lead to *amenorrhea* (absence of menstruation) in some women.

Education Needed

Women may fail to use contraception because they do not understand their risk for pregnancy. They may not be familiar with the variety of methods available or the risks and benefits of the different types. Some methods such as condoms involve very little education, whereas others are more complicated. Women using natural family planning methods need extensive education about body changes that indicate ovulation to practice these methods successfully.

Benefits

Some methods have special benefits that should be discussed. For example, OCs have many noncontraceptive benefits such as reduction in acne, decreased bleeding during periods, and decreased menstrual cramps. Natural family planning methods and the copper IUD offer freedom from exposure to hormones. Condoms provide better protection against human immunodeficiency virus (HIV) compared with other contraceptives.

Side Effects

Some methods of contraception have bothersome side effects that should be explained clearly in advance and when educating women about the advantages and disadvantages of each method. When women know what to expect, they often are more willing to tolerate the side effects and continue using the method, especially if they know that they do not pose a health risk.

Effect on Spontaneity

Contraceptive methods related to **coitus** (sexual intercourse) such as chemical or mechanical barrier methods, withdrawal, and periodic abstinence must be used just before sexual intercourse. They require skill and motivation near the time of intercourse and may be more likely to be used inconsistently or incorrectly. The fact that these methods must be readily available and interrupt lovemaking increases the chance that they will not be used. Some couples remedy this problem by including application of the contraceptive device such as a condom as a part of foreplay. Others prefer methods such as OCs or LARCs that do not interrupt sexual activity.

Availability

Condoms and spermicides are readily available without prescriptions. They can be purchased anonymously at any time without a visit to a health care provider. This may be important to an adolescent who wants to hide her sexual activity or to women who are embarrassed to discuss contraception with a health care provider.

Expense

The cost of family planning methods is important. Less effective contraceptives are often chosen by some couples to save money. These methods may be less expensive but more likely to result in pregnancy, which costs more than the yearly expense of any contraceptive method.

The "per use" cost of methods can be compared with long-term expense. The price of condoms or spermicides is relatively low, but frequent use makes them expensive over a period of years. Couples may find them economical for occasional sexual intercourse or until they can afford a more expensive method. Methods that depend on periodic visits to a health care provider are more costly than over-the-counter methods. However, the visits provide an opportunity for teaching that may enhance contraceptive effectiveness. Such visits also provide an opportunity for health screening and discussion of other health concerns. LARC methods are very cost effective over a 3- to 10-year period because their failure rate is so low.

Publicly funded family planning clinics may provide free or low-cost contraceptives as well as counseling about all contraceptive methods and follow-up services. However, women who attend these clinics may have a long wait and may see a different health care provider at each visit. Family planning is covered by many state Medicaid programs and most insurance companies. As of September, 2017, the Patient Protection and Affordable Care Act, designates a list of preventive services that must be covered, without out-of-pocket costs to the consumer. Those services include provision of all FDA-approved contraceptive methods, along with sterilization procedures and contraceptive counseling to all women (Health Resources and Services Administration, Women's Preventive Services: required health plan coverage guidelines, www.hrsa.gov/womensguidelines).

Preference

The woman usually makes the final decision about her contraceptive method, and her satisfaction with her choice is crucial. Consistent use of any method depends on whether it meets the needs of the woman and her partner. If the woman feels pressured to choose a certain method or if the chosen method fails to live up to her expectations, use is more likely to be inconsistent. The opinion of the woman's partner and her friends also may influence her choice of method.

Religious and Personal Beliefs

Religious or other personal beliefs affect the choice of contraceptives. Certain religions may not believe in the use of any contraceptives other than natural family planning.

Culture

Culture may influence the method chosen. Some cultures place a high value on large families and especially on male children. A woman may have more pregnancies than she might otherwise desire in an effort to have sons. Asian and Hispanic women are often very modest and do not talk about sexuality with others. They need to feel very comfortable with the nurse before talking about sexual matters. Taking time to establish rapport before discussing intimate subjects is important.

Some cultures and religions restrict a woman's activities during menses. Methods that cause increased bleeding or breakthrough bleeding as a side effect may not be acceptable to these couples. If there is a cultural taboo against a woman touching the genital area, sponges, diaphragms, spermicides, the female condom, or the contraceptive ring would not be acceptable.

Other Considerations

Women also consider factors other than those discussed previously when choosing a contraceptive. The length of time before a pregnancy is desired will determine whether a long-acting contraceptive is appropriate. The breastfeeding woman must choose a method that will not harm the baby or reduce milk production. The woman at risk for acquiring or transmitting an STD should use condoms either alone or with another more effective method of preventing pregnancy.

Women in a situation of intimate partner violence often have inconsistent use or problems with their contraceptive method. These women are often at risk for unintended pregnancy because of their partner's interference with their use of contraceptives (Fontenot & Fantasia, 2011).

Informed Consent

Some methods have potentially dangerous side effects. Every woman should receive information about the chosen contraceptive method and its proper use, its risks and benefits, and alternative methods available. The nurse should thoroughly document that the woman received and understands this information. Some methods such as permanent sterilization and LARC methods require written consent.

KNOWLEDGE CHECK

1. Why does the woman usually choose the method of contraception a couple uses?
2. What is the role of the nurse in helping women with contraceptive choices and use?
3. What are some important considerations in choosing a contraceptive technique?
4. Which contraceptive methods require that the woman sign an informed consent form?

ADOLESCENTS AND CONTRACEPTION

In 2013, 47% of high school students reported that they had experienced sexual intercourse, 34% that they were currently sexually active in the last 3 months, and 41% said they did not use a condom the last time they had sex (CDC, 2016d). Although the rate of adolescent pregnancies has decreased in recent years, adolescent pregnancy is still a major problem. Because of the serious impact of pregnancy on adolescents, the U.S. *Healthy People 2020* goals include the following (DHHS, 2010);

- Increasing condom use at first intercourse to 73.6% of adolescent females and 88.6% of males
- Increasing the number of sexually active adolescents ages 15 to 17 years who used a condom and hormonal or intrauterine contraception at first and most recent intercourse

Adolescent Knowledge

Many adolescents have little knowledge about their own anatomy and physiology, including how and when conception occurs. They are likely to learn about contraception from other teenagers, who often pass on incorrect information. Adolescents have higher failure rates with all methods of contraception. Contraceptive failure is almost twice as likely in teenagers as in women age 30 years or more (Ochalski & Sanfilippo, 2011).

Misinformation

Misinformation and erroneous beliefs about contraception are common among teens. Some teenagers assume they cannot become pregnant the first time they have intercourse. Others believe they must have an orgasm or must have been menstruating a certain length of time to become pregnant. Even adolescent mothers are more likely to be inconsistent in contraceptive use or to use ineffective methods (Speroff & Darney, 2011). Although many adolescents have anovulatory menstrual cycles shortly after menarche, they cannot depend on absence of ovulation to avoid pregnancy because some will ovulate before their first menses and a pregnancy can result from any intercourse near ovulation.

Teenagers may *douche* (insert a solution into the vagina) after intercourse to "wash away the sperm" and prevent pregnancy. However, douching is ineffective because sperm may enter the cervix very soon after ejaculation. **Coitus interruptus** (withdrawal) is used by some teenagers, but it is unreliable. It requires more control over timing of ejaculation than most adolescent boys have, and it is important to educate adolescents that there is a small amount of sperm present in the preejaculate fluid.

Risk-Taking Behavior

Adolescents often have a feeling of invincibility. They are more likely than adults to take risks in sexual activity because they believe their chances of becoming pregnant are low. They often do not plan intercourse and therefore are not prepared with contraceptives. This behavior may lead to STDs and pregnancy. Most teenagers wait at least 6 months after becoming sexually active to begin using contraception (Ochalski & Sanfilippo, 2011).

Some adolescents have ambivalent feelings about becoming pregnant. Although they do not plan to become pregnant, they do not have a firm commitment to avoid pregnancy during their teenage years. Discussing how pregnancy may affect them and their life goals may help determine their true feelings about becoming pregnant.

Counseling Adolescents

Nurses who counsel adolescents about sexuality should be sensitive to their feelings, concerns, needs and different communication styles (Fig. 25.2). They should put aside their own personal feelings about adolescent sexuality.

For an adolescent to seek information about contraception, she must admit that she is, and plans to continue to be, sexually active. She may be afraid to ask about contraception because she does not want anyone to know she is sexually active (such as with the use of a parent's health insurance) or she fears she will be lectured or judged about her behavior. Her need for secrecy may cause her to miss appointments for family planning. The nurse should be adept at determining the adolescent's needs and reassure her that her visits are confidential and what is discussed will not be shared with others.

Each contact with the health care system provides an opportunity for counseling that should not be missed. Visits to a health care provider for well-woman checkups, minor

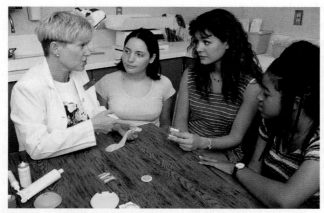

FIG 25.2 Although many adolescents choose oral contraceptives, the nurse emphasizes the need to use condoms for protection against sexually transmitted diseases. Demonstrating with actual contraceptives increases understanding.

illnesses, or pregnancy testing provide such opportunities. If an adolescent thinks she might be pregnant but the pregnancy test result is negative, she can be asked about her desire to become pregnant. She may be particularly interested in pregnancy prevention at that time. The nurse can assess the adolescent's use of contraception and the adequacy of her knowledge and can provide information and resources as appropriate.

Although nurses should encourage adolescents to discuss contraception with their parents, many teenagers will forgo contraception rather than talk to their parents about it. Therefore they need other reliable sources of information. Schools have helped increase birth control use among adolescents by offering information about family planning and prevention of STDs.

Contraceptive services also are available on some school campuses. School nurses and classroom discussions supply information about abstinence as well as contraception. Encouragement to delay becoming sexually active and discussion of the effect pregnancy might have and ways to remain abstinent are included. Some family planning clinics are open after school, during evenings, and on weekends and have staff who are especially skilled in working with adolescents.

The pelvic examination, a source of great anxiety for many young women, is not necessary for a prescription for most forms of contraception in healthy women and may be postponed. Current recommendations from the National Cancer Institute state that cervical cancer screening (Papanicolaou [Pap] tests) should occur every 3 years from ages 21 to 29 years, regardless of the age of sexual debut (National Cancer Institute, 2016). Adolescents and young women who forego speculum or pelvic examinations may be tested for chlamydia and gonorrhea from a urine sample, without an invasive examination. During the first counseling visit, the adolescent should receive information about all appropriate contraceptive methods. Taking this extra time to explain different methods helps dispel misinformation and allays the common concerns of adolescents about potential adverse health effects of contraceptives. It also helps the teenager feel comfortable in the clinic setting and with her nurse.

Because of her youth and possible lack of knowledge about anatomy and physiology, the adolescent often needs more extensive teaching than does the older woman. Liberal use of audiovisual materials such as pictures, anatomic models, and samples of various methods helps the young adult understand the information more easily. For example, giving her a patch, a vaginal ring, and a condom to manipulate or showing her the packet of pills she will be using are important aids.

Using understandable terminology is especially important when teaching adolescents. The nurse should know street terms for body parts and sexual intercourse because they may be the only words that are familiar to the teenager.

Adolescents are most successful when they choose contraceptive methods that are easy to use and seem unrelated to coitus. The most popular contraceptives for adolescents are OCs and condoms (Speroff & Darney, 2011). Teenagers often choose OCs because they are safe, have few contraindications, seem unrelated to sex, and are not difficult or messy. In addition, they increase bone density, regulate menses, reduce menstrual flow and cramping, and may decrease acne (Cunningham et al., 2014; Speroff & Darney, 2011).

Adolescent girls may, however, be quite inconsistent with daily pill ingestion. A method such as a ring used once a month or a patch used once a week may be more useful. Use of LARCs is particularly effective in adolescents and is recommended by the American College of Obstetricians and Gynecologists (2012, 2015b. 2015c) as first-line contraception for adolescents.

Teens are more likely than older women to discontinue any method for side effects such as spotting. Their concerns should be taken seriously, and attempts should be made to alleviate side effects. Otherwise, they are likely to stop using the method, often without notifying their health care provider, with pregnancy a possible result. They should understand all aspects of management of their contraceptive method and when a backup method is necessary.

Adolescents may use condoms alone to prevent pregnancy and STDs, especially at the beginning of a relationship or with casual partners. With long-term partners, they may discontinue condom use and use only hormonal methods. Some may use condoms, with or without hormonal methods, only if they have casual partners or if they are very concerned about both pregnancy and STDs.

Condom use should be encouraged to prevent STDs, even when another contraceptive method is used (see Fig. 25.2). Discussing perceived barriers to using condoms helps dispel misconceptions about pregnancy and STDs. Many young women are uneasy about asking their partners to use condoms. Discussing how to negotiate condom use with a partner can be particularly helpful. Teaching should include signs of STDs and what to do if they should occur, in addition to the current CDC recommendation of annual screening for chlamydia and gonorrhea for all sexually active women ages 25 and under. Using condoms and an OC or LARC method provides highly effective contraception along with protection from STDs and should be encouraged.

CRITICAL THINKING EXERCISE 25.1

A 15-year-old girl approaches the nurse with questions about contraception. She says she does not want to become pregnant, but her boyfriend does not want to use condoms. She says she is too embarrassed to go to a physician for other methods because she is afraid of the examination.

Questions

1. How should the nurse begin the discussion?
2. What should the nurse tell her about visiting a health care provider for contraception?
3. What should the nurse discuss about condom use?

CONTRACEPTION USE IN PERIMENOPAUSAL WOMEN

Pregnancy is uncommon after the age of 50 years. However, perimenopausal women may continue to ovulate as long as they have regular menstrual periods, and some ovulate even when indications of menopause are present. Therefore contraceptive counseling regarding the continued use of contraception until a women is 12 months past her last period is important for these women (Barry, 2011).

Fertility begins to decline when women reach 35 to 40 years, but they are still at risk for an unintended pregnancy (Nelson, 2011b). In fact, more than 30% of pregnancies in women over the of age 35 years are unintended (Godfrey et al., 2011). Therefore the nurse should offer these women contraceptive counseling whenever possible. Permanent sterilization is a very common method used by women who are older than 30 years. Healthy, nonsmoking women in their 40s can use combined hormonal contraceptives (COCs; ring, patch) to provide contraception and help regulate the irregular bleeding that often accompanies perimenopause. Women who smoke and are over the age of 35 years should not use estrogen-containing contraceptives (CDC, 2016c). Barrier methods, progestin-only contraception such as the contraceptive injection, progestin-only OCs, or LARC methods are safe choices for the perimenopausal woman who may smoke or have other health concerns that make other methods unsafe.

Perimenopausal women should have regular physical examinations to identify any conditions that would necessitate a change of contraceptive method.

KNOWLEDGE CHECK

5. What are some erroneous beliefs about contraception commonly held by adolescents?
6. Why might teenagers be hesitant to seek contraceptive information?
7. How can the nurse increase effectiveness in teaching adolescents about contraception?
8. What considerations are necessary in contraception for perimenopausal women?

METHODS OF CONTRACEPTION

Sterilization

Sterilization, both male and female, provides nonreversible, permanent contraception. Couples considering sterilization need counseling to ensure they understand all aspects of the procedure and its permanence. When this procedure is planned immediately after childbirth, the decision should be made well before labor begins and ideally during the third trimester of pregnancy. Future marriage, divorce, or death of a child may cause couples to regret their decision. The greatest risk for later regret occurs in women younger than 30 years of age at the time of sterilization, when there is pressure from a spouse, when there is a medical indication, or when the couple did not receive enough information (Beckmann, Herbert, Laube, Ling, & Smith, 2013).

Complications of sterilization are similar to those of any surgery, such as hemorrhage, infection, and anesthesia complications. Although pregnancy is rare after sterilization, the risk for failure should be discussed. Pregnancies occurring after tubal sterilization are more likely to be ectopic.

Tubal Sterilization

Tubal sterilization is widely used throughout the world. The procedure involves cutting or occluding the fallopian tubes to prevent fertilization and can be performed at any time. Many couples choose surgical tubal sterilization, tubal ligation, at the time of a cesarean birth or before hospital discharge after a vaginal birth. The first 48 hours after vaginal birth is an optimal time for the surgery because the fundus is located near the umbilicus and the fallopian tubes are directly below the abdominal wall. When performed after childbirth, regional (spinal or epidural) anesthesia is most commonly used. Interval sterilization, not associated with childbirth, is generally performed as outpatient surgery under general anesthesia.

Interval sterilization, tubal ligation, is usually performed in one of three ways. A mini-laparotomy incision may be made near the umbilicus in the postpartum period or just above the symphysis pubis at other times. Surgery also can be performed through a laparoscope inserted via a small incision. The third method is performed during other surgery, generally with cesarean birth. With each method, the surgeon blocks the tubes with clips, bands, or rings; removes a piece of the tubes and ties the ends; or uses electrocoagulation to destroy a portion of the tubes. If portions of the tubes are removed, they are sent for pathologic examination to ensure the tissues are actually fallopian tubes. Surgical tubal ligation is approximately 99% to 99.5% effective.

After sterilization, the woman avoids intercourse, strenuous exercise, or lifting heavy objects for 1 week. Mild analgesics may be needed for pain. The woman should call her health care provider if she has a fever over 38°C (100.4°F), fainting, severe pain, or bleeding or discharge from the incision sites (Roncari & Hou, 2011).

Nonsurgical sterilization is also possible. Essure involves the insertion of a small nickel coil through the cervix, vagina, and uterus and then into each fallopian tube. This procedure can be performed in a physician's office with local anesthesia or as an outpatient surgery. The tubes become permanently blocked during the next 3 months as tissue grows in and around the inserts. During this time, another contraceptive method is necessary. A hysterosalpingogram to confirm bilateral tubal occlusion is performed at the end of 3 months. The ACOG (2010) emphasizes the importance of the hysterosalpingogram at 3 months to ensure the tubes are completely blocked. Essure is over 99% effective but should be avoided for those women who have a nickel allergy. There is continued surveillance of the safety of Essure.

Vasectomy

Vasectomy, male sterilization, involves making a small incision or puncture in the scrotum to cut, tie, cauterize, or remove a section of the vas deferens, which carries sperm from the testes to the penis. After vasectomy, sperm no longer pass into the semen.

Although performed less frequently than female sterilization, vasectomy is a very popular method of contraception. It involves a lower morbidity rate and has a lower failure rate compared with tubal sterilization. Because it can be performed in a physician's office using a local anesthetic, it may be less expensive as well. Vasectomy is approximately 99.9% effective.

After surgery the man rests and then wears a scrotal support for 48 hours. He applies ice to the area for 4 hours and takes a mild analgesic, if needed. He should avoid bathing for 24 hours. Strenuous activity should be avoided for 1 week. The health care provider should be notified of fever, severe pain, bleeding or discharge at the site, swelling greater than twice the normal size, or a painful nodule (Roncari & Hou, 2011).

Intercourse may be resumed in 1 week, but the man is not sterile at that time (CDC, 2016c). Sperm may be present in the ductal system, distal to the ligation of the vas deferens, and the man may be able to impregnate a woman until sperm are no longer present in the semen. The couple should understand that complete sterilization may not occur for 3 months or more. The man should submit a semen specimen for analysis at 8 to 16 weeks to be sure that sperm are no longer present.

Long-Acting Reversible Contraceptives
Intrauterine Devices

Intrauterine devices (IUDs) are long-acting contraceptives that are inserted into the uterus to provide continuous pregnancy prevention. The Copper T 380A (ParaGard) and the levonorgestrel intrauterine systems (LNG-IUS, or Mirena, Skyla, and Liletta) are all shaped like the letter "T" (Fig. 25.3). ParaGard is effective for 10 years, Mirena is effective for 5 years, and Skyla and Liletta are effective for 3 years. IUDs are more effective than any other contraceptive method except Nexplanon and male sterilization.

IUDs can be inserted at any time the woman is not pregnant and does not currently have an STD or pelvic infection. Insertion immediately after delivery of the placenta and

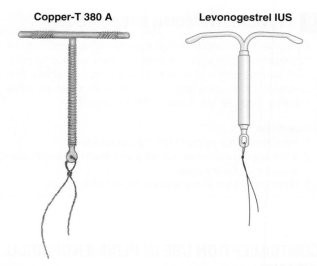

Copper-T 380 A   **Levonogestrel IUS**

FIG 25.3 The Copper T 380A (ParaGard) intrauterine device (IUD) and the levonorgestrel intrauterine system (LNG-IUS or Mirena). Currently, IUDs are considered a very safe method for preventing pregnancy.

during lactation are safe (Jensen & Mishell, 2012). ParaGard is effective immediately, and no backup is required. If Mirena, Skyla, or Liletta is inserted within 5 days of the start of the last menses, no backup contraceptive is needed. If it is inserted later, a backup contraceptive should be used for 7 days (ACOG, 2015c). Fertility returns promptly when the device is removed. ACOG recommends increased usage of IUDs in women of all ages and regardless of previous pregnancy history because they are a long-term, cost-effective means of lowering the risk for unintended pregnancy (ACOG, 2015b, 2015c). A large proportion of women have free or low-cost access to IUDs because of the Affordable Care Act.

Many women have misperceptions regarding the safety and effectiveness of IUDs (Hladky et al., 2011). Although safety was a concern with very different, early models in the 1970s, IUDs are considered very safe at this time. IUDs are convenient long-term, continuous contraceptive methods and eliminate the need to take pills, have injections, or perform other tasks on a daily basis or just before intercourse.

IUDs can be used by some women who cannot use other estrogen-containing hormonal contraception. They are considered safe for adolescents, nulliparas, and, if they use condoms, for women at risk for STDs (Dean & Schwarz, 2011).

Action. All IUDs create a sterile inflammatory response in the uterus that results in a spermicidal intrauterine environment. They do *not* cause abortion (Speroff & Darney, 2011). Progestin is continuously released from the LNG-IUS devices (Mirena, Skyla, and Liletta), which also thickens cervical mucus and prevents transport of sperm into the endometrial cavity and fallopian tubes. Only a small amount of progestin is absorbed systemically, leading to lower blood levels than those in users of other progestin-containing contraceptives.

The copper-covered ParaGard produces a spermicidal intrauterine environment by the release of copper ions into the uterus. This makes the uterus inhospitable to sperm transport and viability.

Side Effects. Side effects include cramping and irregular bleeding after insertion. *Menorrhagia* (increased bleeding during menstruation) and *dysmenorrhea* (painful menstruation) are common side effects of the copper-containing ParaGard. Irregular bleeding or spotting may occur with any IUD in the early months, but is less common with the LNG-IUS and may be followed by amenorrhea. The LNG-IUS may be used in women who had menorrhagia before using an IUD as a nonsurgical way to manage heavy menstrual bleeding. Ibuprofen or another nonsteroidal antiinflammatory drugs may reduce bleeding and cramping. Some women will require iron supplementation to treat anemia that is related to ParaGard.

Complications include perforation of the uterus at the time of insertion, as well as expulsion, which occurs in 1% to 5% of users (Beckmann et al., 2013). Although the rate of ectopic pregnancies in IUD users is much less than that in women not using contraceptives, pregnancies that do occur are more likely to be ectopic or result in spontaneous abortion or preterm birth. Women with recent or recurrent pelvic infections, a history of ectopic pregnancy, bleeding disorders, or abnormalities of the uterus should choose another contraceptive method.

There is a small risk for infection from contamination at the time of insertion, and this can be mediated by strict sterile technique during insertion. The IUD should not be inserted if a woman has mucopurulent cervical discharge (that is suspicious for STD) or a current infection such as chlamydia, gonorrhea, or pelvic inflammatory disease.

Teaching. Teaching the woman about side effects and what to expect in terms of potential change in bleeding patterns is very important. It is also a good idea for a woman to check for the presence of the plastic threads or strings extending from the IUD into the vagina. Expulsion, though uncommon, may occur during menses. Therefore the woman should feel for the threads weekly for the first 4 weeks, then monthly after menses, and if she has signs of expulsion (cramping or unexpected bleeding). If the threads are longer or shorter than they were previously, she should see her health care provider.

Signs and symptoms of infection such as unusual vaginal pain, foul-smelling discharge, pelvic pain, or fever should prompt a call to the health care provider. Any signs of pregnancy should be reported to rule out ectopic pregnancy or spontaneous abortion. The IUD should be removed promptly if pregnancy is confirmed.

KNOWLEDGE CHECK

9. What factors should a couple consider in deciding which method of sterilization to use?
10. What education is important for women choosing an IUD?

Contraceptive Implant

The contraceptive implant Nexplanon is a single rod implant that is inserted subcutaneously into the upper inner arm with the use of a local anesthetic. It is 2 mm thick and 4 cm (1.6 in) long and releases progestin continuously to provide 3 years of contraception. It acts to inhibit ovulation, thickens cervical mucus to prevent sperm penetrability, and thins out the endometrium making it unfavorable for implantation. As with IUDs, increased use of hormone implants is recommended by ACOG as a means of offering effective, long-acting, reversible contraception (ACOG, 2015b, 2015c). Implants can be inserted at any time, including immediately postpartum.

Side effects of the contraceptive implant include irregular menstrual bleeding, as with other progestin-only contraceptives, acne, and minimal weight gain. Bleeding is expected and not a sign of abnormality, but irregular bleeding is the most common reason for discontinuation of this method. Amenorrhea may occur with longer use. Fertility returns immediately, and pregnancy can occur at normal rates when the implant is removed (Speroff & Darney, 2011). The implant is often an appealing method for women who desire long-acting contraceptives, but who may fear the discomfort related to an IUD insertion.

Hormone Injections

Depo-Provera (medroxyprogesterone acetate [DMPA]) is an injectable progestin available in intramuscular (IM) and subcutaneous (SubQ) forms. It prevents ovulation for 15 weeks, although injections should be scheduled every 13 weeks (CDC, 2016c). It is convenient and contains no estrogen. The action and side effects are similar to those of other progestin contraceptives.

The IM form of Depo-Provera is given by deep IM injection. The SubQ form is given in the anterior thigh or abdomen. The site should not be massaged after injection because massage accelerates absorption and decreases the period of effectiveness. No backup method of contraception is necessary after the first injection if it is given within 7 days of the beginning of a menstrual period. A backup method of contraception is used for 7 days if the first injection is given at another time or if the woman is more than 2 weeks late returning for a subsequent injection (CDC, 2016c). It also can be given on the day it is prescribed if it is certain the woman is not pregnant and that she will use backup for the first week.

Menstrual irregularities are the major reason for discontinuation, and women should be informed about this before beginning the method. Although spotting and breakthrough bleeding are common, amenorrhea occurs in 80% of women using the IM form at 5 years and in 55% of women using the SubQ form after 1 year (Speroff & Darney, 2011). Other side effects include weight gain, headaches, depression, hair loss, nervousness, decreased **libido** (sexual desire), breast discomfort, and depression.

A decrease in bone density occurs with Depo-Provera. Although there is an increase in bone density after the drug is discontinued, the effect on peak bone mass and risk for osteoporosis is not known. Therefore current prescribing information states that Depo-Provera should not be used for longer than 2 years unless other methods of contraception are not suitable. It may be more of a problem for women who begin the drug during adolescence or young adulthood However, the World Health Organization considers the advantages of use of Depo-Provera in adolescents under age 18 years to generally outweigh the theoretical risk for bone density decrease (CDC, 2016c). Women using this method should obtain adequate amounts of calcium and vitamin D from diet or supplementation and should increase weight-bearing exercises.

Depo-Provera can be started in the immediate postpartum period and will not have a negative impact on milk supply in lactating women. The effectiveness is not changed by a woman's weight. There is a delay in return to fertility after the drug is discontinued. Approximately 59% of women resume menses in 6 months, and 25% do not resume menses for a year or more (Beckmann et al., 2013).

Oral Contraceptives

Oral contraceptives (OCs) are drugs that inhibit ovulation. They are the leading reversible contraceptive method in the United States (AGI, 2016b). They are available as COCs, which contain both estrogen and **progestin** (a natural or synthetic form of progesterone), and "minipills," which contain only progestin. Both types have much lower hormone levels than the original OCs from many decades ago, and therefore the risk for long-term side effects is decreased. If OCs are used perfectly, 3 women in 1000 become pregnant in the first year.

Combination Oral Contraceptives

Estrogen and progestin combinations (COCs) are the most common OCs. COCs prevent pregnancy primarily by suppressing production of luteinizing hormone and follicle-stimulating hormone, thus inhibiting maturation of the follicle and ovulation, COCs also may cause thickening of cervical mucus, which prevents sperm from entering the upper genital tract. In addition, tubal motility is slowed and interferes with sperm and ova transport.

Monophasic or multiphasic dosages are available. Monophasic pills have estrogen and progestin content, which remains constant throughout the cycle. With multiphasic pills, the estrogen dose and progestin levels may vary at different times of the cycle. Because the dosage changes throughout the phases, women must take the pills in the proper order to maintain effectiveness.

Patterns of pill use vary. Most COCs are available in packets of 21 or 28 tablets. With 21-tablet packets, the woman takes 1 pill daily for 3 weeks and then stops for 1 week, during which time menstruation occurs. Packets of 28 tablets include 21 active tablets and 7 tablets made of an inert substance that the woman takes during the fourth week. In some types, the "placebo" pills contain iron. The extra pills avoid disrupting the everyday routine of taking pills. Some formulations contain 24 active tablets with only 4 inactive tablets. Women using COCs have shorter, lighter withdrawal bleeding. Other COCs are designed to provide 84 days of active pills and 7 placebo pills or 7 pills with a just a small amount of estrogen—this allows women to have menses only four times a year.

Some women prefer continuous extended cycles in which menses is delayed or does not occur. Women may wish to regulate their cycle for a special event or for preference of not having a withdrawal menses. These women take two or more pill packs without taking the placebo pills for several packs or indefinitely. Breakthrough bleeding and spotting are a common problem with extended or continuous use, but this usually lessens over time. A potential disadvantage is that a woman might not recognize an early pregnancy if it occurred.

COCs can be used in the postpartum period, but according to the CDC should be avoided in the first month postpartum because of the increased risk for thrombotic event (CDC, 2016b).

Progestin Only

Progestin-only pills (POPs) are taken daily with no hormone-free days. POPs are less effective at inhibiting ovulation but cause thickening of cervical mucus to prevent penetration by sperm. They also make the endometrial lining unfavorable for implantation. These pills avoid the side effects and risk factors associated with estrogen and are useful for women who cannot take estrogen.

If a woman misses any pills or does not take them at the same time each day, the chances of pregnancy increase. Another method of contraception should be used for the first 2 days of the first cycle unless the woman starts the method during the first 5 days of her cycle or immediately after stopping another hormonal method. Backup contraception also should be used for 2 days if the woman is more than 3 hours late in taking a pill or has vomiting or diarrhea (Raymond, 2011).

Breakthrough bleeding and higher risk for pregnancy have made POPs less popular than the COCs. Amenorrhea occurs in some women.

Benefits, Risks, and Cautions. When OCs are chosen, the balance between benefits and risks must be weighed for each individual (Table 25.4). Women often think the risks are higher than they actually are, yet OCs are safer for most women than pregnancy (Beckmann et al., 2013). The method has many benefits in addition to safe, reliable contraception. OCs result in regular menses and decreased flow, premenstrual syndrome, and dysmenorrhea; reduced acne; and improved bone density. COCs also provide a lifetime risk reduction for ovarian and uterine cancer.

OCs should not be used by women who have certain medical complications (see "Critical to Remember: Cautions in Using Combined Oral Contraceptives"). Smoking significantly increases complications for women of all ages. Women who smoke and are over the age of 35 years should not use estrogen-containing contraceptives (CDC, 2016b; Daniels, 2015). Women who have previously smoked must abstain from all sources of nicotine for at least 6 to 12 months to be considered a nonsmoker (Speroff & Darney, 2011). Taking any COC increases the risk for venous thromboembolism (VTE), and therefore their use should be avoided in women with risk factors for that condition.

TABLE 25.4 Potential Benefits, Disadvantages, and Risks of Oral Contraceptives

Benefits	Disadvantages	Risks*

• Unrelated to coitus
• Highly effective
• Regulates menstrual cycles and reduces dysmenorrhea, menstrual blood loss, and associated anemia
• Amenorrhea (may be seen as a disadvantage)
• Fertility usually returns within 3 months
• Decreased incidence of:
  • Premenstrual dysphoric disorder symptoms
  • Benign breast disease
  • Pelvic inflammatory disease
  • Salpingitis
  • Ectopic pregnancy
  • Ovarian, endometrial, and colorectal cancer
• Improves:
  • Acne
  • Endometriosis
  • Many premenstrual symptoms
  • Dysmenorrhea
  • Bleeding from fibroids (leiomyomas)
  • Bone mass (COCs only)
  • Hirsutism (excessive hair growth)
  • Rheumatoid arthritis
	• Must be taken every day near same time, especially POPs
	• Side effects may include:
	  • Breakthrough bleeding
	  • Nausea
	  • Headache
	  • Breast tenderness
	  • Amenorrhea (may be seen as an advantage)
	  • Chloasma
		• No protection against STDs
		• May increase risk of cervical cancer
		• Increased incidence of:
		  • Deep and superficial vein thrombosis
		  • Pulmonary embolism
		  • Myocardial infarction
		  • Stroke (in smokers)
		  • Hypertension
		  • Migraines
		  • Chlamydial infection
		  • Gallbladder disease

COC, Combined oral contraceptive; *POP,* progestin-only contraceptive pills; *STD,* sexually transmitted disease.
*Incidence of many risks is significantly reduced with low-dose oral contraceptives (OCs) presently used. Avoiding OC use in women who smoke or have other risk factors lowers risk for cardiovascular disease significantly.

CRITICAL TO REMEMBER

Cautions in Using Combined Oral Contraceptives

Combined oral contraceptives should not be used by women with a history of any of the following:
• Thrombophlebitis and thromboembolic disorders
• Cerebrovascular or cardiovascular diseases
• Estrogen-dependent cancer or breast cancer
• Benign or malignant liver tumors
• Hypertension (unless well controlled by medication)
• Migraines with aura or migraines in women older than 35 years of age
• Diabetes longer than 20 years or with vascular or other organ involvement

Combined oral contraceptives should not be used by women who currently have any of the following:
• Any of the previously listed conditions
• Impaired liver function
• Suspected or known pregnancy
• Undiagnosed vaginal bleeding
• Cigarette smoking in women older than 35 years
• Major surgery requiring prolonged immobilization

Data from Nelson, A. L., & Cwiak, C. (2011). Combined oral contraceptives. In R. A. Hatcher, J. Trussell, A. L. Nelson, et al., (Eds.), *Contraceptive technology* (20th ed., pp. 249–341). New York: Ardent Media.

Hazards are decreased by careful screening for risk factors in each woman and the nurse's familiarity of the CDC MEC. Obese women may have a higher risk for thromboembolic problems, but this is not considered a contraindication to OC use. Evidence is inconsistent about whether body weight affects OC effectiveness (CDC, 2016b). Women with diabetes of less than 20 years' duration, who do not smoke, and are in good health may use OCs with adequate supervision of their condition (CDC, 2016b).

OCs provide no protection against STDs. A woman should be advised to have her partner use condoms and spermicide if he may be infected or the relationship is not monogamous.

Side Effects. Approximately 33% of women who do not wish to become pregnant discontinue COCs within the first year, usually because of side effects (Trussell, 2011). Most side effects are minor and include signs and symptoms often seen in pregnancy. Using a different formulation of hormones may reduce some side effects. For example, decreasing the amount of estrogen helps relieve nausea and breast tenderness. Breakthrough bleeding occurs most often in the first 3 months and then usually subsides. If it is a problem, a COC with a different level or type of hormones can be used to decrease bleeding. Some women complain of weight gain while taking OCs, but studies have not shown it to be caused by the pills (Beckmann et al., 2013). Other side effects include fluid retention, amenorrhea, and melasma. Side effects often decrease after the first few months of use and are less frequent in low-dose OCs.

Teaching. Many unintended pregnancies result from failure to carefully follow instructions for the use of OCs. However, education about proper use greatly increases effectiveness. Teaching should be extensive when the woman begins to use the hormones. Follow-up is necessary to ensure her questions are answered and unanticipated problems resolved. Because the instructions can be complex, they should be written clearly and simply in her own language, if she can read.

Teaching about when to start taking OCs is especially important. Methods of beginning OC use include the following:
- *Quick start:* The woman takes the first pill on the day the pills are prescribed (if it is reasonably certain that she is not pregnant). A backup method is needed for the first 7 days of the first cycle unless her period started 5 days ago or less. This method is preferred because it provides immediate protection and may improve continuation. It avoids a delay during which a pregnancy might occur.
- *First-day start:* The first pill is taken on the first day of the next menstrual period. No backup method is needed.
- *Sunday start:* The pills are begun on the first Sunday after menses begins. With this method, the woman avoids having a period on the weekend. A backup method is used for the first 7 days of the first cycle.

The nurse should listen carefully to the woman's concerns about side effects and help her find methods of management. One study showed that women who did not fully understand the advantages of OCs and had low confidence in their ability to use them were less likely to continue use at 6 months (Dempsey et al., 2011).

When women discontinue OCs because of the side effects, they may not use another contraceptive or may use one that is less effective and become pregnant as a result. Women should be instructed to keep a backup contraceptive method or emergency contraception readily available in case they decide to stop taking their OCs.

It is essential that nurses be honest about the side effects that should be expected with all contraceptives. Teaching about temporary side effects may help the woman endure them until they are no longer present. Women should know that spotting is a common side effect of many hormonal contraceptive methods, particularly in the beginning. Over time, spotting may diminish or amenorrhea may develop. If changes in bleeding patterns or irregularity are unacceptable to the woman, she should choose another contraceptive method.

Consistent Daily Ingestion. Maintaining a constant blood hormone level is important for effectiveness, especially with POPs. Therefore the woman must take the pills near the same time each day. Many women make them a part of their bedtime routine, others take their OCs with a meal to avoid nausea, and some take their OCs when they brush their teeth

in the morning. Breakthrough bleeding is more likely when a significant time variation occurs between doses.

Women should understand that some pills must be taken in a certain order and that changing the order will decrease the effectiveness of the method. Illness may affect the blood hormone levels. A woman who experiences vomiting or diarrhea should use a backup method of contraception for 7 days because the hormones may not have been properly absorbed.

Missed Doses. Instructions for the woman who misses one or more doses should be provided. Women who frequently miss OCs should be counseled about other contraceptive methods that might be more effective for them.

The woman should follow instructions from her provider if she misses doses of her OC. Instructions may vary according to the type of OC used, the number of doses missed, and the time in the cycle the OC is missed. The woman who misses pills early in the cycle is at higher risk for ovulating. Different health care providers may use different regimens. See "Patient Teaching: What to Do if an Oral Contraceptive Dose Is Missed" for an example of instructions.

PATIENT TEACHING

What to Do If an Oral Contraceptive Dose Is Missed

Instructions for missed oral contraceptives include the following (CDC, 2016c):

General
Missing inactive tablets at any time will not increase the risk for pregnancy. Discard the missed pills.

Combined Oral Contraceptives
One Missed Pill
- Take one active pill as soon as possible. Take the next dose at the usual time.
- Continue the pack as usual.
- No backup contraceptive is necessary.

Two or More Missed Pills in the First 2 Weeks
- Take two pills as soon as possible, then one tablet daily.
- Use backup contraception for the next 7 days.

Two Missed Pills in the Last Week of Active Pills
- Take one active pill each day until they are finished.
- Discard the inactive pills.
- Start a new package the next day.
- Use backup contraception for 7 days if unable to start a new pack of pills.

Centers for Disease Control and Prevention. (2016c). U.S. Selected Practice Recommendations for Contraceptive Use, 2016. *Morbidity and Mortality Weekly Report, 65*(4), 1–66.

If a woman misses a period and thinks she may be pregnant because she missed one or more doses, she should take a pregnancy test immediately. Using another contraceptive method during this time is essential. However, there is no association between inadvertently taking OCs when pregnant and fetal complications.

Postpartum and Lactation. COCs increase the risk for VTE and reduce milk production in lactating women, and very small amounts may be transferred to the milk. All postpartum women should avoid COCs for 3 weeks after giving birth, and lactating women should avoid COCs for 4 weeks. Progestin-only OCs may be a better choice if a woman wishes to use a hormonal contraceptive because these OCs do not affect milk quantity or quality. There is no evidence of adverse effects on the infant, and no waiting period is required (CDC, 2016c).

Medications. OCs may interact with other medications, and the effectiveness of each may be changed. Some may increase or decrease estrogen or progesterone levels. OCs may interact with some anticonvulsants (which may be used for seizure disorder or psychiatric illnesses) antiretroviral drugs, and rifampin for tuberculosis. Over-the-counter drugs should also be considered. For example, St. John's wort, which some women take for depression, interferes with OC effectiveness (Renner & Jensen, 2012). Because of these various interactions, the woman should always tell her health care providers and her pharmacist about other drugs or supplements she is taking.

Follow-Up. The only essential follow-up for women who take OCs is yearly blood pressure measurement. It is not necessary for women to have yearly pelvic examinations, Pap tests, or breast examinations to receive prescriptions for OCs. Women using OCs should follow the same recommendations as those for women who do not take OCs.

During the follow-up visit, the woman's ability to remember to take a pill every day should be evaluated. Other methods should be discussed if remembering is a problem or if she wants to change methods.

Return of fertility is rapid after the pills are discontinued (Nelson & Cwiak, 2011). A woman may wish to wait until her menstrual cycle is reestablished before conceiving so that she can date the beginning of her pregnancy more accurately. She should be advised to take folic acid for several months before becoming pregnant to help prevent neural tube defects in the fetus.

The woman should report any signs of adverse reactions immediately. Use of the acronym *ACHES* may help the woman remember signs that may indicate complications (Table 25.5).

Emergency Contraception

Emergency contraception (EC), often called the "morning-after pill," is a method to prevent pregnancy after unprotected intercourse. EC may be used after contraceptive failure such as a condom breaking during intercourse or when a woman misses too many OCs. It also may be used after rape or in other situations in which contraceptives were used incorrectly or not at all.

Three forms of EC (Plan B One-Step, Next Choice, Next Choice One Dose) contain the progestin levonorgestrel. In the past, EC was available at pharmacies without a prescription for women age 17 years and older but those younger than 17 years needed a prescription (FDA, 2009). In 2013 a federal court decision declared Plan B One-Step should be available to women and men of all ages without a prescription (FDA, 2013).

The progestin-only ECs work by delaying or inhibiting ovulation, thickening cervical mucus and interfering with the function of the corpus luteum. The treatment is ineffective if implantation has already occurred, and it does not harm a developing fetus (Trussell & Schwarz, 2011).

Another form of EC is ulipristal acetate (Ella), which requires a prescription for all ages. Ella acts to delay or block the surge of luteinizing hormone and ovulation. It also may inhibit implantation and requires a pregnancy test before use, because it may disrupt an early pregnancy (AAP, 2012; ACOG, 2015a).

The most common method of EC involves taking one (Plan B One-Step, Next Choice One Dose) or two (Next Choice) tablets (taken together) that contain a high dose of progestin. The pills should be taken as soon as possible or up to 120 hours after unprotected intercourse (Trussell & Schwarz, 2011). EC will not prevent pregnancy if unprotected intercourse occurs after EC is used.

COCs may also be used in larger-than-usual doses to prevent pregnancy. The number of tablets varies according to the specific COC used and this method should only be used under the guidance and recommendation of a health care provider. This method may cause nausea, so women are often advised to take an antiemetic before taking the pills.

Insertion of the Copper T 380A IUD within 5 days of intercourse also may be used and provides 99% effectiveness (Trussell & Schwartz, 2011). It has the added advantage of

	TABLE 25.5 ACHES*: Warning Signs of Oral Contraceptive Complications	
	Warning Sign	**Possible Complication**
A	Abdominal pain (severe)	Mesenteric or pelvic vein thrombosis
		Benign liver tumor, gallbladder disease
C	Chest pain, dyspnea, hemoptysis, cough	Pulmonary emboli or myocardial infarction
H	Severe headache, weakness or numbness of extremities, hypertension	Stroke, migraine
E	Eye problems (complete or partial loss of vision), headache	Retinal vein thrombosis, stroke, migraine
S	Severe leg pain or swelling (calf or thigh), swelling, heat, redness	Deep vein thrombosis

*The acronym *ACHES* can be used to help women remember warning signs that may indicate complications when using oral contraceptives. Other signs include jaundice, a breast lump, and depression. The woman should contact her health care provider if any of these signs develops. Data from Nelson, A. L., & Cwiak, C. (2011). Combined oral contraceptives. In R. A. Hatcher, J. Trussell, A. L. Nelson, et al. (Eds.), *Contraceptive technology* (20th ed., pp. 249–341). New York: Ardent Media.

providing long-term (10 years) protection from pregnancy for those who choose this method.

Although EC is available, use is suboptimal. Many women are unaware of the availability of EC, and those who are do not always use it to prevent unintended pregnancies. Women may not know how or where to get it. Information about EC and how to obtain it should be included whenever education about contraception is offered to women in case they might later wish to use it. The Association of Women's Health, Obstetric and Neonatal Nurses (AWHONN, 2012) states that nurses should ensure that women receive information about all types of contraception, including how to obtain emergency contraception.

Women who need EC should receive counseling about their regular contraceptive method. They may not understand how to use their method correctly or may wish information about other, more effective options. Because of the short timeframe during which EC is effective, some health care providers give women prescriptions to use at a later date if they should need it. Information about where EC can be obtained is available on the Internet at www.NOT-2-LATE.com. Women who use EC have not been shown to be more likely to have risky sex, future unplanned pregnancies, or STDs (Jurrow, 2011).

Transdermal Contraceptive Patch

The **transdermal contraceptive patch** (Ortho Evra) releases small amounts of estrogen (ethinyl estradiol) and progestin (norelgestromin), which are absorbed through the skin to suppress ovulation and thicken cervical mucus. It also regulates menstrual cycles.

The contraceptive patch is as effective as OCs, or it even may be more effective because it is used once a week instead of daily. A nonhormonal contraceptive should be used during the first week of use, unless the patch is started within the first 5 days of the menstrual period (CDC, 2016c). For most users, fertility returns quickly, with hormone levels back to normal within 1 month of discontinuing the patch (Nanda, 2011).

The patch is applied to clean, dry, nonirritated skin on the abdomen, buttock, upper outer arm, or upper torso, excluding the breasts. Areas where clothing such as straps or waistbands may rub the patch should not be used. The woman should avoid using oils or lotions in the area because the patch may not stick. Adherence to the skin is good even in the shower or when exercising or swimming. The patch should not be cut or altered, and no more than one patch should be worn at a time.

A new patch is applied to a different site weekly on the same day of the week for 3 weeks and worn continuously for 7 days. Then the patch is removed for 1 week. During the patch-free week, the woman has a period. After 7 patch-free days, she applies a new patch and begins the cycle again. Women can have extended cycles without menses by using patches for several cycles or continuously.

Side effects include spotting, breast tenderness, headaches, and skin reactions. Other side effects and risks are similar to those for COCs. The patch has been found to be less effective in women who weigh more than 198 lb (90 kg) (Nanda, 2011).

The risk for VTE is higher with patch use than with OC use because total exposure to estrogen is greater. However, studies have had conflicting results (Cunningham et al., 2014). The risk for VTE is less than that for pregnancy, but women with risk factors for VTE should discuss the risks and benefits of patch use with their health care provider (Nanda, 2011).

Because the patch must be applied only once a week, it may be easier than OCs for women who have difficulty remembering to take a pill every day. However, it is visible on the skin, which may be a problem for adolescents who do not want their contraceptive use known by others.

If a patch detaches, the woman should try to reattach it. If it will not adhere again, she should replace it with a new patch. She should not use tape to keep it on, because the contraceptive is in the glue of the patch. No backup contraception is necessary. If the patch is off 2 or more days or she is 2 or more days late in changing the first or second patch, the woman should apply a new one and use backup for 7 days. If the woman is 2 or more days late in changing the patch in the third patch week, a new one should be applied, she should omit the patch-free week, and start a new patch cycle (CDC, 2016c).

Contraceptive Vaginal Ring

Women using the **vaginal contraceptive ring** (NuvaRing) insert a soft, flexible vinyl ring into the vagina and leave it in place for 3 weeks. The ring, which measures 5 cm (2 inches) in diameter and is 4 mm thick, releases small amounts of progestin and estrogen continuously to prevent ovulation (Fig. 25.4). The woman removes the ring at the end of the third week, and withdrawal bleeding occurs. A new ring is inserted to begin the next cycle 1 week after the old ring was removed.

Although a prescription is required, no fitting or particular placement in the vagina is necessary. There is no need to think about contraception except twice a month when the ring is being placed or removed.

Women must be comfortable inserting the device into the vagina. Placement and removal are quick and easy. Allowing a woman to try placing the ring in the provider's office where

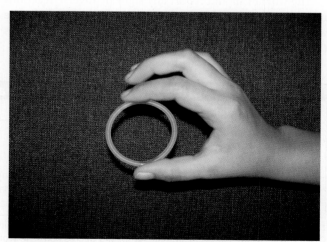

FIG 25.4 The vaginal contraceptive ring (NuvaRing) is 5 cm (2 inches) across and 4 mm thick.

help is available often increases confidence. For the woman who does not want her contraceptive use known by others, the fact that the ring is not visible to others is appealing.

Use can begin during the first 5 days of the menstrual cycle, even if the woman is still bleeding or on any other day. A backup contraceptive is necessary for the first 7 days of the first cycle if the ring is inserted on any day but the first 5 days of menses.

The most common side effects are headaches, breast tenderness, and nausea—similar to those with COCs. Other side effects include vaginitis, expulsion, or vaginal discharge or discomfort. Although some women or their partners can feel the ring during intercourse, it is generally not a problem. Breakthrough bleeding is less common than with OCs. Women who should not use hormonal contraceptives also should not use the vaginal ring.

The ring may be removed for up to 3 hours without loss of effectiveness. If 48 or more hours without the ring occurs in the first 2 weeks, the ring should be reinserted and a backup method used for 7 days. If the ring is out of the vagina for 48 or more hours in the third week, the woman can leave it out and have a withdrawal bleed or insert a new ring, omit the ring-free week, and start a new cycle of ring use (CDC, 2016c; Nanda, 2011). If the woman desires extended cycles, she can insert a new ring when she removes the old one and avoid the withdrawal bleeding.

KNOWLEDGE CHECK

11. What is the mechanism of action of hormonal contraceptives?
12. What side effect is most likely to cause some women to discontinue use of some hormonal contraceptives?
13. What do women taking OCs need to know about this contraceptive method?
14. How soon after unprotected intercourse should EC be used?

Barrier Methods

Barrier methods of contraception involve chemicals or devices that prevent sperm from entering the cervix. The method may kill the sperm or place a temporary partition between the penis and the cervix. All barrier methods are coitus related and may interfere with spontaneity. They avoid the use of systemic hormones, however, and provide some protection from STDs.

Chemical Barriers

Chemicals that kill sperm are called **spermicides** and are available in many forms. Creams and gels are generally used with mechanical barriers such as the diaphragm or the cervical cap. Foams, foaming tablets, suppositories, and vaginal film may be used alone or with another contraceptive. They are inserted deep into the vagina about 15 minutes before sexual intercourse so they are in contact with the cervix. Vaginal films and suppositories must melt before they

become effective, which takes approximately 15 minutes. Spermicides are generally effective for less than 1 hour. They should be reapplied if intercourse is repeated. Women should not douche for at least 6 hours after intercourse (Cates & Harwood, 2011; Taylor, 2011).

Spermicides are readily available without a prescription, inexpensive, and easy to use. Using spermicides increases lubrication, which decreases the risk for condom breakage. This is an advantage, especially during lactation or in menopause when vaginal secretions are decreased. Effectiveness is increased when spermicides are used with a mechanical barrier method.

Some women and their partners think spermicides are messy and interfere with sensation during intercourse. Some women also may experience a vaginal sensitivity to spermicide that may cause burning. Frequent use (two or more times a day) or sensitivity to the products may cause genital irritation, which could increase susceptibility to infections, including HIV infection. Spermicides do not protect against STDs and should not be used for that purpose.

Mechanical Barriers

Mechanical barriers are devices placed over the penis or the cervix to prevent passage of sperm into the uterus. They include the condom, sponge, diaphragm, and cervical cap.

Male Condom. Condoms, the only male contraceptive device currently available, are the third most popular method of contraception in the United States and are used by almost 9 million couples (Warner & Steiner, 2011). They cover the penis to prevent sperm from entering the vagina.

Condoms are most often made of latex and may be coated with a lubricant. Latex condoms provide the best protection available (other than abstinence) against STDs, including HIV infection. For this reason, condoms should be used during any possible exposure to an STD, even if another contraceptive technique is practiced or the woman is pregnant.

People who are allergic to latex should avoid the use of latex condoms because severe reactions are possible. They may use polyurethane or natural membrane condoms instead. Polyurethane condoms are thinner than latex but may require lubrication to avoid breakage and are more likely to slip off. Natural membrane condoms do not prevent passage of organisms that may cause STDs.

Condoms are readily available, are inexpensive, and can be carried inconspicuously by the man or the woman. The typical failure rate can be decreased by combining condom use with another method such as a vaginal spermicide. Reservoir tips and water-based lubricants help prevent breakage. The slippage and breakage rate is approximately 5% to 8% (Beckmann et al., 2013).

Because condoms must be applied just before intercourse, some couples object to the interference with spontaneity. Others think condoms interfere with sensation. Men with erectile dysfunction may have problems with condom slippage (Nelson, 2011a). Condoms may be affected by vaginal medications or lubricants, and they should not be used concurrently. Only water-based lubricants should be used for latex condoms because oil-based lubricants will cause deterioration of the latex.

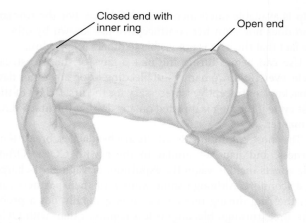

FIG 25.5 The Female Condom. A woman can protect herself from sexually transmitted diseases without relying on use of the male condom.

PATIENT TEACHING

What Is the Proper Way to Use Male Condoms?

Although condoms are easy to use, proper use increases their effectiveness.

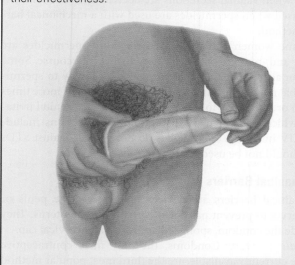

- Condoms are available in a variety of colors, textures, and materials, but those made of latex or polyurethane are most effective. Natural membrane condoms may help protect against pregnancy but not against sexually transmitted diseases.
- Check the expiration dates on packages because condoms may deteriorate after 5 years. Open the package carefully and check the condom to see that it is not torn or damaged before using it.
- Lubrication may increase comfort for the woman and reduce the risk for breakage. Use a water-soluble lubricant or a spermicide because oil-based products (such as petroleum jelly or baby oil) cause deterioration of latex condoms.
- Always apply the condom before there is any contact of the penis with the vagina.
- Squeeze the air out of the end of the condom, and leave half an inch of space at the tip as the condom is unrolled to the base of the erect penis. This space allows a place for sperm to collect and helps prevent breakage.
- Withdraw the erect penis from the vagina while holding the condom at the base so it does not slip off and no semen spills into the vagina.
- Use a new condom each time intercourse is repeated.

Female Condom. The female condom (also called a *vaginal pouch*) is a polyurethane sheath inserted into the vagina. A flexible ring inside the closed end of the condom fits over the cervix like a diaphragm. Another ring extends outside the vagina to partially cover the perineum (Fig. 25.5). The female condom is the first contraceptive device that allows a woman some protection from STDs without relying on the male condom. Male and female condoms should not be used together because they may adhere to each other.

Sponge. The contraceptive sponge (Today) is made of soft polyurethane that traps and absorbs semen and contains the spermicide nonoxynol-9. The sponge is approximately 5 cm (2 inches) in diameter and provides contraception for 24 hours without the need to add spermicide for repeated intercourse. It does not require a prescription, contains no hormones, is easy to use, and can be inserted just before intercourse or hours ahead of time.

To use the sponge, the woman washes her hands and wets the sponge with about two tablespoons of water, squeezing the sponge until it becomes sudsy. She then folds the sponge, with the concave ("dimple") area inside and the loop on the outside of the fold, and inserts it into the vagina. When the sponge is released, the "dimple" covers the cervix and helps keep the sponge in place during intercourse. To eliminate interference with spontaneity, some women insert the sponge hours in advance when intercourse is anticipated.

Repeated intercourse does not require added spermicide or a new sponge. It should remain in place for at least 6 hours after the last intercourse. It is removed by inserting a finger into the loop and pulling slowly. The sponge should not be used during menstruation or left in the vagina for more than 24 to 30 hours because of an increased risk for toxic shock syndrome (Cates & Harwood, 2011). It should not be used by women with a history of toxic shock syndrome, and it does not protect against STDs. The sponge may cause irritation or be difficult to remove for some women.

Diaphragm. The **diaphragm** is a latex dome surrounded by a spring or coil. The woman places spermicidal cream or gel into the dome and around the rim and then inserts the diaphragm over the cervix. Because it covers the cervix, the diaphragm prevents passage of sperm while holding spermicide in place for additional protection.

Traditional diaphragms must be fitted by a health care provider, but in most cases they are no longer available in the United States. Currently, a one size fits "most women" diaphragm, Caya, is commercially available and is covered under most insurance plans. All diaphragms should not be used for the first 6 weeks after delivery (AAP & ACOG, 2012).

Pressure on the urethra from a diaphragm may cause irritation and urinary tract infections. Voiding after intercourse may help prevent infections. An allergy to latex or a history of toxic shock syndrome precludes use. The diaphragm may be damaged by oil-based lubricants and some medications used for vaginal infections.

Cervical Cap. The **cervical cap** (FemCap) is a cuplike device placed over the cervix to prevent sperm from entering. It is similar to the diaphragm but smaller and must be fitted by a health care provider. The flexible silicone cap is inserted over the cervix after placing spermicide on both sides. It stays in place by suction. The cap does not cause pressure on the bladder and can remain in place for 48 hours. More spermicide is inserted into the

PATIENT TEACHING

How to Use a Diaphragm

- Follow instructions carefully when using your diaphragm. Skill at insertion and removal increases with practice.
- Plan to insert the diaphragm up to 6 hours before intercourse. Empty your bladder before insertion.
- Spread about a tablespoon of spermicidal cream or gel inside the dome and around the rim.

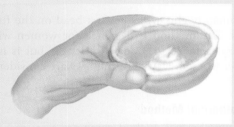

- Insert the diaphragm into the vagina with the spermicide toward the cervix. A squatting position or placing one foot on the tub or toilet seat makes insertion and removal easier.

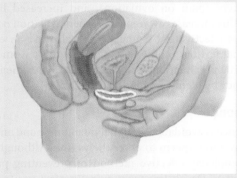

- Be sure that the front rim fits behind your pubic bone and that you can feel the cervix through the center of the diaphragm.

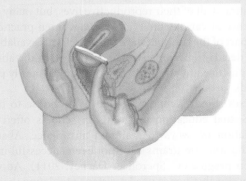

- If more than 6 hours passes between insertion and intercourse or if you have intercourse again, insert more spermicide into the vagina without removing the diaphragm.
- Leave the diaphragm in place for at least 6 hours after the last intercourse. Leaving it in place for more than 24 hours increases the risk for toxic shock syndrome.
- Using the diaphragm during menstrual periods increases the risk for toxic shock syndrome.
- Douching with the diaphragm in place is unnecessary and lessens the effectiveness.
- To remove the diaphragm, assume a squatting position and bear down. Hook a finger around the front rim to break the suction, and pull down.

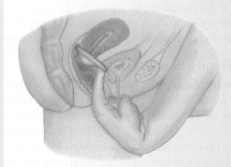

- Wash the diaphragm with mild soap and dry well after each use. Inspect it for holes by holding it up to a light or filling it with water. If you find a hole, use another contraceptive method and go to your health care provider for a new diaphragm.

TABLE 25.6   Natural Family Planning Methods

Method	Application	Comments
Calendar method	Subtract 18 days from shortest cycle and 11 days from longest cycle to determine fertile period.	*Example:* 28- to 32-day cycle = fertile between days 10 and 21.
Standard days method	Intercourse is safe only on days 1 through 7 and day 20 to the end of the cycle. Use a barrier method or abstain on days 8 through 19.	Ineffective if cycle length is shorter than 26 days or longer than 32 days.
Basal body temperature method	See "Patient Teaching: How to Assess Cervical Mucus and Basal Body Temperature."	Avoid intercourse until night of third day after temperature rise. Unreliable if used alone. Affected by illness, lack of sleep, stress.
Cervical mucus (ovulation or Billings) method	Assess mucus at vaginal orifice daily. Avoid intercourse during menses and from time mucus appears until 4 days after clear, slippery, stretchy mucus ends.	Intercourse is safe only every other day, because semen interferes with assessment of mucus.
2-Day method	Check for mucus each day. Fertility is determined by presence of cervical mucus on current or previous day.	Intercourse is avoided if woman notices any secretions at all.
Symptothermal method	Combine all above methods and assess weight gain, libido, bloating, and mittelschmerz.	Requires much education and motivation.

vagina without removing the cap if intercourse is repeated. The nurse should teach the woman to feel her cervix to check placement before and after intercourse because the cap can become dislodged.

Cervical caps should not be removed for 8 hours after the last intercourse (Speroff & Darney, 2011). The cap has a loop to assist in removal. Caps should not be used during menses or in women with a history of toxic shock syndrome. Cap sizes are based on whether the woman has had past pregnancies and births.

Natural Family Planning Methods

Natural family planning methods, also called *fertility awareness* or *periodic abstinence methods,* use physiologic cues to predict ovulation so women can determine when conditions are favorable for fertilization (Table 25.6). These methods can help women who wish to become pregnant (see Chapter 26) or avoid it.

Natural family planning helps women learn about how their bodies change throughout the menstrual cycle. It is acceptable to most religious groups and avoids the use of drugs, chemicals, and devices. Couples must be highly motivated to use these methods because they must abstain from intercourse during as much as half the menstrual cycle. The method is very unforgiving, and errors in predicting ovulation may lead to pregnancy from intercourse during the fertile time. Some women use the method to determine when they are fertile and use a barrier contraceptive at that time.

Calendar

The calendar method is based on the timing of ovulation approximately 14 days before the onset of menses. The couple must abstain or use another method during the days calculated to be fertile. The method is unreliable because many factors such as illness or stress can affect the time of ovulation.

Standard Days Method

This method uses a string of color-coded beads to help keep track of the fertile and infertile days of each cycle.

The woman begins with the first bead on the first day of menses. The method is designed for women with cycles that vary from 26 to 32 days in length but is ineffective for other women. Days 8 through 19 are considered fertile days.

Symptothermal Method

The symptothermal method combines assessment of **basal body temperature (BBT)** (body temperature at rest) and cervical mucus daily. In addition, symptoms that occur near ovulation, such as weight gain, abdominal bloating, **mittelschmerz** (pain on ovulation), and increased libido are noted. This increases awareness of when ovulation occurs and increases effectiveness. Some women also use an electronic hormonal fertility monitor. It is designed for women trying to become pregnant but also can be used by women to avoid pregnancy by identifying fertile times.

Abstinence

Abstinence is avoidance of sexual intercourse and any activity that may allow sperm to enter the vagina. Although it is the only completely effective method of preventing pregnancy and most STDs, abstinence requires perfect use to be effective. Depending on the time within the menstrual cycle it occurs, intercourse without the use of a contraceptive has up to an 85% chance of resulting in pregnancy. Most women are not abstinent all of their reproductive lives, but many practice abstinence at various intervals. Some women practice abstinence part of the time but have other methods available to use if they decide to become sexually active. Periodic abstinence is also practiced by women using the natural family planning methods.

Nurses should support women who choose to be abstinent. Sexual education programs in schools often include information on ways to maintain abstinence. Abstinence-only education programs have not been successful in reducing teen pregnancy (Speroff & Darney, 2011). Adolescents who choose abstinence need assistance to define their values

PATIENT TEACHING

How to Assess Cervical Mucus and Basal Body Temperature

Cervical Mucus Assessment

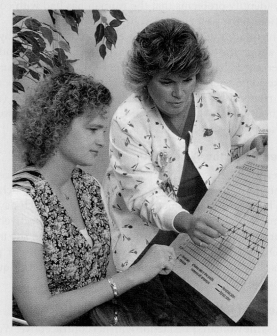

Your cervical mucus normally changes throughout your menstrual cycle. If you check the mucus each day, you can estimate when ovulation occurs. Before and after ovulation, the mucus is scant, thick, sticky, and whitish. It stretches less than 6 cm (2.3 inches). Just before and for 2 to 3 days after ovulation, cervical mucus is thin, slippery, and clear and is similar to raw egg white. It stretches 6 cm (2.3 inches) or more, a quality called *spinnbarkeit*. When this mucus is present, you have probably ovulated and could become pregnant.

Use a tissue to obtain a small sample of mucus each day from just inside your vagina. Note the following:
- The general sensation of wetness (around ovulation) or dryness (not near ovulation) on your labia.
- The appearance and consistency of the mucus: thick, sticky, and whitish, or thin, slippery, and clear or watery.
- The distance the mucus will stretch between your fingers.

Your cervical mucus may be thicker if you take antihistamines. Vaginal infections, contraceptive foams or jellies, sexual arousal, and semen can make the mucus thinner even if ovulation has not occurred. Keep a record of the type of mucus present each day and anything that might affect it.

To use cervical mucus assessment as a method of contraception, avoid intercourse from the time secretions first occur until 4 days after the slippery mucus ends. Intercourse is safe only every other day when there is no mucus because semen interferes with mucus assessment.

As a method to enhance conception, you should have intercourse every 2 days during the period of ovulatory mucus. Ovulation predictors available over the counter provide added information that may be helpful if you are trying to conceive.

Basal Body Temperature

Basal body temperature (BBT) is the lowest, or resting, temperature of the body. It is assessed to detect the slight elevation in temperature that occurs near the time of ovulation. During the first half of your menstrual cycle, your temperature is lower than it is during the second half of the cycle. The BBT may drop slightly just before ovulation, but not all women experience this fall in temperature.

Progesterone is secreted during the second half of the cycle, its level rising just after ovulation. This causes an increase in BBT. The BBT rises near ovulation and remains higher during the second half of the cycle. However, some women do not have a temperature rise even when they ovulate. BBT remains higher if conception occurs and falls about 2 to 4 days before menstruation if conception does not occur.

An electronic thermometer digitally displays temperature in tenths of a degree. You should place the thermometer under your tongue as soon as you awaken each morning and before any activity. It should remain in place until the electronic signal sounds. Record your BBT on a chart.

Also note events that may alter your BBT, such as menstrual periods, intercourse, illness, or other occurrences. BBT may be altered by illness, restless or inadequate sleep (fewer than 6 hours), waking later than usual, traveling across time zones (jet lag), alcohol intake the evening before, sleeping under an electric blanket, or performing any activity before taking the temperature.

As a method to avoid pregnancy, you should not have intercourse from the onset of your menstrual period until the night of the third day of elevated temperature. However, relying on cervical mucus is a better indicator of when intercourse is safe.

To enhance the chances of conception, this method has limited value because the rise in temperature indicates that ovulation has already occurred. It is helpful as a screening method to identify whether the woman is likely to be ovulating and if progesterone is secreted to prepare the endometrium for implantation.

---

and learn practical methods of reaching their goal. They need to consider just what this entails and when it might be difficult to maintain abstinence. Role playing often is used to help them work through what to do and say before it becomes necessary.

Abstinence has no cost, avoids the use of hormones, and has no side effects or medical risks. It is important that users understand that abstinence must include all forms of sexual contact, including oral and anal intercourse, to avoid exposure

to most STDs. Women using abstinence should know where to get information and contraception if they decide to become sexually active at a later time.

KNOWLEDGE CHECK

15. How do barrier methods of contraception work?
16. What are the advantages and disadvantages of natural family planning methods?

Least Reliable Methods of Contraception

The methods of contraception discussed in the following section are not considered reliable but are used by women who lack information about their risks and other options or who do not wish to use other methods for medical or personal reasons. The nurse needs to be familiar with these methods to help women understand the risks involved.

Lactational Amenorrhea

Breastfeeding inhibits ovulation because suckling and prolactin interfere with secretion of gonadotropin-releasing hormone and luteinizing hormone. During lactation the ovarian response to follicle-stimulating hormone and luteinizing hormone may be altered. The frequency, intensity, and duration of suckling are very important in inhibiting ovulation.

Women who breastfeed fully with no supplementary feedings may avoid ovulation and resumption of menstrual cycles. However, use of formula or solid foods decreases the frequency and duration of breastfeeding, increases the length of time between feedings, and reduces night feedings. This may lead to ovulation and a return of menses. The menstrual cycle generally resumes by 6 months, even in women who breastfeed fully. Another method of contraception should be used by that time or earlier if menses has resumed or supplementary feedings are used.

Coitus Interruptus

Also called *withdrawal,* coitus interruptus is the removal of the penis from the vagina before ejaculation. The method requires great control by the man and may be unsatisfying to both partners. Even a man who wishes to use the method may misjudge the timing and withdraw too late. It is important to remember that preejaculate fluid may contain sperm and that sperm spilled near the vaginal opening may enter the vagina and cause pregnancy.

◆ APPLICATION OF THE NURSING PROCESS: CHOOSING A CONTRACEPTIVE METHOD

Contraceptive failure often occurs because women lack knowledge about how to use their contraceptive methods correctly or choose methods unsuited to their needs. When contraception fails, the woman is exposed to the physical, psychological, and social consequences of unintended pregnancy. Lack of understanding also may expose her to unnecessary side effects, possible complications, or STDs.

◆ Assessment

Because contraception is a very private matter, approach it in a sensitive manner. Perform the assessment in a quiet area where interruptions are unlikely, and keep voices low to increase the woman's comfort. Assure the woman that her confidentiality will be maintained.

Introducing the Subject

In the postpartum setting, introduce the subject by asking the woman if she plans to have more children. Most women indicate a desire to wait a certain period before the next pregnancy. Ask the woman, "What method of family planning are you thinking about using now?" or "How did you feel about the method you used before pregnancy?" These questions may identify problems that the woman has had with contraception in the past.

Introduce the topic during well-woman checkups by asking about the woman's current contraceptive method and if her needs have changed. In other settings, a woman may make some reference to her contraceptive method. The nurse can respond by asking her, "How do you like using (name method)?" This shows the nurse is interested if the woman wishes to pursue the topic.

Determining the Woman's Understanding

Determine the woman's understanding of her contraceptive technique. For example, ask where she places her patch or if it is hard for her to remember to take her OC each day. The woman should know how to use her technique effectively and what to do in special circumstances such as when she misses an OC pill. Explore any misinformation, concerns, or problems she may have with regard to effectiveness, technique, or common side effects of the method.

Assessing the Woman's Satisfaction

Assess the woman's satisfaction with her contraceptive. Women may be unsure about their method in the early months until they gain comfort from repetitive use. Satisfaction and effectiveness increase with greater familiarity with the method. Side effects also affect satisfaction. They may be severe enough to cause the woman to consider another method, or they may be relieved by simple techniques. Talking about side effects helps differentiate serious complications from minor effects and leads to a discussion of relief methods.

Assessing Appropriate Choices

If the woman is considering a change in contraceptive method, assess factors that would help determine the best method for her. Include a history of medical conditions that might eliminate certain methods, childbearing history, cultural and religious beliefs, and intensity of her desire to prevent pregnancy. The woman's ability to understand and follow complex directions is important as well.

The couple's relationship is important in terms of contraceptive choice and protection against STDs. If the relationship is mutually monogamous and neither partner is infected, STDs may not be a risk. If there is a possibility that either member of the couple is infected or has more than one partner, condom use is essential, even if the woman uses another type of contraceptive.

Frequency of coitus may help determine the best choice of contraception. For occasional sexual intercourse, a barrier method may be most satisfactory. If intercourse is frequent, the woman may desire a method that is always in place, such as an IUD or a hormone implant. Explore her past experience with other methods, what she considers important, and her individual preferences.

◆ Identification of Patient Problems

Inadequate knowledge about family planning is common. Many women will have a need for patient teaching due to lack of understanding about contraceptive methods.

◆ Planning: Expected Outcomes

Expected outcomes for this diagnosis are that the woman will do the following:

- Correctly describe how to use her contraceptive method, including solving common problems
- Describe common side effects, signs of complications, and correct follow-up
- Report that she and her partner are satisfied with their contraceptive method or explore choosing another method

◆ Interventions

Interventions involve teaching about contraceptive techniques and follow-up of problems that may interfere with the woman's ability to maintain health.

Increasing Understanding of the Chosen Method

Fill in gaps in the woman's knowledge about how her contraceptive method works, its effectiveness, advantages and disadvantages, common side effects and complications, and when to seek help. Use demonstrations (such as applying a patch or inserting a vaginal ring) and return demonstrations for using the method. Give suggestions for managing side effects and common problems. Understanding common side effects and how to manage them often helps women continue to use a method.

Teaching about Other Methods

Provide information about other forms of contraceptives, if the woman wishes. Discuss characteristics of methods that are most important to the woman and her lifestyle. Compare other methods with the one she is currently using. Talk about benefits, disadvantages, and risks so that she can make an informed choice. If a prescription, insertion, or fitting is needed for a new method, discuss what may happen during the visit. Provide written information she can take home to review and discuss with her partner, if she wishes, before making a final decision.

Protecting against Sexually Transmitted Diseases

Address defense against STDs, particularly if the woman is using a method that does not provide protection. A way to approach it might be to say, "The method you are using is very effective against pregnancy but does not protect you against diseases such as HIV infection that you might catch from a partner. If there is any chance that you or your partner might have sex with someone other than each other or that your partner might have an infection, you should protect yourself by using condoms along with your regular contraceptive."

Including the Woman's Partner

Invite the woman to include her partner in the discussions, if possible. He may influence the woman's choice of contraception and whether she actually uses it and uses it correctly. If the partner understands the proper method of use, he may be more cooperative and willing to help ensure contraceptive success.

Providing Ongoing Teaching

Instruct the woman to call if she has any questions or difficulties. If she chooses a new contraceptive, suggest that she visit again in 1 to 2 months to discuss her satisfaction with it. Make a note in the chart to discuss contraception at her next visit, even if the visit is for another reason.

◆ Evaluation

The woman should explain her contraceptive method, including ways to solve common problems and when to seek help for side effects or complications. At later visits, evaluate continued understanding, compliance with proper use, and satisfaction with the method. The woman who wishes to change her contraceptive method should describe other contraceptives available and how they should be used. She should choose a new method and, if necessary, visit a health care provider for further discussion, examination, fitting, or prescription.

▌ SUMMARY CONCEPTS

- The average woman must consider use of contraception for more than 30 years.
- The nurse helps women with family planning by providing current, accurate information about contraception and assisting them to find methods that best meet their needs.
- Important issues in choosing contraceptives include safety, protection from STDs, effectiveness, acceptability, convenience, education needed, benefits, side effects, effect on spontaneity, availability, expense, preference, and religious and cultural beliefs.
- Because some methods have potentially serious complications, a written informed consent form may be necessary.
- Adolescents may lack knowledge about their own bodies, conception, and methods of contraception. Risk-taking behaviors are common.

- Adolescents feel more comfortable talking about contraception with nurses who have an accepting attitude, provide extra time to teach, and use understandable terms and visual aids.
- The most successful methods of contraception for adolescents are those unrelated to coitus.
- Women over 35 years who smoke and women who have other risk factors should not use combined oral contraceptives.
- Sterilization offers permanent contraception. A tubal ligation can be performed soon after childbirth or at any time. Vasectomy is less expensive and can be performed in the physician's office using local anesthesia. Surgery to reverse sterilization is possible but expensive and not always successful.

- Intrauterine devices are very effective and safe for all women regardless of age or parity.
- Hormonal contraceptives include implants, injections, oral contraceptives, emergency contraception, patches, and vaginal rings. Side effects and complications make these unsuitable for some women.
- Oral contraceptives, the patch, and the ring may be used on a monthly basis, for extended cycles, or indefinitely to decrease menstrual periods.

- Emergency contraception helps protect against pregnancy if taken within 5 days after unprotected intercourse.
- Barrier methods may be chemical or mechanical. They kill or prevent sperm from entering the cervix and provide some protection against sexually transmitted diseases.
- Natural family planning methods involve avoidance of coitus when physiologic cues suggest ovulation is likely. Women need high motivation and extensive education about their bodies to be successful with these methods.

REFERENCES & READINGS

Alan Guttmacher Institute (AGI). (2016). *Facts on unintended pregnancy in the United States*. Retrieved from www.guttmacher.org.

Alan Guttmacher Institute (AGI). (2016). *Fact sheet: Contraceptive use in the United States*. Retrieved from www.guttmacher.org.

American Academy of Pediatrics (AAP). (2012). Emergency contraception. *Pediatrics, 130*(6), 1174–1182.

American Academy of Pediatrics & American College of Obstetricians and Gynecologists (AAP & ACOG). (2012). *Guidelines for perinatal care* (7th ed.). Elk Grove Village, IL: Author.

American College of Obstetricians and Gynecologists (ACOG). (2010). *Use of hysterosalpingography after tubal sterilization (ACOG Committee Opinion No. 458)*. Washington, DC: Author.

American College of Obstetricians and Gynecologists (ACOG). (2012). *Adolescents and long-acting reversible contraception: Implants and intrauterine devices (ACOG Committee Opinion No. 539)*. Washington, DC: Author.

American College of Obstetricians and Gynecologists (ACOG). (2015a). *Emergency contraception. (ACOG Committee Opinion No. 112)*. Washington, DC: Author.

American College of Obstetricians and Gynecologists (ACOG). (2015b). *Increasing use of contraceptive implants and intrauterine devices to reduce unintended pregnancy (ACOG Committee Opinion No. 642)*. Washington, DC: Author.

American College of Obstetricians and Gynecologists (ACOG). (2015c). *Long-acting reversible contraception: Implants and intrauterine devices. (ACOG Practice Bulletin No. 59)*. Washington, DC: Author.

American College of Obstetricians and Gynecologists (ACOG). (2016). *Over-the-counter access to oral contraceptives. (ACOG Committee Opinion No. 544)*. Washington, DC: Author.

Association of Women's Health, Obstetric and Neonatal Nurses. (2012). Position statement: Emergency contraception. *Journal of Obstetric, Gynecologic, and Neonatal Nursing, 41*(5), 711–713.

Barry, M. (2011). Preconception care at the edges of the reproductive life span. *Nursing for Women's Health, 15*(1), 68–74.

Beckmann, C. R. B., Herbert, W., Laube, D., Ling, F., & Smith, R. (2013). *Obstetrics and gynecology* (7th ed.). Philadelphia, PA: Wolters Kluwer Lippincott Williams & Wilkins.

Cates, W., & Harwood, B. (2011). Vaginal barriers and spermicides. In R. A. Hatcher, J. Trussell, A. L. Nelson, et al. (Eds.), *Contraceptive technology* (20th ed.) (pp. 391–408). New York: Ardent Media.

Center for Disease Control and Prevention. (2016a). *Sexual risk behaviors: HIV, STD, & teen pregnancy prevention*. Retrieved from www.cdc.gov/healthyyouth/sexualbehaviors/.

Centers for Disease Control and Prevention. (2016b). U.S. medical eligibility criteria for contraceptive use, 2016: Adapted from the World Health Organization Medical Eligibility Criteria for Contraceptive Use (4th ed.). *MMWR Morbidity and Mortality Weekly Report, 65*(3), 1–104.

Centers for Disease Control and Prevention. (2016c). U.S. Selected Practice Recommendations for Contraceptive Use, 2016. *Morbidity and Mortality Weekly Report, 65*(4), 1–66.

Centers for Disease Control and Prevention. (2016d). Youth risk behavior surveillance—United States, 2015. *MMWR Morbidity and Mortality Weekly Report, 65*(1), 1–180.

Cunningham, F. G., Leveno, K. J., Bloom, S. L., et al. (2014). *Williams obstetrics (24th)*. New York: McGraw-Hill.

Daniels, K., Daugherty, J., & Jones, J. (2015). *Current contraceptive status among women aged 15–44: United States, 2011–2013, National Health Statistics Reports, No. 173*. www.cdc.gov/nchs/data/databriefs/db173.pdf.

Dean, G., & Schwarz, E. B. (2011). Intrauterine contraceptives. In R. A. Hatcher, J. Trussell, A. L. Nelson, et al. (Eds.), *Contraceptive technology* (20th ed.) (pp. 147–191). New York: Ardent Media.

Dempsey, A. R., Johnson, S. S., & Westoff, C. L. (2011). Predicting oral contraceptive continuation using the transtheoretical model of health behavior change. *Perspectives on Sexual and Reproductive Health, 43*(1), 23–29.

Finer, L. B., & Zolna, M. R. (2016). Declines in unintended pregnancy in the United States, 2008-2011. *New England Journal of Medicine, 374*, 843–852.

Fontenot, H. B., & Fantasia, H. C. (2011). Do women in abusive relationships have contraceptive control? *Nursing for Women's Health, 15*(3), 239–243.

Godfrey, E. M., Chin, N. P., Fielding, S. L., et al. (2011). Contraceptive methods and use by women aged 35 and over: A qualitative study of perspectives. *BMC Women's Health, 11*, 5.

Hladky, K. J., Allsworth, J. E., Madden, T., et al. (2011). Women's knowledge about intrauterine contraception. *Obstetrics & Gynecology, 117*(1), 48–54.

Jennings, V. H., & Burke, A. E. (2011). Fertility awareness-based methods. In R. A. Hatcher, J. Trussell, A. L. Nelson, et al. (Eds.), *Contraceptive technology* (20th ed.) (pp. 417–434). New York: Ardent Media.

Jensen, J. T., & Mishell, D. R. (2012). Family planing: contraception, sterilization, and pregnancy termination. In G. M. Lentz, R. A. Lobo, D. M. Gershenson, et al. (Eds.), *Comprehensive gynecology* (6th ed.) (pp. 215–272). Philadelphia, PA: Mosby.

Jones, J., Mosher, W. D., & Daniels, K. (2012). Current contraceptive use in the United States, 2006–2010, and changes in patterns of use since 1995. *National Health Statistics Reports, 2012*. No. 60. Retrieved from www.cdc.gov/nchs/data/nhsr/nhsr060.pdf.

Jurrow, R. (2011). Emergency contraception. In D. Shoupe (Ed.), *Contraception* (pp. 123–132). Hoboken, NJ: Wiley-Blackwell.

Nanda, K. (2011). Contraceptive patch and vaginal contraceptive ring. In R. A. Hatcher, J. Trussell, A. L. Nelson, et al. (Eds.), *Contraceptive technology* (20th ed.) (pp. 343–369). New York: Ardent Media.

National Cancer Institute. (2016). *Cervical cancer screening.* Retrieved from www.cancer.gov.

Nelson, A. L. (2011a). Male condoms. In D. Shoupe (Ed.), *Contraception* (pp. 114–122). Hoboken, NJ: Wiley-Blackwell.

Nelson, A. L. (2011b). Perimenopausal, menopause, and postmenopause: Health promotion strategies. In R. A. Hatcher, J. Trussell, A. L. Nelson, et al. (Eds.), *Contraceptive technology* (20th ed.) (pp. 737–777). New York: Ardent Media.

Nelson, A. L., & Cwiak, C. (2011). Combined oral contraceptives. In R. A. Hatcher, J. Trussell, A. L. Nelson, et al. (Eds.), *Contraceptive technology* (20th ed.) (pp. 249–341). New York: Ardent Media.

Nichols, M. I. (2010). Ulipristal acetate: A novel molecule and 5-day emergency contraceptive. *Obstetrics & Gynecology,* 116(6), 1252–1253.

Ochalski, M. E., & Sanfilippo, J. S. (2011). Adolescents: compliance, ethical issues, and sexually transmitted infections. In D. Shoupe (Ed.), *Contraception* (pp. 158–167). Hoboken, NJ: Wiley-Blackwell.

Raymond, E. G. (2011). Progestin-only pills. In R. A. Hatcher, J. Trussell, A. L. Nelson, et al. (Eds.), *Contraceptive technology* (20th ed.) (pp. 237–247). New York: Ardent Media.

Renner, R., & Jensen, J. T. (2012). Progestin-only contraceptive pills. In G. M. Lentz, R. A. Lobo, D. M. Gershenson, et al. (Eds.), *Comprehensive gynecology* (6th ed.) (pp. 40–56). Philadelphia, PA: Mosby.

Roncari, D., & Hou, M. Y. (2011). Female and male sterilization. In R. A. Hatcher, J. Trussell, A. L. Nelson, et al. (Eds.), *Contraceptive technology* (20th ed.) (pp. 435–482). New York: Ardent Media.

Sonfield, A., et al. (2013). *The social and economic benefits of women's ability to determine whether and when to have children.* New York: Guttmacher Institute.

Speroff, L., & Darney, P. D. (2011). *A clinical guide for contraception* (5th ed.). Philadelphia, PA: Lippincott Williams & Wilkins.

Taylor, D. L. (2011). Spermicides. In D. Shoupe (Ed.), *Contraception* (pp. 103–106). Hoboken, NJ: Wiley-Blackwell.

Trussell, J. (2011). Contraceptive failure in the United States. *Contraception,* 83(5), 307–404.

Trussell, J., & Guthrie, K. A. (2011). Choosing a contraceptive: Efficacy, safety, and personal considerations. In R. A. Hatcher, J. Trussell, A. L. Nelson, et al. (Eds.), *Contraceptive technology* (20th ed.) (pp. 45–74). New York: Ardent Media.

Trussell, J., & Schwarz, E. B. (2011). Emergency contraception. In R. A. Hatcher, J. Trussell, A. L. Nelson, et al. (Eds.), *Contraceptive technology* (20th ed.) (pp. 113–145). New York: Ardent Media.

US Food and Drug Administration (FDA). (2009). *Updated FDA action on Plan B (levonorgestrel) tablets [press release].* Retrieved from www.fda.gov.

US Food and Drug Administration (FDA). (2013). *FDA News release: FDA approves Plan B One-Step emergency contraceptive without a prescription for women 15 years of age or older.* Retrieved from www.fda.gov.

US Department of Health & Human Services. (2010). *Healthy People 2020.* Washington, DC: Author.

Warner, L., & Steiner, M. J. (2011). Male condoms. In R. A. Hatcher, J. Trussell, A. L. Nelson, et al. (Eds.), *Contraceptive technology* (20th ed.) (pp. 371–389). New York: Ardent Media.

Zieman, M. (2016). *Managing contraception.* Tiger, GA: Bridging the Gap Foundation.

Infertility

Susan Peck

OBJECTIVES

After studying this chapter, you should be able to:

1. Describe settings in which the nurse may encounter couples with infertility problems.
2. Explain factors that can impair a couple's ability to conceive.
3. Explain factors that may cause repeated pregnancy losses.
4. Specify evaluations that may be done when a couple seeks help for infertility.
5. Explain procedures and treatments that may aid a couple's ability to conceive and carry the fetus to viability.
6. Analyze ways in which infertility can affect a couple and other family members.
7. Summarize the nurse's role in caring for couples experiencing problems with fertility.

Infertility nursing is a specialty, but general practice nurses also encounter couples who are seeking help or have had treatment for infertility in varied settings. A nurse may be a source of information to friends and family if they have challenges conceiving. Nurses working in the perioperative area may care for these couples during diagnostic or therapeutic surgery. Nurses in urology settings often see men who are being evaluated or treated for infertility. In the emergency department, nurses may care for women who are having a spontaneous pregnancy loss or a complication of an infertility procedure.

Nurses in antepartum, intrapartum, and postpartum settings often encounter women with high-risk pregnancies or couples who have a new baby after infertility therapy. In addition, parenthood after infertility may be particularly challenging, and nurses in pediatric and psychosocial settings may counsel families about parenting and changes in their personal relationships.

EXTENT OF INFERTILITY

The extent of infertility depends on its definition. Infertility is not an absolute condition but is a reduced ability to conceive. Infertility is defined as the inability to conceive after 1 year of unprotected intercourse (6 months if the woman is older than 35 years of age) or the inability to carry a pregnancy to live birth. A more workable definition does not specify a time limit but recognizes that infertility is any involuntary inability to conceive when desired. The definition is commonly expanded to include couples who conceive but repeatedly lose a pregnancy (pregnancy wastage) before the fetus is mature enough to survive. Couples with primary infertility

have never conceived. Couples with secondary infertility may have conceived before but are unable to conceive again.

One in eight couples (or 12% of married women) have trouble getting pregnant or sustaining a pregnancy (Martinez, Daniels, & Chandra, 2012). This number may increase as women and couples intentionally delay childbearing. The National Survey of Family Growth (Martinez, et. al., 2012) reported that about 36% of married women and 9% of cohabiting women were involuntarily childless. Couples who delay childbearing until their mid to late 30s or later may feel pressured by the approaching end of their reproductive capacity. A woman without a male partner may seek infertility treatment before the end of her reproductive potential. For older couples, delay in achieving pregnancy or having a living baby may be more time sensitive than for younger couples, who—from an age perspective—have more time to pursue pregnancy and make treatment decisions. As new methods of diagnosis and treatment emerge, couples who once accepted childlessness may have new options for infertility therapy or resume therapy they previously abandoned (Mahomed, 2011; Martinez, Daniels, & Chandra, 2012; Morgan, Merrell, Rentschler, & Chadderton, 2012).

FACTORS CONTRIBUTING TO INFERTILITY

Conception depends on the normal reproductive function of each partner. For some couples, identification and treatment of infertility are simple, but others require complex evaluation and treatment. Some couples delay childbearing until their mid to late 30s, when a natural decline in fertility begins. About one-third of infertility cases are male factor, one-third are female factor, and one-third are a combination of the two (American Society for Reproductive Medicine [ASRM], 2014a).

Because some factors contributing to infertility remain unknown, treatment of an identified problem does not always result in a successful pregnancy. About 20% of infertile couples have no identified problem, yet some never conceive despite having undergone all available treatments.

Male Infertility Factors

The test of a man's fertility is his ability to initiate pregnancy in a fertile woman. Few absolute criteria exist to distinguish normal from abnormal male fertility, although an adequate number of sperm having normal structure and function must be deposited near the woman's cervix. Problems may exist with the sperm itself, ability to achieve or maintain an erection, or ejaculation of **semen** or the seminal fluid that carries the sperm into the woman's reproductive tract. One or more findings may be abnormal, and further complicating evaluation of a man's fertility are the normal daily variations in semen.

Abnormalities of the Sperm

Evaluation of the semen via a semen analysis may reveal that the man has **azoospermia** (sperm absent in semen) or **oligospermia** (decreased sperm in semen). The average number of sperm released at ejaculation is 35 million to 200 million but varies between 150 million and 600 million in a typical ejaculate. Twenty million sperm per milliliter of semen is considered the minimum number adequate for unassisted fertilization (Hall, 2016; Jones, 2016b). Liquefaction of the semen occurs within approximately 20 to 30 minutes, allowing motile sperm to move into the uterus without the seminal fluid. A sufficient number of normal sperm must move in a purposeful direction to reach the ovum in the fallopian tube. Semen analysis (Table 26.1) is used to evaluate whether the quantities and qualities of sperm and the seminal fluid are likely to result in successful conception, assuming that the woman's studies are normal. Abnormal sperm structure or movement may reduce fertility, regardless of the actual number of sperm (Fig. 26.1). Inflammatory processes in the man's reproductive organs may cause the sperm to clump, inhibiting their motility and fertilizing ability. Other sperm may have a normal appearance but may not be able to penetrate the ovum.

Factors that can impair the number and function of the sperm include the following:

- Abnormal hormonal stimulation of sperm production
- Acute or chronic illness such as mumps, cirrhosis, or renal failure
- Infections of the genital tract
- Anatomic abnormalities such as a varicocele or obstruction of the ducts that carry sperm to the penis
- Exposure to toxins such as lead, pesticides, or other chemicals
- Therapeutic treatments such as antineoplastic drugs or radiation for cancer
- Excessive alcohol intake
- Use of illicit drugs such as marijuana or cocaine
- An elevated scrotal temperature resulting from febrile illness, repeated use of saunas or hot tubs, or sitting for prolonged periods
- Immunologic factors, produced by the man against his own sperm (autoantibodies) or by the woman, causing the sperm to clump or be unable to penetrate the ovum

Abnormal Erections

The inability to achieve or maintain an erection may reduce the man's ability to deposit sperm-bearing seminal fluid in the woman's upper vagina. Erections are influenced by physical and psychological factors. Central nervous system dysfunction, which may be caused by drugs, psychiatric disturbance, or chronic illness, can interfere with erections. Surgery and disorders affecting the spinal cord or the autonomic nervous system also may disrupt normal erectile function. Peripheral vascular disease, from cardiovascular disease or diabetes, reduces the amount of blood entering the penis and thereby reduces the ability to maintain an erection. Drugs such as antihypertensives or antidepressants may reduce the erection or shorten its duration.

Abnormal Ejaculation

Abnormal ejaculation prevents deposition of the sperm in the upper vagina to achieve pregnancy. **Retrograde ejaculation** is the release of semen backward into the bladder rather than forward through the tip of the penis. Conditions that may cause retrograde ejaculation are diabetes, neurologic disorders, surgery that impairs function of the sympathetic nerves, and drugs such as antihypertensives and psychotropics. Men who have suffered spinal cord injury may retain the ability to ejaculate, depending on the level of cord damage.

Anatomic abnormalities such as hypospadias (urethral opening on the underside of the penis) may cause deposition of semen near the vaginal outlet rather than near the cervix.

Excessive alcohol intake or use of some therapeutic or illicit drugs can adversely affect ejaculation as well as sperm number and function. Ejaculation may be slow, absent, or retrograde when a man takes drugs that affect neurologic coordination of this event. Premature ejaculation is usually related to psychological disorders such as performance anxiety or unresolved relationship conflicts.

Abnormalities of Seminal Fluid

The seminal fluid nourishes, protects, and carries sperm into the vagina until they enter the cervix. Only sperm enter the cervix; the seminal fluid remains in the vagina. Semen coagulates immediately after ejaculation but liquefies within 20 to 30 minutes, permitting forward progression of sperm. Seminal fluid that remains thick traps the sperm, impeding their movement into the cervix. The pH of seminal fluid is slightly alkaline to protect the sperm from the acidic secretions of the vagina. Adequate fructose, citric acid, and other nutrients must be present to provide energy for the sperm.

TABLE 26.1   Selected Diagnostic Tests on Infertility

Test and Purpose	Nursing Implications
Male	
Semen Analysis	
Evaluates structure and function of sperm and composition of seminal fluid. Semen volume: ≥2 mL. pH: 7.2–7.8. Sperm concentration: ≥20 million/mL. Motility: ≥50% with normal forms. Morphology: ≥30% with normal forms. Viability: ≥50% live. Liquefaction: Within 30 min. Leukocytes (white blood cells): <1 million/mL.	Explain purpose of semen analysis: three or more specimens are usually collected over several weeks for improved accuracy. Explain to the man that he should collect the specimen by masturbation after a 3-day abstinence; semen may be collected in a condom if masturbation is unacceptable. Teach him to note the time the specimen was obtained so the laboratory can evaluate liquefaction of the semen. To maintain warmth, the specimen should be transported near the body and should arrive in the laboratory within 30 min.
Endocrine Tests	
Evaluate function of hypothalamus, pituitary gland, and response of testicles. Assays are made to determine testosterone, luteinizing hormone (LH), and follicle-stimulating hormone (FSH) levels. Additional tests may be done based on history, physical findings, and results of other tests.	Teach the man about the relationship between hypothalamic and pituitary function and sperm formation. LH stimulates testosterone production by Leydig cells of the testes, and FSH stimulates Sertoli cells of the testes to produce sperm.
Ultrasonography	
Evaluates structure of prostate gland, seminal vesicles, and ejaculatory ducts by use of a transrectal probe.	Teach the man that ultrasonography uses sound waves to evaluate these structures; no radiation is involved.
Testicular Biopsy	
An invasive test for obtaining a sample of testicular tissue; identifies pathology and obstructions.	Explain the purpose of the test; a local anesthetic is used, and there should be little discomfort. Ask the man questions to confirm that he understands the test.
Sperm Penetration Assay	
Evaluates fertilizing ability of sperm; assesses ability of sperm to undergo changes that allow penetration of a hamster ovum from which the zona pellucida has been removed. Infrequent use.	Explain the purpose of the test and that abnormal penetration of the hamster ovum does not necessarily mean that the sperm cannot fertilize a human ovum.
Female	
Ovulation Prediction	
Identifies the surge of LH, which precedes ovulation by 24-36 hr; improves ability to time intercourse to coincide with ovulation and identifies the absence of ovulation. Common prediction methods include commercial ovulation predictor kits and cervical mucous assessment (see "Patient Teaching, What to Expect with Infertility Evaluation and Treatment"). Basal body temperature (BBT), or temperature at rest, may be used to identify if ovulation has occurred and the timing of intercourse in relation to probable ovulation.	Explain the purpose of the assessments. Teach the woman to follow the instructions on commercial ovulation predictor. Teach her how to do the basal body temperature and cervical mucous assessment if that is used. Teach her to indicate days on which she and her partner had intercourse to identify frequency during the menstrual cycle and intercourse near ovulation.
Ultrasonography	
Evaluates structure of pelvic organs. Evaluates cyclic endometrial changes. Identifies ovarian follicles and release of ova at ovulation. Evaluates for presence of ectopic or multifetal pregnancy.	Teach the woman that ultrasonography uses sound waves to evaluate these structures; no radiation is involved. Explain preparations needed for specific evaluations.
Hysterosalpingogram	
Gentle injection of contrast medium into the cervix while imaging the pelvis to visualize passage of the dye through the uterus and fallopian tubes.	Review purposes of the imaging test to determine whether the woman understands the procedure. Ultrasound imaging will use a different contrast medium from that used in radiographic imaging.

TABLE 26.1 Selected Diagnostic Tests on Infertility—cont'd	
Test and Purpose	**Nursing Implications**
Postcoital Test Evaluates characteristics of cervical mucus and sperm function within that mucus at time of ovulation. Ultrasonography ensures proper timing for test.	Explain that the test is performed 6-12 hr after intercourse; the woman may have to rearrange her personal or work commitments each time this test is done. Use is infrequent because of stress on the woman and her partner.

Data from Lobo, R. A. (2016). Infertility. In R. A. Lobo, D. M. Gershenson, G. M. Lentz, & F. A. Valea (Eds.), *Comprehensive gynecology* (7th ed.). St. Louis, MO: Elsevier; and Pagana, K. D., & Pagana, T. J. (2015). *Diagnostic and laboratory test reference* (12th ed.). St. Louis, MO: Mosby.

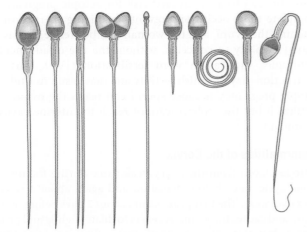

FIG. 26.1 Abnormal infertile sperm compared with a normal sperm on the left. (From Hall, J. E. [2016]. *Textbook of medical physiology* [13th ed.]. Philadelphia, PA: Saunders.)

The specific abnormality found in the seminal fluid suggests the cause of the abnormality, such as obstruction or infection in a specific area of the genital tract. Seminal fluid that is abnormal in amount, consistency, or chemical composition suggests obstruction, inflammation, or infection. The presence of large numbers of leukocytes suggests infection.

🄿 KNOWLEDGE CHECK

1. How is infertility defined? What is the difference between primary and secondary infertility?
2. What are normal characteristics of sperm and the seminal fluid that carries sperm into the woman's vagina?
3. What problems in the man can occur with erection? With ejaculation of semen?
4. What can cause abnormalities in the sperm, ejaculation, and seminal fluid?

Female Infertility Factors

A woman's fertility depends on the following:
- Regular production of normal ova
- An open path from her cervix through the uterus and fallopian tube to permit fertilization and movement of the embryo into the uterus for implantation
- A uterine endometrium that supports the pregnancy after implantation

Disorders of Ovulation

Normal ovulation depends on delicately timed and balanced hormonal interactions between the hypothalamus and pituitary gland and on an ovarian response to cause maturation and release of an ovum. The hypothalamus secretes gonadotropin-releasing hormone (GnRH) beginning even before the obvious changes of puberty. GnRH stimulates the pituitary to release follicle-stimulating hormone (FSH) and luteinizing hormone (LH). FSH stimulates maturation of several follicles in the ovary. As the follicles mature, the ovary secretes estrogen to thicken the endometrium. About 24 to 36 hours before ovulation, a marked increase of LH level occurs, which stimulates final maturation and release of one ovum from its follicle. The other follicles regress permanently. The collapsed follicle from which the ovum was released, now called a *corpus luteum,* produces progesterone and estrogen, which further prepare the endometrium for implantation and nourishment of the fertilized ovum.

Ovulation can be disrupted by many factors, including the following:
- A dysfunction in the hypothalamus or pituitary gland that alters the secretion of GnRH, FSH, and LH
- Failure of the ovaries to respond to FSH and LH stimulation, preventing maturation and release of the ovum

Disruption of hormone secretion or of the ovarian or endometrial responses to hormone secretion can be caused by many factors, such as cranial tumors, stress, obesity, anorexia, systemic disease, and abnormalities in the ovaries or other endocrine glands. Women with polycystic ovarian syndrome (PCOS) often have challenges conceiving, in addition to other problems from abnormal hormone and ovarian function. One percent of women experience premature ovarian failure (POF), also known as *early menopause,* before the age of 40. Autoimmune disorders, genetic disorders, and family history may play a role in the development of POF; however, most cases do not have an identifiable cause.

As a woman approaches the end of her reproductive life, also known as the **climacteric**, she ovulates and menstruates more erratically as her pool of ova diminishes and fewer are available for successful fertilization. This is called a *decreased ovarian reserve.* Oocytes are produced only during prenatal life and are vulnerable to cumulative toxic effects of therapeutic drugs, abused substances, and environmental agents.

In addition to normal aging of oocytes and menstrual cycles, factors that may impair normal ovulation include cancer chemotherapeutic agents, excessive alcohol intake, and cigarette smoking.

Women with ovulation disorders often have abnormal menses because hormone levels do not permit normal development and shedding of the endometrium. The woman may have absent, scant, or heavy menstrual periods. However, other women may have no identifiable menstrual, ovarian or hormonal disorders, and the inability to conceive may be their only complaint.

Abnormalities of the Fallopian Tubes

At least one patent fallopian tube is required for natural conception and implantation to occur (Fig. 26.2). Tubal obstruction may occur because of scarring and adhesions after reproductive tract infections. Infections such as chlamydia, gonorrhea, and other sexually transmissible diseases (STDs) are responsible for many cases of infertility from tubal obstruction. Prevention or prompt treatment and eradication of pelvic infections can reduce the incidence of fallopian tube damage.

Endometriosis (uterine lining tissue growing and shedding outside the uterine cavity) may cause tubal adhesions, painful menstrual periods, and painful intercourse. Small lesions are unlikely to affect tubal function, but large lesions can distort tubal anatomy and lead to scarring, tubal occlusion, and subsequent infertility.

Tubal obstruction may occur if adhesions develop after pelvic surgery, a ruptured appendix, peritonitis, or ovarian cysts. In addition, the fallopian tubes and other reproductive organs may have congenital structural anomalies that disrupt normal function.

The conditions that cause obstruction may interfere with normal motility within the fallopian tube. Poor movement of the fimbriated (distal) end of the tube may prevent the ovum from being picked up at the ovarian surface after ovulation. Abnormal action of the cilia within the tube prevents normal transport of the ovum toward the uterine cavity.

Depending on the extent and location of the blockage, fallopian tube obstructions can prevent fertilization of the ovum or lead to an increased risk for ectopic pregnancy. Complete tubal occlusion prevents fertilizing sperm from reaching the ovum, and the woman will be **sterile**, or have a total inability to conceive, without the use of advanced techniques such as in vitro fertilization (IVF). Partial obstruction may diminish fertility and may result in a tubal ectopic pregnancy because sperm can reach the ovum to fertilize it but the embryo cannot reach the uterine cavity to implant.

Abnormalities of the Cervix

Estrogen levels from the ovary peak twice during the menstrual cycle, once before ovulation and again about 1 week after ovulation. The first peak occurs about 2 days before ovulation and causes the woman's cervix to dilate slightly and produce a clear, thin, slippery mucus that is similar to egg white in consistency (**spinnbarkeit**). This mucus facilitates forward progression of sperm into the uterus and capacitation to prepare one sperm for fertilization. Low estrogen levels prevent development of this mucus and are usually associated with **anovulation** (menstrual cycles that occur irregularly without ovulation).

Polyps or cervical os scarring from past surgical procedures such as cauterization or conization (for cervical dysplasia) may obstruct the woman's cervix. Abnormal cervical mucus caused by estrogen deficiency, surgical destruction of the mucus-secreting glands, and cervical damage secondary to infection or other factors prevent normal capacitation and movement of the sperm through the cervix into the uterus and fallopian tubes for fertilization.

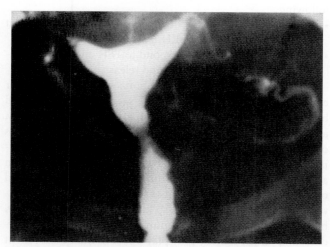

FIG. 26.2 A radiographic hysterosalpingogram evaluates patency of fallopian tubes. Contrast medium that was injected through the cervix spills out of the fallopian tubes into the peritoneal cavity if tubes are open. Sonohysterographic technique with ultrasound is becoming more common and uses contrast medium with hypoechoic effects. (From Gambone, J. C., & Rodi, I. A. [2015]. Infertility and assisted reproductive technologies. In N. F. Hacker, J. C. Gambone, & C. J. Hobel [Eds.], *Hacker & Moore's essentials of obstetrics and gynecology* [6th ed.] Philadelphia, PA: Saunders.)

> ### ? KNOWLEDGE CHECK
>
> 5. What factors can result in abnormal ovulation?
> 6. Why does a woman with ovulation problems often have abnormal menstrual periods?
> 7. What are some causes of fallopian tube obstruction?
> 8. How do abnormalities of cervical mucus contribute to infertility?

Recurrent Pregnancy Loss

Early pregnancy loss is common—approximately 20% of pregnancies may end in first-trimester miscarriage. However, repeated losses may result from abnormalities in the chromosomes, fetal structure, placenta, or from maternal factors.

Abnormalities of the Fetal Chromosomes

Errors in the fetal chromosomes may result in spontaneous abortion, usually in the first trimester. Chromosomal abnormalities often severely disrupt development, and the embryo or fetus does not survive. Maternal advanced age–associated chromosome abnormalities in the ova increase spontaneous abortions and decrease live births in older women who conceive.

Most chromosome abnormalities are sporadic, occurring randomly. Others occur because one parent has a balanced chromosome translocation that is passed on to the offspring. The parent with the balanced translocation has a normal total amount of chromosome material, but the chromosome material is rearranged. When the chromosomes are divided during **gametogenesis** (development and maturation of sperm and ova), the resulting sperm or ovum may receive too much or too little chromosome material, or it may receive a balanced translocation like the parent. The sperm or ovum also may receive a normal chromosome complement with no translocation. (See Chapter 4 for more information about chromosome abnormalities that may affect fertility.)

Abnormalities of the Cervix or Uterus

Stenosis or congenital or structural malformations of the cervix or uterine cavity may cause repeated loss of a normal embryo or fetus (Fig. 26.3). These malformations may prevent normal implantation of the fertilized ovum or normal prenatal growth of the placenta or fetus. Others may increase the risk for miscarriage or birth before the fetus is viable.

Women who were exposed prenatally to diethylstilbestrol (DES), prescribed to pregnant women in the early 1970s to prevent several pregnancy complications, were more likely to

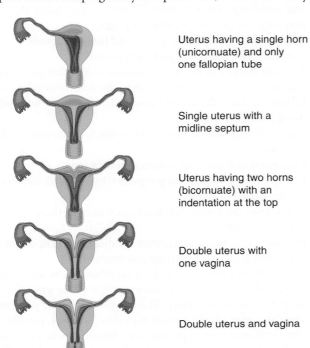

Uterus having a single horn (unicornuate) and only one fallopian tube

Single uterus with a midline septum

Uterus having two horns (bicornuate) with an indentation at the top

Double uterus with one vagina

Double uterus and vagina

FIG. 26.3 Types of uterine malformations that may cause infertility or repeated pregnancy loss.

have uterine malformations or an **incompetent cervix** (will not remain closed). Cervical or uterine abnormalities and possibly hysterectomy may result from trauma associated with a previous birth. Painless and premature cervical dilation and shortening, often early in the second trimester, is characteristic in women with an incompetent cervix. Although the woman may conceive, she may be unable to carry the pregnancy to viability.

Uterine myomas (benign fibroid tumors of the uterus) and adhesions may cause repeated fetal losses if they occur within the uterine cavity. These problems can alter the blood supply to the developing fetus or cause uterine irritability that results in preterm labor and birth. Myomas on the outer surface of the uterus are often obvious but may not cause the complications that inner myomas may cause.

Endocrine Abnormalities

Inadequate progesterone secretion by the corpus luteum (luteal phase defect) prevents normal thickening of the endometrium for implantation and establishment of the placenta. The embryo may not implant, or it may implant poorly. In other cases, the corpus luteum may develop and function properly but the woman's endometrium may not respond to its progesterone secretion.

Uncontrolled or untreated hypothyroidism and hyperthyroidism may be associated with the inability to conceive and recurrent pregnancy loss. Poorly controlled diabetes can result in repeated pregnancy loss and many other complications of pregnancy because of its effects on maternal blood glucose levels and the vascular system.

Immunologic and Thrombotic Factors

Immunologic factors are implicated in some cases of recurrent pregnancy loss, although not all are established conclusively. The embryo has antigens different from those of the mother and ordinarily would be rejected like any other foreign tissue. However, the mother's body normally blocks this rejection response and tolerates the developing baby. Some women's bodies respond inappropriately to the embryo, rejecting it as any other foreign tissue. These women often have recurrent spontaneous abortions.

Women with autoimmune disease such as systemic lupus erythematosus (SLE) are more likely to experience fetal loss. Pregnancy loss in these women appears related to thrombosis or other damage in placental blood vessels. Women with SLE often have other complications during pregnancy, such as exacerbation of their symptoms, fetal heart block, nonreassuring fetal status on antepartum tests or labor monitoring, and fetal death.

Women who have clotting disorders, either inherited or acquired, may be more susceptible to pregnancy loss resulting from thrombosis. These women may require anticoagulation in pregnancy.

Environmental Agents

Some environmental agents have a well-established relationship to impairment of fertility and pregnancy loss.

Others are believed to be damaging but do not show a conclusive link to pregnancy loss. In addition, the amount of exposure (dose) relates to the pregnancy outcome in most cases.

Examples of established toxins are ionizing radiation, alcohol, and isotretinoin (Accutane). Suspected or known toxins are numerous—for example, cigarette smoke, anesthetic gas, chemicals such as organic solvents or pesticides, and lead and mercury in occupational settings. These agents may be directly toxic to the embryo or fetus, causing its death, or they may interfere with the normal placental function necessary to sustain the pregnancy.

Infections

Infections of the reproductive tract are associated with general complications of pregnancy, and they also may be related to early pregnancy losses. These infections often are asymptomatic, making their diagnosis and link to pregnancy loss difficult to establish.

 KNOWLEDGE CHECK

9. How can anatomic abnormalities of a woman's uterus or cervix cause her to lose a normal pregnancy?
10. What endocrine factors can cause repeated pregnancy loss?
11. What known immunologic factors may cause loss of a normal fetus?

EVALUATION OF INFERTILITY

Couples are often anxious for definitive therapy to achieve pregnancy, but a thorough assessment of their problem is essential for effective and financially sound treatment. Some tests, such as semen evaluation, must be repeated sequentially for an accurate picture. Even a targeted, or focused, evaluation is frustrating to many couples, especially those who are approaching advanced reproductive age. In addition, the usefulness and well-accepted normal values are not well established for some tests and other diagnostic tests are investigational. Despite many examinations and tests, infertility may remain unexplained in couples who seek care (Lobo, 2017).

Women's health care providers and infertility specialists use histories, physical examinations, and diagnostic tests to identify the best course of treatment. The proposed treatments will consider the couple's ages, especially female; medical histories; physical examinations; and diagnostic testing. Therapy often requires a series of steps and procedures, rather than one single treatment.

The evaluation and care of infertile couples may involve numerous professionals: nurses, physicians specializing in reproductive medicine, gynecologists, genetic counselors, urologists, microsurgeons, embryologists, and ultrasonographers. In addition, general and specialized laboratory and radiologic facilities may provide diagnostic services. Nutrition counseling may be needed to support therapy.

Because anxiety, depression, and relationship discord are common in couples experiencing infertility, psychological counseling should be offered to help the couple deal with associated personal and family issues. Nurses working in infertility settings often coordinate communication among the many providers and help the couple negotiate the maze of evaluation and treatment.

Preconception Counseling

Couples may be offered preconception counseling to help evaluate their risk for autosomal recessive disorders and birth defects and perhaps reduce their risk for bearing a child with an anomaly. Many women seeking infertility care are older than 35, an age at which having an infant with a chromosome defect increases. A thorough history and physical examination of both members of the couple, including their family histories, may identify increased risk for having a child with a single-gene defect. Preconception counseling also can help the woman understand the importance of an adequate diet and avoidance of teratogens that can harm the developing fetus before she knows she is pregnant.

History and Physical Examination

A thorough history and physical examination of each partner can help identify the appropriate diagnostic tests and therapy and identify risks for birth defects in the couple's offspring.

History

A reproductive history including the following is obtained for both the man and woman:

- The woman's menstrual pattern, including age at onset, and menstrual characteristics (frequency, regularity, duration, amount of flow, presence of pain)
- Any pregnancies, complications, and their outcomes
- Contraceptive methods, past and present
- Previous fertility of the man or woman with other partners
- Pattern of intercourse in relation to the woman's cycles
- Length of time the couple has had intercourse without using contraception
- Exposure to potential toxins, including tobacco and illicit drug use
- Prescribed and over-the-counter medications
- Family history of multiple pregnancy losses, birth defects, or intellectual disability.
- Home tests the couple has used, such as over-the-counter ovulation predictor kits
- Past surgeries, pelvic inflammatory disease, STDs, abnormal cervical cancer screening and treatment

The medical history, including childhood illnesses and surgery, and a history of exposure to toxins may give clues about the cause of infertility. The couple's past and present occupations may identify toxin exposure, stresses, or other adverse influences on reproduction. Investigation of their usual frequency and timing of intercourse may identify the need for a change to promote conception at the time of ovulation.

Physical Examination

Couples who seek help for infertility are often healthy. However, a thorough physical examination of each partner may identify endocrine disturbances, cranial tumors, or undiagnosed chronic disease. Examination of the reproductive organs may reveal structural defects, infection, cysts, or other abnormalities. Chromosomal analysis or maternal blood clotting studies may be done for couples experiencing repeated pregnancy loss.

Diagnostic Tests

Each couple's evaluation is individualized, but, based on the history and physical examinations, testing generally proceeds from tests that are simple, less invasive, and less expensive to more complex and expensive diagnostics. Simple evaluations can be done simultaneously, but more complex tests are often delayed until their need is established.

Early evaluation for the couple may include the following:

- Ovulation monitoring kit to identify if ovulation has occurred
- Evaluation of the cervical mucus to identify changes that occur with ovulation
- Hormone evaluations such as estrogen, progesterone, LH, FSH, antimüllerian hormone (AMH), and thyroid function
- Ultrasound imaging of internal reproductive organs
- Radiographic imaging (hysterosalpingogram) to visualize uterine cavity and patency of the fallopian tubes
- Semen analysis
- Testicular examination to include an ultrasound and/or a biopsy
- Postcoital examination

Table 26.1 describes diagnostic tests that may be offered to an infertile couple and the nursing care associated with each.

THERAPIES TO FACILITATE PREGNANCY

Evaluation of the couple identifies whether therapy might improve their chances to conceive and complete a pregnancy. A variety of procedures may be used, depending on the couple's initial and ongoing evaluations and their personal choices. Some therapy is simple, such as timing intercourse to better coincide with ovulation. Other procedures may involve considerable expense, discomfort, or unpleasant side effects. Many infertile couples need a combination of treatments to improve their chances of conception.

Identification of appropriate infertility therapy is not always straightforward. Many factors should be considered, including the couple's history, medical evaluations, financial resources, ages and other time constraints, as well as religious and cultural values. Simple treatments are indicated before more complex ones, but the needs of each couple are considered individually. More aggressive diagnostic testing and therapy may be appropriate if the woman is approaching the end of her reproductive years or if it is determined that conception is unlikely to occur spontaneously.

Statistical success rates for various procedures often are difficult for couples to evaluate and vary widely among facilities. Factors that affect a center's success rate for a procedure are numerous. For example, a referral center that is willing to help couples with long-standing infertility may have lower success rates than one that accepts only couples with less severe problems.

Pharmacologic Management

Hormones and other medications may be given to either the man or the woman. A medication may be given to improve semen quality, induce ovulation, prepare the uterine endometrium, or support the pregnancy once it is established. Medications may be given to correct infections or endometriosis. Others may help men for whom **erectile dysfunction** (also known as **impotence** or the consistent inability to achieve or maintain a sufficiently rigid penis) is the primary problem. Table 26.2 summarizes many of the medications used in infertility therapy.

Medications to induce ovulation may be prescribed for the woman who does not ovulate or who ovulates erratically. Medications may be given to provide multiple ova if a woman plans to have intrauterine insemination (IUI), IVF, gamete intrafallopian transfer (GIFT), or tubal embryo transfer. Progesterone vaginal suppositories or clomiphene citrate (Clomid) is often used to stimulate follicle development. Human chorionic gonadotropin (hCG) can then be given to induce release of several ova. Human menopausal gonadotropin (hMG) may be injected in small regular pulses for pituitary insufficiency of LH and FSH, similar to use of an insulin pump.

PATIENT TEACHING

What to Expect with Infertility Evaluation and Treatment

General

Both members of the couple are evaluated systematically to identify the most individualized and time- and cost-effective therapy.

Simpler evaluations and therapies are completed before more complex efforts.

Evaluations and therapy proceed more quickly if the woman is in her mid-30s or older.

Costs may be partially covered by insurance; couples are advised to consult with their insurance carriers. The Patient Protection and Affordable Care Act does not cover infertility treatment.

Difficult decisions may be required at different times during evaluation and treatment. Decisions might include whether to proceed to more complex and expensive tests and therapies, to take a break from treatment, or to abandon treatment altogether. Infertility treatment can be stressful and time intensive, and it requires a substantial commitment to self-care.

Internet resources for infertility include the Centers for Disease Control and Prevention (www.cdc.gov), American Society for Reproductive Medicine (www.asrm.org), and Society for Assisted Reproductive Technology (www.sart.org).

Continued

PATIENT TEACHING—cont'd

What to Expect with Infertility Evaluation and Treatment

Male Factor Infertility Evaluation

Semen analysis may be the first test because it is noninvasive, easy, and inexpensive. More than one sample may be needed for the best evaluation.

Depending on the man's medical history, physical examination findings, and semen analysis, other diagnostic tests may be done (hormone assay, an ultrasound of the reproductive organs, a biopsy of the testicles, and specialized tests of sperm function).

Corrective measures may include medications, surgery, and methods to reduce the scrotal temperature.

Female Factor Infertility Evaluation

The first evaluation usually is to determine whether and how regularly the woman is ovulating each month. In addition to a detailed review of her cycles and premenstrual physical changes, an ovulation predictor kit also may be helpful for the woman to recognize ovulation. Self-assessment of basal body temperature and cervical mucus also may be taught. These assessments are often done at the same time as other tests.

Other common evaluations include ultrasound or x-ray imaging of the uterus and fallopian tubes (hysterosalpingogram) to determine their patency. Contrast media specific to the imaging technique help identify obstructions or malformations in the reproductive tract.

For some tests and therapies, an operative procedure is required (e.g., hysteroscopy, laparoscopy, laser surgery, and microsurgery).

Typically, infertility evaluations and treatments require more of the woman's time, energy, physical discomfort, and risk than the man's.

Corrective measures depend on the problem identified. Examples include medications, surgery, and advanced reproductive techniques, such as in vitro fertilization.

⬥ DRUG GUIDE

Clomiphene Citrate (Clomid, Serophene)

Classification

Ovarian stimulant.

Action

Stimulates pituitary gland to increase secretion of luteinizing hormone (LH) and follicle-stimulating hormone (FSH). LH and FSH stimulate maturation of the ovarian follicle, ovulation, and development of the corpus luteum.

Indications

Female infertility in which estrogen levels are normal, including polycystic ovary syndrome (PCOS)

Dosage and Route

Female sterility: First course: 25 to 50 mg PO daily for 5 days (usually days 3 to 7 of the menstrual cycle). Second course: Same dose if ovulation occurred with first course. If ovulation did not occur, increase dose to 100 mg daily for 5 days. Some women require up to 250 mg daily. A higher dose is not beneficial if ovulation is triggered with a lower dose.

Absorption

Readily absorbed from the gastrointestinal tract. Time to peak effect is 4 to 10 days after last day of treatment.

Excretion

Excreted in the feces.

Contraindications and Precautions

Pregnancy, liver disease, abnormal bleeding of undetermined origin, ovarian cysts, neoplastic disease. Therapy is ineffective in women with ovarian or pituitary failure.

Adverse Reactions

Ovarian enlargement; symptoms similar to those of premenstrual syndrome. Ovarian hyperstimulation syndrome. Multiple gestations, if more than one ovum is released. Visual disturbances. Abdominal distention, discomfort, nausea, vomiting. Abnormal uterine bleeding. Breast tenderness. Insomnia, nervousness, headache, depression, fatigue, lightheadedness, dizziness. Hot flashes, increased urination, allergic symptoms, weight gain, reversible alopecia. Dry cervical mucus.

Nursing Considerations

Obtain the history to determine whether the woman has a history of liver dysfunction or abnormal uterine bleeding. Rule out the possibility of pregnancy. Teach the woman to report abdominal distention, pain in the pelvis or abdomen, and visual disturbances. Teach her to avoid tasks requiring mental alertness or coordination because the drug can cause lightheadedness, dizziness, and visual disturbances. Instruct her to stop taking clomiphene and report to the physician if she suspects she might be pregnant. Teach the woman and her partner that she may notice irritability, mood swings, and other symptoms similar to those in premenstrual syndrome but that these are temporary.

Ovulation induction, also known as *superovulation*, increases the risk for multiple births because several ova may be released and fertilized. A serious complication is *ovarian hyperstimulation syndrome*, which involves marked ovarian enlargement with exudation of fluid and protein into the woman's peritoneal and pleural cavities. Adjustment of medication dosage and serial ultrasound examinations to determine the number of mature follicles reduce the occurrence of high-order multifetal pregnancy (triplets or more) and ovarian hyperstimulation syndrome.

Surgical Procedures

Endoscopic procedures may be used to correct obstructions with minimal invasiveness in either the man or the woman.

TABLE 26.2 Selected Medications Used in Infertility Therapy

Drug	Primary Use
Bromocriptine (Parlodel); cabergoline (Dostinex)	Corrects excess prolactin secretion by anterior pituitary, improving gonadotropin-releasing hormone (GnRH) secretion, in turn, normalizing release of follicle-stimulating hormone (FSH) and luteinizing hormone (LH). These drug actions increase ovulation and support early pregnancy by stimulating progesterone secretion by the corpus luteum.
Chorionic gonadotropin, human (hCG; [Novarel, Pregnyl]); recombinant deoxyribonucleic acid (DNA) origin (r-hCG; [Ovidrel])	Used in conjunction with gonadotropins to stimulate ovulation in the female or sperm formation in the male. Stimulates progesterone production by corpus luteum.
Clomiphene citrate (Clomid) Letrozole (Femara)	Induction of ovulation in women who have specific types of ovulatory dysfunction. Drug increases frequency of GnRH secretion from the hypothalamus, thus increasing FSH and LH release, maturing the ovarian follicle, and causing release of the ovum.
FSH, recombinant DNA origin (follitropin [Gonal-F])	Stimulation of ovarian follicle growth; ovulation-induction gonadotropin.
GnRH antagonists (e.g., cetrorelix [Cetrotide], ganirelix [Antagon])	Reduces endometriosis; adjunct to drugs given to stimulate ovulation by suppressing LH and FSH, reducing ovarian hyperstimulation.
GnRH agonists (goserelin [Zoladex], leuprolide [Lupron], nafarelin [Synarel])	Stimulates release of FSH and LH from the pituitary gland in men and women who have deficient GnRH secretion by their hypothalamus. FSH and LH, in turn, stimulate ovulation in the female and stimulate testosterone production and spermatogenesis in the male.
Gonadotropins (Bravelle, Humegon, Pergonal, Repronex)	Induction of ovulation with human-derived FSH and LH; brands may differ in the proportions of FSH to LH; recombinant DNA preparations are becoming more common because of their greater purity.
LH, recombinant DNA origin	Replacement of LH via subcutaneous pump; promotes ability of mature ovarian follicle to rupture and luteinize when hCG is secreted.
Progesterone (parenteral or vaginal preparations)	Luteal phase support; prepares uterine lining and promotes implantation of embryo.
Metformin (Glucophage)	Adjunctive treatment for ovulation induction in women with polycystic ovary syndrome.
Erectile agents (sildenafil [Viagra], tadalafil [Cialis], vardenafil [Levitra])	Increase blood flow to the penis, improving erectile function.

Data from Lobo, R. A. (2015). Infertility. In R. A. Lobo, D. M. Gershenson, G. M. Lentz, & F. A. Valea (Eds.), *Comprehensive gynecology* (7th ed.). St. Louis, MO: Mosby.

The woman may need a laparotomy to relieve pelvic adhesions and obstructions caused by endometriosis, infection, or previous surgical procedures, if these cannot be corrected via laparoscopy. Laser surgical techniques may be used to reduce adhesions because they are minimally invasive, precise, and less likely to cause new adhesions. Correction of a **varicocele**, an abnormal dilation or varicosity, by ligating or embolizing the dilated vein may improve sperm quality and quantity, although there is not a consensus on its usefulness. Microsurgical techniques may be attempted for correction of obstructions in the fallopian tubes or male tubal structures.

Transcervical balloon tuboplasty is a minimally invasive method to unblock the fallopian tubes. A thin catheter is threaded through the cervix and uterus into the fallopian tube. The balloon is then inflated to clear the blockage.

Therapeutic Insemination

Therapeutic insemination may use either the partner's semen or that of a donor to overcome a low or absent sperm count. Donor insemination also may be used if the woman's partner carries a genetic defect or if a woman desires a biologic child without having a relationship with a male partner. IUI is a variation of therapeutic insemination that allows sperm to be placed directly into the uterus, thus bypassing the cervical mucus and reducing some immunologic incompatibilities. This process also removes many of the antibodies that interfere with sperm motility and ability to penetrate the ovum.

Sperm for therapeutic insemination or IUI are obtained from semen collected by masturbation or donation. The sperm are washed in laboratory solutions to remove prostaglandins that cause uterine cramping and then concentrated before insemination. Washing also removes many of the antibodies that interfere with sperm motility and ability to penetrate the ovum. If the man has retrograde ejaculation, he may take sodium bicarbonate 2 hours before obtaining the semen to render the urine alkaline. The urine is collected in a sterile container and washed with a medium to separate sperm from urine.

Men who donate semen for insemination are screened to reduce the risk for transmitting diseases or genetic defects. They are questioned about their personal and family health history, including genetic disorders or birth defects. Questions about their social habits and personality can disclose high-risk behaviors and give recipient parents information about potential traits of their child. Physical and laboratory examinations are performed to evaluate the man's general health, determine his blood type and Rh factor, and screen for infections such as STDs or human immunodeficiency virus (HIV). Carrier testing for specific genetic defects, such as sickle cell and Tay-Sachs diseases, reduces the risk for passing on these disorders. To reduce the risk for transmitting diseases that may not be apparent at the initial screening, donor semen is frozen and held for 6 months before use. The man is retested for diseases such as HIV several times during the 6 months.

Inadvertent **consanguinity** (blood relationship) can occur because half-siblings from two families may not know they were conceived with donor gametes. They may later conceive a child who shares a larger number of genes, both normal and abnormal, than the general population. For this reason, the number of sperm donations may be limited.

Egg Donation

Use of donor oocytes may be an option for some women who do not produce ova because of POF, who do not respond to ovarian stimulation, or whose ova are not successfully fertilized despite apparently normal sperm. It is less successful if used for women who have a birth defect such as Turner's syndrome, in which the ova regress early in life, or for women who have had radiation therapy to the pelvis (Lobo, 2017).

As in use of donor semen, egg donation carries the risk for infecting the recipient, the fetus, and possibly the male partner of the recipient. The egg donor is routinely screened for genetic problems that are more prevalent in her race and for hereditary problems that may exist in the donor or her first-degree relatives (parent, sibling, child). Other tests may be available before conception such as chromosome analysis that may show fragile-X carrier status or an abnormal arrangement of her chromosomes. Chromosome analysis may not indicate a problem in the woman who donates the egg, but it might increase the possibility of an abnormality in the conceptus. Decisions about whether to pursue available testing of the fetus should be made by the recipient, however.

Surrogate Parenting

A **surrogate mother** may enter the picture if the woman is infertile or cannot carry a fetus to live birth. The surrogate mother may supply her uterus only (**gestational carrier**), with the infertile couple supplying the sperm and ovum. Or she may be inseminated with the male partner's sperm and carry the fetus to birth, thus supplying both the genetic component and the gestational component. Surrogacy is different from therapeutic insemination with donor sperm because it is not anonymous. In addition, the woman who carries the child may form bonds with the fetus and male/female during the months of pregnancy. For these reasons, extensive interviews and counseling of both the infertile couple and the surrogate mother are required.

Money paid to the surrogate mother can raise ethical issues. Could a poor but fertile woman feel compelled to provide her body for a more well-to-do couple? However, not compensating a woman for the real physical and emotional risks of this undertaking can be construed as coercive as well.

It also should be considered that the male/female partners will likely need to provide insurance coverage to the surrogate or gestational carrier.

Unfortunately, custody of the resulting child has been the issue in several court cases involving surrogate mothers. In the *Baby M* case, a woman who was inseminated with the man's sperm refused to relinquish the baby as stated in the contract between the birth mother and the infertile couple. Ultimately, custody was awarded to the man providing the sperm and his spouse, but visitation rights were granted to the surrogate mother.

Custody issues when the birth mother is a gestational surrogate are clearer than when she also donates her ovum to the child. Courts have more often recognized the genetic parents as the legal parents and upheld the contracts between them and the gestational surrogate.

Assisted Reproductive Technologies

More than 1% of births in the United States each year are brought about by **assisted reproductive technologies (ARTs)**. The definition used by the Centers for Disease Control and Prevention (CDC) is specific: surgically removing eggs from a woman's ovaries, combining them with sperm in a laboratory, and returning them to the woman's body or donating them to another woman. ART involves medical, surgical, laboratory, and micromanipulation techniques used with ova and sperm to improve the chance of conception. Simpler evaluations and other treatments often precede or accompany ART therapy. Annual National Summary and Fertility Clinic Success Rates are available in ART Reports and Resources at the www.cdc.gov website.

In Vitro Fertilization

IVF may be done to bypass blocked or absent fallopian tubes, for male factor infertility, or for unexplained infertility in either the man or the woman. The physician removes the ova by ultrasound-guided transvaginal retrieval, or occasionally laparoscopy, and mixes them with prepared sperm from the woman's partner or a donor. The ova are examined to determine whether fertilization has occurred about 18 hours after addition of the sperm. The fertilized oocytes are then returned to the uterus or may be cultured for 48 to 96 more hours, allowing cell division for a total of 5 days (Fig. 26.4). The number of fertilized ova returned is individualized, but single embryo transfer is slowly lowering the rate of multiple births from the implantation of multiple embryos, without compromising success rates. Older women may have more ova transferred than younger women to improve their chances of pregnancy without greatly increasing the risk for having a triplet or higher pregnancy. IVF is the most common of current ART procedures. IVF is used to do preimplantation genetic diagnosis for fertile couples having a high risk for a baby with a genetic disorder (Hershberger & Schoenfeld, 2011; Lobo, 2017).

Embryo transfer (ET), combined with IVF (IVF-ET), has become more common. Gamete intrafallopian transfer (GIFT) and zygote intrafallopian transfer (ZIFT) are

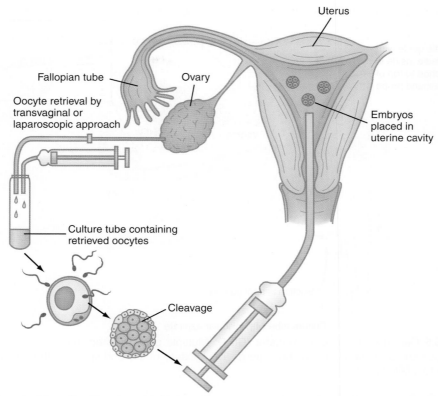

FIG. 26.4 In Vitro Fertilization. Multiple oocytes are obtained by using a transvaginal or laparoscopic approach. The retrieved oocytes are mixed with prepared sperm and incubated 1 to 2 days. Embryos are then transferred to the uterine cavity to allow implantation and continued development.

modifications in which sperm and ova are placed in open fallopian tubes. Variations of ZIFT include tubal embryo transfer (TET), also known as tubal embryo stage transfer (TEST), which places the conceptus in the fallopian tube later than GIFT. Ultrasound guidance targets the best location to obtain the ova. Intracytoplasmic sperm injection (ICSI) is a technique in which a single spermatozoon, obtained with microsurgical techniques, is injected into the cytoplasm of an ovum (Lobo, 2017).

Most ART procedures are done in an outpatient setting. Each procedure begins with ovulation induction to permit retrieval of several ova to improve the likelihood of a successful pregnancy. Sperm are prepared and concentrated in a specialized laboratory as they are for therapeutic insemination.

Supplemental progesterone is given to the woman to promote implantation and support the early pregnancy (luteal phase support). Because of the supplemental progesterone, the woman will not have a menstrual period even if she is not pregnant. Transvaginal ultrasounds are used to identify whether one or more gestational sacs have implanted with IVF and to identify if an ectopic (tubal) pregnancy occurred after methods such as IUI, GIFT, or ZIFT.

IVF success rates vary among infertility centers. Not every ovum is successfully fertilized when IVF or its modifications are used, and embryos transferred to the woman's uterus may not always implant. Although twins are the most common

multifetal pregnancy, triplets or more may occur, raising issues related to the physical and emotional well-being of the mother and babies.

Intrafallopian Transfer

The woman must have at least one patent fallopian tube for GIFT to be an option. The procedure begins in a manner similar to that of IVF, with retrieval of multiple ova and washed sperm. The retrieved ova are drawn into a catheter that also carries prepared sperm. The mix of sperm and ova is injected into each fallopian tube through a laparoscope. Additional prepared sperm may be injected into the uterus through the cervix to improve the chance of successful fertilization. Progesterone is given as it is in IVF (Fig. 26.5).

Zygote Intrafallopian Transfer

ZIFT, often called *tubal embryo transfer (TET),* is a hybrid of IVF and GIFT. The woman's ova are fertilized outside her body, but the resulting fertilized ova are placed in the fallopian tubes and enter the uterus naturally for implantation. The woman must have at least one patent fallopian tube.

Comparison of In Vitro Fertilization, Gamete Intrafallopian Transfer, and Tubal Embryo Transfer

The primary advantage of GIFT and ZIFT over IVF is that more people and religious groups may find GIFT and ZIFT

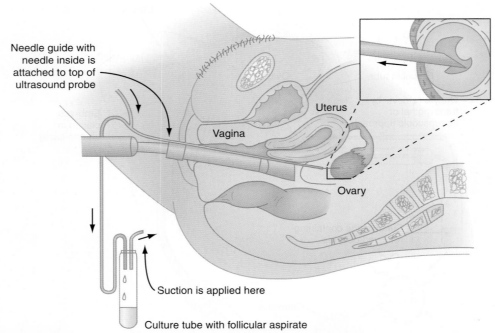

Needle guide with needle inside is attached to top of ultrasound probe

Uterus

Vagina

Ovary

Suction is applied here

Culture tube with follicular aspirate

FIG. 26.5 Gamete Intrafallopian Transfer (GIFT). Multiple ova aspirated from the ovary in this illustration are combined with washed sperm. The mixture of ova and sperm is then transferred directly to a fallopian tube.

more natural and therefore more acceptable than IVF. With IVF or ZIFT, evidence of fertilization exists before placement in the uterus or tubes. The GIFT and ZIFT procedures are more invasive, requiring a laparoscopy to place the gametes or fertilized ova in the distal fallopian tube. Tubal pregnancy may result if embryos cannot reach the uterine cavity to implant. For these reasons IVF is used about 99% of the time if a couple requires ART (CDC, 2013).

Intracytoplasmic Sperm Injection

Microsurgical techniques, combined with IVF, may help couples conceive despite severe male factor infertility. Men who have obstructions to their epididymis or absence of an epididymis may be able to father children with the use of percutaneous or microsurgical sperm aspiration. The sperm are retrieved from the epididymis by percutaneous aspiration of a single spermatozoon with a small-gauge needle. Alternatively, a microsurgical incision may be made to aspirate the sperm if the percutaneous approach cannot be used. The sperm obtained are then used to fertilize ova by ICSI.

Preimplantation Genetic Testing

Couples with concerns about a specific genetic defect in the family may be offered preimplantation genetic testing of their fertilized ova. As in other types of prenatal screening, preimplantation genetic testing cannot rule out every potential abnormality in the offspring. Rather, the testing allows parents to make informed decisions about whether to implant the fertilized ova into the uterus.

KNOWLEDGE CHECK

12. What elements are included in the history and the physical examination for an infertility workup?
13. What medications may be used to induce ovulation?
14. What screening tests are performed if donor sperm is used for therapeutic insemination or GIFT?
15. What are the differences in technique among IVF, GIFT, and ZIFT? What is done in ICSI?

EMOTIONAL RESPONSES TO INFERTILITY

Many couples desire natural childbearing. Even if they delay childbearing, many couples expect to have a child before the end of the woman's reproductive years. Those who chose childlessness earlier in life may reevaluate their decision as they age. If a couple does not achieve pregnancy or produce a living child as expected, the man and the woman may experience psychological distress and a threat to their self-images. Either or both partners may feel like they have failed themselves or each other. Their marital and family relationships may be stressed, and they may withdraw from relationships they previously found satisfying. Every couple is unique, and many reactions depend on the importance attached to having biologic children.

Assumption of Fertility

Most couples practice contraception for a number of years before they decide to become pregnant. They may want to first establish a career and financial security, acquire a comfortable home and lifestyle, or perhaps travel and live freely without the responsibility of a child. They usually assume they are fertile and must take steps to avoid pregnancy until ready.

When they do desire pregnancy, they discontinue contraception and assume that pregnancy will occur within a few months at most. They may plan conception so that the baby will be born at a certain time of year (such as not during the hottest weather) or to avoid major holidays.

Either or both partners may experiment with the role of parent as they anticipate pregnancy. They develop a heightened awareness of children and parenting. Being with others who are expecting or already have children is exciting because they plan to join their ranks shortly. They may discuss issues such as full-time parenting by one partner, child care, and imminent lifestyle changes. They may begin acquiring toys and furnishings that a child will need. Both partners may develop a fantasy child or a concept of what their baby will be like.

Growing Awareness of a Problem

As time goes on without successful conception, the couple gradually becomes concerned about the inability to conceive. If the woman is older, they may feel the urgency of her limited reproductive capacity. The plan to have a baby at a certain time of year is often replaced by the desire for a baby any time—and soon.

The couple may feel uneasy with child-related activities because they are uncertain when or if they will be parents. They may feel hurt when other family members or friends have babies. Events focusing on infants or small children may become melancholy rather than joyful occasions. Family members and friends who are having children may feel guilty when they are around the couple who cannot conceive (Paterno, 2008).

The potential grandparents may think their children are waiting too long to start a family or even that they are selfish. If they are aware the couple is trying to conceive, they become even more worried as the months pass without the longed-for announcement of a pregnancy. They are twice saddened—by the lack of a grandchild and the hurt their adult children are enduring.

Seeking Help for Infertility

Eventually, couples must decide whether to seek help to conceive. They may reach this point after only a few menstrual cycles or, at the opposite extreme, may never seek help. Many factors enter into their decision, such as their ages (especially in older women), how long they have been unable to conceive, how much they desire a biological child, how they regard adoption, and how they feel about a life without children. If they have a biological child but are unable to conceive another, the couple may consider adoption sooner.

Identifying the Importance of Having a Baby

Each partner may place a different priority on having a baby. Conflicts may arise when one partner wants help to conceive sooner than the other. In addition, cultural or religious beliefs influence the way each feels about procreation and whether

options such as assisted reproductive procedures or adoption are acceptable. The way in which the couple resolves these differences is crucial to the stability of the relationship.

Men and women often differ in their reactions to infertility, although they are equally affected. Women may want to talk about their feelings and frustrations, but men often internalize their feelings or think they must be strong for their partners. The woman may interpret her partner's stoicism and reluctance to express his feelings as disinterest or lack of concern and care for her (Paterno, 2008).

Sharing Intimate Information

Evaluation and treatment for infertility require that both partners reveal information about their sexual relationship, such as the frequency and timing of intercourse. This may be difficult for those who regard this information as intimate. In addition, infertile couples may think the evaluation calls their sexual adequacy into question. They may feel defensive if they perceive a threat to their self-image (Paterno, 2008).

Considering Financial Resources

Financial concerns enter into the couple's decision about whether to seek treatment and how far to carry it. Techniques such as ovulation predictor kits are inexpensive but have limited usefulness in achieving successful pregnancy. Advanced techniques such as IVF are expensive and may have a low likelihood of success for some couples. Health insurance may or may not cover infertility treatment or may cover only certain procedures or medications. Investigational treatments are usually not covered. The drugs that must be taken to achieve pregnancy are often quite expensive. Expense and restricted coverage limit treatment choices for many couples. Those who seek and pursue infertility treatment may have greater financial resources than those who do not seek treatment.

Committing to Involvement in Care

Infertility evaluation and treatment require a great commitment from the couple in terms of time, emotional and physical energy, and money. Couples can be involved in this process for several years if they do not set a limit on when they want to stop. They participate daily as they do home assessments, take medications, and keep detailed records similar to what they might do in their jobs. The physical effects of drugs that induce ovulation and support conception can result in many side or adverse effects. For infertility diagnosis and therapy to be most effective, couples should consider their ability and desire to be directly involved in the process over what may be a long time.

Reactions during Evaluation and Treatment

Couples undergoing infertility evaluation and treatment have different reactions to the process. Although early evaluations often result in simple treatment and quick response, a couple's reactions may change as treatment becomes more complex, demanding, and lengthy.

Influences on Decision Making

If their evaluation shows that a treatment or procedure may enable them to conceive, the couple must then decide whether to proceed. The decision-making process begins early and must be repeated during therapy if pregnancy does not occur. A complex array of factors enters into their decisions about beginning and continuing treatment or whether to end their pursuit of pregnancy. Although discussed separately, these factors interact dynamically as the couple makes each decision. The nurse helps them examine each factor and arrive at a decision that is best for them.

Social, Cultural, and Religious Values. Some medically appropriate options are not acceptable to every couple within their personal, social, cultural, and religious frameworks. Surrogate parenting, IVF, and therapeutic insemination (especially with donor sperm or egg) are not consistent with the personal or religious beliefs of some people. If a procedure offers the partners hope for a child but is incompatible with their beliefs, their choices are two: use the technology despite their beliefs or be willing to accept childlessness. Adoption may be a third alternative for some couples if the desire for a biologic child is not absolute. Adoption of a foreign child may be necessary, with associated international implications. As in other decisions, couples must work out conflicting personal values about what therapy is acceptable.

Difficulty of Treatment. The couple must consider how difficult, risky, and physically and/or emotionally uncomfortable therapy may be. The level of difficulty involves physical, psychological, geographic, and time factors. Employment constraints also may affect treatment decisions.

Several diagnostic tests and treatments for infertility involve invasive procedures or surgery. The person who undergoes the procedure should be the one who ultimately decides whether to do it. That person alone, with input from his or her partner, can decide whether the hope for a child is worth the risks and discomfort of the procedure.

Infertility treatment is stressful. Often partners feel or are willing to tolerate different levels of stress. To reduce the stress, they may abandon treatment completely or take a break for a few months from the constant preoccupation with conceiving. Women nearing or in their 40s often do not feel they have the luxury of skipping a treatment cycle.

Some couples encounter geographic difficulties if they must travel a long distance for therapy. Time stresses are substantial, and one or both partners may spend many hours every week in pursuit of pregnancy. Employment constraints may be a barrier to infertility therapy because of the time required for treatment

Probability of Success. Couples often have a biased interpretation of their statistical probability of success, especially when they begin treatment with a new procedure. For example, if a procedure has a 20% likelihood of success with each cycle, they tend to expect they will be in the successful group rather than in the 80% who do not meet with success. As time goes by, however, they must weigh the likelihood of success of any therapy against financial concerns and their own willingness to accept the discomfort and

difficulty associated with it. Again, the woman's age imposes an inescapable limit.

Financial Concerns. Some couples, particularly those with ample resources and a strong desire for a biologic child, pursue expensive treatments and do so longer than others of more limited means, despite a low probability of success. Couples with financial limitations find they must abandon treatment sooner than they want. Other couples go heavily into debt, adding financial strain to the other stresses of treatment in their quest for a biologic child.

Psychological Reactions

A couple's initial reaction to infertility often is one of shock and sadness because the partners are usually healthy and did not expect to have problems conceiving. Their reactions vary according to how easily their infertility is alleviated, their personality and self-image, and the strength of their relationship.

Guilt. A partner having the only identified problem might feel that he or she is depriving the other of children. This feeling may be compounded if the "normal" partner has children from another relationship. It may be difficult for this person to understand that not all factors affecting fertility are known and what seems like the problem of only one partner is often the couple's problem.

Either partner may feel guilty about past choices that now affect fertility. A woman with adhesions resulting from a sexually transmitted infection may regret her past sexual choices. The man who wanted to delay pregnancy longer than the woman may feel guilty if her age is now reducing her fertility.

Isolation. Infertile couples may withdraw from friends and relatives who have children to insulate themselves from painful reminders of their infertility. Some couples develop supportive relationships with others who are infertile, which somewhat diminishes their sense of isolation.

Depression. One or both partners may experience depression as their sense of competence and control over their bodies is challenged, especially if therapy is not successful quickly. They often feel as though they are on a roller coaster of hope alternating with despair when the woman has her menstrual period each month. The couple may feel envy toward those who conceive easily.

Stress on the Relationship. Because infertility can challenge a person's identity and self-esteem, partners may find less satisfaction in their relationship.

The man may have difficulty ejaculating on demand for semen specimens or postcoital tests, feeling that others will judge his sexual function. The fact that semen samples are best obtained by masturbation in an office setting is unacceptable or uncomfortable to some men. Both partners may be stressed when intercourse must be scheduled to coincide with specific evaluations or ovulation. Intercourse can become a chore more than an expression of love. It may come to be associated with failure rather than fulfillment if a pregnancy is not forthcoming.

If sperm from an anonymous donor is used for therapeutic insemination or other techniques, the man may feel that his masculinity is further threatened. He does not want to deprive his wife of a child, but he may be ambivalent about use of sperm from a third party. He may have difficulty distinguishing between fatherhood as a biologic achievement and fatherhood as a relationship.

The couple may find their relationship strained if they disagree on which treatments are appropriate and how long they should be pursued. One partner may want to keep trying "one more month," and the other may want to abandon treatment. If they are considering adoption, their relationship again may be strained if they differ on whether to adopt and what kind of child they are willing to accept.

KNOWLEDGE CHECK

16. What factors do couples consider when they are deciding whether to seek help for their infertility?
17. What factors should couples consider when they reach decision points during infertility evaluation and treatment?
18. What are possible psychological reactions to infertility?

OUTCOMES AFTER INFERTILITY THERAPY

After infertility therapy, three outcomes are possible. A pregnancy may occur and continue to a live birth, may end in pregnancy loss, or may not occur. If pregnancy loss occurs or if infertility therapy is unsuccessful, the couple must decide whether to pursue adoption or to remain childless.

Pregnancy Loss after Infertility Therapy

Couples who suffer pregnancy loss after infertility therapy may interpret the experience with mixed feelings of loss and gain. Couples undergoing infertility evaluation and treatment often are aware of a pregnancy much earlier than fertile couples. They want to hope yet expect to be disappointed again. If a spontaneous abortion occurs, they may grieve profoundly for what they achieved and then lost.

Yet despite their grief about the pregnancy loss, the partners may be encouraged because they have achieved a pregnancy. They may feel that if they succeeded once, they can become pregnant again. A miscarriage may give them the courage to continue or restart treatment.

If a pregnancy results in an ectopic pregnancy, the woman may lose a fallopian tube, although earlier diagnosis reduces the risks for damage or loss of the affected tube. These couples may have an added threat to their fertility because of the increased risk for ectopic pregnancy in future conceptions.

Parenthood after Infertility Therapy

Couples who conceive experience varied emotions. If they have been disappointed before, they may be hesitant to be optimistic about this pregnancy. They will be happy but still anxious about whether they can complete the pregnancy and realize the dream of taking home a baby. Pregnancy after infertility therapy is emotionally tentative for many infertile couples, especially those who have been trying to conceive for a long time or have lost a pregnancy. They may distance themselves from the reality of the pregnancy until much later in gestation than normally fertile couples.

The woman has learned to sense and report every symptom and may interpret normal changes of pregnancy as a threat. Preterm labor may stir greater anxiety in the previously infertile couple. The woman may assume that intermittent periods of fetal quiet are abnormal rather than naps that are normal for every fetus.

The previously infertile couple may find little support from those who do not understand their fear of investing in the pregnancy. Other infertile couples who have been a source of mutual support may either withdraw from the couple who achieve a pregnancy or rejoice in their success.

The parents' anxiety may be heightened during labor. They may be afraid that something will go wrong at the last moment. Even after the birth of a healthy infant, some parents need time to relax and grasp the fact that their baby is really alive and well.

Choosing Adoption

Not every couple who seeks treatment for infertility achieves a biologic pregnancy. Some couples discontinue treatment sooner than others, depending on their age and tolerance for the fatigue, stress, and expense. Some couples investigate adoption early in infertility treatment if a nonbiologic child is acceptable to them. A single parent may choose adoption. Agencies that coordinate international adoptions are often consulted.

Couples who consider adoption must confront their personal preferences, limitations, and prejudices. As much as they want a child, many couples are not willing to adopt a child with special needs, one of a mixed or different race, or a group of siblings.

Some couples fear adopting a child because the woman might then spontaneously become pregnant. Although pregnancy has been their goal for a long time, they may worry that they would love their adopted child differently from their biologic child. If the couple plans to continue trying for a biologic child, they also must come to grips with this issue.

Couples who decide to adopt face further scrutiny of their personal lives. Agencies investigate their home, financial means (which may have been seriously drained), and fitness as parents. Once again, they may feel their personal competence is questioned. International adoptions often have many additional requirements that the couple does not encounter in their home country.

The couple who decides on adoption may have emotions similar to those who achieve a pregnancy. They may be slow to invest in the process emotionally because they expect disappointment again. In addition, the adopted child often arrives suddenly and unexpectedly. A delay in the adoption process may occur, bringing further uncertainty to the couple. Although they may have been waiting months for this happy event, the couple may have little time to adjust to the reality of their new roles as parents.

Menopause after Infertility

A woman or couple may decide when to stop unsuccessful infertility treatment, or natural biologic aging may make that decision for her. After many attempts to conceive and carry a child to term, her ovarian reserve may be exhausted and she may become perimenopausal or menopausal.

◆ APPLICATION OF THE NURSING PROCESS: CARE OF THE INFERTILE COUPLE

Nurses may encounter couples facing infertility in many different settings and identify numerous nursing care needs. Regardless of the setting, the nurse often addresses the couple's emotional needs associated with infertility evaluation, treatment, and outcomes of therapy.

◆ Assessment

In many instances, infertile couples previously have had a positive self-image and feelings of competence about themselves. The diagnosis of infertility may alter this positive view. The nurse should be aware that these feelings may be present, regardless of the practice setting in which the couple is encountered.

The nurse should determine at what point the couple is in their infertility treatment journey. Couples who have just discovered they may have difficulty conceiving may be shocked yet optimistic that therapy will result in a baby. Other couples for whom simple treatments were unsuccessful may face shock again if the more complex treatments such as IVF or ICSI are recommended, particularly if these treatments may result in financial hardship. Listen for remarks that are negative, expressing guilt or helplessness.

Evaluate the way infertility has affected the partners' relationship with each other. Are there conflicts or differences in values between the two? Observing their body language, such as eye contact, may provide clues about similarities and differences in their commitment to diagnosis and treatment. Ask them how their relationship has changed. Are they more or less satisfied with their marital relationship than they were before they had problems conceiving? How is each member of the couple adjusting to the situation?

Ask about support systems. Couples suffering from infertility often withdraw from old relationships yet do not form new supportive ones. Do others who are significant in the partners' lives know that they are trying to conceive? Are family members and friends nearby, and are they supportive? Have they sought the counsel of a therapist trained in infertility? Ask whether they have encountered assumptions by others that infertility is the "fault" of one partner or the other. Are they subjected to questions that invade their privacy, such as "When are you two going to have a baby?"

Determine how the couple's culture or religion views infertility and the impact of these values on therapy. Are some therapies unacceptable to one or both partners? The partners may have differing views that can cause conflict during treatment, and they may need help to work these out.

Determine how the couple is coping with the stresses of treatment. How much has infertility cost them in terms of time, money, and discomfort? Identify the successes and failures they have experienced as well as outcomes that have provided them hope or comfort. Their ages, especially the woman's, add another stressor that cannot be ignored in their decisions.

If the woman is pregnant or has given birth recently or the couple has adopted a child recently, observe for high levels of anxiety in either or both parents. Assess them for negative behaviors and comments, such as reluctance to feel joy or a sense that they will "fail" again.

◆ Identification of Patient Problems

Infertility can result in a patient feeling anxious, hopeless and a sense of loss. An appropriate patient problem is altered self-confidence resulting from a loss of control.

◆ Planning: Expected Outcomes

Three expected outcomes are appropriate for this patient problem during the early days of evaluation and decision making. The outcomes may apply to the man, the woman, or both partners. The person(s) will do the following:

- Express feelings about infertility and its evaluation and treatment.
- Explore ways to increase control within the situation of infertility.
- Identify aspects of self that are positive.

◆ Interventions
Assist Communication

Therapeutic communication is the primary technique for assessment and intervention related to this patient problem. Recognize that either partner may be reluctant to express his or her feelings as openly as his or her partner. A variety of communication techniques such as active listening and exploration may encourage the partners to express their feelings honestly. Provide privacy and acceptance of their feelings. Nurses should recognize the validity of the couple's views and emotions, even if they differ from the nurse's own feelings.

Encourage the partners to accept their feelings, both positive and negative. The partners may act elated because they believe they should feel happy, yet inside they are cautious and hesitant about becoming attached to their baby. Explain that feelings are not right or wrong but simply exist. Opening the subject of negative feelings (fear of attachment) within a successful situation (pregnancy or birth) may be helpful to reinforce the normality of their emotions. This technique gives them the opportunity to talk about emotional reactions that they or others feel are inappropriate and might otherwise be reluctant to discuss.

Discuss possible differences in ways the man and the woman communicate. For example, explain that the woman may feel more comfortable than the man in talking about their problem and concerns about treatment. Explain that these differences in communication style can cause misunderstandings because one partner believes that the other does not care as much about their problem. Encourage them to be open with each other for the best mutual support. Support groups provide another means for communication and ventilation of feelings among those who are most likely to understand what an infertile couple is experiencing.

Increase the Couple's Sense of Control

Explore how the couple has dealt with stressors in the past and how these techniques might be used to cope with the present crisis. A couple's pattern of dealing with stress in other parts of life is likely to carry over into infertility diagnosis and treatment and throughout pregnancy and parenthood. Reinforce positive coping skills such as learning more about infertility and the proposed therapy for it.

Couples who experience undue stress may benefit from relaxation techniques such as visualization and moderate exercise. Frequent strenuous exercise may reduce the woman's ability to ovulate. Although a hot tub is relaxing for many people, it should be avoided because the high temperatures may inhibit spermatogenesis. In addition, the woman could become pregnant with any cycle, and high maternal body temperatures may be associated with fetal anomalies.

Discuss behaviors that enhance the ability to handle stress and provide a good environment for a pregnancy that might occur. Reinforce healthy choices such as good nutrition and a balance between exercise and rest. Teach the couple ways to enhance general health if deficiencies are identified.

Explain any procedures and their purpose in language the couple can understand. Reinforce any medical explanations that may have been given. Encourage questions so the couple is fully informed. Have the partners restate what was explained to reduce misunderstandings.

Help the couple explore options at each decision point. The couple must decide the best course of action, but the nurse can help identify pros and cons of each choice so the partners can arrive at a decision appropriate for them. Be nondirective so the choices are theirs and do not reflect the biases of the nurse or other caregivers.

Reduce Isolation

Because couples often distance themselves from friends and family relationships that they find painful, they may have little social support. Refer them to available support groups to provide emotional outlets, a sense of belonging, and a source of information.

Couples who achieve pregnancy or adopt a child may again find themselves isolated if infertile couples in their circle of support are no longer comfortable with them. Encourage them to take the initiative to reestablish ties with relatives and friends, who can be an important source of aid during pregnancy and child-rearing. Help them identify ways they can improve communication with these significant others. Remind them that they have undergone significant shifts in self-image, which also have affected those around them.

Promote a Positive Self-Image

Because infertility work often is such a dominant factor in their lives, a continuing inability to conceive erodes the partners' perception of themselves. Explore with them other areas of competence and activities that make them feel good about themselves. Reinforce positive attitudes and self-evaluations. Encourage them to maintain activities such as hobbies, sports, or volunteer work. The career of either partner may be a source of stress that needs relief, or it may be an avenue that fosters a positive self-perception.

Encourage them to avoid activities that involve infants or children if these events make them sad. Help them identify the best way to cope with these activities if they do not want to avoid them.

Some people benefit from self-improvement activities such as continuing education courses or enhancement of appearance. Encourage these activities if they help the individuals feel better about themselves. If the activity might impair fertility treatments, such as strict dieting, also inform the person of this fact.

◆ Evaluation

The goals established are achieved if the individual or both partners can do the following:
- Express their feelings about their situation, usually over time.
- Explore ways to increase personal control over their lives, as evidenced by expressing feelings of reduced helplessness and dependence.
- Identify one or more aspects of self that are perceived as positive and identify areas of competence.

▌ SUMMARY CONCEPTS

- Nurses may encounter persons having infertility problems in a variety of settings other than infertility clinics, such as maternity and gynecology services, urology services, the perioperative area, and the emergency department. Friends and family members also see the nurse as an information resource about infertility care.
- About 20% of infertile couples have no identified problem that is explained by current evaluation techniques.

- Because many unknown factors in reproduction exist, identification and correction of problems in one or both partners does not necessarily resolve their infertility.
- A variety of structural and functional abnormalities may contribute to a couple's infertility. The man may have abnormalities of the sperm or the seminal fluid or with ejaculation. The woman may have ovulation disorders, anatomic problems such as fallopian tube occlusion, or physiologic disorders such as hormone imbalances.

- A systematic evaluation of both partners, proceeding from simple to more complex, identifies therapy that is most likely to be successful and cost-effective. The couple may decide to stop evaluation or therapy at any point.
- Infertility is a crisis for the couple and often for the extended family. Either or both partners may think the inability to conceive represents a personal failure. They may have a variety of psychological reactions.
- Infertile couples must make choices at many points before and during evaluation and therapy. Some major factors that

enter into their decisions involve personal, social, cultural, and religious values; difficulty of treatment; probability of success; financial resources; and age, particularly the woman's.
- The possible outcomes after infertility therapy may present new challenges to the couple and their families, such as unsuccessful therapy and the choice of whether to pursue adoption, pregnancy loss after infertility, and parenthood after infertility.
- Many nursing care needs may be identified as the couple negotiates infertility evaluation and treatment.

REFERENCES & READINGS

American College of Obstetricians and Gynecologists (ACOG). (2009). *Preimplantation genetic screening for aneuploidy.* (ACOG Committee Opinion No. 430). Washington, DC: Author .

American College of Obstetricians and Gynecologists (ACOG). (2013). *Multifetal pregnancy reduction.* (ACOG Committee Opinion No. 553). Washington, DC: Author.

American College of Obstetricians and Gynecologists (ACOG). (2016). *Age-related fertility decline.* (ACOG Committee Opinion No. 413). Washington, DC: Author.

American Society for Reproductive Medicine (ASRM). (2006). *Patient's fact sheet: Ovulation detection.* Retrieved from www.reproductivefacts.org.

American Society for Reproductive Medicine (ASRM). (2008). *Patient's fact sheet: Diagnostic testing for male factor infertility.* Retrieved from www.reproductivefacts.org.

American Society for Reproductive Medicine (ASRM). (2014a). *Frequently asked questions about infertility.* Retrieved from www.reproductivefacts.org.

American Society for Reproductive Medicine (ASRM). (2014b). *Patient's fact sheet: What is intracytoplasmic sperm injection (ICSI).* Retrieved from www.reproductivefacts.org.

American Society for Reproductive Medicine (ASRM). (2015). *In vitro fertilization (IVF): What are the risks?* Retrieved from www.reproductivefacts.org.

Baker, V. L., Rone, H. M., & Adamson, G. D. (2008). Genetic evaluation of oocyte donors: Recipient couple preferences and outcome of testing. *Fertility and Sterility, 90*(6), 2091–2098.

Blackburn, S. T. (2013). *Maternal, fetal, and neonatal physiology: A clinical perspective* (4th ed.). St. Louis, MO: Saunders.

Centers for Disease Control and Prevention (CDC). (2013). *What is assisted reproductive technology?* Retrieved from www.cdc.gov.

Chandra, A., Copen, C. E., & Stephen, E. H. (2013). Infertility and impaired fecundity in the United States, 1982–2010: Data from the National Survey of Family Growth. *National health statistics reports; no 67.* Hyattsville, MD: National Center for Health Statistics.

Cunningham, F. G., Leveno, K. J., Bloom, S. L., et al. (2014). *Williams obstetrics* (24th ed.). New York: McGraw-Hill.

Gambone, J. C., & Rodi, I. A. (2015). Infertility and assisted reproductive technologies. In N. F. Hacker, J. C. Gambone, & C. J. Hobel (Eds.), *Hacker & Moore's essentials of obstetrics and gynecology* (6th ed.). Philadelphia, PA: Saunders.

Hall, J. E. (2016). *Guyton and Hall textbook of medical physiology* (13th ed.). Philadelphia, PA: Saunders.

Hershberger, P. F. E., & Schoenfeld, C. (2011). Unraveling preimplantation genetic diagnosis for high-risk couples: Implication for nurses at the front line of care. *Nursing for Women's Health, 15*(1), 36–45.

Jones, E. E. (2016a). The female reproductive system. In W. F. Boron & E. L. Boulpaep (Eds.), *Medical physiology* (3rd ed.). Philadelphia, PA: Saunders.

Jones, E. E. (2016b). The male reproductive system. In W. F. Boron & E. L. Boulpaep (Eds.), *Medical physiology* (3rd ed.). Philadelphia, PA: Saunders.

Lobo, R. A. (2012). Infertility. In R. A. Lobo, D. M. Gershenson, G. M. Lentz, & F. A. Valea (Eds.), *Comprehensive gynecology* (7th ed.). St. Louis, MO: Mosby.

Mahomed, K. (2011). Nonmalignant gynecology. In D. K. James, P. J. Steer, C. P. Weiner, & B. Gonik (Eds.), *High risk pregnancy: Management options* (4th ed.). Philadelphia, PA: Saunders.

Martinez, G. M., Daniels, K., & Chandra, A. (2012). *Fertility of men and women aged 15–44 years in the United States: National Survey of Family Growth, 2006–2010. National Health Statistics Reports, No. 51.* Hyattsville, MD: National Center for Health Statistics. Retrieved from www.cdc.gov.

Morgan, P. A., Merrell, J. A., Rentschler, D., & Chadderton, H. (2012). Triple whammy: Women's perceptions of midlife mothering. *MCN: American Journal of Maternal/Child Nursing, 37*(3), 156–162.

Pagana, K. D., & Pagana, T. J. (2015). *Diagnostic and laboratory test reference* (12th ed.). St. Louis, MO: Mosby.

Paterno, M. T. (2008). Families of two: Meeting the needs of couples experiencing male infertility. *Nursing for Women's Health, 12*(4), 300–306.

Women's Health

Mary Suzanne White

OBJECTIVES

After studying this chapter, you should be able to:

1. Explain examinations and screening procedures recommended to maintain the health of women.
2. Explain benefits of indicated immunization(s) to a woman.
3. Explain benign disorders of the breast and discuss diagnostic procedures used to rule out breast cancer.
4. Describe the incidence, risks, pathophysiology, management, and nursing considerations related to malignant breast tumors.
5. Discuss cardiovascular disease in women, including risk factors, signs and symptoms, and prevention measures.
6. Discuss common menstrual cycle disorders.
7. Explain premenstrual syndrome, management options, and nursing considerations.
8. Discuss medical termination of pregnancy in terms of procedures, possible complications, and follow-up care.
9. Describe the physical and psychological changes associated with menopause and options to alleviate uncomfortable changes.
10. Discuss measures to reduce severity of osteoporosis.
11. Describe the major disorders associated with pelvic relaxation in terms of cause, treatment, and nursing considerations.
12. Discuss the most common benign and malignant disorders of the reproductive tract in terms of signs and symptoms, management, and nursing considerations.
13. Describe care of the woman with an infectious disorder of the reproductive tract, including sexually transmitted diseases, pelvic inflammatory disease, and toxic shock syndrome.

PREVENTIVE HEALTH CARE

There is an increasing demand for women's health care providers as more is learned about health risks specific to women and their need for preventive care. Certified nurse-midwives (CNMs) and women's health nurse practitioners (WHNPs) often provide basic preventive health care to nonpregnant women. This chapter focuses on examinations and screening procedures recommended to maintain the health of women. It also will include information as it relates to immunizations, benign and malignant disorders of the breast, cardiovascular disease, menstrual cycle disorders, premenstrual syndrome (PMS), medical termination of pregnancy, menopause, osteoporosis, pelvic floor dysfunction, common benign and malignant disorders of the reproductive tract, and infectious disorders of the reproductive tract.

NATIONAL EMPHASIS ON WOMEN'S HEALTH

Two national programs have had a major impact on women's health. The Women's Health Initiative (WHI) of the National Institutes of Health (NIH) was a major 15-year research program to address the most common causes of death, disability, and poor quality of life in postmenopausal women: cardiovascular disease, cancer, and osteoporosis. *Healthy People 2020* continues to have a health promotion and disease prevention agenda coordinated by the U.S. Department of Health and Human Services. For more information about these programs, see www.nhlbi.nih.gov/whi.

Healthy People 2020 Goals

The *Healthy People 2020* home page may be found at www.healthypeople.gov/2020. Several ***Healthy People 2020* goals** relate to women's health, and many address the goals in the WHI, as follows:

- Increase the proportion of adults, 20 years and older, who are at a healthy weight from 30.8% (2005 to 2008) to 33.9%.
- Lower breast cancer deaths from 22.9 per 100,000 women in 2007 to no more than 20.6 per 100,000 women.
- Reduce deaths from cancer of the cervix from 2.4 per 100,000 women in 2007 to 2.2 per 100,000 women.
- Increase cervical cancer screening, according to the most recent 2008 guidelines, from 84.5% of women to 93%.

- Increase the proportion of adults who receive a colorectal screening, based on the most recent guidelines, from 52.1% in 2008 to 70.5%.
- Increase the proportion of cancer survivors who are living 5 years or longer after diagnosis from 66.2% in 2007 to 72.8%.
- Reduce hip fracture hospitalizations among women, 65 years and older, from 823.5 hospitalizations per 100,000 women to 741.2 per 100,000 women.
- Reduce the incidence of gonorrhea in women between the ages of 15 and 44 from 285 cases per 100,000 women in 2008 to 257 cases per 100,000.
- Reduce the prevalence of *Chlamydia trachomatis* infections among women 15 to 24 years old who attended a family planning clinic in the past 12 months from 7.4% to 6.7%.
- Reduce congenital syphilis from 10.1 per 100,000 live births in 2008 to no more than 9.1 per 100,000 live births.
- Reduce coronary heart disease deaths from 126 per 100,000 (2007) to 100.8 per 100,000.
- Reduce stroke deaths from 42.2 per 100,000 (2007) to 33.8 per 100,000.

HEALTH MAINTENANCE

Health maintenance refers to measures that can be taken for prevention or early detection of specific diseases. Unfortunately, many women do not take advantage of recommended health maintenance procedures and choose to seek care only once a problem exists. For others, the only health care they receive comes from a gynecologist or nurse practitioner, often with their annual checkup. Therefore it is important that those who provide health care for women are familiar with principles of screening and counseling in areas that are not traditionally associated with gynecology, such as assessing risk factors for colon cancer and heart disease.

Health History

The health history identifies risk factors for a variety of conditions and may be obtained from sources such as questionnaires, interviews, and records. The focus of a health history depends on the woman's age, but some topics should be discussed with all women. Box 27.1 provides a summary of information to obtain. These topics include dietary intake, physical activity, habits, and sexual practices. Discussions of drugs should include long-term use of prescription and over-the-counter (OTC) medications. Illicit drugs also should be discussed to provide the safest care for the woman. Questions about use of **complementary and/or alternative medicine (CAM)** should be included in the woman's history. A woman's health history often identifies actions she takes to promote her health.

Many people take herbal or other botanical preparations but do not mention them because they do not consider them drugs. The nurse should specifically ask about use of these preparations or any therapies the woman may use in addition

---

BOX 27.1 Health History

Personal History
Demographic data (name, age, marital status or whether living with a partner)
Reason for seeking medical care (chief complaint)
Current and past state of health, previous surgeries
Height, weight, vital signs
Allergies (drugs, food, environmental allergens)
Medications, usual and the reason for taking (over-the-counter, prescribed, illicit)
Use of complementary or alternative therapies, such as herbal or botanical preparations, acupressure, chiropractic treatment
Habits (smoking, use of alcohol, drugs)
Appetite, usual dietary intake
Exercise pattern (type, frequency, duration)
Patterns of elimination (current or chronic problems)
Sleep and rest patterns
Degree of stress and stress management techniques

Menstrual History
Age of menarche
Regularity, duration of menstrual cycle
Menstrual discomfort (time during cycles, intensity, relief measures)
Age at menopause, if applicable

Obstetric History
Gravida, para, length of gestation, weight of infant at birth
Labor experience, medical interventions, and method of delivery

Sexual History
Sexual activity (how many partners, age when first sexually active)
Method of contraception (satisfaction with method, adverse reactions, accuracy of use)
Previous sexually transmitted infection and treatment
Knowledge or practice of measures to protect self from sexually transmitted diseases, including human immunodeficiency virus (HIV)

Family History
Cardiovascular problems (anemia, hypertension, clotting disorders, stroke, heart attacks)
Cancer (breast, uterine, ovarian, bowel, lung, other)
Osteoporosis

Psychosocial History
Primary language, additional languages spoken or understood, ability to read
Marital status, employment, occupation, education (relevant to determine financial, social, and emotional support)
Evaluation for possible domestic violence

---

to medically prescribed interventions to obtain the most complete information for the medical history.

Family history identifies many risk factors that cannot be modified. History of diabetes mellitus, hyperlipidemia, heart disease, osteoporosis, and thyroid disease suggests the best choice of screening tests. A list of family members who had cancer, the type of cancer they had, and their ages when it was discovered provides important information about the woman's risk for cancer, particularly breast and colon cancer.

A family history of heart disease is especially important when the woman is postmenopausal because the level of estrogen, which provides some protection against coronary artery disease (CAD), decreases after menopause and obesity may increase. If family history, obesity, or other factors increase the woman's risk for heart disease, a baseline electrocardiogram, stress test, and analysis of cholesterol and lipid profiles may identify other risk factors.

A psychosocial assessment helps caregivers determine the best way to teach the woman health promotion behaviors. Inquiry can help identify her means of support and also possible risks to her well-being such as domestic (intimate partner) violence.

❓ KNOWLEDGE CHECK

1. Why is a family history an important part of a health history?
2. What are some important psychosocial assessments in a health history?
3. What questions should be asked when taking a sexual history?

Physical Assessment

A complete physical examination is essential to detect general health problems and to identify positive aspects of health. (Refer to physical assessment textbook for a full explanation of the process of physical examination.) Blood pressure, temperature, pulse, respirations, and weight are measured at each visit. Height is taken at the initial examination and yearly after that. Loss of height, abnormal curvature of the vertebral column (dorsal kyphosis or scoliosis), and a thickening waistline in the absence of weight gain are important observations in identifying **osteomalacia** (softening of bones) or **osteoporosis** (increased spaces [porosity] of bone).

The heart is auscultated to determine rate and rhythm and detect heart murmurs or irregularities. Auscultation of the lungs identifies abnormal sounds that may suggest the presence of fluid secondary to heart dysfunction or malignancy. The extremities are observed for varicosities or edema, and pedal pulses are palpated for strength and equality. Reduced sensation when palpating legs and feet may indicate circulation problems often associated with diabetes. The abdomen is palpated for tenderness, masses, or distention that may indicate the presence of benign or malignant tumors.

Additional assessments are necessary if the woman is in a high-risk group. For instance, if she has a family history of diabetes mellitus, tests such as a glucose tolerance test or hemoglobin A1C (Hgb A1C) may be indicated. If she has a history of multiple sexual partners or a sexual partner with multiple contacts, testing for sexually transmitted diseases (STDs), including human immunodeficiency virus (HIV) infection, is indicated.

Preventive Counseling

Physical examination provides an excellent opportunity to counsel women about preventive measures that often reduce their physical problems. Major preventable problems are overweight and obesity, inactivity, and smoking. Overweight and obesity are associated with numerous health problems such as diabetes, hypertension, stroke, and CAD, as well as some cancers of the breast and reproductive organs. Some of these obesity-related conditions are leading causes of preventable death. Non-Hispanic blacks have the highest age-adjusted rates of obesity (48.1%), followed by Hispanics (42.5%), non-Hispanic Whites (34.5%), and non-Hispanic Asians (11.7%). Obesity is higher among middle-aged adults of 40 to 59 years (40.2%) and older adults aged 60 and over (37.0%) than among younger adults aged 20 to 39 (32.3%) (Ogden, Carroll, Kit, & Flegal, 2014).

Counseling about self-care measures to improve health should be offered. Positive health behaviors, such as adequate physical activity or making the decision to stop smoking, should be reinforced. Use of latex condoms should be emphasized for high-risk women with multiple sexual partners or those whose partner has multiple sexual partners.

Counseling about diet may identify measures that improve multiple problems. For example, a weight reduction diet can include measures to improve calcium intake to slow osteoporosis, to lower cholesterol, and to reduce diabetes mellitus severity. Achieving adequate exercise can reduce diabetes effects, lower weight, reduce cholesterol levels, and slow osteoporosis. A woman often feels better physically and emotionally as she achieves her personal goals, and the nurse can provide consistent encouragement.

The history or physical examination may identify other areas for patient counseling. These include the dangers of malignant melanoma with repeated exposure to ultraviolet rays of the sun. In addition, counseling and referral for alcohol and other substance abuse may be needed for some women. Domestic violence may be discovered, requiring counseling for the woman to deal with this complex social problem.

Immunizations

Determining the woman's need for immunization is becoming more common at her annual well-woman checkup. Immunization needs will vary with the time of year, the patient's age, and history of infections. Fear of adverse effects from immunizations may become evident. Updated information about recommended immunizations is available from www.cdc.gov.

Influenza vaccine is often offered during the fall and winter. It is not unusual to hear people say they had the "flu shot" last year and "got the flu anyway," so teaching is important to encourage the vaccine. The composition of annual flu vaccines must be determined well before the infections start to emerge so they may be more effective in one year compared with another year. People often do not realize that their annual vaccines require about 2 weeks to become effective and that they will show signs of the infection if they have already acquired it at the time of their vaccination.

Hepatitis B vaccine may be offered if the woman has not had it. Rubella vaccine may be given if the woman has never had the infection or vaccine and is not pregnant. Pregnancy testing is done and rubella immunization is delayed until after birth if she is pregnant.

Adults should receive a dose of tetanus and diphtheria (Td) every 10 years. One dose of tetanus, diphtheria, and acellular pertussis vaccine (Tdap) should be given to adults, ages 19 through 64, as a substitute for one of their Td immunizations. Tdap is especially important for health care professionals and anyone having close contact with an infant younger than 12 months. Pregnant women should get a dose of Tdap during every pregnancy, to protect the newborn from pertussis (CDC, 2015b).

 DRUG GUIDE

Human Papillomavirus Quadrivalent Vaccine (Gardasil)

Classification
Vaccine against human papillomavirus (HPV), types 6, 11, 16, 18.

Indications
Prevention of infections caused by HPV types 16 and 18 that may cause cervical, vaginal, and vulvar cancer. Prevention of genital warts caused by HPV types 6 and 11.

Dosage and Route
Intramuscular (IM) injection: Prefilled syringe of 0.5 mL of vaccine suspension at the following schedule: first dose; 2 months after first dose; 6 months after first dose.

Contraindications
Hypersensitivity to any component, including yeast.

Adverse Reactions
Headache is the most common adverse reaction. Others are fever, nausea, dizziness, pain, edema, itching, and bruising of the injection site. Fainting has occurred.

Nursing Considerations
Teach the woman that HPV vaccine is not treatment for existing genital warts or cervical, vaginal, or vulvar cancers and that regular cervical cancer screening should continue as recommended by her care provider. Cervical, vaginal, or vulvar cancers are not always caused by the HPV viral strains in this vaccine. Observation for 15 minutes after vaccine administration is recommended to reduce risk for fall if fainting occurs.

The HPV vaccine, a series of three injections, is available and currently recommended for females and males from 11 to 12 years old, although the series may be started at age 9 to 26 years. Some strains of HPV are known to cause cervical cancer and genital warts, and the recent HPV vaccine is effective against these strains. The ideal time to immunize is before any sexual activity. As might be expected, parents must grapple with uncomfortable issues when making the decision about immunizing a preteen or adolescent girl or boy, an age younger than age of legal consent, against this STD. Cost of the three injections may be beyond the family's ability to pay if not covered by insurance or through Medicaid or other public funding. For more information about possible federal and manufacturer funding, see www.gardasil9.com or www.cdc.gov.

? KNOWLEDGE CHECK

4. What issues may have an impact on recommendations for HPV immunization?

BOX 27.2   Risk Factors for Coronary Artery Disease in Women

Cigarette smoking
Hypertension (including isolated systolic hypertension)
Serum lipids (dyslipidemia)
    Elevated total cholesterol (normal: ≤199 mg/dL; borderline: 200-239 mg/dL; elevated: ≥240 mg/dL)
    Low levels of high-density lipoprotein (HDL) cholesterol: <39 mg/dL (<40 mg/dL men; <50 mg/dL women)
    Cholesterol ratio: The ratio of cholesterol to HDL cholesterol is often used instead of total blood cholesterol. The goal is to keep the ratio lower than 5 (total cholesterol) to 1 (HDL cholesterol), with an optimum ratio of 3.5:1.
    Triglyceride levels: >150 mg/dL
Diabetes mellitus
Overweight and obesity
Sedentary lifestyle
Poor nutrition, especially a diet high in saturated fat and cholesterol but low in fiber and fruit
Age older than 60
Postmenopause status
Family history of coronary artery disease

Data from American Heart Association (2014). *What your cholesterol levels mean.* Retrieved from www.heart.org.

SCREENING AND SELF-EXAMINATIONS

The value of screening procedures is based on two assumptions: (1) prevention is better than cure, and (2) early diagnosis allows early treatment while the pathologic process is most curable.

Some screening procedures are recommended for all women of reproductive age, including some screening procedures for early detection of breast cancer as well as vulvar self-examination and screening for cervical cancer. Additional tests depend on the age, history, and risk assessment of the woman and might include the following:

- Testing for STDs, such as gonorrhea, chlamydia, syphilis, and HIV
- Testing for rubella immunity, which is particularly important in the childbearing years, although the overall incidence of the disease is very low in the United States
- Tuberculosis skin testing or chest x-ray examination
- Cholesterol and other lipid profile testing of women at risk for CAD (particularly important after menopause) (Box 27.2)
- Fasting glucose testing or other tests to identify development of diabetes, recommended every 3 years after age 45 or earlier if the woman has high-risk factors such as family history or being overweight
- Urinalysis to detect signs of urinary tract infection (UTI)

TABLE 27.1   Screening Procedures

Procedure	Purpose
Breast self-awareness	To assess breasts so that women become aware of their normal appearance and feel
Mammography with additional imaging, such as ultrasonography, as needed for ≥40 - 45 years (routine screening mammography) Diagnostic mammograms and other imaging may be started at a younger age for women having a higher risk for breast cancer or previous breast cancer or other disorders	To detect breast lumps before they become palpable, promoting long-term survival
Cholesterol test	To detect blood levels that raise risk for heart disease; usually combined with additional tests for high-quality screening (lipid profile), such as triglyceride level, high-density (HDL), and low-density (LDL) lipoprotein (see Box 27.2)
Vulvar self-examination	To detect signs of precancerous conditions or infection
Pelvic examination	To confirm that no disease exists or for early detection if disease does exist
Pap test	To detect abnormal cervical cytology as early as possible
Rectal examination	To check for hemorrhoids and lesions and to evaluate sphincter control
Fecal occult blood test (FOBT)	To detect blood in stool, an early sign of colon cancer
Urinalysis	To screen for diabetes and urinary tract infections

Additional Procedures May Be Based on Risk Factors

Procedure	Risk Factors
Bone density every 2 yr starting at 65 yr Begin bone density screening earlier than 65 yr for high-risk women	Family history, fracture history, estrogen deficiency, fall history, physically inactive, underweight, poor nutrition, tobacco or alcohol abuse, chronic steroid use, dementia, European or Asian ancestry
Sexually transmitted disease (STD) testing; human immunodeficiency virus (HIV) testing	Multiple sexual partners of the woman or her partner, history of STDs; seeking treatment for STDs, injection drug use, sexual partner who is HIV-positive or bisexual or injects drugs, recurrenor persistent episodes of infections such as candidiasis and herpes
Lipid profile	Diabetes, smoking, no estrogen use after menopause, family history of high cholesterol or coronary artery disease
Fasting glucose test	Overweight, history of gestational diabetes, family history of diabetes
Rubella antibodies	To determine immunity to rubella
Thyroid-stimulating hormone (TSH)	Signs or strong family history of thyroid disease
Blood tests to evaluate risk for reproductive cancers (see Box 27.9)	To determine the degree of higher risk influenced by genetic alterations, improving options for therapy
Transvaginal ultrasound examination	Family history of ovarian cancer
Sigmoidoscopy (every 5 yr) or colonoscopy (every 10 yr)	Family history of bowel cancer or older than 50 yr
Tuberculosis testing	To determine infection in a person at higher risk for tuberculosis

- Thyroid function tests, which may be indicated if the woman exhibits signs of thyroid dysfunction, such as heart palpitations and heat intolerance
- Serum testing for genes associated with specific cancers, such as the *BRCA1, BRCA2,* or *p53* genes associated with breast and some other cancers
- Serum testing for CA-125, a tumor marker that may be elevated with ovarian cancer
- Transvaginal ultrasonography, which may be recommended for women who are at increased risk for malignant disorders of the reproductive tract
- Fecal occult blood test yearly
- Bone density test every 2 years starting at age 65; an earlier start to bone density screening may be recommended for women at higher risk for osteoporosis

- A colonoscopy (every 10 years after age 50); a yearly colonoscopy may be recommended if the woman has a family history of colon cancer
  See Table 27.1 for a summary of recommended procedures.

Screening for Breast Cancer

Because of the lack of evidence that indicates a clear benefit of physical breast examinations done by either a health professional or self-examinations performed by women, the American Cancer Society (ACS) no longer recommends them. Still, all women should be familiar with how their breasts normally look and feel and report any changes to a health care provider right away (ACS, 2015b).

Most women have an average risk for breast cancer and should begin yearly mammograms at age 45. Women should

Female

Age: For a woman living in the United States, a lifetime risk of 1 in 8

Race: White women are more likely to develop breast cancer, but Black women are more likely to die because they tend to develop breast cancer at an age younger than 40 years and in a more aggressive form. Asian, Hispanic, and Native American women have a lower risk for developing and dying from breast cancer.

Early menarche (<12 years), late menopause (>55 years)

Nulliparity or first pregnancy after 30 years

Personal history of breast cancer

Genetic risk factors

  Family history in first-degree relatives (mother, sister, daughter)

  Family history of other cancer

  Mutations in the *BRCA1* and *BRCA2* genes

  Mutations in other genes: *CHEK-2* gene, *ATM* (ataxia-telangiectasia mutated) gene, *PTEN* gene

Previous irradiation of the chest area as a child or a young woman as treatment for another cancer (such as Hodgkin's disease or non-Hodgkin's lymphoma)

Previous abnormal breast biopsy results

  Atypical hyperplasia increases the risk four to five times.

  Fibrocystic changes without proliferative changes do not change breast cancer risk.

Long-term hormone replacement therapy with estrogen and progesterone

Excessive alcohol consumption

Overweight or obesity

Physical inactivity

Data from American Cancer Society. (2015). *Breast cancer facts and figures, 2015 to 2016.* See www.cancer.org.

be able to start the screening as early as age 40 if desired and agreed upon by the health care providers regarding when to begin screening. At age 55, women should have mammograms every other year, though women who want to keep having yearly mammograms should be able to do so. Regular mammograms should continue for as long as a woman is in good health. These guidelines are for women at average risk for breast cancer. Women at high risk—because of family history, a breast condition, or another reason—need to begin screening earlier and/or more often (Box 27.3).

Despite the known value of mammography, many women have never had a mammogram. Reasons for this include lack of a health care professional's recommendation, expense, fear that radiation exposure will cause cancer, fear of pain, and reluctance to hear "bad news." Nurses provide information and reassurance whenever possible and, in this way, help the woman overcome her objections to the use of this valuable screening tool. Mammography is relatively expensive, but part of its cost is usually covered by health insurance, Medicaid, or Medicare. Screening mammograms may be offered by community agencies at low cost. Acknowledge that brief discomfort occurs when the breast is compressed between two plates while the image is obtained. Scheduling the mammography

after a menstrual period, when the breasts are less tender, reduces discomfort. Knowing that mammography has minimal to nonexistent risks, because very-low-dose exposure to radiation is used, may help women overcome some of their fear.

Vulvar Self-Examination

Vulvar self-examination should be performed monthly by all women older than 18 and by those younger than 18 who are sexually active. Vulvar self-examination is visual inspection and palpation of the female external genitalia to detect signs of precancerous conditions or infections.

The woman should sit in a well-lighted area and use a hand mirror to see her external genitalia. She is taught to examine the vulva in a systematic manner, starting at the mons pubis and progressing to the clitoris, labia minora, labia majora, perineum, and anus. Palpation of the vulvar area should accompany visual inspection. She should report to her health care provider as soon as possible the presence of any new moles, warts, or growths of any kind; ulcers; sores; changes in skin color; or areas of inflammation or itching. Increasing rates of HPV are associated with increased incidence of vulvar intraepithelial neoplasia (VIN).

Pelvic Examination

The complete gynecologic assessment includes a pelvic examination. The woman should schedule the examination between menstrual periods and should not douche or have sexual intercourse for at least 48 hours before the examination. She also is advised not to use vaginal medications, sprays, or deodorants that might interfere with interpretation of specimens that are collected.

The procedure is carefully explained before the examination, and the woman empties her bladder. Although pelvic examinations are relatively painless, most women dislike them and welcome sensitive, considerate support. Women who have undergone female genital mutilation (Box 27.4) need extra consideration. A pediatric vaginal speculum may be needed for these or other women with a very small vaginal opening. Routine preventive pelvic examinations may be impossible for women who have only a tiny opening left for drainage of urine and menstrual blood.

The pelvic examination is done usually with the woman in the lithotomy position, with a pillow under her head. If she wishes, she may be placed in a semi-sitting position and offered a hand mirror so she can observe the external genitalia and the examination and learn more about her body. She is draped so only the parts being examined are exposed.

Women who cannot tolerate a lithotomy position, such as a frail elderly woman, may benefit from a side-lying pelvic examination. The pelvic examination also can be done with the woman in a semi-Fowler's position, with her knees bent and feet on the examination table, rather than using the stirrups and having her hips at the edge of the table. The paraplegic woman, with no control over her lower extremities, usually can be examined with her legs separated in a V shape without her knees being bent. Necessary equipment to

BOX 27.4 Female Genital Mutilation

Female genital mutilation (FGM), sometimes called *female circumcision* or *female genital cutting*, is the ritual disfigurement and the partial or total removal of a girl's external genitalia or other injury to her external genitalia for cultural, religious, or other nontherapeutic reasons.

Between 100 and 140 million girls and women are estimated to have undergone female genital mutilation, and another 3 million are at risk annually. About 200 million girls are estimated to have undergone FGM (World Health Organization [WHO], 2016).

The age at which the procedure is performed varies from a few days old to adult. Most are done between infancy and 15 years, an age at which the girl cannot give informed consent for a procedure with lifetime consequences for her health.

FGM may be done by a village practitioner using crude tools, such as knives, razor blades, broken glass, thorns, or scissors, and without anesthesia. Parents in more developed countries may obtain the procedure from a physician to ensure pain relief and sterility. However, the increasing trend for performance of FGM by health professionals is strongly discouraged.

Female genital mutilation is considered a part of the coming-of-age ceremonies in some societies, and a girl may not be considered marriageable unless she has undergone the procedure. Some societies think the practice enhances female chastity and increases male sexual pleasure. Other societies consider the external female genitalia to be unsightly and dirty. Therefore they are removed to promote hygiene and the woman's attractiveness.

FGM is illegal and subject to criminal prosecution in several countries, including the United States.

Four major types of female genital mutilation exist (WHO, 2016):

- Clitoridectomy: Partial or total removal of the clitoris and sometimes the prepuce that surrounds the clitoris
- Excision of part or all of the clitoris and the labia minora, with or without excision of the labia majora
- Infibulation: Narrowing of the vaginal opening with the creation of a covering seal
- Other nonmedical practices of pricking, piercing, incising, scraping, and cauterizing the genitals

Genital mutilation has no benefits and many associated problems. Health consequences may include the immediate results of severe pain, shock, hemorrhage, ulceration, urinary retention, and infection. Tetanus, bacterial sepsis, and human immunodeficiency virus infection are concerns if unsterile materials are used or if the vaginal opening is so small that anal intercourse is used as an alternative to vaginal intercourse. Infibulation may result in scar formation that causes dyspareunia, difficulty urinating, difficulty with menstruation, recurrent urinary tract infections, and infertility. Painful intercourse and reduced sexual sensitivity may have consequences on psychological health (WHO, 2016).

From World Health Organization (2016). *Female genital mutilation fact sheet updated February 2016.* Retrieved from http://www.who.int/en/.

be assembled before the examination begins includes gloves, speculum (several sizes, including pediatric, should be available), slides, cotton swabs, a fixative agent, and a Cytobrush and spatula for obtaining material for the cytology specimen, or Pap test (see later in this chapter). A stool specimen may be obtained by the examiner during the rectal examination, and a slide for this specimen should be available. Equipment for specimens to identify vaginal infections should be available.

External Organs

The pelvic examination is conducted systematically and gently. The external organs are inspected for the degree of development or atrophy of the labia, the distribution of hair, and the character of the hymen. Any cysts, tumors, or inflammation of Bartholin's glands is noted. The urinary meatus and Skene's glands are inspected for discharge. Perineal scarring resulting from childbirth is noted.

Speculum Examination

A bivalve speculum of the appropriate size is used to inspect the vagina and cervix. The speculum is warmed with tap water and gently inserted into the vagina. Plastic speculums do not get as cold as metal ones. Lubrication other than water or water-based lubricant on the cervix interferes with accurate cytology results. The size, shape, and color of the cervix are noted. Samples are taken for the Pap test. Routine testing for gonorrhea and chlamydia is common because of the increased incidence of these two STDs. Additional samples of any unusual discharge are obtained for microscopic examination or culture.

Bimanual Examination

The bimanual examination provides information about the uterus, fallopian tubes, and ovaries. The labia are separated, and the gloved, lubricated index finger and middle finger of one hand are inserted into the vaginal introitus.

The cervix is palpated for consistency, size, and tenderness to motion. The uterus is evaluated by placing the other hand on the abdomen with the fingers pressing gently just above the symphysis pubis so that the uterus can be felt between the examining fingers of both hands. The size, configuration, consistency, and mobility of the uterus are evaluated (Fig. 27.1).

Feeling the fallopian tubes is usually impossible, although the ovaries may be palpated between the fingers of both hands. Because ovaries atrophy after menopause, palpating the ovaries of a postmenopausal woman may not be possible.

Cervical Cytology or Papanicolaou Test
Purpose

It is known that, in virtually all cases, changes occur in cells of the cervix before cervical cancer develops. These changes have variously been called *cervical intraepithelial neoplasia, dysplasia, squamous intraepithelial lesions (SILs),* and *carcinoma in situ.* Cervical cytology, or the **Pap test,** often combined with a test for HPV, is the most useful procedure for detecting precancerous and cancerous cells that may be shed by the cervix. As Pap testing became routine in this country during the past half-century, preinvasive lesions (precancers) of the cervix became far more common than invasive cancer (ACOG, 2016).

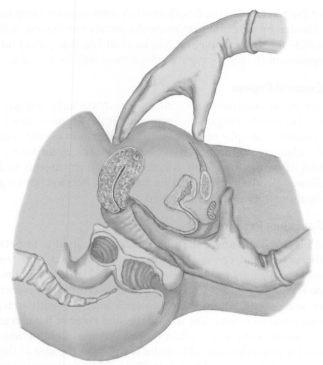

FIG. 27.1 Bimanual palpation provides information about the uterus, fallopian tubes, and ovaries

Current Guidelines

According to the most recent guidelines from the ACS, cervical cancer testing should start at age 21. Women under age 21 should not be tested. Women between the ages of 21 and 29 are recommended to be tested every 3 years. HPV testing should not be used in this age group unless it is needed after an abnormal Pap test result. Women between the ages of 30 and 65 should have a Pap test plus an HPV test (called "cotesting") done every 5 years. Women over age 65 who have had regular cervical cancer testing in the past 10 years with normal results should not be tested for cervical cancer. Once testing is stopped it should not be started again. Women with a history of a cervical precancer should continue to be tested for at least 20 years after that diagnosis, even if testing goes past age 65. A woman who has had her uterus and cervix removed for reasons not related to cervical cancer and who has no history of cervical cancer or precancer should not be tested. All women who have been vaccinated against HPV should still follow the screening recommendations for their age groups. Some women may need different screening schedules based on medical issues. Examples might include HIV infection, organ transplant, and exposure to diethylstilbestrol (DES) (ACS, 2016a).

Procedure

With the speculum blades open and the cervix in view, samples of the superficial layers of the cervix and endocervix are obtained. Samples are best obtained with a spatula and a Cytobrush or with a broom-type sampling device.

Specimens obtained with the broom-type device, such as those in the liquid-based ThinPrep or AutoCyte tests for cervical cancer, are stirred into the liquid that preserves the cells for analysis. The liquid-based tests use image processing to select the slides that need additional preparation by a technician for best analysis.

Classification of Cervical Cytology

A great deal of variation existed in how cervical cytology findings were reported until recently. The Bethesda system was devised to offer standard terminology and give a narrative, descriptive diagnosis. It consists of three elements: (1) a statement of specimen adequacy, (2) a general categorization (normal or abnormal), and (3) a descriptive diagnosis regarding abnormal cytologic findings. Additional interpretations not related to cancer include presence of infecting organisms (such as *Trichomonas vaginalis*); changes that may be associated with inflammation, radiation, intrauterine contraceptives, or atrophy of the cervical cells.

Categories for epithelial cell abnormalities include the following:
- Atypical squamous cells of undetermined significance (ASCUS)
- Squamous intraepithelial lesion, which is subdivided into (1) low-grade SIL (including cellular changes of HPV) and (2) high-grade SIL (previously categorized as carcinoma in situ). High-grade SIL is more likely to become cancerous without definitive treatment.
- Squamous cell cancer
  Glandular cell abnormalities are categorized as follows:
- Atypical glandular cells of unknown significance (AGCUS)
- Adenocarcinoma

The woman's follow-up depends on the nature of the abnormality and whether it is persistent. Pap tests that have persistent ASCUS findings after a 3- to 6-month interval are also usually evaluated by colposcopy. Suspicious lesions are examined with colposcopy and biopsy.

Rectal Examination

The anus is inspected for hemorrhoids, inflammation, and lesions. The examiner's lubricated index finger is gently inserted, and sphincter tone is noted. A slide may be prepared to test for the presence of occult blood in stool.

High-sensitivity fecal occult blood testing (FOBT) is a useful yearly screening measure for colorectal cancer beginning at age 50. Only high-sensitivity forms of guaiac-based tests should be used for this purpose. A newer test, the fecal immunochemical test (FIT), may be done, requiring only two samples and having a high-quality stool-based screening and a lower risk for false-positive results (ACS, 2015a).

Special instructions are necessary to prevent false test results when the woman is given materials for a FOBT. She should be instructed to do the following:
- Avoid aspirin and nonsteroidal antiinflammatory drugs (NSAIDs) such as ibuprofen or naproxen for at least 7 days before collecting the specimen
- Avoid red meat, raw fruits and vegetables, horseradish, and vitamin C for 72 hours before testing
- Collect a specimen from three consecutive stools
- Return slides as directed within 4 to 6 days after the specimens are collected

WOMEN'S HEALTH PROBLEMS

CARDIOVASCULAR DISEASE

Cardiovascular diseases (CVDs) include disorders of the heart and blood vessels, such as myocardial infarction (MI), congenital abnormalities, and stroke. Those discussed here primarily relate to diseases of the blood vessels, particularly CAD. The topic is extensive, and only an overview will be presented in this text. A medical-surgical text should be consulted for more extensive information about CVD and associated nursing care.

CVD is the leading global cause of death, accounting for more than 17.3 million deaths per year, a number that is expected to grow to more than 23.6 million by 2030. Annual direct and indirect costs of CVDs and stroke total more than $316.6 billion. CVD is the number one killer of women, taking more lives than all forms of cancer combined and accounted for killing 289,758 women in 2013. Nearly half of all African-American adults have some form of CVD, 48% of women and 46% of men. Sometimes CVDs may be silent and progress undiagnosed until a woman experiences signs or symptoms of a heart attack, heart failure, an arrhythmia, or stroke. Whereas some women have no symptoms, others often experience symptoms with CVD that are atypical of men: unusual fatigue, upper back pain, nausea and/or vomiting, loss of appetite, dizziness, palpitations, jaw pain, and neck pain. These may occur during rest, begin during physical activity, or be triggered by stress (American Heart Association [AHA], 2016; Centers for Disease Control and Prevention [CDC], 2016d).

Stroke can be ischemic if a cerebral artery is blocked or hemorrhagic if a cerebral artery ruptures. Almost 90% of strokes are ischemic. Women in the 45- to 74-year age group have a lower mortality rate than men in this age group. However, women older than 85 years have a higher stroke mortality rate than men in their age group. Metabolic syndrome (abdominal obesity, dyslipidemia, hypertension, and hyperglycemia) doubles the stroke risk in women but does not affect the stroke risk in men. Migraine, particularly with an aura, is associated with risk for stroke in women younger than 45 and has been associated with increased CVD risk. Symptoms of ischemic stroke appear to have few gender differences. Traditional symptoms include arm and/or leg weakness and speech disturbance. Less common symptoms include facial weakness, loss of sensation in arm and/or leg, headache, and nonorthostatic dizziness.

Nurses should maintain awareness to identify possible risk factors in the women they encounter in care so appropriate teaching and referrals can be made if needed. The nurse should also share knowledge about risk factors and symptoms of CVD with the health care provider so referrals to specialists or appropriate laboratory tests are done. An environment of collaborative and participatory care may help women adopt health-promoting behaviors and receive specialized care when needed and may help women achieve better health with weight control and exercise.

Risk Factors

Many factors increase risk for CVD, but common ones include hypertension, inadequate physical activity, overweight and obesity, and poor nutrition. These and other risk factors often contribute to development of other problems that further increase the risk for CVD, such as type 2 diabetes. Each risk factor may add to the risk for developing another of the problems listed here.

Risk factors may be fixed or may be factors that can or cannot be changed. Aging is a major risk factor, because the woman loses the protection that estrogen, secreted before menopause, exerts on the blood vessels. Estrogen's protective effect delays onset of CVD, making most women older at the onset of the disease than men. Other risk factors are listed in Box 27.2 and are similar to those for men. Several risk factors deserve additional discussion in this chapter.

The leading preventable cause of CAD and other diseases in women and men is smoking. Cigarette smoking adds to the burden of heart, blood vessel, and respiratory disorders; cancers; and many other diseases in women. Smoking is often more attractive to a woman if her family and friends smoke, she thinks smoking helps control her weight, or she thinks smoking reduces her anxiety.

Both systolic and diastolic blood pressure elevations are associated with CAD and other vascular disorders. Adequate control of hypertension reduces death and disability from MI, stroke, and other blood vessel disorders. The person may not consider hypertension a problem because no symptoms are present. Smoking, overweight, and diabetes further contribute to hypertension. Hypertension is more prevalent in African-Americans than in Whites.

Inadequate exercise contributes to many of the risk factors listed. Overweight and obesity are more likely when a person is sedentary, and these weight problems increase the likelihood that diabetes and hypertension will occur. **Dyslipidemia** (abnormal fat and cholesterol levels) is more likely in both women and men who do not get adequate exercise, adding further to the risk.

Prevention is the key to reducing death and illness from all CVDs among women. Although once thought to reduce a woman's risk for CVD, estrogen's benefits for this have not proved true when hormone replacement therapy (HRT) is chosen after natural estrogen levels decline at menopause.

Health Promotion Activities to Reduce the Risk for Coronary Artery Disease

Risk for CAD can be lowered with the following health promotion activities:

- Stop smoking
- Maintain a normal weight
- Eat right

- Limit alcohol to 1 drink per day if you are a woman
- Control high blood pressure
- Exercise
- Control diabetes

To learn more about CVD and its prevention, visit these websites: the American Heart Association, www.heart.org, and the Academy of Nutrition and Dietetics (formerly the American Dietetic Association), www.eatright.org.

Hypertension

People may be unaware of current definitions for the levels of blood pressure and do not seek the information because hypertension can be a disease that causes subtle damage over long periods. Current standards that define hypertension are lower than what many people expect (CDC, 2016b):

- Normal: Less than 120 mm Hg systolic; less than 80 mm Hg diastolic
- Prehypertension: 120 to 139 mm Hg systolic; 80 to 89 mm Hg diastolic
- Hypertension: 140 mm Hg or greater systolic; 90 mm Hg or greater diastolic

Lowering hypertension, including isolated systolic hypertension in older women, to levels less than 140 mm Hg systolic and less than 90 mm Hg diastolic reduces the risk for CAD and stroke. Even borderline, or prehypertension, can be dangerous. Medication should be considered if regular aerobic exercise, weight reduction, improved nutrition, and stress management do not lower the blood pressure adequately (DeMartinis, 2009). The Dietary Approaches to Stop Hypertension (DASH) diet plan from the National Heart, Lung, and Blood Institute (NHLBI) of the National Institutes of Health (NIH) is often recommended to maintain good blood pressure control and can be retrieved at www.nhlbi.nih.gov.

Diet and Glucose Control

Women with diabetes have a relatively greater risk for CAD than men, so maintaining weight and glucose levels within normal limits is especially important. Diet is the primary means to control the lipid profile. Diet recommendations should be individualized, but general guidelines are that fat intake should be a maximum of 30% of daily calories and that no more than 10% of daily calories should come from saturated fat (found in foods such as meat, butter, cream, and cheese). Cholesterol intake maintained lower than 200 mg/day is ideal. Increased evidence shows that fish, especially fatty fish, confers cardiovascular benefits, and at least two servings per week is recommended. Eating a diet high in vegetables, fruits, and low-fat dairy products and limiting salt intake to under 6 g/day and alcohol to a maximum of one drink per day have shown to be beneficial at reducing blood pressure in women (AHA, 2014; Keresztes & Wcisel, 2009).

Increased Activity

Aerobic exercise helps control weight, blood pressure, lipid profile, and glucose level. It reduces body fat while increasing muscle mass and improving muscle tone, making it easier to maintain a healthy body weight or reduce weight if overweight or obese. Additionally, it reduces stress and depression. As described by the Physical Activity Guidelines for Americans, adults should engage in at least 150 minutes of moderate-intensity activity each week (U.S. Department of Health and Human Services [DHHS], 2014).

Aspirin

Low-dose aspirin therapy (81 mg, or "baby aspirin") is well accepted as an agent for the secondary prevention of cardiovascular events, and current guidelines also define a role for aspirin in primary prevention. Low-dose aspirin therapy each day has been shown to be beneficial to inhibit platelet aggregation, which can increase clot formation and lead to CAD. Acute chest pain should be treated with a single adult-dose tablet (325 mg, equivalent to four baby aspirin tablets) as soon as MI is suspected to reduce clot formation and increase the chances of full recovery. Aspirin use in males is primarily intended for the prevention of CAD, whereas in females, stroke prevention is the focus area. For those unable to tolerate aspirin or who have recent gastrointestinal (GI) bleeding, prescription drugs such as clopidogrel (Plavix) may be prescribed. Individual needs are based on age, risk factors, and history (Ittaman, VanWormer, & Rezkalla, 2014.)

> ### ❓ KNOWLEDGE CHECK
> 8. What are the symptoms of CAD, such as an MI, in a woman?
> 9. List appropriate measures to reduce the risk for CAD.

DISORDERS OF THE BREAST

Benign Disorders of the Breast

Four relatively common benign disorders of the breast tend to occur at different ages.

Fibrocystic Breast Changes

Fibrocystic breast changes are common breast changes during the reproductive years before **menopause**, or permanent cessation of menstruation. Fibrosis, or thickening of the normal breast tissue, occurs in the early stages. Cysts may form in the latter stages and are felt as multiple, smooth, well-delineated nodules that have a tender, movable character. The lumpy, rubbery, or ropelike nodules often vary in size, from less than 1 cm to several centimeters. Fibrocystic changes are not cancerous, although atypical hyperplasia of the terminal breast ducts or lobules is associated with a greater risk for breast cancer. Tissue specimens obtained by fine needle aspiration (FNA) or from an open surgical biopsy are examined to identify the tissue type and any malignant changes (Katz & Dotters, 2012).

The most common symptom of fibrocystic breast changes is pain and tenderness. The pain is often bilateral and most noticeable during the premenstrual phase of the normal cycle. Women with large breasts may have pain associated with stretching of the breast ligaments. Premenstrual pain is believed to be the result of an imbalanced estrogen-to-progesterone ratio. Women with fibrocystic breast changes improve dramatically during pregnancy and lactation because the large amounts of progesterone present during pregnancy block the excess amounts of estrogens present when the woman is not pregnant.

The initial therapy varies with the age of the woman and her risk for breast cancer. Aspiration of cysts may relieve pain, with follow-up needed only if the cyst recurs or fluid aspirated is suspicious. The bilateral nature of the changes and pain suggests that the condition is benign, but definitive studies such as **mammogram** (study of breast tissue with low-dose radiography) and ultrasound imaging, FNA of the cysts, or surgical biopsy may be needed to identify malignancy. Fibrocystic breast changes may fall into the following three categories:

- Nonproliferative lesions
- Hyperplasia without atypical cells
- Atypical hyperplasia

Hyperplastic lesions with atypical cellular changes have an increased risk to become malignant, but most women with fibrocystic breast changes do not have a greater risk for breast cancer.

Specific symptom relief for fibrocystic disease has not proved beneficial, but some methods may be worth trying. Wearing a support bra is a simple way to reduce pain from large breasts that stretch ligaments. Avoiding caffeine and other stimulants (coffee, tea, chocolate, and some soft drinks) reduces levels of methylxanthines, which may increase discomfort during the last half of the menstrual cycle. Oral contraceptives taken during the secretory phase (second half) of the menstrual cycle have been successful, but pain returns if the contraceptives are discontinued. Danazol (Danocrine), an androgenic medication that suppresses estrogen production, may be given for severe pain but for no longer than 4 to 6 months. Other possible drugs include bromocriptine (a prolactin inhibitor) and tamoxifen (an estrogen inhibitor that is usually given in breast cancer treatment).

Fibroadenoma

Fibroadenomas are common benign tumors of the breast, and although they may occur at any age, they are most common during the teenage years and the 20s. Fibroadenomas are composed of both fibrous and glandular tissue. They are firm, freely mobile nodules that may or may not be tender when palpated. Fibroadenomas do not change during the menstrual cycle. They are generally located in the upper, outer quadrant of the breast, and more than one is often present.

Treatment may involve careful observation for a few months to determine whether the mass is stable. FNA or core biopsy of the tumor is done if the mass continues to enlarge. The mass may be excised and the specimen analyzed to rule out malignancy if results of other diagnostic tests are not conclusive (Katz & Dotters, 2012).

Ductal Ectasia

Ductal ectasia usually occurs as a woman approaches menopause. It is characterized by dilation of the collecting ducts, which become distended and filled with cellular debris. This initiates an inflammatory process resulting in the following:

- A mass near the areola that feels firm and irregular
- Enlarged axillary nodes
- Nipple retraction and discharge

These signs and symptoms are similar to those of breast cancer, and accurate diagnosis through biopsy is vital. Although ductal ectasia is benign, the ducts may be excised to prevent further discharge or remove an abscess that results from infection (Katz & Dotters, 2012).

Intraductal Papilloma

Intraductal papilloma develops most often just before or during menopause. It occurs when papillomas (small elevations or protuberances) develop in the epithelium of the ducts of the breasts, often under the areola. As the papilloma grows, it causes trauma and erosion within the ducts that result in serous or bloody discharge from the nipple. Ultrasonography and diagnostic mammography aid in the diagnosis of the intraductal papilloma. Treatment consists of excision of the mass and ductal area, plus analysis of nipple discharge to rule out a malignant tumor. Long-term follow-up is essential to identify any malignancy early (Katz & Dotters, 2012).

Nursing Considerations

The nurse should acknowledge the anxiety that all women feel when a breast disorder is discovered. Furthermore, the apprehension continues for most women while they await a final diagnosis. Some women may find it helpful to learn that most breast disorders are benign. Some benign disorders do increase the risk for later occurrence of cancer, however. For others, the most helpful intervention is to encourage them to express their concerns.

Diagnostic Procedures

Differentiating between benign and malignant breast disorders may require diagnostic procedures. Ultrasound examination can be used to discriminate fluid-filled cysts from solid tissue, which is more likely to be malignant. Fine-needle aspiration (FNA) biopsy can be done to remove fluid or small tissue fragments for analysis of the cells. Core biopsy uses a larger needle to obtain a cylinder of tissue from an area of questionable breast tissue. Open, or surgical, biopsy is performed to remove all or part of the lump of breast tissue if the following other conditions exist:

- Suspicious mass that persists through a menstrual cycle
- Bloody fluid aspirated from a cyst
- Failure of the mass to disappear completely after fluid aspiration
- Recurrence of the cyst after one or two aspirations
- Solid dominant mass not diagnosed as fibroadenoma
- Serous or serosanguineous nipple discharge
- Nipple ulceration or persistent crusting
- Skin edema and erythema suspicious for inflammatory breast carcinoma (IBC)

- Suspicious mammography or ultrasound findings
- Known or possible genetic abnormality that increases a woman's risk for breast cancer

---

? KNOWLEDGE CHECK

10. How is fibrocystic breast disease treated?
11. What diagnostic procedures are used to determine whether a breast disorder is benign or malignant?

Malignant Tumors of the Breast
Incidence

The lifetime risk for a woman to develop breast cancer in the United States is 1 in 8. In 2016 an estimated 246,660 new cases of invasive breast cancer are expected to be diagnosed in women in the United States, along with 61,000 new cases of noninvasive (in situ) breast cancer. Deaths in women are expected to be approximately 40,500. Breast cancer in men is rare, with an expected 2600 new cases in men and 440 expected to result in death in 2016. The lifetime risk in men is estimated to be 1 in 1000 (ACS, 2015c).

Breast cancer is a major type of cancer among women of all races. Breast cancer incidence rates are highest in non-Hispanic White women, followed by African-American women, and are lowest among Asian/Pacific Islander women. In contrast, breast cancer death rates are highest for African-American women, followed by non-Hispanic, White women. Breast cancer death rates are lowest for Asian/Pacific Islander women. Breast cancer incidence and death rates also vary by state (ACS, 2015c; Katz & Dotters, 2012).

Risk Factors

Although the actual cause of breast cancer remains unknown, several factors are known to increase the risk for the development of breast and ovarian cancer or other diseases (see Box 27.3). Mutations in two genes (*BRCA1* and *BRCA2*) thought to be responsible for most cases of familial breast and ovarian cancer, including breast cancer in men, continue to be studied. Mutation of the *CHEK-2* gene has shown higher risk for development of breast cancer in both women and men. Mutation of the *p53* tumor suppressor gene has been associated with breast and other cancers. Study of genetic links to many types of cancers and nonmalignant diseases is ongoing. Because research has linked these and other genes to an increased risk for breast or other cancers, testing is offered to the woman having a higher risk or who has developed cancer at a younger age than expected (Katz & Dotters, 2012; NCI & NIH, 2016).

Knowing risk factors is important to guide breast cancer screening and treatment processes so a cancer is diagnosed at the earliest stage possible. It is also important for the nurse to convey to women that many breast cancers develop in women with no known risk factors, whereas other women with one or more risk factors do not develop breast cancer.

Pathophysiology

Approximately 65% to 80% of breast cancers are infiltrating ductal carcinoma, which originates in the epithelial lining of the mammary ducts. The cancer becomes invasive when it is no longer confined to the duct and spreads to surrounding breast tissue. Another 10% to 14% of invasive breast cancers are infiltrating lobular cancer that originates in the milk-secreting pockets of breast tissue. Most breast cancers grow in irregular patterns and invade the lymphatic channels, eventually causing lymphatic edema and the dimpling of the skin that resembles an orange peel (**peau d'orange**). Several types of breast tumors may be present at the same time.

Inflammatory breast carcinoma (IBC) has cutaneous findings with invasive involvement in the dermis. IBC is rare, occurring in 1% to 2% of U.S. women and more likely to occur in younger or African-American women. IBC is aggressive and may manifest as a pink or red skin rash rather than a distinct lump that might show on imaging. Tenderness, itching, or breast edema may be present. These characteristics are typical of infection, so antibiotics are often prescribed. A woman should promptly contact her health professional for follow-up testing if antibiotics do not quickly clear the infection; then the true cause for the woman's signs and symptoms can be determined and cancer treatment can be started, if needed.

Cancer cells are carried by the lymph channels to the lymph nodes, and 40% to 50% of patients have involvement of axillary lymph nodes at the time of diagnosis. By the time a patient consults a physician, breast cancer already may be a systemic disease rather than being confined to the local tissue. Metastasis occurs when the malignant cells are spread by both blood and lymph systems to distant organs. Distant metastases include the lungs, liver, bones, and brain.

Staging

Confirmation of malignancy is the first step in evaluating the woman with cancer, and staging is necessary to understand the severity of the cancer and plan the best therapy. Staging is based on the tumor, node, and metastasis (TNM) system used to describe the cancer's anatomic extent. Stages of breast cancer progress from stage 1, indicating a small tumor without lymphatic involvement in the local area or metastases, to stage 4, which indicates spread to lymph nodes and metastases to distant organs. The stages are used to guide treatment and help provide a prognosis. The type of cancer cell, the presence of hormone receptors, and the proliferative rate of the breast cancer cells are also important factors in the rate of recurrence and determination of the most appropriate treatment.

Management

Many new treatments have emerged. A combination of surgical excision of the tumor and locally involved lymph nodes and **adjuvant therapy** (added treatment to enhance action) is recommended. The combination of therapies is individualized for each patient. New techniques, medications, and management emerge frequently, and the nurse who cares for women with cancer should stay informed about changes in therapy.

Surgical Treatment. The surgical procedure depends on the type, stage, and location of the disease. The most common surgeries are the following (Katz & Dotters, 2012):

- Breast conservation treatment, which involves wide local excision (lumpectomy) of the tumor to microscopically clean margins for tumors that are small relative to the breast size. The excision can be performed without major cosmetic deformity. Varying numbers of axillary lymph nodes are usually removed to identify the stage of the woman's breast cancer.
- *Quadrantectomy* is a more extensive surgery for a breast tumor, removing a quadrant of tissue. Removal of the tumor involves resection of the skin and other tissue in the area to reach a microscopically clear margin of healthy tissue. Analysis of lymph nodes removed during the quadrantectomy allows staging of the cancer.
- Simple mastectomy, which is removal of the entire breast. Axillary dissection is omitted, although some lymph nodes may be removed for staging purposes. It may be recommended for selected cases in which prophylactic removal of the breast is considered for a woman at high risk for development of breast cancer. Simple mastectomy in the absence of cancer does not eradicate the risk for later breast cancer, however, because a small amount of breast tissue remains.
- Modified radical mastectomy, which involves removal of breast tissue, axillary nodes, and some chest muscles; however, the pectoralis major muscle is preserved. This surgical procedure may be recommended when a single large primary lesion or multiple lesions exist in a relatively small breast because cosmetic results may be less than satisfactory with the other methods described. Other factors include whether the woman can undergo radiation therapy. Radiation therapy after surgery may not be possible if she is pregnant, has had prior breast or chest radiation, or has an autoimmune disease such as systemic lupus erythematosus.

Sentinel lymph node (SLN) biopsy is a technique to remove a few key lymph nodes to evaluate cancer spread rather than removing most of the nodes in the area (**axillary dissection**). A radioisotope suspension or a special dye is injected near the tumor site, where it is transported by the lymphatics toward the axillary nodes and trapped by the first one or two lymph nodes, or the "sentinel" nodes. The nodes identified by one or both of these techniques are excised for evaluation. If cancer has not spread to a sentinel node, the surgeon does not need to remove a large number of lymph nodes for staging of the cancer. Reducing the number of lymph nodes removed helps avoid some of the problems caused by lymphedema.

Adjuvant Therapy. Adjuvant therapy is supportive or additional therapy that is usually recommended after the surgical procedure. Radiation, chemotherapy, hormone therapy, and immunotherapy are adjuvant therapies that are often recommended. The decision about adjuvant therapy is based on the woman's age, the stage of the disease, the woman's preference, and the hormone receptor status of the lesion. Radiation and chemotherapy are known to improve the chance of long-term survival, and one or both are usually recommended after surgical excision of the tumor. Research continues to determine the best uses for these adjuvant therapies when treating breast cancer.

Radiation Therapy. Radiation uses high-energy rays to destroy cancer cells that remain in the breast, the chest wall, and the underarm area after surgery. The lymph nodes above the clavicle and the internal mammary lymph nodes are also irradiated. Radiation may be used to reduce the size of a large tumor before surgery. A radiation oncologist directs use of radiation in cancer therapy. The skin in the treated area may have a reaction similar to sunburn. Lymphedema is more likely to occur if the axillary lymph nodes are treated. A newer technology to limit the adverse effects of radiation on normal tissues while giving a maximum dose of radiation to the tumor site is intensity-modulated radiation therapy.

Chemotherapy. Chemotherapy drugs are designed to kill the proliferating cancer cells. The specific combination of drugs and the number of treatment cycles are individualized for factors such as type of cancer cells, the woman's age, the hormone receptor status of malignant cells, whether she is postmenopausal, and other important factors such as medications she needs for nonmalignant disorders. Chemotherapy may both precede and follow tumor removal. Depending on the specific drugs, chemotherapeutics often kill normal cells, especially rapidly dividing cells such as those in the mucosa, the blood cells, and the platelets. For this reason, the woman often has sore, bleeding gums or other bleeding tendencies and may be more susceptible to infection during treatment. Loss of head and body hair or menstrual irregularities are common side effects during treatment. Anemia, with resulting fatigue, is common because erythrocyte production is impaired. Antiemetic drugs control nausea for most women.

Hormone Therapy. Medications to reduce production of estrogen are prescribed because many breast tumors are estrogen and/or progesterone receptor–positive, meaning that their growth is stimulated by estrogen. Estrogen receptor–positive tumors may occur in both premenopausal and postmenopausal women. Risks and benefits of proposed estrogen-blocking medications are discussed with the oncologist, particularly in premenopausal women because their estrogen and progesterone levels are coordinated with their menstrual cycles.

Tamoxifen is one of the oldest estrogen-blocking drugs given for breast cancer to prevent recurrence. However, tumors in some women become resistant to tamoxifen, and the cells actually use the drug to stimulate growth. Laboratory values for calcium, cholesterol, and triglycerides may be elevated with tamoxifen.

Anastrozole (Arimidex), exemestane (Aromasin), and letrozole (Femara) are aromatase inhibitors that hinder production of estrogen because they block conversion of androgens to estrogen in postmenopausal women. Aromatase inhibitors are being studied as alternatives to tamoxifen because they inhibit estrogen in a different way.

Raloxifene (Evista) is an estrogen modifier used to reduce osteoporosis by binding to estrogen receptors; therefore this drug also blocks estrogen effects on the breast. Raloxifene lowers levels of low-density lipoproteins and cholesterol.

Immunotherapy. Trastuzumab (Herceptin) is a biologically based therapy that targets cell pathways that promote cancer growth. Some tumors produce excessive amounts of the HER-2 protein, promoting tumor cell growth. Trastuzumab blocks the effect of this protein to inhibit growth of the cancer cells. Research is ongoing into other immunotherapy for breast and other cancers.

Breast Reconstruction

Timing. Breast reconstruction is often an option in breast cancer treatment, and the timing of reconstruction should be discussed with the woman before surgical treatment. Immediate reconstruction has a psychological appeal, but expected therapy after surgery may have aspects that make later reconstruction the best option. The prospect of having life-threatening breast cancer and simultaneously facing the loss of a breast may be overwhelming for many women. Conversely, delayed reconstruction may give a woman time to learn about the procedure, to heal from the mastectomy, and to consider her values and desires for added surgery.

Methods. Several methods of breast reconstruction are available. The tissue expansion method uses an empty silicone prosthesis fitted with a valve that can be accessed by percutaneous needle puncture. The bag is filled with saline in small increments to slowly expand the tissue. When the desired volume is attained, the incision is reopened, the device is removed, and the expander is exchanged for the appropriate implant. In some models, only the valve must be removed and the expander serves as the permanent implant (ACS, 2016b; Craft, 2009).

Tissue flap procedures move **autogenous** tissue from the back, abdomen, or buttocks to create a breast mound. Although these procedures do not always involve implants of a foreign substance as the tissue expansion method does, they involve at least two incisions: one at the breast and one at the site of the woman's donor tissue. Not all women are suitable for muscle flap grafts, particularly those with diabetes or connective tissue disorders and those who smoke, because these procedures involve altering the blood supply to the transplanted tissue, with the possibility of poor wound healing for these women. Thin women may not have sufficient tissue for transplant to the breast (ACS, 2016b; Craft, 2009).

Psychosocial Consequences of Breast Cancer

The time from discovery to treatment of breast cancer is the most stressful time for many women. Factors that contribute to presurgical distress include a sense of uncertainty, incomplete information, the need to make difficult treatment decisions, and scheduling problems. Surgery may be preceded by chemotherapy or adjuvant therapy, or these therapies also may follow surgery. Because of the many complexities to be considered for treatment to be most effective, consultations with several specialists, including a surgeon, a radiation oncologist, a plastic surgeon, and a medical oncologist, are needed. Scheduling difficulties arise when women must travel significant distances for treatment. The many appointments with unfamiliar specialists and studies to determine best treatment often result in frustration and confusion for a woman and her family.

Concerns frequently expressed during treatment for breast cancer include fear of death, uncertainty about the quality of life, changes in body image, the effect on sexuality, and side effects of recommended therapy. For most women the knowledge that they will lose their hair as a result of chemotherapy creates one of the most difficult situations in therapy, adding yet another assault on their body image.

Breast cancer has psychological consequences not only for women but also for their significant others. Women who are diagnosed in their 30s may have young children who cannot understand why their parents are so worried. Difficulties reported include sleep disturbances, eating disorders, and problems with work responsibilities. The marital relationship may be strained, primarily in the areas of sexual relations and communication about matters related to the illness. Women and their partners sometimes differ in regard to how much they want to discuss the illness. Some women have a great need to discuss their diagnosis, treatment, and fears of recurrence. Other women and many men view discussion of such fears as negative thinking that delays adjustment.

Nursing Considerations

The woman who is diagnosed with breast cancer depends on the nurse for emotional support and accurate information. The woman needs time to express her feelings, and the nurse should convey a sense of empathetic understanding by quiet presence, touch, and close attention to the woman's concerns. Many women feel a sense of loss of control and that their lives have been taken over by cancer and the recommended treatments. Some women are concerned about family relationships and how their sexual partner or children will respond. Each woman should be encouraged to express her fears and worries. In addition to providing time and demonstrating genuine interest in the woman's concerns, the nurse should use communication techniques such as clarifying, paraphrasing, and reflecting feelings, so the woman can participate in decisions about her care.

Most women with a clear understanding of procedures and care experience a reduction in anxiety. Preoperative teaching should include significant others to increase their ability to support the woman. Teaching should include the length of the hospital stay and what will happen during that time. The nurse should describe the dressings, drainage tubes, and appearance of incisions for the breast procedure or procedures being planned (lumpectomy, mastectomy, reconstruction). Specific exercises such as arm lifts and pulley exercises may be necessary to promote flexibility in surgical areas.

Lymphedema, caused by blocked drainage of the lymphatic system in the arm on the side of the mastectomy, is possible if most axillary lymph nodes must be removed. Lymphedema may not occur for many years and is not anticipated for women who do not require an extensive lymphatic tissue removal in the axilla. Compression arm sleeves, similar to thromboembolism deterrent (TED) hose, are an available treatment to control lymphedema if needed.

Discharge teaching focuses on self-care and the need for continued care and treatment. Some areas of concern are how to reduce the risk for wound infection, care of the arm on the affected side, side effects of postoperative and adjuvant medications, and signs and symptoms that should be reported to the physician. If the woman will be discharged with the drains in place, she should be taught how to empty them. Most women also benefit from information about groups such as Reach to Recovery through the American Cancer Society (www.cancer.org) that provide support, information, and guidance after mastectomy. Support groups associated with the hospital and oncology center may offer additional support. The Internet may be a resource for community and online support groups. Printed information about local support groups is usually provided at discharge.

 KNOWLEDGE CHECK

12. Why is staging for breast cancer important?
13. What is meant by *adjuvant therapy,* and why is it used?
14. When should breast reconstruction take place and by what methods?
15. What should preoperative teaching include?
16. What should discharge planning emphasize?

MENSTRUAL CYCLE DISORDERS

The four most common menstrual cycle disorders are absence of menses (**amenorrhea**), abnormal uterine bleeding, pain associated with the menstrual cycle, and cyclic mood changes, including premenstrual syndrome (PMS). Although most of the disorders are benign, all require comprehensive gynecologic assessment. Nurses should be knowledgeable about underlying processes, diagnostic procedures, and expected treatment to fulfill the basic core of nursing activities, which include patient advocacy, education, and supportive counseling.

Amenorrhea

Amenorrhea can indicate either normal physiologic processes or pathologic issues in the reproductive system. Amenorrhea before **menarche** (onset of menstruation), during pregnancy, during the puerperium and lactation, and after menopause is normal. Amenorrhea at other times is abnormal, and it is called either *primary* or *secondary amenorrhea,* depending on when it occurs.

Primary Amenorrhea

Absence of menses may create a great deal of concern for the young woman and her family. Amenorrhea is a symptom, not a diagnosis, and they may worry that it indicates a serious disease. Menstruation is a unique function of women, and absence of menstruation may provoke concerns about femininity and the ability to have children. Concern

increases if a cause cannot be found or medical treatment is not successful.

Menstrual periods should begin within 2 years of breast development, between the ages of about 9 and 15 years. Lack of breast development or other secondary sexual development or a shortened growth spurt in addition to the absence of menstruation provides additional diagnostic clues. Primary amenorrhea may be suspected if the girl is more than 1 year older than the ages at which her mother and sisters had menarche. Although amenorrhea may result from a number of different conditions, a systematic evaluation including a detailed history, physical examination, and laboratory assessment of selected serum hormone levels can usually identify the underlying cause. Pregnancy should be excluded in all cases (Cromer, 2011; Klein & Poth, 2013; Lobo, 2012d).

Ovarian failure may occur in girls who have Turner's syndrome, in which only one of the normal two X chromosomes is present. They have a total of 45 chromosomes, with a single X chromosome. If secondary sex characteristics are present, incomplete development of internal reproductive organs may be the cause of amenorrhea. Other causes may include hormonal imbalances, systemic disease such as cancer with its associated therapy, and abnormalities of the hypothalamic-pituitary axis that result in hormone imbalance.

Primary amenorrhea, which by definition is failure to reach menarche, is often the result of chromosomal irregularities leading to primary ovarian insufficiency or anatomic abnormalities. A common systemic cause of primary amenorrhea is low body weight for height. This may occur in competitive athletes and dancers but also occurs in girls with eating disorders, such as anorexia nervosa, who have a very low body weight. If a girl began sexual development and then restricted calories (or began an intense exercise program), her sexual development may be arrested at the point of the calorie restriction. Other systemic causes of primary amenorrhea include chronic stress, hypothyroidism, abnormal steroid secretion, central nervous system diseases, and drug use (therapeutic or illicit). Obesity is often associated with insulin resistance and chronic anovulation related to high androgen levels (Cromer, 2011; Lobo, 2012d).

Abnormalities in the uterus, vagina, or hymen can obstruct the outflow of the menstrual flow. Congenital enzyme abnormalities may disable different aspects of the reproductive cycle.

Medical management depends on the cause identified in a diagnostic workup. Counseling for eating disorders, such as anorexia nervosa, and reducing excessive exercise to allow adequate weight gain may prove helpful. Hormone therapy may establish normal menses if the cause is hormone imbalance. However, some conditions cannot be successfully treated. For example, if the cause is reproductive tract or congenital anomalies, normal menses and fertility may not be possible, and psychological support becomes the most important therapy.

Secondary Amenorrhea

Secondary amenorrhea is the cessation of menstruation for 6 months or more in a woman who has established a pattern of menstruation, or absence for the duration of three normal cycles. In addition to pregnancy, there may be a variety of causes, including systemic diseases such as diabetes mellitus, tuberculosis, hypothyroidism, or central nervous system lesions. Polycystic ovary syndrome (PCOS), hormonal imbalances, strenuous aerobic exercise, poor nutrition, use of hormonal contraceptives, and ovarian tumors also may be causes. Most cases of secondary amenorrhea can be attributed to polycystic ovary syndrome (PCOS), hypothalamic amenorrhea, hyperprolactinemia, or primary ovarian insufficiency. Events such as divorce, death of a close friend or family member, moving, or a job change often result in stressors that occur with secondary amenorrhea (Klein & Poth, 2013; Lobo, 2012a, d).

Assessment includes a thorough medical and obstetric history and questions about eating habits, history of dieting, and current exercise pattern. Women are also questioned about their use of drugs, such as oral contraceptives, phenothiazines, and antihypertensives, which can cause secondary amenorrhea.

Medical treatment aims at identifying and correcting the underlying cause after ruling out pregnancy and determining whether the woman wants children. Pregnancy testing is done for a sexually active woman, and medications that are potentially teratogenic should be withheld until pregnancy is ruled out. Other treatment may include testing levels of hormones related to the menstrual cycle, therapy to improve timing of the cycle, treatment of anovulation, and identification of other abnormalities that may be related to the disorder. Excess androgen levels may cause PCOS, characterized by acne and excess weight and body hair, as well as the anovulation that results in amenorrhea.

Nursing Considerations

Emotional support is essential if medical diagnostics are needed to evaluate the cause of absent menses, particularly if the problem is primary amenorrhea. Adolescence is a time when being different from peers is often painful, especially if a correctable cause for the difference cannot be identified. Teaching includes the importance of adequate nutrition and discouragement of rigorous dieting. The nurse should explain that although exercise is beneficial, strenuous workouts or aerobic training can cause amenorrhea. Effective weight control may reduce factors related to PCOS. Referral for psychological counseling may be needed for eating disorders.

Abnormal Uterine Bleeding

The normal menstrual cycle was described in Chapter 3. Dysfunctional bleeding includes prolonged or heavy bleeding (**menorrhagia**), bleeding that occurs irregularly and often between menstrual periods (**metrorrhagia**), or bleeding that occurs irregularly and more frequently (**menometrorrhagia**), which is essentially a combination of the other two terms. Complications of an unrecognized pregnancy, such as spontaneous abortion, should be considered when making the diagnosis.

Etiology

The most common causes of abnormal bleeding fall into the following five basic categories:

1. Pregnancy complications, such as spontaneous abortion
2. Anatomic lesions, either benign or malignant, of the vagina, cervix, or uterus
3. Drug-induced bleeding, such as breakthrough bleeding that may occur in women taking hormonal contraceptives
4. Systemic disorders, such as diabetes mellitus, uterine myomas (fibroids), and hypothyroidism
5. Failure to ovulate

Management

Evaluation of abnormal uterine bleeding may include a sensitive pregnancy test, coagulation studies, and tests to determine whether ovulation is occurring. Hormone and liver function tests, plus tests to determine whether the woman is anemic, often are done. Ultrasonography or hysteroscopy may be used to look for polyps and check the condition of the uterine lining.

A common hormone treatment is progestin-estrogen combination oral contraceptives that suppress ovulation and allow a more stable endometrial lining to form. Surgical therapy may include dilation and curettage (D&C) to remove polyps or to diagnose **endometrial hyperplasia** (excess normal uterine lining cells), which may be treated with progesterone to suppress excess uterine lining. Hysterectomy may be performed if the uterus is enlarged as a result of fibroids or adenomyosis (benign invasive growth of the endometrium into the muscular layer of the uterus) and if the woman does not want more children. Laser ablation may be used to permanently remove the endometrial lining without hysterectomy. Treatment of iron-deficiency anemia is needed by many women with excessive vaginal bleeding (Lobo, 2012a).

Nursing Considerations

Nurses should encourage women to seek medical attention promptly when irregular or prolonged bleeding occurs. Nurses also help the woman keep a record of the bleeding episodes and the amount of blood lost. This involves keeping a calendar and noting any vaginal bleeding (spotting, menses) that occurs in addition to the number of pads and tampons saturated each day.

The nurse teaches the importance of nutrition and methods to reduce stress and promote relaxation. Nurses should provide support for women who fear that irregular bleeding indicates a serious disease, such as cancer. Offering false reassurance is unwise, but information about diagnostic procedures, such as pelvic examination, the Pap test, and other tests, is helpful.

❓ KNOWLEDGE CHECK

17. How does primary amenorrhea differ from secondary amenorrhea in terms of onset, cause, and treatment?
18. What are possible causes of dysfunctional uterine bleeding, and why should it not be ignored?

Cyclic Pelvic Pain

Cyclic pelvic pain should be distinguished from acute pelvic pain. Acute pelvic pain is sudden in onset and is not experienced with each menstrual cycle. It may indicate a serious disorder, such as ectopic pregnancy or appendicitis. Cyclic pelvic pain occurs repetitively and predictably in a specific phase of the menstrual cycle. The most common causes of cyclic pelvic pain are mittelschmerz, primary **dysmenorrhea** (painful menstruation), and **endometriosis** (tissue resembling endometrium outside uterine cavity). Secondary dysmenorrhea, or pelvic pain that is not cyclic, is usually related to pelvic pathologic processes.

Mittelschmerz

Mittelschmerz ("middle" pain) is pelvic pain that occurs midway between menstrual periods at the time of ovulation. The pain results from growth of the dominant follicle within the ovary or rupture of the follicle and subsequent spillage of follicular fluid and blood into the peritoneal space. The pain is fairly sharp and is felt on the right or left side of the pelvis. It generally lasts from a few hours to 2 days, and slight vaginal bleeding may accompany the discomfort. Generally, women do not need medical treatment beyond simple explanation of the discomfort or mild analgesics.

Primary Dysmenorrhea

Primary dysmenorrhea is menstrual pain without identified pathologic cause. Its onset is usually 1 to 3 years after menstruation begins, when ovulatory menstrual cycles are well established, and it is most common in young, nulliparous women. Commonly called "cramps," primary dysmenorrhea causes significant loss of school or work hours. The pain begins within hours of the onset of menses, and it is spasmodic or colicky because of increased prostaglandins secreted at this time. It is felt in the lower abdomen but often radiates to the lower back or down the legs. Nausea, vomiting, loose stools, or dizziness may also occur. The duration of the pain is usually 48 to 72 hours.

Two recommended treatments of primary dysmenorrhea provide marked relief: oral contraceptives and prostaglandin inhibitors. Oral contraceptives decrease the amount of endometrial growth that occurs during the menstrual cycle and thereby reduce the production of endometrial prostaglandins. For women who do not wish to take oral contraceptives, prostaglandin inhibitors offer relief. The most effective prostaglandin inhibitors are NSAIDs such as ibuprofen (Motrin, Advil) and naproxen (Naprosyn, Anaprox). To be effective, the NSAID should be taken around the clock for at least 48 to 72 hours beginning when menstrual flow starts. Other possible therapies include the levonorgestrel-releasing intrauterine system (LNG-IUS), with greatest pain relief early in the life of the contraceptive device (Lentz, 2012b).

Simple relief measures supplement medical interventions and may be sufficient for a woman. Rest in a comfortable position and application of warmth often provide additional relief.

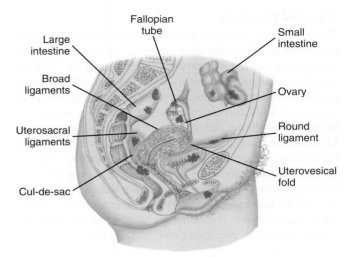

FIG. 27.2 Common Sites of Endometriosis.

Endometriosis
Pathophysiology

Endometriosis is defined as the presence outside the uterus of tissue that resembles the endometrium in both structure and function. The response of this tissue to the stimulation of estrogen and progesterone during the menstrual cycle is identical to that of the endometrial tissue. That is, it grows and proliferates during the follicular and luteal phases of the cycle and then sloughs during menstruation. However, the menstruation from endometriosis lesions occurs in a closed cavity, which causes pressure and pain on adjacent tissue. In addition, prostaglandins secreted by the endometriosis lesions irritate nerve endings and stimulate uterine contractions that further increase pain. Cyclic bleeding into the pelvic cavity can cause chronic inflammatory changes that may make conception and implantation difficult. The most common sites of endometriosis lesions are illustrated in Fig. 27.2.

The estimated incidence of endometriosis is about 10%, but the true prevalence is unknown. Some women with significant endometriosis may be asymptomatic, and endometrial tissue is found on pelvic organs during an unrelated surgery. The cause remains unknown. One theory is that reflux of the menstrual flow through the fallopian tubes allows the endometrial cells to attach to nearby structures and proliferate, creating spots of endometrial tissue. Endometrial tissue has been found in distant sites such as the lungs, raising the possibility that the cells are spread by blood circulation. Spread of the endometrial cells by the lymphatic system has been implicated. Endometriosis of the anterior abdominal wall has been found after a cesarean delivery near the incision line, leading to the theory that microscopic endometrial tissue may have been implanted during the cesarean and then stimulated to grow with later menstrual cycles. Studies have also shown a familial predisposition (Bloski & Pierson, 2008; Lobo, 2012b).

Most women with endometriosis are in their 30s and nulliparous, and many have had infertility problems. Signs and symptoms of endometriosis usually regress after menopause unless a woman takes estrogen supplementation.

Signs and Symptoms

The two major problems associated with endometriosis are cyclic pain and infertility. Endometriosis should be considered in a woman seeking infertility treatment even if she does not have the typical pain. Pain of endometriosis differs from that of primary dysmenorrhea. Endometriosis pain is deep, unilateral or bilateral, and either sharp or dull. It is constant, as opposed to the spasmodic or colicky pain of primary dysmenorrhea. **Dyspareunia** (painful intercourse) may occur, usually with deep penetration. Rectal pain may occur during defecation. Diarrhea, constipation, and sensations of rectal pressure or urgency are other symptoms of endometriosis. Although causes of infertility may not be known, some factors may be retrograde menstruation, endometrium transplant via lymphatics, immunologic changes, or familial predisposition (Lobo, 2012b).

Management

Treatment may be either medical or surgical. A woman must often weigh her need for pain relief and the desire to maintain fertility against the side effects that accompany many treatment regimens when choosing therapy. Growth and bleeding of displaced endometrial tissue depends on adequate production of ovarian hormones during the menstrual cycle. Other factors to be considered include symptom severity, desire for future fertility, the woman's age, and the effect of the endometriosis on nearby organs, such as obstruction of the urinary or GI tracts (Lobo, 2012b).

Continuous oral contraceptives for 6 to 12 months suppress endometrial tissue proliferation, particularly in a woman who desires pregnancy after medical treatment. Both the testosterone derivative danazol and gonadotropin-releasing hormone (GnRH) agonists such as leuprolide acetate (Lupron) and nafarelin (Synarel) interfere with hormones needed for ovulation and the menstrual cycle, creating a "pseudomenopause" while taken. The woman may have hot flashes, vaginal dryness, insomnia, decreased libido, and reduced bone density. In addition, danazol may produce masculinizing effects, such as deepening of the voice, facial and body hair, and weight gain. The woman takes the drug for a varying time, often between 3 and 6 months, depending on the drug and the degree of her endometriosis. Surgical treatment of endometriosis may have different options because of the varied size, number, and location of lesions; the age of the affected woman; and whether endometriosis contributes to her infertility. **Laparoscopy** (insertion of an illuminated tube into the abdominal cavity) may be performed for lysis of adhesions and laser vaporization of the lesions of endometriosis. This procedure is used especially when infertility is a problem. For women with severe pain who no longer wish to have children, a hysterectomy, sometimes including removal of one or both ovaries and fallopian tubes, and removal of all lesions offer relief. The appendix is often removed at the same time, and pathologic examination often finds endometrial tissue attached. Removal of both ovaries causes loss of their hormone production, resulting in an early menopause. Postoperative HRT may be recommended if most endometrial lesions are removed (Lobo, 2012b).

Nursing Considerations

Dysmenorrhea varies from mild "menstrual awareness" to incapacitating pain that affects the quality of life for several days each month. Too often the pain is belittled ("It's just cramps"). One of the most important nursing actions is to acknowledge the pain: "I understand this is really uncomfortable, and you are concerned that you have this much pain every month." Infertility may be accompanied by the cyclic increase in pain of endometriosis.

The nurse should suggest nonpharmacologic pain-relief measures, such as frequent rest periods, application of heat to the lower abdomen, moderate exercise, and a well-balanced diet. The woman should avoid scheduling stress-provoking situations during the menstrual period if possible. The nurse should counsel the woman about expected effects of OTC or prescribed medications. The woman also should be instructed about side or adverse effects specific to the medications recommended that should be reported.

The nurse should allow time for the woman to express her concerns about the therapy. The woman is taught expected effects of drugs given for endometriosis and about each drug's precautions and side or adverse effects that may occur. Some women benefit from information about measures that promote sleep and relaxation and, most importantly, from the knowledge that someone is available to provide support and guidance when needed. A woman may demonstrate emotional distress if she has not had all the children she desires but must decide whether to have a hysterectomy to reduce physical pain that simpler measures have not relieved.

> ### ? KNOWLEDGE CHECK
>
> 19. What causes primary dysmenorrhea, and how may it be treated?
> 20. How does endometriosis cause dysmenorrhea, and how can it be treated?
> 21. What are the major side effects of danazol? Of the GnRH agonists?

Premenstrual Syndrome

Many women notice some minor physical and emotional changes related to their menstrual cycles. However, some women have severe problems associated with these cyclic changes. PMS, also called *premenstrual dysphoric disorder* (PMDD), affects about 5% to 10% of women severely enough to cause significant disruption with their daily lives. Although PMDD is the official diagnostic name for the diagnostic criteria, PMS is now a term ingrained in lay culture and will be used in this chapter. After exclusion of other diagnoses, the following criteria must be met for the condition to be diagnosed as PMS (Lentz, 2012b):

- The signs and symptoms must be cyclic and recur in the luteal phase (after ovulation) of the menstrual cycle.
- The woman should be free of symptoms during the follicular phase (before ovulation) of the menstrual cycle, and the cycle must include 7 symptom-free days.

BOX 27.5 Symptoms of Premenstrual Syndrome

Physical Symptoms
Headaches, dizziness
Abdominal bloating or swelling; swelling of the extremities
Breast tenderness
Hot flashes
Abdominal cramps
Generalized muscle and joint pain
Fatigue
Appetite changes: Binge eating, cravings
Sleep changes: Excessive sleep or insomnia
Reduced sexual interest

Behavioral Symptoms
Depressed mood
Feelings of hopelessness
Marked anxiety
Confusion, forgetfulness, poor concentration
Accident proneness
Irritability and anger
Emotional lability: Tearfulness or readiness to cry, loneliness, mood instability
Reduced interest in activities of living
Social avoidance
Lethargy or high energy

- Symptoms must be severe enough to have an impact on work, lifestyle, and relationships.
- Diagnosis should be based on the woman's *prospective* symptom recording or charting of symptoms as they occur rather than recall of symptoms that occurred in the past.

Some women who have medical or psychiatric disorders have an increased intensity of symptoms during the last half of their cycles, often leading them to assume they have PMS. Examples of these are depression, panic disorder, and generalized anxiety disorder. A psychiatric illness such as bipolar disorder may have symptoms unrelated to PMS, but the two disorders may coexist. Occupational or personal stress may worsen PMS.

Numerous symptoms have been ascribed to PMS, but a relatively small number make up the majority of complaints. They can be divided into behavioral and physical symptoms. Box 27.5 lists those that are most common. Several PMS diaries with varied amounts of detail are available for the woman to record her symptoms and their severity, lifestyle impact, and medications.

Etiology

Although the cause of PMS is unknown, several theories or predisposing factors have been proposed. The current theory of the cause of PMS is that normal fluctuations in gonadal hormones during a cycle, chiefly estrogen and progesterone, trigger central biochemical responses, specifically serotonin. The premenstrual fall in serotonin levels occurs in most women, but a susceptible woman may show psychiatric symptoms as her estrogen, progesterone, and serotonin levels fall during the luteal phase. Most women show a rapid postmenstrual return to a feeling of well-being.

Impact on Family

PMS puts a consistent strain on family relationships because symptoms recur monthly. The episodes of PMS affect the functioning of the entire family. Clinical descriptions of severe family disruptions include increased family conflict, disrupted communication, and decreased family cohesion. Of particular concern is the group of women who report symptoms of loss of control, child battering, self-injury, and increased accidents. Work and social relationships may suffer.

PATIENT TEACHING

How to Relieve Symptoms of Premenstrual Syndrome

Diet
Decrease consumption of caffeine (coffee, tea, colas, chocolate), which increases irritability, insomnia, anxiety, and nervousness.
Avoid simple sugars (cookies, cake, candy) to prevent high blood glucose levels followed by a rapid decline and a period of low blood glucose levels (hypoglycemia).
Decrease intake of salty foods (chips, pickles) to reduce fluid retention.
Drink at least 2000 mL (2 quarts) of *water* per day, and do not include other beverages in this total.
Eat six small meals a day to prevent hypoglycemia. Meals should be well balanced, with emphasis on fresh fruits and vegetables, complex carbohydrates, and nonfat milk products.
Avoid alcohol, which aggravates depression.

Exercise
Increase physical exercise to relieve tension and decrease depression. Aerobic activity, such as jogging or walking, several times a week is recommended.

Stress Management
During the time when there are no symptoms of PMS, acknowledge the effect of PMS on daily life and make plans to avoid stressful situations during the premenstrual period when symptoms are acute.
Use guided imagery, conscious relaxation techniques, warm baths, and massage to reduce stress.

Sleep and Rest
To reduce fatigue and combat insomnia do the following:
Adhere to a regular schedule for sleep.
Drink a glass of milk, which is high in tryptophan and known to promote sleep, before bedtime.
Schedule exercise in the morning or early afternoon rather than late afternoon.
Engage in relaxing activities, such as reading, before bedtime, and avoid excitement at this time.

Management

Treatment of PMS is based on the symptom profile of each woman after ruling out other problems, especially psychiatric diagnoses such as depression. Supportive therapy such as reassuring the woman that PMS is a common problem that has a physiologic basis may reduce her anxiety and should be part of other treatments. Relaxation therapy has shown benefits to women with the more severe PMS symptoms. Exercise has been shown to reduce PMS symptoms and also has many other benefits to a woman's health. Modifying the diet to reduce salty foods, caffeine, chocolate, red meat, dairy products, and alcohol may be helpful. Small and frequent meals may reduce mood swings.

Clinical trials have shown that supplementation with calcium (1200 mg/day) has some effectiveness and that magnesium supplementation (200 to 400 mg/day) is minimally effective. Carbohydrate-rich foods and beverages may improve the mood and reduce food cravings in some women. Reducing caffeine intake and taking vitamin E (400 international units [IU]/day) during the luteal phase of the cycle may reduce breast pain (mastalgia) in some women. Evening primrose oil also may have some benefit in reducing breast pain. See Box 27.6 for other complementary and alternative therapies. Women with physical, emotional, and cognitive symptoms may be prescribed antidepressant medications, oral contraceptives to suppress ovulation, or both. Estrogen therapy may relieve premenstrual migraines. Danazol taken in low doses may relieve breast pain and other symptoms. Bromocriptine (Parlodel) during the luteal phase may relieve breast pain. Selective serotonin reuptake inhibitors (SSRIs) taken at lower doses than those used to treat depression—such as fluoxetine (Sarafem), sertraline (Zoloft), or paroxetine (Paxil)—have been shown to be very effective for most women with correctly diagnosed PMS. The SSRI may be initially prescribed for the luteal phase only; however, if ineffective, it can then be prescribed for continuous intake (Lentz, 2012b).

Nursing Considerations

Many women experience some of the symptoms and diagnose themselves as having PMS. Nurses should discourage this practice because serious systemic disease can be missed if the criteria for diagnosis are ignored. Instead of self-diagnosis, nurses should recommend that the woman consult with her health care provider so a complete history and physical examination can be performed to rule out other causes or a problem that may coexist with PMS. Psychoactive drugs may be ineffective or contraindicated if a woman's true problem is not PMS.

Once the diagnosis of PMS is confirmed, nurses can educate the family about lifestyle changes that may help. Nurses should acknowledge that dietary changes are particularly difficult because many women crave salty or sweet foods, which should be restricted. Women also benefit from education about expected cyclic changes. As they learn to predict the

pattern of symptoms and gain a sense of control over them, the symptoms often diminish.

Education and support should be expanded to include the family. When the woman exhibits symptoms of PMS, family members often respond by withdrawing or confronting the woman. Family members also should be encouraged to express their feelings so anger and resentment within the family can be minimized.

Nurses should help the woman make concrete arrangements to obtain relief when she feels she is losing control or when she fears that she may harm herself or a child. A neighbor, friend, or family member should be identified to provide immediate relief, without questions or explanations, when the woman feels she is losing control.

It is more helpful if the family acknowledges feelings they believe the woman is experiencing. For instance, saying, "It must be disturbing to feel so irritable. What can I do to help?" provokes a different emotional response than comments that are confrontational or blaming.

ELECTIVE TERMINATION OF PREGNANCY

Elective termination of pregnancy, also called *induced abortion,* is a voluntary method of ending a pregnancy at the request of the woman but not for reasons of impaired maternal health or fetal disease. Therapeutic termination is usually performed to preserve the health of the mother, to prevent the birth of an infant with severe birth defects, or to end a pregnancy caused by rape or incest. A woman may choose elective termination of pregnancy for a variety of reasons, possibly economic or social. Therapeutic and elective abortions involve many social and ethical issues (Crandell, 2012). Recent abortion surveillance may be found at www.cdc.org (Pazol et al., 2015).

Methods of Elective Termination of Pregnancy

The technique used to terminate a pregnancy depends on the length of gestation. Abortion techniques based on medications may be options within 7 weeks of the woman's last menstrual period. Inducing uterine contractions with specific medications to end pregnancy early makes the process more private, eliminates risks such as uterine trauma or perforation, and does not require anesthesia.

Drugs that may be used in medical abortion regimens to terminate a pregnancy up to 9 weeks include the following:

- Mifepristone (Mifeprex, or RU-486), an antiprogesterone drug, followed by misoprostol (Cytotec), a prostaglandin drug commonly used to reduce gastric acid secretion. Oral or vaginal use of misoprostol in medical abortion is unlabeled by the manufacturer. The woman usually expels the early pregnancy within 14 days of her first visit (Jensen & Mishell, 2012).
- Methotrexate (Folex, Mexate) is an antimetabolite also used to treat certain types of cancer. Although not approved by the U.S. Food and Drug Administration for medical abortion, individualized doses have been successfully used for medical pregnancy termination. Misoprostol may be prescribed to enhance expulsion of uterine contents.

Surgical abortion techniques are needed if the woman has been pregnant for more than 7 weeks or if her medical abortion failed and she still desires pregnancy termination. Through 12 weeks of gestation, vacuum aspiration with curettage is the method of choice. The cervix is dilated after locally injecting anesthetic in the area, and a plastic cannula is inserted into the uterine cavity. The contents are aspirated with negative pressure, and the uterine cavity may be scraped with a curet to ensure the uterus is empty. Cramping may last 20 to 30 minutes after the procedure is completed. Complications may include uterine perforation, hemorrhage, cervical lacerations, and adverse reactions to the anesthetic agent.

For second-trimester abortions, cervical dilation with removal of the fetus and placenta is generally performed. The procedure is similar to vacuum curettage but requires greater cervical dilation and a larger aspirator because the products of conception have grown in size and should be removed gradually. Dilation begins with insertion of laminaria—rounded, cone-shaped materials that absorb water—into the cervix 24 hours before the procedure. Other osmotic dilators include Dilapan and Lamicel. The laminaria draw fluid from the cervical canal and expand, causing the cervix to dilate slowly and with minimal trauma. If needed, before aspiration and removal of the products of pregnancy, additional cervical dilation is done.

Medical methods exist for abortion in the second trimester, but these involve labor. Retention of the placenta often occurs, requiring a D&C to fully clean the uterus. Laminaria are inserted about 12 hours before the procedure to start cervical dilation. Prostaglandin E_2, which stimulates contractions, may be given via vaginal suppository or intraamniotic infusion. Oxytocin is not effective at starting labor because of the early gestation, but it may shorten labor after it has been established by other methods. Because of the emotional distress caused by the longer procedure and the increased risks involved, medical termination of pregnancy is not often chosen in the second trimester (Jensen & Mishell, 2012).

PATIENT TEACHING

Guidelines for Self-Care after Elective Termination of Pregnancy

Normal activities may be resumed, but strenuous work or exercise should be avoided for a few days.

Bleeding or cramping may occur for 1 or 2 weeks. If either becomes severe, medical advice should be sought. Light "spotting" may occur for about a month.

Sanitary pads should be used instead of tampons for the first week after the abortion to avoid possible infection.

Intercourse should be curtailed for 1 week after the abortion because of the possibility of infection until the uterine lining heals.

Birth control measures should be used if sex is resumed before menstruation begins because it is possible to become pregnant during this time. Menstruation usually resumes in 4 to 6 weeks.

Temperature should be taken twice a day to detect possible infection; a temperature above 37.8°C (100°F) should be reported to the health care provider.

It is important to keep the follow-up appointment in 2 weeks or as recommended.

Nursing Considerations

The nurse's role in caring for women seeking elective abortion is one of providing physical and emotional support and information. History taking and collection of laboratory data depend on the routine of the health care setting in which the nurse is functioning. Counseling and lending emotional support are nursing responsibilities, although a designated counselor also may perform these services.

Nurses are also responsible for providing information about self-care after an elective abortion. Self-care is similar to that after spontaneous abortion or miscarriage: observation for excessive bleeding or signs of infection (temperature greater than 37.8°C [100°F], foul-smelling vaginal drainage). Nurses also provide information about follow-up visits and contraception. The Rh-negative woman should receive Rho(D) immune globulin (RhoGAM).

KNOWLEDGE CHECK

22. What are the criteria for diagnosing PMS?
23. What should the nurse teach the patient and family regarding lifestyle changes that may reduce the symptoms of PMS or increase patient and family coping?
24. What drugs may be used in an early elective termination of pregnancy?
25. What discharge teaching is appropriate after termination of pregnancy?

MENOPAUSE

Menopause means the end of menstruation. However, most people use the term to include the array of endocrine, somatic, and psychic changes that occur at the end of the reproductive period. The entire process, often called the "change of life," is correctly termed the **climacteric**. *Premenopause* refers to the early part of the climacteric, before menstruation ceases but after the woman experiences some of the climacteric symptoms, such as irregular menses. Perimenopause includes premenopause, menopause, and at least 1 year after menopause. *Postmenopause* refers to the phase after menopause, when menstrual periods have ceased.

Unexpected postmenopausal bleeding should be investigated as soon as possible because it suggests endometrial cancer. Conversely, planned or scheduled postmenopausal bleeding is generally not a cause for concern. It occurs when the woman who takes estrogen and progesterone sequentially stops taking the drugs, usually once a month. This allows the uterine lining to be sloughed and prevents endometrial hyperplasia.

Age of Menopause

The average age for natural menopause is 51.5 years (Lobo, 2012c). The natural climacteric takes place over 3 to 5 years. Menopause can be induced or created artificially, however, at any age. Surgical removal of the ovaries or destruction of the ovaries by radiation or chemotherapy causes abrupt, permanent cessation of ovarian function, including the production of estrogen. The most common reason for performing these procedures is treatment of cancer or endometriosis. Young women who experience artificial menopause often have more symptoms associated with menopause than do women who go through the process naturally because theirs is not a gradual process as it is for the older woman.

Women can now expect to live another 30 years or more after natural menopause. During this period they must deal with physical, psychological, and social changes that often require a reevaluation of their primary roles and restructuring of personal goals.

Physiologic Changes

During the normal reproductive cycle, the ovaries respond to gonadotropins (follicle-stimulating hormone and luteinizing hormone) in a predictable pattern: (1) a follicle matures, (2) the ovary secretes estrogen, (3) ovulation occurs, and (4) the corpus luteum produces progesterone. During the premenopausal period, however, the ovaries are less responsive to gonadotropins, and, although increased amounts of follicle-stimulating hormone are secreted, ovulation is sporadic and menstrual periods are irregular. With progressive aging, the ovaries become unresponsive, even to high levels of gonadotropins, and ovulation, menstruation, and the secretion of ovarian hormones (estrogen and progesterone) cease.

Estrogen is responsible for the secondary sex characteristics of women. When estrogen levels decline, the organs of reproduction undergo regression. The labia become thin and pale. The vaginal mucosa atrophies, and vaginal tissue loses its lubrication and therefore is easily traumatized. Dyspareunia is common, and bacterial invasion of the epithelium may occur and lead to frequent vaginal infections. This entire process is referred to as **atrophic vaginitis**. Breasts become smaller, and atrophy of the uterus and ovaries occur. However, a concurrent benefit is that uterine myomas (fibroids) and endometriosis lesions also atrophy. Estrogen deficit can result in atrophic changes in the bladder and urethra that may cause loss of urethral tone and frequent atrophic cystitis.

In addition, absence of estrogen is associated with an adverse change in serum lipids. Serum levels of low-density lipoproteins (LDLs), which carry cholesterol to blood vessels, increase. At the same time, levels of high-density lipoproteins (HDLs), which are known to carry cholesterol to the liver and protect against the development of CAD, decrease.

Many menopausal women experience hot flashes or flushes, which are the result of vasomotor instability. The cause of vasomotor instability is not known, but it is closely associated with increased secretion of gonadotropins. Hot flashes are characterized by a sudden feeling of heat or burning of the skin, followed by perspiration. They occur more frequently during the night, and fatigue as a result of interrupted sleep is a major problem for some women. Hot flashes are often more frequent and severe in younger women who undergo the climacteric, particularly if loss of ovarian function was abrupt because of medical therapy. Many women in the climacteric have few annoyances from the hot flashes, however.

Psychological Responses

It is easy to understand why menopause is called the "change of life." It is accompanied by physical, psychological, and social changes, and individual responses vary widely. Many women are relieved that their childbearing and child-rearing tasks are ending. They see this as an exciting time, when they can pursue personal development. Other women grieve that the possibility of childbearing is past. This may be particularly true for women who have never had a child, whether because of infertility or because of lack of a male partner. However, artificial reproductive techniques have blurred the line that defines the age at which it is and is not possible to bear a child (see Chapter 26).

Menopause requires a woman to come to terms with aging. It may be difficult to accept aging in a society that reveres youth, and many women become extremely concerned with measures that slow the signs of aging. Many women become grandmothers at this time, which also confirms aging and requires a major adjustment in how the woman views herself. A large population of "baby boomers"—those born from 1946 to 1964—have entered menopause. These women are likely to change many of society's ideas about menopause because of the sheer size of their group and because they have changed the social fabric of the United States dramatically as they have grown up and matured.

Some symptoms do not have a physiologic explanation, but they are no less real to women who experience them. Depression, mood swings, irritability, and agitation are common climacteric complaints. Insomnia and fatigue are often mentioned as major problems.

One of the most puzzling aspects of menopause is the wide variation in both physical and psychological symptoms that women experience. For some women, the only changes are mild, infrequent hot flashes and amenorrhea. Other women experience severe, debilitating hot flashes; atrophic vaginitis; and multiple psychological symptoms, such as irritability and prolonged depression.

Therapy for Menopause

Although many women comfortably undergo the age-associated changes of menopause, others seek relief for discomforts such as hot flashes, interrupted sleep, or vaginal dryness. The psychological perception that increasing reproductive hormones might slow the aging process and promote a more youthful appearance has strengthened use of HRT during the climacteric. Additional beneficial effects were thought to be a reduction in CVD, colorectal cancer, breast cancer, and osteoporosis, as well as other medical-surgical conditions associated with aging.

As greater research emerged, risk factors as well as benefits of hormone therapy emerged. Two groups of perimenopausal women were included in the hormone studies of the WHI research, as follows:

- Estrogen and progesterone were given to women with a uterus. Combining progesterone with estrogen therapy prevents uterine hyperplasia, a precursor to uterine cancer, in this group.

- Estrogen therapy alone was given to women who have had a hysterectomy because uterine hyperplasia is not a risk.

The combination of estrogen and progesterone replacement is usually called *hormone replacement therapy (HRT)*, whereas the estrogen-only replacement therapy may be called *estrogen replacement therapy* (ERT). It is common to see HRT used for either or both therapies, however.

The WHI and other hormone replacement studies showed increasing evidence that estrogen plus progesterone therapy significantly increased risks for some disorders, primarily breast cancer and heart disease. The estrogen-progesterone arm of the WHI study was stopped in 2002. A woman enrolled in the estrogen-progesterone arm was not obligated to stop taking estrogen-progesterone therapy, but she had to make choices based on both the benefits and the unexpected risks that emerged with the early results. Rather than receive estrogen-progesterone supplements through the study, the women could continue the combined hormones via prescription from their health care provider. The estrogen-only arm of the study continued until 2004, when an increase in strokes among this group was identified.

Although once routinely prescribed to reduce the annoying changes of menopause for many women, the decision about hormone therapy is more complex because both the benefits and the risks associated with a prescribed hormonal drug should be considered. In addition, complementary therapy often has a greater usefulness for women having mild menopausal changes (Boxes 27.7 and 27.8).

PATIENT TEACHING

Hormone Replacement Therapy

Hormone replacement therapy (HRT) is highly individualized owing to research findings about possible unfavorable cardiovascular effects of estrogen-progesterone supplementation during the climacteric. However, women may continue using the estrogen-only HRT or the estrogen-progesterone HRT for significant discomforts that are unrelieved by other methods or for beneficial effects such as reduction in osteoporosis. The woman and her health care provider should consider both benefits and risks of HRT to make the decision about whether to use the hormone replacement.
Take the medication with meals to reduce nausea.
If you miss a dose, take the medication as soon as you remember, but not immediately before the next scheduled dose. *Do not take double doses.*
Expect withdrawal bleeding (if your uterus is present) when estrogen and progestin are temporarily discontinued.
Report unexpected bleeding to your health care provider.
Stop smoking to reduce the risk for thromboembolism.
Use sunscreen and protective clothing to prevent increased pigmentation.
Continue follow-up physical examinations, including blood pressure measurements, Pap tests, and examinations of breasts, abdomen, and pelvis.

BOX 27.7 Contraindications and Cautions Related to Estrogen Replacement Therapy

Previous episode of breast or ovarian cancer or other estrogen-dependent tumor
Close family history of breast cancer (first-degree relative)
Uterine cancer
Active thromboembolic disease or prior thromboembolic disorder when taking estrogen
Risk for cardiovascular disease
Stroke
Acute or chronic liver disease
Undiagnosed abnormal vaginal bleeding
Gallbladder or pancreatic disease
Diabetes mellitus
Conditions that may be aggravated by fluid retention, such as migraine, epilepsy, cardiac or renal dysfunction, depression

Risks

HRT was not considered safe for all women before the WHI findings. For example, women who have had estrogen receptor–positive or progesterone receptor–positive breast cancer or blood coagulation disorders influenced by estrogen or progesterone do not qualify. A woman who has had breast cancer may take a drug to block the effects of estrogen and reduce the risk for recurrence. Likewise, a woman who has a close family history of breast cancer might not want to take it. Unexplained uterine bleeding and endometrial cancer are contraindications. Smoking, hypertension, diabetes, CVD, and renal or liver disease are often contraindications for hormone therapy, whether therapy includes both estrogen and progesterone or estrogen only. Other possible contraindications include seizure disorders, migraines, and gallbladder or pancreatic disease.

Nursing Considerations

Nursing care focuses on helping women understand the physical and psychological changes that may occur during perimenopause. If the woman chooses hormone therapy, nurses should reinforce the prescribed regimen and the risks and benefits of the therapy. For instance, women should be told that although HRT effectively treats atrophic vaginitis and reduces dyspareunia, it may not correct the loss of libido that some women experience.

If HRT is contraindicated, nurses are often the primary source of information about measures that reduce problems and promote comfort, as follows:

- Using water-soluble lubricants such as K-Y Liquid, K-Y Silk-E, Lubrin, or Replens to relieve vaginal dryness and dyspareunia. Oil-based lubricants should not be used because they adhere to the mucous membrane for long periods and provide a medium for bacterial growth.

BOX 27.8   Complementary and Alternative Therapy for Menopause

All patients should be asked about their use of complementary and alternative therapy methods, and their response should be documented.

"Natural" should not be assumed to be safe or therapeutic.

Errors are possible with natural products because of non-standardized dosing, inconsistent quality control, errors in compounding, and incorrect labeling of the actual plant compound in a container.

Many biologic products should not be used by a woman considering becoming pregnant or during pregnancy and lactation. Natural biologic products cannot be assumed to be safe for children.

Botanical products that may be used for hot flashes, although effectiveness is not yet well supported by research, include the following:

Black cohosh: Reduced sweating; suppression of luteinizing hormone; no influence on endometrial thickness, levels of follicle-stimulating hormone, estrogenic or prolactin levels; should not be used with estrogen therapy, anticoagulants, and antihypertensives.

Soy products: Contain **phytoestrogens** that may serve as weak estrogenic compounds, stimulating estrogen receptors; no convincing evidence that soy products reduce hot flashes more than placebos in some studies; should be avoided in women with estrogen-dependent tumors such as breast, ovarian, or endometrial cancer because tumor growth may be stimulated; possible interaction between estrogen replacement therapy or the drug tamoxifen; should be avoided in pregnant or lactating women.

Dong quai: May be used with other herbal products; contains coumarin products that have vasodilation and antispasmodic effects; more study needed to determine effects on hot flashes, although it is a traditional Chinese medicine product.

Vitamin E: A fat-soluble vitamin supplement having antioxidant properties; inhibits platelet aggregation and low-density lipoprotein (LDL) oxidation, possibly interfering with therapeutic effects of anticoagulant chemotherapy, or statin drugs designed to normalize levels of lipids; has been associated with gastrointestinal disturbances; recent results have shown an association with heart failure.

Chasteberry: Possible reduction in premenstrual symptoms of mood alteration and menopausal symptoms; the National Center for Complementary and Alternative Medicine is funding research.

From American College of Obstetricians and Gynecologists (ACOG). (2012d). *Use of botanicals for management of menopausal symptoms.* Practice Bulletin No. 28. Washington, DC: Author; and National Center for Complementary and Alternative Medicine. (2009a). *Herbs at a glance: Evening primrose oil;* National Center for Complementary and Alternative Medicine. (2009b). *Herbs at a glance: Chasteberry;* National Center for Complementary and Alternative Medicine. (2009c). *Get the facts: Menopausal symptoms and CAM.* Bethesda, MD: Author

- Discussing alternatives to estrogen, such as botanical preparations, if the woman does not want ERT. The woman should discuss these with her health care provider, because some have side or adverse effects or interactions with other drugs. Research is often minimal for these therapies. The website for the National Center for Complementary and Alternative Medicine of the NIH, www.nccam.nih.gov, contains updated information (see Box 27.7).
- Doing Kegel exercises to increase muscle tone around the vagina and urinary meatus and counteract the effects of genital atrophy.
- Drinking at least eight glasses of water a day decreases the concentration of urine, flushes urine from the bladder, and reduces bacterial growth, thereby preventing atrophic cystitis.
- Wiping from front to back after urination and defecation reduces the transfer of bacteria from the anus to the urinary meatus and helps prevent cystitis.

? KNOWLEDGE CHECK

26. What are the effects of estrogen depletion at menopause (either natural or artificial) on the body?
27. What are the major psychological symptoms associated with menopause?
28. How does hormone replacement affect menopausal and postmenopausal women? What concerns were raised by the WHI research?

OSTEOPOROSIS

Osteoporosis is one of the greatest hazards of the postmenopausal years. It is characterized by decreased bone density, leaving the bones porous, fragile, and susceptible to fractures. The vertebrae, wrists, and hips are the most common sites of fractures, with forearms, feet, and toes also susceptible. More than 53 million people in the United States today either already have osteoporosis or are at high risk because of low bone mass. Osteoporosis can occur at any age, although the risk for developing the disease increases with age. Osteoporosis is most common in non-Hispanic White women, but the disease affects many older Americans of any race or sex. Hip fractures increase the risk for reduced mobility and death in the elderly (National Institute of Arthritis and Musculoskeletal and Skin Diseases [NIAMS], 2016).

Risk Factors

The combination of peak bone density and the rate of bone loss influences the severity of osteoporosis. Small-boned, fair-skinned White women of Northern European descent and Asian women are at greatest risk for osteoporosis, but African-American and Hispanic women also are at risk. Other risk factors may include a family history of the disease, late menarche, early menopause, and a sedentary

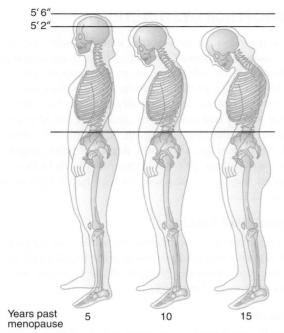

5'6"
5'2"

Years past menopause   5   10   15

FIG. 27.3 With progression of osteoporosis, the vertebral column collapses, causing loss of height and back pain. *Dowager's hump* is the term used for this curvature of the upper back.

lifestyle. Women who smoke, drink alcohol, or consume excessive amounts of caffeine have an increased risk for osteoporosis. Drug intake such as corticosteroids, some anticonvulsants, or aromatase inhibitors for breast cancer may reduce bone density. Inadequate lifetime intake of calcium or vitamin D is a risk factor. Women usually reach their peak bone mass between 18 and 25 years. Bone loss in women usually accelerates with menopause. Osteoporosis occurs as a woman loses too much bone, makes too little bone, or both (National Osteoporosis Foundation [NOF], 2016).

Signs and Symptoms

Osteoporosis has been called the "silent thief" because bone mass is lost over many years with no signs or symptoms. The first noticeable evidence is loss of height and back pain that occurs when the vertebrae collapse. Later signs include the "dowager's hump," which occurs when the vertebrae can no longer support the upper body in an upright position. Secondary to this, the waistline disappears and the abdomen protrudes as the rib cage moves closer to the pelvis. Depending on the number of fractures, several inches of height may be lost. Fig. 27.3 illustrates progressive changes in posture associated with osteoporosis.

Diagnosis of osteoporosis requires a thorough history, physical examination, and bone mineral analysis. Dual-energy x-ray absorptiometry (DEXA or DXA) is a highly accurate, fast, and relatively inexpensive method for measuring bone mineral density and involves low exposure to radiation. Results can be evaluated with risk factors to

direct management. Bone density examination can not only confirm the presence of osteoporosis but also detect low density before a fracture and predict the risk for fracture. Repeating bone density imaging helps determine the rate of bone loss and monitor treatment effectiveness (NIAMS, 2015).

Prevention and Medical Management

The major goal of treatment is to prevent or slow osteoporosis and stabilize remaining bone mass. Although research has upheld estrogen therapy to reduce osteoporosis by inhibition of bone resorption, fewer women are choosing hormone therapy because of its potential adverse effects. In addition, many breast cancer survivors take medications such as aromatase inhibitors that suppress or block estrogen because of its effects on tumor cells.

Drug Therapy. Drug categories to reduce osteoporosis include the following (NIAMS, 2015; NOF, 2016):

- Calcitonin (Calcimar, Miacalcin, Fortical), a synthetic hormone, is usually prescribed as a daily nasal spray to reduce factors that cause loss of calcium and increase reabsorption of calcium in the GI tract.
- Bisphosphonates inhibit osteoclasts, reducing bone turnover. Alendronate (Fosamax), risedronate (Actonel), and ibandronate (Boniva) are used to prevent and treat postmenopausal osteoporosis. Oral bisphosphonates may be contraindicated for women with ulcers or an inflammatory GI disease such as dysphagia or esophagitis. Alendronate and risedronate are also approved to treat bone loss that results from glucocorticoids and to treat men with osteoporosis. Zoledronic acid (Reclast) is approved for treatment of postmenopausal osteoporosis and is given by intravenous (IV) infusion yearly. Headache or flulike pain in muscles or joints may occur for 2 or 3 days after zoledronic acid infusion.
- Raloxifene (Evista), a selective estrogen receptor modulator (or SERM), binds to estrogen receptors to reduce bone loss. Because of the combined estrogen agonist and estrogen antagonist effects of SERMs, raloxifene is being studied to see if its effects also improve cardiac health without raising breast or uterine cancer incidence.
- Teriparatide (Forteo) is an injectable parathyroid hormone approved for postmenopausal women and men at high risk for fracture. Current approved duration of use is a maximum of 24 months. Teriparatide stimulates new bone formation, reducing the risk for both vertebral and nonvertebral fractures. Nausea, dizziness, and leg cramps are side effects.
- Denosumab (Prolia) is a recently approved receptor activator of nuclear factor-kappa β (RANK) ligand (RANKL) inhibitor that inhibits osteoclasts. Increased RANKL in postmenopausal women results in greater bone resorption with the osteoclasts. Denosumab reduces bone loss by inhibiting osteoclasts produced by higher RANKL levels (NIAMS, 2015; NOF, 2016).

Calcium and Vitamin D. Although calcium does not prevent bone loss, other therapies cannot be effective if calcium is deficient. A woman 50 years of age and younger needs 1000 mg of calcium daily, and a woman 51 years or older needs 1200 mg/day. Daily calcium supplements are recommended because it is difficult to ingest these quantities through food intake only. Vitamin D is necessary for calcium to be absorbed from the intestine. Supplemental vitamin D, 400 to 800 units, is often recommended for women under 50 years of age; 800 to 1,000 units is recommended for those 50 years of age or older (National Osteoporosis Foundation, 2017)

Exercise. Weight-bearing and resistance exercise has been shown to be beneficial in slowing loss of bone mass to maintain density if there is adequate calcium and vitamin D intake. Most of the bone mass is acquired by age 18, but muscle-strengthening exercise may continue to build bone into the 30s. High-impact exercise improves bone mineral density but should be avoided in a person who already has fragile vertebrae from osteoporosis. At least 30 minutes of daily therapeutic exercise is needed. Other exercises, such as swimming or water-based exercises, often improve cardiovascular and respiratory fitness while managing weight, although their primary use is not to limit bone loss.

Nursing Considerations

Nurses often counsel women about lifestyle factors that contribute to bone loss, such as cigarette smoking, excessive alcohol or caffeine intake, and the importance of following the recommended medical regimen. Adolescents and young women should be counseled about factors that impair as well as promote their ideal amount of peak bone density. Nurses are also concerned about how to prevent falls and thereby reduce the risk for fractures, particularly in older women or those with mobility impairments. A major responsibility is to help the woman make her environment as safe as possible. Lighting should be ample, with switches easily accessible. Loose electrical cords should be kept out of the way, and area rugs should have nonskid backing. The bathtub should have nonskid devices, and grab bars should be installed near toilets and tubs. Stairways should have handrails, and loose items should be kept out of the walking pathways. Consultation with an occupational or physical therapist may be needed if the woman has serious mobility problems. See www.niams.nih.gov/bone for added information.

> ### 🄯 KNOWLEDGE CHECK
>
> 29. Why is osteoporosis called the "silent thief"?
> 30. How can osteoporosis be prevented?
> 31. What can nurses do to help women with osteoporosis prevent fractures?

PELVIC FLOOR DYSFUNCTION

Pelvic floor dysfunction occurs when muscles, ligaments, and fascia that support the pelvic organs are damaged or weakened. This relaxation of pelvic support allows the pelvic organs to prolapse into, and sometimes out of, the vagina. Pelvic disorders generally occur in the perimenopausal period and may be the delayed result of traumatic childbirth or the effects of aging. Although 50% of women over 50 years of age have some degree of pelvic organ prolapse, fewer than 20% seek treatment. Pelvic floor dysfunction may occur in a woman who had a hysterectomy (Lentz, 2012a, c).

Vaginal Wall Prolapse

The vagina may prolapse at either the anterior or the posterior wall. Anterior wall prolapse involves the bladder and urethra and is called **cystocele**. Prolapse of the posterior wall produces enterocele or **rectocele**.

Cystocele

When the weakened upper anterior wall of the vagina is no longer able to support the weight of urine in the bladder, cystocele develops. The bladder protrudes downward into the vagina, resulting in incomplete emptying of the bladder. Cystitis is likely to occur because of the stagnant urine. Urethral displacement, formerly termed *urethrocele,* may occur when the urethra bulges into the lower anterior vaginal wall, producing stress urinary incontinence (Fig. 27.4, *A*).

Stress incontinence is the loss of urine that occurs with a sudden increase in intraabdominal pressure, such as that generated by sneezing, coughing, laughing, lifting, or sudden jarring motions. The two most common causes of stress incontinence are damage to the normal supports of the bladder neck and urethra that occurs during pregnancy and childbirth and tissue atrophy that occurs after menopause.

Enterocele

Enterocele is prolapse of the upper posterior vaginal wall between the vagina and rectum. This is almost always associated with herniation of the pouch of Douglas (a fold of peritoneum that dips down between the rectum and the uterus) and may contain loops of bowel. Enterocele often accompanies uterine prolapse (see Fig. 27.4, *B*).

Rectocele

Rectocele occurs when the posterior wall of the vagina becomes weakened and thin. Each time the woman strains at defecation, feces are pushed against the thinned wall, causing further stretching, until finally the rectum protrudes into the vagina. Many rectoceles are small and produce few symptoms. If the rectocele is large, the patient may have difficulty emptying the rectum. Some women facilitate bowel elimination by applying digital pressure along the posterior vaginal wall to keep the rectocele from protruding during a bowel movement (see Fig. 27.4, *C*).

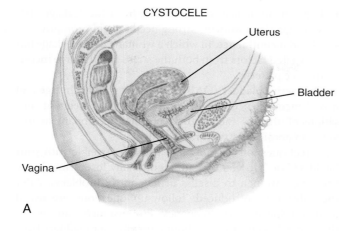

CYSTOCELE

Uterus

Bladder

Vagina

A

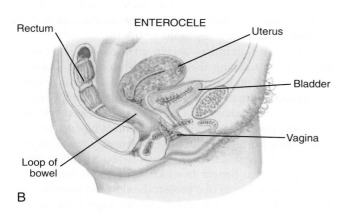

ENTEROCELE

Rectum

Uterus

Bladder

Vagina

Loop of bowel

B

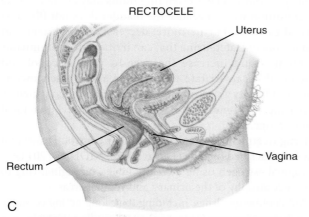

RECTOCELE

Uterus

Vagina

Rectum

C

FIG. 27.4 Three Types of Vaginal Wall Prolapse. A, Cystocele: Note bulging of bladder into the vagina. **B,** Enterocele: Note loop of bowel between rectum and uterus. **C,** Rectocele: Note bulging of rectum into vagina.

Uterine Prolapse

Uterine prolapse occurs when the cardinal ligaments, which support the uterus and vagina, are unduly stretched during pregnancy and do not return to normal after childbirth. This allows the uterus to sag backward and downward into the

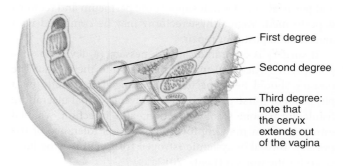

First degree

Second degree

Third degree: note that the cervix extends out of the vagina

FIG. 27.5 Three Degrees of Uterine Prolapse.

vagina. Uterine prolapse is less common than in the past, largely because of a reduction in traumatic vaginal deliveries. The condition continues to exist, however, particularly when the woman has had many vaginal deliveries or when the infants were large. Fig. 27.5 illustrates three degrees of uterine prolapse from first degree, in which the uterus remains in the vagina, to third degree, in which the cervix protrudes from the vagina (Lentz, 2012a).

Symptoms

Symptoms of pelvic floor dysfunction generally become obvious during the menopausal period. This is because estrogen diminishes at this time, resulting in atrophic changes in the supporting structures. The most common symptoms of vaginal wall prolapse are feelings of pelvic fullness, a dragging sensation, pelvic pressure, and fatigue. Low backache and a feeling that "everything is falling out" are sometimes described. Sexual problems related to arousal, orgasm, and painful vaginal intercourse may occur with pelvic floor dysfunction.

Symptoms relate to the structures involved and the level at which support has decreased. For instance, urinary frequency and urgency and urinary incontinence are seen in patients with cystocele because support of the urethra and lower vaginal wall has decreased. Constipation, flatulence, and difficulty defecating are major symptoms of rectocele. Regardless of the location or structure involved, symptoms become worse after prolonged standing and are relieved by lying down.

Symptoms of uterine prolapse are produced by the weight of the descending structures and may include sensations of pelvic pressure, backache, and fatigue. Cervical ulceration and bleeding occur if the cervix protrudes from the vaginal introitus.

Management

Treatment of disorders related to pelvic floor dysfunction depends on the woman's age, physical condition, sexual activity, and degree of prolapse. Surgical procedures provide the most satisfactory therapy for women who have significant discomfort. The most common procedures are the anterior and posterior colporrhaphy, often called an A&P repair. The anterior colporrhaphy involves suturing the pubocervical fascia to support the bladder and urethra when a cystocele exists. If a rectocele exists, a posterior colporrhaphy (suturing the fascia and perineal muscles that support the perineum and rectum) is performed. Vaginal hysterectomy may be combined with anterior and posterior repair.

If surgery is contraindicated, a pessary (a device to support pelvic structures) may be inserted into the vagina. The pessary should be inspected and changed frequently by a physician or nurse practitioner to prevent vaginal ulceration, fistula formation, stool impaction, and infection. Vaginal estrogen cream may improve the woman's tolerance of the pessary. Topical or systemic estrogen treatment may be indicated for the woman (Lentz, 2012a).

Nursing Considerations

Pelvic Exercises. Pelvic floor muscle training is directed toward strengthening the levator ani and pubococcygeal muscles that affect urethral closure and pelvic floor support. Kegel exercises are isometric, and one possible application is for the woman to consciously contract and relax these muscles slowly 8 to 12 times for a count of 6 to 8 seconds each and repeat this series for three sets. Before teaching pelvic floor muscle training, determine whether the woman can contract the muscles by asking her to sit with her legs apart while she urinates and to squeeze the muscles to stop the stream of urine. If she can accomplish this, the muscles are contracted and it is possible for her to perform the exercise. Muscles of abdomen, thighs, and buttocks should *not* tighten during pelvic floor muscle training. Women should be taught to exhale and keep the mouth open to avoid bearing down when contracting their pelvic muscles, and then gradually relax the muscle contraction. Variations exist about how frequently to repeat pelvic muscle contractions each day. To maintain pelvic muscle tone, the woman should continue pelvic floor or Kegel exercises for the rest of her life (Lentz, 2012a; National Institute of Diabetes and Digestive and Kidney Diseases [NIDDKD], 2016, 2014).

Graduated weight cones may be used as an adjunct to pelvic muscle exercise. Incrementally weighted cones are inserted into the vagina, and the woman attempts to hold the weights in place. As the weight of the cones increases, the resistance against which the pelvic muscles contract increases, thereby strengthening the pelvic muscles (Lentz, 2012c).

Measures that help reduce the symptoms of pelvic relaxation also may prove helpful. These include lying down with the legs elevated for a few minutes several times a day. Some women are relieved by assuming a knee-chest position for a few minutes. In addition, teaching may include measures to prevent constipation.

Urinary Incontinence. Evaluation of the characteristics of a woman's urinary incontinence guides treatment. The following are three major patterns (Lentz, 2012c; NIDDKD, 2014):

- Stress incontinence, with urine leakage occurring as the woman increases her intraabdominal pressure. Examples of times when intraabdominal pressure may increase sufficiently include coughing, sneezing, laughter, or physical exertion such as picking up a full shopping bag or heavier load.

- Urge incontinence, characterized by urine leakage that accompanies a woman's strong need to void promptly.
- Mixed incontinence, in which a woman's urine leakage has associated factors from both the stress and the urge incontinence patterns.

Overactive bladder (OAB) may occur with both urge and mixed incontinence. OAB is characterized by frequent sensations of urgency and nocturia and may accompany neurologic, anatomic, or structural disorders.

Direct questions such as "Do you have trouble with your bladder?" or "Do you ever unintentionally lose urine?" may encourage women to discuss urine control problems. After the subject is introduced, follow-up questions are asked to determine urinary frequency. For instance, can she sit through a 2-hour movie without emptying her bladder? How many times does she get up to urinate each night? Does she often feel she must hurry to empty her bladder and that she will lose urine while going to the restroom?

Nursing research has shown that continence can be improved by teaching specific health promotion activities, such as pelvic floor exercises and bladder training, which involves adhering to a prescribed schedule for emptying the bladder. Women who cannot execute even a weak pelvic muscle contraction or are unable to implement bladder training may benefit from biofeedback or electrical stimulation provided by a skilled practitioner (Lentz, 2012c; NIDDKD, 2014).

Women often benefit from knowing about some of the commercial products that protect the skin and prevent odor. These products are made of material that traps urine and prevents constant contact with the skin.

Women often restrict fluids, thinking this will decrease urinary incontinence. Restricting fluids may actually make the condition worse because the bladder does not fill to its normal capacity. Furthermore, decreased fluid intake can lead to concentrated urine that can irritate bladder mucous membranes and increase the urge to void. Alcohol and caffeine also can irritate the bladder and worsen incontinence. Obesity is associated with urinary incontinence, increasing the benefits for a woman to achieve her ideal weight range.

Drug treatment may enhance bladder control. Drugs that may be prescribed include (Lentz, 2012c; NIDDKD, 2014):

- Vaginal estrogen using a cream, tablet, or vaginal ring to reduce atrophy of the urinary and vaginal areas.
- Anticholinergic drugs, including their long-acting versions, such as oxybutynin (Ditropan) or tolterodine (Detrol).
- Other drugs are being studied for possible use in improving bladder control.

❓ KNOWLEDGE CHECK

32. How does cystocele differ from rectocele in terms of location? Symptoms?
33. What causes uterine prolapse, and how is it treated?
34. What are nursing actions to alleviate problems associated with pelvic floor relaxation? Urinary incontinence?

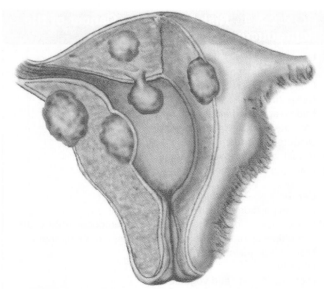

FIG. 27.6 Sites within the uterus where fibroids commonly occur.

DISORDERS OF THE REPRODUCTIVE TRACT

Benign Disorders

The most common benign conditions of the reproductive tract include cervical polyps, uterine leiomyomas (fibroids), and ovarian cysts.

Cervical Polyps

Polyps are small tumors, usually only a few millimeters in diameter, that are generally on a pedicle (a stalk or stem-like structure). They are caused by proliferation of cervical mucosa and often cause intermittent vaginal bleeding.

Cervical polyps are surgically removed in an outpatient setting, and the specimen is sent for pathologic examination to rule out malignancy.

Uterine Leiomyomas

Leiomyomas, also called *fibroids,* are one of the most common gynecologic conditions encountered. Although the cause is unknown, they develop from uterine smooth muscle cells and are estrogen dependent. As a result, they grow rapidly during the childbearing years, when estrogen is abundant, but shrink during menopause unless growth is maintained by HRT for menopausal symptoms. Fibroids may occur throughout the muscular layer of the uterus and may be prominent near the end of pregnancy as the estrogen levels are high and the uterus is large (Fig. 27.6).

Uterine fibroids do not often cause symptoms. Uterine size is sometimes increased, and excessive menstrual bleeding may occur. Excessive bleeding may result in anemia, weakness, and fatigue. Infertility may be related to uterine fibroids. Additional symptoms include feelings of pelvic pressure, bloating, and urinary frequency that occur when the tumor applies pressure on the bladder. Pressure on the ureter may cause hydroureter (dilation of the ureter). Many symptoms of fibroids depend on the location of the benign uterine tumors.

Treatment depends on multiple factors, including the size, number, and location of the fibroids; the symptoms experienced; whether future childbearing is desired; and how near the woman is to natural menopause. In the absence of symptoms, treatment may consist of observation only. If abnormal bleeding is a problem, surgical intervention may be necessary. Hysterectomy may be appropriate for the woman who does not desire future childbearing. Myomectomy, or removal of the fibroid from uterine muscle, may be an option for the woman who desires future children. Uterine artery embolization (UAE) is a procedure focused on reducing the fibroid size by introducing obstruction in the arteries that supply the fibroid. Pregnancy after UAE is often more likely to have intrauterine growth restriction or preterm birth (Katz, 2012a).

Medical treatment with progesterone-only or combination estrogen-progesterone oral contraceptives may reduce excess menstrual flow. Short courses of GnRH agonists may be effective in reducing the size of myomas and lessen symptoms before surgical removal. GnRH agonists cause hot flashes, vaginal dryness, and other discomforts similar to those of menopause and therefore are not tolerated well by some women. Loss of bone mineral density is an adverse effect of long-term therapy (Katz, 2012a).

Ovarian Cysts

An ovarian cyst may be either follicular or luteal. If the ovarian follicle fails to rupture during ovulation, a follicular cyst may develop. These cysts are usually asymptomatic and may be an incidental finding on an ultrasound. They generally regress during the subsequent menstrual cycle. A lutein cyst may develop if the corpus luteum becomes cystic and fails to regress. A lutein cyst is more likely to cause pain and delay in the next menstrual cycle. Occasionally, an ovarian cyst can rupture or twist on its pedicle and become infarcted, causing pelvic pain and tenderness (Katz, 2012a).

Treatment depends on differentiating a cyst from a solid ovarian tumor that is more likely to indicate cancer. If the woman is in her childbearing years, when the risk for ovarian cancer is less, the physician may wait until after the next menstrual cycle and examine the woman again. Transvaginal ultrasound examination is useful to determine whether it is a fluid-filled cyst or a solid tumor. Laparoscopy may be helpful in ruling out endometriosis. **Laparotomy** (visualization of abdominal or pelvic organs through incision) may be necessary to remove the cyst from the ovary for examination by a pathologist.

Malignant Disorders

The primary sites for cancer in the female reproductive organs are the uterus, ovaries, and cervix. Cancer of the vagina, vulva, and fallopian tubes is relatively uncommon.

CRITICAL TO REMEMBER

Symptoms That Always Should Be Investigated

Irregular vaginal bleeding
Unexplained perimenopausal or postmenopausal bleeding
Unusual vaginal discharge
Dyspareunia
Persistent vulvar or vaginal itching
Elevated or discolored lesions of the vulva
Persistent abdominal bloating or constipation
Persistent anorexia or vomiting
Blood in stools

Although cancer can occur at any age, the incidence increases with age.

Signs and Symptoms

Cancer of the reproductive organs may not be diagnosed until it is advanced because few symptoms are experienced in the early stages. When symptoms occur, they are often nonspecific and could be caused by infection or other benign conditions. Cancer of the ovaries is particularly difficult to diagnose because it may remain "silent" until far advanced, when the chance of long-term survival is greatly reduced.

Risk Factors

Risk factors vary according to the site of the cancer. Risk factors for cervical cancer include a history of STDs, particularly **condyloma acuminatum**, also known as genital warts, caused by the HPV. Prolonged use of unopposed ERT (estrogen-only) predisposes to overgrowth (hyperplasia) of endometrial tissue and is a significant risk factor for uterine cancer. See Box 27.9 for a summary of risk factors for cancer of the reproductive organs.

Diagnosis

Early diagnosis is strongly associated with long-term survival. Many screening and diagnostic tests are useful. Screening tests include periodic pelvic examinations, Pap tests, ultrasonography, and serum tests for tumor markers such as CA-125, which may be increased with ovarian or other cancers. Genes linked to other cancers, such as *BRCA1* or *BRCA2* mutations, may lead to more diagnostic procedures than if the genetic risk is not apparent. Significant family history of specific cancers of the reproductive organs or linked cancers such as breast and ovarian cancers may alter the risk for a woman's development of cancer. Diagnostic procedures such as endometrial biopsy for endometrial cancer and **colposcopy** (examination with a colposcope to magnify cells) can identify patterns of abnormality near the cervical os, where most cancers of the cervix develop. Specific strains of HPV infection are a significant risk factor for cervical cancer even if the original infection has healed.

BOX 27.9   Risk Factors for Cancer of the Reproductive Organs

Uterus
African-Americans: Higher risk for leiomyosarcoma
Obesity
Nulliparity
Middle-aged and elderly
Late menopause (>52 years old)
Diabetes mellitus
Breast, colon, or ovarian cancer
Estrogen replacement therapy

Cervix
Human papillomavirus (HPV) infection
Sexual risks: Young age at start of intercourse (<20 years), multiple sexual partners, uncircumcised male partners
Many pregnancies
Obesity
Diet low in fruits and vegetables
Smoking
Lower socioeconomic status (may be related to infrequent gynecologic examinations)
History of sexually transmitted diseases, such as chlamydia or human immunodeficiency virus (HIV) infection

Ovaries
Menses started at younger than 12 years of age
No child or first child after 30 years of age
Late menopause (>55 years old)
Infertility, infertility drugs
Family history of ovarian, breast, or colorectal cancer
Personal history of breast cancer

Management

Treatment of cancer of the reproductive organs is based on the location and extent of the disease and the age and desire of the woman to have children. The extent of surgical treatment for these cancers varies with the tumor size, degree of malignancy, and extent of spread beyond the primary tumor site. Chemotherapy and radiation oncology therapy supplement surgical treatment for many invasive cancers.

Treatment of one type of cancer may be based on previous cancer treatment in the same or related organs. For instance, treatment of previous breast cancer with the chemotherapy drug Adriamycin often means that the woman has reached the maximum lifetime amount that she can take because of the drug's effects on her heart. Drugs such as anastrozole (Arimidex) and exemestane (Aromasin), aromatase inhibitors, may reduce estrogen secretion that increases cancer growth in most breast and reproductive organs.

Cervical Cancer. Testing for HPV often reveals the cervical infection that contributes to cancer. A biopsy of the suspicious area and an endocervical curettage are done for diagnosis if the woman is not pregnant. A vaccine against the HPV strains that are most likely to cause genital warts and cervical cancer (Gardasil) has been released. HPV vaccine is most likely to be effective before sexual activity begins, with the first dose of three being given at 13 to 26 years or as young as 9 years.

A lesion of early cervical cancer is usually a squamous intraepithelial lesion (SIL). Early treatment of cervical cancer may consist of cryosurgery, destruction of abnormal tissue by laser, loop electrosurgical excision procedure (LEEP), or surgical conization to remove the central cervix. Regular surveillance after cervical cancer therapy is recommended to identify recurrence, particularly in the woman who had a high-grade SIL, whose risk for repeated cervical cancer is greater.

Treatment for advanced cervical cancer usually consists of a total abdominal hysterectomy and bilateral salpingo-oophorectomy. Removal of the uterus and ovaries and **sentinel lymph node (SLN) biopsy** may be done via laparoscopy. Adjuvant therapy with radiation and chemotherapy is likely (Jhingran & Levenback, 2012).

Endometrial Cancer. Abnormal vaginal bleeding, usually near or after menopause, is the most common presentation for endometrial cancer. Cancer of the endometrium is the most common cancer of the female reproductive organs. The American Cancer Society (2016c) estimates for cancer of the uterus in the United States for 2016 are that approximately 60,050 new cases of cancer of the body of the uterus (uterine body or corpus) will be diagnosed and about 10,470 women will die of cancers of the uterine body. Although endometrial cancer occurs more often in a postmenopausal woman, about one-fourth of the cases may occur in premenopausal women. However, endometrial cancer in the older woman is likely to be more advanced. The highest cure rate is with surgery (hysterectomy and salpingo-oophorectomy) followed by adjuvant chemotherapy and/or radiation therapy. Poor surgical candidates may be treated with only chemotherapy or radiation (Soliman & Lu, 2012).

Ovarian Cancer. Women with ovarian cancer may be asymptomatic, or they may seek care for abdominal or pelvic pain, increased abdominal girth, and sometimes abnormal bleeding. Total abdominal hysterectomy, bilateral salpingo-oophorectomy, and removal of ovarian tissue in the pelvis may be curative for women in the earliest stages of ovarian cancer. Surgery for more advanced ovarian cancer improves diagnostic information, allows more accurate staging, and permits surgical reduction of the cancer. Ovarian cancer is usually treated by surgery followed by chemotherapy. However, it may be treated by chemotherapy to reduce the tumor's size, followed by hysterectomy and bilateral salpingo-oophorectomy. A second surgery may be done to determine whether more surgical or adjuvant treatment is needed. Chemotherapy is required after surgery for all but the very early cancers. The 5-year survival rate varies with the stage at diagnosis and response to chemotherapy (Coleman, Ramirez, & Gershenson, 2012).

❓ KNOWLEDGE CHECK

35. What are the signs and symptoms of leiomyomas (uterine fibroids), and how are they treated?
36. Why is ultrasonography used to evaluate ovarian cysts?
37. What signs and symptoms suggest possible cancer of the reproductive organs and should always be investigated?
38. How may cancer of the following reproductive organs be treated: Cervix? Endometrium? Ovary?

INFECTIOUS DISORDERS OF THE REPRODUCTIVE TRACT

Infections of the reproductive tract may cause a variety of problems for women of all ages. Although some (such as candidiasis) are mostly annoying, others (such as HIV) may be lethal. Some infections are seldom associated with sexual activity, whereas others are almost exclusively spread in this way. Infections may spread silently in the reproductive organs, allowing damage to the organs before the woman has symptoms.

Candidiasis

Candidiasis, also known as *moniliasis* and *yeast infection,* is the most common form of vaginitis. The cause is believed to be related to a change in vaginal pH that allows accelerated growth of *Candida albicans,* a yeastlike fungus commonly found in the digestive tract and on the skin. Some conditions, such as pregnancy, diabetes mellitus, oral contraceptive use, and systemic antibiotic therapy, result in changes in vaginal pH and flora that favor accelerated growth of *C. albicans.* Although not considered an STD (also abbreviated STI for sexually transmitted infections), recurrent candidiasis in sexually active women may occur. A small number of male partners may have erythema and itching of their glans penis (balanitis).

The main symptoms for candidiasis are vaginal and perineal itching. Vulvar and vaginal tissues are inflamed, causing burning on urination. Vaginal discharge is white with a typical "cottage cheese" appearance. Diagnosis is made by identifying the spores of *C. albicans.*

Treatment may consist of nonprescription or prescription medications. Medications available without prescription include butoconazole, miconazole, clotrimazole, terconazole, and tioconazole by vaginal application. The duration for most of the nonprescription medications for candidiasis ranges from 3 to 7 days, depending on the specific medication. Women should be advised to seek medical attention with the first infection or if the infection persists or recurs frequently. Oral fluconazole is a prescription medication for treatment of candidiasis with a single dose. Patients with more severe candidiasis may need another dose of fluconazole in 4 days. Recurrent yeast infections that resist treatment are associated with diabetes mellitus or HIV infection.

Sexually Transmitted Diseases

Many diseases can be transmitted through sexual activity. For some diseases, such as syphilis, gonorrhea, and chlamydial infection, sexual activity is almost the only method of transmission. For other diseases, such as bacterial vaginosis, sexual activity may or may not be the mode of transmission.

Incidence

STDs are most frequent among adolescents and young adults. Because the vagina and microscopic tears in mucosa from intercourse provide favorable conditions for infection, women are twice as likely as men to get an STD. The number of untreated infected individuals with no symptoms is most likely immense. For many reasons these infections remain a major health problem despite advancements in the development of antibiotics. The age of the first sexual experience has been declining steadily, and sexual activity is high among adolescents and young adults. The immature vaginal mucosa of the young adolescent is more easily injured during sexual activity. Multiple sexual partners, inadequate knowledge of transmission and prevention, and feelings of invincibility are common among this age group (CDC, 2015a).

Methods of contraception have a significant impact on the risk for STDs. Barrier methods, such as condoms and female condoms, offer the best protection from infection. Diaphragms, cervical caps, and spermicidal foams and jellies do not offer the same protection as condoms, although they can decrease the risk for cervical and upper genital tract infections. When counseling teen girls and boys, nurses should emphasize that oral contraceptives can prevent pregnancy but do nothing to prevent exposure to STDs.

Major concerns include the following:

- The vulnerability of women, especially teens, to STDs
- The resistance of some organisms to antibiotics
- The relationship between HIV infection and other STDs
- Failure of asymptomatic persons to seek treatment when their sexual partner is infected

See Chapter 10 for information on the impact of STDs on pregnancy and the fetus.

Types of Sexually Transmitted Diseases

Trichomoniasis. Trichomoniasis is caused by *Trichomonas vaginalis,* a protozoon that thrives in an alkaline environment. The presenting symptoms include a purulent vaginal discharge that is thin or frothy, malodorous, and yellow-green or brownish-gray. The pH of the discharge is usually greater than 4.5. Vulvar itching, edema, and redness may be present. The diagnosis is made by identifying the organism in a wet mount preparation.

Treatments of choice are metronidazole (Flagyl) 2 g or tinidazole (Tindamax) 2 g in a single oral dose. *Alcohol ingestion when taking metronidazole may result in a disulfiram-like (Antabuse) reaction.* Women should be advised to avoid using alcohol during treatment with metronidazole and for 24 hours after treatment is complete.

Sexual partners should refrain from intercourse until a cure is established. Reinfection may result when the woman's partner is not treated. In particular, emphasize that all sexual partners should be treated and that condoms should be used with a new partner (CDC, 2015a; Eckert & Lentz, 2012).

Bacterial Vaginosis. This infection, previously referred to as *nonspecific vaginitis,* is associated with organisms that replace normal lactobacilli with *Gardnerella vaginalis* or *Mycoplasma hominis* or with anaerobic bacteria, such as *Prevotella* or *Mobiluncus.* Causes of the bacterial proliferation are not known, although tissue trauma and vaginal intercourse have been identified as contributing factors. Multiple partners, douching, and lack of vaginal lactobacilli are associated with bacterial vaginosis.

Chief signs and symptoms are a thin, grayish-white vaginal discharge that typically exudes a fishy odor. The diagnosis is made by preparing a saline wet mount and identifying characteristic clue cells (epithelial cells with numerous bacilli clinging to their surface).

Treatment for bacterial vaginosis is directed toward reestablishing the balance of flora in the vagina. Metronidazole has been shown to relieve symptoms and improve vaginal flora. Clindamycin is an alternative treatment. The woman should refrain from sexual intercourse until cured, or her partner should use a condom. Treatment of her partner has not proved beneficial (CDC, 2015a; Eckert & Lentz, 2012).

Chlamydial Infection. The most common STD in Western countries is caused by the gram-negative bacterium *C. trachomatis.* The incidence is particularly high in sexually active teens and young adults. Chlamydial infection is often asymptomatic in women, which makes diagnosis and control of the disease difficult. It should be suspected when the male sexual partner is treated for nongonococcal urethritis and when the culture results for gonorrhea are negative, yet the woman exhibits symptoms similar to those of gonorrhea, such as a yellowish vaginal discharge and painful urination. Gonorrhea and chlamydial infections often coexist.

Diagnosis of chlamydial infection can be made by isolating the bacterium in tissue culture, by enzyme-linked immunosorbent assay (ELISA), or by direct fluorescent monoclonal antibody. Tissue culture of the organism is most accurate but requires more time.

Untreated, chlamydial infection ascends from the cervix to involve the fallopian tubes and is one of the chief causes of tubal scarring that results in pelvic inflammatory disease (PID), infertility, or ectopic pregnancy. Treatment is usually directed to eradicate both chlamydia and gonorrhea because the two often coexist. Treatment options include azithromycin (Zithromax), doxycycline (Vibramycin), ofloxacin (Floxin), levofloxacin (Levaquin), and erythromycin. Treatment of all sexual partners is essential to prevent recurrence and further spread. Use of condoms until a cure is established is essential as well.

Gonorrhea. Gonorrhea is an infection of the genitourinary tract that is caused by the gonococcus *Neisseria gonorrhoeae.* Gonorrhea may be asymptomatic in women, but when symptoms do occur, they usually include purulent discharge, **dysuria,** or painful urination, and dyspareunia. Diagnosis is based on a positive culture for the gonococcus. Gonorrhea is associated with PID (which increases the risk for tubal scarring and can result in infertility or ectopic pregnancy), as is chlamydial infection.

Dual treatment of gonorrhea and chlamydial infections is often routine. Additional drugs to those previously discussed for chlamydia with gonorrhea infections include cefixime (Suprax), ceftriaxone (Rocephin), and ciprofloxacin (Cipro). All sexual partners should be treated simultaneously, and intercourse should be avoided or the man should use a condom until a cure is confirmed.

Syphilis. Syphilis is caused by the spirochete *Treponema pallidum,* and it is divided into primary, secondary, and tertiary stages. The first sign of primary syphilis is a painless chancre that develops on the genitalia, anus, or lips or in the oral cavity. At this time, diagnosis is made by identifying the spirochete on dark-field microscopy in material scraped from the base of the chancre. Serologic test results are generally negative in the primary stage. If untreated, the chancre heals in about 6 weeks. The disease is highly infectious at the primary stage.

Although the chancre disappears, the spirochete lives and is carried by the blood to all parts of the body. About 2 months after the initial infection, infected people exhibit symptoms of secondary syphilis, including enlargement of the spleen and liver, headache, anorexia, and a generalized maculopapular skin rash. Skin eruptions, called *condylomata lata,* may develop on the vulva during this time. Condylomata lata resemble warts; they contain numerous spirochetes and are highly contagious. Serologic test results are generally positive at this time.

If untreated, the disease enters a latent phase that may last for several years. Tertiary syphilis, which follows the latent phase, may involve the heart, blood vessels, and central nervous system. General paralysis and psychosis may result.

In addition to identification of the spirochete in material scraped from a chancre, diagnosis is also made by serology. The usual screening test is the Venereal Disease Research Laboratory (VDRL) serum test, which is based on the presence of antibodies produced in response to the infection. The rapid plasma reagin (RPR) and fluorescent treponemal antibody absorption (FTA-ABS) tests are more specific and are often done to confirm a positive VDRL test.

The best treatment of all stages of syphilis is with parenteral penicillin G. A woman who is allergic to penicillin can be admitted to the hospital for desensitization to penicillin followed by administration of the drug (CDC, 2015a).

Herpes Genitalis. Herpes genitalis is an STD caused by the herpes simplex virus (HSV). Two types of HSV have been identified: type 1 and type 2. HSV-2 usually causes genital lesions, and HSV-1 usually causes oropharyngeal infection. However, either organism may infect the less-frequent location. Transmission occurs through direct contact with an infected person. A person infected with HSV-1 develops antibodies that may reduce the severity of the first HSV-2 infection. A primary HSV-2 infection is one in which the person had no preceding HSV-1 infection and therefore has no antibodies. Transmission may occur from a partner who

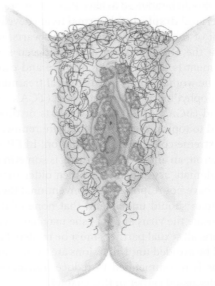

FIG. 27.7 Condylomata acuminata, also called *venereal* or *genital warts,* are caused by the human papillomavirus (HPV).

is infected but has no visible lesions or symptomatic viral shedding.

Within 2 to 12 days after the primary infection, vesicles (blisters) appear in a characteristic cluster on the vulva, perineum, or perianal area. The initial lesions may cause severe vulvar pain and tenderness as well as dyspareunia. Lesions also may occur on the cervix or in the vagina. With primary infection, the woman may experience flulike symptoms, including fever, general malaise, and enlarged lymph nodes. The vesicles rupture within 1 to 7 days and form ulcers that take an average of 7 to 10 days to heal.

When symptoms abate, the virus remains dormant in the nerve ganglia and periodically reactivates, particularly in times of stress, fever, and menses. Recurrent episodes are seldom as extensive or painful as the initial episode, but they are just as contagious. Diagnosis is often based on clinical signs and symptoms and confirmed by viral culture of fluid from the vesicle.

No cure exists, but antiviral drugs reduce or suppress symptoms, shedding, and recurrent episodes. Antiviral drugs include acyclovir (Zovirax), famciclovir (Famvir), and valacyclovir (Valtrex). Women should be advised to abstain from sexual contact while the lesions are present to avoid transmission to their partner. If it is an initial infection, they should continue to abstain until they become culture-negative, because prolonged viral shedding may occur in such cases.

Human Papillomavirus. Condylomata acuminata, also known as venereal or genital warts, are caused by HPV. The dry, wartlike growths may be small and discrete, or they may cluster and resemble cauliflower (Fig. 27.7). Common sites include the vagina, labia, cervix, and perineal area.

Condylomata acuminata are of particular concern because of the association of HPV with cervical cancer. Colposcopy, examination by a magnifying instrument called the colposcope, is generally recommended to evaluate abnormal cervical tissue and to identify HPV. Women with condylomata acuminata should be advised to have Pap tests more frequently to detect cervical **dysplasia** (abnormal tissue development).

The goal of treatment is to remove the warts, which easily transmit the HPV back and forth between sexual partners. Treatment is determined by the site and extent of the warts and the woman's preference. Topical treatment options include podophyllin, trichloroacetic acid (TCA), and bichloroacetic acid (BCA). More extensive warts or those that do not respond to topical therapy may require removal by **cryotherapy** (extreme cold), laser vaporization, LEEP, or conization. Interferon, an antineoplastic drug, is sometimes used to treat condylomata acuminata in women older than 18 years of age who have not responded to conventional therapy.

The woman should understand that none of these treatments eradicate the virus and that she may have recurrences. Furthermore, all sexual partners must be treated. Sexual contact should be avoided until all lesions are healed, and the use of condoms is recommended to reduce transmission. HPV vaccine is discussed earlier in this chapter.

Acquired Immunodeficiency Syndrome. Acquired immunodeficiency syndrome (AIDS), caused by HIV, remains the most devastating STD in the world today, although new treatments have improved the outlook considerably. HIV has been isolated from blood, semen, vaginal secretions, urine, saliva, tears, cerebrospinal fluid, amniotic fluid, and breast milk. The primary modes of transmission are intimate contact with infected bodily secretions, exposure to infected blood and blood products, and perinatal transmission from mother to infant.

HIV testing is routine for all pregnant women so treatment can be started if needed, possibly avoiding transmission to the fetus. A woman's risk for infection through a heterosexual relationship has surpassed the risk that her HIV infection stems from injectable drug use. Diagnosis of another STD is an indication for HIV testing, as is the patient who has repeated infections such as herpes virus or candidiasis. The health care provider should address concerns if a pregnant woman refuses testing or if she refuses retesting with subsequent pregnancies because the first test was negative. Consent for HIV testing should be incorporated into the plan of care (verbally or written). Patients also have the right to decline or "opt-out" of routine HIV testing (CDC, 2016a).

No medications have been shown to cure HIV and AIDS. Research continues about the benefits and safety of drug regimens that interrupt production of the virus. See Chapter 10 for a discussion of HIV and AIDS management in pregnant women and neonates. Updated guidelines for HIV and AIDS treatment in the pediatric, adult, and perinatal groups may be found at the AIDS Info website, a service of the NIH, at www.aidsinfo.nih.gov.

PATIENT TEACHING

Sexually Transmitted Diseases

What are the most common signs and symptoms of sexually transmitted diseases (STDs)?

Unexpected nonbloody vaginal discharge (increased amount, unusual color, or odor) or vaginal bleeding.

Vulvar itching or swelling.

Pelvic pain, including painful intercourse, painful urination, and abdominal tenderness.

Skin eruptions or changes (rashes, ulcers, warts, blisters).

Flulike symptoms (fever, swollen or painful lymph glands, loss of appetite, nausea or vomiting).

Presence of symptoms in a sexual partner, even if symptoms are absent in the woman.

What are the common methods of diagnosis?

Culture (vaginal discharge, cervix, lesions) to identify organism.

Blood test (serology) to determine whether antibodies for specific diseases are present.

VDRL, RPR, or FTA-ABS test for syphilis; HIV test for human immunodeficiency virus.

How can STDs be prevented?

Establish monogamous relationship with uninfected partner.

Limit number of sexual partners.

Use mechanical and chemical barriers such as a latex condom with every act of intercourse.

Remember that one episode of an STD offers no protection from future infection.

Make sure partner is simultaneously treated to prevent reinfection.

What are the most important things to know about the treatment?

The entire course of medication should be completed even if symptoms subside.

Comply with follow-up evaluation as recommended by the health care provider.

Curtail sexual intercourse until free of infection.

Partner should be examined and treated and a follow-up evaluation done before sexual intercourse is resumed.

Side effects of medications, such as skin rashes, difficulty breathing, or headaches, should be reported.

Not all STDs can be cured (herpes, AIDS, venereal warts), treatment is aimed at slowing the disease and preventing complications.

Are there measures that provide comfort and prevent secondary infections?

Keep the vulva clean but avoid strong soaps, creams, and ointments unless prescribed by the health care provider.

Keep the vulva dry; using a hair dryer on low heat is helpful.

Wear absorbent cotton underwear and avoid pantyhose and tight pants as much as possible.

Take analgesics (aspirin or acetaminophen) as directed by the health care provider.

Cool or tepid sitz baths may provide relief from itching.

Wipe vulva from front to back after urination or defecation, and then carefully wash hands.

AIDS, Acquired immunodeficiency syndrome; *FTA-ABS,* fluorescent treponemal antibody absorption; *HIV,* human immunodeficiency virus; *RPR,* rapid plasma reagin; *VDRL,* Venereal Disease Research Laboratory.

Nursing Considerations

As teachers and counselors, nurses can play a major part in preventing the spread of STDs and treating specific infections. Women must often be encouraged to use preventive measures to avoid infection, including HIV infection, from a man who does not want to use condoms as a barrier to infection. To fulfill this role, nurses should be prepared to do the following:

- Teach the signs and symptoms that require medical attention.
- Explain diagnostic or screening tests and follow-up testing needed for some infections.
- Teach preventive measures and follow-up care.
- Identify STD preventive measures that are compatible with age, language, male-female relationships in the woman's culture, values for her own well-being, frequency of intercourse, number of partners, and many other factors that may be identified when the woman seeks care.
- Refer the woman to support groups and HIV specialists for best treatment options and follow-up if she has HIV infection.

KNOWLEDGE CHECK

39. What conditions may change the normal flora of the vagina and result in *C. albicans* vaginitis?
40. How does the vaginal discharge of candidiasis differ from that of trichomoniasis?
41. Why are barrier-type contraceptives recommended to prevent STDs?
42. How do primary and secondary syphilis differ in terms of signs and symptoms and potential for transmitting the disease?
43. How are condylomata acuminata associated with cervical cancer?

Pelvic Inflammatory Disease

Pelvic inflammatory disease (PID) infection of the upper genital tract, is a serious health problem in the United States. About 1 million women develop PID each year in the United States, and many of them have ectopic pregnancy or infertility as added complications. Women who are under 25 years of age are more likely to develop PID because the cervix is not fully matured, increasing their susceptibility to infectious organisms that ascend into the uterus, fallopian tubes, ovaries, and other pelvic organs. Exposure to multiple sexual partners increases the risk for acquiring an infection that causes PID. Douching increases the risk for PID because it changes the natural vaginal flora that helps resist infection and pushes infectious organisms toward the uterine cavity (CDC, 2016c; Eckert & Lentz, 2012).

Etiology

Most PID cases are caused by *C. trachomatis* and *N. gonorrhoeae* infections. The remainder are caused by a variety of aerobic and anaerobic organisms such as *Escherichia coli*, *G. vaginalis*, *Streptococcus*, group B *Streptococcus*, *Peptostreptococcus*, *Peptococcus*, *Bacteroides* species, *Prevotella*, *Mycoplasma genitalium*, *Ureaplasma*, and cytomegalovirus (CMV) (CDC, 2016c). These organisms invade the endocervical canal, where they cause cervicitis. Microorganisms ascend and infect the endometrium, fallopian tubes, and pelvic cavity. The chronic inflammatory response results in tubal scarring and peritubal adhesions, which interfere with conception or with transport of the fertilized ovum through the obstructed fallopian tubes to the uterus. Inadequate treatment of a vaginal infection increases the risk that the organisms will ascend into the uterus, infecting deeper reproductive structures and causing PID.

Symptoms

Signs and symptoms of PID vary widely. Some women are asymptomatic or have subtle symptoms, whereas others experience pelvic pain, fever, purulent vaginal discharge, nausea, anorexia, and irregular vaginal bleeding. Findings during physical examination may include abdominal or **adnexal** (accessory organs) tenderness and tenderness of the uterus and cervix when they are moved during bimanual examination (cervical motion tenderness). Laboratory evaluation may reveal a marked leukocytosis and increased sedimentation rate. A urinalysis is needed to rule out UTI. Cultures for *N. gonorrhoeae*, *C. trachomatis*, or other suspected infectious organisms help diagnose and best treat PID.

Management

Women with serious infection, as manifested by fever, abdominal pain, and leukocytosis, may be admitted to a hospital. They are most often treated with IV administration of broad-spectrum antibiotics such as ceftriaxone plus azithromycin or doxycycline, or cefixime plus azithromycin or doxycycline. IV antibiotic treatment usually can be changed to oral treatment after 48 hours, and the total duration of antibiotic therapy should be 14 days. Laparoscopy may be required to rule out surgical emergencies such as appendicitis or ectopic pregnancy, which have similar signs and symptoms, and to obtain specimens for culture. Pelvic abscess often requires surgical treatment. Outpatient treatment is appropriate for some women who are not as ill and will comply with the recommended regimen (CDC, 2015a; Fantasia, 2013).

Nursing Considerations

Nurses can play an important role in preventing PID by teaching women how to prevent STDs in themselves and in their partners. Prevention can be thought of as occurring on two levels: primary and secondary. Primary prevention involves avoiding exposure to these diseases or preventing acquisition of infection during exposure. Primary preventive measures include limiting the number of sexual partners and avoiding intercourse with those who have had multiple partners or other high-risk behaviors such as injectable drug use, which is associated with HIV infection. Barrier methods (latex condoms) used consistently and correctly during all sexual activity help prevent STDs.

Secondary prevention involves keeping a lower genital tract infection from ascending to the upper genital tract or from being further transmitted within the community. This involves seeking medical attention promptly after having unprotected sex with someone who is suspected of having an STD and when vaginal discharge or genital lesions are apparent. Periodic medical assessment is necessary if a woman is not in a mutually monogamous relationship, even if she is asymptomatic. Additional measures include taking medication as prescribed and returning for follow-up evaluation.

Toxic Shock Syndrome

Although **toxic shock syndrome** is rare, it is a potentially fatal condition caused by toxin-producing strains of *Staphylococcus aureus*. The toxin alters capillary permeability, which allows intravascular fluid to leak from the blood vessels, leading to hypovolemia, hypotension, and shock. The toxin also causes direct tissue damage to organs and precipitates serious defects in coagulation.

If toxin-producing strains of *S. aureus* inhabit the vagina, certain factors increase the risk that the toxin will gain entry into the bloodstream. These include the use of high-absorbency tampons during menstruation and barrier methods of contraception (cervical cap or diaphragm), both of which may trap and hold bacteria if left in place for a prolonged time. However, about 50% of cases are not related to menses. Persons having had nasal surgery or previous *S. aureus* wound infections also have a greater risk.

Symptoms of toxic shock syndrome include a sudden spiking fever (38.9°C [102°F]) and flulike symptoms (headache, sore throat, vomiting, diarrhea), hypotension, a generalized rash resembling sunburn, and skin peeling from the palms of the hands and the soles of the feet 1 and 2 weeks after the onset of the illness.

Treatment consists of fluid replacement, administration of vasopressor drugs, and antimicrobial therapy. Corticosteroids may be used to treat skin changes.

Nurses are often responsible for providing information that may help prevent toxic shock syndrome. Nurses should instruct women to do the following:

- Tampon use
  - Wash the hands thoroughly to remove bacteria before inserting tampons.
  - Change tampons at least every 4 hours to prevent excessive bacterial growth on a tampon that is left in place for a longer time.
  - Do not use superabsorbent tampons at any time because they may be left in the vagina for a prolonged period, allowing bacteria to proliferate.
  - Use pads rather than tampons during hours of sleep, which usually exceeds 4-hour segments of tampon use.
- Diaphragm or cervical cap use
  - Wash hands thoroughly before inserting a diaphragm or cervical cap.

- Do not use a diaphragm or cervical cap during menstrual periods.
- Remove a diaphragm or cervical cap within the time recommended by the health care provider.

> ### ❓ KNOWLEDGE CHECK
> 44. What organisms cause PID?
> 45. How can the risk of toxic shock syndrome be reduced?

◆ APPLICATION OF THE NURSING PROCESS: PROMOTING WOMEN'S HEALTH

Nurses may find themselves having the pleasure of promoting a woman's health rather than mostly finding problems with it. Promoting health can improve outcomes for families, not just individual women. This Application of the Nursing Process is slightly different from the previous ones in that it uses a case study to demonstrate use of the nursing process but also involves the woman in the process. Our reader should consider what he or she might do as a nurse.

◆ Assessment

Consider a 36-year-old woman who arrives for her annual well-woman examination (WWE). She is overweight and states that she eats too much food and "the kind that's bad for you." When giving her annual history, she states that many members of her family have diabetes. She also tells the nurse, "I don't want to be sick all the time like most of my family" and asks, "Can I change anything?"

This single mother also describes her 6- and 10-year-old children as "sitting around too much" and says that they are also overweight. She states that she wants her children not only to stay in school but also to be more active. She is aware that increasing her children's activity level will help prevent excess weight gain.

The woman is being seen for her WWE in an outpatient teaching clinic, and her care is provided by medical residents. She works at a fast food restaurant for varying hours per week. Health insurance is offered by the restaurant chain, but she cannot afford the premiums. She does qualify for Medicaid, so that is her major source of funding for medical care.

◆ Identification of Patient Problems

Although the woman has some obvious health problems and has financial limitations, she has indicated a personal desire to have better health for herself and her children. Her statements indicate that she is aware of the need to improve her actions but does not know the best way. An appropriate patient problem for the woman is "Opportunity for patient teaching due to a desire to take charge of her own health and influence the health of her children in a positive way."

◆ Planning: Expected Outcomes

Expected outcomes for this brief clinic visit are that the woman will do the following:

- Describe foods that she likes, can afford, and will help her lose weight.
- Explore how she might increase her own activity level and how she could include her children.

◆ Interventions

Reinforce the Woman's Desire for Change

Recognizing that the nurse values her desire to improve her health and that of her children helps motivate the woman to search for ways to make the changes she can accomplish over time. Explain how her actions to improve her own health set a positive example for her children, despite the family's financial limitations. Explain that she will have setbacks but that she does not need to abandon her positive change to improve her health and that of her children.

Identify Food Preferences

Determining what the woman eats regularly and what she enjoys the most helps the nurse identify beneficial aspects of her current diet and changes that might benefit her desire for better health. Ask her about food she eats during an average day, including the frequency and timing of meals. Ask her what foods she eats where she works. Identify what vegetables and fruits she eats and in what form (e.g., fresh or canned fruits or fruit snack cakes that have very little actual fruit and may be more costly). Describe what is good about her choices and basic changes that she should consider. Help her identify beneficial changes from what she says about her personal preferences and explore ways to make those changes within her limited budget.

Ask her if she eats breakfast and what she eats. Is it cereal with milk or is it leftover pizza? Explain to her that a nourishing breakfast for her and her children might be food that she had not considered. If she starts her day with adequate, nourishing food, even if it is leftovers, explain that she is less likely to overeat or eat nonnourishing food later in the day.

Drinking fewer soft drinks or bottled water might reduce an expense that the woman has not considered. If she says her vegetables are canned, ask her if they are brand name or generic and if she has considered using generic brands of food and other household products.

Teach the woman that information about good nutrition is often available by computer and that computers are available without charge at most public libraries.

Financial Assistance

Ask the woman if she receives any public assistance such as the Supplemental Nutrition Assistance Program (SNAP) (www.nutrition.gov), formerly the Food Stamps program. Refer her to the appropriate source for information about qualifications and application if she does not receive public assistance. Referral to a social worker may identify other sources for food such as a free lunch program for her children on school days or church or neighborhood groups that feed hungry people.

Activity

Explain that daily activity helps her burn calories and can improve her energy level. Explore ways she might increase her activity such as walking to work, the grocery store, or the post office. Help her evaluate whether it is realistic for her children to walk to school if she or another adult walks with them. What active games can she play with her children, perhaps at a nearby park?

◆ Evaluation

Although this encounter with the woman is brief, it is an opportunity for the nurse to reinforce her ability to achieve better health. As the woman lists foods she often eats during a day, the nurse can promote those that are good for her health and/or the health of her children but also help her find alternatives to less nutritious foods. Finding that the woman has discovered ways to increase her family's activity level meets the second outcome and can motivate the woman to seek more opportunities that might be possible.

SUMMARY CONCEPTS

- The Women's Health Initiative was a 15-year national study to address the best prevention and treatment for three major diseases that affect women as they age: cardiovascular disease, breast cancer, and osteoporosis.
- *Healthy People 2020* goals are health targets for the United States. Many goals address women's issues.
- Many women do not have a primary health care provider, such as a family physician or family nurse practitioner, and depend on their reproductive health provider for their regular health checks.
- A health history helps identify a woman's health problems and risks for specific problems, actions she can take to promote her health, and other measures needed to further improve her health.
- A complete physical assessment can identify general health problems and guide further testing that should be done.
- Major preventable problems that can create other problems are overweight and obesity, inactivity, and smoking.
- Screening procedures may prevent problems and/or identify a problem early, when it is most curable. Some screenings are monthly or annually, some age-based, and others risk-based procedures.
- Disorders of the breast may be benign, such as fibrocystic changes that occur in relation to the menstrual cycle, or malignant. The discovery of any breast disorder creates anxiety in women, and nurses should be prepared to explain diagnostic procedures, such as mammogram,

ultrasound, fine needle aspiration biopsy, core needle biopsy, and surgical biopsy.

- One in eight women in the United States develops breast cancer. Besides gender, the greatest risk factors are advancing age, a prior history of breast cancer, and genetic mutations in the *BRCA1, BRCA2,* and *p53* genes. Additional factors include family history (mother, sister, daughter) of breast cancer and previous uterine, ovarian, or colon cancer. Lifestyle factors such as a high intake of dietary fat, smoking, and consumption of alcohol are also suspected to increase risk.
- Management of breast cancer includes surgical removal of the tumor plus varying amounts of surrounding tissue and lymph glands. Adjuvant therapy includes radiation, chemotherapy, hormone therapy, and immunotherapy.
- Breast reconstruction is an integral part of the surgical management of breast cancer. Methods include tissue expansion and autogenous grafts. Reconstruction at the time of surgical tumor removal or a later reconstruction are options for many women.
- Nursing care for women with breast cancer focuses on providing emotional support and accurate information.
- Cardiovascular disease kills more women than breast cancer. Preventive measures include modifying risk factors, such as maintaining a normal weight and stopping smoking. Added preventive measures include controlling hypertension, diet, and glucose level; increasing activity; and, for many women, using low-dose aspirin on a daily basis.
- Pap tests can identify early changes in cervical tissue that may lead to cervical cancer.
- Human papillomavirus vaccine is designed to prevent infection with four strains of human papillomavirus that can result in genital warts or cervical cancer. The best time for immunization is before the girl engages in any sexual activity, although it can be started after sexual activity.
- Fecal occult blood testing is a yearly test that may identify colon or rectal cancer early.
- Menstrual cycle disorders include amenorrhea, abnormal uterine bleeding, cyclic pelvic pain, and premenstrual syndrome. Some of the disorders, such as premenstrual syndrome, may respond to lifestyle alterations such as changes in diet, exercise habits, and stress management.
- Elective termination of pregnancy may be performed by medical or surgical methods, and each method is associated with social and ethical conflicts.

- The climacteric is a combination of endocrine, somatic, and psychic changes that occur at the end of the reproductive cycle. Menopause is the final menstrual period, although most people use the term interchangeably with *climacteric.* Women's responses to menopause vary widely, but all women are in a permanent state of estrogen deficit after menopause that can result in bone loss (osteoporosis), increased risk for coronary artery disease, and atrophic vaginitis.
- Hormone replacement therapy may be prescribed to manage the symptoms of estrogen deficit, such as hot flashes and atrophic vaginitis, and to decrease bone mineral loss that results in osteoporosis. Each woman and her health care provider should individually evaluate whether hormone replacement therapy is beneficial.
- Hormone replacement therapy has risks and benefits and is contraindicated for women who have thromboembolic disease, undiagnosed vaginal bleeding, previous episodes of breast cancer or untreated uterine cancer, or chronic liver disease. For these women, alternative measures are needed to control the symptoms of menopause.
- Relaxation of pelvic support structures occurs as a delayed result of traumatic childbirth and becomes troublesome when a deficiency in estrogen hastens genital atrophy as menopause nears.
- Many infections of the reproductive tract are transmitted by sexual contact. The incidence of sexually transmitted diseases is reduced by barrier methods of contraception, particularly the condom, which prevents contact between infected skin or mucosal surfaces and prevents potentially infected ejaculate from entering the woman's lower genital tract.
- Pelvic inflammatory disease is often a complication of untreated sexually transmitted diseases, and a large number of cases are caused by chlamydial or gonorrheal infections. Pelvic inflammatory disease can cause infertility or ectopic pregnancy because of scarring of fallopian tubes resulting from inflammatory processes in the pelvic cavity.
- Toxic shock syndrome is a life-threatening condition resulting from infection with toxin-producing strains of *Staphylococcus aureus.* Some infections may be related to use of high-absorbency tampons that trap and hold bacteria in nutrient-rich menstrual blood for an extended time. Tampons and other items that trap bacteria, such as cervical caps and diaphragms, should be removed as directed by the health care provider.

REFERENCES & READINGS

American Cancer Society (ACS). (2015a). *American Cancer Society FluFOBT Program Implementation Guide for Primary Care Practices.* Retrieved from www.cancer.org.

American Cancer Society (ACS). (2015b). *American Cancer Society releases new breast cancer guideline.* Retrieved from www.cancer.org.

American Cancer Society (ACS). (2015c). *Breast cancer facts & figures 2015-2016.* Retrieved from www.cancer.org.

American Cancer Society (ACS). (2016a). *American cancer society guidelines for the early detection of cancer.* Retrieved from www.cancer.org.

American Cancer Society (ACS). (2016b). Breast reconstruction after mastectomy. Retrieved from www.cancer.org.

American Cancer Society (ACS). (2016c). *Endometrial (uterine) cancer: Overview.* Retrieved from www.cancer.org.

American College of Obstetricians and Gynecologists (ACOG). (2012). *Use of botanicals for management of menopausal symptoms.* Practice Bulletin No. 28. Washington, DC: Author.

American College of Obstetricians and Gynecologists (ACOG). (2016). *Cervical Cancer Screening. Frequently Asked Questions Special Procedures.* Retrieved from www.acog.org.

American Heart Association (AHA). (2014). What your cholesterol levels mean. Retrieved from www.heart.org.

American Heart Association (AHA). (2016). Heart attack prevention in women. Retrieved from www.americanheart.org.

Bloski, T., & Pierson, R. (2008). Endometriosis: Understanding the mystery behind this complex condition. *Nursing for Women's Health, 12*(5), 382–395.

Centers for Disease Control and Prevention (CDC). (2015a). Sexually transmitted diseases treatment guidelines, 2015. *MMWR: Morbidity and Mortality Weekly Report, 64*(RR3), 1–137.

Centers for Disease Control and Prevention (CDC). (2015b). *Vaccine information statement.* tdap vaccine. Retrieved from www.cdc.gov.

Centers for Disease Control (CDC). (2016a). An opt-out approach to HIV screening. Retrieved from www.cdc.gov.

Centers for Disease Control and Prevention (CDC). (2016b). High blood pressure. Retrieved from www.cdc.gov.

Centers for Disease Control (CDC). (2016c). Pelvic inflammatory disease fact sheet. Retrieved from www.cdc.gov.

Centers for Disease Control and Prevention (CDC). (2016d). Women & heart disease. Retrieved from www.cdc.gov.

Coleman, R. L., Ramirez, P. T., & Gershenson, D. M. (2012). Neoplastic diseases of the ovary. In G. M. Lentz, R. A. Lobo, D. M. Gershenson, & V. L. Katz (Eds.), *Comprehensive gynecology* (6th ed.) (pp. 731–771). Philadelphia, PA: Mosby.

Craft, M. (2009). Management of clients with breast disorders. In J. M. Black & J. H. Hawks (Eds.), *Medical-surgical nursing: Clinical management for positive outcomes* (8th ed.) (pp. 940–971). St. Louis, MO: Saunders.

Crandell, L. (2012). Psychological outcomes of medical versus elective first trimester abortion. *Nursing for Women's Health, 16*(4), 291–307.

Cromer, B. (2011). Menstrual problems. In R. M. Kliegman, B. F. Stanton, J. W. St. Geme, III, N. F. Schor, & R. E. Behrman (Eds.), *Nelson textbook of pediatrics* (19th ed.) (pp. 685–692). Philadelphia, PA: Saunders.

DeMartinis, J. E. (2009). Management of clients with hypertensive disorders. In J. M. Black & J. H. Hawks (Eds.), *Medical-surgical nursing: Clinical management for positive outcomes* (8th ed.) (pp. 1290–1306). Philadelphia, PA: Saunders.

Eckert, L. O., & Lentz, G. M. (2012). Infections of the lower and upper genital tract. In G. M. Lentz, R. A. Lobo, D. M. Gershenson, & V. L. Katz (Eds.), *Comprehensive gynecology* (6th ed.) (pp. 519–559). Philadelphia, PA: Elsevier.

Fantasia, H. C. (2013). Updated treatment guidelines for gonorrhea infections. *Nursing for Women's Health, 17*(3), 231–235.

Ittaman, S. V., VanWormer, J. J., & Rezkalla, S. H. (2014). The role of aspirin in the prevention of cardiovascular disease. *Clinical Medicine & Research, 12*(3-4), 147–154. Retrieved from www.clinmedres.org.

Jensen, J. T., & Mishell, D. R. (2012). Family planning: Contraception, sterilization, and pregnancy termination. In G. M. Lentz, R. A. Lobo, D. M. Gershenson, & V. L. Katz (Eds.), *Comprehensive gynecology* (6th ed.) (pp. 215–272). Philadelphia, PA: Mosby.

Jhingran, A., & Levenback, C. (2012). Malignant diseases of the cervix. In G. M. Lentz, R. A. Lobo, D. M. Gershenson, & V. L. Katz (Eds.), *Comprehensive gynecology* (6th ed.) (pp. 667–684). Philadelphia, PA: Mosby.

Katz, V. L. (2012a). Benign gynecologic lesions. In G. M. Lentz, R. A. Lobo, D. M. Gershenson, & V. L. Katz (Eds.), *Comprehensive gynecology* (6th ed.) (pp. 383–432). Philadelphia, PA: Mosby.

Katz, V. L. (2012b). The interaction of medical diseases and female physiology. In G. M. Lentz, R. A. Lobo, D. M. Gershenson, & V. L. Katz (Eds.), *Comprehensive gynecology* (6th ed.) (pp. 129–136). Philadelphia, PA: Mosby.

Katz, V. L., & Dotters, D. (2012). Breast diseases: Diagnosis and treatment of benign & malignant disease. In G. M. Lentz, R. A. Lobo, D. M. Gershenson, & V. L. Katz (Eds.), *Comprehensive gynecology* (6th ed.) (pp. 301–334). Philadelphia, PA: Mosby.

National Cancer Institute & National Institutes of Health (NCI & NIH). (2016). *Breast cancer.* Retrieved from www.cancer.gov.

Keresztes, P. A., & Wcisel, M. (2009). Management of clients with functional cardiac disorders. In J. M. Black & J. H. Hawks (Eds.), *Medical-surgical nursing: Clinical management for positive outcomes* (8th ed.) (pp. 1410–1449). Philadelphia, PA: Saunders.

Klein, D. A., & Poth, M. A. (2013). Amenorrhea: An approach to diagnosis and management. *American Family Physician, 87*(11), 781–788.

Kupferer, E. M., Dormire, S. L., & Becker, H. (2009). Complementary and alternative medicine use for vasomotor symptoms among women who have discontinued hormone therapy. *Journal of Obstetric, Gynecologic, and Neonatal Nursing, 38*(1), 50–59.

Lentz, G. M. (2012a). Anatomic defects of the abdominal wall and pelvic floor. In G. M. Lentz, R. A. Lobo, D. M. Gershenson, & V. L. Katz (Eds.), *Comprehensive gynecology* (6th ed.) (pp. 453–474). Philadelphia, PA: Mosby.

Lentz, G. M. (2012b). Primary and secondary dysmenorrhea, premenstrual syndrome, and premenstrual dysphoric disorder. In G. M. Lentz, R. A. Lobo, D. M. Gershenson, & V. L. Katz (Eds.), *Comprehensive gynecology* (6th ed.) (pp. 791–803). Philadelphia, PA: Mosby.

Lentz, G. M. (2012c). Urogynecology. In G. M. Lentz, R. A. Lobo, D. M. Gershenson, & V. L. Katz (Eds.), *Comprehensive gynecology* (6th ed.) (pp. 475–502). Philadelphia, PA: Mosby.

Lobo, R. A. (2012a). Abnormal uterine bleeding. In G. M. Lentz, R. A. Lobo, D. M. Gershenson, & V. L. Katz (Eds.), *Comprehensive gynecology* (6th ed.) (pp. 805–814). Philadelphia, PA: Mosby.

Lobo, R. A. (2012b). Endometriosis. In G. M. Lentz, R. A. Lobo, D. M. Gershenson, & V. L. Katz (Eds.), *Comprehensive gynecology* (6th ed.) (pp. 452–453). Philadelphia, PA: Mosby.

Lobo, R. A. (2012c). Menopause and care of the mature woman. In G. M. Lentz, R. A. Lobo, D. M. Gershenson, & V. L. Katz (Eds.), *Comprehensive gynecology* (6th ed.) (pp. 273–299). Philadelphia, PA: Mosby.

Lobo, R. A. (2012d). Primary and secondary amenorrhea and precocious puberty. In G. M. Lentz, R. A. Lobo, D. M. Gershenson, & V. L. Katz (Eds.), *Comprehensive gynecology* (6th ed.) (pp. 815–836). Philadelphia, PA: Mosby.

National Center for Complementary & Alternative Medicine (NCCAM): National Institutes of Health. (2009a). *Herbs at a glance: Chasteberry.* Retrieved from www.nccam.nih.gov.

National Center for Complementary & Alternative Medicine (NCCAM): National Institutes of Health. (2009b). *Herbs at a glance: Evening primrose oil.* Retrieved from www.nccam.nih.gov.

National Center for Complementary & Alternative Medicine (NCCAM): National Institutes of Health. (2009c). *Get the facts: Menopausal symptoms and CAM.* Retrieved from www.nccam.nih.gov.

National Institute of Diabetes and Digestive and Kidney Diseases & National Institutes of Health (NIDDKD & NIH). (2014). National Kidney and Urologic Diseases Clearinghouse. *Kegel exercise tips.* Retrieved from www.kidney.niddk.nih.gov.

National Institute of Diabetes and Digestive and Kidney Diseases & National Institutes of Health (NIDDKD & NIH). (2016). *Urinary incontinence in women.* Retrieved from www.kidney.niddk.nih.gov.

National Institutes of Health & National Institute of Arthritis and Musculoskeletal and Skin Diseases (NIH & NIAMS). (2015). *Osteoporosis overview.* Retrieved from www.niams.nih.gov.

National Institutes of Health & National Institute of Arthritis and Musculoskeletal and Skin Diseases (NIH & NIAMS). (2016). *Osteoporosis: handout on health.* Retrieved from www.niams.nih.gov.

National Osteoporosis Foundation (NOF). (2016). *Bone basics.* Retrieved from www.nof.org.

National Osteoporosis Foundations (NOF). (2017). *Calcium/Vitamin D.* Retrieved from www.nof.org.

Ogden, C. L., Carroll, M. D., Kit, B. K., & Flegal, K. M. (2014). Prevalence of obesity in the United States, 2011-2012. *JAMA,* *311*(8), 806–814. http://dx.doi.org/10.1001/jama.2014.732.

Pazol, K., Creanga, A. A., Zane, S. B., et al. (2015). Abortion surveillance—United States, 2012. *Morbidity and Mortality Weekly Report (MMWR),* *64*(SS10), 1–40.

Soliman, P. T., & Lu, K. H. (2012). Neoplastic diseases of the uterus. In G. M. Lentz, R. A. Lobo, D. M. Gershenson, & V. L. Katz (Eds.), *Comprehensive gynecology* (6th ed.) (pp. 713–730). Philadelphia, PA: Mosby.

US Department of Health & Human Services. (2014). *Active living.* Retrieved from www.surgeongeneral.gov.

World Health Organization (WHO). (2016). *Female genital mutilation fact sheet updated February 2016.* Retrieved from www.who.int/en/.

Answers to Knowledge Check

CHAPTER 1

1. High rates of maternal and infant mortality among poor women led to federal programs to improve the health of mothers, infants, and young children. Distribution of health care remains inequitable between poor women and more affluent women because many health care providers practice in an area in which payment for care is more certain, limiting access to prenatal care and information.

2. Family-centered care provides safe, quality care that adapts to both the physical and the psychological needs of the entire family during reproduction and greatly increases the responsibilities of nurses providing care. Family-centered care and support are often part of women's health care in nonchildbearing years as well.

3. Birthing centers provide professional care during pregnancy and childbirth in a homelike environment for women with low-risk pregnancies. They are associated with a nearby hospital to which the woman can be transferred in case of unexpected complications. Although the home setting provides comfort and closeness, it may not have adequate equipment or personnel to handle unexpected developments. Family members and friends must assist with care of other children, the mother, and her new infant. Labor, delivery, and recovery (LDR) and labor, delivery, recovery, and postpartum (LDRP) rooms offer a comfortable setting that promotes family involvement for birth but within the hospital, where emergencies can be handled more easily.

4. Interprofessional education can improve patient safety and quality of care by promoting interprofessional team-based patient care.

5. A patient safety bundle is a set of evidence-based practices performed together to improve patient outcomes. Maternal safety bundles have been developed for maternal mental health, including depression and anxiety, obstetric hemorrhage, severe hypertension in pregnancy, venous thromboembolism, safe reduction of primary cesarean birth, reduction of peripartum racial/ethnic disparities, and support after a severe maternal event.

6. The Association of Women's Health, Obstetric and Neonatal Nurses (AWHONN's) Nursing Care Quality Measures are currently being tested for feasibility, validity, and reliability, but currently include triage of a pregnant woman and her fetus(es); second stage of labor: mother-initiated, spontaneous pushing; skin-to-skin contact initiated immediately after birth; duration of uninterrupted skin-to-skin contact; eliminating supplementation of breastfed, healthy, term newborns; protection of maternal milk volume for premature infants admitted to the neonatal intensive care unit (NICU); initial contact with mothers after a neonatal transport; perinatal grief support; women's health and wellness coordination throughout the life span; labor support/partial labor support; and freedom of movement during labor.

7. Safety is the major concern with the use of complementary and alternative medicine because these modalities are largely unregulated. Additionally, patients usually refer themselves to practitioners and either may delay care from a conventional health care provider or may not tell the conventional provider about substances they are taking that may be harmful when combined with other medications. Some organic substances have active pharmacologic ingredients of varying strengths.

8. Infant mortality has decreased because of improved health of the general population, application of basic principles of sanitation, and increase in medical knowledge. Improvements in health care, including widely available antibiotics, public health facilities, and increased prenatal care, further reduced infant mortality.

9. The infant mortality rate in the United States ranked twenty-sixth among developed countries, much lower than expected given the resources available.

10. The roles of the nurse include communicator, teacher, collaborator, researcher, advocate, and manager. In addition nurses with advanced education and licensure may be clinical nurse specialists or primary care providers such as nurse midwives and nurse practitioners.

11. Therapeutic communication is purposeful, goal directed, and focused.

12. Many factors, including the family's developmental level, primary language, cultural orientation, and previous experiences, influence learning. In addition, the nurse should be aware that the physical environment and the organization and skill of the instructor will also affect learning.

13. The purpose of critical thinking is to help nurses make the best clinical judgments and to identify and overcome habits or impulses that result in poor decisions or inappropriate actions.

14. Steps that may be helpful in learning or refining critical thinking can be organized into an "ABCDE" pattern. They include recognizing **a**ssumptions; examining possible

personal **b**iases; determining the need for **c**losure; developing the ability to collect, organize, and analyze **d**ata in an expert manner; and acknowledging how **e**motions or **e**nvironmental factors may interfere with the ability to think critically.

15. Reflective skepticism means to suspend judgment to avoid making decisions in haste or with insufficient data.

16. The screening assessment gathers information about all aspects of the patient's health. The focused assessment gathers information about an actual health problem or one for which the patient appears to have a higher risk. A woman's desire to improve health may be identified during both types of assessment.

17. Actual patient problems reflect health problems that can be validated by the presence of defining characteristics. Risk patient problems indicate that risk factors are present that make the person vulnerable to the development of a particular problem that has not yet developed.

18. The terms *goals* and *expected outcomes* (*outcome criteria*) are often used interchangeably to describe desired endpoints of care, but they are different. Broad goals do not have the specific criteria of outcome criteria. Expected outcomes should (1) be stated in terms of the patient, (2) be observable and measurable, (3) have a time frame, (4) be realistic, and (5) be worked out with the woman and family.

19. Nursing interventions that are not specific and do not identify exactly what is to be done are difficult to implement. Clearly written interventions that provide detailed, objective instructions correct the problem.

CHAPTER 2

1. Characteristics of a functional family include open communication, flexibility in role assignments, agreement of adults on the basic principles of parenting, and resiliency and adaptability.

2. Factors interfering with healthy family functioning include lack of financial resources, absence of adequate family support, birth of an infant who requires specialized care, presence of unhealthy habits such as substance abuse or lack of anger management, and the inability to make mature decisions that are necessary to provide care to an infant.

3. Differing cultures and lack of understanding of cultures (between the nurse and the childbearing family) may create difficulties related to communication style, decision making, touch, spirituality and religiosity, and time orientation. Nurses should attempt to reconcile these differences by taking the opportunity to learn about the uniqueness of each woman and her cultural beliefs and practices.

4. Integrating harmless traditional cultural practices into the care of the childbearing woman demonstrates respect for her culture.

5. Nurses should examine their own cultural values and beliefs to determine ways in which their beliefs may generate conflict with those who hold different cultural beliefs.

6. Cultural negotiation involves providing information while acknowledging that the woman may hold views that are different from those of the nurse.

7. Poverty is the underlying factor that causes problems such as inadequate access to health care. The lack of access to health care includes the inability to pay for it, lack of transportation, lack of care for other children, inaccessible hours for appointments, and language barriers.

8. An important barrier to health care results from the unsympathetic attitude of some health care workers toward those who are unable to pay for prenatal care. Poor families may experience long delays, hurried examinations, rudeness, and arrogance from some members of the health care team. Staff may be overworked and frustrated with the workloads they carry. Women may wait hours for an examination that lasts only a few minutes. Many never see the same health care provider more than once. These women may not keep clinic appointments because they do not see the importance of the hurried, impersonal examinations.

9. Poverty is the underlying factor that causes problems such as inadequate access to health care. The lack of access to health care is a major reason for the large number of low-birth-weight infants and the high infant mortality rate.

10. Health care disparities in the United States across racial, geographic, socioeconomic status, age, and gender result in differences in the health outcomes for different groups of people.

11. Battering may start or become worse during pregnancy. The face, arms, buttocks, abdomen, and breasts are frequent targets for battery. Women may start prenatal care late and miss appointments. They have an increased risk for uterine rupture, placental abruption, preterm birth, low-birth-weight infant, maternal and fetal death, sexually transmitted diseases (STDs), and postpartum depression.

12. Nurses can examine their own biases to determine whether they accept a common myth that blames the victim. In addition, nurses can consciously practice in ways that empower women and make it clear that the woman owns her body and no one deserves to be beaten.

13. The physically abused woman often appears hesitant, embarrassed, or evasive. She may avoid eye contact and appear ashamed, guilty, or frightened. Signs of present and past injury may be present, such as bruising, swelling, lacerations, burns, scars, and old fractures, as well as genital injuries.

14. Nurses can help establish short-term goals by helping the woman acknowledge the abuse, develop a plan for protecting herself and her children, and identify community resources that provide protection.

15. Victims of human trafficking may have a pattern of "red flags." One red flag may not be indicative of the patient being a victim of trafficking in persons (TIP); the nurse should assess for the patterns of possible

indicators, which include being accompanied by an individual who insists on answering all questions for the woman; reluctance or inability of the victim to reveal their true situation; signs and symptoms of physical and mental abuse; evidence of being controlled; fearfulness; submissiveness; fear of authority figures; lack of identification documents; the woman cannot communicate her physical address; inconsistencies in stories and/or histories; a woman who is foreign or non-English speaking; homelessness; a history of previous and/or current prostitution charges or sexual abuse; possession of expensive electronics, jewelry, and other luxury items; a history of substance abuse; markings on the body that appear to be branding; and a high number of sex partners relative to age.

16. Ethics examines conduct and distinctions between right and wrong to determine the best course of action. Bioethics applies specifically to the ethics of health care.

17. The deontologic model applies ethical principles to determine what is right. It does not vary the solution according to individual situations. The utilitarian model analyzes the benefits and burdens to determine a course of action that provides the greatest amount of good in a given situation. Belief that every patient has basic human rights is the basis for the human rights model.

18. Ethical principles may conflict when the application of one principle violates another.

19. Assessment is used to gather data from all concerned persons. Ethical theories and principles are analyzed to determine whether an ethical dilemma exists. Planning involves identifying as many options as possible and choosing a solution. Interventions must be identified to implement the chosen solution, and the results are evaluated.

20. The Supreme Court decision in *Roe v. Wade* declared that abortion was legal anywhere in the United States and that existing state laws prohibiting abortion were unconstitutional because they interfered with a woman's right to privacy. Stipulations in terms of the trimester of pregnancy were part of *Roe v. Wade*.

21. The belief that abortion is a private choice conflicts with the belief that abortion is taking a life.

22. Punitive approaches are against the ethical principles of autonomy, bodily integrity, and personal freedom. Although the intended plan may be to protect the fetus, such a plan can have unexpected outcomes, causing the woman to avoid prenatal care or be dishonest with care providers, causing greater harm to her fetus.

23. Problems involved in the use of advanced reproductive techniques include high cost, low success rate, limitation to the affluent, control of unused embryos, and problem or unexpected pregnancy outcomes.

24. Log off of computer terminals when access is complete. Maintain secret identity codes that access private information. Maintain a low volume in phone reports. Direct reports to another professional should be done on a "need to know" basis rather than reporting to those who do not need to know. Verbal reports should be done in a private area. Care must be taken not to violate patient or institutional confidentiality when having any discussion on the Internet.

25. State boards of nursing administer the individual states' nurse practice acts, which establish what the nurse is allowed and expected to do when practicing nursing in that state.

26. Standards of care and agency policies influence judgment about malpractice because they describe the level of care that can be expected from practitioners at the time of care.

27. Nursing actions that help defend malpractice claims include securing informed consent appropriately, keeping documentation that provides evidence that the standard of care has been maintained, acting appropriately as a patient advocate in terms of taking a problem through the chain of command, and maintaining expertise.

28. Concerns about the use of unlicensed assistive personnel include whether this use compromises the quality of care and if the high workload of the nurse restricts the time available to supervise unlicensed personnel adequately.

29. Short lengths of stay lead to concerns about the woman's ability to care for herself and her infant, potential complications that new parents may not identify, and the fact that parents will not have had time to absorb the necessary teaching. Follow-up phone calls help alleviate some concerns and identify some problems that develop after discharge. In nonmaternity medical situations, many older women are often discharged early from the hospital. Because the cognitive abilities of a woman may decline with advanced age, in these situations it is important to also provide teaching to the woman's care provider.

30. Facilities that use phone call follow-up should have regularly reviewed and updated protocols, good documentation forms, and specific instructions to the patient about actions to take if further problems develop.

CHAPTER 3

1. Development of the breasts is the first sign of puberty in girls. In boys, growth of the testes is the first sign, followed by growth of the penis about 1 year later.

2. The female pelvis has a wide, rounded, basinlike shape that favors efficient passage of the fetus during birth. The male pelvis is heavier and narrower and structurally suited for tasks requiring load bearing.

3. Males generally attain a greater adult height than females because they begin their growth spurt about 1 year later than girls and continue growing for a longer period.

4. Female secondary sex characteristics include round hips and breasts, pubic hair, finer skin texture, and a higher-pitched voice. Male secondary sex characteristics include facial and

pubic hair, a deeper voice, broader shoulders, and greater muscle mass.

5. The female external reproductive organs are collectively called the *vulva*. The labia majora extend from the mons pubis to the perineum. The labia minora are within and parallel to the labia majora. The clitoris is at the anterior junction of the labia minora. The urinary meatus and vaginal introitus are found within the vestibule (the area enclosed by the labia minora). The hymen partially closes the vaginal opening. The perineum extends from the fourchette (posterior rim of the vaginal opening) to the anus.

6. The three divisions of the uterus are the corpus (body), isthmus (transition zone between corpus and cervix), and cervix (neck). The uterine fundus is the part of the corpus that lies above the entry points of the fallopian tubes.

7. The myometrium is the middle layer of thick uterine muscle between the perimetrium and endometrium. The myometrium includes three types of muscle fibers: (1) longitudinal fibers, mostly in the fundus, to expel the fetus during birth; (2) interlacing figure-eight fibers to compress bleeding blood vessels after birth; and (3) circular fibers to provide constrictions near the fallopian tubes and the internal cervical os, enabling the proper implantation of the fertilized ovum and preventing the reflux of menstrual blood into the fallopian tubes.

8. The fallopian tubes are lined with cells with cilia that beat rhythmically toward the uterine cavity to propel the ovum through the fallopian tube. The fertilized ovum undergoes its early cell divisions in the fallopian tube so that implantation is most likely to occur in the uterine fundus.

9. The two functions of the ovaries are to produce hormones (primarily estrogen and progesterone) and mature an ovum for release during each reproductive cycle.

10. The pelvis is located at the lower end of the spine. The true pelvis is located below the linea terminalis. The true pelvis is most relevant during birth.

11. Pelvic muscles enclose the lower pelvis and support internal reproductive, urinary, and bowel structures. Ligaments maintain internal reproductive organs and their nerve and blood supplies in the proper positions in the pelvis.

12. The ripening follicle secretes estrogen to form new endometrial epithelium and endometrial glands. After ovulation, the follicle (now called the *corpus luteum*) secretes large amounts of both estrogen to continue thickening of the endometrium and progesterone to cause the endometrium to secrete substances to nourish a fertilized ovum.

13. Three ovarian phases of the female reproductive cycle are the follicular (maturation of an ovum), ovulatory (release of the mature ovum), and luteal (secretion of estrogen and progesterone by the corpus luteum). The length of the follicular phase varies more among women than the other two phases.

14. The three endometrial phases are the proliferative, secretory, and menstrual phases. The proliferative phase occurs during the first half of the cycle, during which the endometrium thickens in preparation for a fertilized ovum. The secretory phase occurs during the second half of the cycle and is characterized by continued growth of the endometrium, growth of blood vessels and glands, and secretion of substances to nourish a fertilized ovum. If pregnancy does not occur, the endometrium becomes ischemic and necrotic as secretion of estrogen and progesterone from the corpus luteum declines. The old endometrium is shed in the menstrual phase.

15. The cervical mucus becomes thin, clear, and elastic during ovulation to facilitate entrance of sperm from the vagina into the uterus and fallopian tube, thereby enhancing the chances for conception.

16. Montgomery's tubercles secrete a substance during pregnancy and lactation that keeps the nipples soft.

17. A woman's breast size is not related to the amount of milk she can produce. Breast size is influenced by the amount of fatty tissue in the breast.

18. Milk secretion does not occur during pregnancy because estrogen and progesterone produced by the placenta inhibit its production. Estrogen and progesterone stimulate the growth of the alveoli and ductal system during pregnancy.

19. As a urinary organ, the penis transports urine from the bladder to outside the body during urination. As a reproductive organ, it carries and deposits semen into the vagina during coitus.

20. The two types of erectile tissue in the penis are the corpus spongiosum that surrounds the urethra and the two columns of corpus cavernosum tissue on each side of the penis. The function of erectile tissue is to facilitate entry of the penis into the female's vagina.

21. The scrotum holds the testes away from the body to keep them cooler than the core body temperature, thus facilitating sperm production.

22. The testes function as endocrine glands to produce testosterone and the male gametes (spermatozoa).

CHAPTER 4

1. DNA is the building block of genes. A varying number of genes makes up each chromosome.

2. Genes are too small to be seen under a microscope. They can be studied by analysis of the products they instruct cells to produce, by direct study of the DNA, or through their close association with another gene that can be studied by one of these other methods.

3. Chromosomes can be seen under a microscope when living nucleated cells are dividing. Cell division during the metaphase is a common time for analysis because each chromosome is compact. Fluorescent in situ hybridization (FISH) identifies chromosomal abnormalities in more than one stage of cell division, allowing rapid test results.

4. 46,XY describes the chromosome makeup of a normal human male. 46,XX describes the chromosomes of a normal human female. Abnormalities are described

beginning with the total number of chromosomes, followed by the sex chromosome complement, and followed by the abbreviation that describes the chromosome abnormality.

5. The child of a parent with an autosomal-dominant disorder has a 50% chance of having the same disorder.

6. Blood relationship (consanguinity) of parents increases the likelihood that both share some of the same abnormal autosomal-recessive genes, increasing the chance that their offspring will be affected with a disorder. The closer the parents' blood relationship, the more genes they are likely to share.

7. If both parents carry an abnormal gene for an autosomal-recessive disorder, each child has a 25% chance of receiving both copies of the defective gene and having the disorder. Each child also has a 50% chance of receiving only one copy of the defective gene and being a carrier like each parent. Each child also has a 25% chance of receiving the normal gene from each parent, thereby being neither a carrier nor affected and having no chance of passing the gene to future generations.

8. Males are more likely to have X-linked recessive disorders because they do not have a compensating X chromosome with a normal gene. Each son of a female carrier has a 50% chance of having the trait and a 50% chance of being unaffected. Each daughter of the female carrier has a 50% chance of being a carrier and a 50% chance of being unaffected.

9. A trisomy exists when each body cell contains an extra copy of one chromosome. Down syndrome is the most common trisomy and involves three copies of chromosome 21, for a total of 47 chromosomes in each cell.

10. A monosomy exists when each body cell is missing a chromosome. Turner syndrome (a female with a single X chromosome) is the only monosomy compatible with postnatal life.

11. Genetic material can be lost or duplicated when a chromosome has a structural abnormality. Also, the position of genes on the chromosome may be altered, preventing them from functioning normally.

12. A parent with a balanced chromosomal translocation may have a child with completely normal chromosomes, or the child may have a balanced chromosomal translocation like that of the parent. The offspring may also receive an unbalanced amount of chromosomal material (too much or too little), which often results in spontaneous abortion or birth defects.

13. Multifactorial disorders are typically present and detectable at birth. They are usually isolated defects rather than being present with other unrelated defects. However, sometimes the primary multifactorial defect alters further development and results in other related defects.

14. Factors that may affect the likelihood that a multifactorial disorder will occur or recur include the following: the number of affected close relatives, severity of the defect in those affected, gender of the affected person, geographic location, and seasonal variations.

15. The woman may be able to prevent exposing her fetus to teratogens by being immunized against infections such as rubella at least 28 days (1 month) before pregnancy, eliminating the use of nontherapeutic drugs such as alcohol and illicit drugs, changing therapeutic drugs to those having a lower risk to the fetus, and avoiding radiation exposure when she may be pregnant.

16. A pregnant woman who has phenylketonuria should return to her low-phenylalanine diet when she is pregnant to prevent buildup of toxic products that would damage the developing fetus.

17. Adequate folic acid intake of at least 0.4 mg (400 mcg) has been associated with a lower incidence of neural tube defects. Because the neural tube begins closure at 4 weeks of gestation, the woman should have adequate intake beginning before conception to ensure the best outcome.

CHAPTER 5

1. Meiosis is a type of cell division that halves the number of chromosomes so that only one of each chromosomal pair goes into each gamete. Meiosis also promotes genetic variation by the process of crossing over, or exchange of chromosomal material between each member of the pair of chromosomes. The union of male and female gametes at conception restores the number of chromosomes to 46 in the offspring.

2. Each oogonium produces one mature ovum after two meiotic divisions. The first meiotic division begins in fetal life and is not completed until shortly before that ovum undergoes ovulation. The second meiotic division begins at ovulation but is not completed unless fertilization occurs.

3. Each spermatogonium undergoes two meiotic divisions to result in four mature spermatozoa. Meiosis begins at puberty, and both meiotic divisions are completed before the sperm mature and are ejaculated.

4. Fertilization usually occurs in the distal third of the fallopian tube (the ampulla), near the ovary.

5. Seminal fluid nourishes and protects the sperm from the acidic environment of the woman's vagina.

6. As sperm approach the ovum, they secrete hyaluronidase to digest a pathway through the corona radiata and zona pellucida. When one spermatozoon finally penetrates the ovum, changes in the zona pellucida prevent other spermatozoa from entering. The cell membranes of the ovum and sperm fuse to allow the sperm to penetrate the ovum. The ovum also completes its second meiotic division.

7. Fertilization is complete and a new human conceived when the nuclei of the ovum and spermatozoon unite.

8. Implantation begins 6 days after conception and is complete by the tenth day.

9. The upper uterus is the ideal location for implantation for three reasons: (1) it has a rich blood supply for fetal gas exchange and nutrition, (2) the thick uterine lining prevents the placenta from attaching too deeply, and (3) the strong interlacing muscle fibers contract to limit blood loss after birth.

10. Nutritive fluids produced in the thick decidua pass to the conceptus by diffusion before a placental circulation is established. Primary chorionic villi, which will form the fetal side of the placenta, extend from the conceptus into the decidua basalis, which will become the maternal side of the placenta, to tap these nutrients.

11. During the first 8 weeks after conception, the embryonic period, all major organ systems develop. The woman may be unaware that she is pregnant and may inadvertently expose the embryo to harmful substances. These substances may damage organs that are developing.

12. At 4 weeks the trachea develops as a bud of the upper digestive tract. After the trachea separates from the upper digestive tract, it branches into the two bronchi, which then divide to form the three lobes of the right lung and the two lobes of the left. Branching continues until terminal air sacs develop.

13. The intestines are contained mostly within the umbilical cord until 10 weeks because they grow more rapidly than the abdominal cavity and the liver and kidneys are relatively large. By 10 weeks after conception, the abdominal cavity has caught up with the growth of its contents and can accommodate them.

14. Gestational age is calculated from the woman's last menstrual period and is about 2 weeks longer than fertilization age which is calculated from conception. Gestational age is most commonly used because the menstrual period provides a specific marker. Ultrasound imaging may further clarify gestational age.

15. The fetus usually assumes a head-down position because this position best fits the egg shape of the uterus. Also, the head is heavier and tends to go downward with gravity in the pool of amniotic fluid.

16. Vernix caseosa protects fetal skin from constant exposure to amniotic fluid. Lanugo helps vernix adhere to the skin. Brown fat helps the infant maintain temperature stability in the cooler external environment after birth. Surfactant keeps the lung alveoli from collapsing with each expiration, thus making breathing easier after birth.

17. The placenta gradually takes over the function of the corpus luteum and secretes estrogen and progesterone.

18. Exchange of oxygen, nutrients, and waste products between the woman and the fetus takes place in the intervillous spaces of the placenta.

19. Maternal and fetal blood may be of incompatible blood types and thus should not mix.

20. The fetus can thrive in a relatively low-oxygen environment because of the following:
    a. Fetal hemoglobin carries more oxygen than adult hemoglobin.
    b. The fetus has a higher hemoglobin and hematocrit level than does the newborn or adult.
    c. Rapid diffusion of carbon dioxide into the maternal blood causes the mother to release oxygen more readily and causes oxygen to combine with fetal blood more readily.

21. Human chorionic gonadotropin (hCG) causes the corpus luteum of the ovary to persist and secrete estrogens and progesterone, which are essential to maintain the uterine lining for implantation. It also facilitates fetal testosterone secretion in the male fetus. Human placental lactogen promotes normal fetal nutrition and growth and maternal breast development. Estrogens cause enlargement of the woman's uterus and genitalia and enlargement and development of the breasts. Progesterone maintains the secretory endometrium and changes the endometrium into the decidua to nourish the conceptus; progesterone also reduces uterine contractions to prevent spontaneous abortion. Progesterone facilitates growth and development of the mother's breasts and the cells that will secrete milk. Progesterone may allow immune tolerance of the conceptus.

22. The fetal membranes contain the amniotic fluid that cushions the fetus and circulation within the umbilical cord, maintains a stable temperature, and promotes normal prenatal structural development.

23. Oxygenated blood enters the fetus through the umbilical vein. Part of the blood goes to the liver, and the rest passes through the ductus venosus to the inferior vena cava. Blood enters the right atrium, where a small amount passes to the right ventricle, and the rest flows through the foramen ovale to the left atrium and then to the left ventricle. Some blood from the right ventricle goes to the lungs to nourish their tissue, and the rest passes through the ductus arteriosus, where it joins blood ejected from the left ventricle. After circulation through the fetal body, deoxygenated blood returns to the placenta through the two umbilical arteries.

24. Monozygotic twins are conceived when one spermatozoon fertilizes one ovum and the resulting conceptus later divides into two inner cell masses that will become two fetuses.

25. The placentas and chorions may fuse before birth, making it difficult to determine whether the twins are monozygotic or dizygotic.

26. Dizygotic twins develop from two ova that are each fertilized by a spermatozoon and are like other siblings in a family.

CHAPTER 6

1. The uterine fundus is midway between the symphysis and the umbilicus at 16 weeks, at the level of the umbilicus by 20 weeks, and to the xiphoid process at 36 weeks of gestation.

2. In late pregnancy, 17% of the cardiac output goes to the uterus and placenta, with almost 90% of it going to the placenta.

3. The cervical mucus plug blocks ascent of bacteria from the vagina into the uterus, thereby providing additional protection of the fetus from possible infection.

4. The major purpose of progesterone in early pregnancy is to stop contractions, help prevent fetal tissue rejection, and, with estrogen, prevent ovulation.

5. During pregnancy the breasts enlarge and become more vascular; the areolae increase in size and become more pigmented; the nipples darken, enlarge, and become more erect; and Montgomery's tubercles become more prominent.

6. Expanded blood volume is needed for the added maternal tissues of pregnancy, to provide blood flow to the placenta, and to allow for loss of blood at childbirth.

7. Physiologic anemia of pregnancy is caused by a greater increase in plasma volume than in red blood cells (RBCs), resulting in a dilution of, but not inadequate, hemoglobin concentration. Iron-deficiency anemia is caused by a true lack of iron that affects hemoglobin levels.

8. In the supine position, the weight of the uterus on the vena cava and aorta impedes blood flow to and from the lower extremities, resulting in decreased cardiac output and supine hypotensive syndrome.

9. During pregnancy, increased circulation through the kidneys is needed to remove metabolic wastes generated by the mother and the fetus. Increased circulation through the skin is necessary to dissipate heat that is generated by accelerated metabolism.

10. Progesterone causes slight hyperventilation and increases sensitivity of the respiratory center to carbon dioxide, leading to a feeling of dyspnea.

11. Flaring of the ribs, widening of the substernal angle, and increased circumference of the chest allow adequate intake of air with each breath.

12. Estrogen causes hyperemia of the gums that may lead to bleeding or gingivitis. Vascular hypertrophy of the gums (epulis) may occur. Excessive salivation (ptyalism) is a problem for some. Progesterone relaxes smooth muscle in the gastrointestinal tract, which slows gastric emptying time and intestinal motility and may lead to heartburn and constipation. Emptying time of the gallbladder is increased, and thicker bile and gallstones may result.

13. Expectant mothers are at increased risk for urinary tract infection because compression of the ureters between the uterus and the pelvic bones and dilation of the ureters and kidney pelvis cause stasis of urine, allowing time for bacteria to multiply.

14. Relaxation of pelvic connective tissue and joints by relaxin and progesterone creates instability and results in a wide stance and "waddling" gait. Lordosis occurs when the large uterus causes the woman to lean backward to maintain her balance.

15. The hormones follicle-stimulating hormone (FSH) and luteinizing hormone (LH) are suppressed during pregnancy by high levels of estrogen and progesterone to prevent ovulation. Progesterone maintains the endometrium and prevents menstruation.

16. Maternal hormones create increasing resistance of maternal tissues to insulin to provide glucose for the fetus. Normally, the mother produces more insulin to meet her needs.

17. Most, but not all, presumptive signs are subjective. Probable signs are objective. Both can have causes other than pregnancy. Positive indicators of pregnancy have no other possible causes.

18. Many things such as gas, peristalsis, or pseudocyesis (false pregnancy) can be mistaken by the woman for fetal movement.

19. Common causes of inaccurate pregnancy test results include a urine specimen that is too dilute or contains protein or blood; maternal ingestion of certain drugs such as some diuretics, anticonvulsants, antiparkinson drugs, hypnotics, or tranquilizers; incorrect testing procedure; or testing too early in the pregnancy.

20. The fetus seems vague and unreal during the first trimester. Gradually, physical changes (uterine growth, weight gain, quickening) confirm that a fetus is developing, and the expectant mother begins to perceive the fetus as a separate though dependent being.

21. The pregnant woman may have increased interest in sex during the first trimester unless she has nausea or fears miscarriage. Interest is often increased in the second trimester because of pelvic vasocongestion and a general feeling of well-being. The discomforts of the third trimester may decrease sexual responsiveness. Some expectant fathers are more interested in sex during pregnancy, but others find the pregnant woman unattractive and fear harming the fetus.

22. The pregnant woman explores the role of mother to develop a sense of herself in the role and selects behaviors that confirm her idea of fulfilling the role.

23. Pregnancy brings the realization that the woman will have to give up certain aspects of her previous life. This causes a temporary sadness and the need for grief work.

24. Seeking safe passage involves going to a health care provider and following recommendations of the provider and of her culture.

25. Reality boosters include seeing the fetus via ultrasound, hearing the fetal heart, and feeling the fetus move. They are important in making the coming child seem real.

26. Nurses can help men gain recognition as parents by focusing on the father as well as the mother, encouraging the father's questions, and including him in the plan of care.

27. Information about infant behavior and care is more relevant and therefore more useful after the infant is born.

28. The age of the grandparents, the number and spacing of other grandchildren, and their perceptions of their role help shape the way grandparents respond to an expected grandchild.

29. Toddlers do not understand that a birth is expected and should be told shortly before the expected date. Preschoolers may expect the infant to be a playmate near their age. School-age children may like to be involved and to help prepare for the birth. Adolescents may be embarrassed by evidence of their parents' sexuality, indifferent to the pregnancy, or very involved in preparations.

30. Parents can make any changes in sleeping arrangements several weeks before the infant is born so that other children do not feel displaced by the newborn. They can

increase time and attention to older children and reassure them of their love and acceptance.

CHAPTER 7

1. A preconception visit identifies factors that may cause harm to the fetus or the mother so that steps can be taken before pregnancy occurs to avoid problems.

2. Medical, surgical, psychological, and obstetric histories are necessary to identify chronic conditions or past difficulties that might affect the outcome of the pregnancy.

3. All caregivers should use the same techniques to measure blood pressure because position and how the blood pressure is taken affect the results. Monitoring changes in blood pressure during pregnancy is an important component of prenatal care.

4. Major risk factors during pregnancy are age under 16 or over 35 years; low socioeconomic status; nonwhite race; multiparity; obesity; previous problem pregnancies; preexisting medical disorders or infections; and use of substances such as alcohol, tobacco, or illicit drugs.

5. The usual schedule of antepartum visits begins in the first trimester and continues every 4 weeks until 28 weeks, then every 2 weeks until 36 weeks, and weekly from 37 weeks to birth.

6. A gradual, predictable increase in uterine size occurs as gestation advances. From approximately 16 weeks until 38 weeks, fundal height in centimeters is nearly equal to gestational age in weeks.

7. In multifetal pregnancies, increased blood volume results in additional work for the heart of the mother. The greatly increased size of the uterus causes greater elevation of the diaphragm and more compression of the large vessels, ureters, and bowel. Nausea and vomiting are more frequent.

8. Relief methods for morning sickness include eating dry carbohydrates (crackers, dry toast, dry cereal) before getting out of bed in the morning. Small frequent meals and high-protein snacks my help alleviate nausea and vomiting during the day. If necessary, the provider may prescribe vitamin B_6 (pyridoxine), doxylamine, or phenothiazines.

9. Correct posture and body mechanics and exercises such as pelvic rocking can help alleviate backache during pregnancy. Wearing low-heeled shoes and application of heat or acupuncture may also help.

10. The goals of perinatal education are to help women and their support persons become knowledgeable consumers; to be active participants in pregnancy and childbirth; and to provide coping techniques for pregnancy, birth, and parenting.

11. Preconception classes generally include information about nutrition before conception, healthy lifestyle, signs of pregnancy, and choosing a caregiver. The emphasis is on the benefits of early and regular prenatal care to reduce risk factors for poor pregnancy outcome. The effects of pregnancy and childbirth on a woman's relationships and career may also be discussed.

Early pregnancy (first trimester) classes cover information on adapting to pregnancy and understanding what to expect. Emphasis is on regular prenatal care and avoiding hazards to promote a healthy pregnancy.

Second-trimester classes focus on changes occurring during middle pregnancy and what to expect during the third trimester. Teachers discuss childbirth choices and information to help students become more knowledgeable consumers.

12. Childbirth preparation classes during the third trimester focus on self-help measures, what to expect during birth, and how to prepare for the birth of the baby. Specific techniques include pharmacologic and nonpharmacologic pain control.

13. Having a support person during labor increases a woman's satisfaction by helping her cope with stress, focus on her learned techniques, and feel that her experience is being shared.

14. Various support roles include active assistance and physical care, verbal encouragement, minimal physical assistance, and presence without active involvement.

CHAPTER 8

1. Maternal weight gain helps determine fetal growth. Too little weight gain may be associated with low neonatal birth weight, and too much gain may be associated with large infants.

2. The average woman should gain 11.5 to 16 kg (25 to 35 lb). Underweight women and those carrying more than one fetus should gain more, and overweight women should gain less.

3. The average woman should gain approximately 0.5 to 2 kg (1.1 to 4.4 lb) the first trimester and 0.35 to 0.5 kg (0.8 to 1 lb) per week in the second and third trimesters.

4. Although no additional calories are needed during the first trimester, the recommendation for the second and third trimesters is 340 calories and 452 calories.

5. Approximately 71 g of protein per day, an increase of 25 g above prepregnancy needs, is recommended during pregnancy.

6. Fat-soluble vitamins (A, D, E, K) are stored in the fat and are available longer than the water-soluble vitamins (such as B_6, B_{12}, folic acid, thiamine, riboflavin, niacin, C), which must be replenished daily. Excessive intake of fat-soluble vitamins is more likely to cause toxicity.

7. Because many pregnancies are not planned and the neural tube forms early in gestation, all women of childbearing age should have 400 mcg (0.4 mg) of folic acid daily to prevent birth of infants with neural tube defects from folic acid deficiency. Once pregnancy occurs, 600 mcg (0.6 mg) of folic acid should be taken daily.

8. Iron, calcium, and folic acid are often below the recommended amounts in the diets of pregnant women.

9. Excessive intake of vitamins and minerals may result in toxicity and interfere with absorption of other vitamins and minerals.

10. During pregnancy a woman should drink 8 to 10 cups (or approximately 3 liters) of fluids (mostly water) daily.

11. During pregnancy the woman should eat 7 to 9 oz of whole grains, 3 to 3½ cups of vegetables, 2 cups of fruits, 3 or more cups or the equivalent from the dairy group, and servings equal to 6 to 6½ oz from the protein group.

12. The nurse should consider traditional foods from the woman's culture, the degree to which she follows the traditional diet, and her inclusion of nontraditional foods in her diet.

13. The nurse should assess the woman's financial resources for food purchase, need for financial assistance, and education about nutrition.

14. The vegan can include nonanimal sources of iron; calcium; zinc; riboflavin; and vitamin B_6, B_{12}, and D and combine incomplete protein foods to ensure intake of all essential amino acids. She may also need to take supplements.

15. Lactose-intolerant women can choose calcium-containing foods such as leafy green vegetables, broccoli, peanuts, tofu, salmon, and sardines.

16. Other nutritional risk factors during pregnancy are excessive nausea and vomiting, anemia, abnormal prepregnancy weight, eating disorders, food cravings and aversions (including pica), multiparity, closely spaced pregnancies, multifetal pregnancy, and substance abuse.

17. The adolescent may skip meals and vitamin-mineral supplements and eat snacks and fast foods of low nutrient value to be like her peers.

18. The lactating woman needs more of many nutrients than does the woman who is not pregnant. She needs to eat 330 more calories than her nonpregnant needs during the first 6 months of lactation, and 170 calories will be drawn from her fat stores. During the second 6 months the lactating woman needs 400 calories daily more than the nonpregnant woman does.

19. The woman who is not breastfeeding should decrease calories to her prepregnant level, continue to eat a well-balanced diet including enough protein and vitamin C, and plan to lose extra weight slowly.

CHAPTER 9

1. The primary objective of prenatal screening and diagnosis is to detect disorders or abnormalities that could affect the woman, fetus, and newborn.

2. The three categories of obstetric ultrasound are standard (or basic), limited, and specialized (detailed or targeted). The two routes used for obstetric ultrasound are transvaginal and transabdominal.

3. Basic obstetric ultrasound provides the following information:
   • Maternal anatomy (cervix, uterus, adnexa)
   • Number of fetuses
   • Biometry (fetal measurements of specific structures) that estimates gestational age and fetal weight or determines whether a structure is a normal or abnormal size

• Survey of fetal anatomy
• Fetal presentation
• Presence of fetal cardiac activity
• Placental location
• Amniotic fluid volume

4. A water-soluble transmission gel or lotion is used to increase transmission of sound waves.

5. Nuchal translucency (NT) is a first-trimester ultrasound measurement of the fluid-filled space measured at the back of the fetal neck. An enlarged NT, often defined as 3.0 mm or greater or above the 99th percentile for gestational age, is associated with trisomy 21 as well as structural abnormalities such as congenital heart defects.

6. Neural tube defects (NTDs) are most commonly associated with elevated alpha-fetoprotein (AFP) levels. Other conditions include underestimation of gestational age, undiagnosed multiple gestation, fetal demise, conditions associated with fetal edema such as cystic hygroma, and abdominal wall defects such as gastroschisis.

7. Multiple-marker screening, sometimes called a *triple or quad screen*, is a maternal blood test for three or four substances (human chorionic gonadatropin [hCG], alpha-fetoprotein [AFP], unconjugated estriol [uE3], and, in the quad screen, inhibin A). It is performed to evaluate a woman's risk for trisomy 21, trisomy 18, and open neural tube defects (NTDs).

8. The major advantage of chorionic villi sampling (CVS) compared with amniocentesis is that it is done in the first trimester (10 to 13 weeks gestation) and provides faster results. This prevents a long delay between screening and diagnosis and provides results before the mother perceives fetal movement. This may ease the decision-making process regarding continuation of the pregnancy and decrease emotional distress on the patient and family.

9. There is an increased risk of limb reduction defects associated with chorionic villi sampling (CVS) when the procedure is performed before 10 weeks gestation.

10. Second trimester indications for amniocentesis include prenatal diagnosis of chromosomal, genetic, and metabolic disorders. Third-trimester indications are to test for fetal lung maturity (FLM), identification of fetal infection, and therapeutic amniocentesis for amniotic fluid volume disorders such as hydramnios and oligohydramnios.

11. Risks of early amniocentesis (before 15 weeks of gestation) include increased degree of difficulty of the procedure with an increased failure rate, inadequate amniotic fluid volume for sampling, increased rates of pregnancy loss, and amniotic fluid leakage that has been linked to talipes equinovarus (clubfoot) deformity in the infant.

12. Surfactant is important for fetal lung maturity because it reduces surface tension on the inner walls of the alveoli, allowing them to stay slightly open during exhalation. Additionally, surfactant stabilizes lung volume, alters lung mechanics, and maintains gas exchange in the lung. Without adequate surfactant, lung walls adhere to one another, making alveoli inflation during inhalation

difficult, which in turn increases the amount of pressure required to keep alveoli open. If this situation is not corrected, impaired oxygenation eventually leads to respiratory distress syndrome (RDS) and other neonatal complications, increasing the rates of neonatal morbidity and mortality.

13. The primary goal of antepartum fetal testing is identification of fetuses at risk for permanent neurologic injury or stillbirth so timely intervention can be done to decrease perinatal morbidity and mortality rates.

14. To explain fetal movement counting to a patient, the nurse should tell her to rest in a quiet location and count distinct fetal movements, such as kicks or rolls. Once 10 movements are perceived, record the number of movements and amount of time on a cell phone app or piece of paper. If you do not feel 10 movements in 1 to 2 hours, or you notice a decrease in the movements, notify your provider.

15. Reactive NSTs contain two or more FHR accelerations within a 20-minute period. Accelerations are defined as visually apparent increases in the FHR that reach a peak of 15 beats per minute (bpm) above the baseline, with the entire acceleration lasting a minimum of 15 seconds but less than 2 minutes ("15 × 15"). Before 32 weeks of gestation, accelerations are defined as visually apparent increases in the FHR that reach a peak of 10 bpm above the baseline with the entire acceleration lasting at least 10 seconds ("10 × 10").

16. Contraction stress tests (CSTs) determine fetal well-being by monitoring FHR responses to contractions. Healthy, well oxygenated fetuses can physiologically tolerate the interrupted placental blood flow which occurs during contractions and maintain FHR with normal characteristics such as a stable baseline rate and accelerations. In compromised fetuses, brief interruptions of oxygen transfer during contractions can result in late decelerations.

17. The interpretation criteria for CST are as follows:
  • *Negative*—No late decelerations
  • *Positive*—Late decelerations are present with a minimum of 50% of the contractions even when fewer than three contractions occur in 10 minutes
  • *Equivocal–suspicious*—Intermittent late decelerations or significant variable decelerations (sudden decreases in the FHR that quickly return to the baseline)
  Equivocal—FHR decelerations in the presence of contractions that are more frequent than every 2 minutes or last longer than 90 seconds
  • *Unsatisfactory*—Fewer than three contractions in 10 minutes or a tracing that cannot be interpreted

18. The four biophysical characteristics evaluated with ultrasound during a biophysical profile (BPP) are fetal movement, fetal tone, fetal breathing movement, and amniotic fluid amount. Biophysical characteristics are a reflection of the central nervous system (CNS) and provide an indirect means of evaluating fetal oxygenation.

19. Amniotic fluid volume is an important parameter in biophysical profiles (BPPs) and modified biophysical profiles (MBPPs) because it is the only long-term indicator of fetal oxygenation.

20. Shunting occurs because the fetus redirects blood from areas not critical to fetal life, such as the kidneys, gastrointestinal tract, and extremities, to the vital organs, which include the heart, brain, and adrenal gland. If changes in oxygenation are prolonged, blood flow to the fetal kidneys ceases. Therefore oligohydramnios in fetuses with normal renal structures and intact amniotic membranes suggests prolonged fetal hypoxia and is a strong indication of fetal compromise.

CHAPTER 10

1. Bleeding is the most common sign of threatened abortion. It may be accompanied by rhythmic cramping, backache, or feelings of pelvic pressure. Gross rupture of membranes and subsequent cervical dilatation and bleeding make the abortion inevitable.

2. Recurrent spontaneous abortions (also called *miscarriages*) most often occur as a result of genetic or chromosomal abnormalities of the embryo or anomalies of the maternal reproductive tract. Additional causes are believed to be hormonal and immunologic factors or systemic diseases or infections.

3. Nurses can facilitate the grief response by being aware that although many couples grieve over an early pregnancy loss, they often feel a lack of support from family, friends, and health care personnel. Grief often includes feelings of guilt and speculation about whether the woman could have done something to prevent the loss. Nurses may help by emphasizing that abortions usually occur as the result of factors or abnormalities that cannot be avoided. When nurses demonstrate empathy and unconditional acceptance of the feelings expressed, they support the grief response. Providing information about the grieving and referrals to additional support groups also may be helpful.

4. Ectopic pregnancy remains a significant cause of maternal death because of hemorrhage, and it can reduce the woman's chance of subsequent pregnancies because of damage to a fallopian tube. Also, the condition that caused the ectopic pregnancy in the tube may be present in the opposite tube.

5. The increase in incidence of ectopic pregnancy may occur as a result of pelvic inflammatory disease that may complicate untreated sexually transmitted infections. Scarring of the fallopian tubes that may result from the infection may make it difficult for the fertilized ovum to pass through the obstructed tube. Ectopic pregnancy is also more likely to occur in women who have assisted reproduction for infertility, ovulation disorders, contraceptive devices, and use of progesterone agents. Treatment for ectopic pregnancy may be medical (chemotherapeutic agent) or surgical (salpingostomy or salpingectomy).

6. Hydatidiform mole is a form of gestational trophoblastic disease that involves abnormal development of the placenta as the fetal part of the pregnancy fails to develop. The first phase of treatment is evacuation of the

molar pregnancy from the uterus. The second phase is follow-up to detect malignant changes in remaining trophoblastic tissue.

7. Painless vaginal bleeding in the latter half of pregnancy is the classic sign of placenta previa. Bed rest, no sexual intercourse, an adult caregiver present at all times, and availability of emergency transportation to the hospital are essential for home care. The woman must also be taught to monitor fetal movement and to report a decrease in movement or increase in vaginal bleeding.

8. The five classic signs of placental abruption are (a) bleeding, which may be evident vaginally or concealed behind the placenta; (b) uterine tenderness; (c) uterine irritability, with poor relaxation between contractions; (d) abdominal pain; and (e) a high uterine resting tone if an intrauterine pressure catheter is being used. Additional symptoms include a "boardlike" abdomen, firm to the touch; "port wine"–colored amniotic fluid, and nonreassuring fetal heart rate (FHR) pattern and signs of hypovolemic shock.

9. Hemorrhagic shock is the major danger of placental abruption for the mother; anoxia, excessive blood loss, and delivery before maturity are major dangers for the fetus.

10. Disseminated intravascular coagulation is a life-threatening disorder in which procoagulation and anticoagulation factors are activated simultaneously, resulting in profuse bleeding from any vulnerable area. It may occur with missed abortion (primarily if the pregnancy had reached the second trimester when fetal death occurred), placental abruption, severe pregnancy-induced hypertension, amniotic fluid embolism, and other conditions such as sepsis.

11. Both morning sickness and hyperemesis gravidarum begin in the first trimester. Morning sickness is self-limiting and causes no serious complications. Hyperemesis is persistent, uncontrollable vomiting that may cause excessive weight loss, dehydration, and electrolyte or acid-base imbalance.

12. Goals of management are to maintain hydration, replace electrolytes and vitamins, maintain nutrition, and provide emotional support.

13. Nurses must use critical thinking to examine personal biases that may result in lack of comfort and support for women with hyperemesis. Helping the woman identify any reluctance to accept her pregnancy may lead to solutions that can reduce the intensity of hyperemesis.

14. Persistent vasospasm of uterine arterioles may result in fetal hypoxemia, intrauterine growth restriction, or even fetal death.

15. Classic signs of preeclampsia include hypertension and possibly proteinuria. Nonspecific edema that is severe and generalized is often seen but is no longer considered a classic sign of preeclampsia. Headache, hyperreflexia, visual disturbances, and epigastric pain indicate the disease is worsening. Rest, especially in a lateral position, increases maternal cardiac return and circulatory volume, thus improving perfusion of vital organs.

16. Vasospasms cause rupture of cerebral capillaries and small cerebral hemorrhages.
Symptoms of arterial vasospasm include headache and visual disturbances such as blurred vision, "spots" before the eyes, and hyperactive deep tendon reflexes (DTRs).

17. Magnesium sulfate prevents seizures by reducing central nervous system irritability and decreasing vasoconstriction. The primary adverse effect is central nervous system depression, which includes depression of the respiratory center.

18. Pulmonary edema, circulatory or renal failure, aspiration of gastric contents, and cerebral hemorrhage are complications of eclampsia. HELLP syndrome, which demonstrates coagulation and liver function abnormalities, is more likely to occur when a woman has severe preeclampsia or eclampsia. Disseminated intravascular coagulation (DIC) may cause unexpected bleeding as levels of coagulation factors decline.

19. Assessments for the woman with preeclampsia include daily weights; location and degree of edema; vital signs; hourly urinary output; urine for protein; deep tendon reflexes; and subjective signs such as headache, visual disturbances, and epigastric pain. The fetal heart rate should be assessed for nonreassuring patterns. Respiratory rate; oxygen saturation level; consciousness level; and laboratory data such as creatinine, liver enzymes, and magnesium levels should be evaluated. Psychosocial assessment should include the reaction of the woman's family and support system. Nursing assessment helps determine whether the condition is responding to medical management, if the condition is stable, or if the disease is worsening.

20. To prevent seizures, maintain a quiet environment, reduce environmental stimuli, and maintain a therapeutic level of magnesium. Nurses must remain with the woman and call for help if a seizure occurs. Attempt to turn the woman on her side before the onset of a seizure. Note the sequence and time of the seizure. Insert an airway after the seizure, and suction the woman's nose and mouth, administer oxygen, administer medications, and prepare for additional medical interventions.

21. To prevent seizure-related injury, the side rails should be padded and raised. The bed should be in the lowest position with the wheels locked. Oxygen and suction should be readily available. Necessary equipment and medications should be immediately available.

22. Signs of magnesium toxicity include respiratory rate below 12 breaths per minute, hyporeflexia, sweating or flushing, altered sensorium (lethargy, drowsiness, disorientation), and serum magnesium level beyond the therapeutic range. If toxicity occurs, discontinue the drug and notify the physician. Calcium gluconate is an antidote for magnesium toxicity and should be immediately available.

23. H, Hemolysis; EL, elevated liver enzymes; LP, low platelets. Major symptoms are pain and tenderness in the right upper quadrant. Additional signs and symptoms may include nausea, vomiting, and severe edema. Laboratory data include a low hematocrit level, abnormal liver

studies, coagulation abnormalities, and often abnormal renal studies. Palpating the liver could cause trauma, including rupture of a subcapsular hematoma.

24. Preeclampsia occurs only during pregnancy and the early postpartum period. Chronic hypertension is present before pregnancy or before the twentieth week of gestation and persists after the postpartum period. Hypertension that remains several weeks postpartum suggests that the woman has chronic hypertension even if her blood pressure measurements were normal when she entered care. Treatment may be similar during pregnancy; however, chronic hypertension may be treated with antihypertensive medications before and during pregnancy. Preeclampsia may further complicate chronic hypertension.

25. Administration of Rho(D) immunoglobulin prevents development of maternal anti-Rh antibodies and is recommended after any procedure that includes the possibility of maternal exposure to Rh-positive fetal blood.

26. A mother who is sensitized has developed antibodies to the Rh antigen. Maternal anti-Rh antibodies cross the placental barrier. If the fetus is Rh positive, the antibodies destroy fetal Rh-positive red blood cells. The fetus becomes anemic, bilirubin concentration increases, and in extreme cases severe neurologic disease can result.

27. Many women with blood type O have anti-A or anti-B antibodies before they become pregnant, so the first pregnancy can be affected. The effects of ABO incompatibility are milder than Rh sensitization because the primary antibodies of the ABO system are IgM, which do not readily cross the placenta.

28. The hormones of pregnancy cause resistance of maternal cells to insulin, which increases the availability of glucose for the fetus.

29. The mother is at risk to develop preeclampsia, urinary tract infections, ketoacidosis, and preterm labor. Possible fetal and neonatal effects include congenital malformations; small or large fetal size, depending on the placental vascular supply; fetal hypoxemia; and polycythemia. Neonatal effects include hypoglycemia, hypocalcemia, hyperbilirubinemia, and respiratory distress syndrome.

30. Insulin needs decrease during the first trimester and increase sharply during the second and third trimesters (when placental hormones initiate insulin resistance). During the muscular exertion and reduced oral intake associated with labor, insulin needs must be determined by frequent checks of blood glucose levels to keep the maternal glucose level within normal limits. In the postpartum period, insulin needs decrease as levels of placental hormones decline.

31. Glycosylated hemoglobin gives an accurate evaluation of blood glucose level for the past 2 to 3 months and is not affected by recent intake or restriction of food.

32. Gestational diabetes mellitus is first diagnosed during pregnancy with none of the classic signs of type 1 diabetes: thirst, heavy urine excretion, and weight loss despite heavy food intake. Type 1 diabetes mellitus usually emerges during childhood or early adulthood and requires insulin for control. Type 2 diabetes usually occurs in adulthood and is usually managed by diet and/or oral hypoglycemics if not pregnant. Gestational diabetes is often managed by diet and exercise, although insulin may be needed if fasting or postprandial capillary blood glucose values are persistently high. Oral hypoglycemics are not commonly used.

33. A glucose challenge test (GCT) is a screening procedure only and requires no fasting before the woman drinks a 50-g glucose solution and has a serum glucose drawn 1 hour later. A 3-hour oral glucose tolerance test (OGTT) is performed to diagnose diabetes mellitus, including gestational diabetes. The OGTT requires measurement of a fasting blood glucose level followed by intake of 100 g of glucose solution. Blood glucose levels are determined hourly after the solution is taken, at 1, 2, and 3 hours.

34. Maternal effects of gestational diabetes mellitus include increased incidence of urinary tract infections, hydramnios (excessive amniotic fluid), premature rupture of membranes, and development of hypertension. Fetal effects may include macrosomia, which can result in shoulder dystocia or cesarean birth. The newborn is at risk for hypoglycemia. Preexisting diabetes has similar maternal effects as gestational diabetes, but fetal and infant effects may be more severe if the disease is not well controlled. The infant may have intrauterine growth restriction (IUGR) if the woman's diabetes has caused vascular impairment, or macrosomia if her glucose level is poorly controlled and no vascular impairment exists. Congenital anomalies are increased in preexisting diabetes, especially if the diabetes is poorly controlled at conception and during early gestation.

35. Increased intravascular volume and increased cardiac output (particularly stroke volume) place an added burden on the heart of a woman who has a cardiac defect.

36. Acquired and congenital heart disease are the two major categories of heart disease during pregnancy. Acute problems such as myocardial infarction or conduction disorders may also occur during pregnancy. Functional classification depends on the person's ability to tolerate activity. Class I indicates no limitation on activity. Class II indicates slight restriction if necessary. Class III is associated with marked limitation. Class IV indicates that the person has symptoms such as dyspnea at rest.

37. Goals of treatment are to prevent anemia with adequate iron and folic acid intake so the supply of red blood cells is adequate to transport oxygen and thus reduce the demands on the heart, limit physical activity so cardiac demand does not exceed the capacity of the heart, and limit weight gain, which would add further demands on the heart.

38. With every contraction, blood is shifted from the uterus and placenta into the central circulation. This can lead to fluid overload if fluids are administered rapidly.

39. An additional 500 mL of blood is returned to the central circulation with delivery of the placenta. Also, the compression of the vena cava that characterized much of

pregnancy is gone. This increases the load on the heart and can lead to further compromise of the heart.

40. The obese woman should gain 11 to 20 lb during pregnancy.

41. During the intrapartum period, the nurse caring for an obese patient should assess for signs of dysfunctional labor (abnormal contraction pattern, slow or no cervical change, inadequate fetal descent).

42. Most women begin pregnancy with marginal iron stores, do not have adequate iron stores to meet the demands of pregnancy, and have difficulty meeting the high iron needs of pregnancy with diet alone.

43. The fetus usually receives adequate iron, even at a cost to the mother. Therefore neonatal effects of moderate maternal anemia are rare. With very severe maternal anemia, however, the fetus may become hypoxic.

44. The fetal and neonatal effects of folic acid deficiency are increased risk of spontaneous abortion, abruption of the placenta, and fetal anomalies, particularly neural tube defects.

45. Pregnancy may worsen sickle cell disease, and the risk of "sickle cell crisis" is increased.

46. Frequent measurements of hemoglobin, blood count, serum iron, and iron-binding capacity, as well as folate, are necessary to determine the degree of anemia. Frequent fetal surveillance and monitoring for signs of sickle cell crisis are also necessary. The nurse should also be aware that the woman's pain could be a pregnancy complication rather than a result of sickle cell crisis.

47. Thalassemia is associated with increased iron absorption and storage, making women with this disorder susceptible to iron overload.

48. The maternal and fetal effects of systemic lupus erythematosus are increased incidence of abortion, fetal death, and preterm delivery. Congenital heart block, often permanent, is a serious complication for the newborn. Pregnancy can exacerbate the disease, and renal complications pose a special risk.

49. Rheumatoid arthritis often markedly improves during pregnancy. However, relapse often occurs soon after childbirth.

50. Hypothyroidism in the woman may cause adverse effects on the mental development of the fetus through birth and childhood. A greater risk for miscarriage, preterm birth, and preeclampsia exists if it is not corrected.

51. Anticonvulsant drugs may be teratogenic. Many have probable or known adverse effects on the fetus. However, generalized seizures may also have adverse fetal effects, so maintaining the anticonvulsant dose as low as possible is important. Newer anticonvulsants have less data related to their possible fetal effects.

52. The recommended supportive care for women with Bell's palsy includes eye patching, applying ointment or drops to prevent trauma to the cornea, facial massage, and psychological support. Corticosteroids may be given.

53. Primary maternal infection is more likely to result in fetal and neonatal infection. About 90% of newborns are not affected, but about 10% will have symptoms at birth. About 10% of this group will show full cytomegalovirus (CMV) inclusion disease. Another 10% of this birth group will show late-onset signs. Problems include enlarged spleen and liver, central nervous system (CNS) abnormalities, developmental delay, dental defects, jaundice, chorioretinitis, hearing loss, and growth impairment.

54. The first trimester is the time of organogenesis, when damage can be done to all developing organ systems.

55. A vaccine is available to prevent rubella, but it cannot be given during pregnancy. During pregnancy a woman can only avoid situations in which she is likely to contract rubella. Rubella immunization should be given to the woman before discharge after birth, and she should be taught that pregnancy should be avoided for 4 weeks (1 month) after the immunization.

56. Immunization with varicella-zoster immune globulin is recommended. Because of viral shedding, infected mothers and infants must be isolated from those who are not immune.

57. Vertical transmission of herpesvirus occurs when organisms ascend after rupture of membranes and during birth when the fetus comes into contact with infectious tissue and secretions.

58. The fetal and neonatal effects of parvovirus B19 infection are failure of red blood cell production, severe fetal anemia, hydrops, and heart failure.

59. Hepatitis B virus is transmitted by contact with infected blood, saliva, vaginal secretions, semen, or breast milk. A newborn whose mother is known to carry the hepatitis B surface antigen should receive hepatitis B immune globulin soon after birth, followed by hepatitis B vaccine. The infant should receive the second and third doses of vaccine at regularly scheduled times.

60. Avoid sexual transmission by abstinence, avoiding intercourse with infected persons, or using recommended barrier methods such as a condom. Intravenous drug users who refuse rehabilitation must avoid transmission that occurs when needles are shared with those who are infected. Use standard precautions to avoid contact with secretions that may carry the virus.

61. Several combinations of antiretroviral medication regimens may be administered to delay replication of the virus. Opportunistic diseases are treated. Good hygiene reduces transmission of infectious organisms to the susceptible person, and nutritious meals reduce the risk for opportunistic infection. Antiretroviral therapy reduces vertical transmission of HIV to the infant and ideally begins during the second trimester of pregnancy. Additional treatment continues after birth for the infant. Individualized maternal therapy may include multiple antiretrovirals.

62. Toxoplasmosis can be prevented by cooking meat thoroughly, not touching mucous membranes while handling raw meat, washing kitchen surfaces and hands thoroughly after handling raw meat, avoiding uncooked eggs and unpasteurized milk, washing vegetables and fruit

before consumption, and avoiding contact with materials that may be contaminated with cat feces.

63. Risk factors for the mother transmitting group B Streptococcus (GBS) to her infant include a prior infant with GBS infection, presence of GBS organisms in the urine in the present pregnancy, preterm birth (before 37 weeks), maternal fever in labor, and prolonged membrane rupture (≥18 hours). Intravenous antibacterial therapy is used to prevent colonization in the newborn of the GBS-positive mother or if her status is unknown.

64. Isoniazid, rifampin, and ethambutol are given for 2 months followed by isoniazid and rifampin daily or twice per week for 7 months to treat tuberculosis in the mother. Pyridoxine (vitamin B_6) is added to prevent neurotoxicity. The infant is skin-tested at birth and may be prescribed isoniazid. Isoniazid is usually continued for the infant until the mother's tuberculosis has been inactive for at least 3 months. Infant tuberculosis medication may stop if the mother and family members are well treated and show no additional disease. If the skin test result shows conversion to positive, a full course of drug therapy should be given to the infant.

CHAPTER 11

1. Pregnancy interrupts developmental tasks such as the achievement of a stable identity, development of a personal value system, completion of educational goals, and achievement of independence from parents.

2. Teenage mothers have an increased chance of perinatal complications, including death, pregnancy-associated hypertension, anemia, preterm labor and birth, depression, substance abuse, intimate partner violence, poor nutrition and self-care, perineal lacerations, and striae gravidarum with itching. They are also at risk for another teenage pregnancy. Infants are at greater risk for preterm birth, low birth weight, and neonatal death.

3. A variety of teaching methods such as visual aids, videos, group classes with other teens, and one-to-one counseling may be effective for teenagers.

4. Prospective teenage parents should be taught that infants develop a sense of trust, which is necessary for future development, when their needs are met promptly and gently. Crying indicates a need and does not mean the infant is "spoiled."

5. Mature gravidas often have maturity, problem-solving skills, and emotional and financial resources that may be unavailable to younger women.

6. The fetus of a mature woman is at increased risk for chromosomal anomalies that may be detected by prenatal screening.

7. The older mother may have less energy than younger mothers, and conserving her energy for care of herself and her infant is important.

8. Neonatal effects of maternal smoking include risk for low birth weight, increased risk for sudden infant death syndrome (SIDS), and an increased risk of colic, asthma, and childhood obesity.

9. Fetal alcohol syndrome is characterized by slow growth, central nervous system impairment, and cranial and facial anomalies.

10. Effects of maternal cocaine use on the infant include increased risk for preterm birth, preterm rupture of the membranes, intrauterine growth restriction, and low birth weight.

11. Pregnant heroin users are placed on methadone to provide a long-acting, steady drug dose to the fetus to avoid the problems of intrauterine overdosage and withdrawal. The dosage is gradually decreased to wean the pregnant woman off of the drug. Buprenorphine may also be used.

12. Prenatal behaviors that suggest substance abuse include prenatal care sought late in pregnancy, failure to keep appointments, inconsistent follow-through with recommended regimens, poor grooming, inadequate weight gain, needle punctures, thrombosed veins, signs of cellulitis, defensive or hostile reactions, and severe mood swings.

13. Signs and symptoms of recent cocaine use include profuse sweating, high blood pressure, tachycardia, irregular respirations, lethargic response to labor, dilated pupils, increased body temperature, sudden onset of severely painful uterine contractions, fetal tachycardia, and excessive fetal activity. Emotional signs include anger, caustic or abusive reactions to the caregiver, emotional lability, and paranoia.

14. Interventions are focused on preventing maternal or fetal injury and may require setting limits in a firm, nonjudgmental manner with a woman who may be abusive and in great pain.

15. Parents experience less anxiety when they are gently told about the condition of the infant and allowed to hold their newborn as soon as possible.

16. Facial, genital, and irreparable defects are likely to affect parenting most.

17. The reaction of parents can be described in terms of a grief response. Initial reactions include shock and disbelief. Denial, anger, and guilt are common.

18. Nurses can promote bonding by handling the infant gently, emphasizing normal traits, helping parents hold and cuddle the infant, and using communication skills to help parents come to terms with their feelings.

19. Discharge planning should include special feeding and other techniques that the infant may require, the follow-up care needed, and referral to agencies and organizations that may be helpful.

20. The way in which the stillborn infant is presented creates memories that the parents will retain. The infant should be washed and taken to the parents while still warm and soft, wrapped in a soft, warm blanket.

21. A memory packet that includes photographs of the baby, handprints, footprints, a birth identification band, crib card, blanket, cap, and, if possible, a lock of hair help parents grieve.

22. Mothers see adoption as an act of sacrifice and love when they give up the infant to those who can provide a better life.

23. Adoptive parents must be taught how to care for an infant and what to expect in terms of growth and development.

24. The symptoms of postpartum depression differ from those of postpartum "blues" in their intensity and persistence. In postpartum depression, the symptoms are present daily for at least 2 weeks. They include anxiety, feelings of guilt, agitation, fatigue, sleeplessness, feeling unwell, irritability, difficulty concentrating or making decisions, confusion, appetite changes, loss of pleasure in normal activities, crying, sadness, depression, suicidal thoughts, and being less responsive to the infant.

25. Nurses can demonstrate caring, provide anticipatory guidance, help the mother verbalize her feelings, and make appropriate referrals.

26. Postpartum psychosis usually requires hospitalization, psychotherapy, and appropriate medication.

CHAPTER 12

1. Effacement and dilation of the cervix occur because contractions pull the cervix upward over the fetus and amniotic sac while pushing the fetus and amniotic sac downward against the cervix. The muscle fibers of the upper uterus become shorter to maintain these forces between contractions. In addition, the uterus changes shape and becomes more elongated and narrow to maintain pressure of the fetus and amniotic sac against the cervix.

2. The cervix of the nullipara effaces more before it dilates. The cervix of a multipara is usually thicker than that of a nullipara during the entire labor.

3. Maternal changes occurring during labor include the following:
   a. Cardiovascular system—A slight increase in blood pressure and decrease in pulse rate occur as each contraction temporarily stops blood flow to her uterus. Supine hypotension may occur if she lies on her back because the heavy uterus compresses her inferior vena cava and reduces blood flow to her heart.
   b. Respiratory system—The depth and rate of respirations increase.
   c. Gastrointestinal system—Gastric motility is reduced during labor, which can result in nausea and vomiting. Controversy exists on whether laboring women should be allowed to eat or drink during labor. Concerns surround the risk for vomiting and aspiration of undigested foods in the event general anesthesia is required. Evidence supports allowing low-risk laboring women some form of oral intake. The American Society of Anesthesiologists supports oral intake of clear liquids in low-risk laboring women.
   d. Urinary system—The sensation of a full bladder is reduced.
   e. Hematopoietic system—Leukocyte counts are as high as 20,000 to 30,000/mm^3, and levels of clotting factors are elevated.

4. Uterine contractions temporarily decrease blood flow to the placenta. If the contractions were sustained, the fetus could not receive freshly oxygenated blood and nutrients and dispose of waste products through the placenta.

5. Labor and vaginal birth primarily benefit the newborn by increasing absorption of fetal lung fluid. They also cause compression of the upper airways, causing some lung fluid to be expelled. These effects reduce the amount of lung fluid remaining in the newborn's respiratory tract when breathing begins. Labor also stimulates the fetus to secrete catecholamines, which help speed clearance of the lung fluid after birth, stimulate cardiac contraction and breathing, and aid in temperature regulation.

6. The power of labor during the first stage involves uterine contractions. Powers during the second stage include uterine contractions, augmented by the woman's voluntary pushing efforts.

7. The three divisions of the true pelvis are the inlet, midpelvis, and outlet.

8. The vertex presentation, in which the fetal head is fully flexed forward, allows the smallest diameter of the fetal head to enter the pelvis. It also more effectively dilates the cervix.

9. ROP: The fetal landmark is the occiput, indicating a vertex presentation. It is located in the mother's right posterior pelvic quadrant. OA: The fetal landmark is the occiput, which is located in the mother's anterior pelvis and is not directed toward her left or her right. This is often the presentation just before birth. RSA: The fetal landmark is the sacrum, indicating that the fetus is in a breech presentation. It is located in the mother's right anterior pelvis. LMA: The fetal landmark is the mentum, or chin, indicating that the fetus is in a face presentation. The chin is in the mother's left anterior pelvis.

10. If the fetus is in the face presentation, the occiput is not accessible to the examiner's fingers during vaginal examination. For this reason the fetal chin (mentum) is used to describe the position (such as RMA [right mentum anterior]).

11. The woman may note several changes as labor approaches: increased strength and frequency of Braxton Hicks contractions, lightening, increased vaginal mucus, bloody show, an energy spurt, and a small weight loss.

12. False labor tends to differ from true labor in three major ways. True labor is characterized by contractions that progressively become more frequent, last longer, and are more intense. The discomfort of true labor begins in the lower back and sweeps to the lower abdomen, whereas the discomfort of false labor is more often in the abdomen or groin and is often simply annoying. In true labor, progressive effacement and dilation of the cervix occur, which is the most significant difference from false labor.

13. The transverse diameter of the pelvic inlet is slightly larger than the inlet's anteroposterior diameter. The

anteroposterior diameter of the fetal head (in line with the sagittal suture) is slightly larger than the transverse diameter. Therefore the fetal head best fits the pelvis if the sagittal suture is aligned with the pelvic transverse diameter at entry.

14. Because the woman's pelvic outlet is usually slightly larger in its anteroposterior diameter than its transverse diameter, the fetal head turns in the mechanism of internal rotation so that the sagittal suture aligns with the anteroposterior diameter as the fetus descends.

15. During the first stage, latent phase, the woman is often sociable, excited, and somewhat anxious. During the first stage, active phase, the woman becomes less sociable and is inwardly focused. During the first stage, transition phase, the woman may become irritable and temporarily lose control. During the second stage, the woman usually concentrates her energy toward pushing her baby out and interacts little with others. She often regains a feeling of control and active participation in the birth during the second stage.

16. Contractions vary among women, but the general pattern includes increasing frequency, duration, and intensity throughout labor. In the first stage, latent phase, contractions gradually increase until they are about 5 minutes apart, lasting for 30 to 40 seconds with mild to moderate intensity. In the first stage, active phase, contractions increase to about 2 to 5 minutes apart with a duration of about 40 to 60 seconds and moderate to strong intensity. In the first stage, transition phase, contractions are strong with a frequency of 1 ½ to 2 minutes apart and a duration of 60 to 90 seconds. In the second stage, contractions are strong and about 2 to 3 minutes apart and have a duration of about 40 to 60 seconds.

17. Signs that the placenta may have separated include a spherical uterine shape, the rising of the uterus upward in the abdomen, protrusion of the umbilical cord farther outward from the vagina, and a gush of blood.

18. Hemorrhage may occur if the uterus does not remain contracted after birth of the placenta because open blood vessels at the site will not be compressed by the interlacing muscle fibers of the uterus.

CHAPTER 13

1. Childbirth pain differs from other painful experiences because it is part of a normal process, the woman has time to prepare for it, it is self-limited and intermittent, and it ends with the birth of the baby.

2. Excessive, unrelieved labor pain may result in a stress response (diverting blood flow from the uterus and compromising fetal oxygenation), maternal acid-base imbalance, and fetal acidosis. It may increase the length of labor. Poor pain relief can lessen the joy of childbirth for the woman and her partner and may have lasting psychological effects.

3. Physical and psychological factors interact to alter the ability to tolerate pain. For example, relaxation and

working with the forces of labor enhance the chance that the woman who has a large baby and a small pelvis will give birth vaginally.

4. Four sources of pain present in most labors are cervical dilation, uterine ischemia, pressure and pulling on pelvic structures, and distention of the vagina and perineum.

5. Physical factors that influence pain include the following:
   a. A short, intense labor may be more painful because dilation, effacement, and fetal descent occur rapidly.
   b. A cervix that does not efface or dilate easily is likely to be associated with a longer and more uncomfortable labor.
   c. An abnormal fetal position may cause a longer labor as the woman's body maneuvers it into a better position. Back pain is especially noticeable if the fetus is in an occiput posterior position.
   d. Variations in the mother's pelvic size or shape may result in abnormal fetal presentations or positions and in a longer labor because the fetus does not fit through the pelvis easily.
   e. Fatigue reduces the woman's pain tolerance and ability to use coping skills.

6. Psychosocial factors that influence labor pain include culture, anxiety and fear, previous experiences, preparation for childbirth, and the mother's support system.

7. The gate control theory of pain assumes that a gating mechanism in the dorsal horn of the spinal cord controls the transmission of painful impulses to the brain for interpretation. Pain impulses are transmitted through small-diameter fibers, whereas other sensations, such as tactile sensations (e.g., massage, heat, cold), are transmitted more quickly through large-diameter fibers. Therefore the impulses transmitted through the large-diameter fibers interfere with, or "close the gate," to transmission of pain impulses. Impulses from the brain, such as responses to auditory stimuli (listening to music, for instance), can also impede pain transmission.

8. Nursing actions to promote relaxation include arranging for environmental comfort, maintaining the woman's general comfort, reducing factors that cause anxiety and fear, and using specific relaxation techniques such as helping the woman focus on relaxing specific tense muscles.

9. Accurate information and a focus on the normal aspects of childbirth help reduce anxiety and fear. Avoid referring to the woman as a client or patient because these words are associated with illness in a hospital. Call her and her partner by the names they requested when admitted. Empowerment of the birthing partners helps them see themselves as competent to give birth successfully.

10. Self-massage might include effleurage, rubbing the hands together, or patting or banging the hands on the rail. Massage by others helps relax tense muscles and aids relaxation. Counterpressure, which may include sacral pressure or other variations, is often used to reduce back pain when the fetus is in an occiput posterior position. Acupressure uses directed pressure for pain management.

Warmth relaxes muscles, promoting relaxation. Warmth may be in the form of a shower, tub bath, or whirlpool. Cool often feels better to the laboring woman who may be hot, or she may want cool only in a local area or ice in her mouth.

11. Hydration must be adequate to offset the diuresis that often occurs with immersion in water. Diuresis could reduce placental perfusion if plasma volume is low. Water temperature must be controlled to prevent hyperthermia or hypothermia, which could raise the mother's metabolic rate, increasing her oxygen and glucose consumption. These changes could reduce oxygen and glucose delivered to the fetus. Hyperthermia in the mother increases fetal body temperature and increases fetal demand for oxygen.

12. The more complex breathing techniques are more effective for greater pain, but they are tiring. Advancing from simpler to more complex breathing techniques too quickly can cause the mother to become fatigued when she most needs to use these methods.

13. The cleansing breath has four purposes: (a) to release tension; (b) to increase oxygen intake to combat myometrial hypoxia; (c) to clear the woman's mind so she can focus on relaxing through the contraction; and (d) to signal her labor partner that a contraction has begun.

14. Lengthy pushing in the second stage has shown greater maternal fatigue, more operative births, and nonreassuring fetal heart rate (FHR) patterns and does not significantly shorten the second stage. Strenuous directed pushing has shown a greater risk for structural and neurogenic injury to a woman's pelvic floor. Closed glottis pushing delivers less blood to the placenta, possibly resulting in fetal hypoxia and nonreassuring fetal heart monitor patterns.

15. Drugs taken by the mother can affect the fetus directly, such as by decreasing fetal heart rate variability, or indirectly, such as by causing maternal hypotension that reduces placental blood flow and fetal oxygen supply.

16. Aortocaval compression should be offset by placing a wedge under the woman's hip if a supine position is required. Tilting the patient table during surgery reduces compression until the infant is born. The woman is more sensitive to general anesthesia and may have a greater fall in oxygenation when general anesthesia is induced. Reduced peristalsis and tone of the sphincter at the junction of the esophagus and stomach can lead to regurgitation and aspiration of gastric contents, primarily with general anesthesia. Lower doses of anesthetic agents will be needed for epidural or subarachnoid blocks.

17. Drugs (prescribed, over the counter, or illicit), botanical preparations, and alcohol may interact with one another. These interactions may be harmful to the woman, the fetus, or both. Knowledge of exactly what drugs she uses allows the safest choices in pharmacologic pain-relief methods.

18. Neonatal respiratory depression is the primary drawback to the use of opioid analgesia. This effect can be reduced by timing the dose to reduce the amount transferred to the fetus (which varies according to the drug) and by giving the narcotic in small, frequent IV doses at the beginning of the contraction. Naloxone (Narcan) is the drug that may be given to reverse opioid-induced respiratory depression in the neonate, with bag-and-mask ventilation being the initial method to oxygenate the infant.

19. Airway management (i.e., bag-and-mask ventilation) takes precedence over use of naloxone for the newborn, and the drug is no longer routinely given to the baby for respiratory depression. Naloxone may be used to reverse opioid-induced respiratory depression in the adult. The respiratory depression may be from systemic or epidural administration of opioids.

20. The two major advantages of regional pain management are that the woman can have pain relief and remain alert.

21. Epidural and subarachnoid blocks can cause maternal hypotension. The fall in blood pressure may result in reduced placental blood flow, compromising fetal oxygen supply. Giving the woman IV fluids before the block reduces this effect. Other less serious adverse effects are bladder distention, prolonged second stage of labor (epidural), and postdural puncture headache (usually only subarachnoid block).

22. Epidural or intrathecal opioid analgesics may cause nausea, vomiting, itching, or a combination of these. They may also result in delayed respiratory depression (up to 24 hours), depending on the drug used. Management includes promethazine for nausea and vomiting; diphenhydramine, naloxone, or naltrexone for itching; and pulse oximetry and monitoring of respirations while the opioid is given and up to 24 hours after administration ends, depending on the drug.

23. Maternal regurgitation with aspiration of acidic gastric contents is the major potential adverse effect of general anesthesia. The risk may be reduced by limiting intake to clear fluids, giving drugs to raise the gastric pH, giving drugs to reduce gastric secretions or speed emptying of the stomach, and using cricoid pressure (Sellick maneuver) to block the esophagus while the endotracheal tube is being inserted. Respiratory depression, primarily in the infant, is minimized by delaying general anesthesia until the surgery team is prepared and by keeping the anesthesia level as light as possible until the umbilical cord is cut.

CHAPTER 14

1. The electronic fetal monitor (EFM) is used to assess fetal heart rate (FHR) and uterine activity (UA) during labor for women. Intermittent auscultation (IA) of the FHR and palpation of uterine contractions is the safe and acceptable low-technology method of assessing the labor in low-risk women.

2. Maternal blood flow to the uterus and placenta originates primarily in the uterine arteries, as well as the internal iliac and ovarian arteries. Maternal arterial blood

pressure maintains oxygen- and nutrient-rich blood flow to the uterus and placenta. Blood enters to the intervillous spaces of the placenta via spiral arteries. The intervillous space allows for exchange of substances, such as oxygen, without mixing of maternal and fetal blood. Simultaneously, maternal blood carrying away carbon dioxide and fetal waste products drains from the intervillous spaces through endometrial veins and returns to maternal circulation for elimination.

3. The two umbilical arteries carry deoxygenated blood from the fetus to the placenta.

4. Intermittent auscultation promotes the laboring woman's mobility and creates a more natural atmosphere. However, assessment of the fetus is intermittent—significant events may not be detected, periodic and nonperiodic changes in fetal heart rate (FHR) cannot be determined, the patient may be intolerant of the clinician's touch during contractions, and contractions cannot be assessed objectively. Continuous electronic fetal monitoring provides more data, is often expected by parents, and can assist the nurse to better observe more than one woman. It allows the nurse to devote more time to coaching the woman and her partner. Its primary drawbacks are reduced maternal mobility, adjustments to the equipment, and its technical atmosphere. When using external transducers (ultrasound/tocotransducer), the FHR may be doubled or halved in cases of fetal bradycardia or tachycardia, the maternal heart rate may be recorded as fetal data if the ultrasound transducer is placed over maternal arterial vessels, obese women and preterm or multifetal gestations may be difficult to monitor, and the tocotransducer does not accurately assess the intensity of contractions or resting tone of the uterus between contractions. Internal monitors (fetal scalp electrode [FSE]/intrauterine pressure catheter [IUPC]) are not usually affected by maternal position changes (although the IUPC needs to be recalibrated with maternal position changes) and accurately measure all parameters of uterine activity. However, they require cervical dilatation, and ruptured fetal membranes can cause trauma and infection.

5. When palpating uterine contractions, the fingertips are used to indent the uterus at the peak of the contraction. The descriptive terms used are *"mild", "moderate"* and *"firm",* or *"strong".* A mild contraction can be compared with the tip of the nose—easily indented. A moderate contraction is compared with the chin—it can be slightly indented. A firm or strong contraction is compared with the forehead—unable to indent.

6. The FHR records on the upper grid of the monitor paper or computer tracing; the uterine activity records on the lower grid.

7. The ultrasound transducer, or external electronic fetal monitor (EFM), detects fetal heart motion to measure fetal heart rate (FHR). A handheld Doppler device uses the same technology. Using a fetoscope or Pinard stethoscope, the listener hears the fetal heart sounds. An internal fetal scalp electrode measures, processes, and records the R to R interval of the fetal QRS complexes.

8. The accuracy of the uterine activity (UA) data from a tocodynamometer may be affected by the position of the toco on the maternal fundus, the amount of maternal tissue (adipose) between the toco and uterus, and the maternal position.

9. Fetal heart rate (FHR) accelerations, whether spontaneous or evoked, are predictive of adequate oxygenation and a fetal pH that rules out acidemia.

10. Late decelerations are visually apparent and usually symmetric in shape, with a gradual decrease and return of the fetal heart rate (FHR) to baseline. Late decelerations occur when the onset of the deceleration to the nadir is equal to or greater than 30 seconds, and the nadir of the deceleration occurs after the peak of the contraction. Late decelerations that occur in the presence of fetal heart rate variability indicate transient fetal hypoxia caused by an interruption along the oxygen pathway. Once corrective measures are initiated, they will typically resolve. Late decelerations are more concerning when they are recurrent and associated with tachycardia and a loss of variability. If uncorrected, hypoxic stress will lead to acidemia and neonatal depression.

Early decelerations are visually apparent, are symmetric in shape, and have a gradual decrease and return to FHR baseline that mirrors a uterine contraction. The deceleration onset, nadir, and recovery coincide with the beginning, peak, and ending of a contraction. The onset of the deceleration to the nadir is equal to or greater than 30 seconds. Early decelerations are thought to represent a vagal response during fetal head compression. Early decelerations are benign and not associated with an interruption of fetal oxygenation.

Variable decelerations are visually apparent, abrupt decreases from onset to nadir of a deceleration. The onset of the deceleration to the nadir is less than 30 seconds. The decrease is at least 15 bpm below the baseline, with the deceleration lasting at least 15 seconds and no longer than 2 minutes from onset to the return to baseline. Deceleration shape, depth, duration, and timing in relationship to contractions may vary. Variable decelerations are suggestive of an interruption of oxygenation at the level of the umbilical cord where cord vessels may be compressed. Generally, variable decelerations are not associated with significant hypoxia or acidosis as long as they are intermittent and accompanied by normal baseline rate and variability. If cord compression is recurrent or prolonged, interruption in fetal oxygenation can progress to hypoxemia, hypoxia, metabolic acidosis, and final metabolic acidemia if corrective measures are not successful.

11. Frequency is the time (minutes) from the onset of one contraction to the onset of the next contraction. Uterine activity may also be quantified as the number of contractions in a 10-minute window of time, averaged over 30 minutes. Duration is the time (sec) from the onset

of one contraction to the end of the same contraction. Intensity is the strength of the contraction at its peak. It is measured by palpation as mild, moderate, strong, or firm. It is quantified in mmHg with the use of an intrauterine pressure catheter (IUPC). Resting tone is the amount of pressure (tone) in the uterus at rest. Normal resting tone is palpated as soft or relaxed or measured with an IUPC as approximately 10 mmHg. Relaxation time is the amount of time from the end of one contraction to the beginning of the next contraction.

12. Category III FHR is an abnormal pattern that is predictive of abnormal fetal acid-base status at the time of observation.

13. The ABCD management approach is a standardized approach to fetal heart rate (FHR) management.
    - **A**—Assess oxygen pathway and identify the cause of FHR changes, both maternal and fetal
    - **B**—Begin corrective measures
    - **C**—Clear obstacles to delivery
    - **D**—Determine a delivery plan

14. Corrective measures that may be considered to correct a category II or III fetal heart rate (FHR) pattern include maternal repositioning, IV fluid bolus, administering oxygen, reducing uterine activity (UA), correcting maternal hypotension, performing amnioinfusion, and modifying second-stage pushing efforts.

15. An IV fluid bolus benefits fetal oxygenation because it improves maternal cardiac output, which improves uteroplacental perfusion, resulting in improved fetal oxygenation.

16. Fetal scalp stimulation should elicit an acceleration of the fetal heart rate (FHR). This confirms fetal oxygenation and a normal fetal acid-base balance at the time of the acceleration.

17. Umbilical cord blood gas sampling is a direct method of assessing the level of oxygenation and fetal acid-base after delivery in situations in which a category II or III pattern is observed. Blood from the umbilical vein is oxygenated, coming from the placenta to the fetus. Blood from the umbilical arteries is deoxygenated, returning from the fetus to the placenta.

18. Potential obstacles to be considered during the "C" part of the ABCD approach include operating room and equipment availability; availability of staff (obstetrician, surgical assistant, anesthesiologist, neonatologist, pediatrician, nursing staff); considerations regarding the mother (consent, anesthesia options, laboratory results, need for blood or blood products, need for an IV, urinary catheter and abdominal prep, what is required for a speedy transfer to the operating room [OR]); considerations regarding the fetus (how many, estimated fetal gestational age and weight, presentation and position, known or anticipated anomalies), and finally, considerations about the monitoring of labor—are adequate data provided to allow appropriately informed management decisions? Measures to overcome these obstacles include preparing the OR; notifying relevant staff; reviewing the mother's medical record for consents, laboratory results, and prenatal data; verifying the status of the patient's IV; inserting a urinary catheter; and prepping her abdomen for surgery if ordered.

CHAPTER 15

1. The nurse should show warmth, concern, and friendliness when the woman and her family enter the hospital or birth center. Determining the woman's and family's expectations about birth, conveying confidence, assigning a primary nurse, and respecting cultural values are specific skills that the nurse can use throughout labor. In addition, a nonjudgmental attitude facilitates communication and shows respect to the woman as an individual.

2. The nurse should try to identify and incorporate beneficial or neutral cultural practices into care during labor and birth by asking about specific practices that are important during birth and facilitating communication by obtaining a fluent interpreter who is acceptable to the woman and her family.

3. The nurse should promptly evaluate the maternal and fetal conditions and the nearness of birth when a woman comes to the hospital or birth center. Prompt assessments should include checking the maternal vital signs, fetal heart rate and patterns, and progress of labor.

4. A lower limit of 110 bpm and an upper limit of 160 bpm with a regular rhythm are normal. When assessing fetal heart rate (FHR) with a continuous electronic fetal monitor, accelerations and the absence of decelerations from the baseline also are normal.

5. Impending birth should be suspected if the woman is grunting, bearing down, sitting on one buttock, or urgently signifying that her baby is about to be born. In that case, the nurse should abbreviate the initial assessment and collect other information after the birth.

6. Women often bring several people with them to the birthing room and want them to stay during admission. Caution is prudent when asking for sensitive information, such as prior pregnancies, sexually transmitted infections (STIs), and potential abuse, when others are present. The woman's partner and other visitors may be unaware of her history. Delay asking intimate information until the woman is alone for confidentiality, safety, and accuracy. A victim of domestic violence is unlikely to answer truthfully when others are around.

7. The current status of the woman's labor is determined by the contraction pattern (frequency, duration, and intensity), status of the amniotic membranes (ruptured or intact), and the cervical exam (dilation, effacement, and fetal station).

8. The woman may specifically request other pain management measures, including epidural analgesia or other medication, express ineffectiveness of nonpharmacologic measures, show muscle tension during and between contractions, have a tense facial expression, and express an inability to tolerate the pain.

9. Three major risks of amniotomy are prolapsed umbilical cord, infection, and placental abruption.

10. The fetal heart rate (FHR) is assessed before the membranes are ruptured to identify whether the fetus has a normal rate and pattern and to establish a baseline. It is checked after the membranes are ruptured to identify patterns that suggest umbilical cord compression and other problems.

11. Signs of chorioamnionitis include fetal tachycardia (often the first sign), elevated maternal temperature, and amniotic fluid that has a foul or strong odor, or a cloudy or yellowish appearance.

12. Greenish, meconium-stained fluid may be seen in response to transient fetal hypoxia, postterm gestation, or placental insufficiency. The newborn may need suctioning at birth if the fluid is stained with meconium. Fluid with a foul or strong odor, cloudy appearance, or yellow color suggests chorioamnionitis (inflammation of the amniotic sac, usually caused by bacterial and viral infections).

13. Frequent vaginal examinations may cause infection because microorganisms from the perineal area can be introduced into the uterus.

14. Hypotension reduces blood flow to the placenta and therefore reduces fetal oxygenation because it diverts blood away from the uterus to better supply the mother's brain, heart, and kidneys. Hypertension may result in vasospasm that can reduce exchange of oxygen, nutrients, and waste products in the placenta. Fetal hypoxia and acidosis can be the ultimate result of maternal hypotension and hypertension.

15. The supine position should be avoided because it causes the woman's uterus to compress her aorta and inferior vena cava (aortocaval compression), reducing blood flow to the placenta. If she must be in the supine position for a procedure such as catheterization, a small pillow or folded blanket under one hip shifts her uterus to maintain placental blood flow.

16. General physical comfort measures during labor include soft, dim lighting; a comfortable temperature; maintenance of cleanliness; mouth care; observations for a full bladder; positions for comfort; and a warm bath or shower. Caring for the support person includes respect for the couple's wishes about partner involvement in the birth process. The nurse should provide support that the partner cannot and should consider physical needs for food and rest.

17. Shortly before birth, the woman's perineum bulges and the fetal head becomes visible as the mother pushes. At this time birth can occur suddenly.

18. The fetal heart rate (FHR) should be monitored before external version to identify abnormal patterns that would preclude the procedure and to establish a baseline. It should be monitored by Doppler or real-time ultrasound as much as possible during and after external version to detect cord compression that can occur if the umbilical cord becomes entangled during change of the fetal presentation.

19. Uterine activity should be observed after external version for possible onset of labor because this procedure may cause uterine irritability or possible placental abruption; therefore the procedure is done near term.

20. Five precautions that promote safe oxytocin induction or augmentation of labor include the following:
    a. Dilution of the oxytocin in an isotonic solution
    b. Piggybacking the oxytocin solution into the port of the primary nonadditive (maintenance) IV line that is nearest the venipuncture site
    c. Starting the oxytocin infusion slowly
    d. Increasing the rate of infusion gradually
    e. Monitoring uterine contractions and fetal heart rate (FHR)

21. Labor may be augmented if it stops or contractions become ineffective. The woman whose labor is augmented with oxytocin usually needs less of the drug than the woman whose labor is being induced, because her uterus is more sensitive to its effects.

22. The fetus may have an adverse reaction to oxytocin, manifested by nonreassuring fetal heart rate (FHR) patterns such as tachycardia, bradycardia, decreased variability, and pathologic (late, variable, or prolonged) decelerations.

23. More than 5 contractions in a 10-min period, increased resting tone of the uterus, and relaxation time of less than 60 seconds between contractions in first-stage labor and 45 to 50 seconds in second-stage labor are signs of increased uterine activity.

24. Administration of oxytocin for a prolonged time may lead to postpartum hemorrhage because the fatigued uterus cannot contract properly to compress bleeding vessels at the placenta site (uterine atony).

25. Forceps and vacuum extraction are used to provide traction to assist the mother in rotation, expulsion, or both of the fetal head. Special forceps (Piper) can be used to deliver the aftercoming head of the fetus in a breech presentation, but a vacuum extractor can be used only with a cephalic presentation. Forceps may cause fetal injury such as facial bruising and nerve injury. The vacuum extractor may create an artificial caput called a *chignon*. No more than three "pop-offs" should be done, and these should not be followed by forceps attempts at vaginal birth.

26. Catheterization before forceps or vacuum extractor are used eliminates a full bladder, which would reduce available room in the pelvis. Emptying the bladder also reduces the risk of bladder injury.

27. Use of cold immediately (for the first 12 hours) after episiotomy reduces pain, edema, and formation of hematomas. The nurse should also observe for continuous, bright red bleeding that suggests a vaginal wall laceration. Warmth after at least 12 hours of cold application promotes resolution of the edema and hematoma.

28. The infant with an asymmetric facial appearance when crying may have facial nerve injury, usually a temporary condition that sometimes occurs when forceps are used to assist birth.

29. The low transverse uterine incision is less likely to rupture during another pregnancy than either of the two vertical incisions. There are, however, valid reasons for the use of vertical incisions.

30. The woman expecting a cesarean birth should be taught about the following regarding the operating room and recovery area:
    a. Preoperative procedures, such as skin preparation and insertion of an indwelling catheter.
    b. Personnel who will be present and their functions.
    c. The narrow table, safety strap, and positioning measures.
    d. When her partner or support person can come in.
    e. If a regional anesthetic is planned, she will be awake and feel pulling and pressure sensations but should not expect pain. If a general anesthetic is planned, all preparations will be made before anesthesia is induced, but the surgery will not begin before she is asleep and she will not awaken during it.
    f. In the recovery area, use of oxygen, pulse oximeter, and automatic blood pressure cuff for vital signs; checking of her fundus, incision, lochia, and pain-relief needs.

31. The woman who has cesarean birth needs care similar to that of the woman who delivers vaginally in terms of vital signs and fundus and lochia assessments. Additional care includes assessment of oxygen saturation and respiratory status, observation of urine output from the indwelling catheter, observation of the incision, pain management, and respiratory care (turning, coughing, deep breathing). Anesthesia-related care includes level of consciousness (primarily if general anesthesia was used) and return of movement and sensation (primarily if epidural or subarachnoid block was used).

CHAPTER 16

1. Labor dystocia usually occurs during the active phase of first-stage labor (6 cm cervical dilation or more). Uterine contractions become weaker, shorter, and less frequent. It is not painful because the contractions decrease, although the woman may become tired. Tachysystole can be either spontaneous or induced and is defined as excessive uterine activity. Tachysystole is more than five contractions in 10 minutes (averaged over 30 minutes). In addition to tachysystole, contractions lasting 2 minutes or longer, contractions with less than 1 minute resting time between, or failure of the uterus to return to resting tone between contractions via palpation, or intraamniotic pressure above 25 mmHg measured by an intrauterine pressure catheter (IUPC) may be of concern. Contractions may be uncoordinated and erratic in their frequency, duration, and intensity. The mother becomes very tired because of nearly constant discomfort.

2. Maternal position changes encourage the fetus to rotate from an occiput transverse or occiput posterior position to an occiput anterior position, similar to nesting two spoons together. The convex surface of the rounded fetal back rotates toward the convex surface of the anterior uterus. The squatting position also increases pelvic diameters and straightens the pelvic curve to facilitate both fetal rotation and descent.

3. A cesarean birth is the usual delivery method of choice for infants in the breech presentation to avoid major complications associated with breech birth, including slow labor, risk for prolapse of the umbilical cord, and the risks associated with possible umbilical cord compression before the head is born.

4. The staff must be prepared for care of multiple infants. Duplicate staff and equipment should be ready for every infant expected.

5. Bladder distention during labor can occupy available room in the woman's pelvis, thus impeding labor progress and fetal descent. In addition, it is a potential source of discomfort.

6. Psychological support reduces stress that otherwise can consume energy the uterus needs, inhibit uterine contractions, reduce placental blood supply, impair the woman's pushing efforts, and increase the woman's pain experience.

7. Based on Friedman's curve, the average nullipara's cervix dilates about 1.2 cm per hour and expected fetal descent is 1 cm per hour. The average parous woman's cervix dilates about 1.5 cm per hour, with minimal descent of 2 cm per hour. Research by Zhang et al found that labor may take over 6 hours to progress from 4 to 5 cm and over 3 hours to progress from 5 to 6 cm of dilation. Nulliparas and multiparas appeared to progress at a similar pace before 6 cm. They concluded that allowing labor to continue for a longer period before 6 cm of cervical dilation may reduce the rate of cesarean deliveries.

8. Nursing care for the woman who has prolonged labor is similar to that for dysfunctional labor. Promoting comfort, energy conservation, position changes, and assessments for related complications such as infection should be done.

9. Trauma is the primary maternal risk of a precipitate labor and may include uterine rupture, cervical lacerations, and hematomas. Fetal risks may include trauma, such as intracranial hemorrhage or nerve damage, and hypoxia due to intense contractions with a short relaxation period, which reduces the time available for gas exchange in the placenta.

10. Premature rupture of the membranes (PROM) occurs before true labor begins and may occur at any gestational age. Preterm premature rupture of the membranes (PPROM) occurs before 37 weeks of gestation and may be accompanied by contractions. PPROM is more likely to be associated with preterm labor and birth.

11. Infection may be both a cause and a result of premature rupture of the membranes, particularly if birth is not desired because of fetal immaturity.

12. Labor may be induced if the woman is at or near term and it does not begin spontaneously. The physician must consider multiple factors such as risk for infection (mother and fetus/newborn) and risk for preterm complications if the fetus is preterm.

13. The nurse should assess the woman's vital signs and fetal heart rate (FHR) and teach her to avoid inserting anything into the vagina, avoid breast stimulation, maintain activity restrictions, and note any uterine contractions or foul odor to vaginal discharge. Teach her how to observe fetal kick counts or other fetal activity. Temperature should be taken at least four times per day.

14. Symptoms of preterm labor often are vague. They include uterine contractions that may often be painless, the fetus "balling up," menstrual-like cramps, backache, pelvic pressure, changed or increased vaginal discharge, abdominal cramps, thigh pain, and a sense of "feeling bad."

15. Early identification of preterm labor enables management that may delay birth and allow further maturation of the fetus or permit transfer to a facility equipped to care for an immature infant. Corticosteroids may be given to the mother of a fetus between 24 and 34 weeks of gestation to accelerate maturation of the lungs before preterm birth.

16. Classifications of drugs to inhibit preterm contractions include magnesium sulfate, calcium channel blockers such as nifedipine, prostaglandin synthesis inhibitors such as indomethacin, and beta-adrenergics such as terbutaline.

17. To accelerate maturation of the fetal lungs, corticosteroids are given to the woman who is likely to deliver prematurely. The greatest benefits occur if steroids are in the mother's system at least 24 hours before birth. The newborn who delivers before 24 hours after the mother receives corticosteroids may also benefit.

18. The three potential fetal or newborn risks are reduced placental function and umbilical cord compression before birth and meconium aspiration after birth.

19. If umbilical cord prolapse occurs, the priority of care is to reduce compression and restore normal blood flow through the cord by elevating the presenting part while giving the mother oxygen to maximize her blood oxygen concentration. At the same time, the nurse should summon help to expedite delivery, usually by cesarean birth.

20. Stimulated contractions are potentially more powerful than natural ones and may cause the pressure in the uterus to exceed the uterine wall's ability to withstand that pressure.

21. Shock and hemorrhage are rapidly developing complications of uterine inversion. They are managed by rapid IV fluid and blood replacement, often using two IV lines. A drug that relaxes the uterus is given to allow uterine replacement to its proper position, and general anesthesia may be needed. Oxytocin is given after the uterus is returned to the proper position. Hemodynamic monitoring may be required to ensure stabilization.

22. For intrapartum emergencies, nursing considerations include the following: *Prolapsed umbilical cord*—Relieve pressure on the cord to restore adequate blood flow through it until the baby can be delivered. *Uterine rupture*—Attempt its prevention by cautious intrapartum use of uterine stimulants and close monitoring of uterine contractions. *Uterine inversion*—Avoid pressure on the poorly contracted fundus after birth; assess for and correct shock. *Amniotic fluid embolism*—Provide cardiorespiratory support and hemodynamic monitoring and observe for coagulation deficits.

23. The fetus may suffer direct injury such as skull fracture or intracranial hemorrhage related to maternal injuries such as pelvic fracture, penetrating wounds, or blunt trauma. Fetal injury from indirect causes includes placental abruption and disruption of placental flow because of maternal hemorrhage or shock.

CHAPTER 17

1. The three processes involved in involution are contraction of muscle fibers, catabolism, and regeneration of uterine epithelium.

2. The fundus is expected to descend 1 cm (approximately 1 fingerbreadth) per day so that by the fourteenth day after birth it cannot be palpated in the abdomen.

3. A multipara is expected to experience afterpains because repeated stretching of the uterus makes continuous uterine contraction more difficult. Overdistention of the uterus and breastfeeding also cause afterpains. Afterpains are treated with analgesics. Lying in a prone position also provides relief.

4. Lochia rubra is red, consists mostly of blood, and lasts for 1 to 3 days. Lochia serosa is pink to brown tinged and usually lasts from the third to tenth days. Lochia alba is white, cream, or yellowish and may last until 3 to 6 weeks after delivery.

5. Menses will resume in about 6 to 8 weeks for 40% to 45% of women who are formula feeding, for 75% by 12 weeks, and for all by 6 months. The breastfeeding woman may begin menses between 12 weeks and 18 months after childbirth.

6. Breastfeeding delays the return of both ovulation and menstruation.

7. The white blood cell (WBC) count is normally elevated to an average of 14,000 to 16,000/mm³ after childbirth, although it may rise to 30,000/mm³. If the woman has a fever or is at increased risk for infection, the nurse should be especially alert for a WBC count that increases over 30% in 6 hours and other signs of infection.

8. The postpartum woman is at risk for urinary retention because her bladder is less sensitive to fluid pressure, decreasing the urge to void even when the bladder is distended. Trauma of childbirth and lingering effects of regional anesthesia may also make it difficult to void. Urinary tract infection is more likely because stasis of urine allows time for bacteria to multiply. Excessive postpartum bleeding may occur because a full bladder displaces the uterus, causing the uterine muscles to relax.

9. Hyperpigmentation decreases because estrogen, progesterone, and melanocyte-stimulating hormone decrease rapidly after childbirth.

10. Women lose approximately 4.5 to 5.8 kg (10 to 13 lb) during childbirth. They often lose another 3.2 to 5 kg (7 to 11 lb) by the end of the first week.

11. Orthostatic hypotension results from engorgement of visceral blood vessels from decreased intraabdominal pressure after delivery. Signs and symptoms include a 15 to 20 mmHg drop in systolic blood pressure, dizziness, lightheadedness, or faintness when the woman moves from lying down to sitting or standing.

12. When tachycardia is noted, assessment of blood pressure (BP), temperature, location and firmness of the fundus, amount of lochia, estimated blood loss at delivery, hemoglobin, hematocrit, and degree of pain are necessary to help identify the cause. Excitement, pain, anxiety, fatigue, dehydration, anemia, infection, or hypovolemia may cause tachycardia.

13. Uterine massage is necessary when the uterus is not firmly contracted. The nurse places the nondominant hand above the woman's symphysis pubis to anchor and support the uterus during massage.

14. A cervical or vaginal laceration may cause excessive bleeding even when the uterus is firmly contracted.

15. Assessment of pain, frequent respiratory assessments, auscultation of breath sounds and bowel sounds, inspection of the surgical dressing and wound, and intake and output are necessary for the postcesarean mother.

16. Hypostatic pneumonia can be prevented by frequent turning, coughing, breathing deeply, and ambulating early and frequently.

17. Early ambulation, tightening and relaxing the abdominal muscles, restriction of carbonated beverages and straws for drinking, pelvic lifts, and simethicone or rectal suppositories as ordered prevent or minimize abdominal distention.

18. Current recommendations include instructing the woman to wear a firm bra 24 hours a day and express only a small amount of milk if absolutely necessary for pain relief. The woman may use cold compresses or gel packs inside the bra for comfort. Cold cabbage leaves also promote comfort. Analgesics may be recommended by the provider.

19. Providing adequate information in a short time is a major problem in preparing parents for discharge.

20. Before discharge, the nurse should be sure that the mother has no complications and all assessments and laboratory work are normal. Ambulation and ability to eat and drink should be normal. The mother should indicate understanding of self-care instructions, signs of complications and proper responses, and infant care. Postpartum follow-up care should be arranged. She should have adequate support during the early days after discharge.

21. Bonding describes the initial attraction felt by the parents for the infant. Attachment is the development of an enduring, loving relationship between parents and child. It is progressive and requires response from the infant.

22. Maternal touch may progress from fingertipping in the discovery phase to stroking, then enfolding the infant, and then to consoling behaviors.

23. Parents progress from referring to the newborn as "it" to "he" or "she" and then to using the given name. Parents who know the sex of the baby before birth may call the infant by name from before birth.

24. The mother is focused primarily on her own needs during the taking-in phase. She often is passive and dependent and repeatedly recounts her birth experience. In the taking-hold phase, she becomes more independent, focuses on the infant, and exhibits a heightened readiness to learn.

25. In the letting-go phase, parents relinquish previous lifestyle patterns to assume the parenting role.

26. The anticipatory stage begins during pregnancy as women prepare for the birth. The formal stage begins with birth as they become acquainted with the baby. During the informal stage, parents respond to their infant's unique cues rather than relying on directions from others. The personal stage is attained when the mothers feel comfortable with their roles as parents.

27. Postpartum blues may be related to emotional letdown, discomfort, fatigue, and anxiety about parenting and body image. It is characterized by irritability, fatigue, tearfulness, mood swings, and anxiety. The symptoms are usually unrelated to events, and the condition does not seriously affect the mother's ability to care for the infant. With postpartum depression, the depression becomes severe, lasts longer than 2 weeks, or interferes with the mother's ability to cope with daily life. Nurses can provide reassurance to the mother and teach the family about postpartum blues and warning signs of postpartum depression. Many facilities or providers conduct a screening for depression before discharge.

28. Fathers who are sometimes ignored and not included in infant care may feel left out and unneeded.

29. Siblings may feel jealousy and fear that they will be replaced by the newborn in the affection of the parents.

CHAPTER 18

1. The nurse examines a woman's previous records to identify factors that would predispose her to complications such as postpartum hemorrhage.

2. Overdistention of uterine muscles from a twin gestation makes the uterine contraction more difficult and excessive bleeding more likely.

3. The nurse cannot be certain that bleeding is controlled because concealed bleeding can occur in soft tissue and produce a hematoma.

4. Initial management of uterine atony focuses on measures to contract the uterus, such as massaging, expressing clots, and emptying the bladder. Pharmacologic measures include fluid replacement and administration of oxytocin, methylergonovine, or other drugs such as carboprost.

5. Large hematomas may require incision and evacuation of clots, as well as ligation of the bleeding vessel. Small hematomas do not require treatment.

6. The major signs of subinvolution are prolonged lochial discharge, irregular or excessive uterine bleeding, pelvic pain and heaviness, backache, fatigue, and malaise.

7. Nurses should teach the mother how to palpate the fundus; estimate fundal height; and report abnormalities of lochia, a foul odor, or pelvic pain.

8. It may be difficult to recognize hypovolemia because of compensatory mechanisms, such as carotid and aortic baroreceptors, which constrict peripheral blood vessels. This shunts blood to the central circulation, maintains blood pressure, and increases the heart rate.

9. Venous stasis increases during pregnancy because of compression of the large vessels by the enlarging uterus. At birth, stasis may occur when the woman is in stirrups. Changes in the coagulation and fibrinolytic systems during pregnancy and the postpartum period elevate the factors that favor coagulation and decrease the factors that favor lysis of clots.

10. Signs and symptoms of superficial venous thrombosis include swelling, tenderness, warmth, and redness.

11. Heparin remains the long-term treatment of the pregnant woman with deep venous thrombosis because warfarin (Coumadin) may be teratogenic and predisposes the fetus to hemorrhage. Heparin is changed to warfarin in the postpartum period.

12. Bed rest is prescribed for the woman with deep vein thrombosis to decrease swelling and to promote venous return from the leg.

13. The nurse assesses mothers receiving anticoagulants for unexplained bruising; petechiae; bleeding from the nose, bladder, or gums; or increased vaginal bleeding. Signs of hemorrhage, such as tachycardia, falling blood pressure, or other signs of shock, also should be noted.

14. The nurse should assess family structure and function that will need to change as a result of prolonged treatment for the mother. The nurse should evaluate mother-infant interaction and determine what support system may be available to provide assistance.

15. Cesarean birth or the use of vacuum extraction or forceps may result in trauma that provides a portal of entry for infectious organisms.

16. All parts of the reproductive tract are connected, and organisms can move from the vagina through the cervix, uterus, and fallopian tubes and into the peritoneal cavity. Alkalinity of the vagina during labor, necrosis of the endometrium, and the presence of lochia encourage bacterial growth.

17. When labor is prolonged, organisms have time and opportunity to ascend from the vagina into the uterus, increasing the risk of infection. Also, there may be more vaginal examinations and ruptured membranes for a longer time.

18. Fever, chills, lethargy, malaise, anorexia, abdominal pain and cramping, uterine tenderness, purulent foul-smelling lochia, tachycardia, and subinvolution are signs and symptoms of endometritis. It usually is treated by IV administration of antibiotics, antipyretics, and oxytocics to promote involution.

19. Wound infection most often occurs in cesarean incisions, episiotomies, and lacerations.

20. Incisions and lacerations should be inspected for redness, tenderness, edema, and approximation of the edges of the wound, which may pull apart with infection.

21. To prevent urinary tract infection, the woman should be advised to drink at least 2500 to 3000 mL of fluid each day, empty her bladder every 2 to 3 hours during the day, and practice meticulous hygiene. Cystitis and pyelonephritis may be treated with oral antibiotics on an outpatient basis. Severe pyelonephritis or infection may require hospitalization and IV antibiotics.

22. Measures to prevent mastitis include correct positioning of the infant during nursing, frequent emptying of the breasts, and avoiding nipple trauma and supplemental feedings. In addition, the woman should avoid continuous pressure on the breasts caused by tight bras or infant carriers.

CHAPTER 19

1. Hypoxia causes decreased PO_2 and pH and increased PCO_2. These, along with cool air and handling at birth, affect chemoreceptors and sensors that stimulate the respiratory center to cause initiation of respirations at birth.

2. Surfactant reduces surface tension in the alveoli and allows them to remain partially open on expiration, reducing the work of breathing.

3. Fetal lung fluid begins to move into the interstitial spaces shortly before birth and when air enters the lungs at birth. It is absorbed from the interstitial spaces by the lymphatic and vascular systems. A small part of the fluid is squeezed out during birth.

4. The ductus arteriosus closes as a result of increases in blood oxygen and decreased prostaglandins from the placenta. The foramen ovale closes when pressure in the left atrium exceeds that in the right atrium. The ductus venosus closes when the vessels of the cord become occluded.

5. At birth, increasing oxygen causes the pulmonary blood vessels to dilate. In addition, movement of fetal lung fluid into the interstitial tissues allows more room for expansion of the pulmonary vessels. The ductus arteriosus constricts because of the increased oxygen in the blood when the neonate begins to breathe.

6. Newborns have thinner skin with less subcutaneous fat than older children and adults. They have blood vessels close to the surface and a larger skin surface area. These all contribute to greater loss of heat than in older children or adults.

7. Newborns respond to low temperatures by increasing activity, flexion, and metabolism; vasoconstriction; and nonshivering thermogenesis. This raises oxygen and glucose consumption and may cause respiratory distress, hypoglycemia, acidosis, and jaundice.

8. Newborns have higher levels of erythrocytes and hemoglobin than adults because the available oxygen is lower before birth than after birth. More red blood cells with fetal hemoglobin are needed to adequately oxygenate the cells in the fetus.

9. Stools progress from thick, greenish-black meconium to loose, greenish-brown transitional stools to milk stools that are frequent, soft, seedy, and mustard-colored if the infant is breastfed, and pale yellow or light brown, firmer, and less frequent if formula fed.

10. Hypoglycemia is a problem for the newborn because glucose is the major source of energy in the brain.

11. Infants have an immature liver and more hemolysis of erythrocytes than adults. Trauma at birth, poor early feeding, and an intestinal enzyme that deconjugates bilirubin also increase jaundice.

12. Physiologic jaundice occurs in normal newborns after the first 24 hours of life as a result of hemolysis of unneeded red blood cells and immaturity of the liver. Nonphysiologic jaundice is generally a result of excessive destruction of erythrocytes, causing bilirubin levels to rise faster and higher than in physiologic jaundice. It begins within the first 24 hours and may necessitate phototherapy. True breast milk jaundice lasts longer than physiologic jaundice and may result from substances in the milk.

13. The newborn's body is composed of a greater percentage of water with more located in the extracellular compartment than in the adult's body.

14. Newborns receive passive immunity to infections when IgG crosses the placenta in utero. After birth, infants produce IgM and IgA to protect against infection. IgM rises in response to infection. IgA helps protect the gastrointestinal and respiratory tracts from infection and is present in breast milk.

15. During both periods of reactivity, newborns are active and alert, may be interested in feeding, may have elevated pulse and respiratory rates, and may have transient signs of respiratory distress.

16. In the deep or quiet sleep state, the infant is in a deep sleep with regular respirations and little response to outside stimuli. In active sleep, infants move about and may have irregular respirations. The drowsy state is the time between sleep and waking. In the quiet alert state, the infant is awake and interested in stimuli. The active alert state is a fussy period that may lead to the crying state if the infant's needs are not met.

CHAPTER 20

1. Focused assessments of the infant immediately after birth help detect serious abnormalities that need immediate attention. They focus on cardiorespiratory status, thermoregulation, and the presence of anomalies. A more complete assessment follows when the infant is stable.

2. The cardiovascular assessment includes evaluation of history, airway, color, heart sounds, and pulses. Blood pressure is assessed if indicated.

3. Taking a rectal temperature is dangerous because it risks perforation of the rectum, which turns sharply to the right after about 3 cm (1.2 inches).

4. Molding of the head is a change in the shape because of normal temporary overriding of bones during birth. Caput succedaneum is localized swelling from pressure against the cervix, which can cross the suture lines. Cephalhematoma is bleeding between the periosteum and the bone that never crosses suture lines. Molding and caput disappear within a few days, but cephalhematoma may last for 2 to 3 months.

5. Measurements of the infant help determine if in utero growth was adequate for gestational age and if complications are present.

6. Some signs of hypoglycemia are jitteriness, poor muscle tone, respiratory distress (tachypnea, dyspnea, apnea, and cyanosis), high-pitched cry, diaphoresis, low temperature, poor suck, lethargy, irritability, seizures, and coma.

7. Using an incorrect site for heel punctures risks injury to the bone, nerves, or blood vessels of the heel.

8. Newborn reflexes provide information about the status of the neonate's central nervous system.

9. The first feeding allows the nurse to evaluate the newborn's ability to suck, swallow, and breathe in coordination and assess for signs of esophageal atresia or tracheoesophageal fistula.

10. Infants should void within 12 to 48 hours. Infants void at least one to two times during the first 2 days and at least 6 times a day by the fourth day.

11. The nurse documents location, size, color, elevation, and texture of marks on the skin; explains marks to parents; and offers emotional support as needed.

12. The gestational age assessment provides an estimate of the infant's age since conception and alerts the nurse to possible complications related to age and development.

13. The periods of reactivity are important because the infant may need nursing intervention for low temperature, elevated pulse and respirations, and excessive respiratory secretions. During the sleep period, the infant will have relaxed muscle tone and no interest in feeding.

CHAPTER 21

1. Newborns receive vitamin K to prevent vitamin K–dependent bleeding. The eyes are treated with an antibiotic ointment to prevent ophthalmia neonatorum.

2. Nurses can prevent heat loss in newborns by keeping them dry, covered, and away from cold objects or surfaces, drafts, and outside windows and walls and by teaching parents.

3. When infants show signs of hypoglycemia, the nurse should follow agency policy to check the blood glucose level and temperature, feed the infant, and watch for signs of other complications.

4. Interventions for preventing jaundice include ensuring the infant is feeding well by working with mothers and infants having difficulty and teaching parents about jaundice and what observations they should make.

5. Nurses can prevent a baby being given to the wrong parents by always checking the infant's identification and parent's identification every time the two are reunited.

6. Nurses and parents can prevent infant abductions by always being alert for suspicious behavior and stopping anyone who might be taking a baby. Nurses must teach parents how to identify hospital staff and that they should never allow anyone without proper identification to remove their infant from them.

7. Scrupulous handwashing by staff and all who come in contact with newborns is the most important way to prevent infections in newborns.

8. Parents choose circumcision because of the decreased incidence of urinary tract infections, penile cancer, and some sexually transmittable diseases; religious dictates; parental preference; and lack of knowledge about care of the foreskin. Parents decide against circumcision because it causes pain and the risk of hemorrhage, infection, poor cosmetic result, stenosis or fistulas of the urethra, adhesions, necrosis, or other injury to the glans penis. They also question the need for surgery to prevent uncommon conditions.

9. Teach parents not to retract the foreskin on an uncircumcised penis until it begins to separate from the glans later in childhood. They can teach the child to retract it to clean after separation occurs. Teach parents of circumcised infants to watch for bleeding and infection and to apply petroleum jelly as instructed unless a Plastibell was used.

10. Planning parent teaching includes coordinating teaching to include all topics, setting priorities based on parents' needs, using a variety of teaching techniques, modeling behavior, including other family members, and considering culture and language.

11. The first hepatitis B vaccine is given at the birth facility to infants of uninfected mothers, as well as to those whose mothers are positive for hepatitis B. Hepatitis B immune globulin is also given to infants of infected mothers.

12. Newborn screening tests should be performed as close to discharge as possible, as the blood tests are more sensitive after the first 24 hours of life. If infants are discharged earlier, they should be retested so that any disorders can be diagnosed early.

13. Parents obtain information about infant care from friends, family, nurses, health care providers, child care classes, television, books, magazines, and the Internet.

14. Nurses may provide follow-up phone calls, home visits, clinic visits, and child care classes.

15. All equipment should be checked for safety, and parts should be inspected to ensure that they are functioning properly.

16. Car seats must be chosen according to the size of the infant and must be used correctly to maintain safety. Newborns should be placed in rear-facing car seats in the back seat of the car.

17. Infants are not "spoiled" by prompt attention to their needs. Prompt, consistent response to crying may decrease overall crying later.

18. Nurses can assist parents of crying infants to determine the cause and teach them appropriate techniques for coping with a crying infant. Therapeutic communication techniques can be used to help parents with negative feelings.

19. Diaper rash can be prevented by keeping the area clean and dry and avoiding products to which the infant seems sensitive. If rash occurs, parents should expose the area to air and apply creams sparingly.

20. Infants should not start solid foods until 6 months old.

21. Regurgitation is expulsion of small amounts of milk, often along with a burp. Vomiting involves larger amounts that are expelled with more force.

22. Understanding the infant's changing capabilities helps parents assess situations and the home environment to prevent accidents.

23. Well-baby checkups allow the health care provider to assess the infant's growth and development, provide parent teaching, and give immunizations.

24. Immunizations prevent infants from becoming infected with very serious communicable diseases.

25. Immediate help should be obtained if infants have difficulty breathing, are cyanotic, or are hard to arouse from sleep.

26. The cause of sudden infant death syndrome (SIDS) remains unknown, but the risk may be increased with sleeping in a prone position or on soft, loose bedding, overheating, maternal smoking, and sleeping with another person or on an adult bed or sofa. Infants should sleep alone in a supine position at all times.

CHAPTER 22

1. Infants lose weight after birth because of insufficient intake and normal loss of meconium and extracellular fluid.

2. Colostrum is rich in protein, vitamins, minerals, and immunoglobulins. Transitional milk has less protein and immunoglobulins but more lactose, fat, and calories than colostrum. Mature milk appears less rich than colostrum and transitional milk, but it supplies all nutrients needed.

3. Breast milk nutrients are in an easily digested form and in proportions required by the newborn. Commercial formulas contain cow's milk adapted to simulate human milk. Infants may develop allergies to modified cow's milk and may need other types of formula, but they are unlikely to be allergic to human milk.

4. Breast milk contains bifidus factor to help establish intestinal flora, leukocytes, lysozymes that are bacteriolytic, lactoferrin to bind iron in bacteria, and immunoglobulins.

5. Commercial formulas include modified cow's milk formula, soy-based or hydrolyzed formulas, and formulas for preterm infants or those with special needs.

6. Support from her partner, family and friends, cultural influences, employment demands, knowledge about each method, and education may influence a woman's choice of feeding method.

7. Suckling causes release of oxytocin, which produces the let-down reflex. Suckling and removal of milk cause the release of prolactin to increase milk production.

Therefore the more frequently the infant breastfeeds, the more milk is produced. Infrequent feedings decrease prolactin output and milk production.

8. During pregnancy, identification of flat and inverted nipples is important. Soap should not be used on the nipples. No other preparation is necessary.

9. The nurse can help the mother establish breastfeeding in the beginning by initiating early feeding, helping position the infant at the breast, and showing the mother how to position her hands. The nurse also can help the infant latch on to the breast, assess the position of the mouth on the breast, check for swallowing, and remove the infant from the breast properly.

10. The mother should feed the infant every 1.5 to 3 hours (8 to 12 times each day) for about 10 to 15 minutes on each side or longer if the infant wishes. Length of feedings may vary but should average at least 20 minutes of effective suckling.

11. To wake up a sleepy infant, unwrap the infant's blankets, talk to the infant, change the diaper, rub the infant's back, place the baby skin to skin with you, and express colostrum onto the breast.

12. Sucking from a bottle requires pushing the tongue against the nipple to slow the flow of milk. Suckling from the breast requires drawing the nipple far into the mouth so that the gums compress the areola.

13. To help the mother with engorged breasts, the nurse can encourage nursing frequently, applying heat and cold, massaging, and expressing milk to soften the areola.

14. The nurse should advise the mother with sore nipples to ensure proper positioning of the infant at the breast, vary the position of the infant, apply colostrum or compresses to the nipples, and expose the nipples to air.

15. The mother who plans to work and breastfeed should be taught use of a breast pump, proper storage of milk, and ways to maintain her milk supply.

16. There is no one right time for weaning. Breastfeeding for at least 1 year is often recommended. Weaning should be done gradually to help the mother avoid engorgement and help the infant adjust.

17. A mother might ask about the types of formula available, how to prepare it correctly, frequency and amount of feedings, and feeding techniques.

18. Propping bottles risks aspiration of milk. Infants who sleep with a propped bottle have more ear infections and may develop cavities when the teeth come in.

CHAPTER 23

1. Preterm infants appear frail and weak and are small, with limp extremities; poor muscle tone; red skin; and immature ears, nipples, areolae, and genitals.

2. Factors that increase respiratory problems in preterm infants include lack of surfactant, poor cough reflex, small air passages, and weak muscles.

3. Nursing responsibilities include working with respiratory therapists to manage equipment, monitoring the infant's changing oxygen needs, positioning infants to promote drainage, and suctioning.

4. Nurses wean infants to the open crib by making gradual changes in the environmental temperature, dressing the infant, and using blankets and a hat when the infant is out of the incubator.

5. To measure intake and output for infants, all fluids (IV and oral), including medications, are measured. Diapers are weighed to calculate urine output, and drainage, regurgitation, and stools are measured.

6. Preterm infants' kidneys do not concentrate or dilute urine well, and they have large insensible water losses. They lack passive antibodies from the mother and have an immature immune system. Pain causes physiologic and behavioral responses and can have long-term effects.

7. Nonpharmacologic methods to manage pain in infants include positioning, swaddling, facilitated tucking, sucking, sucrose, skin-to-skin positioning, and breastfeeding.

8. The nurse can diminish overstimulation by organizing care to provide for rest periods, reducing environmental stimuli, minimizing pain, and discussing the plan of care with others.

9. Feeding tolerance is assessed by checking gastric residual volume before gavage feedings, measuring abdominal girth, testing stools for reducing substances and blood, and observing for regurgitation. During nipple feedings, the nurse watches for signs of respiratory difficulty, decreased oxygenation, and fatigue.

10. When allowed to set the pace of feedings, infants can stop to rest to conserve energy, regulate breathing, and control the flow of milk. Moving the nipple in the infant's mouth may cause fatigue and choking.

11. The nurse can help breastfeeding mothers of preterm infants by helping them pump and store milk, by teaching breastfeeding techniques adapted to the preterm infant's needs, and by providing support and encouragement.

12. The nurse can help parents feel comfortable with preterm infants by providing warm support, realistic encouragement, and information about the neonatal intensive care unit (NICU) environment, the infant's condition and characteristics, and the equipment and care. Involving the parents in care also helps.

13. Beginning early in hospitalization, the nurse should help parents take on gradually increasing responsibility for care of the infant, which will help them prepare for discharge. Helping them prepare their home for the infant is also important.

14. Postmature infants may be thin and may have loose skin folds, cracked and peeling skin, minimal vernix, long nails, and meconium staining.

15. Postmature infants may have polycythemia, meconium aspiration, hypoglycemia, and poor temperature regulation.

16. In symmetric growth restriction, all body parts are proportionately small. In asymmetric growth restriction, the head is normal in size but seems large for the body, the weight is decreased, and the length is generally normal.

17. Large-for-gestational-age (LGA) infants may have birth injuries such as fractures, nerve injury, cephalhematoma, hypoglycemia, and polycythemia.

CHAPTER 24

1. Effective ventilation is the most important element in resuscitation. Chest compressions and medications are rarely needed. Although most newborns have no difficulty with breathing at birth, up to 10% require some help to begin respirations and 1% require extensive resuscitative measures.

2. The nurse's role in the care of the infant with asphyxia is to begin resuscitation promptly, assist the team, and provide follow-up and parental support.

3. Transient tachypnea of the newborn is caused by failure of fetal lung fluid to be absorbed completely in infants who are usually full-term or late preterm. Respiratory distress syndrome occurs in preterm infants as a result of inadequate surfactant.

4. Meconium staining is most likely to occur when infants are postterm, small for gestational age (SGA), have decreased amniotic fluid, and have cord compression.

5. Infants with persistent pulmonary hypertension of the newborn (PPHN) have constriction of the pulmonary blood vessels from inadequate oxygen levels. This increases resistance to blood flow from the heart into the lungs and causes blood to flow through the foramen ovale and patent ductus arteriosus.

6. Kernicterus can be prevented by identifying women whose infants are at risk for blood incompatibilities, giving Rh-negative mothers Rh immune globulin, recognizing infants with bilirubin levels that are not normal, and instituting phototherapy when it is needed.

7. Nurses can help reduce bilirubin in an infant receiving phototherapy by ensuring that the lights or blankets are functioning and positioned properly; reducing the infant's time out of phototherapy; ensuring adequate milk intake to increase removal of bilirubin by frequent stools; preventing cold stress or hypoglycemia, which would decrease albumin-binding sites for bilirubin; and turning the infant frequently to expose all areas to the lights.

8. The role of the nurse in sepsis is to use infection prevention methods, identify infants at risk, watch for early signs, notify the physician, coordinate treatment, observe for change, and support the family.

9. Macrosomia occurs in infants of diabetic mothers (IDMs) because of excessive transfer of glucose, amino acids, and fatty acids from the mother to the fetus. This results in fetal production of insulin and excessive growth in the fetus.

10. Infants of diabetic mothers (IDMs) may develop hypoglycemia after birth because they have high levels of insulin even though they no longer receive glucose from the mother. Infants may need early feeding as a result.

11. The nurse can help the drug-exposed infant rest by minimizing stimulation, swaddling in a flexed position, organizing care to avoid interruptions, and providing a pacifier.

12. The nurse can promote bonding in cases of prenatal drug abuse by helping the mother feel welcome, encouraging her to participate in infant care, teaching her how to respond to the infant's behavior and about the infant's care, and modeling parenting behaviors.

CHAPTER 25

1. Almost all contraceptive methods are used by women, and failure will most affect women.

2. The nurse's role in helping women with contraception is to provide information to help women choose contraceptives appropriately and use them correctly.

3. Important considerations in choosing contraceptive techniques include safety, protection from sexually transmitted diseases (STDs), effectiveness, acceptability, convenience, education needed, benefits, side effects, effect on spontaneity, availability, expense, preference of the woman and her partner, religious and personal beliefs, and culture.

4. Sterilization and LARC methods may require signed informed consents.

5. Adolescents may have incorrect beliefs, such as that they cannot conceive during first intercourse, without orgasm, or without having menstruated a certain length of time or that douching will prevent pregnancy.

6. Adolescents may not seek contraception because they may fear lack of acceptance, loss of sexual privacy, pelvic examination, or adverse effects of contraception on their health.

7. The nurse can teach adolescents effectively by showing sensitivity to their feelings, being accepting, providing extensive teaching without hurry, and using understandable terms and audiovisual materials.

8. Women who are over age 35 and who smoke should not use estrogen-containing contraceptives. Healthy women in their forties who do not smoke and are not obese can use combined hormonal contraceptives.

9. Important factors to consider when choosing a method of sterilization include time involved, cost, need for hospitalization, and feelings of each partner about a permanent end to the ability to have more children.

10. Education for women choosing intrauterine devices includes information about side effects, when and how to check the threads, and when to seek medical treatment.

11. Hormonal contraceptives alter normal hormone changes, preventing ovulation and making the cervical mucus thicker.

12. Menstrual changes and spotting are the reason some women stop using some hormonal contraceptives.

13. Women using oral contraceptives (OCs) need to know that the pills must be taken consistently and in the right

order every day, what to do if pills are missed, common side effects, and signs that may indicate a problem.

14. Emergency contraception (EC) should be taken as soon as possible after unprotected intercourse and within 120 hours.

15. Barrier methods kill sperm or prevent them from entering the cervix or both.

16. Natural family planning methods avoid drugs, chemicals, and devices; are inexpensive; and are acceptable to most religions. Couples need extensive education and high motivation, however, and they risk pregnancy if they make an error.

CHAPTER 26

1. Infertility is strictly defined as the inability to conceive after 1 year of unprotected regular intercourse. A more workable definition that considers the age and other individual factors is the inability of a couple to conceive when desired. Primary infertility is that which occurs in couples who have never conceived. Secondary infertility occurs in those who have conceived before and cannot conceive again.

2. The normal average number of sperm released at ejaculation is 35 to 200 million. Twenty million per milliliter is probably the minimum required for unassisted fertility. Seminal fluid should liquefy within 30 minutes, allowing motile sperm to move into the uterus without the seminal fluid.

3. Erection problems exist if the man cannot initiate and maintain a penile erection that is sufficient to allow intercourse and deposit of seminal fluid with sperm near the woman's cervix. Ejaculation abnormalities may result from retrograde ejaculation, hypospadias, or abnormal ejaculation response (premature, slow, or absent).

4. Abnormalities of the sperm, ejaculation, or the seminal fluid can result from factors such as abnormal hormone stimulation, systemic illness, infections or abnormalities of the reproductive tract, anatomic abnormalities of the reproductive system, exposure to toxins, therapeutic medications, excessive alcohol intake, illicit drug use, elevated scrotal temperature, obstruction, and immunologic factors.

5. Abnormal ovulation can occur because of hormone disruptions caused by cranial tumors, stress, obesity, anorexia, systemic disease, and abnormalities in the ovaries or other endocrine glands.

6. Hormone abnormalities associated with ovulation problems interfere with normal buildup and decline of the endometrium. Menstrual periods may be absent, scant, or very heavy.

7. Fallopian tube obstruction may be caused by scarring or adhesions secondary to infections, endometriosis, or pelvic surgery. Congenital anomalies of the reproductive structures also can cause mechanical interference with successful pregnancy.

8. Abnormal cervical mucus can trap sperm and prevent them from entering the uterus and fallopian tube or prevent their preparation (capacitation) for fertilization.

9. Anatomic abnormalities of the woman's reproductive tract may prevent normal fertilization or implantation. They also may prevent normal placental or fetal growth, or they may increase the risk for miscarriage or previable birth.

10. Endocrine abnormalities associated with repeated pregnancy loss include inadequate progesterone secretion, inadequate endometrial response to progesterone, hypothyroidism and hyperthyroidism, and maternal diabetes.

11. Immunologic causes of repeated pregnancy loss include an intolerance of the embryo's foreign tissue and systemic lupus erythematosus.

12. Elements included in the history and physical examination include a reproductive history; a medical history; and an examination for undiagnosed endocrine disturbances, tumors, chronic disease, and abnormalities of the reproductive organs. Chromosome analysis is sometimes done. Imaging studies are done if structural abnormalities are suspected.

13. Medications used to induce ovulation include clomiphene citrate, chorionic gonadotropins, gonadotropin-releasing hormone, and human gonadotropins. Clomiphene is a common drug for this purpose. Additional drugs may be given to increase the formation and release of ova and to support a resulting pregnancy.

14. Screening tests related to use of donor sperm include those for blood type and Rh factor, possible genetic abnormalities, and infection. In addition, the man's history, physical examination, and lifestyle are reviewed for possible problems that might not be revealed by standard tests. Donor sperm are frozen for 6 months to allow identification of infections or other problems that are not evident at the time of collection.

15. In vitro fertilization mixes the male and female gametes outside the body and places embryos back into the uterus. Gamete intrafallopian transfer retrieves ova and then places the ova and sperm into the fallopian tubes, where fertilization occurs. Zygote intrafallopian transfer mixes male and female gametes to allow fertilization and places the fertilized ova into the fallopian tubes. Intracytoplasmic sperm injection (ICSI) is used to retrieve sperm from the epididymis by using percutaneous aspiration or a microsurgical incision to aspirate a single sperm. The sperm obtained are then used to fertilize ova.

16. Factors that couples consider when seeking infertility help include their age, the length of their attempt to conceive, their desire for a biologic child, and their feelings about adoption or a child-free life. Financial constraints and difficulty coordinating work or travel and treatment may be other considerations.

17. When deciding about infertility evaluations and treatments, the couple considers their personal, social, cultural, and religious values; how difficult treatment may be; the probability of success with treatment; and financial concerns.

18. Psychological reactions to infertility may include guilt, isolation, depression, or stress on the relationship.

19. Parenthood after infertility may be marked by anxiety about the pregnancy, loss of support from infertile couples, or unrealistic expectations about their parenting abilities.

20. Couples considering adoption must confront their personal preferences, limitations, and prejudices.

21. Couples who lose a pregnancy after a period of infertility often experience grief, but sometimes the grief is mixed with optimism because they were able to achieve pregnancy, even if completion was not possible.

CHAPTER 27

1. Family history is an important part of a health history to assess risk factors for conditions such as heart disease, breast and colon cancers, osteoporosis, and other health problems that should be studied.

2. A psychosocial evaluation helps caregivers identify the best teaching approaches for the individual woman. Evaluating the woman's family and other support helps determine stresses in her life and may identify if counseling regarding domestic violence is needed.

3. When taking a sexual history, the nurse should ask about sexual activity, number of partners, age when sexual activity began, method of contraception, and knowledge about and measures used for protection from sexually transmitted diseases (STDs).

4. Human papillomavirus (HPV) vaccine is ideally started at 11 to 13 years, an age younger than the age of legal consent. Therefore the adult who is qualified to give permission, usually a parent, must face the issue of possible sexual activity at a young age.

5. Vulvar self-examination is recommended to detect signs of precancerous conditions or infections.

6. A Pap test is a cytology specimen of the superficial layers of the cervix and endocervix to detect precancerous and cancerous cells of the cervix.

7. Fecal occult blood testing is important to screen for colon or rectal cancer.

8. Although a woman may have the "classic" crushing chest pain that is associated with a myocardial infarction, she is more likely to have atypical pain that often is confused with other conditions. These symptoms include fatigue or weakness, upper back pain, nausea and/or vomiting, loss of appetite, dizziness, palpitations, jaw pain, and neck pain. These symptoms may occur at rest or begin during physical activity.

9. Measures to reduce the risk for coronary artery disease include smoking cessation and control of hypertension; diet and glucose control to maintain normal weight and optimum fat and cholesterol intake; increase in activity level; and, for many women, daily aspirin therapy.

10. The initial therapy for fibrocystic breast disease varies with the age of the woman and her risk for breast cancer. Aspiration of cysts may relieve pain, with follow-up needed only if the cyst recurs or fluid aspirated is suspicious. Specific symptom relief for fibrocystic breast disease has not proved beneficial, but some methods that may be worth trying include wearing a supportive bra to reduce pain from large breasts that stretch ligaments and reducing the intake of caffeine and other stimulants. Other medications that may be tried include oral contraceptives during the second half of the menstrual cycle. Danazol, bromocriptine, and tamoxifen are other possibilities, but their use is temporary.

11. Ultrasound examination, fine-needle aspiration biopsy, core biopsy, or surgical biopsy is used to determine whether a breast disorder is benign or malignant.

12. Staging of breast cancer is important to determine the extent of the breast cancer and to plan appropriate therapy.

13. Adjuvant therapy is supportive or additional therapy recommended after surgery to improve the chance of long-term survival. Adjuvant therapy may include radiation therapy, chemotherapy, hormonal therapy, and immunotherapy.

14. Breasts may be reconstructed during the initial surgery or later. Two major methods are the tissue expansion method and autogenous grafts from another area of the woman's body. Tissue grafting cannot be done in every woman.

15. Teaching should include the length of the hospital stay and what will happen during that time, dressings, drainage tubes, and appearance of incisions for the expected procedures (lumpectomy, mastectomy, reconstruction). Lymphedema may occur in the immediate postoperative period, but it usually does not appear until well after discharge. Specific exercises such as arm lifts and pulley exercises will be taught as needed before discharge.

16. Discharge planning after breast cancer treatment should emphasize the need for continued care, methods to reduce the risk of infection on the affected side, postoperative medications that should be taken, and signs and symptoms that should be reported to the physician. Referral to local support groups also may be helpful.

17. Primary amenorrhea is menstruation that fails to occur within 2 years of breast development and within 1 year after onset of menses of her mother and a sister. Causes include hormonal imbalances, congenital anomalies, chromosomal defects, systemic diseases, and rigorous dieting and exercise. Treatment is aimed at identifying and treating the underlying cause. Secondary amenorrhea is cessation of menstruation for a period of at least 6 months in a woman who has an established pattern of menstruation. Pregnancy is the most common cause. Other causes include systemic disorders; hormonal imbalances; low weight for height; stress, poor nutrition; drug therapy for other disorders; and tumors of the ovary, pituitary, or adrenal gland. Once pregnancy is ruled out, treatment may include correction of the underlying cause, hormonal replacement therapy, and ovulation stimulation.

18. Possible causes of dysfunctional uterine bleeding include complications of pregnancy; benign or malignant lesions of the vagina, cervix, or uterus; drug-induced bleeding; systemic diseases, which require prompt treatment; and failure to ovulate.

19. Primary dysmenorrhea has no identified pathology. High levels of endometrial prostaglandin diffuse into endometrial tissue, causing spasmodic or colicky pain often called *cramps*. Effective treatment includes rest, application of warmth, oral contraceptives, and prostaglandin inhibitors.

20. Endometriosis lesions grow and proliferate during the follicular and luteal phases of the menstrual cycle and then slough during menstruation. The menstruation from endometriosis lesions occurs in deeper tissue, causing pressure or pain that is deep, bilateral or unilateral, and dull or sharp. Treatment varies with the woman's age, whether she is nearing menopause, her desire for children, her willingness to take the drugs that inhibit excessive tissue growth, and the problems caused to nearby organs by endometriosis. In addition to delaying pregnancy, drug therapy may induce menopausal symptoms.

21. Side effects of danazol include masculinizing effects and weight gain. The most common side effects of gonadotropin-releasing hormone (GnRH) agonists are hot flashes, vaginal dryness, decreased libido, and loss of bone mineral density.

22. Symptoms of premenstrual syndrome (PMS) must be cyclic and recur in the luteal phase of the menstrual cycle; the woman should be symptom free during the follicular phase; symptoms must be severe enough to alter the work, lifestyle, and relationships of the woman; and the diagnosis must be based on the woman's charting of her symptoms in a diary as they occur rather than by recall.

23. Common nursing education includes planning exercise therapy, incorporating dietary measures to reduce fluid retention and other symptoms (such as restricting salty or sweet foods, chocolate, caffeine, and others), educating the family about how to relate to a woman who is very irritable, and helping the woman make arrangements so that she can avoid harming her child if she becomes very agitated.

24. Mifepristone, methotrexate, and misoprostol are drugs that may be used for elective termination of pregnancy.

25. The nurse should teach the woman self-care measures, similar to self-care after spontaneous abortion or miscarriage: observation for excessive bleeding or signs of infection, information about follow-up visits, and contraception information.

26. Without estrogen, the reproductive organs begin to atrophy and the vagina and labia are thinner and more fragile. The breasts become smaller and atrophy. Bladder changes associated with atrophy make the woman more vulnerable to cystitis. Levels of total cholesterol and low-density lipoproteins ("bad" cholesterol) increase, whereas levels of high-density lipoproteins ("good" cholesterol)

decrease, increasing the woman's risk for coronary artery disease. Hot flashes occur because of vasomotor instability. Bone mineral loss accelerates in the first few years of the climacteric.

27. Depression, mood swings, and irritability are common psychological symptoms of menopause as the woman comes to term with aging. A woman may also greet menopause as freedom from earlier obligations in life as she shifts responsibility to her adult children.

28. Estrogen replacement controls hot flashes, alleviates genital atrophy, and protects against osteoporosis. Estrogen replacement must begin early in perimenopause to provide significant protection against osteoporosis. If the woman has a uterus, progesterone is given for part of the cycle to prevent excessive buildup of the endometrium. Although once thought to reduce the incidence of cardiovascular disease and breast cancer, estrogen-progesterone replacement showed the opposite effect in the Women's Health Initiative study. At this time a woman must make a careful choice after weighing the benefits and risks of hormone replacement therapy (HRT). Women with a history of estrogen- and/or progesterone-positive breast cancer should not take HRT.

29. Osteoporosis is called the *silent thief* because no signs or symptoms may be apparent until posture changes as the vertebrae collapse or fractures occur.

30. Osteoporosis can be prevented by medications to enhance calcium absorption and inhibit calcium loss (such as calcium and vitamin D supplementation) and by weight-bearing exercises that strengthen muscles and increase bone mass. HRT also enhances calcium retention, but potential problems with HRT limit its usefulness for many women.

31. Nurses can help women with osteoporosis prevent fractures by teaching them how to avoid falls by making their environment as safe as possible and to strengthen their bones with medication compliance and load-bearing exercise programs. Adolescents and young women can also be taught the value of exercise in maintaining long-term bone health.

32. With a cystocele, the weakened upper anterior wall of the vagina cannot support the weight of urine, and the bladder protrudes downward into the vagina, resulting in incomplete emptying of the bladder and consequent cystitis and stress incontinence. With a rectocele, the rectum protrudes into the vagina as the upper posterior wall of the vagina becomes weakened, which may result in difficulty emptying the rectum.

33. Uterine prolapse is caused when the cardinal ligaments are stretched excessively, often with pregnancy, and do not return to normal. This condition is usually treated surgically according to severity and coexisting pelvic floor disorders.

34. Pelvic exercises and bladder training may alleviate symptoms of pelvic floor relaxation and urinary incontinence. Additional measures include teaching about the need

to maintain hydration and restrict alcohol and caffeine intake, adherence to weight control programs to reach optimal weight, and use of commercial products to protect the skin and prevent odor. Teaching about any prescribed medications may be indicated.

35. Signs and symptoms of leiomyomas are increased uterine size and excessive vaginal bleeding, which often results in anemia. Other symptoms are pelvic pressure, bloating, and urinary frequency, depending on the size and location of the fibroids. Treatment depends on size, symptoms, and whether the woman desires more children. Surgical treatment options include removal of the fibroids (myomectomy) or hysterectomy. Uterine artery embolization may be an option for the woman who does not want surgery.

36. Ultrasound is used to distinguish a fluid-filled ovarian cyst from a solid tumor, which requires additional evaluation to determine if the solid tumor is malignant.

37. Signs and symptoms that may indicate cancer of the reproductive organs are irregular vaginal bleeding, unexplained postmenopausal bleeding, unusual vaginal discharge, dyspareunia, persistent vaginal itching, elevated or discolored lesions of the vulva, abdominal bloating, persistent constipation, anorexia, or nausea. Reproductive organ cancers such as ovarian cancer may have no symptoms in the early stages.

38. Cervical cancer may be treated by cryosurgery, destruction of tissue by laser, loop electrosurgical excision procedure (LEEP), electrocoagulation surgical conization, or hysterectomy with chemotherapy for more advanced cases. Endometrial cancer is best treated with hysterectomy and bilateral salpingo-oophorectomy plus radiation. Radiation only may be used if the woman is a poor surgical candidate. Ovarian cancer is usually treated by surgery followed by chemotherapy; however, chemotherapy to reduce tumor size followed by surgery to remove malignancy may also be done. A second surgery may be performed to determine if more treatment is needed.

39. Pregnancy, diabetes mellitus, oral contraceptive use, and antibiotic therapy may result in vaginitis caused by *Candida albicans*.

40. Candidiasis causes a thick, white discharge, often with "cottage-cheese" characteristics. Trichomoniasis causes a thin or frothy, malodorous, and yellow-green or gray discharge.

41. Barrier methods of contraception (particularly condoms) prevent potentially infected ejaculate from entering the genital tract and prevent contact between the penis and vagina.

42. The major symptom of primary syphilis is a painless chancre that disappears in about 6 weeks; the disease is highly infectious during the primary stage. Symptoms of secondary syphilis are enlargement of the liver and spleen, headache, anorexia, and skin rash. Condylomata lata that contain numerous spirochetes and are highly contagious may develop.

43. Condylomata acuminata (genital warts) are caused by human papillomavirus (HPV), which is associated with cervical cancer.

44. *Chlamydia trachomatis* and *Neisseria gonorrhoeae* cause most cases of pelvic inflammatory disease (PID). Other pathogens, including *Escherichia coli*, *Gardnerella vaginalis*, *Streptococcus*, *Peptostreptococcus*, *Bacteroides*, *Prevotella*, *Mycoplasma*, *Ureaplasma*, and cytomegalovirus, may cause PID. Other aerobic and anaerobic microorganisms may also cause PID.

45. The risk of toxic shock syndrome can be reduced by changing tampons at least every 4 hours, avoiding use of superabsorbent tampons, and using pads rather than tampons during hours of sleep. The diaphragm or cervical cap should not be used during menstruation, and the device should be removed within the time limits recommended. Careful handwashing should be done before and after use of tampons, pads, diaphragm, or cervical cap for all women.

Answers to Critical Thinking Exercises

CHAPTER 2

Critical Thinking Exercise 2-1

1. The nurse may have assumed that the husband's behavior indicated concern for his wife. Instead, it may have been a manifestation of hovering husband syndrome, which occurs in the honeymoon phase of the cycle of violence.
2. Facial injury, signs of previous bruising that resemble "grab marks," and abdominal bruising should make the nurse question Mandy's explanation. Mandy's story of falling and hurting herself is not congruent with the location of abdominal injury and injuries on her arms. Mandy's lethargy and avoidance of eye contact also suggest that she is afraid.
3. The nurse should not question Mandy's explanation of the injury in the presence of the husband because this can increase the danger of escalating violence when the mother and the infant are discharged.
4. The nurse should respond, "No one deserves to be hurt and it's not your fault. You have a right to be respected and safe. There are resources to help you." Nurses should examine their own thinking to be certain that they do not accept a common bias that physical abuse is deserved by the victim.
5. Mandy needs information about protecting herself and the coming infant from future harm. This is not, however, the appropriate time to give her this information. The nurse must inform the physician and the postpartum staff of the problem and must make the necessary referrals to the hospital's social service department for follow-up.

Critical Thinking Exercise 2-2

1. The deontologic view is that taking organs necessary for life from one human being to give to another is wrong, even when the donor cannot survive. Maintenance of life at all costs is the goal.
2. The utilitarian view is that anencephalic infants cannot survive, but that their organs could benefit other infants (beneficence). Because this family feels strongly that helping other infants allows good to come from their own tragedy, the greatest good would be for an organ transplant.
3. The human rights view disapproves of aggressive treatment necessary to maintain perfusion to the organs until a recipient is located, because treatment does not help the dying infant and may increase suffering.

4. This concern invokes the principle of nonmaleficence. Despite the inability of this infant to survive, the human rights view is that his or her care and comfort needs are primary. Problems that could arise from such transplantations result from the conflict between ethical principles held by different groups of people: the patient, family, health care team, and society.

CHAPTER 6

Critical Thinking Exercise 6-1

1. The nurse should use therapeutic communication techniques to encourage each woman to talk more about her concerns. This shows interest and may identify other concerns as well.
2. These multiparas will have more concerns about lack of time and increased fatigue than a primigravida. In addition, they will have concerns about the effect of another baby on their other children and the time and energy required to meet the needs of all children.
3. Although both have 2-year-olds, Ruth will be concerned about her son's response to sharing her time and attention. Elisa has experienced this before and may be more worried about the effect of another baby on her economic situation and her ability to manage yet another child.
4. Suggest that any changes in sleeping arrangements be made early so that the other child(ren) will not feel displaced by the infant. Recommend that they plan ways to have time alone with the older child(ren) when the baby arrives, and review measures to reduce sibling rivalry. Ask Elisa about measures that were helpful when her last two children were born, and suggest that she involve the older children in preparing for the new baby.

CHAPTER 7

Critical Thinking Exercise 7-1

Liz and her support person should attend classes because they may have forgotten some information, especially because it has been over 5 years since the last class. Birthing care and options may have changed since the last birth. Couples often have concerns and questions about their last experience, and the nurse can discuss these issues and help them feel more positive about the impending birth. The needs of other children can also be addressed, including practical suggestions about easing the transition.

CHAPTER 8

Critical Thinking Exercise 8-1

1. Cheryl has gained an excessive amount of weight for this point in pregnancy. If she continues to gain weight at this rate, she will have a large amount of weight to lose after giving birth, and that may be difficult. Excessive weight gain in pregnancy can lead to obesity, gestational diabetes, labor complications, and postpartum weight retention. It can also cause increased birth weight of the infant and complications such as asphyxia, low Apgar scores, and hypoglycemia.

2. The nurse should look at Cheryl's eating habits and identify what may be leading to the excessive weight gain. The negative effects on the fetus of severe diet restrictions should be explained to Cheryl. The nurse should discuss a plan for limiting calories while still meeting the recommendations for calories and nutrients in pregnancy. If Cheryl is sedentary, a plan for moderate daily exercise may also be helpful.

CHAPTER 10

Critical Thinking Exercise 10-1

Nurses often assume that patients possess and know how to use a thermometer and that they know the signs of infection. Many nurses assume that patients realize the connection between blood loss and the tendency to develop infection. As a result, nurses may not emphasize the need for a diet that is high in nutrients that increase hemoglobin and hematocrit (iron and vitamin C). Nurses also may assume incorrectly that women know foods that contain these nutrients.

Critical Thinking Exercise 10-2

1. Many people wrongly assume that early pregnancy loss does not produce the grieving that accompanies loss at a later stage. Telling a woman that she is lucky when this happens ignores her feelings and invalidates any grief she feels.

2. The nurse also mistakenly assumes that little cause for grief exists over the loss of this pregnancy if later children are possible. However, a unique relationship exists between the woman and this fetus. She may experience an emotional upheaval when this special relationship comes to an abrupt end. Another pregnancy is not guaranteed to any woman.

3. It would be beneficial if the nurse examined her assumptions before having the interaction with a woman experiencing early fetal loss. The patient might feel free to express her feelings and acknowledge the grief that she is feeling. A statement such as "I'm sorry this happened to you" may be appropriate.

Critical Thinking Exercise 10-3

1. The team has apparently assumed many things about this woman, such as that she knows the importance of frequent follow-up for gestational diabetes and that she has the transportation and available time off from work to return

weekly. The team has assumed that the diet has food that is affordable and fits with her food preferences.

2. To improve compliance and identify specific patient needs, the team needs to ask the woman about her food preferences with the diet and possibly its affordability. Lack of transportation and time off from work may present another need. The team should ask questions that may reveal other needs for diabetes-related pregnancy care.

3. The nurse could agree that a large baby might be a normal family trait, but emphasize that measures to keep glucose normal are important to the well-being of her baby, regardless of size.

4. These tests provide reassurance that the pregnancy is progressing well and identify problems that need to be addressed.

CHAPTER 11

Critical Thinking Exercise 11-1

1. The nurse assumed that Aricella's feelings are the transient, self-limiting moods of sadness that occur in many women who give birth. The nurse fails to obtain additional data that may indicate whether Aricella is experiencing postpartum depression (PPD) that requires additional therapy. She could quickly screen for PPD by asking: (a) do you feel down, depressed, or hopeless; and (b) do you feel little interest or pleasure in doing things?

2. The nurse's response is not helpful because it minimizes the feelings Aricella has expressed and it offers no measures for coping with them. Aricella is unlikely to tell the nurse more about her feelings because the nurse has implied that they are unimportant.

3. The nurse should acknowledge Aricella's feelings and ask follow-up questions that allow Aricella to express her feelings fully.

4. The nurse should convey genuine interest and caring. She can do this best by:
   a. Indicating awareness that something may be wrong.
   b. Sharing as much time as Aricella needs to express her feelings.
   c. Providing hope by reassuring Aricella that these feelings are common, that the condition is not her fault, that it can be cured, and that it is acceptable to talk about these feelings and seek help.
   d. Making appropriate referrals to provide as much continuity of care as possible. Provide Aricella phone numbers and Internet addresses for a crisis center and support groups.

CHAPTER 12

Critical Thinking Exercise 12-1

1. Additional information is needed. Ask to talk to Heather and find out the following:
   a. Is there any leaking or gush of fluid? If so, what did it look like, and what color was it?
   b. Is there any vaginal bleeding other than spotting or pinkish mucus?

c. Has the baby's activity level been "normal"?

d. Are the contractions regular? How often do they occur? Is this closer together or further apart than earlier in the day?

e. How long do the contractions last? Is this longer or shorter than earlier in the day?

f. Has the strength of the contractions increased, or does it vary? Other than not being able to sleep, how are you coping?

g. Have you had other children/labor? How does this compare? How long was your labor with other children?

h. How far away from the hospital do you live?

You want to speak with Heather. By putting her on the phone, you can assess her anxiety level and how she responds to any contractions that she has while you are talking to her.

Questions a, b, and c: If there is possible rupture of the amniotic membranes, vaginal bleeding, or decreased fetal activity, Heather needs to come in for an assessment, regardless of whether or not she is in labor.

Questions d, e, and f: You are trying to determine if the contractions are labor or Braxton Hicks. Labor contractions will be regular with increasing frequency, duration, and intensity. Braxton Hicks contractions will be irregular in timing, duration, and intensity. If the contractions are regular, you need to know the current frequency, duration, and intensity to anticipate whether she is in latent or active phase. You also need to assess Heather's coping ability.

Questions g and h: If Heather has had other labors, you need to know if they were usually fast. If so, you may want her to come in earlier in the labor than someone who has a history of longer labors. Multigravida women typically labor faster than primigravida women do. You may instruct her to come in a little earlier in the labor so that she will have time to arrive at the hospital without undue anxiety.

2. Recommend that Heather stay home if you determine that her membranes are intact, she is not bleeding, and the fetus is active; that she is either primigravida or does not have a history of rapid labors; and that she lives near the hospital and is either having Braxton Hicks contractions or is in latent phase of first-stage labor. Explain to Heather that she is most likely having Braxton Hicks contractions. Some of them may feel very intense, but others will not. However, they are important to prepare her body for active labor. Suggest that she walk around for a while, stay well hydrated, and take a warm bath or shower to relax. Instruct her to come to the hospital when the contractions are regular and every 5 minutes for 1 hour (every 10 minutes if she is a multigravida), if she has a gush or leaking of fluid or bright red vaginal bleeding, if the baby's movements substantially decrease, or if she is not able to cope effectively with the contractions.

Critical Thinking Exercise 12.2

1. Carmelita is in the latent phase of first-stage labor. The occiput of the baby's head is toward the right side of her spine.

This fetal position is typically associated with slower, more painful labors. Nursing interventions should include activities to promote rotation of the fetus to an OA position. You would expect Carmelita to be excited and sociable at this time. She will probably complain of back pain, which may begin to encircle her abdomen. An increase in frequency, duration, and intensity of contractions indicates that she is making rapid progress. If she becomes serious, with an inward focus, anxious, or expresses feelings of hopelessness, she has probably progressed to the active phase of labor. If she progresses very rapidly to transition, she may become irritable and lose control.

CHAPTER 13

Critical Thinking Exercise 13-1

1. Truc's labor progress and pattern of contractions, plus her tension, suggest that she may need medication. However, the nurse should not assume that she needs or wants medication. Breathing techniques or other nonpharmacologic measures may be adequate for Truc. The nurse must not assume that Truc does not need pain relief just because she smiles and has not requested pain medication. Asian women often value stoicism and are concerned with harmonious relationships. Truc may be smiling to please the nurse rather than because she is comfortable. In addition, Truc may not fully understand what the nurse says about pain relief if she is not comfortable speaking and understanding the nurse's language.

2. The nurse needs additional data about Truc's needs and plans for pain relief.

3. The nurse can share observations about Truc's body posture during contractions. If Truc does not speak English well, an interpreter may improve assessment of her need for pain relief. The nurse can demonstrate nonpharmacologic actions, such as breathing techniques, for Truc to use with or without medication or regional block analgesia.

CHAPTER 14

Critical Thinking Exercise 14.1

The pattern described is one of early decelerations, caused by fetal head compression. The fetal heart rate (FHR) pattern described is Category I, normal. It is strongly predictive of normal fetal acid-base balance at this time. Therefore no corrective actions are needed; the nurse should continue heightened surveillance (every 15 minutes) due to Margaret's history of gestational diabetes and oxytocin induction of labor.

Critical Thinking Exercise 14.2

Eleanor's pattern is a Category II, indeterminate pattern. Although the baseline rate is within normal limits and there is moderate variability, recurrent variable decelerations are described. Variable decelerations are caused by umbilical cord compression. Although the fetus is currently not acidotic (as evidenced by the moderate variability and normal baseline rate), if the umbilical cord compression is recurrent or prolonged, interruption in the fetal oxygenation can progress to hypoxemia, hypoxia, and acidosis. The first corrective action would be a vaginal exam to rule out a prolapsed umbilical cord and assess the progress of labor. If the examiner does not palpate an umbilical cord and birth of the baby is not imminent, the next action is maternal repositioning. Repositioning the mother to lateral or hands and knees will alter the relationship between the uterine wall, amniotic fluid, fetus, and umbilical cord. In many cases, this will resolve the variable deceleration pattern. The provider may consider an amnioinfusion to replace amniotic fluid volume and relieve umbilical cord compression. If the pattern worsens with a loss of variability, an IV fluid bolus and administration of oxygen will maximize uteroplacental perfusion.

CHAPTER 15

Critical Thinking Exercise 15.1

1. The woman is either insulted that the nurse asked such a question or has indeed used drugs or herbal preparations.
2. In either case, it may be beneficial for the nurse to stop the interview and explain that the question is asked of all women who are admitted and why the information is important to the care of a woman in labor and her baby. If other people are in the room, the nurse should continue the interview when the patient is alone. Assure her of the confidentiality of her medical record, but be honest with her if any drug tests will be performed on her or her baby.

Critical Thinking Exercise 15.2

The most important nursing action at this time is assessment of the fetal heart rate (FHR). When the membranes rupture, the umbilical cord may be washed into the vagina with the fluid. The fetal head may then compress the cord and cut off its own blood supply. This is an obstetric emergency known as a *prolapsed umbilical cord.* If the cord is prolapsed, the FHR will be low (<110 bpm, probably much lower than that). If the FHR has dropped, the nurse should perform a vaginal exam to feel for the cord and elevate the presenting part off of the cord until an emergency cesarean birth can be performed.

Critical Thinking Exercise 15.3

1. Fetal heart rate (FHR) is elevated from the usual range of 110 to 160 bpm, possibly because the fetal temperature may be one degree more than the mother's temperature, making it near 38.3°C (101°F). The amount of amniotic fluid is normal, but the pale yellow color and strong odor suggest chorioamnionitis, or infection of the amniotic sac. The risk for chorioamnionitis increases as the duration of ruptured membranes increases, but it can be apparent at any time, including at initial rupture. Accelerations with fetal movement are a reassuring sign of fetal well-being. The maternal temperature, pulse, and respirations are slightly elevated. Epidural analgesia is sometimes associated with temperature elevation. Accurately interpreting

these values is difficult, because the baseline values at the time of admission are not stated. The contractions are typical for a woman entering the active phase of first-stage labor.
2. Notify other medical staff of the woman's present situation, who were not involved in the amniotomy, such as anesthesia professionals. Observe temperature at least every 2 hours for elevation to 38°C (100.4°F) or higher. The nurse should continue to assess the fetus for tachycardia, which often precedes maternal fever, and for signs of fetal compromise that may occur with maternal infection. Report abnormalities to the physician.

Critical Thinking 15.4

1. The nurse must consider that the fetal heart rate (FHR) and pattern and contractions are externally monitored. The frequency of contractions is not yet excessive at every 2 minutes (no more than five in a 10-minute time span). The duration of contractions is within the normal limits of 90 to 120 seconds. However, the relaxation time of the uterus is inadequate because it never fully relaxes. Inadequate uterine relaxation can be identified in two ways: (a) contractions with a frequency of every 120 seconds and a duration of 100 seconds means that only 20 seconds of timed uterine relaxation occur; (b) palpation by the nurse identifies that the uterus never fully relaxes before the next contraction begins.
2. Although the fetus is tolerating labor now, fetal oxygenation may be compromised if the excessive contractions and lack of full uterine relaxation continue. Appropriate nursing interventions with normal fetal heart rate patterns include the following:
   - Position the woman on her side.
   - Administer an IV fluid bolus of at least 500 mL.
   - If the resting tone does not improve in 10 to 15 minutes, the oxytocin infusion rate should be decreased by half.
   - If tachysystole/increased resting tone persists after another 10 to 15 minutes, the oxytocin infusion should be stopped until the uterine activity is normal.

If the FHR pattern becomes abnormal, the nurse should stop the oxytocin infusion, continue with the listed interventions, and consider oxygen administration at 10 L/min via a nonrebreather face mask until the FHR pattern improves, and notify the provider; anticipate an order for terbutaline (Brethine 0.25 mg subcutaneously) if no improvement occurs with other interventions.

CHAPTER 16

Critical Thinking Exercise 16-1

1. When the fetus is in one of the occiput posterior positions, back pain is usually persistent because the fetal head presses on the mother's sacrum with each contraction, often called *back labor.* Additionally, the fetal head has to rotate internally through a wider arc to ultimately reach an occiput anterior position for birth. This process prolongs labor in most women.

2. The nurse should take actions to make the woman more comfortable and promote rotation of the fetal head to an occiput anterior position. The nurse should encourage the woman to change positions regularly. Positions that cause her uterus to fall forward reduce pressure on her sacrum and straighten the pelvic curve somewhat to encourage fetal rotation. Examples of these are leaning forward while sitting, kneeling, or standing or a hands-and-knees position. Lunging toward her right side provides slightly more room on that side of her pelvis. If she wants to lie in bed, a left side-lying position favors fetal rotation toward an occiput anterior position. Analgesia may be helpful.

CHAPTER 17

Critical Thinking Exercise 17-1

1. Any time a patient has more pain than would be expected, further assessment is necessary to determine the cause. Ask Lani to rate her pain. Exactly where is the pain located? What type of pain is it: burning, pressure, dull ache? Ask her whether she urinated a large or small amount. How did the amount compare with her usual voidings? How much lochia does she have compared with previous assessments?

2. Regardless of the amount she thinks she voided previously and Lani's lack of the sensation of needing to void, assist her to the bathroom to see if she can void. If she urinates, measure the amount to see if it is adequate (approximately 300 mL) and determine if she feels relief after voiding. If she is unable to void and an order is available, catheterize her. If no order exists, call the health care provider to obtain an order.

3. A distended bladder is the most likely cause of Lani's pain. However, she may have a very low pain tolerance or need a different kind of analgesic. In this case, however, Lani had surgery yesterday and has received pain medication since that time. A low pain tolerance would already have been noted. Some surgical complication may exist. If the pain continues, refer the problem to the provider.

Critical Thinking Exercise 17-2

1. Callie's priority needs are for physical care and comfort. She also needs to make the experience of childbirth part of her reality and does this by recounting the details of the birth and trying to fill in the missing pieces about the cesarean birth.

2. Callie is in the taking-in phase. She is getting acquainted with her "real" baby by exploring with her fingertips. This usually is the first maternal touch observed.

3. Callie's priorities are to assume control of her own body functions and manage her care so that she can "take hold" and assume care of the baby.

4. Callie has become more independent and now initiates breastfeeding. She demonstrates readiness to learn by requesting the assistance of the lactation consultant.

5. Anticipatory guidance should focus on ways she can manage the care of the infant while still getting adequate rest and nutrition. Keeping a flexible schedule, resting while the infant rests, and preparing easy, nutritious meals are some of the most important items to emphasize.

6. Assisting her in identifying friends and neighbors who might provide some support while her husband is away would be most helpful. If this is not possible, she should have telephone numbers for community resources such as the hospital "baby line." A follow-up home visit, visit to a postpartum clinic, or telephone call initiated by the nurse would be very helpful. The nurse could assess the mother and infant, reinforce teaching, and provide encouragement.

CHAPTER 18

Critical Thinking Exercise 18-1

1. Her history of multiparity, birth of a large infant, and rapid labor and delivery indicate that Dawn is at risk for postpartum hemorrhage. The nurse should increase the frequency of her assessments of the fundus, lochia, vital signs, and skin temperature and color.

2. Massage the fundus and express clots that may have accumulated in the uterus. Massage stimulates uterine contractions that compress torn myometrial blood vessels and stop excessive bleeding. If any clots have formed inside the uterus, they must be expelled to allow the uterus to contract. Continued assessment of the fundus and lochia is imperative to determine whether the uterus relaxes again, leading to resumption of bleeding.

3. Assist Dawn to void, because a distended bladder lifts the uterus, making contraction more difficult and resulting in excessive bleeding.

4. Continue to massage the fundus and turn on the call light to ask a colleague for help. Ask that another nurse notify the health care provider, because excessive bleeding requires the combined efforts of primary health care providers and nurses to prevent postpartum hemorrhage. Start IV fluids or increase the flow rate of an existing IV, and give medications according to orders or hospital protocol. Insert a catheter to ensure that urine output can be measured easily and the bladder does not interfere with uterine contraction.

CHAPTER 19

Critical Thinking Exercise 19-1

If an opening were present between the right and left atria after birth, blood would flow from the left atrium, where pressures are high after birth, into the right atrium, where pressures are low after birth. This is the reverse of the blood flow through the foramen ovale during fetal life. The blood would then flow to the right ventricle, the pulmonary artery, and the lungs. This would cause an increased workload on the lungs and could lead to serious complications.

Critical Thinking Exercise 19-2

Some sources of heat loss are:

- Evaporation—liquid on the body at birth or during bathing, contact with wet towels or blankets, regurgitation, urine on the skin, increased insensitive water loss while under a radiant warmer or under phototherapy lights
- Conduction—cool blankets, clothing, mattress, scale, stethoscope, circumcision restraint board, hands of caregivers
- Convection—air conditioning or fans, drafts, movement of people around the infant, open windows, cold oxygen
- Radiation—placement of crib or being held near an outside wall or window (open or closed), cool walls in a poorly heated room

CHAPTER 20

Critical Thinking Exercise 20-1

Failure of the reflexes to fade on schedule may interfere with normal development. For example, the palmar grasp reflex must disappear so that the infant can learn to grasp voluntarily and later to release objects at will. Persistence of the plantar reflex would interfere with walking. Retention of reflexes beyond the age at which they should disappear indicates pathology and should prompt further investigation.

Critical Thinking Exercise 20-2

Begin by expanding your assessment of the facts. First, check through the chart to be sure that no stool is recorded. Did the infant pass meconium at delivery? Check the delivery notes. Ask the mother if she has changed a diaper with stool in it. Instruct her to inform the nurse if she does. If agency policy permits, carefully taking a rectal temperature may stimulate peristalsis and passage of meconium and verifies that the anus is patent. However, even with a patent anus, obstruction of the intestine above the anus is possible.

Consider the infant's intake. How often is the infant feeding, and how well are feedings being taken? If the infant has been sleepy and has fed poorly, increase the feedings. Asking the nursing mother to feed more often or offering extra formula to the formula-fed neonate may make the difference.

Alert other caregivers to watch for a stool, and let the mother know that the infant is being watched for stools without alarming her. Although some infants do not have a stool until nearly 48 hours after birth, the primary caregiver may wish to know about the situation at 24 hours.

CHAPTER 21

Critical Thinking Exercise 21-1

1. Determine whether Nicholas is showing signs of inadequate thermoregulation, hypoglycemia, or both. Reassure and teach Vicki as assessments and interventions are completed.
2. While taking the infant's temperature, assess for skin temperature, jitteriness, and general behavior. Check the blood glucose level if indicated. Also assess the environment for possible causes of heat loss.
3. If the baby's temperature is slightly low, change any wet linens, double-wrap him in warm blankets, and put a hat on his head. Or place him skin to skin with Vicki with a blanket over both of them. Have Vicki feed him if it is near a feeding time or if the blood glucose level is low. Recheck the temperature in 30 minutes. If it is still low, place Nicholas under a radiant warmer. Notify the physician if the infant continues to have difficulty maintaining temperature.
4. Sue should praise Vicki for being so observant of her son. If the temperature is normal and Nicholas is not jittery, discuss the fact that peripheral circulation is sluggish in newborns and that their hands and feet tend to be cool. If the "shakiness" is the Moro reflex or normal newborn behavior, discuss the reflex and the immaturity of the central nervous system. Show Vicki how to wrap Nicholas so he stays warm and the Moro reflex is not elicited. Discuss methods of temperature control, and be sure that Vicki knows how to read a thermometer. Explain all interventions.
5. Sue should explain to the grandmother and the parents that although infants have slept on the abdomen without harm, research has shown that infants sleeping in this position have a higher chance of dying from sudden infant death syndrome (SIDS) than those who sleep on the back. To prevent flattening of the head, babies should spend time on the abdomen every day while they are awake. "Tummy time" helps keep the head rounded and helps develop the infant's muscles. The infant should always be supervised when lying prone. Occasionally placing the infant at alternate ends of the crib changes the pressure on the head because an infant is more likely to look toward the door.

Critical Thinking Exercise 21-2

1. The major priorities are to support the parents in their new role and to determine if Susan is progressing normally.
2. Use therapeutic communication techniques to allow Mary and Skip to express their feelings adequately. If Susan appears to be progressing normally, emphasize that she is doing well. Point out that the problems they are encountering are quite common for both biologic and adoptive parents.
3. Information should be based on the parents' concerns. Explain normal characteristics and behaviors of the newborn. Determine if Mary and Skip need more information about basic infant care, such as feeding, cord care, and signs of illness. Provide frequent opportunities for them to ask questions.
4. Obtain more information about Susan's sleep patterns. Discuss normal sleep in newborns and methods of helping infants sleep. Offer suggestions for methods of coping with crying. Help Mary and Skip work out a plan for sharing the burdens and the joys of parenthood.

CHAPTER 23

Critical Thinking Exercise 23-1

Compared with the full-term infant, Giovanni will need more frequent feedings with special formula in smaller amounts. He will start by having tube feedings in very small amounts. Gradually the amount will increase. When he shows signs of readiness for feeding from a bottle, he will be given a small amount of feeding by bottle and will finish with tube feedings. After a while he will be able to take all of his feeding by bottle.

Critical Thinking Exercise 23-2

1. The mother may be intimidated by the equipment and fear she might break it or cause it to malfunction if she touches it. If alarms sound frequently, she may be especially uneasy. She may be frightened of the infant's small size and afraid she might cause harm by touching her baby. She may be experiencing anticipatory grieving because her infant may not survive. She may also be too overwhelmed to be able to participate in touching her infant at this time and may need more time.

2. To assist the mother, the nurse can use therapeutic communication techniques to help her express her feelings and fears. The purpose of equipment and reasons for alarms should be explained. Involving the mother in small tasks, such as handing the nurse a blanket or holding a bottle of formula, may help her feel more a part of her baby's care. The nurse should continue to suggest that the mother touch the baby and to suggest ways it might be appropriate. For example, the nurse might ask the mother to hold the infant's hand to comfort the infant during minor procedures. As she becomes more comfortable, she might be amenable to holding the baby in kangaroo care.

Critical Thinking Exercise 23-3

Explain the concept of corrected or developmental age to the mother. Because the infant was born 10 weeks early, the corrected age at this time is 4 weeks. This is the chronological age (14 weeks) minus the number of weeks the infant was born early (10 weeks). Therefore the infant can be expected to turn from prone to supine at 6½ to 7½ months chronological age, which is 4 to 5 months corrected or developmental age.

CHAPTER 24

Critical Thinking Exercise 24-1

Patches hide the eye area, and an irritation or infection might not be noticed with patches in place. The warm, dark, moist area under the patches provides a good breeding ground for organisms to grow. Removal of the patches at feedings allows inspection for signs of infection such as redness, edema, and drainage. Removal also allows a time of visual sensory stimulation for the infant. Parental visits should be coordinated with feedings, if possible, so parents can see the infant's whole face while they visit. This will help the infant appear more normal to them and enhances attachment.

CHAPTER 25

Critical Thinking Exercise 25-1

1. Find a private place to talk without interruption. Use therapeutic communication techniques to explore her feelings further. Help her think through the ways in which a pregnancy might change her life and how she would feel about those changes.

2. Explore what the teenager feels would be most embarrassing about seeing a provider. Would a female nurse practitioner, nurse-midwife, or physician be more acceptable? Discuss what happens when a woman is examined during a visit for contraceptive counseling. Let her know that a pelvic examination is not necessary if she is not having any problems and that the provider may prescribe contraceptives without an examination. Discuss common contraceptive methods and determine her understanding and concerns about them.

3. Discuss negotiation skills for condom use because condoms are important for prevention of sexually transmitted diseases (STDs) as well as pregnancy. Try role playing, with the adolescent acting in the role of her partner and the nurse taking the role of the adolescent.

ΔOD450 (delta OD 450) A test used to measure the change (delta, or δ) in optical density of the amniotic fluid caused by staining with bilirubin.

abortion A spontaneous or elective termination of pregnancy before the twentieth week of gestation. Spontaneous abortion is frequently called *miscarriage*.

abruptio placentae See *Placental abruption*.

abstinence syndrome A group of signs and symptoms that occurs when a person who is dependent on a specific drug withdraws or abstains from taking that drug.

acidosis Condition resulting from accumulation of acid (hydrogen ions) or depletion of base (bicarbonate); acid-base balance measured by pH.

acme Peak, or period of greatest strength, of a uterine contraction.

acrocyanosis Bluish discoloration of the hands and feet caused by reduced peripheral circulation.

adjuvant therapy Additional treatment that increases or enhances the action of the primary treatment.

adnexa Accessory parts or organs, such as the fallopian tubes and ovaries, associated with the uterus.

afterpains Cramping pain after childbirth caused by alternating relaxation and contraction of uterine muscles.

agonist Substance that causes a physiologic effect.

allele An alternative form of a gene.

alpha-fetoprotein (AFP) Plasma protein produced by the fetus.

ambiguity (ambiguous) Lack of clarity or certainty; having more than one meaning.

ambivalence Simultaneous conflicting emotions, attitudes, ideas, or wishes.

amenorrhea Absence of menstruation. Primary amenorrhea is a delay of the first menstruation, and secondary amenorrhea is cessation of menstruation after its initiation.

amniocentesis Transabdominal puncture of the amniotic sac to obtain a sample of amniotic fluid that contains fetal cells and biochemical substances for laboratory examination.

amnioinfusion Infusion of a sterile isotonic solution into the uterine cavity during labor to reduce umbilical cord compression; may also be done to dilute meconium in amniotic fluid and reduce the risk that the infant will aspirate thick meconium at birth.

amniotic fluid embolism An embolism in which amniotic fluid with its particulate matter is drawn into the pregnant woman's circulation, lodging in her lungs.

amniotic fluid index (AFI) An ultrasound examination in which the vertical depth of the largest fluid pocket in each of the four quadrants of the uterus is measured and totaled.

amniotomy AROM—artificial rupture of the fetal membranes (i.e., the amniotic sac).

analgesic Systemic agent that relieves pain without causing loss of consciousness.

anaphylactoid syndrome A disorder in which amniotic fluid with its particulate matter enters the pregnant woman's circulation, lodging in her lungs. Previously called *amniotic fluid embolism*.

anesthesia Loss of sensation, especially to pain, with or without loss of consciousness.

anesthesiologist Physician who specializes in administration of anesthesia.

angina pectoris Myocardial pain usually caused by physical activity or stress; usually called simply *angina*.

anorexia nervosa Refusal to eat because of a distorted body image and feeling of obesity.

anovulation Menstrual cycles that occur without ovulation.

antagonist Substance that blocks the action of another substance or of body secretions.

antepartum Pertaining to the time during pregnancy before the onset of labor.

apnea A pause in breathing lasting 20 seconds or more or accompanied by cyanosis, pallor, bradycardia, or decreased muscle tone.

apneic spells Cessation of breathing for more than 20 seconds or accompanied by cyanosis, pallor, bradycardia, or hypotonia.

asphyxia Insufficient oxygen and excess carbon dioxide in blood and tissues.

aspiration pneumonitis Chemical injury to the lungs that may occur with regurgitation and aspiration of acidic gastric secretions.

assisted reproductive technologies (ART) Medical, surgical, laboratory, and micromanipulation techniques used with ova and sperm to improve chances of conception.

assumptions Beliefs taken for granted without examination.

atony Absence or lack of usual muscle tone.

atrophic vaginitis Inflammation that occurs when the vagina becomes dry and fragile, usually as a result of estrogen deficit after menopause.

attachment Development of strong affectional ties as a result of interaction between an infant and a significant other (such as mother, father, sibling, caretaker).

attitude Relationship of fetal body parts to one another.

augmentation of labor Artificial stimulation of uterine contractions that have become ineffective.

autogenous Tissue that is moved from one part of the body to another part of the same person's body.

autosome Any of the 22 pairs of chromosomes other than the sex chromosomes.

axillary dissection Removal of most of the axillary lymph nodes for staging and treatment of breast cancer.

azoospermia Absence of sperm in semen.

baroreceptors Cells that are sensitive to blood pressure changes.

basal body temperature Body temperature at rest.

baseline data Information that describes the status of the client before treatment begins.

baseline risk The risk, usually in reference to birth defects or spontaneous abortion, of the general population of pregnant women who have no identified high-risk factors or invasive procedures.

bias A prejudice that sways the mind.

bicornuate (bicornate) uterus Malformed uterus with two horns.

bilirubin Unusable component of hemolyzed (broken down) erythrocytes.

bilirubin encephalopathy Acute manifestation of bilirubin toxicity occurring in the first weeks after birth.

bioethics Rules or principles that govern right conduct, specifically those that relate to health care.

biophysical profile (BPP) Method for evaluating fetal status during the antepartum period based on five variables originating with the fetus: fetal heart rate, breathing movements, gross body movements, muscle tone, and amniotic fluid volume.

birth defect An abnormality of structure, function, or body metabolism present at birth that results in physical or mental disability or is fatal.

birth plan A plan describing a couple's preferences for their birth experience. (Also called a *family preference plan*.)

bloody show Mixture of cervical mucus and blood from ruptured capillaries in the cervix; often precedes labor and increases with cervical dilation.

body image Subjective view of one's physical appearance and capabilities; derived from one's own observations and the evaluation of significant others.

bonding Development of a strong emotional tie of a parent to a newborn.

Braxton Hicks contractions Irregular, usually mild uterine contractions that occur throughout pregnancy and become stronger in the last trimester.

breast self-awareness Women's awareness of the normal appearance and feel of their breasts; can include breast self-examination as part of it.

breast self-examination (BSE) Organized monthly evaluation by the woman of her breasts; supplements clinical breast examination.

bronchopulmonary dysplasia Chronic pulmonary condition in which damage to the infant's lungs requires prolonged dependence on supplemental oxygen. (Also called *chronic lung disease*.)

brown fat Highly vascular specialized fat that provides more heat than other fat when metabolized.

bulimia Eating disorder characterized by ingestion of large amounts of food followed by induced vomiting, fasting, or use of laxatives or diuretics.

café-au-lait spots Light-brown birthmarks.

CAM Abbreviation for complementary and/or alternative medicine.

caput succedaneum Area of edema over the presenting part of the fetus or newborn resulting from pressure against the cervix; often called simply *caput.*

carcinoma in situ Malignant neoplasm in surface tissue that has not extended into deeper tissue.

catabolism Destructive process that converts living cells into simpler compounds; process involved in involution of the uterus after childbirth.

caudal regression syndrome A malformation that results when the sacrum, lumbar spine, and lower extremities fail to develop.

cephalhematoma Bleeding between the periosteum and skull from pressure during birth; does not cross suture lines.

cephalopelvic disproportion Fetal head size that is too large to fit through the maternal pelvis at birth. (Also called *fetopelvic disproportion.*)

cerclage Encircling the cervix with sutures to prevent recurrent spontaneous abortion caused by early cervical dilation.

cervical cap A small cuplike device placed over the cervix to prevent sperm from entering.

cervical incompetence or cervical insufficiency An anatomic defect that results in painless dilation of the cervix in the second trimester.

cesarean birth Surgical birth of the fetus through an incision in the abdominal wall and uterus.

Chadwick's sign Bluish-purple discoloration of the cervix, vagina, and labia during pregnancy as a result of increased vascular congestion.

chemical dependence Physical and psychological dependence on a substance such as alcohol, tobacco, or drugs, either legal or illicit.

chemoreceptors Cells that are sensitive to chemical changes in the blood, specifically changes in oxygen and carbon dioxide levels, and changes in acid-base balance.

chignon Newborn scalp edema created by a vacuum extractor.

choanal atresia Abnormality of the nasal septum that obstructs one or both nasal passages.

chordee Ventral curvature of the penis.

chorioamnionitis Inflammation of the amniotic sac (fetal membranes); usually caused by bacterial and viral infections. (Also called *amnionitis* or Triple I-intrauterine infection or inflammation or both.)

chorionic villus sampling (CVS) Transcervical or transabdominal procedure to obtain a sample of chorionic villi (projections of the outer fetal membrane) for analysis of fetal cells.

chromosomes Organization of DNA of specific genes into strings within the cell nucleus.

cilia Hairlike processes on the surface of a cell that beat rhythmically to move the cell or to move fluid or other substances over the cell surface.

climacteric Endocrine, body, and psychic changes occurring at the end of a woman's reproductive period. (Also informally called *menopause,* although this term does not encompass all changes.)

clinical breast examination (CBE) Breast examination by a professional that may identify problems that the woman has not identified with breast self-examination (BSE).

closure Reaching a decision.

coitus Sexual union between a male and a female.

coitus interruptus Withdrawal of the penis from the vagina before ejaculation.

colostrum Breast fluid secreted during pregnancy and the early days after childbirth.

colposcopy Examination of the vaginal and cervical tissue with a colposcope for magnification of cells.

complementary and alternative medicine (CAM) Nonmainstream or unconventional health care treatments and practices that are generally not used in hospitals and often not reimbursed by insurance companies.

complete protein food Food containing all the essential amino acids.

compliance Stretchability or elasticity of the lungs and thorax that allows distention without resistance during respirations.

conceptus Cells and membranes resulting from fertilization of the ovum at any stage of prenatal development.

condyloma acuminatum A wartlike growth of the skin seen on the external genitalia, in the vagina, on the cervix, or near the anus; may be caused by human papillomavirus (condyloma acuminatum) or by syphilis (condyloma latum).

congenital Present at birth.

congenital anomaly Abnormal intrauterine development of an organ or structure.

congestive heart failure Condition resulting from failure of the heart to maintain adequate circulation; characterized by weakness, dyspnea, and edema in body parts that are lower than the heart.

consanguinity Blood relationship.

containment A method of increasing comfort in infants by swaddling or other means to keep the extremities in a flexed position near the body.

contraception Prevention of pregnancy.

contraction stress test (CST) Method for evaluating fetal status during the antepartum period by observing response of the fetal heart to the stress of uterine contractions that may induce recurrent episodes of fetal hypoxia.

corpus luteum Graafian follicle cells remaining after ovulation that produce estrogen and progesterone.

corrected age Gestational age that a preterm infant would be if still in utero; the chronologic age minus the number of weeks the infant was born prematurely. (May also be called *developmental age.*)

couvades Pregnancy-related rituals or a cluster of symptoms experienced by some prospective fathers during pregnancy and childbirth.

craniosynostosis Premature closure of the sutures of the infant's head.

crowning Appearance of the fetal scalp or presenting part at the vaginal opening.

cryotherapy Destruction of tissue using extreme cold.

cryptorchidism Failure of one or both testes to descend into the scrotum.

cultural values Principles or standards which guide the thinking, decisions, and actions of a group, particularly during pivotal life events.

culture Sum of values, beliefs, and practices of a group of people that is transmitted from one generation to the next.

cystocele Prolapse of the urinary bladder through the anterior vaginal wall.

decidua Name applied to the endometrium during pregnancy. All except the deepest layer are shed after childbirth.

decrement Period of decreasing strength of a uterine contraction.

deontologic model Ethical model stating that the right course of action is the one dictated by ethical principles and moral rules.

developmental task A step in growth and maturation that one must complete before additional growth and maturation are possible.

diabetes mellitus A disorder of carbohydrate metabolism caused by a relative or complete lack of insulin secretion; characterized by glycosuria (glucose in the urine) and hyperglycemia.

diabetogenic Refers to a condition such as pregnancy that produces the effects of diabetes mellitus.

diaphragm A latex dome that covers the cervix and prevents entrance of sperm; must be used with a spermicide to be effective.

diastasis recti Separation of the longitudinal muscles of the abdomen (rectus abdominis) during pregnancy.

dietary reference intakes A label for several terms that estimate nutrient needs; includes recommended dietary allowance, adequate intake, tolerable upper intake level, and estimated average requirement.

dilation Opening.

dilation and curettage (D&C) Stretching of the cervical os to permit suctioning or scraping of the walls of the uterus. The procedure is performed to obtain samples of endometrial tissue for laboratory examination during the postpartum period to remove retained fragments of placenta.

dilation and evacuation (D&E) Wide cervical dilation followed by mechanical destruction and removal of fetal parts from the uterus. After complete removal of the fetus, a vacuum curette is used to remove the placenta and remaining products of conception.

diploid Having a pair of chromosomes that represents one copy of every chromosome from each parent; the number of chromosomes (46 in humans) normally present in body cells other than gametes.

dominant Gene for which a single copy on either the maternal or paternal chromosome can cause the trait to be expressed.

doula A trained labor support person who provides labor or postpartum support, or both.

duration Period from the beginning of a uterine contraction to the end of the same contraction.

dyslipidemia Abnormal fat and cholesterol levels.

dysmenorrhea Painful menstruation.

dyspareunia Difficult or painful coitus in women.

dysplasia Abnormal development of tissue.

dystocia Difficult or prolonged labor; often associated with abnormal uterine activity and cephalopelvic disproportion.

dysuria Painful urination often associated with urinary tract infection.

eclampsia Form of hypertension of pregnancy complicated by generalized (grand mal) seizures.

ectopic pregnancy Implantation of a fertilized ovum in any area other than the uterus; the most common site is the fallopian tube.

EDD Estimated date of delivery; may also be abbreviated EDB (*estimated date of birth*).

effacement Thinning and shortening of the cervix.

effleurage Light stroking or massage of the abdomen or another body part performed during labor contractions.

egocentrism Interest centered on the self rather than on the needs of others.

ejaculation Expulsion of semen from the penis.

emancipated minor An adolescent younger than the age of majority (usually 18 years) who is considered developmentally competent to make certain medical decisions independent of a parent or guardian.

embolus A mass that may be composed of a thrombus (blood clot) or amniotic fluid released into the bloodstream which may cause obstruction of pulmonary vessels.

embryo The developing baby from the beginning of the third week through the eighth week after conception.

en face Position that allows eye-to-eye contact between the newborn and a parent.

endometrial hyperplasia Excessive proliferation of normal cells of the uterine lining; may be caused by administration of estrogen during the postmenopausal period.

endometriosis Presence of tissue resembling the endometrium outside the uterine cavity.

endometritis Infection of the inner lining of the uterus.

endometrium Lining of the uterus.

endomyometritis Infection of the muscle and inner lining of the uterus.

endoparametritis Infection of the muscle and inner lining of the uterus, as well as the surrounding tissues.

endorphin Substance similar to opioids that occurs naturally in the central nervous system and modifies pain sensations; related to enkephalins.

engagement Descent of the widest diameter of the fetal presenting part to at least a zero station (the level of the ischial spines in the maternal pelvis).

engorgement Swelling of the breasts resulting from stasis and distention of the vascular and lymphatic circulations and accumulation of milk as lactation is established.

engrossment Intense fascination and close face-to-face observation between the father and newborn.

enkephalin Substance similar to opioids that occurs naturally in the central nervous system and modifies pain sensations; related to endorphins.

enteral feeding Nutrients supplied to the gastrointestinal tract orally or by feeding tube.

entrainment Newborn movement in rhythm with adult speech, particularly high-pitched tones, which are more easily heard.

epidural space Area outside the dura, between the dura mater and the vertebral canal.

episiotomy Surgical incision of the perineum to enlarge the vaginal opening.

epispadias Abnormal placement of the urinary meatus on the dorsal side of the penis.

erectile dysfunction Consistent inability of a man to achieve or maintain an erection of the penis that is sufficiently rigid to permit successful sexual intercourse. (Also called *impotence.*)

erythema toxicum Benign rash of unknown cause in newborns, with blotchy red areas that have white or yellow papules or vesicles in the center.

erythroblastosis fetalis Agglutination and hemolysis of fetal erythrocytes resulting from incompatibility between maternal and fetal blood.

esophageal atresia Condition in which the esophagus is separated from the stomach and ends in a blind pouch.

essential amino acids Amino acids that cannot be synthesized by the body and must be obtained from foods.

ethical dilemma A situation in which no solution seems completely satisfactory.

ethics Rules or principles that govern right conduct and distinctions between right and wrong.

ethnic Pertaining to religious, racial, national, or cultural group characteristics, especially speech patterns, social customs, and physical characteristics.

ethnicity Condition of belonging to a particular ethnic group; also refers to ethnic pride.

ethnocentrism Opinion that the beliefs and customs of one's own ethnic group are superior.

extremely-low-birth-weight infant An infant weighing 2 lb, 3 oz (1000 g) or less at birth.

extrusion reflex Automatic nervous system response that causes an infant to push anything solid out of the mouth.

familial Presence of a trait or condition in a family more often than would be expected by chance alone.

fantasies Mental images formed to prepare for the birth of a child.

fern test Microscopic appearance of amniotic fluid resembling fern leaves when the fluid is allowed to dry on a microscope slide. (Also called *ferning.*)

fertilization age Prenatal age of the developing baby, calculated from the date of conception. (Also called *postconceptional age.*)

fetal alcohol spectrum disorders All disorders resulting from maternal use of alcohol during pregnancy; includes fetal alcohol syndrome.

fetal alcohol syndrome A group of physical, behavioral, and mental abnormalities that are the most severe effects of fetal alcohol exposure.

fetal growth restriction Failure of a fetus to grow as expected for gestational age (also called intrauterine growth restriction, or IUGR).

fetal lie Relationship of the long axis of the fetus to the long axis of the mother.

fetal lung fluid Fluid that fills the fetal lungs, expanding the alveoli and promoting lung development.

fetus The developing baby from 9 weeks after conception until birth.

fingertipping First tactile (touch) experience between the mother and newborn in which the mother explores the infant's body, mainly with her fingertips.

first period of reactivity Period beginning at birth in which newborns are active and alert. It ends when the infant first falls asleep.

fontanel Space at the intersection of sutures connecting fetal or infant skull bones.

foremilk First breast milk received in a feeding.

fornix (Pl. fornices) An arch or pouchlike structure at the upper end of the vagina. (Also called a *cul-de-sac.*)

fourth trimester First 12 weeks after birth; a time of transition for parents and siblings.

frequency Period from the beginning of one uterine contraction to the beginning of the next.

gamete Reproductive cell or germ cell; in the female an ovum and in the male a spermatozoon.

gametogenesis Development and maturation of the sperm and ova.

gastroschisis Protrusion of the intestines through a defect in the abdominal wall. The intestines are not covered by a peritoneal sac or skin.

gate-control theory A theory about pain based on the premise that a gating mechanism in the dorsal horn of the spinal cord can open or close a "gate" for transmission of pain impulses to the brain.

gene Segment of DNA that directs the production of a specific product needed for body structure or function.

general anesthesia Systemic loss of sensation with loss of consciousness.

genetic Pertaining to the genes or chromosomes.

genetic sex Sex determined at conception by union of two X chromosomes (female) or an X and a Y chromosome (male). (Also called *chromosomal sex.*)

genotype Genetic makeup of an individual.

gestational age Prenatal age of the developing baby (measured in weeks) calculated from the first day of the woman's last menstrual period; approximately 2 weeks longer than the fertilization age. (Also called *menstrual age.*)

gestational carrier (or gestational surrogate) A woman who carries the embryo of an infertile couple and relinquishes the child to the couple after birth.

gestational trophoblastic disease Spectrum of diseases that includes both benign hydatidiform mole and gestational trophoblastic tumors such as invasive moles and choriocarcinoma.

gluconeogenesis Formation of glycogen by the liver from noncarbohydrate sources such as amino and fatty acids.

glycosuria Glucose in the urine.

gonad Reproductive (sex) gland that produces gametes and sex hormones. The female gonads are ovaries, and the male gonads are testes.

gonadotropic hormones Secretions of the anterior pituitary gland that stimulate the gonads, specifically follicle-stimulating hormone and luteinizing hormone. Chorionic gonadotropin is secreted by the placenta during pregnancy.

Goodell's sign Softening of the cervix during pregnancy.

graafian follicle A small sac within the ovary that contains the maturing ovum.

gravida A pregnant woman; also refers to a woman's total number of pregnancies, including the one in progress, if applicable.

gynecologic age The number of years since menarche (first menstrual period).

habituation Decreased response to a repeated stimulus.

haploid Having one copy of a chromosome from each pair (23 in humans, or half the diploid number); normal for gametes.

***Healthy People 2020* goals** National health promotion and disease prevention goals.

Hegar's sign Softening of the lower uterine segment that allows it to be easily compressed at 6 to 8 weeks of pregnancy.

hematoma Localized collection of blood in a space or tissue.

heme iron Iron obtained from meat, poultry, or fish sources; the form most usable by the body.

heterozygous Having two different alleles for a genetic trait.

hindmilk Breast milk received near the end of a feeding; contains higher fat content than foremilk.

homologous Chromosomes that pair during meiosis, one received from the person's mother and one from the father.

homozygous Having two identical alleles for a genetic trait.

human rights model Ethical model based on the belief that every person has human rights.

hydramnios Excessive volume of amniotic fluid, more than about 2000 mL at term. (Also called *polyhydramnios*.)

hydrops fetalis Heart failure and generalized edema in the fetus secondary to severe anemia resulting from destruction of erythrocytes.

hyperbilirubinemia Excessive amount of bilirubin in the blood.

hypercapnia Excess carbon dioxide in the blood, evidenced by an elevated Pco_2.

hyperemia Excess blood in an area of the body.

hypospadias Abnormal placement of the urinary meatus on the ventral side of the penis.

hypovolemia Abnormally decreased volume of circulating fluid in the body.

hypovolemic shock Acute peripheral circulatory failure resulting from loss of circulating blood volume.

hypoxemia Reduced oxygenation of the blood, evidenced by a low Po_2.

hypoxia Reduced availability of oxygen to the body tissues.

iatrogenic Term used to describe an adverse condition resulting from treatment.

impotence See *Erectile dysfunction.*

incomplete protein food Food that does not contain all the essential amino acids.

increment Period of increasing strength of a uterine contraction.

independent nursing interventions Nurse-prescribed actions used in both nursing diagnoses and collaborative problems.

induction of labor Artificial initiation of labor.

infant mortality rate Number of deaths per 1000 live births that occurs within the first 12 months of life.

inference The act of drawing a conclusion or making a deduction.

infertility Inability of a couple to conceive after 1 year of regular intercourse (two to three times weekly) without using contraception; also, the involuntary inability to conceive and produce viable offspring when the couple chooses. Primary infertility occurs in a couple who has never conceived; secondary infertility occurs in a couple who has conceived at least once before.

intensity Strength of a uterine contraction at its peak.

intermittent monitoring Variation of electronic fetal monitoring in which an initial strip is obtained on admission. If patterns are reassuring, the woman is remonitored for 15 minutes at regular intervals (such as every 30 minutes).

interval Period between the end of one uterine contraction and the beginning of the next.

intrapartum Time of labor and childbirth.

intrauterine device Long-acting contraceptives that are inserted into the uterus to provide continuous pregnancy prevention.

intraventricular hemorrhage Bleeding around and into the ventricles of the brain. (Also called *germinal matrix hemorrhage* and *periventricular-intraventricular hemorrhage.*)

introversion Inward concentration on the self and body.

involution Retrogressive changes that return the reproductive organs, particularly the uterus, to their nonpregnant size and condition.

jaundice Yellow discoloration of the skin and sclera caused by excess bilirubin in the blood.

judgment An opinion.

kangaroo care A method of providing skin-to-skin contact between infants and their parents.

karyotype A display of a cell's chromosomes, arranged from largest to smallest pairs, with sex chromosomes displayed as a separate pair.

Kegel exercises Alternate contracting and relaxing of the pelvic floor muscles to strengthen the muscles surrounding the urinary meatus and vagina.

kernicterus Staining of brain tissue caused by accumulation of unconjugated bilirubin in the brain. Bilirubin encephalopathy is the brain damage that results from these deposits.

ketosis Accumulation of ketone bodies (metabolic products) in blood; frequently associated with acidosis.

kilocalorie A unit of heat; used to show the energy value in foods (commonly called *calorie*).

lactation Secretion of milk from the breasts; also describes the period during which a child is breastfed.

lactogenesis The production of milk.

lacto-ovovegetarian A vegetarian whose diet includes milk products and eggs.

lactose intolerance Inability to digest most dairy products because of a deficiency of the enzyme lactase.

lactovegetarian A vegetarian whose diet includes milk products.

lanugo Fine, soft hair that covers the fetus.

laparoscopy Insertion of an illuminated tube into the abdominal cavity to visualize contents, locate bleeding, and perform surgical procedures.

laparotomy Incision through the lower abdominal wall to examine the abdominal or pelvic organs or perform other surgical procedures.

large-for-gestational-age infant An infant whose size is above the ninetieth percentile for gestational age.

latch Attachment of the infant to the breast.

late deceleration The slowing of the fetal heart rate after the onset of a uterine contraction and persisting after the contraction ends.

late preterm infant An infant born between 34⁴⁄₇ and 36⁶⁄₇ weeks of gestation.

lecithin/sphingomyelin ratio (L/S ratio) Ratio of two phospholipids in amniotic fluid used to determine fetal lung maturity; ratio of 2:1 or greater usually indicates fetal lung maturity.

let-down reflex See *Milk-ejection reflex.*

letting-go A phase of maternal adaptation that involves relinquishment of previous roles and assumption of a new role as a parent.

libido Sexual desire.

lightening Descent of the fetal head into the pelvic cavity before labor.

linea nigra Pigmented line extending in the midline of the abdomen from the fundus to the symphysis pubis.

linear salpingostomy Incision along the length of a fallopian tube to remove an ectopic pregnancy and preserve the tube.

lipogenic Substance such as insulin that stimulates the production of fat.

lochia Vaginal drainage after birth.

lochia alba White, cream-colored, or light yellow vaginal discharge that follows lochia serosa. Occurs when the amount of blood is decreased and the number of leukocytes is increased.

lochia rubra Reddish or red-brown vaginal discharge that occurs immediately after childbirth; composed mostly of blood.

lochia serosa Pink or brown-tinged vaginal discharge that follows lochia rubra and precedes lochia alba; composed largely of serous exudate, blood, and leukocytes.

low-birth-weight infant An infant weighing less than 5 lb, 8 oz (2500 g) at birth.

maceration Discoloration and softening of tissues and eventual disintegration of a fetus that is retained in the uterus after its death.

macrosomia Infant birth weight above the ninetieth percentile for gestational age. Some sources use more than 4000 g (8 lb, 13 oz) or 4500 g (9 lb, 15 oz).

malpractice Negligence by a professional person.

mammogram Study of breast tissue using very-low-dose radiography; primary tool in the diagnosis of breast tumors.

Marfan syndrome A hereditary condition that involves weakness in connective tissue, bones, and muscles; the vascular system is affected, particularly the aorta.

mastitis Infection of the breast.

maternal mortality rate Number of maternal deaths from births and complications of pregnancy, childbirth, and puerperium (the first 42 days after the pregnancy ends) per 100,000 live births.

mature milk Breast milk that replaces transitional milk.

meconium aspiration syndrome Obstruction and air trapping caused by meconium in the infant's lungs, which may lead to severe respiratory distress.

meiosis Reduction cell division in gametes that halves the number of chromosomes in each cell.

melasma Brownish pigmentation of the face during pregnancy. (Also called *chloasma* and "*mask of pregnancy*.")

menarche Onset of menstruation, usually between 10 and 16 years of age or within 2 years of the start of breast development.

meningocele Protrusion of the meninges through a defect in the vertebrae; a form of neural tube defect.

menometrorrhagia Uterine bleeding that is irregular in frequency and excessive in amount.

menopause Permanent cessation of menstruation during the climacteric.

menorrhagia Excessive bleeding at the time of menstruation in number of days' duration, amount of blood lost, or both.

methadone A synthetic compound with opiate properties; used as an oral substitute for heroin and morphine in the opiate-dependent person.

metritis Infection of the decidua, myometrium, and parametrial tissues of the uterus.

metrorrhagia Bleeding from the uterus at any time other than during the menstrual period.

milia White cysts, 1 mm in size, on the face.

miliaria (prickly heat) Rash caused by heat.

milk-ejection reflex Release of milk from the alveoli into the ducts. (Also known as the *let-down reflex*.)

mimicry Copying the behaviors of other pregnant women or mothers as a method of "trying on" the role of advanced pregnancy or motherhood.

mitosis Cell division in body cells other than the gametes.

mittelschmerz Low abdominal pain that occurs at ovulation.

molding Shaping of the fetal head during movement through the birth canal.

Mongolian spots Bruiselike marks that occur mostly in newborns with dark skin tones.

monosomy Presence of only one of a chromosome pair in every body cell.

Montevideo unit Method to quantify intensity of labor contractions with uterine activity monitoring. The baseline intrauterine pressure for each contraction in a 10-minute period is subtracted from the peak pressure.

mortality rate Number of deaths that occur each year by different categories.

morula Fertilized ovum that resembles a mulberry when it contains 12 to 16 cells.

motor block Loss of voluntary movement caused by regional anesthesia.

multifetal pregnancy A pregnancy in which the woman is carrying two or more fetuses. (Also called *multiple gestation*.)

multigravida A woman who has been pregnant more than once.

multipara A woman who has delivered two or more pregnancies at 20 or more weeks of gestation.

multiple-marker testing/screening Sometimes called a triple or quad screen; a maternal blood test for three or four substances (human chorionic gonatropin, alpha fetoprotein, unconjugated estriol, and in the quad screen, inhibin A). It is performed to evaluate a woman's risk for trisomy 21, trisomy 18, and open neural tube defects.

mutation Alteration in DNA sequence in a gene, usually one that adversely affects its function.

mutual recognition Nurse licensure that allows nurses to hold licenses in their states of residence and practice in other states that also recognize the home state's license. (Also known as a *multistate licensure compact*.)

myelomeningocele Protrusion of the meninges and spinal cord through a defect in the vertebrae; a form of neural tube defect.

nadir Lowest point, such as the lowest pulse rate in a series.

narcissism Undue preoccupation with oneself.

natural family planning Method of predicting ovulation based on normal changes in a woman's body.

necrotizing enterocolitis Serious inflammatory condition of the intestines.

negligence Failure to act in the way a reasonable, prudent person of similar background would act in similar circumstances.

neonatal abstinence syndrome A cluster of physical signs exhibited by the newborn exposed in utero to maternal use of substances such as heroin. (See also *Abstinence syndrome*.)

neonatal mortality rate Number of deaths per 1000 live births occurring at birth or within the first 28 days of life.

neural tube defect A congenital defect in the closure of the bony encasement of the spinal cord or skull. Includes defects such as anencephaly, spina bifida, meningocele, myelomeningocele, and others.

neutral thermal environment Environment in which body temperature is maintained without an increase in metabolic rate or oxygen use.

nevus flammeus Permanent pink to dark reddish-purple birthmark. (Also called *port-wine stain*.)

nevus simplex Flat, pink area on the nape of the neck, on the midforehead, or over the eyelids resulting from dilation of the capillaries. (Also called *stork bites, salmon patches,* or *telangiectatic nevi*.)

nevus vasculosus Rough, red collection of capillaries with a raised surface that disappears with time. (Also called *strawberry hemangioma*.)

nidation Implantation of the fertilized ovum (zygote) in the uterine endometrium.

noncompliance Resistance of the lungs and thorax to distention with air during respirations.

nonheme iron Iron obtained from plants and fortified foods.

nonnutritive sucking Sucking during which little or no milk flow is obtained or sucking on an object such as a pacifier or finger.

nonshivering thermogenesis Process of heat production, without shivering, by oxidation of brown fat.

nonstress test A method for evaluating fetal status during the antepartum period by observing the response of the fetal heart rate to fetal movement.

nuchal cord Umbilical cord around the fetal body, often the neck.

nullipara A woman who has never completed a pregnancy beyond 20 weeks' gestation.

nurse anesthetist A registered nurse who has advanced education and certification in administration of anesthetics; also, certified registered nurse anesthetist (CRNA).

nurse practice acts Laws that determine the scope of nursing practice in each state.

nutrient density The quality and quantity of protein, vitamins, and minerals per 100 calories in foods.

nutritive suckling (sucking) Steady, rhythmic suckling at the breast or sucking at a bottle to obtain milk.

occult prolapse See *Prolapsed cord*.

oligohydramnios Abnormally small amount of amniotic fluid, less than about 500 mL at term.

oligospermia A decreased number of sperm in semen, usually considered to be under 20 million per milliliter.

omphalocele Protrusion of the intestines into the base of the umbilical cord.

oogenesis Formation of gametes (ova) in the female.

opiate Any narcotic-containing opium or a derivative of opium.

oral contraceptive Drug that inhibits ovulation; contains progestins alone or in combination with estrogen.

osmotic diuresis Secretion and passage of large amounts of urine as a result of increased osmotic pressure that can result from hyperglycemia.

osteomalacia Softening of bones; precedes osteoporosis.

osteoporosis Increased spaces (porosity) of bone; process usually accelerates after menopause.

ovovegetarian A vegetarian whose diet includes eggs.

ovulation Release of the mature ovum from the ovary.

pain threshold (or pain perception) The lowest level of stimulus one perceives as painful; relatively constant under different conditions.

pain tolerance Maximum pain one is willing to endure. Pain tolerance may increase or decrease under different conditions.

Pap test Evaluation of cells taken from the cervix for evaluation of possible cervical cancer.

para A woman who has given birth after a pregnancy of at least 20 weeks of gestation; also designates the number of a woman's pregnancies that have ended after at least 20 weeks of gestation.

paroxysmal nocturnal dyspnea Respiratory distress occurring when lying down; often associated with congestive heart failure.

peau d'orange Dimpled skin condition in which skin resembles an orange peel; associated with lymphatic edema and often seen over the area of breast cancer.

pedigree A graphic representation of a family's medical and hereditary history and the relationships among the family members. (Also called a *genogram*.)

percutaneous umbilical blood sampling (PUBS) Procedure for obtaining fetal blood through ultrasound-guided puncture of an umbilical cord vessel to detect fetal problems such as inherited blood disorders, acidosis, or infection. (Also called *cordocentesis*.)

perinatologist Physician who specializes in the high-risk pregnancy care of the mother and fetus during the perinatal period (from approximately the twentieth week of pregnancy to 4 weeks after childbirth). (Also known as a *maternal-fetal medicine specialist*.)

periodic breathing Cessation of breathing lasting 5 to 10 seconds followed by 10 to 15 seconds of rapid respirations without changes in skin color or heart rate.

persistent pulmonary hypertension Vasoconstriction of the infant's pulmonary vessels after birth; may result in right-to-left shunting of blood flow through the ductus arteriosus, the foramen ovale, or both.

pH test A paper or commercial swab used to test pH; helps determine whether the amniotic sac has ruptured. Nitrazine test.

phenotype The outward expression of a person's genetic makeup; observed characteristics produced by the interaction of genes and environment.

phimosis Tightening of the prepuce (foreskin) of the penis.

phosphatidylglycerol (PG) A major phospholipid of surfactant whose presence in amniotic fluid indicates fetal lung maturity.

phosphatidylinositol (PI) A phospholipid of surfactant that is produced and secreted in increasing amounts as the fetal lungs mature.

physiologic anemia of pregnancy Decrease in hemoglobin and hematocrit values caused by dilution of erythrocytes from expanded plasma volume rather than by an actual decrease in erythrocytes or hemoglobin.

phytoestrogen Estrogen substance of plant origin.

pica Ingestion of nonnutritive substances such as laundry starch, clay, or ice.

placenta Fetal structure that provides nourishment and removes wastes from the developing baby and secretes hormones necessary for the continuation of pregnancy.

placenta accreta A placenta that is abnormally adherent into the uterine wall. If the condition is more advanced, it is called *placenta increta* (the placenta extends into the uterine muscle) or *placenta percreta* (the placenta perforates through the uterine muscle).

placenta previa Abnormal implantation of the placenta in the lower uterus at or very near the cervical os.

placental abruption Premature separation of a normally implanted placenta. Also called abruptio placentae.

plagiocephaly Flattening or asymmetry of the back of the head.

point of maximum impulse Area of the chest in which the heart sounds are loudest when auscultated.

polycythemia Abnormally high number of erythrocytes.

polydactyly More than 10 digits on the hands or feet.

polydipsia Excessive thirst.

polyhydramnios See *Hydramnios*.

polymerase chain reaction (PCR) A technique to rapidly analyze sequences of genes for in vitro diagnosis of infections; many hereditary characteristics can also be analyzed by the technique.

polymorphism Alternative form of a gene found in the population at a frequency greater than 1%.

polyphagia Excessive ingestion of food.

polyploidy Having additional full sets of chromosomes, such as 69 (triploidy) or 92 (tetraploidy).

polyuria Excessive excretion of urine.

position Relation of a fixed reference point on the fetus to the quadrants of the maternal pelvis.

postictal Unresponsive state after a seizure.

postmaturity syndrome Condition in which a postterm infant shows characteristics indicative of poor placental functioning before birth. (Also called *dysmaturity syndrome*.)

postpartum Refers to the first 6 weeks after childbirth.

postpartum blues Temporary, self-limited period of tearfulness experienced by many new mothers beginning the first week after childbirth.

postterm infant An infant born after 42 weeks of gestation.

precipitate birth A birth that occurs without a trained attendant present.

precipitate labor An intense, unusually short labor (less than 3 hours).

preeclampsia A hypertensive disorder of pregnancy characterized by new onset of hypertension after 20 weeks gestation and multisystem involvement.

pregnancy-related mortality rate Death of a woman during pregnancy or within 12 months after the end of the pregnancy from any cause related to or worsened by the pregnancy, but not due to accidental or incidental causes.

premature rupture of the membranes Spontaneous rupture of the membranes before the onset of labor (term, preterm, or postterm gestation).

presentation Fetal part that enters the pelvic inlet, or the presenting part.

preterm birth A birth that occurs after the twentieth week and before the beginning of the thirty-seventh week of gestation.

preterm infant An infant born before the beginning of the thirty-eighth week of gestation. (Also called *premature infant*.)

preterm labor Onset of labor after 20 weeks and before the beginning of the thirty-seventh week of gestation.

preterm premature rupture of the membranes Rupture of the membranes before the onset of labor in a pregnancy after 20 weeks and before the beginning of the 37th week of gestation.

primigravida A woman who is pregnant for the first time.

primipara A woman who has given birth after a pregnancy of at least 20 weeks of gestation; also used informally to describe a pregnant woman before the birth of her first child.

progestin Any natural or synthetic form of progesterone.

prolapsed cord Displacement of the umbilical cord in front of or beside the fetal presenting part. An occult prolapse is one that is suspected on the basis of fetal heart rate patterns; the umbilical cord cannot be palpated or seen.

pseudomenstruation Vaginal bleeding in the newborn resulting from withdrawal of placental hormones.

psychoprophylaxis Method of prepared childbirth that emphasizes mental concentration and relaxation to increase pain tolerance.

psychosis Mental state in which a person's ability to recognize reality, communicate, and relate to others is impaired.

puberty Period of sexual maturation accompanied by the development of secondary sex characteristics and the capacity to reproduce.

puerperal infection A temperature of 38°C (100.4°F) or higher after the first 24 hours and occurring on at least 2 of the first 10 days after childbirth.

puerperium Period from the end of childbirth until involution of the reproductive organs is complete; approximately 6 weeks.

pulmonary embolus A potentially fatal complication that occurs when the pulmonary artery is obstructed by a blood clot that was swept into circulation from a vein or by amniotic fluid.

pulse oximetry Method of determining the level of blood oxygen saturation by sensors attached to the skin.

pulse pressure The difference between systolic and diastolic blood pressures.

quickening The first movements of the fetus felt by the mother.

recessive Gene that requires two copies, one from the maternal and one from the paternal chromosome, for the trait to be expressed.

reciprocal attachment behaviors Repertoire of infant actions that promotes attachment between the parent and newborn.

recommended dietary allowance (RDA) Level of nutrient intake considered to meet the needs of healthy individuals.

rectocele Herniation (protrusion) of the rectum through the posterior vaginal wall.

REEDA Acronym for redness, ecchymosis, edema, discharge, and approximation; useful for assessing wound healing or the presence of inflammation or infection.

reflection Meditation, attentive consideration.

regional anesthesia Anesthesia that blocks pain impulses in a localized area without loss of consciousness.

respiratory distress syndrome Condition caused by insufficient production of surfactant in the lungs; results in atelectasis (collapse of the lung alveoli), hypoxia (decreased oxygen [O_2] concentration), and hypercapnia (increased carbon dioxide [CO_2] concentration).

retinopathy of prematurity Condition in which injury to blood vessels may cause decreased vision or blindness in preterm infants.

retrograde ejaculation Discharge of semen into the bladder rather than from the end of the penis.

ripening Softening of the cervix as labor nears as the result of an increase in water content and the effects of relaxin on the connective tissue of the cervix.

role transition Changing from one pattern of behavior and one image of self to another.

ruga (Pl. rugae) Ridge or fold of tissue, as on the male's scrotum and in the female's vagina.

salpingectomy Surgical removal of a fallopian tube.

seborrheic dermatitis (cradle cap) Yellowish, crusty area of the scalp.

second period of reactivity Period of 4 to 6 hours after the first sleep after birth when the newborn may have an elevated pulse rate and respiratory rate and excessive mucus.

secondary sex characteristics Physical differences between mature males and females that are not directly related to reproduction.

semen Spermatozoa with their nourishing and protective fluid; discharged at ejaculation.

sensory block Loss of sensation caused by regional anesthesia.

sentinel lymph node (SLN) biopsy Technique to remove a minimal number of key lymph nodes to determine spread of the tumor.

seroconversion Change in a blood test result from negative to positive, indicating the development of antibodies in response to infection or immunization.

servocontrol Mechanism on a radiant warmer or incubator to regulate the amount of heat produced.

sex chromosome The X or Y chromosome; females have two X chromosomes and males have one X and one Y chromosome.

short bowel syndrome A condition caused by a bowel that is shorter than normal.

shoulder dystocia Delayed or difficult birth of the fetal shoulders after the head is born.

skepticism Doubt in the absence of conclusive evidence.

small-for-gestational-age infant An infant whose size is below the tenth percentile for gestational age.

somatic cells Body cells other than the gametes, or germ cells.

somatic sex Gender assignment as male or female on the basis of form and structure of the external genitalia.

spermatogenesis Formation of male gametes (sperm) in the testes.

spermicide A chemical that kills sperm.

spina bifida Defective closure of the bony spine that encloses the spinal cord; a type of neural tube defect.

spinnbarkeit Clear, slippery, stretchy quality of cervical mucus during ovulation.

standard of care Level of care that can be expected of a professional as determined by laws, professional organizations, and health care agencies.

standard procedures Procedures determined by nurses, physicians, and administrators that allow nurses to perform duties usually part of the medical practice.

station Measurement of fetal descent in relation to the ischial spines of the maternal pelvis. (See also *Engagement.*)

sterility Total inability to conceive.

strabismus A turning inward ("crossing") or outward of the eyes caused by poor tone in the muscles that control eye movement.

striae gravidarum Irregular pink to purple streaks on the woman's abdomen, breasts, or buttocks resulting from tears in connective tissue.

subarachnoid space Space between the arachnoid mater and the pia mater containing cerebrospinal fluid.

subinvolution Delayed return of the uterus to its nonpregnant size and consistency.

suckling Giving or taking nourishment from the breast. Sometimes used interchangeably with *sucking,* which refers only to drawing into the mouth with a partial vacuum, as with a bottle or pacifier.

sudden infant death syndrome (SIDS) Sudden death of an infant that is unexplained by history, autopsy, or examination of the scene of death.

surfactant Combination of lipoproteins produced by the lungs of the mature fetus to reduce surface tension in the alveoli, thus promoting lung expansion after birth.

surrogate mother A fertile woman who is inseminated with the purpose of conceiving and relinquishing a child to an infertile couple.

suspend To delay or bring to a stop temporarily.

sutures Narrow areas of flexible tissue that connect fetal skull bones, permitting slight movement during labor.

syndactyly Webbing between fingers or toes.

tachypnea Respiratory rate greater than 60 breaths per minute in the newborn after the first hour of life.

taking-hold Second phase of maternal adaptation during which the mother assumes control of her own care and initiates care of the infant.

taking-in First phase of maternal adaptation during which the mother passively accepts care, comfort, and details about the newborn.

telemetry Wireless transmission of electronic fetal monitoring data to the bedside or central monitor unit.

teratogen An environmental agent that can cause defects in a developing baby during pregnancy.

term Refers to the period of time a pregnancy is expected to last. (Also known as *full term.*)

thermogenesis Heat production.

thermoregulation Maintenance of body temperature.

thrombophlebitis Occurs when the vessel wall develops an inflammatory response to the thrombus. This further occludes the vessel.

thrombus Collection of blood factors, primarily platelets and fibrin, that may cause vascular obstruction.

tocolytic Drug that inhibits uterine contractions.

total parenteral nutrition Intravenous infusion of all nutrients known to be needed for metabolism and growth.

toxic shock syndrome Rare, potentially fatal disorder usually caused by a toxin produced by *Staphylococcus aureus;* has been associated with improper use of tampons.

tracheoesophageal fistula Abnormal connection between the esophagus and the trachea.

transcultural nursing Concerned with the provision of nursing care in a manner that is sensitive to the needs of individuals, families, and groups.

transdermal contraceptive patch Adhesive patch containing estrogen and progestin, which are absorbed through the skin to prevent pregnancy.

transducer Device that translates one physical quantity to another, such as fetal heart motion into an electrical signal for rate calculation, generation of sound, or a written record.

transient tachypnea of the newborn Condition of rapid respirations caused by inadequate absorption of fetal lung fluid.

transitional milk Breast milk that appears between secretion of colostrum and mature milk.

translocation Exchange of genetic material between nonhomologous chromosomes.

trimester One of three equal, 13-week parts of a full-term pregnancy.

Triple I Intrauterine infection or inflammation or both. See *Chorioamnionitis.*

trisomy Presence of three copies of a chromosome in each body cell.

tubal sterilization Cutting or mechanically occluding the fallopian tubes to prevent passage of ova or sperm, thus preventing pregnancy. (May also be called *tubal ligation.*)

ultrasound Use of sound waves for visualizing deep structures of the body by recording the reflections (echoes) of high-frequency sound waves directed into the tissue.

uterine inversion Turning of the uterus inside out after birth of the fetus.

uterine resting tone Degree of uterine muscle tension when the woman is not in labor or during the interval between labor contractions.

uterine rupture A tear in the wall of the uterus.

uteroplacental insufficiency Inability of the placenta to exchange oxygen, carbon dioxide, nutrients, and waste products properly between the maternal and fetal circulations.

utilitarian model Ethical model stating that the right course of action is the one that produces the greatest good.

vacuum curettage (vacuum aspiration) Removal of the uterine contents by application of a vacuum through a hollow curette or cannula introduced into the uterus.

vaginal contraceptive ring Flexible ring releasing small amounts of estrogen and progesterone to prevent pregnancy.

validate To make certain that the information collected is accurate.

varicocele Abnormal dilation or varicosity of veins in the spermatic cord.

vasa previa Branching of umbilical cord vessels in the amniotic sac rather than inserting into the placenta.

vasectomy Cutting or occluding the vas deferens to prevent passage of sperm, thus preventing pregnancy.

VBAC Acronym for vaginal birth after cesarean.

vegan A complete vegetarian who does not eat any animal products.

vegetarian An individual whose diet consists wholly or mostly of plant foods and who avoids animal food sources.

vernix caseosa Thick, white substance that protects the skin of the fetus.

version Turning the fetus from one presentation to another before birth, usually from breech to cephalic.

very-low-birth-weight infant An infant weighing 3 lb, 5 oz (1500 g) or less at birth.

vibroacoustic stimulation Use of sound stimulation to elicit fetal movement and acceleration (speeding up) of the fetal heart rate.

well-woman exam Verbal history, physical examination, and screening tests for a woman with no complaints of serious diseases, usually done annually. Often abbreviated WWE.

zygote The developing baby from conception through the first week of prenatal life.

Page numbers followed by *f* indicate figures; *t*, tables, *b*, boxes.

825